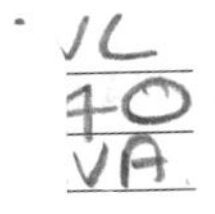

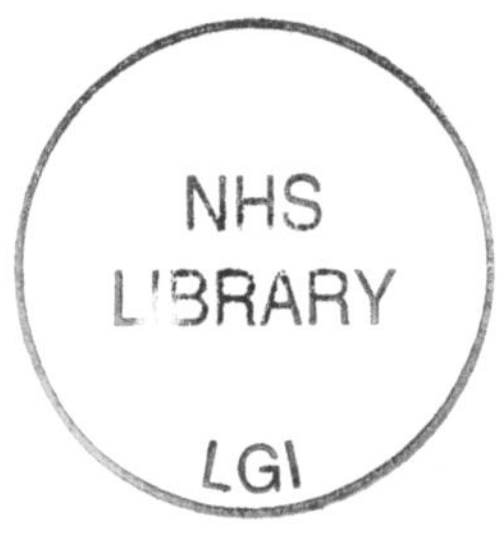
NHS
LIBRARY
LGI

Neurology and Trauma

NEUROLOGY AND TRAUMA

Second Edition

RANDOLPH W. EVANS, M.D.

OXFORD
UNIVERSITY PRESS
2006

OXFORD
UNIVERSITY PRESS

Oxford University Press, Inc., publishes works that further
Oxford University's objective of excellence
in research, scholarship, and education.

Oxford New York
Auckland Cape Town Dar es Salaam Hong Kong Karachi
Kuala Lumpur Madrid Melbourne Mexico City Nairobi
New Delhi Shanghai Taipei Toronto

With offices in
Argentina Austria Brazil Chile Czech Republic France Greece
Guatemala Hungary Italy Japan Poland Portugal Singapore
South Korea Switzerland Thailand Turkey Ukraine Vietnam

Published by Oxford University Press, Inc.
198 Madison Avenue, New York, New York 10016

www.oup.com

Library of Congress Cataloging-in-Publication Data
Neurology and trauma / [edited by] Randolph W. Evans. — 2nd ed.
p. ; cm.
Includes bibliographical references and index.
ISBN-13: 978-0-19-517032-0
ISBN 0-19-517032-6
1. Nervous system—Wounds and injuries. 2. Central nervous system—Wounds and injuries.
[DNLM: 1. Trauma, Nervous System—complications. 2. Trauma, Nervous System—diagnosis. 3. Trauma, Nervous System—therapy. 4. Iatrogenic Disease—prevention & control. WL 140 N9425 2006] I. Evans, Randolph W.
RD593.N4156 2006
617.4'8044—dc22 2005018932

9 8 7 6 5 4 3 2 1

Printed in the United States of America
on acid-free paper

To my family with love
My parents, Dr. Richard I. Evans and the late Zena A. Evans
My wife, Marilyn, and my children, Elliott, Rochelle, and Jonathan

Preface to the Second Edition

I have been delighted with the enthusiastic reception given to the first edition of *Neurology and Trauma* since its publication in 1996. This second edition reviews the many advances in basic and clinical research and practice over the past decade. Twenty-two of the first edition's chapters have been revised and updated, eight with new coauthors, and 20 new chapters have been added.

The book features completely new sections on sports and neurologic trauma and iatrogenic trauma to complement existing sections on head trauma, spinal trauma, plexus and peripheral nerve injuries, environmental trauma, and posttraumatic sequelae and medicolegal aspects. *Neurology and Trauma, second edition* remains a unique compilation of topics that will be of value to neurologists, neurosurgeons, physiatrists, occupational medicine physicians, orthopedic surgeons, emergency medicine physicians, psychiatrists, and neuropsychologists.

I am grateful to our 68 contributors for their outstanding chapters and I am pleased to have this edition published by Oxford University Press, the world's largest university press, which originated in 1668. I appreciate the advice and encouragement of our senior editor, Fiona Stevens, and our executive editor, William Lamsback as well as the excellent work of our managing editor, Nancy Wolitzer, and our copy editor, Helen Greenberg.

Preface to the First Edition

Many disorders due to head, spine, and peripheral nerve injuries are among the most common seen by neurologists and neurosurgeons. Other sequelae, such as reflex sympathetic dystrophy, post-traumatic movement disorders, and decompression sickness, are uncommon but important in the practice of neurology. The impact of these injuries can be devastating for individuals and society.

The impetus for this book is the November, 1992 issue of "Neurological Clinics" which I edited, *The Neurology of Trauma*. The original 15 articles have all been revised and updated. An additional 24 new chapters have been added. The book is divided into seven sections, head trauma; spinal trauma; plexus and peripheral nerve injuries; post-traumatic pain syndromes; environmental trauma; post-traumatic sequelae; and medicolegal aspects. Common and uncommon topics which will be of interest to the neurologist have been selected.

Unfortunately, many neurologists are indifferent about seeing patients with trauma-associated disorders. During residency training, there is often cursory formal education about these disorders. Once in practice, the frequent medicolegsal and workers' compensation aspects are discouraging. I hope this volume will help to alter this attitude favorably. These disorders encompass an important, controversial, and fascinating spectrum that should be part of the mainstream of neurologic thought and research. The book may also be of interest to colleagues in neurosurgery, physical medicine and rehabilitation, occupational and industrial medicine, orthopedics, emergency medicine, psychiatry, and neuropsychology.

I am grateful to our outstanding contributors. I also appreciate the encouragement and advice of our editor at W.B. Saunders Company, William R. Schmitt, and the fine work of the entire Saunders production team including that of Berta Steiner, Director of Production.

Randolph W. Evans

Contents

Part II Spinal Trauma

Part III Plexus and Peripheral Nerve Injuries

Part IV Posttraumatic Pain Syndromes

Part V Sports and Neurological Trauma

Part VI Environmental Trauma

Contributors

Michael J. Aminoff, M.D., D.Sc., F.R.C.P.
Professor
Department of Neurology
University of California-San Francisco
San Francisco, California

Joshua M. Ammerman, M.D.
Resident in Neurosurgery
George Washington University Medical Center
Department of Neurological Surgery
Washington, D.C.

Charles E. Argoff, M.D.
Director
Cohn Pain Management Center
North Shore University Hospital
Manhasset, New York

Robert W. Baloh, M.D.
Professor of Neurology
Department of Neurology
Los UCLA Medical Center
Los Angeles, California

David Baskin, M.D., F.A.C.S.
Professor
Department of Neurosurgery
The Methodist Hospital Neurological Institute
Houston, Texas

Ralf W. Baumgartner, M.D.
Head
Division of Neuroangiology and Stroke Unit
Department of Neurology
University Hospital
Zürich, Switzerland

Nikolai Bogduk, M.D.
Professor of Pain Medicine
Department of Clinical Research
Royal Newcastle Hospital
Newcastle, New South Wales, Australia

Susan R. Borgaro, Ph.D.
Staff Neuropsychologist
Department of Clinical Neuropsychology
Barrow Neurological Institute
St. Joseph's Hospital and Medical Center
Phoenix, Arizona

M. Capelli-Schellpfeffer, M.D., M.P.A.
Principal
CapSchell, Inc.
Chicago, Illinois

Daniel X. Capruso, Ph.D., A.B.P.P.
Diplomate in Clinical Neuropsychology
Kirby Forensic Psychiatric Center
Ward's Island, New York

Andrew Chennelle, M.D.
Private Practice Neurosurgery
Hinsdale, Illinois

Michael Cherington, MD
Emeritus, Professor of Clinical Neurology
University of Colorado School of Medicine
Lightning Data Center
St. Anthony Hospital
Denver, Colorado

Keith D. Cicerone, Ph.D.
Clinical Professor
Department of Physical Medicine and Rehabilitation
University of Medicine and Dentistry of New Jersey
New Brunswick, NJ
Director of Neuropsychology and Rehabilitation Psychology
JFK-Johnson Rehabilitation Institute
Edison, New Jersey

Valeria Conte, M.D.
Post-Doctoral Fellow
Department of Neurosurgery
University of Pennsylvania Medical Center
Philadelphia, Pennsylvania

Randolph W. Evans, M.D.
Clinical Professor of Neurology
Department of Neurology and Neuroscience
Weill Medical College of Cornell University and Department of Neurology
The Methodist Hospital
Chief of Neurology
Park Plaza Hospital
Houston, Texas

Mavis D. Fujii, M.D.
Associate Clinical Professor
The University of Texas Medical Branch at Galveston
Houston, Texas

Daoying Geng, M.D.
Visiting Professor of Radiology
Division of Neuroradiology
Department of Radiology
University of Southern California Keck School of Medicine
Los Angeles, California

John L. Go, M.D.
Professor of Radiology and Otolaryngology
Division of Neuroradiology
Department of Radiology
University of Southern California Keck School of Medicine
Los Angeles, California

Christopher G. Goetz, M.D.
The United Parkinson Foundation Professor of Neurology
Department of Neurological Sciences
Section of Movement Disorders
Rush University Medical Center
Chicago, Illinois

Douglas S. Goodin, M.D.
Professor
Department of Neurology
University of California-San Francisco
San Francisco, California

David I. Graham
Professor
Academic Unit of Neuropathology
Division of Clinical Neuroscience
University of Glasgow
Glasgow, Scotland, UK

Nidhi Gupta, B.A.
Medical Student
George Washington University School of Medicine
Washington, D.C.

H. Bruce Hamilton, M.D.
Private Practice Neurosurgery
Waco, Texas

James F. Howard, Jr., M.D.
Professor
Neuromuscular Disorders Section
Department of Neurology
The University of North Carolina at Chapel Hill
Chapel Hill, North Carolina

Ilia Itin, M.D.
Former Fellow
Department of Neurological Sciences
Section of Movement Disorders
Rush University Medical Center
Chicago, Illinois

S. Taylor Jarrell, M.D.
Resident in Neurosurgery
George Washington University Medical Center
Department of Neurological Surgery
Washington, D.C.

Bashar Katirji, M.D., F.A.C.P.
Professor
EMG Laboratory and Neuromuscular Division
Department of Neurology
University Hospitals of Cleveland and Case Western Reserve University
School of Medicine
Cleveland, Ohio

James R. Keane, M.D.
Professor
Department of Neurology
Los Angeles County-USC Medical Center
Los Angeles, California

Paul E. Kim, M.D.
Assistant Professor of Radiology
Division of Neuroradiology
Department of Radiology
University of Southern California Keck School of Medicine
Los Angeles, California

David G. Kline, M.D.
Boyd Professor and Chairman
Department of Neurosurgery
School of Medicine
Louisiana State University Health Sciences Center
New Orleans, Louisiana

Douglas Kondziolka, M.D., F.R.C.S. (C), F.A.C.S.
Professor of Neurological Surgery and Radiation Oncology
Department of Neurological Surgery
University of Pittsburgh and Center for Image-Guided Neurosurgery
University of Pittsburgh Medical Center
Pittsburgh, Pennsylvania

Jess F. Kraus, M.P.H., Ph.D.
Professor of Epidemiology
Southern California Injury Prevention Research Center
School of Public Health
University of California-Los Angeles
Los Angeles, California

Harvey S. Levin, Ph.D.
Professor
Department of Physical Medicine, Rehabilitation, and Neurosurgery
Baylor College of Medicine
Houston, Texas

L. Dade Lunsford, M.D., F.A.C.S.
Professor and Chairman
Department of Neurological Surgery
University of Pittsburgh and Center for Image-Guided Neurosurgery
University of Pittsburgh Medical Center
Pittsburgh, Pennsylvania

James F. Malec, Ph.D.
Professor and Co-chair
Division of Therapy Psychiatry and Psychology
Mayo Clinic College of Medicine
Rochester, Minnesota

Niklas Marklund, M.D.
Post-Doctoral Fellow
Department of Neurosurgery
University of Pennsylvania Medical Center
Philadelphia, Pennsylvania

Shaden Marzouk, M.D.
Spine Fellow
Northwestern Memorial Hospital
Chicago, Illinois

E. Wayne Massey, M.D.
Professor Department of Neurology
Duke University Medical Center
Durham, North Carolina

David L. McArthur, Ph.D., M.P.H.
Epidemiologist
Department of Surgery
Division of Neurosurgery
David Geffen School of Medicine
University of California-Los Angeles
Los Angeles, California

John W. McDonald, M.D., Ph.D.
Associate Professor
Spinal Cord Injury Program
Department of Neurology
Washington University in St. Louis School of Medicine
St. Louis, Missouri

Tracy K. McIntosh, Ph.D.
Former Professor and Director
Department of Neurosurgery
University of Pennsylvania
Philadelphia, Pennsylvania

Harold Merskey, D.M., F.R.C.P. (C), F.R.C.Psych
Emeritus Professor of Psychiatry
University of Western Ontario
London, Ontario, Canada

Timothy M. Miller, M.D., Ph.D.
Clinical Instructor and Research Fellow
Neurosciences Department
University of California, San Diego
La Jolla, California

Diego Morales, B.A.
Technician
Department of Neurosurgery
University of Pennsylvania Medical Center
Philadelphia, Pennsylvania

Anil Nanda, M.D., F.A.C.S.
Professor and Chairman
Department of Neurosurgery
LSU Health Sciences Center in Shreveport
Shreveport, Louisiana

Richard S. Polin, M.D.
Chief of Neurosurgery
Northwest Permanente
Portland, Oregon

George P. Prigatano, Ph.D.
Department of Clinical Neuropsychology
Newsome Chair of Clinical Neuropsychology
Barrow Neurological Institute
St. Joseph's Hospital and Medical Center
Phoenix, Arizona

F. Clifford-Rose, F.R.C.P.
Consultant Neurologist
London Neurological Centre
London, England

Nicolas Royo, Ph.D.
Post-Doctoral Fellow
Department of Neurosurgery
University of Pennsylvania Medical Center
Philadelphia, Pennsylvania

Satish Rudrappa, M.D.
Visiting Faculty
Department of Neurosurgery
LSU Health Sciences Center Shreveport
Shreveport, Louisiana

Kathryn E. Saatman, Ph.D.
Associate Professor
Department of Physiology, University of Kentucky College of Medicine
Lexington, Kentucky

Robert J. Schwartzman, M.D.
Professor and Chairman
Department of Neurology
Drexel University College of Medicine
Philadelphia, Pennsylvania

Michael Sharpe, M.D., F.R.C.P., F.R.C. Psych.
Professor of Psychological Medicine and Symptoms Research
Division of Psychiatry
School of Molecular and Clinical Medicine
University of Edinburgh
Western General Hospital
Edinburgh, Scotland

Jon Stone, M.B., Ch.B., M.R.C.P.
Consultant Neurologist
Division of Clinical Neurosciences
School of Molecular and Clinical Medicine
University of Edinburgh
Western General Hospital
Edinburgh, Scotland

Cory Toth, M.D., B.Sc., F.R.C.P.C.
Associate Member
Division of Neurology
Department of Clinical Neurosciences
University of Calgary
Heritage Medical Research Building
Foothills Hospital
Calgary, Alberta, Canada

Hakan Tuna, M.D.
Fellow
Department of Neurosurgery
LSU Health Sciences Center in Shreveport
Shreveport, Louisiana

Allan R. Tunkel, M.D., Ph.D.
Professor of Medicine
Drexel University College of Medicine
Chair, Department of Medicine
Monmouth Medical Center
Long Branch, New Jersey

Alan R. Turtz, M.D.
Associate Professor of Surgery
UMDNJ-Robert Wood Johnson Medical School
Department of Surgery-Division of Neurosurgery
Cooper Hospital
Camden, New Jersey

Prasad Vannemreddy, M.D., M.Ch.
Associate Professor of Neurosurgery Research
Department of Neurosurgery
LSU Health Sciences Center in Shreveport
Shreveport, Louisiana

Joseph L. Voelker, M.D.
Associate Professor
Department of Neurosurgery
West Virginia University School of Medicine
Morgantown, West Virginia

Oksana Volshteyn, M.D.
Associate Professor
Department of Neurology
Spinal Cord Program
Washington University in St. Louis School of Medicine
St. Louis, Missouri

Yakov Vorobeychik, M.D.
Assistant Professor of Neurology
Drexel University College of Medicine
Philadelphia, Pennsylvania

Michael I. Weintraub, M.D., F.A.C.P., F.A.A.N.
Clinical Professor of Neurology and Internal Medicine
New York Medical College
Briarcliff, New York

Anthony H. Wheeler, M.D.
Private Practice
Pain and Orthopedic Neurology
Charlotte Spine Center
Charlotte, North Carolina

Asa J. Wilbourn, M.D.
Director
EMG Laboratory
Neurology Department
The Cleveland Clinic Foundation
Associate Clinical Professor of Neurology
Case Western Reserve University Medical School
Cleveland, Ohio

L. James Willmore, M.D.
Professor of Neurology and Pharmacology and Physiology
Associate Dean
Saint Louis University School of Medicine
St. Louis, Missouri

Alison M. Wilson, M.D.
Associate Professor
Department of Trauma
Department of Surgery
West Virginia University School of Medicine
Morgantown, West Virginia

Chi-Shing Zee, M.D.
Professor of Radiology and Neurosurgery
Director of Neuroradiology
University of Southern California Hospital
Department of Imaging
Los Angeles, California

Part I

Head Trauma

Chapter 1
Epidemiology of Brain Injury

JESS F. KRAUS AND
DAVID L. MCARTHUR

Injury has been the fourth leading cause of mortality in the United States for the past 50 years and is the foremost cause of death among persons aged 1–44.[12] In 2001, 157,078 persons died of acute traumatic injury in the United States—a rate of 55 per 100,000 persons per year. This number is only 6460 fewer than the total number of persons who died from stroke in the same year.[59] Injury is the most rapidly increasing cause of death in developing countries, resulting from the combination of increased urbanization and motor vehicle use, along with reductions in deaths due to infectious diseases.[23] From the mid-1950s to the mid-1960s, for example, injury fatalities increased 600% in Mexico, 450% in Thailand, 243% in Venezuela, and 200% in Chile.[89] Proportional mortality rates from injury in Latin America, Asia, Africa, and Oceania range as high as 10%.[4,6,9,19,46,60,64,89] For most developing countries, the mortality rate from injury is substantially greater than the rate in the United States.

The exact number or percentage of injury deaths with significant brain involvement is not known but can be estimated using published data. In 2000, for example, the U.S. population was about 275 million, and various U.S. reports on mortality rates from traumatic brain injury (TBI) range from about 14 to 30 per 100,000 population per year.[41] If the average mortality rate of 22 per 100,000 from published U.S. reports is applied to the 2000 U.S. population, a figure of 60,720 deaths is calculated, representing about 43% of all acute traumatic fatal injuries per year.

The objective of this review is to assemble basic epidemiological evidence on brain injury occurrence, persons at risk, circumstances of exposure, severity and outcomes following injury, and preventive measures using available published accounts. For the purposes of this review, the studies selected for evaluation are U.S.-based, published since about 1980, except for an occasional published account in the foreign literature (or country) to illustrate a substantial difference in finding or an exceptional study.

Methodological Issues in TBI Research

While the clinical aspects of brain injury have been widely studied, population-based assessments of TBI are still relatively new and limited, and the methodologies used across the published studies have not yet been completely standardized. A central issue in comparing findings from earlier reports is the definition of (or criteria for) *brain injury* used by researchers, a term often used synonymously with head injury. For research purposes, the former must be considered a subset of the latter. Many injuries classified by some researchers (e.g., Refs. 2, 20), as *head injury* or *head trauma* may or may not include neurological involvement. For example, it is well recognized clinically that skull fracture per se, while a head injury, may not necessarily involve trauma to the brain, but skull fracture has been used in some studies as a criterion for brain injury study group inclusion.

Another methodological concern in identifying the brain-injured patient is assessment of the initial severity of the injury, which is often the product of a set of negative rather than positive clinical findings. Another concern in past years is that many less serious brain injuries never come to the attention of a hospital inpatient or outpatient service, and therefore are easily missed by researchers who rely on conventional hospital admission only case-finding methods.[24] More recently, however, patients with mild traumatic brain injury (MTBI) are being identified and evaluated epidemiologically.[37] Despite this recent focus on emergency department (ED) patients, a substantial percentage of "head"-injured persons treated in EDs or admitted to hospitals may not have neurological involvement.[43] In addition, many mildly or trivially brain-injured persons may not seek medical treatment or may obtain care through clinics or physicians' offices.[24] This could result in a significant undercount of true brain injuries, mostly those with milder forms of brain trauma. To help correct this situation, researchers from the World Health Organization (WHO)[87] and the Centers for Disease Control and Prevention (CDC)[81] developed standardized administrative and clinical criteria for traumatic brain injury (TBI), including MTBI. When fully adopted, these criteria should serve to minimize false-positive and false-negative diagnoses of TBI, especially MTBI.

When research studies are conducted using clinical criteria alone, three factors are critical in differentiating head injury without neurological involvement from brain injury: loss of consciousness, posttraumatic amnesia (PTA), and mental disorientation. Brain injuries without cognitive impairment but with vomiting, headaches, and/or dizziness are often diagnosed as concussion.[61] A diagnosis of TBI should include loss of consciousness, either at the scene of the injury or later, PTA, or demonstrated mental impairment. Some studies have considered skull fracture a necessary and sufficient finding.[2] However, as mentioned above, a significant proportion of skull fractures are not associated with concurrent brain injury, and the positive predictive value of skull fracture for intracranial injury is only about 22%.[51] Even when brain injury is properly defined, population-based ascertainment of cases can be difficult. For example, all hospitals or other sources of emergency care in a given study area must be included in the case ascertainment plan, the population base must be known (catchment area counts are not accurate enough), rates must be adjusted for age (and other confounders) if rates are to be compared, and all specific causes of injury must be considered (with both penetrating and blunt causes).[20,24,25,40,41,48,86]

One form of misclassification of brain injury can occur when deaths that should be attributable to brain trauma are coded to another cause. This may be seen when the deaths are not autopsied or when they are due to multiple severe injuries. Whether brain injury is the primary cause of death or one of several secondary causes, for research purposes the evidence of injury to the brain must be recorded. Frequently, however, secondary diagnoses of brain injury are often excluded from the hospital record or autopsy report. The extent of this phenomenon in head injury–associated deaths has been examined in a study of multiple-cause-of-death data; findings suggest underestimation of as much as 44%.[41,69,70]

Findings from epidemiological studies of brain injury occurrence, risk factors, and outcomes are difficult to compare because of significant differences both in the lengths of follow-up phases and in the types of patients who are included for follow-up. Additionally, outcome assessments are difficult to interpret when tests of cognitive, psychosocial, or physical outcomes are applied inconsistently.

Mortality and Case Fatality Rates

Slightly over 157,000 U.S. deaths (6.5% of all deaths) were attributed to injury causes in 2001.[59] If 43% of these deaths were attributable to brain injury (see above), there were approximately 62,830 brain injury deaths—an overall brain injury–associated death rate of about 22 per 100,000 per year, a rate which has remained stable over the past two decades.[69,70]

Case fatality rates (CFRs) may be used to measure extreme outcomes for groups of patients who are admitted to a hospital and diagnosed with brain injury. Reported CFRs obtained from population-based studies vary by a factor of more than 5 among the reports (see Table 1.1).[2,20,24–27,40,66,78,85,86] This variation in the data may reflect a combination of differential admission criteria at different treatment facilities, differences in severity distributions of patients across hospitals, and differences in the quality of medical management. Ideally, CFRs for various institutions should be compared only after controlling for (1) TBI severity distributions across hospitals; (2) age; (3) comorbid and premorbid conditions; (4) extent and site of injury; and (5) availability of medical care. Data on factors 1, 2, and 4 are easily obtainable and should be used in adjusting CFRs.

Hospital Admissions

The exact number of persons admitted annually to hospitals for brain injury is not known for the United States or for most other countries in which admission statistics are kept. Reasons are similar with respect to death certificate diagnoses; for example, brain injury may not have been the principal diagnosis and hence may have been listed only after other more severe injuries. One estimate has been derived for the United States using National Hospital Discharge data.[79] The estimated average number of TBI admissions for 1994–1995 is about 241,100 persons. The estimating procedure used data on detailed diagnoses and procedures from the U.S. National Hospital Discharge Survey (NHDS) and required selection of appropriate International Classification of Disease (ICD) codes.[18] Investigators at CDC used ICD codes 800.0–801.9, 803.0–804.9, and 850.0–854.1 to arrive at their estimate of 241,100. Another estimate of annual hospitalized occurrences of TBI[53] was derived from the Healthcare Cost and Utilization Project (HCUP), operated by the Public Health Service's Agency for Healthcare Research and Quality.[73] This inpatient database contains selected demographic, clinical disposition, and diagnostic/procedural information. ICD–9th Revision–Clinical Modification. (ICD-9-CM) diagnostic codes were examined for each of the 21.5 million persons in the 1998, 1999, and 2000 HCUP datasets, along with age and death in hospital. Possible head injuries were found in 346,000 cases, or 1.6% of total admissions. Within this sample were 31,500 deaths recorded in hospital (a CFR of 9.1 per 100 admissions). The discrepancy between the CDC estimate (241,000) and that from the HCUP (346,000) may be due to a gross difference in case-finding algorithms. It is difficult to imagine that the difference of about 100,000 TBI admissions between the two sources could be accounted for by a 5-year difference in time period. Differences between these values and earlier published estimates [41,43] could reflect declines in hospital admissions in the 1990s compared with earlier years,

Table 1.1. Traumatic Brain Injury (TBI) Case Fatality Rates (CFRs) from Population-Based U.S. Studies

Location, Year(s) (Reference)	Source of Data	Study Group Size	CFR	95% CI
Chicago area 1979–80 (86)	Hospital/medical examiner records	782	7.9	6.0–9.8
Rhode Island 1979–80 (25)	Hospital records	2969	4.9	4.1–5.9
Bronx, NY 1980–82 (20)	Hospital/medical examiner records	1209	24.9	23.4–29.4
San Diego Co., CA 1981 (40)	Hospital/medical examiner records/death certificates	3359	16.7	15.4–18.0
Seattle 1980–81 (27)	Medical center admissions	451	19.0	15.4–22.6
Maryland 1986 (48)	Hospital records	5938	4.4	3.9–4.9
Oklahoma 1989 (35)	Hospital/medical examiner records	3672	23.0	21.6–25.4
Massachusetts 1990 (66)	Hospital/medical examiner records	5778	10.1	9.3–10.9
Colorado 1991–92 (26)	Colorado surveillance system	6010	7.6	6.9–8.3
Alaska 1991–93 (85)	Alaska trauma registry	2178	5.6	4.6–6.6
Seven states 1994 (78)	Hospital records	26, 669	5.6	5.3–5.9
Total U.S. 1994–95 (79)	National Hospital Discharge Survey	NR	5	

NR = not reported.

especially for less seriously injured persons, which in turn may be due in part to changes in health care financing and increasing use of outpatient facilities. However, among those who are hospitalized and survive, one in five will suffer significant long-term disability.[41]

The number of ED-attended head injuries has been estimated in two recent reports.[31,37] In both reports, the data were derived from the National Hospital Ambulatory Medical Care Survey (NHAMCS) for 1992–1994[31] and 1995–1996.[37]

The NHAMCS is a national probability survey of visits to EDs and outpatient departments of noninstitutional, general, and short-stay hospitals located in the 50 states and the District of Columbia. All diagnoses are coded to the ICD-9-CM, and both reports used the same diagnostic codes: 800.0–801.9, 803.0–804.9, and 850.0–854.1. The estimate of ED/outpatient visits for head injury in 1992–1994 was 1,144,807 (a rate of 444 per 100,000) per year for 1995–96 was 1,027,000 (a rate of 392 per 100,000 per year). A more recent estimate for 1995–2001 provided by the CDC gives an average annual number of ED TBI visits of 1,351,000 or a rate of 403 per 100,000.[44] These rates are about five to six times higher than the U.S. estimated hospitalized TBI rate of 85 per 100,000 per year for 1995–2001.[44] If a conservative average value for ED/outpatient visits (a rate of 400 per 100,000) is added with the TBI hospitalization rate of 85 per 100,000 and the estimated annual TBI mortality rate of about 18 per 100,000, then an overall annual estimate of 503 per 100,000 population per year is derived. Applying this rate to the estimated U.S. population in late 2005 of 298 million yields a total of nearly 1.5 million new TBI cases per year of all severities.

Another perspective on brain injury occurrences is provided in Figure 1.1, where hospital discharge rates for the leading neurological conditions are compared. Except for diagnoses of occlusion of cerebral arteries (stroke) and schizophrenia disorders, brain injury is a more common diagnosis than hemorrhagic stroke, epilepsy, Alzheimer's disease, migraine, brain cancer, Parkinson's disease, and multiple sclerosis.

With all available data, it is then possible to estimate the ratios of fatal to nonfatal hospital admissions to nonfatal medically treated and released brain-injured persons per year—1:4.4:20; that is, for each fatality there are about 4 or 5 persons hospitalized and about 20 persons are examined and released for a brain injury in the United States each year (Fig. 1.2).

Incidence Studies

Incidence is defined as the number of newly diagnosed cases in a specified period of time. When such cases occur in a defined (known) population, an incidence rate can be derived. The incidence

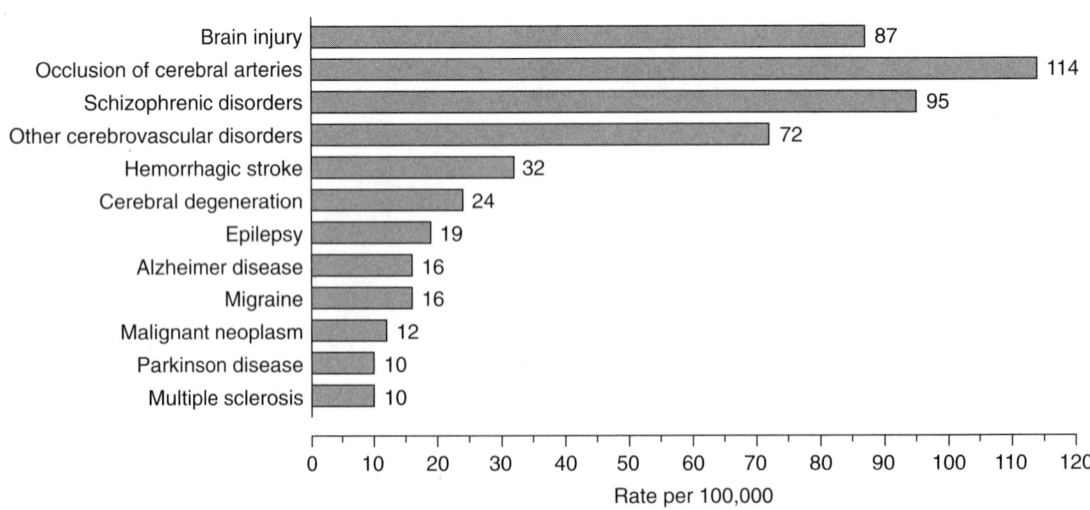

Figure 1.1. Brain injury hospital discharge rate compared with rates of 11 leading neurological diagnoses. (Source: reference 12)

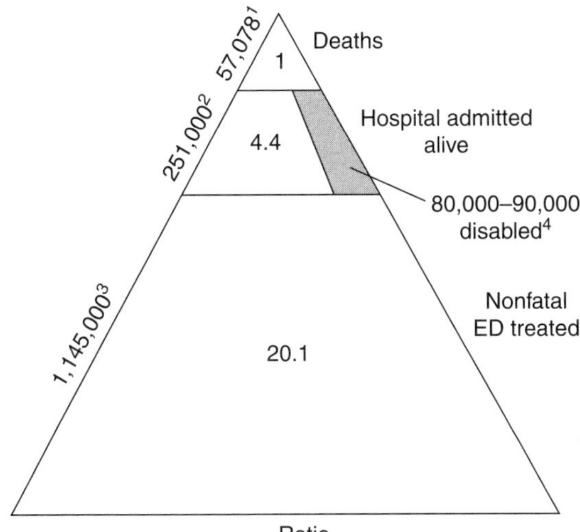

Figure 1.2. Number and ratio of brain injury deaths to nonfatal brain injuries, United States, 2001. ED, emergency department.

[1]Based on a U.S. brain injury death rate of 22 per 100,000 in 2001

[2]Based on Centers for Disease Control and Prevention hospitalized discharge data of 241,000 with any listed traumatic brain injury diagnosis[13]

[3]Based on reference 37

[4]Based on reference 78

group cannot contain previously diagnosed cases, repeat diagnoses by a second physician, or readmission to a health care facility. The incidence rate is a gross approximation of the risk or probability of an event. These parameters probably explain why so few incidence studies of TBI have been attempted. Since about 1980, only 15 such studies have been attempted for a subset of the U.S. population. Early studies were limited to counties[40] or cities.[20,86]

Methods used for incidence studies have also varied. Some studies [40] relied on hospital or coroner record–based case finding using specific discharge codes. In addition, the original institutional records were reviewed and pertinent data abstracted. Later studies used hospital administrative discharge records and electronic file information for descriptive purposes. In a few instances, a trauma registry was the source of data on TBI.[85] Figure 1.3 summarizes incidence (and mortality) rates per 100,000 population for these studies. Using the rate data available from these studies (since about 1980), the average rate of fatal and nonfatal hospitalized TBI is about 140 per 100,000 per year. Excluding the highest reported rate (367/100,000) and the lowest reported rate (69/100,000) leaves an average U.S. rate of *hospitalized* (plus immediately fatal) TBIs of about 130 per 100,000 per year. These estimates do not include ED-based studies reporting rates of 444 per 100,000, as reported by Jager et al.,[37] or 392 per 100,000, as reported by Guerrero et al.[31] The rates presented in Figure 1.3 represent three different case-finding methods: (1) hospitalized cases and those identified from medical examiner records (N = 10), (2) only hospital discharge records (N = 3), and (3) trauma registry files (N = 2). Because of this difference in case-finding approaches and other methodological differences, the average rates given here must be used with caution.

External Causes of Brain Injury

Data from many studies (Fig. 1.4) suggest that the most frequent exposure associated with brain injury is transport.[1,2,10,20,25,26,31,35,37,40,48,66,78,80,85,86] This category includes riders of automobiles and trucks, bicycles, motorcycles, aircraft, watercraft, and road farm equipment, as well as pedestrians hit by vehicles. The distributions of these external causes can vary significantly across most studies but do illustrate vast differences within general causes. For example, in the two ED-based studies, the most important exposure reported is falls, compared with hospital-based studies, where transport is the most frequent cause of brain injury. In raw numbers, the next most significant single exposure after transport is falls, especially among the very young and the elderly. In many areas of the world, injury from assault is quickly becoming one of the leading causes of brain trauma. Additional significant exposures are sports and recreation. Misclassifications are likely, however; for example, sports-related events may account for up to 10% of TBI deaths but might be reported as falls or being struck by an object.[86]

Risk Markers for Brain Injury

Age and Gender

Age groups at highest risk vary, depending on the brain injury level selected for analysis. For example, the very young (aged 0–4) and the very old

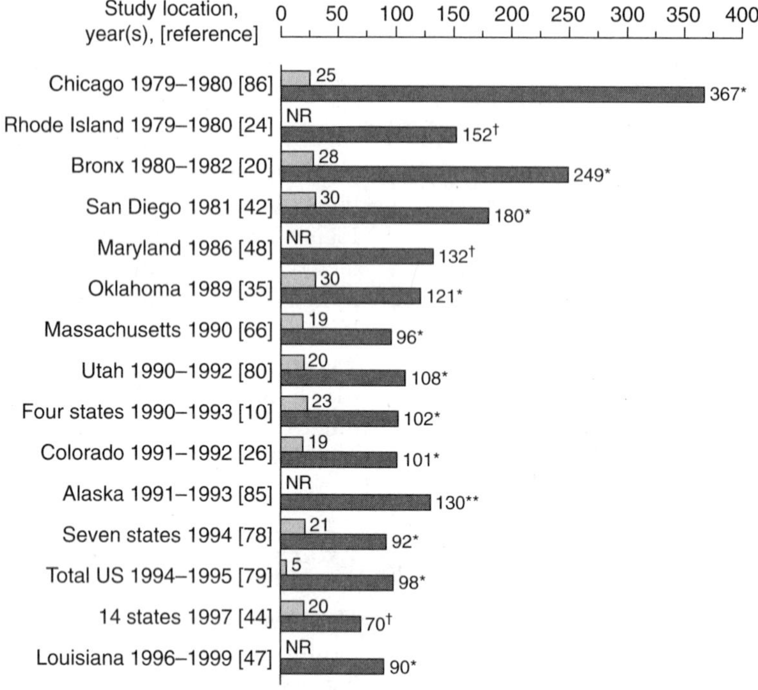

Figure 1.3. Brain injury incidence and fatality rates from selected U.S. studies.
= Mortality rate per 100,000
= Incidence rate per 100,000
° = rate includes hospitalized patients and coroner cases
°° = source is trauma registry
† = hospital discharge records only

(aged 85+) are the two most frequent groups presenting to an ED with a brain injury, while those aged 15–25 and over age 65 are most frequently hospitalized. The mortality rates from TBI are highest after age 76 (Fig. 1.5). The age-specific rate patterns tend to reflect differences in exposure, particularly to motor vehicle crashes and falls. Males are at greater risk for TBI than females at all ages in all incidence studies. This may reflect differences in risk taking or differential exposure to hazards in specific activities. For example, the male/female rate ratio of TBI due to falls from ladders and scaffolds is 28 times higher in males compared with females.[4] Under similar circumstances (i.e., climbing a ladder), females may characteristically elect to use less risky maneuvers than males; females may also be less likely to be on a ladder in the first place due to sometimes profound differences in the ratio of the sexes in occupations that normally have such high-risk exposures. Population-based U.S. studies show that the incidence rate ratio of TBI varies from 1.4:1 to 2.5:1 in comparing males with females. Mortality gender-specific rate ratios are approximately 3.5:1, strongly indicative of more severe injuries among males.[1]

Ethnicity and Socioeconomic Status

Centers for Disease Control data show that African Americans have the highest overall injury death rate of any racial/ethnic group in the United States. In 2000, the injury rate for African Americans was 124.7 per 1000, while the rates for white non-Hispanics (84.6 per 1000), and Hispanics (70.0 per 1000) were significantly lower.[14] The excess deaths and injuries may be related to increased exposure to firearms and violence as well as to residential fires, pedestrian injuries, drownings, and spinal cord injuries.[58] The excess in overall injury rates from all causes or types is also seen in the findings for TBI (Fig. 1.6). For example, the TBI death rate

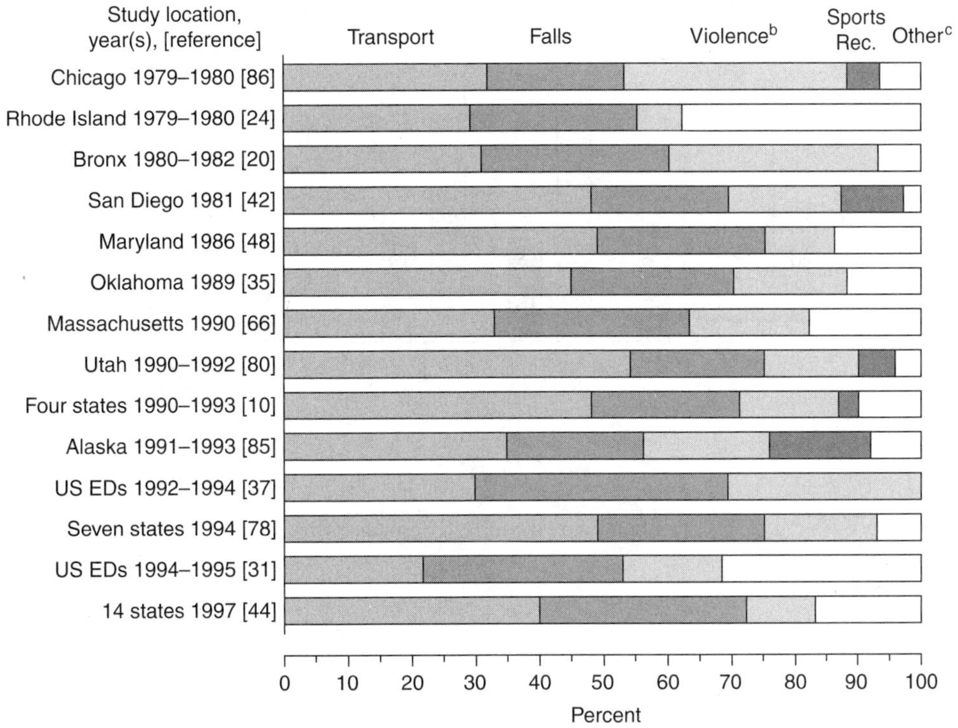

Figure 1.4. Percent distribution of traumatic brain injury external causes, selected U.S. studies. ED, emergency department.

[a]values rounded to whole numbers; hence, percentages may be slightly less or more than 100

[b]includes intentional firearms and assaults

[c]includes others plus no E-coded available cases

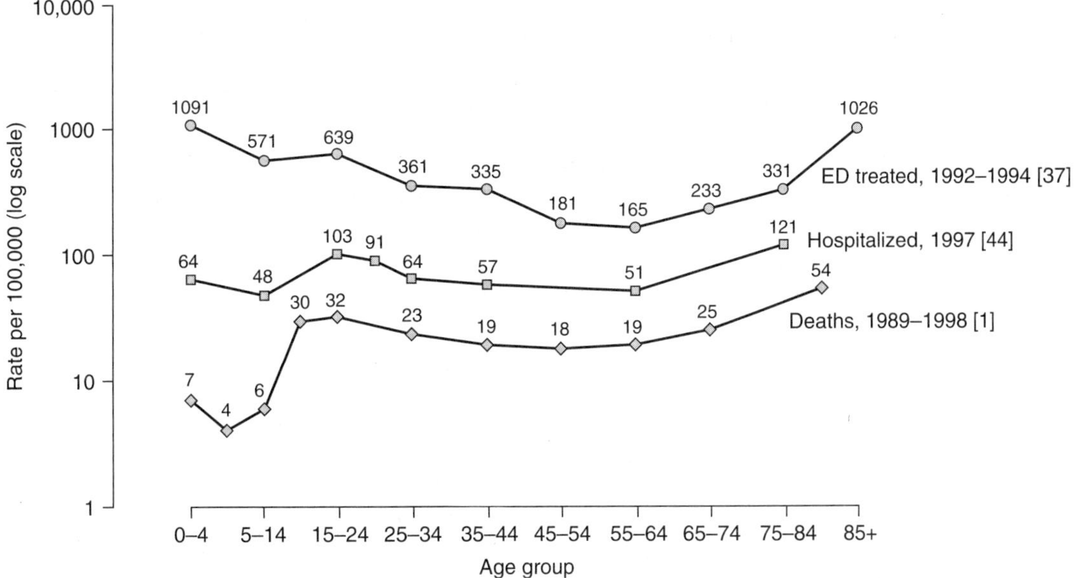

Figure 1.5. Brain injury incidence rates by age group: three U.S. estimates (references 1, 31, 44).

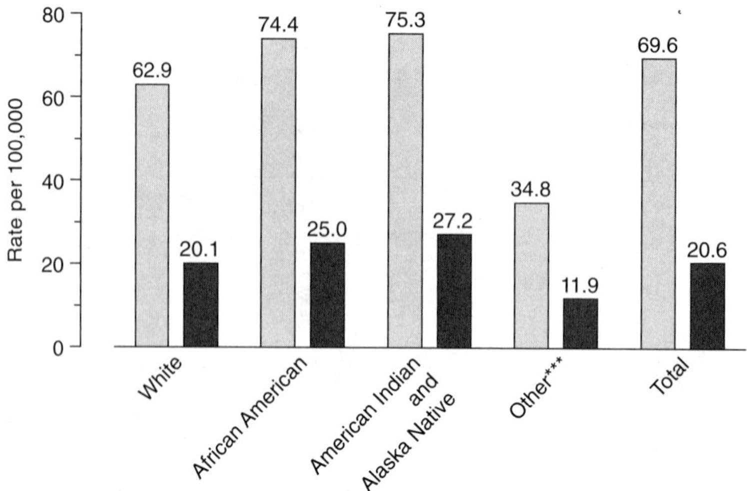

Figure 1.6. Race-specific traumatic brain injury death[1] and hospital discharge[2] rates per 100,000, United States.
▒ = hospital discharge rate
■ = mortality rate
[1]Source: reference 1
[2]Source: reference 44
°°° = includes Asian/Pacific Islanders

was 24.0 per 100,000 for African Americans compared with whites (20.1 per 100,000), and the nonfatal TBI hospitalization rate was 74.4 per 100,000 for African Americans and 76.3 per 100,000 for American Indian/Alaskan Natives compared with 62.9 per 100,000 for whites. Emergency department studies of TBI show similar results, albeit often lacking complete racial/ethnic categories. For example, the report by Jager et al.[37] shows the ED-treated TBI rate for blacks at 502 per 100,000, while the rates for whites and all others were 408 and 333 per 100,000, respectively. The basis for the excess in TBI injuries and deaths also appears to relate to differential exposures to various external causes of injury such as firearms.

For some ethnic and socioeconomic groups, risk exposure for traumatic injury may be systematically elevated. Lower socioeconomic status in large American cities may mean an elevated risk in at least three ways: increased exposure to physically demanding or unsafe employment settings (e.g., manual labor); increased exposure to violence (assault, gunshot, etc.); and increased exposure to older domiciles and vehicles (e.g., falling as a result of a domestic hazard, being a passenger in an older car; being more exposed as a pedestrian to cars in high-density urban settings. Thus, the overall risk pattern for a member of an economically disadvantaged group may be elevated compared with the risk pattern for someone who works at a desk job, lives in a modern house in a safer part of town, and drives a late-model car.[22,34,49]

In the United States, families at the lowest income levels have been shown to incur the highest numbers of injuries of all types on a per capita basis.[17] This was also found for TBI in a closely controlled study of San Diego County residents,[42] in two communities in Chicago,[86] and in Rhode Island.[25] The San Diego study demonstrated that the link between injury and low socioeconomic status was not modified when race or ethnicity was controlled for in the analysis.

Cultural differences and human ecology have long been known to have profound effects on patterns of disease and death.[7,65] Because, in general, minority populations of the urban United States are often of lower socioeconomic status, epidemiologically they may have an elevated risk for injury.[52] A relationship between ethnicity and head injury was identified—but inconclusively—in a complex analysis of cognitive impairment in blacks, Mexican-Americans, and whites by Molgaard et al.[57]

TBI Severity

Level of consciousness is the most commonly reported parameter used for evaluating brain injury severity, and the most widely used measure for level of consciousness is the Glasgow Coma Scale (GCS), despite a variety of methodological and scientific concerns. Developed in 1974 by Teasdale and Jennett,[75] the GCS uses a simple integer scoring of eye opening, verbal response, and motor function. Many treatment centers continue to use the original 14-point version instead of the authors' subsequent modification,[76] which allows a maximum total of 15 points. The opposite ends of the scale represent the best and worst neurological status and are relatively obvious. Immediately adjacent points on the scale (e.g., 8/9), however, are subject to varying degrees of professional judgment. Further difficulties in comparability of the GCS measured at different medical locations stem from incomplete or improper assessments and different timing. For example, intubation and sedation of the head-injured patient while being transported from the scene of the injury to the hospital will profoundly affect the person's apparent verbal and motor abilities and eye responses. Assessment of the person's neurological condition will also be affected by such factors as psychological stress, injuries to other parts of the body (especially the face), alcohol and drug use, and a variety of preexisting conditions.

For research purposes, differences in timing of the administration of any measurement tool are undoubtedly critical. Teasdale and Jennett[76] urged that GCS measurements be standardized at 6 hours postinjury. However, because a patient's apparent neurological condition may be closely linked to ED procedures like intubation and sedation or to acute surgical intervention, one score may be superseded by another score within a matter of minutes or hours. Thus, no single time period is the ideal candidate of choice. The later the GCS measurement is made, the better its prognostic value with respect to long-term mortality and total disability. However, GCS measurements days or weeks postinjury have little predictive value. Assessments are often made at the scene of injury and/or at the ED. However, which assessment constitutes the "best" indicator of a patient's neurological status remains controversial.[50] Table 1.2 compares selected predictors (including GCS) that have been used to assess a number of different outcomes following TBI.

The distribution of severity of brain injury as assessed by the GCS (or other parameters) is shown in Figure 1.7. Across all studies, the majority of hospital-admitted brain injuries are classified as *mild* (generally, a GCS score of 13–15 or an abbreviated injury score (AIS) of 1 or 2). However, *mild* is a highly imprecise description of brain trauma and is conceived differently by various researchers, some of whom use *mild* to describe any GCS score above 7, while others refer to GCS scores above 8, above 10, above 13, or 15 only.[41] The studies of the 1980s, with the exception of the report from Oklahoma, showed a ratio of mild to moderate to severe (as defined by the respective researchers) of about 8:1:1. A study from Oklahoma[35] reported 6%, 63%, and 30% for mild, moderate, and severe levels of TBI, respectively. More recently, two reports[79,80] showed significant declines in mild TBI levels for hospital admissions.

In the Utah report,[80] TBI severity was assessed using the GCS, while in the U.S. 1994–1995 report, severity assessment was accomplished using the International Clarification of Diseases-MAP (ICD-MAP), which converts ICD nature-of-injury codes to the AIS.

Other scales, among which are the Comprehensive Level of Consciousness,[71] the Reaction Level Scale,[72] the Clinical Neurological Assessment,[21] and the Innsbruck Coma Scale,[5] have been put forward as both practical and statistical improvements, in some cases, over the GCS. Some of these have generally been designed to be more sensitive than the GCS to neurological impairments across the continuum of consciousness; others have more specialized goals (see Table 1.3). Detailed psychometric studies indicate that the GCS fails as a reliable and valid measure of change in levels of consciousness for those patients in the middle range between full alertness and complete coma.[67] However, the GCS remains the scale that is easiest to administer while still retaining good interobserver reliability,[5] and itself has been incorporated into other indicators such as the Trauma Score and APACHE.[88]

Problems arise when designers of an assessment instrument increase the number of scoring criteria within a domain or add additional factors to be evaluated. The first and most obvious problem is time: The time needed to make an assessment

Table 1.2. Predictors of Outcome Following Brain Injury—Selected Studies

Reference	Predictors	Outcome Measured As:
van der Naalt et al.[83]	Duration of PTA	1, 3, 6 and 12 month GOS; complaints and return to work
Nissen, et al.[62]	Glasgow Head Injury Outcome Program (age, GCS, pupil response, CT scan findings, other clinical factors)	1. Dead or vegetative 2. Severely disabled 3. Moderately disabled or good recovery
Signorini et al.[68]	GCS score, pupil reactivity, hematoma on CT	Survival to 1 year
Asikainen et al.[3]	GCS, level of consciousness, duration of PTA	5-year status: GOS, occupational outcome
Gollaher et al.[30]	GCS, DRS, age, education, preinjury productivity	1–3 years employment status
Cifu et al.[16]	Disability Rating Scale, FIM, RLAS, GCS, NRS and neuropsychological tests	1-year return to work
Bullock et al.[8]	Age, hypotension, CT scan irregularities, abnormal papillary responses, GCS of 3–5	Mortality
Gerber et al.[28]	Graded scale composed of neurological status and CT results within 96 hours of admission	3-month status: full recovery, good, poor, death
Jeret et al.[38] 1993	Age, race, basilar skull fracture, mechanism of injury	Abnormal CT findings
Michaud et al.[55]	ISS and pupillary response at admission, GCS motor response 72 hours postadmission	Survival to discharge Discharge status: GOS
Wärme et al.[84]	GCS motor score, systemic hypotension, duration of hyperventilation, epilepsy	6-month status: GOS
Tompkins et al.[82]	GCS, history of psychological, physical, cognitive disorders	Language, memory, visual-motor skills
Pal et al.[63]	GCS	GOS
Choi et al.[15]	Hospital admission, GCS motor score, age, pupillary response	6-month status: good outcome, moderately disabled, severely disabled, dead
Lewin et al.[45]	Age at injury, worst state of neurological responsiveness in hospital, duration of PTA	10- to 25-year status: disability minimal, mild or moderate, severe or worse
Stewart et al.[74]	Age, pattern of consciousness	Mortality, length of hospital stay

CT, computed tomography; DRS, Disability Rating Scale; FIM, Functional Independence Measure; GCS, Glasgow Coma Scale; GOS, Glasgow Outcome Scale; NRS, Neurobehavioral Rating Scale; PTA, posttraumatic amnesia; RLAS, Rancho Los Amigo Scale.

often proves the inverse of the instrument's practical utility. Only slightly more subtle is a problem of training: The more a given scale or subscale depends on the assessor's depth of knowledge, the fewer the persons who will be qualified to give reliable estimates. Third is a problem of escalating alternatives: If the number of scoring possibilities exceeds an intuitively good fit to the reality that is being assessed, the likelihood of the instrument's results being incorporated into ongoing clinical practice begins to diminish. Though all of the assessment tools put forward as alternatives to the GCS use simple integer scoring, some raise the number of distinct variations by which a set of subscale scores describes a given patient into the tens of thousands or more (see Table 1.3). This is the product of the number of available scores times the number of independent components assessed within a given body region or behavior times the number of separate body regions or behaviors studied. At some point, this product becomes excessive and results in so many possible scoring variations that data cannot be readily interpreted. However, to rely on a single summary value (usually the sum of the subscale scores) is to obviate the goal of the instruments' authors: to design sensitive and discriminating assessment tools.

Prediction of Outcome

The question of accurate prediction of the outcome has been pursued by a variety of investigators. Their results show that no single set of indicators has been uniformly demonstrated to be useful in predicting patient outcomes (see Table 1.2). Thatcher et al.[77] found that electroencephalography and the GCS scores were excellent predictors of outcome if only those with dichotomous outcomes of *good recovery* or *dead* were considered, but the success of prediction dropped if patients with intermediate outcomes were also included. Wärme et al.[84] found

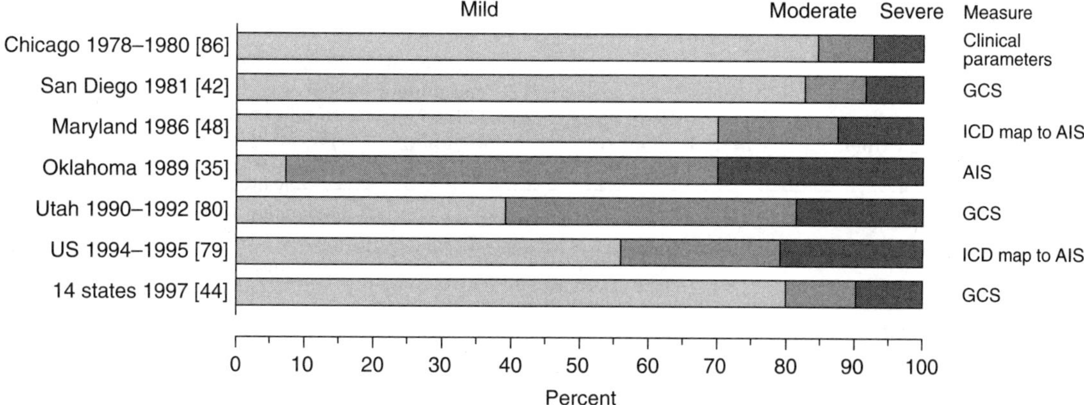

Figure 1.7. Distribution of brain injury severity distributions, selected U.S. studies. ICD, International Classification of Disease.

that the GCS motor score, systemic hypotension, and duration of hyperventilation were able to predict good recovery, as determined by the Glasgow Outcome Scale (GOS). Choi et al.[15] and Meredith et al.[54] showed that the GCS motor score alone was as good or better at predicting patient outcome as the entire GCS. Tompkins et al.[82] and Kilaru et al.[39] found that GCS and other markers of psychological, physical, or cognitive disorders prior to injury were successful in predicting cognitive performance after injury. Lewin et al.[45] found that age, PTA, and the worst neurological response score obtained soon after injury were the best predictors of the patient's cognitive capacity up to 24 hours following the injury. Gerber et al.[28] used neurological grade and computed tomography (CT) scan results to successfully predict 3-month outcomes. Michaud et al.[55] used a complex model of prediction and outcome to show that brain injury severity, extracranial injury severity, and pupillary response in the ED were predictive of long-term survival; brain injury severity, extracranial injury severity, and GCS scores obtained 72 hours after injury were predictive of long-term disability levels.

More than half of all TBI deaths occur at the scene of the injury event.[40] Among those who survive, outcomes appear to depend on two general phenomena: tear necrosis or nerve tissue degeneration and swelling of brain tissues that leads to nerve tissue necrosis. Unless both of these general categories of damage are prevented, permanent brain damage and resulting permanent disabilities can follow. Since secondary brain damage can begin within hours of the initial injury, early assessment is crucial to successful management. This is particularly true for those occasional persons who present initially with quite mild symptoms, only to deteriorate relatively quickly.

The Public Health Impact of Intervention

Primary prevention of injury is premised on reducing the frequency or degree of exposure to potential hazards. For example, improvements in road conditions and vehicle design act to prevent crashes and thus reduce all types of injury. Countermeasures like seat belts, bicycle and motorcycle helmets, and air bags are secondary and do not reduce the chances of a crash but act to interpose a barrier at the time of impact, resulting in reductions in the number and severity of injuries. Hence the countermeasures still prevent damage at the point of primary prevention. Some estimates of the effectiveness of countermeasures can be synthesized. For example, when motorcyclists use helmets, mortality has been shown to be reduced by about 38%, and both frequency of hospitalization and severity of injuries also decline significantly.[41]

Secondary prevention focuses on reducing mortality and morbidity following an acute exposure to some level of energy. Evidence suggests that mortality is reduced by up to 43% in brain-injured persons with timely surgical intervention and case monitoring.[56] Secondary (clinical) prevention begins

Table 1.3. Some Outcome Measures of Neurological Conditions

Instrument, Design Goal, Reference	Body Regions or Behaviors	Number of Components within Body Region or Behavior	Range of Total Scores within Body Region or Behavior (Lowest Value to Highest Value*)	Number of Possible Scoring Combinations†
GCS, "depth and duration of impaired consciousness and coma"[75]	Eye	1	1..4	
	Verbal	1	1..5	
	Motor	1	1..6	120
Comprehensive Level of Consciousness Scale (CLOCS), "assess a wider range of behavior [than GCS]"[71]	Posture	1	0..4	
	Eye	4	0..23	4,939,200
	General motor functioning	1	0..6	
	General responsiveness	1	0..8	
	Best communicative effort	1	0..7	
Reaction Level Scale (RLS85), "scale by which even intubated patients and patients with swollen eyelids could be reliably assessed"[72]	Alertness	1	8..1	8
Clinical Neurologic Assessment, "more sensitive to subtle changes in level of consciousness"[21]	Response after verbal stimulation	2	2..10	
	Response after tactile stimulation	3	3..17	9.48×10^{13}
	Following commands	3	3..14	
	Muscle tone	4	4..17	
	Body and extremity movement/position	5	5..24	
	Chewing, yawning, verbalization	4	4..16	
Innsbruck Coma Scale, "ability to predict death, even before initial treatment"[5]	Reaction to stimuli	2	0..6	49,152
	Body posture	1	0..3	
	Eye	4	0..12	
	Oral automatisms if vegetative	1	0..2	
Coma Recovery Scale, "to assess subtle changes in neurologic responsiveness over time"[29]	Arousal and attention	6	0..6	
	Hearing	5	0..5	35,290
	Eye	7	0..7	
	Motor	7	0..7	
	Oromotor	2	0..2	
	Verbalization	6	0..6	
	Initiates behavior	2	0..2	

Lowest = score reflecting most impairment; *highest* = score reflecting least impairment; where applicable, both are sums of individual component scores.

†Product of scores within scales, under assumptions of complete independence between components within the instrument.

with the arrival of emergency medical service (EMS) personnel who can maintain the patient's airway, enhance respiration, and start treatment for shock. However, half of the fatalities among brain injury victims occur within 10 minutes of the incident. Data from San Diego County, California, showed that EMS staff need a median of 20 minutes to reach the scene; thus, half of the fatalities may not be readily preventable by early EMS intervention.[40] Another 20% of TBI deaths occur within 2 hours of the incident; these are potentially prevented by the actions taken by EMS and ED staff. Thus, establishing a trauma center with an EMS system to transport patients may reduce TBI deaths by up to 20%. For communities with trauma centers, some reduction in mortality may occur by increasing the amount and quality of patient monitoring and by preventing secondary brain damage in those patients suspected of having TBI. A mean case fatality rate of about 5–6 per 100 admitted patients appears to be consistent with existing technology and community organization. Unfortunately, until rigorous clinical guidelines for prevention of secondary brain damage are standardized and widely implemented, the full effects of such efforts will not be achieved. The development of clinical guidelines for the management of severe head injury[8] are now available and should improve the quality of outcomes following TBI, but unfortunately, there has not been widespread implementation.[33]

Tertiary prevention includes physical, psychological, and vocation rehabilitation for patients suffering the residual effects from TBI. Although the impact on mortality at this stage is nil, the greatest tasks regarding functional restoration remain future challenges.

Intervention Feasibility

Numerous primary prevention strategies are possible for TBI.[11,32] A variety of preventive measures can be imagined, some of which address persons at risk specifically, while others address environmental improvements or legislative changes (see Table 1.4). The key topics, which appear to be subject to modification through these means, are vehicles and transport, falls, firearms, and sports. The expected reduction in TBI deaths can be estimated from existing data for some preventive measures. The economic and technical feasibility of each measure can be rated on a simple scale from low to high, and the general tenor of the public response to each possibility can be roughly approximated.

A technically feasible strategy does not automatically imply that the intervention will succeed, as the public response may be poor or the cost may be too high. A low-cost strategy may have no hope of succeeding for more than a minute fraction of the possible exposures. A publicly acceptable strategy may have no viability for strictly technical reasons. For example, the evidence is unmistakable that the likelihood of a fatal vehicle crash doubles for every increase of 0.02 gm/dl of blood alcohol in the driver, yet public acceptance of a zero alcohol prevention program would be minimal and enforcement would be exceptionally costly. There is growing acceptance, however, of zero alcohol tolerance with enforcement for younger drivers, as evidenced by laws in several states (Alaska, Arizona, the District

Table 1.4. Feasibility and Impact of Different Traumatic Brian Injury (TBI) Preventive Measures

	Expected Reduction in TBI Deaths*				
Examples of Preventive Action	**Exposed**	**All E-Causes**	**Economic Feasibility**	**Technical Feasibility**	**Public Response**
Improve roads	Unknown	Unknown	Low	Moderate	High
Medical checkup of drivers	<1%	≈0%	Moderate	Low	Low
"Safe Ride" Program	<1%	≈0%	High	Low	Low
Continuing driver education	Unknown	Unknown	Moderate	Low	Low
Seat belts for all occupants	32–54%	12–45%	High	Low	Low
Air bags for all vehicles	45–55%	23%	High	High	Low
Helmets for all bicyclists and motorcyclists	30%	7%	Moderate	Moderate	High
Zero BAC level for all drivers	9–72%	46%	Low	High	Low
BAC <.05 gm/dl for all drivers	50%	36%	High	High	Low
Ban handguns	30	12	High	High	Moderate
Changes in architectural design to prevent falls	10–69%	3–18%	Moderate	Low	Low
Changes in medical management and referral practices	10–50%	Unknown	Low	Moderate	High
Use CT/MRI in cases of suspected brain injury	<5%	n/a	Low	Low	High
Changes in rehabilitation practices	Unknown	Unknown	Low	Low	High

**Exposed* = all persons whose actions places them at specified risk, that is, persons receiving direct benefit of preventive action.

All e-causes = all persons, regardless of exposure.

BAC, blood alcohol concentration; CT, computed tomography; MRI, magnetic resonance imaging.

of Columbia, Illinois, North Carolina, Oregon, Utah, and Wisconsin[4,36]).

Educational approaches have been attempted for many years, many focusing on educating adolescents in the school system, especially in driver training and education for crash reduction or avoidance. Unfortunately, few demonstrations of the educational effectiveness of these programs are available, and those few tend to have limited success in modifying actual behaviors even when attitudes and knowledge have been modified. Legislation coupled with environmental measures, rather than educational measures, will probably continue to have a substantially larger overall effect on TBI reduction. For example, an intervention such as an air bag or a motorcycle helmet can be implemented across large groups of persons at risk with maximum benefit.

ACKNOWLEDGMENTS

We acknowledge with appreciation the library research of Candace Edamura, MPH. Work on this chapter was supported by the Southern California Injury Prevention Research Center.

REFERENCES

1. Adekoya N, Thurman DJ, White DD, Webb KW: Surveillance for traumatic brain injury deaths—United States, 1989–1998. MMWR 51:1–14, 2002.
2. Annegers JF, Grabow JD, Kurland LT, Laws ER Jr: The incidence, causes and secular trends of head trauma in Olmsted County, Minnesota, 1935–74. Neurology 30:912–919, 1980.
3. Asikainen I, Kaste M, Sarna S: Predicting late outcome for patients with traumatic brain injury referred to a rehabilitation programme: A study of 508 Finnish patients 5 years or more after injury. Brain Injury 12:95–107, 1998.
4. Australian Injury Prevention Bulletin: National Injury Surveillance Unit—issue 6, National Injury Surveillance Unit, Bedford Park, South Australia, 1994.
5. Benzer A, Mitterschiffthaler G, Marosi M, et al: Prediction of non-survival after trauma: Innsbruck Coma Scale. Lancet 338:977–978, 1991.
6. Bouraga P: Road traffic accidents and the role of the police. Papua New Guinea Med J 23:58, 1980.
7. Brown PJ, Inhorn MC: Disease, ecology, and human behavior. In: Johnson TM, Sargent CF (eds): Medical Anthropology: A Handbook of Theory and Method. New York, Greenwood Press, 1990, chap. 11.
8. Bullock R, Chestnut RM, Clifton G, et al: Guidelines for the management of severe head injury. J Neurotrauma 11:639–734, 1996.
9. Butchart A, Nell V, Yach D, Johnson K, Radebe B: Epidemiology of non-fatal injuries due to external causes in Johannesburg—Soweto. Part II: Incidence and determinants. S Afr Med J 79:472–479, 1991.
10. Centers for Disease Control: Traumatic brain injury—Colorado, Missouri, Oklahoma and Utah 1990–1993. MMWR 46:8–11, 1997.
11. Centers for Disease Control, National Committee for Injury Prevention and Control. Injury prevention: Meeting the challenge: The National Committee for Injury Prevention and Control. Am J Prev Med 5:3 (suppl), 1989.
12. Centers for Disease Control and Prevention: National Vital Statistics Report 52, 2003. www.cdc.gov/nchs/fastats/lcod.htm (November 2005).
13. Centers for Disease Control and Prevention: NCIPC home page, WISQARS, Atlanta, GA, 2004.
14. Centers for Disease Control and Prevention: Web-based Injury Statistics Query and Reporting Systems (WISQARS) [online]. 2003. National Center for Injury Prevention and Control, Centers for Disease Control and Prevention (procedures). Available from URL: www.cdc.gov/ncipc/wisqars (November 2005).
15. Choi SC, Narayan RK, Anderson RL, Ward JD: Enhanced specificity of prognosis in severe head injury. J Neurosurg 70:381–385, 1988.
16. Cifu D, Keyser-Marcus L, Lopez E, et al: Acute predictors of successful return to work 1 year after traumatic brain injury: A multicenter analysis. Arch Phys Med Rehabil 78:124–131, 1997.
17. Collins JG. Types of injuries by selected characteristics: United States, 1985–1987. Vital Health Stat. Series 10. 176:1–68, 1990.
18. Commission on Professional and Hospital Activities: The International Classification of Diseases, 9th Revision, Clinical Modification (ICD-9-CM). Ann Arbor, MI, 1978.
19. Committee on Trauma Research, Commission of Life Sciences, National Research Council and the Institute of Medicine: Injury in America. Washington, DC, National Academy Press, 1985.
20. Cooper KD, Tabaddor K, Hauser WA, et al: The epidemiology of head injury in the Bronx. Neuroepidemiology 2:69–88, 1983.
21. Crosby L, Parsons LC: Clinical Neurologic Assessment Tool: Development and testing of an instrument to index neurologic status. Heart Lung 18:121–128, 1989.
22. Cubbina C, Le Clereb FB, Smith GS: Socioeconomic status and injury mortality: Individual and neighborhood determinants. J Epidemiol Commun Health 54:517–525, 2000.
23. Feachem R, Kjellsotm T, Murray CJL, et al: The Health of Adults in the Developing World. New York, Oxford University Press, 1992.
24. Fife D: Head injury with and without hospital admission: Comparisons of incidence and short-term disability. Am J Public Health 77:810–812, 1987.
25. Fife D, Faich G, Hollinshead W, Boynton W: Incidence

and outcome of hospital-treated head injury in Rhode Island. Am J Public Health 75:773–778, 1986.

26. Gabella B, Hoffman RE, Marine WW, Stallones L: Urban and rural traumatic brain injuries in Colorado. Ann Epidemiol 7:207–212, 1997.
27. Gale JL, Dikmen S, Wyler A, et al: Head injury in the Pacific Northwest. Neurosurgery 12:487–491, 1983.
28. Gerber CJ, Lang DA, Neil-Dwyer G, Smith PWF: A simple scoring system for accurate prediction of outcome within four days of a subarachnoid haemorrhage. Acta Neurochir 122:11–22, 1993.
29. Giacino JT, Kezmarsky MA, DeLuca J, Cicerone KD: Monitoring rate of recovery to predict outcome in minimally responsive patients. Arch Phys Med Rehabil 72:897–901, 1991.
30. Gollaher K, High W, Sherer M, et al: Prediction of employment outcomes one to three years following traumatic brain injury (TBI). Brain Injury 12:245–263, 1998.
31. Guerrero JL, Thurman DJ, Sniezek JE: Emergency department visits associated with traumatic brain injury: United States 1995–1996. Brain Injury 14:181–186, 2000.
32. Haddon W Jr: Advances in the epidemiology of injuries as a basis for public policy. Public Health Rep 95:411–421, 1980.
33. Hesdorffer D, Ghajar J, Iacona L: Predictors of compliance with evidence-based guidelines for traumatic brain injury care: A survey of United States trauma centers. J Trauma 52:1202–1209, 2002.
34. Hoofien D, Vakil E, Gilboa A, Donovick PJ: Comparison of the predictive power of socioeconomic variables, severity of injury and age on long-term outcome of traumatic brain injury: sample-specific variables versus factors as predictors. Brain Injury 16:9–27, 2003.
35. Injury Epidemiology Division: Traumatic brain injuries Oklahoma, 1989. Oklahoma City, Oklahoma State Department of Health, 1991.
36. Insurance Institute for Highway Safety: State Law Facts 1994. Alexandria, VA, Insurance Institute for Highway Safety, 1994.
37. Jager TE, Weiss HB, Coben JH, Pepe PE: Traumatic brain injuries evaluated in U.S. emergency departments, 1992–1994. Acad Emerg Med 7:134–143, 2000.
38. Jeret JS, Mandell M, Anziska B, et al: Clinical predictors of abnormality disclosed by computed tomography after mild head trauma. Neurosurgery 32:9–16, 1993.
39. Kilaru S, Garb J, Emhoff T, et al: Long-term functional status and mortality of elderly patients with severe closed head injuries. J Trauma 41:957–963, 1996.
40. Kraus JF, Black MA, Hessol N, et al: The incidence of acute brain injury and serious impairment in a defined population. Am J Epidemiol 119:186–201, 1984.
41. Kraus J, Chu L: Epidemiology. In: Silver J, Yudofsky S, Hales R (eds): Neuropsychiatry of Traumatic Brain Injury. Washington, DC, American Psychiatric Press, 2004, chap. 1.
42. Kraus J, Fife D, Ramstein K, et al: The relationship of family income to the incidence, external causes, and outcomes of serious brain injury, San Diego County, California. Am J Public Health 75:1345–1347, 1986.
43. Kraus JF, McArthur DL: Epidemiology of head injury. In: Cooper P (ed): Head Injury, 4th rev. Baltimore, Williams & Wilkins, 2002, chap. 1.
44. Langlois J, Rutland-Brown W, Thomas K: Traumatic brain injury in the United States: Emergency department visits, hospitalizations and deaths. Atlanta, Georgia, Centers for Disease Control and Prevention, National Center for Injury Prevention and Control, 2004.
45. Lewin W, Marshall TFD, Roberts AH: Long-term outcome after severe head injury. BMJ 15:1533–1537, 1979.
46. Li GH, Baker SP: A comparison of injury death rates in China and the United States, 1986. Am J Public Health 81:605–609, 1991.
47. Louisiana Office of Public Health, Injury Research and Prevention Section: Traumatic Brain and Spinal Cord Injury in Louisiana: 1996–1999. Cumulative Report. Baton Rouge: Louisiana Department of Health and Hospitals, Office of Public Health, May 10, 2004.
48. MacKenzie EJ, Edelstein SL, Flynn JP: Hospitalized head-injured patients in Maryland: Incidence and severity of injuries. Maryland Med J 38:724–732, 1989.
49. Marcin JP, Schembri MS, He J, Romano PS: A population-based analysis of socioeconomic status and insurance status and their relationship with pediatric trauma hospitalization and mortality rates. Am Public Health 93; 461–466, 2003.
50. Marion DW, Carlier PM: Problems with initial Glasgow Coma Scale assessment causedby prehospital treatment patients with head injuries: Results of a national survey. J Trauma 36:89–95, 1994.
51. Masters SJ, McClean PM, Arcarese JS, et al: Skull x-ray examinations after head trauma. N Engl J Med 316:84–91, 1987.
52. Maurer JD, Rosenberg HM, Keemer JB: Deaths of Hispanic origin, 15 reporting states, 1979–81. Vital and Health Statistics Series 20, No. 18, 1979–82. Washington, DC, National Center for Health Statistics, 1990.
53. McArthur DL, Chute DJ, Villablanca JP: Moderate and severe traumatic brain injury: Epidemiologic, imaging and neuropathologic perspectives. Brain Pathol 14: 185–194, 2004.
54. Meredith W, Rutledge R, Hansen A, et al: Field triage of trauma patients based upon the ability to follow commands: A study in 28,573 injured patients. J Trauma 38:128–135, 1995.
55. Michaud LJ, Rivara FP, Grady MS, Reay DT: Predictors of survival and severity of disability after severe brain injury in children. Neurosurgery 31:244–264, 1992.
56. Miller JD: Head injury. J Neurol Neurosurg Psychiatry 56:443–444, 1993.
57. Molgaard CA, Standford EP, Morton DJ, et al: Epidemiology of head trauma and neurocognitive impairment in a multi-ethnic population. Neuroepidemiology 9:233–240, 1990.
58. National Center for Injury Prevention and Control: Injury Fact Book 2001–2002. Atlanta. Centers for Disease Control and Prevention, 2001.
59. National Center for Injury Prevention and Control: Injury

Mortality Report, 2001, United States. All Injury Deaths and Rates per 100,000. WISQARS, www.cdc.gov/ncipc/wisqars (November 2005).

60. National Institute of Mental Health and Neurosciences: Bangalore, India, Epidemiology of Head Injuries: Summary Project Report, 1993.

61. Nestvold K, Lundar T, Blikra G, Lonnum A: Head injuries during one year in a central hospital in Norway: A prospective study. Neuroepidemiology 7:134–144, 1988.

62. Nissen JJ, Jones PA, Segnorini DF, et al: Glasgow Head Injury Outcome Prediction Program: An independent assessment. J Neurol Neurosurg Psychiatry 67:796–799, 1999.

63. Pal J, Brown R, Fleiszer D: The value of the Glasgow Coma Scale and Injury Severity Score: Predicting outcome in multiple trauma patients with head injury. J Trauma 28:746–748, 1989.

64. Pan American Health Organization: Mortality from accidents and violence in the Americas. Epidemiol Bull 15(2):1–2, 1994.

65. Polendak AP: Racial and Ethnic Differences in Disease. New York, Oxford University Press, 1989.

66. Schuster M: Traumatic Brain Injury in Massachusetts. Boston, Massachusetts Department of Public Health, Bureau of Family and Community Health, Injury Prevention and Control Program, 1994.

67. Segatore M, Way C: The Glasgow Coma Scale: Time for change. Heart Lung 21:548–557, 1992.

68. Signorini D, Andrews PJD, Jones PA, et al: Predicting survival using simple clinical variables: A case study in traumatic brain injury. J Neurol Neurosurg Psychiatry 66:20–24, 1999.

69. Sosin DM, Sacks JJ, Smith SM: Head injury-associated deaths in the United States from 1979 to 1986. JAMA 262:2241–2245, 1989.

70. Sosin DM, Sniezek JE, Waxweiler RJ: Trends in deaths associated with traumatic brain injury, 1979 through 1992. JAMA 273:1778–1780, 1995.

71. Stanczak DE, White JG 3d, Gouview WD, et al: Assessment of level of consciousness following severe neurological insult. J Neurosurg 60:955–960, 1984.

72. Starmark J-E, Stålhammar D, Holmgren E: The Reaction Level Scale (RLS85) manual and guidelines. Acta Neurochir 91:12–20, 1988.

73. Steiner C, Elixhauser A, Schnaier J: The healthcare cost and utilization project: An overview. Effect Clin Pract 5:142–151, 2002.

74. Stewart WA, Litten SP, Sheehe PR: A prognostic model for head injury. Acta Neurochir 45:199–208, 1979.

75. Teasdale G, Jennett B: Assessment of coma and impaired consciousness. A practical scale. Lancet 2:81–84, 1974.

76. Teasdale G, Jennett B: Assessment and prognosis of coma after head injury. Acta Neurochir 34:45–55, 1975.

77. Thatcher RW, Cantor DS, McAlaster R, Geisler F, Krause P: Comprehensive predictions of outcome in closed head-injured patients. Ann NY Acad of Sci 620:82–101, 1991.

78. Thurman DJ, Alverson C, Dunn K, et al: Traumatic brain injury in the U.S.: A public health perspective. J Head Trauma Rehabil 14:602–615, 1999.

79. Thurman DJ, Guerrero, JL: Trends in hospitalization associated with traumatic brain injury. JAMA. 292:954–957, 1999.

80. Thurman DJ, Jeppson L, Burnett CL, et al: Surveillance of traumatic brain injuries in Utah. West J Med 165:192–196, 1996.

81. Thurman DJ, Sniezek JE, Johnson D, et al: Guidelines for Surveillance of Central Nervous System Injury. Atlanta, Centers for Disease Control and Prevention, 1995.

82. Tompkins CA, Holland AL, Ratcliff G, et al: Predicting cognitive recovery from closed head-injury in children and adolescents. Brain Cognition 13:86–97, 1990.

83. van der Naalt J, van Zomeren AH, Sluiter WJ, Minderhoud JM: One-year outcome in mild to moderate head injury: The predictive value of acute injury characteristics related to complaints and return to work. J Neurol Neurosurg Psychiatry 66:207–213, 1999.

84. Wärme PE, Bergström R, Persson L: Neurosurgical intensive care improves outcome after severe head injury. Acta Neurochir 110:57–64, 1991.

85. Warren S, Moore M, Johnson MS: Traumatic head and spinal cord injuries in Alaska (1991–1993). Alaska Med 37:11–19, 1995.

86. Whitman S, Coonley-Hoganson R, Desai BT: Comparative head trauma experiences in two socioeconomically different Chicago-area communities. Am J Epidemiol 119:569–590, 1984.

87. WHO, Advisory Committee on Neurotrauma Prevention: Standards for Surveillance of Neurotrauma. Geneva, World Health Organization, 1996.

88. Yates DW: Scoring systems for trauma. Br Med J 301:1090–1093, 1990.

89. Zwi A: The public health burden of injury in developing countries: A critical review of the literature. Trop Dis Bull 90:R5–R45, 1993.

Chapter 2
The History of Cerebral Trauma

F. CLIFFORD ROSE

Though we should not refuse to give modem authors due credit for their discoveries or happy imitations, it is none the less just to restore to the ancients what properly belongs to them.
Celsus, *Liber Medicinae Secundus*, Cap. XIV

A murder committed over 1 million years ago provides the first evidence of brain injury. At that time, the human's predecessor was a semierect hominid now named *Australopithecus africanus*. A damaged skull from this species found in South Africa revealed two posterior fractures close together that fit the condyles of an antelope humerus discovered nearby, which was therefore presumed to be the instrument used for the clubbing to death from behind.[10]

Such fractured skulls have been found in later hominids who walked more erectly (*Homo erectus*), such as Java man (more than 300,000 years ago), Peking man (more than 100,000 years ago), and Neanderthal man (more than 40,000 years ago). "The literature of trepanation is large, well over 1000 references."[24] "Not all holes in skulls were made by human hands and these have been grouped as pseudo-trephination. The earliest known trephined skulls date from 10,000 BC and were found in North Africa. A distinction is made between the trephined skulls found in Europe which date from about 3000 BC, and those found in South America which are from the two millennia between 500 BC and 1500 AD."[24a]

Brain injuries had a reputation for being fatal, and Younge[27] in 1682 "reviewed the entire medical literature back to Galen—more than 1,500 years—and was able to find reports of only a hundred individuals who survived a brain wound." In the nineteenth century, this view was challenged because of the findings of skulls on which surgery had been performed.[24b]

Trepanation

There is often confusion between *trepanation* and *trephination*, as the two terms have been used interchangeably. The word *trepanation* is derived from the Greek *trypanon*, meaning a borer, and this is the operation done in neolithic times, where the head was kept still by "a frame or brace similar to, and used in the manner of, the carpenter's wimple" (p. 11).[25] Trephination "implies using a cutting instrument rotating around a centre."[25] The term is of more recent French origin, but both terms imply more than making a depression or perforation of the calvarium since they entail removing a piece of bone with a saw-like instrument. [22]

When the ancient Greeks performed trepanation, they used either an instrument called a *terebra*, a drill that was rotated using a strap around its center, or a *trepanon*, which was operated by a bow. A third instrument was a *serrata terebra*, a cone-shaped piece of metal with a circular edge at the bottom that was serrated and kept in place by a central pin. That pin was removed after the drill, rotated by rolling its large handle by hand or with a bow, had made an initial hole. Hippocrates described the trepan, which was used for contusions, fissure fractures, and indentations of the skull, but rarely for depressed fractures.[26] Celsus disagreed, advising trepanation for depressed fractures. Heliodorus (c. 100 A.D.), in recommending trepanation near a fracture site, advised cooling the instrument by dropping water onto the wound.

The New World

The first illustration of a trepanned skull was in 1839 in an anthropological atlas by S.G. Morton of the United States. However, he did not recognize the results of trepanation, thinking that the hole in the skull was due to an injury from a blunt instrument, probably the back of a war axe. The first perforated skull to be recognized as the result of surgery was revealed by Ephraim George Squires, who was the U.S. Commissioner to Peru and, according to Broca, the "foremost archaeologist in American Indian matters."[6] Squires left Peru in 1865, and in the following year this skull was demonstrated to the New York Academy of Medicine, where it can now be found, as a "supposed case of trephining [sic] of the calvarium of one of the tribes of South America." Squires noted that the skull had a quadrilateral trepanation: "the most notable proof of surgical knowledge among the natives that has been discovered in this context, as trepanation is one of the most difficult of surgical procedures. . . ." He took the skull to Paris for a second opinion, and Broca showed it to both the Société d'Anthropologie and the Académie de Médicine in 1867.[6]

Broca was confident that since the outline of the hole was regular, it was not due to trauma but was surgical in origin. Furthermore, there were signs of postoperative inflammation indicating survival (he estimated from 7 to 8 days). A square of bone 15 × 17 mm had been removed, and the outline differed from the oval and serrated one of later Greek times. Since there was no evidence of trauma he concluded that trepanation had been performed "to evacuate an epidural hematoma."

Broca became fascinated by this procedure and, using pieces of cut silex, made a perforation in the skull of a dog in just over 8 minutes. Using a piece of glass, he did the same in an adult human in about 1 hour, but took only 4 minutes using the skull of a 2-year-old child. In 1888 Broca discussed a dozen skulls with man-made perforations that were oval in shape, the long axis being in the anteroposterior plane and mostly in the parietal area and found twice as often on the left as on the right.

Since the 1860s, many such skulls have been discovered, particularly in Peru, where they range in date from 3000 years ago to the immediate pre-Columbian Inca civilization based in Cuzco less than 1000 years ago. At this site, nearly half of the skulls found have man-made openings, whereas in other areas of Peru, such as south of Lima among the Paracas Indians, the frequency is just over 5%. These latter skulls were found in burial caverns of sandy beaches and were excavated in the 1920s. The perforations were made using metallic instruments of bronze or copper called *tumi*, and since the vast majority of patients survived, it is likely that the operation was stopped when the dura was reached.

The indications for the operation are uncertain, but initially Broca thought it was performed for ritualistic rather than therapeutic purposes. Although the skulls came from humans of all ages, there were four times as many men as women, so that it is likely that the operation was performed in cases of depressed fracture due to trauma.

Albucasis (936–1013 A.D.) copied the trepanation techniques of Paulus Aeginata by using a drill that would not penetrate the brain. He described the operation as follows: "you cut through the bone in the confident knowledge that nothing inward can happen to the membrane even though the operator be the most ignorant and cowardly of men; yes even if he be sleepy," but if the dura turned black, "you may know that he is doomed" (p. 420).[14]

It is unknown whether patients were anesthetized or comatose at the time of the operation or, more remotely possible, conditioned to withstand great pain. Possible anesthetics would have been cocoa leaves and alcohol, prepared as *chicha* (fermented maize). In addition, such locally acting drugs from the belladonna family as scopolamine, hyoscyamic acid, and atropine were probably applied to the head. Infection may have been prevented by the use of mercury salts, arsenic, copper sulfate, or cinnamic-acid-rich substances, whereas bleeding was stopped by tannic acid found in Pumaca, a common plant in the Peruvian Andes. Scalp wounds were approximated by tying groups of hair or cotton sutures, and examples have been found of the head bandaged with cloth.

Europe

Although trepanned skulls in South America date back to 5000 years ago, in Europe they are at least 10,000 years old, from the Paleolithic period, as dated by the objects found with them. The first such skull was discovered in France as early as 1685 A.D., but its significance was not appreciated until 1816 A.D., when the next such skull was found in the same country; however, its advanced age was not recognized.[14]

On May 21, 1868, Louis Lartet read a paper to the Societe d'Anthropologie on Troglodytes in the Perigord ("Skulls of Les Eyzies"). The skulls were found at Cro-Magnon, near the railroad station of the borough of Les Eyzies, where widening of the railway tracks revealed the caves containing the skulls. One of the most complete skeletons was that of a woman, aged about 35 years, whose skull had a left frontal perforation measuring 33 × 12 mm. She survived the injury, which was thought to have been due to a blow with a flint axe, since there were signs of formation of new bone. These Cro-Magnon finds were the first and best-described prototype of *Homo sapiens* from the Paleolithic period (from about 350,000 to 100,000 years ago).

Five years later, Prunières, a consultant physician, was the first to suggest that the holes in the skulls found in a prehistoric burial grave near Lazère were man-made,[25] and in the following years, skulls with scalloped edges were excavated in central France. These skulls were from the Neolithic period; some were healed and others unhealed. Some of the holes were made postmortem, presumably for the making of religious amulets. Since then, such skulls have been found in many European countries and share common characteristics. Varying in size from a few centimeters to 13 × 10 cm (i.e., half of the skull), the holes are mostly located in the parietal region; although occipital and frontal holes are also seen, they are rare in the temporal region. These operations were done with polished stones and were grouped "over the motor and epileptogenic region of the surface of the brain."[18] Horsley argued that trephination would have been performed over the motor cortex, but probably not for Jacksonian epilepsy, and that it could cure convulsions and perhaps some other conditions, such as a depressed fracture.

The Broca Museum of Anthropology in Paris contains 60 specimens of perforated skulls, 10 of which are fairly complete, yet the number in the rest of Europe "could be counted on the fingers."[24a]

Asia

Victor Horsley[18] raised the question of whether trepanation originated in Asia. Certainly, the operation was not universally popular. For example, a Chinese surgeon, Hua To (190–265 A.D.), recommended trepanation for the headaches of his prince, who rewarded his medical advisor by executing him.

In the twentieth century, primitive societies performed the operation for insanity, epilepsy, and headaches and to "let the devils out." South Sea islanders have treated headaches and dizzy spells by scraping the cranium down to the dura.

Ancient Egypt

In the Edwin Smith Papyrus,* there is no mention of the trepan. Although it has been claimed that the ancient Egyptians did not perform trepanation,[11]

*Edwin Smith (1822–1906) was an American Egyptologist who settled in Luxor in 1858. Four years later, he was approached by an Egyptian merchant who had a papyrus that he had found in a tomb and wished to sell. Although Edwin Smith recognized its medical content, he noted that the outside of the roll was tattered, as if some layers had been stripped off. He declared his interest, and a few months later the same vendor came with another roll, the outside layers of which had come from the first roll and had been pasted around a dummy; these fragments contained a discussion of the heart and its vessels. Edwin Smith eventually obtained eight fragments, which are now known by his name. Although he put five together approximately, Breasted was asked in 1920 to translate the whole text, which he published 10 years later.

The Edwin Smith Papyrus dates from the time when the pyramids "were being built—3000–2500 B.C.—and could even recent evidence suggests that they did.[21] The first written evidence of brain injuries about 5000 years ago is to be found in the Egyptian papyri.

Of all the Egyptian papyri, seven are of medical interest—those of Edwin Smith, Ebers, Hearst, Berlin 3038, London, Carlsberg VIII, and Chester Beatty VI. Only the Edwin Smith Surgical Papyrus, which antedates by several centuries the Ebers Papyrus, makes a significant contribution to the history of treatment of brain injuries. Because the causes of injuries are self-evident, the descriptions are accurate, in contrast to those of the later Ebers Papyrus, which was concerned mainly with medical disorders for which the causes were unknown and were considered to be due to visitations from the gods and treated irrationally. It is to Breasted[5] that we owe a debt for his decade of work translating the Edwin Smith Papyrus. Not a physician, he could not recognize its importance for neurology, but he did realize "the treatise to be unique by way of content, philosophy and form."[7]

The Edwin Smith Papyrus contains the first written records of head injuries, of which there were 27. However, only 13 of these case histories concern skull fractures with neurological features, the others being soft tissue injuries only. The prognosis is divided into three categories: Verdict I, "an ailment which I will treat"; Verdict II, "an ailment with which I will contend"; and Verdict III, "an ailment not to be treated." The approach to injuries is anatomical from above downward, and the case reports are systematized into these sections: Title, Examination, Diagnosis, Treatment, and Definitions of Terms Used. Skull fractures are divided into: (1) splits (i.e., fissures), (2) smashes (i.e., comminuted), (3) compound comminuted, and (4) comminuted and depressed. There are also cases of fractures of the skull base, as evidenced by bleeding from one or both ears.

Observation and palpation are emphasized. Head posture is important, as is skin color. With palpation, the patient's brain may be felt to be "throbbing [and] fluttering like the weak place of an infant's crown before it becomes whole" (Case 6), and the physician can feel and count the pulse of the head, neck and extremities.[17] (Although this is the first note of pulse counting, the first done with a time measure was by Herophilus [c. 330–260 B.C.].[5]) The physician also elicits signs by asking the patient to rotate the neck and move the limbs. Speechlessness is an ominous sign.

Case 6 describes a gaping head wound with a comminuted fracture and rupture of the meningeal membranes that reveals the brain surface, which is compared to the surface of cooling molten copper. This was the first time that words meaning *brain*, *meninges*, and *cerebrospinal fluid* were used.[5] The commentator compares what he sees with what is familiar; not only is the brain surface compared to molten slag, but a fractured skull is likened to a broken pottery jar and the mandibular ramus to a two-toed bird. In addition, this Papyrus provides the first mention of the cranial sutures, "which the ancient Arabs believed were the patient's destiny written by the hands of Allah" (p. 276).[12]

Case 8 is also a comminuted fracture, but without any visible external injury. The patient had a "smash in his skull under the skin of his head, there being no wound upon it." The statement, "his eye on that side was askew," suggests an ipsilateral ocular palsy possibly due to an orbital fracture, rather than the facial palsy suggested by Elsberg.[12] There was also an ipsilateral hemiparesis, as evidenced by "shuffling with his feet . . . walking with his sole dragging"; "the presence of nails in the middle of his palm" suggests contractures, and the ipsilateral paralysis suggests a contrecoup injury. Several days after a head injury, the patient was "unable to look at his shoulders and his breast"—a clear reference to the nuchal rigidity of meningeal irritation. Other cases of neck stiffness are due to tetanus[6] or injured cervical muscles or vertebrae. The Papyrus also includes the first written description of tetanus: the patient had a drooping head posture, weeping facies with drawn eyebrows, thick saliva, a tightly closed mouth, and clammy skin; symptomatic treatment was heat to the clamped jaw "until [the patient] is comfortable."

Case 20, of a temporal wound with a speech disturbance, is considered to be the first description of a cranial injury causing aphasia.[12]

Case 22, entitled "Compound comminuted frac-

be the work of Imhotep. Polymath, architect, statesman, and physician to the court of Pharoah Zoser, the author of the Papyrus was possibly a military surgeon who knew about weapons and the injuries they inflict." In 69 discussions, he explained anatomical terms and injuries, which give a good idea of the state of medical knowledge at that time. Although the original documents were lost, a second contributor modernized the script several centuries later, and a third contributor, a Theban scribe, not knowing any medicine, wrote it down by hand around 1600 B.C.

ture of the temporal bone," is the most serious of five cases of temporal injuries. The surgeon had to probe the ear and remove bone splinters. After this assessment, the prognosis was Verdict III—no treatment recommended.

In ancient Egypt, head wounds were treated by application of a piece of meat on the first day, followed by a linen cloth soaked in honey or fat. With skull fractures, the patient was advised to maintain a sitting position, supported by bricks on either side—good advice to keep the intracranial pressure lower and help prevent intracranial bleeding. The treatment of penetrating injuries of the brain was the application of grease, but bandages were avoided to allow drainage. The fats applied, according to the Ebers Papyrus, were a mixture taken from snake, crocodile, ibex, lion, and hippopotamus. Oral feeding was recommended through "a wooden brace put into the mouth"; "a draught of fruit" was given to pale and exhausted patients.

Herodotus of Halicarnassus (c. 484–420 B.C.) relates that when he traveled to Egypt, medical practice was based on specialization, so that there were different doctors for the eyes, teeth, or head. However, treatments were irrational. According to the Leiden Papyrus, charms were applied to the painful area or, for headaches, were hung around the neck or even the hand or foot.

The Bible

There are biblical references (c. 1300 B.C.) to brain injuries, such as when Joel slew the enemy King Sisera by driving "a metal tent stake through his temples while he slept" and Goliath (c. 1050 B.C.) was rendered unconscious by a stone that sunk into his forehead. Goliath had put on his helmet of brass but suffered a concussion, presumably with a depressed frontal fracture in the unprotected frontal region.

Ancient Greece

Homer

It has been estimated that, of 140 penetrating wounds of the body reported in Homer's works, the mortality rate was over 75%. Mortality was higher with spear and sword wounds than with those caused by arrows because, in the latter, if the vital structures were injured, there could be healing without infection once the arrow was removed.

Cerebral trauma in animals was also recorded—for example, Nestor's horse: "In agony the horse sprang into the air as the missile passed into the brain. The man was thrown into confusion by the rolling of the wounded horse on the ground" (*Iliad*). Presumably the arrow would have entered from the front and traveled by the side of the falx to reach the cerebellum, which is larger in the horse than in humans. It entered "where the first hairs of a horse grow upon the cranium"; Greek horses had no forelock, and this would therefore have been the vertex or top of the crown.

Hippocrates

Hippocrates was the son of the physician Heraclides and was taught not only by him, but also by Herodotus and Democritus. He practiced in Thessaly, Abdera, and Argos. He was said to have brought the plague under control in Athens, and a monument was erected to his memory. Artaxerxes, the king of Persia, wanted him as his court physician, but he refused. The Sydenham Society commissioned Frances Adams, a Scottish surgeon, to translate his works, which were first published in 1849, and later in 1886 and 1929.

The Hippocratic Corpus consists of 76 Treatises, one of which is "On Injuries of the Head."[20] In it he states:

> Apart from the examination you shall have done yourself, whatever aspect the bone may present, you shall enquire about the circumstances of the injury (these give you indications as to the degree of gravity), and if the injured person was confused, if darkness gathered around him, if he became giddy, if he fell down. . . .
>
> A bone may be injured in a different part of the head from that on which the person has received the wound. . . . And for this misfortune, . . . there is no remedy; there is no means of ascertaining by any examination whether or not it has occurred, or on what point of the head.
>
> In the first place, one must examine the wounded person, in what part of the head the wound is situated. . . . These things one should say from a distant inspection, and before laying a hand on the man; but on a close examination one should endeavour to ascertain clearly whether the bone be denuded of flesh or not; and if the denuded bone be visible to the eyes, this will be enough; but of course an examination

> must be made with the sound. . . . One should also enquire of the wounded how and in what way he sustained the injury. . . .
>
> When a person has sustained a mortal wound of the head, which cannot be cured, nor his life preserved, you may form an opinion of his approaching dissolution, and foretell what is to happen from the following symptoms which such a person experiences. . . . Fever will generally come on before the fourteenth day if in winter, and in summer, the fever usually seizes after seven days. And when this happens, the wound loses its colour. . . . But when suppuration is fairly established in it, small blisters form on the tongue and he dies delirious. And, for the most part, convulsions seize the other side of the body; for, if the wound be situated on the left side, the convulsions will seize the right side of the body; or if the wound be on the right side of the head, the convulsion attacks the left side of the body. And some become apoplectic.

Hippocrates makes many comments on *brain trauma*, which Adams translated as *concussion*. In cerebral concussion, whatever the cause, the patient becomes speechless.

> Sufferers from brain concussion, whether by a blow or from any other cause, fall down immediately, lose their speech, cannot see and hear; most of them will die.

> Those who have sustained an injury to the temple will have convulsions on the side opposite the injury.

> When concussion of the brain is caused by a blow, the victim loses his speech and cannot see or hear.

> If one is in doubt about a fracture of the skull, the injured man should be asked to chew a piece of wood and to state whether he observes a cracking sound in his bone.

Whereas the Edwin Smith Surgical Papyrus classifies cranial fractures into *splits* (linear fractures) and *smashes* (comminuted and perhaps depressed fractures), Hippocrates categorizes them as fissures, contusions of bone, compressed fractures, indentations (*hedra*) with or without fracture, and fractures by contrecoup.

Other Greek and Roman Physicians

In ancient Greece and Rome, unconsciousness, paralysis, and convulsions indicated a torn dura, and contralateral exploration was often performed. Mortality was high, although not inevitable, in injury to the meninges. The signs of injury to both brain and meninges include bleeding from the nose or ears, vomiting, visual disturbances, loss of speech, falling level of consciousness, wandering eyes, and, a few days later, delirium and convulsions. Celsus thought the most severe brain injury was that affecting the brainstem. He was familiar with an extradural hematoma, even in the absence of a skull fracture.

Paulus Aeginata (625–690) did not believe in contrecoup injuries:

> Some also add that by repercussion, what happens, say they, when a fracture of the cranium takes place opposite to the part which received the blow. But they are in mistake, for what happens to glass vessels does not, as they say, happen here; for, this happens to them from being empty, but the skull is full and otherwise strong.

Arabia

Although it had been known from the time of Celsus in the second century A.D. that bleeding into the brain could occur even without obvious skull damage, it was not until 800 years later (Rhazes, 850–923) that it was recognized that *concussion* (a term first used by Rhazes) could occur without skull injury. Rhazes also exposed the quack treatment of removing a stone from a circular opening of the skull.

Abul-Qasim AI-Zahran was known in the West as Albucasis; he was born near Cordoba in AI-Zahra and wrote 30 medical treatises, the final one containing three books, one of which concerns neurosurgery. He divides skull fractures into crushing and penetrating types, the former being subdivided into those that are superficial and those that penetrate the meninges. Ominous prognostic features are "vomiting, seizures, mental derangement, loss of speech, fainting, high fever, and protrusion and inflammation of the eyes" (p. 93).[10] With headaches, he suggests cutting and ligating the superficial temporal artery with silk or the string from a lute.

Medieval Times

Roger of Salerno (c. 1170) was the first European to write about surgery of the head:

> On the Treatment of the Skull: If the wound is small it should be enlarged unless bleeding or other complication prevents. The trephine should be cautiously

> applied close to the fissure on each side and as many perforations made as seem necessary. Then with a chisel a cut is made from one hole to another, so that the opening reaches from end to end of the fissure and exudation can escape and should be carefully cleaned away with strips of the finest linen inserted by means of a feather between the brain and the skull. After introducing a fold of linen between the bone and the dura, the injured bone should be removed. (p. 51)[3]

Although this was written 600 years ago, the advice is modern.

Another associate of the Salerno school, but probably a Frenchman, was Walter of Agilon, who also emphasized the importance of applying clean dressings to the meninges: "A fracture of the skull is known thus: there is low fever from the first day with headache, which gets a little worse each day; there is a squint, the cheeks are flushed. . . . A wound in any part of the head which reaches the brain substance is mortal."[3]

The earliest French medical school in Paris was taught by Lanfrancus (1296), who had been driven out of Milan by the civil wars in 1295. He stated that symptoms after a head injury could rapidly disappear and were a result of a transitory paralysis of cerebral function caused by the brain's being shaken. Lanfrancus was familiar with the crossed effects of brain lesions. He thought that there was only one indication for trepanation: dural irritation by depressed bone fragments. He also believed that if both fever and convulsions occurred after a head injury, the prognosis was hopeless, but if only one occurred, then survival was possible.

In the thirteenth to fifteenth centuries, trephining was also performed by Guy de Chauliac (1363), Ambroise Paré (1561), and Andrea dellla Cruce (1573).

Guy de Chauliac (born c. 1300) criticized Theodoric (1205–1298) because he went against Galenic principles of humors and because of the latter's belief that the fourth ventricle was important for memory. One of the first to remove successfully a part of the brain, he recommended trepanation for removal of foreign bodies, but only with severe fractures on the most dependent site and avoiding sutures. (He also believed in astrology and would not operate when the moon was full.)

There was little progress in the treatment of head injuries in the fifteenth century until the work of Berengaria da Carpi (c. 1465–1527), who noted that damage to the dura caused pain, vomiting, fever, and conjunctival injection, whereas damage to the pia caused paralysis, numbness, tremor, fits, diminished state of consciousness, and speech disturbances, clearly because the brain was also involved. He termed brain damage with no skull fracture or obvious brain hemorrhage *cerebrum commotum*. He also noticed personality changes after head injuries, as well as hyperphagia and hypersexuality.[4] Andrea della Cruce (fl. 1560) published a work illustrating the different types of surgical instruments used, one being a cannula made of gold or silver for draining fluid from the cranial cavity in epilepsy.[11]

In the classification of cerebral trauma, the terms *commotio*, *contusio*, and *compressio* have been used for many centuries but differently in various countries. Books of case reports, or *consilia*, were common at that time; for example, Ambroise Paré 1510–1590) produced many case reports of head injuries. Paré had no university education and was initially a barber surgeon famed for his aphorism "Guérir rarement, soulager souvent, aider toujours" ("Cure rarely, soothe often, help always"). He advised surgeons to remove any bone spicules from the brain.

Paré considered *commotio* to be a disorder of brain movement with brain swelling and hemorrhage as epiphenomena. He called the *cerebellum commotum* of Berengaria *concussion* or *commotion du cerveau*, and it was after this time that concussion began to feature in the medical literature. He advised "straining with the nose and mouth closed to force out sanious matter and filth" (p. 146).[26]

The distinction of *commotio* from *contusio* and *compressio* began with Boviel (1674) and continued with Jean Louis Petit (1674–1750). The actual mechanism for concussion was first postulated by Petit,[7] who felt that the vibrations of the skull produced by the injury were transmitted to the brain. It was in fact Petit (1750) who first described the injury and increased intracranial pressure due to an extradural hemorrhage, for which he advised trepanation to evacuate the clot. Petit considered that immediate loss of consciousness was due to concussion, whereas such a state occurring after a delay was due to compression from extravasation. In 1705, Alexis Littré (1658–1725) performed a postmortem examination on a patient who had dashed his head into a wall, fell down unconscious, and died a few minutes later. No damage to the brain was visible to the naked eye,[23] Although Littré used the term *contusio* for lesions of the skull, it was Dupuytren (1777–1835) who introduced the concept of cerebral contusion (*contusio cerebri*). Dupuytren gave extensive descriptions of these three terms but pointed out that they often occurred together. Other causes for concussion included cerebral anemia, molecular or metabolic disturbances, cerebral edema, cerebrospinal shock, medullary pressure, separation of gray from white matter, stretching of nerve fibers. hypothalamic pressure, and shock to the nerve cells.[7]

Such luminaries as Berengaria (1518), Ambroise Paré (1561), and Fallopius (c. 1566) emphasized the frequency of contrecoup lesions opposite the site of the blow.

Known as Fallopius, Gabriele Fallopio (1523–1562), while professor of anatomy at the Universitv of Padua, wrote two books on head injuries. However, his successor in the chair, Heironymus Fabricius da Acquapendente (1537–1619), was more original, recommending conservative management rather than surgical intervention.

In the second half of the seventeenth century, the standard surgical text was written by Johann Schulthes (1595–1645), one illustration of which was a comb-like saw-*serrula versatilis*, used for the skull in preference to a burr hole or even trephination. He illustrated how craniotomies should be done from experience gained in the Thirty Years' War (1618–1648). At this period, trephining was done to evacuate blood and pus, but it was also performed prophylactically to prevent compression and inflammation after a head injury.

A famous case of trepanning was that of Prince Rupert, who was shot in the head in 1649 in Armentières. Although he recovered, this injury troubled him further, and the wound broke down after a minor accident many years later. Pepys records the trepanation in his diary dated February 3, 1677:

> Hear that the work is done to the Prince in a few minutes without any pain at all to him, he not knowing when it was done. . . . Having cut the outward table, as they call it, they find the all corrupted, so as it comes out without any force; and their fear is, that the whole inside of the head is corrupted like that. (p. 170)[24b]

As he recovered and died 5 years later of an unrelated illness, it is clear that the brain was not corrupted.

Andreas Vesalius, the anatomist, performed craniotomies and, when physician to the court of Philip the Second of Spain, treated the king's son, who had tripped while chasing the kitchen maid. An operation was recommended to remove an epidural clot, and the patient recovered.

Richard Wiseman (1621–1675) worked as a military surgeon in the English, Spanish, and Dutch armies and had a great deal of experience with battle wounds. He not only removed epidural hematomas but recommended incising the dura to remove subdural hematomas, even though he did not think survival was possible if the meninges had been perforated by gunshot.[14]

The Eighteenth Century

According to Mettler and Mettler,[22] "Scarcely a year of the 18th century passed without the publication of at least one treatise on head injury" (p. 27).

One of the first to do experimental work on head injuries was François Gigot de Lapeyronie (1678–1747). He considered that the *vital factors* were located in the corpus callosum.

During the eighteenth century, gunshot wounds became more common and were thought to be poisonous because of the sulfur, saltpeter, and charcoal contained in the gunpowder. However, this thesis was soon dismissed by, among others, Benjamin Bell (1749–1806). He classified three posttraumatic syndromes—concussion, compression, and inflammation—and used the pulse and respiration rate to differentiate between concussion and compression, since they could be distinguished only by these features.

Throughout the eighteenth century there was much controversy about the management of concussion. Some argued for radical prophylactic trephining if there were such localizing signs as pain, whereas others advocated conservative treatment. John Abernethy of England pointed out that compression can occur slowly and can resolve without therapy. The radicals did not know that intracranial pressure could be raised even without a skull fracture. This view permeated the laity, so that murder by blows to the head was not punishable unless there was an associated skull fracture. This was in spite of a case report by Alexis Littré (1658–1725) of a convict who committed suicide by striking his head against the wall without sustaining a fracture.

Born in 1694 on a small farm in France, François Quesnay (1694–1774) was unable to read until the age of 16. Apprenticed to a barber-surgeon, he became self-taught and read all he could find, learning Latin and Greek. While studying in Paris, he learned the art of engraving, which he later used to illustrate his anatomical works. He became the first secretary of the newly founded Académie Royale de Chirurgie, but gave up the position at the age of 34, when his wife died and he had to look after his two children. In 1723 he was appointed the royal physician and saved the life of Louis XV in 1744, later being honored as a Fellow of the Royal Society. Madame de Pompadour, the king's mistress, was frigid, and Quesnay, a highly moral man who did not indulge in the frivolities of the Versailles court, gave good advice. He later switched to economics, fell from grace, and died in poverty at the age of 80.

Quesnay was one of the first to believe that brain injury was not necessarily fatal. He treated brain injuries successfully, stating that "wounds of this organ . . . heal almost as rapidly as wounds of other viscera." He showed that a dog could survive even though nails had been driven into its brain. He recognized that the brain was insensitive to pain and recommended seeking in the brain substance for a foreign body "when the circumstances require it."[2]

Quesnay took particular interest in trepanation, stating, "As a general rule, we should apply the trepan whenever there is a fracture." This view is not generally held but, in order to avoid infection, he preferred to do the operation in the patient's home rather than in a hospital, "on account of the unwholesome state of the air." He was much criticized by the British surgeon John Bell for these views.

Antoine Louis (1723–1792) was another French surgeon interested in head trauma, and he convened meetings on contrecoup injuries where a prize was given to the best contributed essay: the prize winner in 1768 suggested that the patient should not lie on the paralyzed side, as the hematoma could migrate to this side. The indication for the use of trepanation in depressed fracture was appreciated in the eighteenth century by such eminent surgeons as Percival Pott (1713–1788) and John Hunter (1728–1793). Pott, who was on the staff of St. Bartholomew's Hospital, London (from 1744), stated that symptoms arising in head injury are not due to a fractured skull but to injury of the brain. He also disproved the idea that extradural or subdural blood would inevitably become pus. Hunter also made accurate observations on concussion, compression, and laceration of the brain, correlating the level of consciousness with variations in pulse and respiration and noting the pupillary light reaction:

> Fractures of the skull of themselves produce no symptoms respecting the brain, only those of broken bone. We do not trepan for concussion alone. In young people a depression fracture may give rise to no symptom at the time, but as the patient grows up bad symptoms may arise. In all cases of depression the trepan is necessary. We must not divide the dura unless we are certain that there is fluid effused under it. (p. 175)[3]

Each of these succinct sentences incorporates years of experience and is typical of the scientific philosophy that characterized John Hunter's work. The famous British surgeon Sir Astley Cooper (1768–1841), a pupil of Hunter, did not perform preventive surgery on the skull except in the case of compound fracture: "It might be thought that it would be time enough to [trephine] when inflammation had appeared, but this is not the case, for if inflammation comes on the patient will die whether you trephine or not." (p. 176)[24b]

The Nineteenth Century

Two army surgeons—one French and one British—gained tremendous experience treating head injuries during the Napoleonic wars. The French surgeon, Baron Larrey (1766–1842), was a great favorite of Napoleon and thought that trephining was indispensable in a depressed fracture. Larrey was aware that a lesion of the cerebellum caused symptoms on the homolateral side.

On the British side was George James Guthrie (1788–1856), who wrote an excellent and eloquent monograph on his experiences with head injuries. A Fellow of the Royal Society and President of the Royal College of Surgeons, Guthrie felt that operative intervention was mandatory for both extradural hemorrhage and epidural abscess, a view prescient of that held today. "In consequence there is no more interesting chapter in the entire history of therapeutics . . . than that of the treatment of cranial injury."

In his book on *Injuries of the Head Affecting the Brain*,[16] Guthrie writes:

> Injuries of the head affecting the brain are difficult of distinction, doubtful in their character, treacherous in their course, and for the most part fatal in their results . . . The rule in surgery is absolute to trepan in extradural hemorrhage. When operation is necessary in fractured skull, it should be done at once-delay is fatal. (p. 25)[16]

Guthrie reports that death from a fractured petrous temporal bone is due to a ruptured carotid artery. He was the first neurosurgical writer to apply the neurophysiological principles of Flourens and Whytt to lesion localization. The three reflexes he uses are eyelash stimulus to provoke eye closure, the anal reflex, and movement of the toes in response to stroking of the sole.

Guthrie considers the most likely explanation of concussion to be "wave-like lines of force which disturb the structural, microscopic continuity of neural tissue and its blood vessels" (p. 36).[22] This observation was supported by the experiments of Jean-Pierre Gama (1775–1861), who filled glass retorts with isinglass jelly, which has the consistency of brain, in which he suspended threads "to study the direction of resultant forces" (p. 35).[22] Guthrie, like others of that time, thought that delirium was a result of inflammation, as was the presence of blood, so that when he spoke of inflammatory changes, the symptoms were the result of cerebral hemorrhage. Although opposed to repeated trepanning that was characteristic of medieval times, Guthrie quotes the case of Philip of Nassau, a grandson of William of Orange, who, when thrown from a horse in August 1664, fractured his skull on a tree stump. Trepanned 27 times, he made a complete recovery and proved this by drinking three of his companions to death.[3]

Probably the first description of posttraumatic hygroma (or hydroma), which Charles Mayo in 1894 called a *brain cyst* and Richter in 1899 called a *hygroma of the dura mater*, is by Thomas Schwencke in 1773.[13] In 1726 General van Keppel hit his head on a branch of a tree while riding and was thrown from the saddle. He recovered but developed drop attacks, dizziness, and convulsions. Two years after the accident, he developed right hemiplegia, from which he recovered, but continued to experience dizziness and transient paresis of his arm, hand, and foot. Seven years after his trauma, he developed another hemiplegia and died. Postmortem examination revealed a "large amount of clear fluid between the pia mater and the left cerebral hemisphere, as much as one pound apothecaries' weight (375 ml). The cerebral cortex under the pool of fluid *Seri collection* was hardened and its surface yellow."[14]

Between the American Revolution and the American Civil War, there were more than 100 wars in which soldiers suffered gunshot wounds of the head. Although considerable experience should have accrued, it was often the case that lessons learned in one war had to be learned again in the next. Consider this quote: "Trephining of itself was not brain surgery but skull surgery. . . . The skull must be dealt with for the sake of the brain: but the less that the surgeon saw of the brain, the better he was pleased."

In the American Civil War, the North lost 360,000 men (225,000 by disease and 110,000 in combat), and the South lost 258,000 men (with similar proportions lost by disease and in combat). Eleven percent of the injuries were to the head and neck. Injuries of the head possess a peculiar significance. All wounds of the head are more or less serious (George Chisholm, 1864, quoted by Kaufman).[19] One treatment strategy was to place the patient with a head injury supine, with the head depressed below the chest level to increase the blood supply to the brain (p. 853).[28] In prolonged coma, catheterization was advised to "avoid poisoning of the blood from the absorption of decomposing urine."

Since the Civil War, the mortality of brain injury has steadily declined in succeeding wars, a trend that is likely to continue.[8,15]

In the introduction to this chapter, the rare recovery from brain injury was attested to by Younge, who in 1682 could find only about 100 such cases in the medical literature of the past 1500 years since Galen. Even his contemporaries doubted his observation, to which Younge responded:

> To my learned and civil antagonist, Dr W. Durston of Plimouth . . . Several modern observations relate, viz. that, on dissection, they found not only sheep . . . without any brain at all. . . . Your death (if your skull is penetrable) will furnish the world with an instance more surprising and incredible viz. a man above fifty years old no better stokt in the noddle than those other addle-headed cattel . . . who but a brainless physician would suppose his single and ungrounded opinion against the sense and observations of a multitude of the best and most reputable authors.[28]

Evidently, a diatribe between professional rivals is not a new phenomenon.

References

1. Al-Rodhan NRF, Fox JG: AI-Zahnmi and Arabian neurosurgery, 936–1013 AD. Surg Neurol 26:92–95, 1986.
2. Bakay L: Francois Quesnay and the birth of brain surgery. Neurosurgery 17:518–521, 1985.
3. Ballance CA: The Thomas Vicary Lecture. A Glimpse into the History of the Surgery of the Brain. London, Macmillan, 1992.
4. Berengario da Carpi G: Tractatus perutilis et completus de fractura cranei. Bologna, JA de Nicolenis de Sabio for JB Pederzanus, Venus, 1535.
5. Breasted JH: The Edwin Smith Surgical Papyrus. Chicago, University of Chicago Press, 1930.
6. Schiller F, Broca P: Explorer of the Brain. New York, Oxford, 1992.
7. Courville CB: Some notes on the history of injury to the skull and brain. Bull LA Neurol Soc 9:1–16, 1944.
8. Crockard HA: Bullet injuries of the brain. Ann R Coli Surg Engl. 5:111–123, 1974.
9. da Acquapendente FG: Lopere chiaugiche del Sign. Gorolomo Fabrizio D·Acquapendente. Bologna, Longi, 1878.
10. Dart RA: The incremental technique of Australopithecus. Am J Phys Anthropol 7:1–38, 1949.
11. della Cruce CA: Churusgia Universalee Perfetto. Venezia, Pizzana, 1661.
12. Elsberg CA: The Edwin Smith surgical papyrus and the diagnosis and treatment of injuries to the skull and spine 5000 years ago. Am Med Hist 3:271, 1931.
13. Endtz LJ: Post-traumatic hygroma in the eighteenth century described by Thomas Schwenke. Surg Neurol 10:305–307, 1978.
14. Finger S: Origins of Neuroscience. New York, Oxford University Press, 1994.
15. Gurdjian ES: The treatment of penetrating wounds of the brain sustained in warfare. A historical review. J Neurol 40:157–167, 1974.
16. Guthrie CJ: On Injuries of the Head Affecting the Brain, 4th ed. London, John Churchill 1842.
17. Helgason CM: Commentary on the significance for modem neurology of the 17th century B.C. surgical papyrus. Can J Neurol Sci 14:560–569, 1987.
18. Horsley V: Brain surgery in the Stone Age. Br Med J 1:582, 1887.
19. Kaufman HK: Treatment of head injuries in the American Civil War. J Neurosurg 78:838–848, 1993.
20. Kelly EC: Hippocrates on injuries of the head. In: Krieger RE (ed): Classics of Neurology. Huntington, NY, 1949.
21. Mazzone P, Bancherot IA, Esposito S: Neurological sciences at their origin: Neurology and neurological surgery in the medicine of ancient Egypt. Pathologica 79:787–800, 1987.
22. Mettler FA, Mettler CC: Historic development of knowledge relating to cranial trauma. Res Nerv Ment Dis 24:1–47, 1945.
23. Ommaya, Rockoff SD, Baldwin M: Experimental concussion. J Neurosurg 21:249–265, 1964.

24a. Rose FC: An overview from Neolithic times to Broca: In: Arnott R, Finger S, and Smith CUM (eds): Trepanation: History, Discovery, Theory. Abingdon, Swets and Zeitlinger, 2003, pp 347–363.

24b. Rose FC: The History of Head Injuries: An overview. J. Hist. Neurosci. 6(2):154–180, 1997.

25. Walker AE: The dawn of neurosurgery. Clin Neurosurg 6:1–38, 1959.
26. West CGH: A short history of the management of penetrating missile injuries of the head. SurgNeurol 16:145–149, 1981.
27. Younge J: Wounds of the Brain. London, Faithborn and Kersey, 1682.
28. Zellech RT: Wounded by bayonet, ball and bacteria: Medicine and neurosurgery in the American Civil War. Neurosurgery 17:850–860, 1985.

Chapter 3

Computed Tomography and Magnetic Resonance Imaging in Traumatic Brain Injury

CHI-SHING ZEE, JOHN L. GO, PAUL E. KIM, AND DAOYING GENG

Head trauma is the major cause of accidental death in the United States, particularly in the juvenile and young adult groups.[11,17,18,32] Severe traumatic brain injury (TBI) accounts for a death rate of 16.9 per 100,000 population per year.[44] Motor vehicle accidents (57%), firearms injuries (14%), and traumatic falls (12%) are the most frequent causes. Males are three times more likely to die from brain injury–associated death than females. Head injuries are responsible for 200 to 300 hospital admissions per 100,000 population per year in the United States.[6] Most of the admissions last only a few days, and the patients are admitted for clinical observation. Head injury is not only a cause of death but also a cause of serious financial burden to the society providing treatment and care to these patients. Lost labor and reduced productivity to the society further add to the negative impact. The cost of head trauma to the society is estimated to be billions of dollars annually. The majority of the patients suffering head injuries are considered to have *mild head injury*. Most patients recover fully from mild TBI, but 15% to 29% of patients with mild TBI may have significant neurocognitive problems.[27] Common symptoms include attention deficit, deficit in working memory and speed of information processing; headaches, dizziness, and irritability.

Computed Tomography in Traumatic Brain Injury

The advent of computed tomography (CT) in the early 1970s revolutionized the diagnosis and management of head trauma patients. The most efficient method for evaluating acute head trauma today remains CT.[52] This technology has evolved from a slow, time-consuming imaging modality to today's multislice helical CT. A whole-head CT scan can be obtained within 1 second.

Computed tomography, is widely available, fast, low-cost, and accurate for detecting acute hemorrhage.[40] It is compatible with the life support devices that are commonly in use. The introduction of multidetector CT allows optimal evaluation of a traumatized patient with a CT scan of the head, neck, chest, abdomen, and pelvis in a few minutes, thus providing critical information for immediate surgical care. Computed tomography angiography can readily provide information on vascular injury without the risks of cerebral angiography. High-resolution CT is excellent for evaluating facial and skull base fractures. Neurosurgically significant lesions, such as epidural hematomas, subdural hematomas, and depressed skull fractures are all readily detected by CT. Computed tomography is excellent for detecting intraventricular hemorrhage, which is commonly associated with shear injuries of the corpus callosum, and white matter (Fig. 3.1).[20]

Computed tomography does have a number of pitfalls when used to evaluate head injuries. Isodense or low-density acute hemorrhages are seen in patients who are severely anemic or suffer from disseminated intravascular coagulopathy. A small subdural or epidural hematoma may not be detected if the appropriate setting for window width and level is not used. This is particularly important when evaluating patients for child abuse. Subtle chronic or subacute extra-axial hematomas may be missed on CT. It is much less sensitive than magnetic resonance imaging (MRI) for detecting diffuse axonal injury, cortical contusion, deep cerebral/brain stem injury, and small subdural hematomas.[24,31,52] The early detection of many surgically significant extra-axial hematomas is made possible with the increase in the number of CT scans performed in head trauma patients. This results in early surgical intervention, with marked improvement in morbidity and mortality in patients with head trauma.[29,30,37,42] *Diffuse axonal injury* (DAI) refers to white matter injury caused by unequal rotation or deceleration of adjacent tissues with differing density and rigidity.[1,45] The most common shearing lesions are seen in the parasagittal white matter. As the shearing force increases, the corpus callosum and dorsolateral brain stem become injured. The internal capsule, the cerebellar hemisphere, and sometimes the basal ganglia and thalami may also be involved.[23] Clinically, patients may present in a comatose state despite having a relatively benign appearance on CT scan. On CT scan, DAI involving the white matter may present as multiple small, focal, low-density lesions or petechial hemorrhage in the white matter.[14,39,54] They tend to be ovoid or elliptical, with the long axis oriented in the direction of injured axons.[22] They are typically less than 1 cm in size and spare the adjacent cortical surface of the brain. Lesions are usually located entirely within the white matter or at the gray matter–white matter junction and are seen in both hemispheres.[21] Cerebral swelling with obliteration of the basal cisterns and compression of the lateral ventricles, third ventricle can be an early finding. After about 3 weeks, enlargement of the cerebral sulci and basal cisterns and dilatation of the ventricles can be seen, with well-defined foci of hypointensity in the white matter.[54] Sasiadek et al. [39] reported that the typical CT findings of DAI were small hemorrhagic lesions in the cerebral white matter, and internal capsule. Hemorrhagic lesions due to shearing injury in the cerebral white matter and at the gray matter–white matter junction are easily identified on CT in the acute stage. However, CT is limited in the evaluation of DAI. Mittl et al.[38] found that abnormalities compatible with DAI were seen on MRI (spin-echo T2-weighted and T2*-weighted gradient echo images) in 30% of patients with normal head CT scans following minor head trauma (Fig. 3.2).

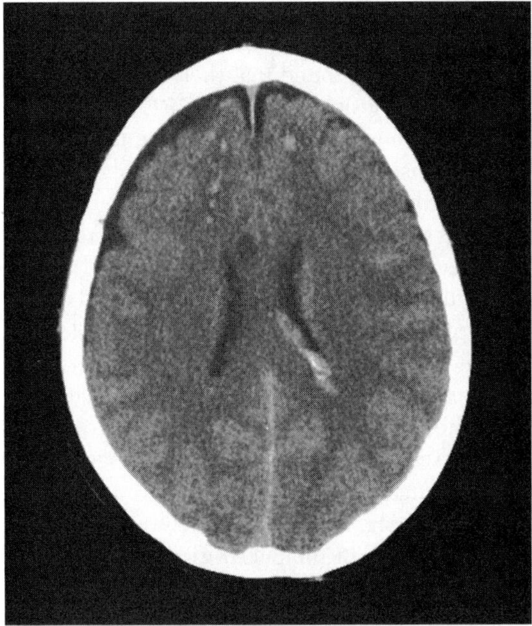

Figure 3.1. Intraventricular hemorrhage and diffuse axonal injury (DAI). An axial computed tomography scan demonstrates the presence of intraventricular hemorrhage in the left lateral ventricle and small petechial hemorrhage in the frontal white matter, consistent with DAI.

Magnetic Resonance Imaging in Traumatic Brain Injury

Magnetic resonance imaging has rapidly become the imaging modality of choice for most neurological

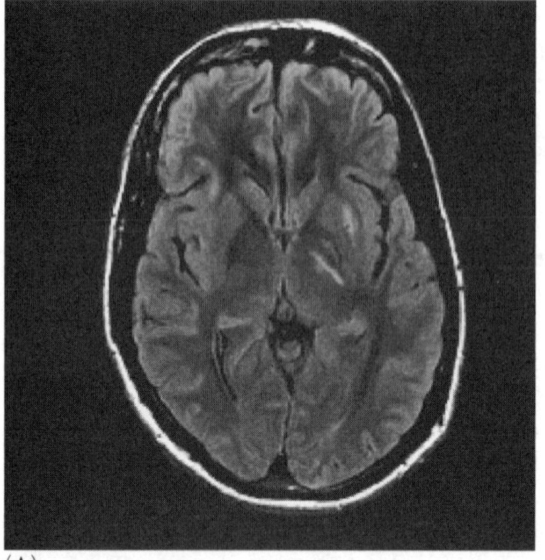

(A)

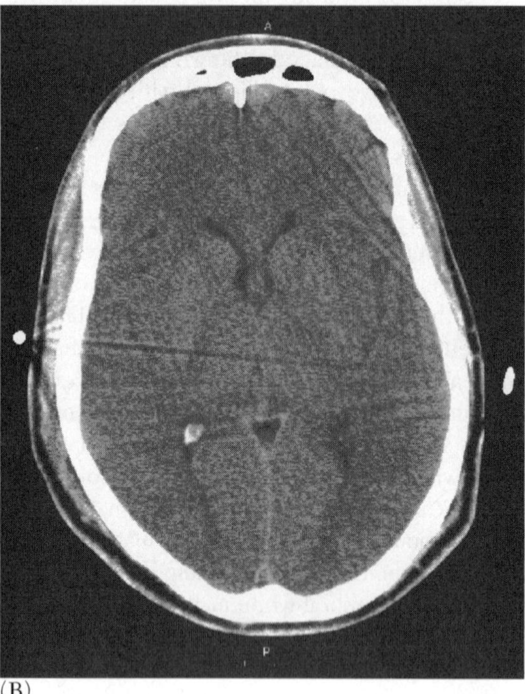

(B)

Figure 3.2. Diffuse axonal injury detected by magnetic resonance imaging with a normal-appearing computed tomography (CT) scan. (*A*) Axial fluid-attenuated inversion-recovery sequence demonstrates shearing injury involving the left internal capsule and external capsule. (*B*) Axial CT scan at the same level reveals no abnormality in the left internal capsule and external capsule.

diseases. In TBI, it become an important adjunct to CT in the evaluation of patients with head trauma.[17] The ability of MRI to detect small extra-axial hematomas in various stages makes it an important tool in the evaluation of child abuse patients.

Several different MRI sequences have been studied in the evaluation of head trauma. The utility of fluid-attenuated inversion-recovery (FLAIR) sequences in head trauma has been reported by several authors, who found the sensitivity of FLAIR images to be equal or superior to that of conventional T2-weighted spin-echo images in the evaluation of patients with head trauma, including DAI.[4] Diffuse axonal injury is better seen on MRI than on CT. Magnetic resonance imaging is indicated when there is a significant discrepancy between the patient's clinical condition and CT findings, which could be unremarkable in some instances. Gradient echo (GRE) images further enhance the sensitivity in detecting hemorrhagic shearing injury in the acute phase (deoxyhemoglobin) and chronic phase (hemosiderin) of the injury (Fig. 3.3). This is due to the shortening of $T2^*$ by the heterogeneous local magnetic field arising from paramagnetic blood breakdown products. These changes can persist for months and even years after the head trauma. $T2^*$-weighted images are critical in the evaluation of patients with chronic head injury. Yanagawa et al.[49] found that there is a correlation between the lesions seen on GRE images, the Glasgow Coma Scale score, and the duration of unconsciousness. They also found that the number of hemorrhagic lesions detected by GRE per patient was significantly higher than those seen by T2 weighted-Fast Spin Echo (T2–FSE).

Magnetization transfer imaging is based on the principle that protons bound in macromolecules exhibit T1 relaxation coupling with protons in the aqueous phase. Application of an off-resonance saturation pulse can effectively saturate bound protons selectively. Subsequent exchange of longitudinal magnetization with free water protons reduces the signal intensity detected from these free protons. The magnetization transfer ratio (MTR) provides a quantitative index of this magnetization transfer effect and may be an indicator as a quantitative measure of the structural integrity of the tissue.[5] Magnetization transfer ratio imaging in experimental models of DAI in pigs showed reduced MTR values in regions of histologically proven axonal injury. McGowen et al.[36]

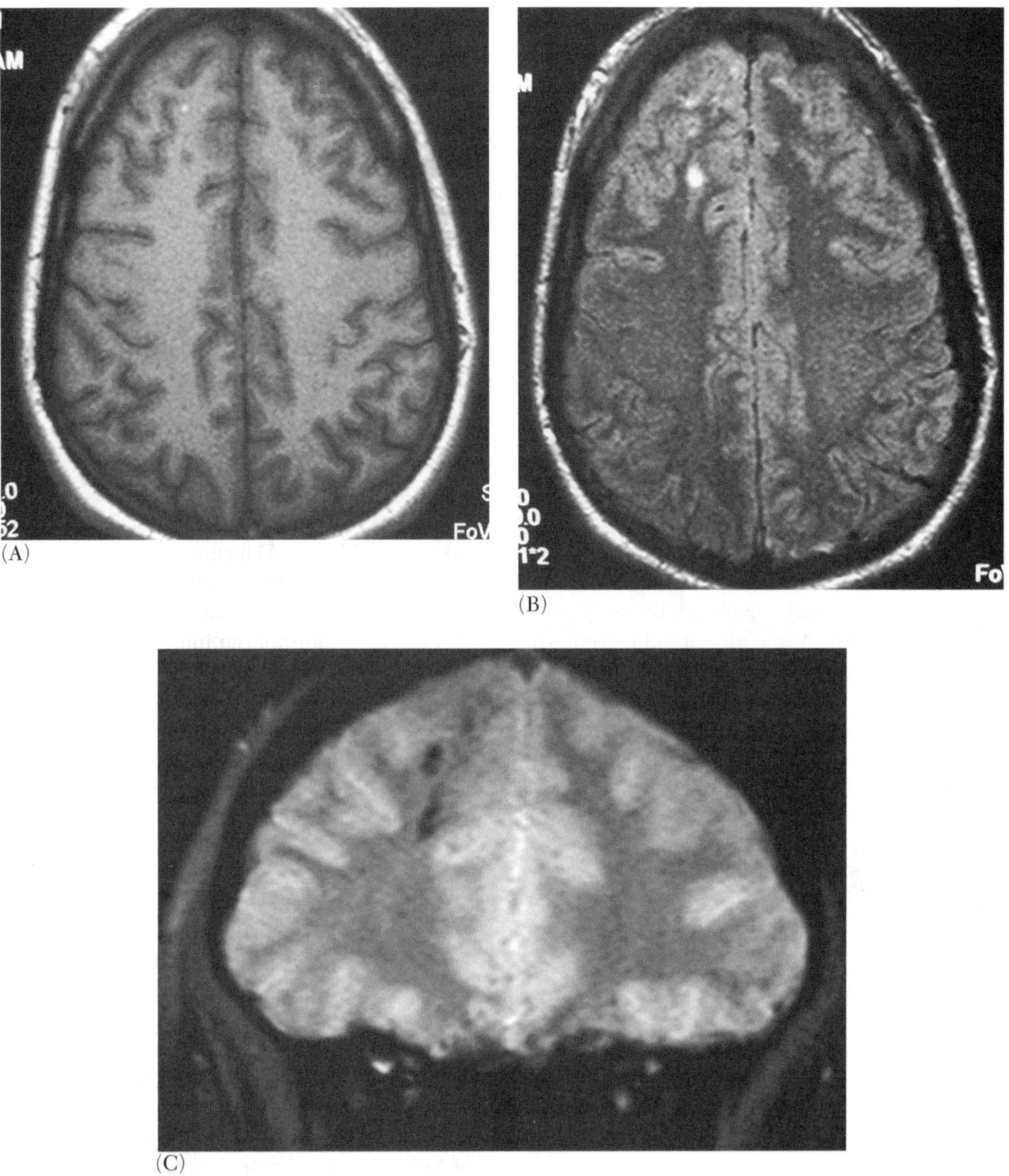

Figure 3.3. Diffuse axonal injury demonstrated by a gradient echo sequence. (*A*) Axial T1-weighted sequence reveals a tiny hyperintense petechial hemorrhage in the right frontal white matter. (*B*) Axial fluid-attenuated inversion-recovery sequence demonstrates small hyperintense areas in the right frontal white matter. (*C*) Coronal gradient echo sequence clearly shows several hypointense areas of petechial hemorrhage consistent with diffuse axonal injury.

found that the MTR in the splenium of corpus callosum was lower in patients who suffered minor head injury compared to those in a control group, but no significant reduction in MTR was found in the pons. All the patients demonstrated impairment on at least three measures of the neuropsychological tests, and in two cases a significant correlation was found between regional MTR values and neuropsychological performance. The authors also found that quantitative magnetization transfer imaging (MTI) can be used to detect lesions of DAI even when conventional T2-weighted MRI is negative. Bagley et al.[5] found that average MTR values were higher in all areas of white matter in patients without persistent neurological deficit than in patients with deficits. They concluded that detection of abnormal MTR in normal-appearing white matter may suggest a poor prognosis.

Magnetic resonance spectroscopy (MRS) is a noninvasive method of evaluating microscopic injury of the white matter in patients with DAI and may help to predict the outcome. Magnetic resonance spectroscopy is a sensitive tool in detecting DAI and may be particularly useful in evaluating patients with mild TBI with unexplained neurological and cognitive deficits. Since DAI disturbs the balance of chemicals that exist in the brain such as *N*-acetyl aspartate (NAA), lactate, choline, and high-energy phosphates, MRS can provide an index of neuronal and axonal viability by measuring levels of NAA. A majority of mildly brain-injured patients, as well as those who were severely injured, showed diminished NAA levels and reduced NAA/creatine ratios in the splenium of the corpus callosum compared to normal controls. Reduced NAA levels, corresponding to neuronal injury, were observed in patients with elevated lactate up to 24 hours following TBI. Marked reduction of NAA in the white matter continues into the subacute phase. However, in some patients, normal NAA levels may be detected 6 months following the trauma.[10] Elevated lactate levels on MRS in normal-appearing tissues on MRI correlate with a poor clinical outcome.[12]

The Extra-Axial Injuries

Epidural Hematoma

Epidural hematoma (EDH) occurs in the potential space between the dura and the inner table of the skull. It occurs most commonly in the region of temporal squamosa where the middle meningeal artery is located. Arterial bleeding from this artery typically causes a hyperdense, biconvex collection along the calvarium. The majority of EDHs are associated with skull fractures.[52] Epidural hematomas in the posterior fossa are usually secondary to rupture of the torcula or transverse sinus. Other venous EDHs are seen in the middle fossa from rupture of the sphenoparietal sinus and at the vertex from disruption of the superior sagittal sinus.[17] The *swirl sign* within the otherwise hyperdense hematoma is manifested as irregular hypodense areas and is thought to be due to active bleeding within the arterial EDH. Differentiation of EDH from subdural hematoma (SDH) is usually straightforward, but there are several imaging features that can help make the distinction. Epidural hematoma is biconvex in shape, limited by suture, and not limited by the falx (crosses the midline) or tentorium. On MRI, the displaced dura can be identified as a low-signal zone surrounding the hematoma. Immediately after head trauma, a lucid interval is seen in approximately 25% to 50% of cases before deterioration of the clinical condition. Computed tomography shows a biconvex, high-density extra-axial mass (Fig. 3.4). Delayed EDHs are uncommon lesions that may arise hours to days after initial injury.[52] The authors reviewed eight cases of delayed EDH at their institution and found that it occurred 8 to 72 hours after the initial injury or subsequent to surgery for decompression of a contralateral EDH, SDH, or intracerebral hematoma. In six of the eight cases, the delayed EDH occurred after surgical decompression of a contralateral traumatic lesion due to reduction of the tamponade effect (Fig. 3.5).

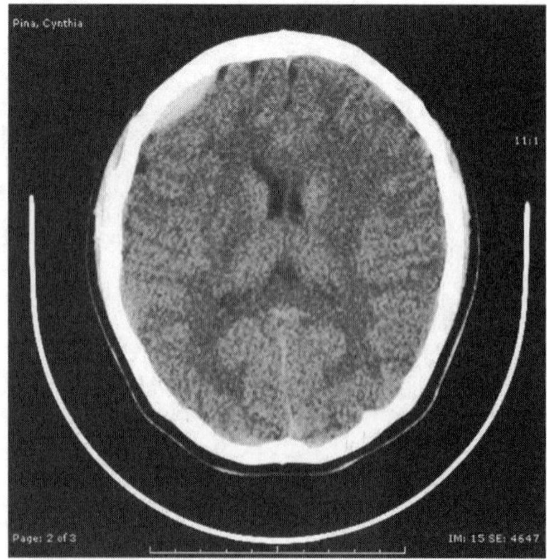

Figure 3.4. Epidural hematoma. Axial computed tomography demonstrates a biconvex extra-axial blood collection in the right frontal region.

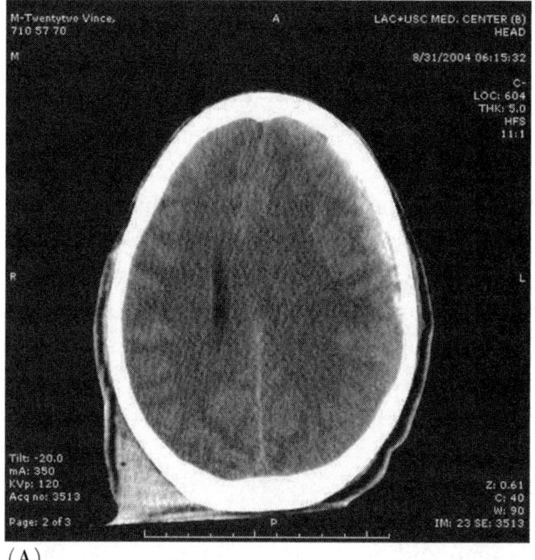

(A)

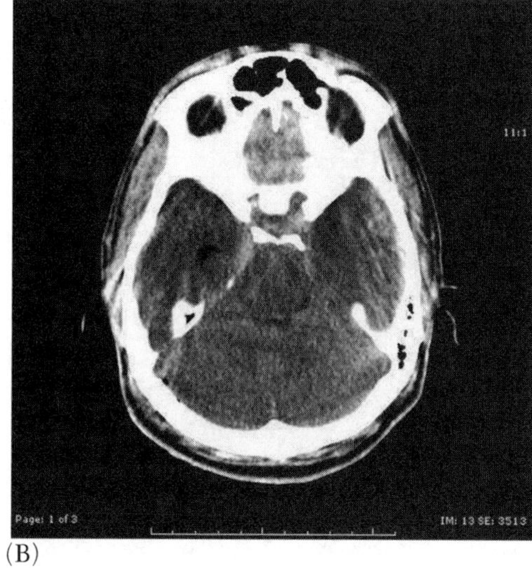

(B)

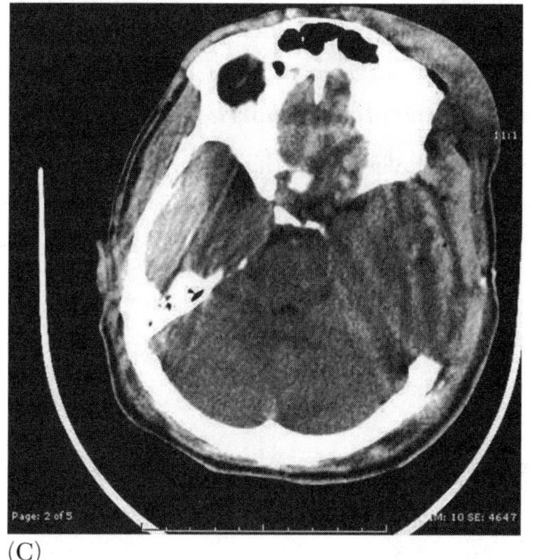

(C)

Figure 3.5. Delayed epidural hematoma (EDH). (*A*) Axial computed tomography (CT) demonstrates the presence of a small subdural hematoma (SDH) in the left frontoparietal convexity. (*B*) Axial CT at the level of the suprasellar cistern shows subarachnoid hemorrhage in the perimesencephalic cistern. No evidence of any extra-axial hematoma is seen in the right temporal fossa. (*C*) Following surgical evacuation of the thin but extensive SDH in the left frontoparietal region, the patient developed an EDH in the right temporal fossa.

Subdural Hematoma

Subdural hematomas are seen in approximately 30% of patients with severe closed head trauma. They are located between the inner dural layer and the arachnoid. Most SDHs are caused by laceration of the bridging cortical veins during sudden head acceleration and deceleration.[52] Rapid decompression of obstructive hydrocephalus after shunt placement can also cause laceration of cortical veins. Traumatic SDHs are often associated with an underlying brain injury, such as intracerebral hematoma or contusion.[19] On CT, SDHs present as a crescentic, extra-axial, hyperdense collection along the surface of the brain (Fig. 3.6). Patients with SDHs often exhibit more mass effect and a greater midline shift on imaging studies than can be explained by the size of the SDH alone. This is because acute SDHs are frequently associated with brain parenchymal hematoma, contusion, and edema. The SDH usually involves a large area along the convexity, resulting in the presence of a large volume of extra-axial blood within the bony calvaria, although the SDH may look *thin* on each image (Fig. 3.5*A*). Subdural hematomas are also seen at interhemispheric fissures and along the tentorium. As an SDH evolves, it gradually shows decreases in density. At some point, an SDH may become isodense to the adjacent brain parenchyma. Bilateral isodense

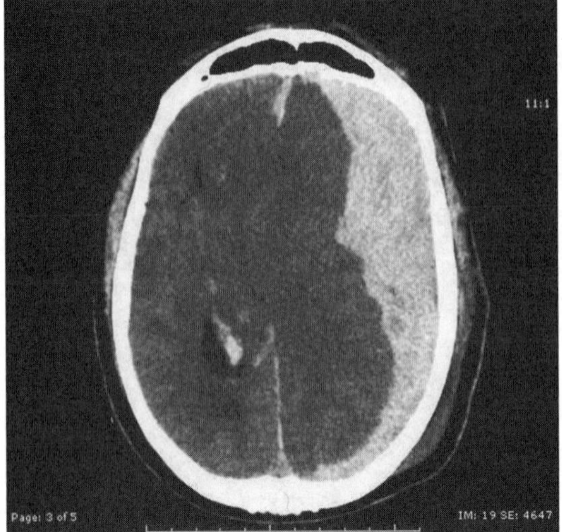

Figure 3.6. Subdural hematoma. Axial computed tomography demonstrate a large, crescentic extra-axial hematoma in the left frontoparietal region. There is marked compression of the left lateral ventricle with a significant shift of the midline structure.

SDHs can pose a diagnostic challenge on CT; however, they are easily detected on MRI. They are usually hyperintense on T1-weighted images and may be hypointense or hyperintense on T2-weighted images, depending on the evolution of the blood by-products. In the chronic stage of SDH, activated fibroblasts and the blood vessels originating from the dura begin to invade the membrane of the hematoma. Because the blood vessels in the fibrovascular granulation tissue are fragile, recurrent hemorrhage is often seen in chronic SDH and in some cases may gradually take a lentiform shape.

Subdural Hygroma

Subdural hygromas are caused by a traumatic tear of the arachnoid, which allows cerebrospinal fluid to leak into the subdural space.[17] Degradation of an SDH results in chronic SDH. An acute subdural hygroma and a chronic SDH can have a similar appearance on CT. They both present as extra-axial fluid collections of low density, whereas a chronic SDH is usually of higher signal intensity than a subdural hygroma on both T1-weighted and T2-weighted images.

Subarachnoid Hemorrhage

Subarachnoid hemorrhage is seen in the majority of patients with head trauma. In fact, the most common cause of subarachnoid hemorrhage is head trauma.[17] There are three sources of subarachnoid hemorrhage: (1) direct injury to the pial vessels, (2) blood from hemorrhagic cortical contusion, and (3) extension of intraventricular hemorrhage into the subarachnoid space. In most instances, subarachnoid hemorrhage is seen in association with other manifestations of head injury. On CT, subarachnoid hemorrhage appears as an area of high density in the sulci and the subarachnoid cisterns (Fig. 3.7). Hyperdense blood in the interpeduncular fossa is unequivocal evidence of subarachnoid hemorrhage. Subarachnoid hemorrhage can interfere with cerebrospinal fluid resorption and cause communicating hydrocephalus.

Intraventricular Hemorrhage

Intraventricular hemorrhage is frequently seen in conjunction with other evidence of head trauma. Hemorrhage can occur as a result of shearing of the subependymal veins, retrograde extension of subarachnoid hemorrhage, and extension of a parenchymal hemorrhage into the ventricular sys-

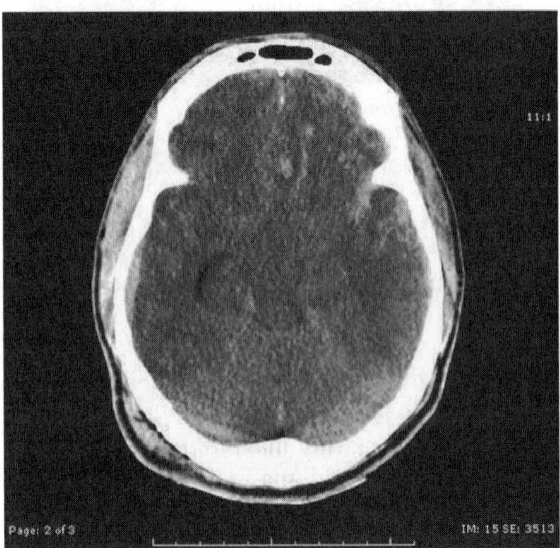

Figure 3.7. Subarachnoid hemorrhage. Axial computed tomography demonstrate blood in the left sylvian fissure as well as petechial hemorrhage in the left frontal region.

tem.[33] On CT, there is a cerebrospinal fluid–blood level, usually seen at the occipital horns of the lateral ventricle. The presence of intraventricular hemorrhage indicates a poor prognosis.

The Intra-Axial Injuries

Cortical Contusion

Cerebral contusion without significant hemorrhage generally is shown as an area of low density on CT. Hemorrhagic contusions usually present as an ill-defined area of high density surrounded by low density. The gyral crests are frequently involved, especially those in contact with roughened inner surfaces of the skull (e.g., the orbital roof, sphenoid ridge, and anterior middle cranial fossa). Acute hemorrhagic contusions are diffusely hypointense on T1-weighted images, and hypointense (deoxyhemoglobin), surrounded by hyperintense edema, on T2-weighted images. Early subacute hemorrhagic contusions are hyperintense (intracellular methemoglobin), surrounded by hypointense edema on T1-weighted images, and hypointense (intracellular methemoglobin), surrounded by hyperintense edema on T2-weighted images. On late subacute hemorrhagic contusions, extracellular methemoglobin exhibits hyperintensity on both T1-weighted and T2-weighted images.

The *coup-contrecoup* mechanism refers to the condition in which the moving skull comes to an abrupt hault while the brain continues to move for another brief moment. The portion of the brain opposite the impact site initially pulls away from the dura, but on recoil it hits the dura forcefully, creating a coup-contrecoup situation.[15,17]

Intracerebral Hematoma

Traumatic cerebral hematoma is located deeper in the brain parenchyma, in contrast to the peripheral location of cerebral contusion. On CT, it appears as a high-density mass lesion with minimal or no surrounding edema in the acute stage; its periphery starts to evolve into low density as the hematoma ages. Eventually, the whole hematoma may exhibit low density on CT. In the subacute stage, the peripheral margin of the hematoma shows ring-like enhancement on both CT and MRI due to the proliferation of new capillaries in the hematoma capsule. Delayed intracerebral hematomas can occur in an area of normal-appearing brain or in an area of previous cerebral contusion (Fig. 3.8). They are most frequently seen 1–4 days after trauma, but can be seen as late as two weeks following the head injury.[52]

Diffuse Axonal Injury

It is most important in the evaluation of patients with TBI to identify DAI, injury, cortical contusion, subcortical white matter injury, and primary brain stem injury.[20] Severe and moderate head injuries, and even some minor head injuries, can often be associated with rotational forces that produce shear stresses on the brain parenchyma. The brain is soft and malleable. Relatively little force is required to distort its shape. There are significant differences in density between the cerebrospinal fluid of the ventricles and the surrounding white matter. Differences in density also exist between gray and white matter to a lesser degree. When the skull is rapidly rotated, it carries along the superficial gray matter but the deeper white matter lags behind, causing axial stretching, separation, and disruption of nerve fiber tracts. Shear stresses are most marked at junctions between tissues of different densities. As a result, shear injuries commonly occur at gray matter–white matter junctions, but they are also found in the deeper white matter of corpus callosum, centrum semiovale, basal ganglia, brain stem (midbrain and rostral pons), and cerebellum.

Gentry et al.[20] studied 63 cases of acute head injury and 15 cases of chronic head injury. Corpus callosal injury was found in 47% of the patients. The corpus callosum is prone to injury because of its rigid attachment to the falx and its relationship to the independently mobile cerebral hemisphere. Because the falx is broader posteriorly, it effectively prevents transient displacement of the splenium of the corpus callosum, causing greater shear to occur within the fibers of the splenium of the corpus callosum. Gentry et al. also found that the diffuse axonal lesions of the lobar white matter and brain stem are usually very small and difficult to detect on CT or MRI, while those in the corpus callosum are larger and readily visible. Pathologically, the diagnosis of DAI depends on the identification of axonal bulbs microscopically. Early injury of axons is best detected immunocytochemically. The most sensitive indicator of injured axons is the presence

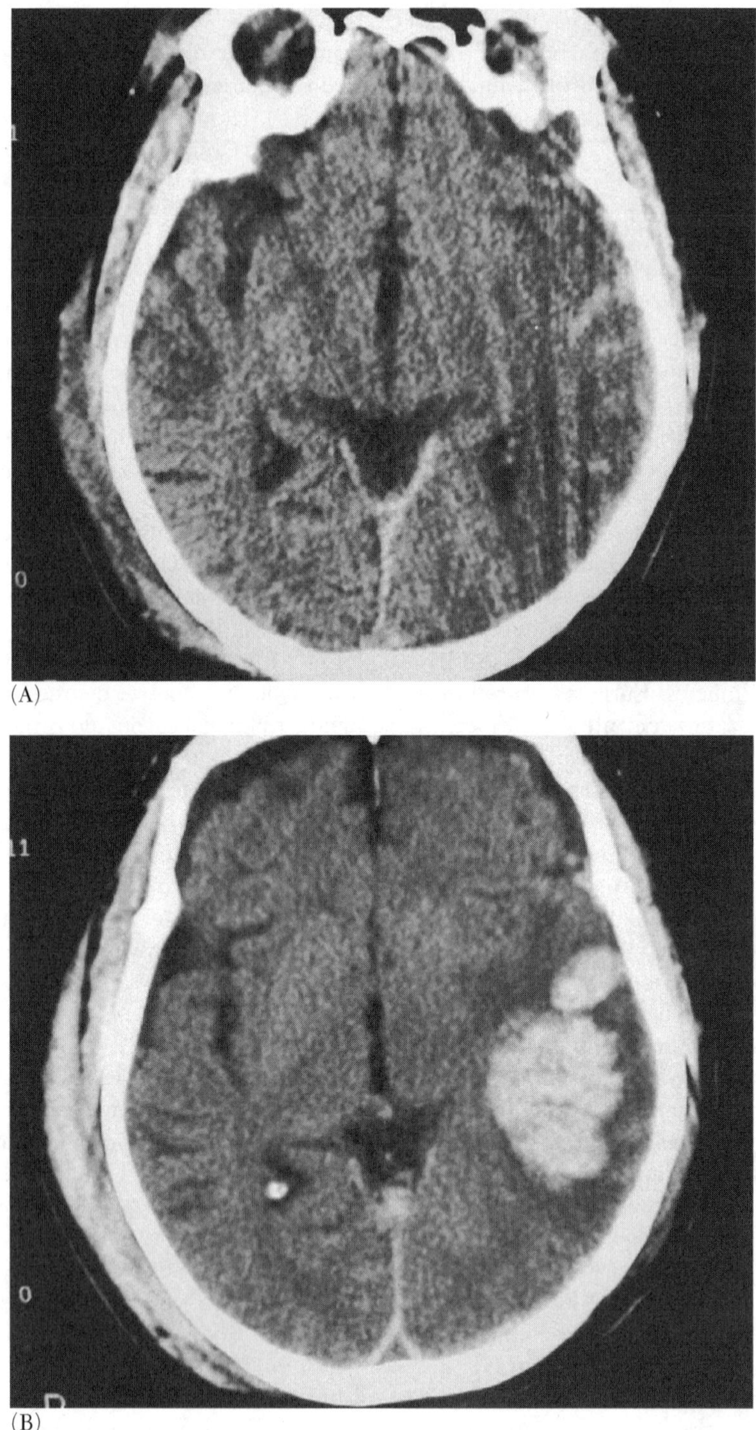

Figure 3.8. Delayed intracerebral hemorrhage. (*A*) Axial computed tomography (CT) shows subarachnoid blood in the left temporal region. (*B*) Axial CT scan obtained 2 days later, following deterioration of the patient's condition, revealed the presence of an intracerebral hematoma in the left temporal region.

of beta-amyloid precursor protein in the damaged axons. Injured axons may be seen within 2–3 hours of injury and as long as 99 days after trauma.[9,26] Diffuse axonal injury most frequently involves the white matter of the frontal and temporal lobes, the corpus callosum, and the corona radiata (Fig. 3.9). Cortical contusions most commonly involve the inferior, lateral, and anterior portions of the frontal and temporal lobes where they are exposed to the rough bony surface of the frontal and temporal fossa. Primary brain stem injury occurs in the dorsolateral aspects of the midbrain.

Animal studies of diffusion-weighted imaging demonstrated conflicting results in the change of the apparent diffusion coefficient (ADC) due to DAI.[2,25,28] Liu et al.[34] reported the first clinical study of diffusion-weighted imaging in DAI. They performed diffusion-weighted imaging in patients with acute and subacute DAI and demonstrated that a significant decrease in ADC values can be seen in areas of DAI up to 18 days following head injury. This probably reflects cellular swelling or cytotoxic edema in the acute stage. The authors hypothesize that very low ADC values, compared to those seen in acute ischemia, might be due to the presence of blood products and ruptured axons with membrane fragmentation, thus increasing the restriction to free movement of the water molecules and producing very low ADC values. In the first few hours following TBI, DAI is characterized by disruption of the cytoskeletal network and axonal membranes. Histological abnormalities seen in association with DAI decrease the diffusion along axons and increase the diffusion in directions perpendicular to them. White matter structures with reduced diffusion anisotropy are detected in the first 24 hours in patients suffering from DAI after TBI. A follow-up study revealed several regions that might have recovered from the injury 1 month later. Diffusion tensor imaging technique may be a tool for early detection of DAI in patients with minor TBI.[3]

Brain Stem Injury

Traumatic brain stem injuries (BSIs) may be classified as primary or secondary, depending on whether the lesion occurred at the time of impact or subsequent to it. Primary lesions include the brain stem contusion, the shearing injury.[13] Secondary lesions include hypoxic/ishemic injury and the Duret hemorrhage.[16] The Duret hemorrhage is always seen in association with transtentorial herniation and is thought to result from damage to the medial pontine perforating branches of the basilar artery. Therefore, the Duret hemorrhage is seen anterior to the pons. Computed tomography is somewhat limited in detecting brain stem lesions. Magnetic resonance imaging is the preferred imaging modality for evaluating these lesions. Diffuse axonal injuries of the brain stem are usually small to microscopic and are frequently located in the midbrain and rostral pons (Fig. 3.10). Gentry et al.[22] reported that MRI demonstrated a significantly higher number of lesions in BSI than CT. Patients with BSI had a significantly higher frequency of corpus callosum and white matter shearing lesions. The authors also found that the mean Glasgow Coma Scale scores at admission were significantly lower in patients with evidence of brain stem injury on MRI. Traumatic injury to the brain stem involving the dentato-rubro-olivary pathway can result in unilateral or bilateral olivary hypertrophy, which is readily detected by MRI as a focal area of enlargement with high signal intensity on T2-weighted images in the region of the inferior olivary nucleus.[8]

Cerebral Swelling

Traumatic cerebral swelling can occur secondary to cerebral hyperemia or cerebral edema. Cerebral hyperemia results from a loss of normal autoregulation of cerebral blood flow, which is secondary to elevation of systemic blood pressure. The cerebral blood flow then passively follows systemic blood pressure. Loss of autoregulation of cerebral blood flow is more common in children than in adults. Cerebral edema results from an increase in water content. Diffuse brain injury can cause generalized cerebral swelling.[50] Infarction secondary to intracranial and extracranical vascular injury is seen with edema. On CT, the edematous brain is hypodense due to increased water content, and there is subsequent loss of the normal differentiation between gray and white matter. Ventricular compression and sulcal effacement are also seen. In children, diffuse cerebral edema and subarachnoid hemorrhage are frequently seen as a result of closed head trauma.[41] When diffuse cerebral swelling is predominantly due to cerebral hyperemia,

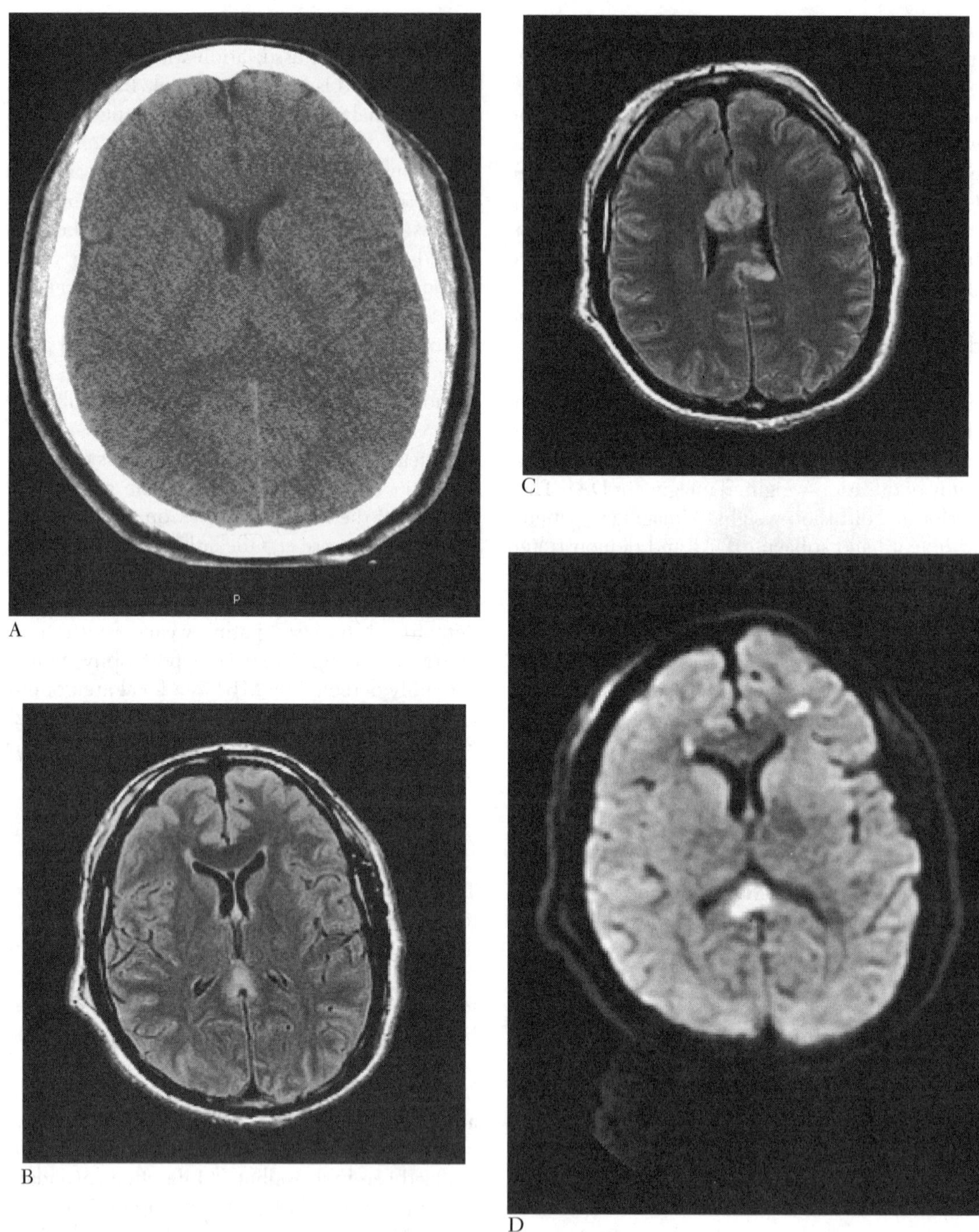

Figure 3.9. Extensive diffuse axonal injury (DAI) involving the corpus callosum. (*A*) Axial computed tomography demonstrate no abnormality in the genu or splenium of the corpus callosum. (*B*, *C*) Axial fluid-attenuated inversion-recovery sequences reveal extensive abnormal signal intensity involving most of the corpus callosum, consistent with diffuse axonal injury. (*D*, *E*) Axial diffusion-weighted images demonstrate abnormal signal intensity involving the majority of the corpus callosum, consistent with restricted diffusion secondary to DAI. In addition, small areas of signal abnormalities are seen in the frontal white matter bilaterally.

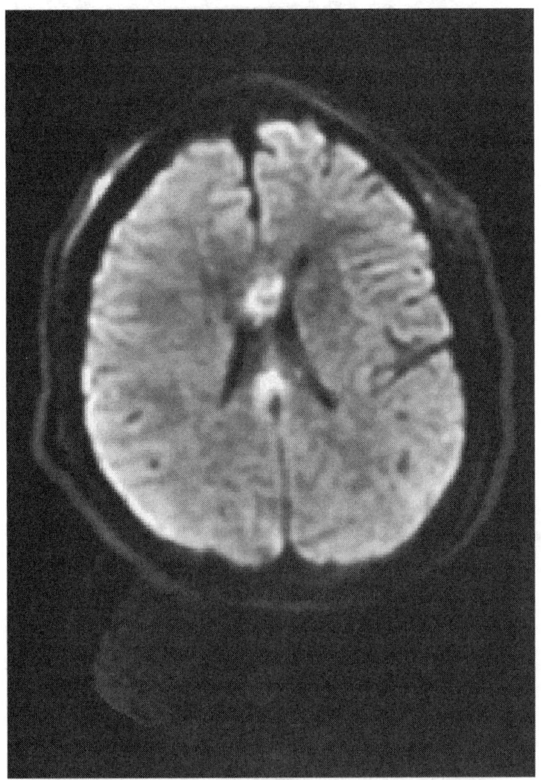

E
Figure 3.9. (*continued*)

initial CT may show a slight increase in the overall density of the brain. This is particularly common in children. Unilateral cerebral swelling is seen frequently with ipsilateral SDH, less frequently in ipsilateral EDH, and occasionally as an isolated finding.[35]

Posttraumatic Atrophy of Cerebrum, Cerebellum, and Corpus Callosum

Atrophy of the cerebrum may occur focally or diffusely in patients with previous head trauma.[6,47] In such cases, both CT and MRI will show widening of the cortical sulci and concordant ventriculomegaly in the affected areas. Cerebellar atrophy is demonstrated by the prominence of the subarachnoid and cisternal spaces in the posterior fossa. Time-dependent atrophic changes occurring after TBI can be quantified using MR volumetric studies, and in chronic stages, these studies, may predict the eventual cognitive outcome.[6] Focal atrophy may present as focal areas of encephalomalacia or as a porencephalic cyst. Sometimes it may be difficult to differentiate encephalomalacia from porencephalic cyst on CT, as both entities show low density. Since porencephalic cyst contains cerebrospinal fluid, it is generally of lower density than areas of encephalomalacia. On MRI, the two conditions can be easily differentiated from each other on the FLAIR sequence, as porencephalic cyst shows low signal intensity, whereas encephalomalacia demonstrates high signal intensity.

In patients with long-standing, severe closed head injury and diffuse white matter injury, atrophy of the corpus callosum can occur. The degree of corpus callosal atrophy correlates significantly with the chronicity of the injury. Magnetic resonance imaging provides an in vivo determination of corpus callosal atrophy which may reflect the severity of diffuse axonal injury. The MRI findings of corpus callosal atrophy following closed head trauma appear to correlate clinically with posttraumatic hemispheric disconnection effects.[7] Reduction in fornix size and hippocampal volume has also been reported in patients with TBI.[46] We have recently observed a case of posttraumatic seizure in a patient with previous temporal lobe injury. Magnetic resonance imaging of the temporal lobe demonstrated temporal lobe encephalomalacia and bilateral mesial temporal sclerosis.

Correlation of Neuroimaging and Neurotraumatic Outcome

The relationship of advanced neuroimaging techniques in TBI management is undergoing a fundamental change. Historically, the radiographic findings in neurotrauma focused on the descriptive anatomy of lesions, with little regard to correlation with the clinical outcome of patients. Given the wide spectrum of traumatic mechanisms and the complexity of neurophysiological autoregulation, prognostication based solely on the location, number, and size of lesions has been poor at best. However, recent advances in neuroimaging have created opportunities for understanding the biology of neurotrauma, as well as for stratifying the clinical outcomes based on physiological, functional, and anatomical imaging correlates. With the growing widespread use of MRI, single-photon emission CT (SPECT), and positron emission tomography (PET) scanning, new techniques are

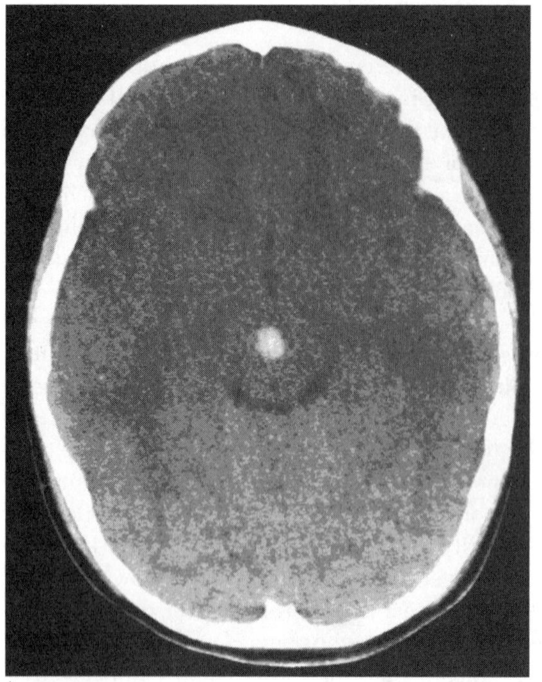
A

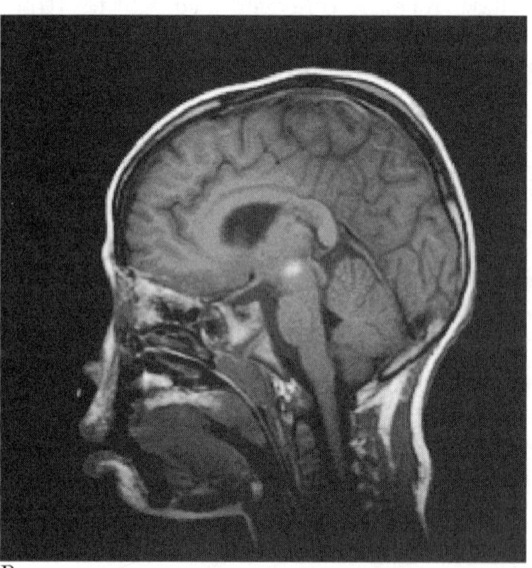
B

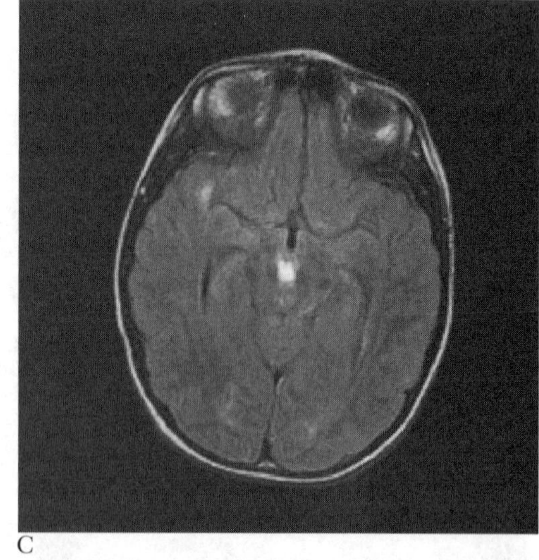
C

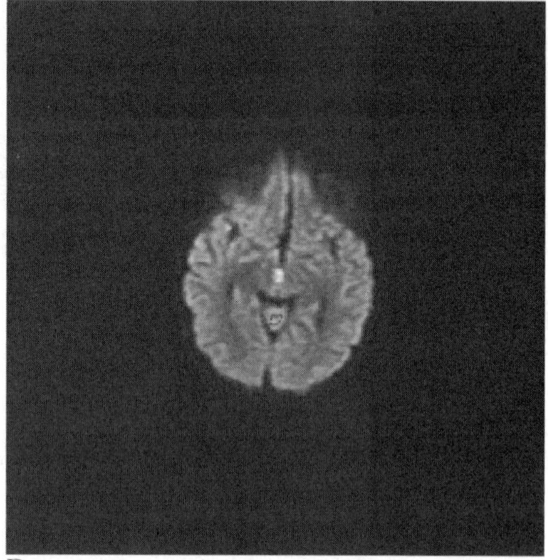
D

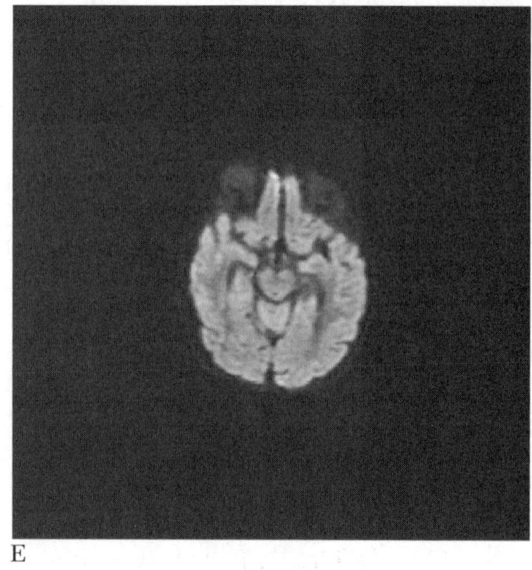
E

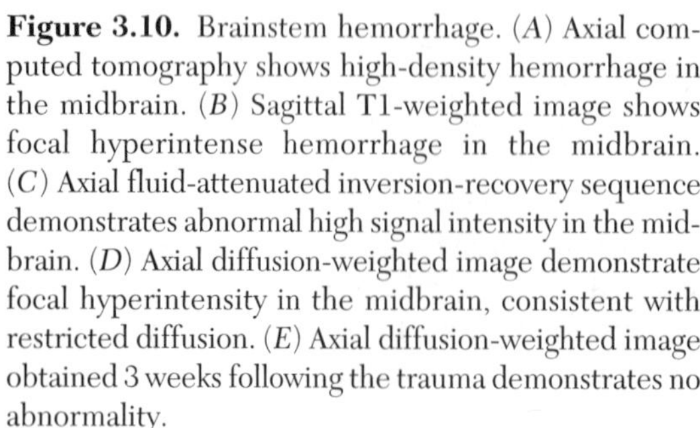

Figure 3.10. Brainstem hemorrhage. (*A*) Axial computed tomography shows high-density hemorrhage in the midbrain. (*B*) Sagittal T1-weighted image shows focal hyperintense hemorrhage in the midbrain. (*C*) Axial fluid-attenuated inversion-recovery sequence demonstrates abnormal high signal intensity in the midbrain. (*D*) Axial diffusion-weighted image demonstrate focal hyperintensity in the midbrain, consistent with restricted diffusion. (*E*) Axial diffusion-weighted image obtained 3 weeks following the trauma demonstrates no abnormality.

being applied to trauma situations with the aim of improving clinical diagnosis and prognosis.

With the widespread adoption of advanced neuroimaging studies, neuroradiologists have gained the ability to correlate subtle changes in neurophysiology and map them anatomically. Magnetic resonance imaging can detect punctate areas of hemorrhage, differentiate between vasogenic and cytotoxic edema, and demonstrate areas of ischemia/infarct with much greater precision and speed than earlier generation neuroimaging modalities. While several studies have examined the link between TBI and routine MRI findings, these investigations have focused primarily on lesional anatomy.[27,46,48] However, with the development of MRS, MTI, diffusion/perfusion imaging, and functional imaging, our understanding of the neurophysiology of TBI has been greatly enhanced.[23] For example, both MRS and MTI have been shown to quantify damage after TBI, as reported by Sinson et al.[43] Posttraumatic differences in NAA/creatine ratios between patients with good and bad outcomes were observed but were not statistically significant. Furthermore, McGowan et al.[36] have reported that quantitative MTI can be utilized to detect abnormalities associated with mild TBI that are not detected on routine CT or MRI. Although there was only a weak correlation between the MRI and neurophysiological data, refinements in the technique may allow the development of a grading system to predict the extent of injury.[51] In fact, mild TBI is becoming an intense area of focus given its high prevalence in the population and the greater sensitivity of advanced MRI techniques. Hofman et al.[27] recently reported the largest prospective study to date correlating neuroimaging findings and neurocognitive test findings in patients with mild TBI.[27] Their results suggest that even mild trauma to the brain results in abnormalities identified on SPECT and MRI that were previously inapparent. Unfortunately, the correlation between the two imaging techniques and neurocognitive test results was poor. Nevertheless, the data support the further application of MRI and SPECT imaging to patients with head trauma given the sensitivity of these techniques to posttraumatic brain lesions.

The future of TBI research and neuroimaging is bright. We are no longer limited to simple anatomical descriptive analysis but can extend our work into the arena of microscopic imaging and the sphere of outcomes research. The role of the neuroradiologist as prognosticator is becoming more important as the tools at our disposal allow better understanding of the link between what we see and what clinicians observe.

References

1. Adams JH et al: Diffuse axonal injury due to non-missile head injury in humans: An analysis of 45 cases. Ann Neurol 12:557–563, 1982.
2. Alsop D et al: Detection of acute pathologic changes following experimental traumatic brain injury using diffusion weighted magnetic resonance imaging. J Neurotrauma 13:515–521, 1996.
3. Arfanakis K et al: Diffusion tensor MR Imaging in diffuse axonal injury. AJNR 23:794–802, 2002.
4. Ashikaga R, et al: MRI of head injury using FLAIR. Neuroradiology 39(4):239–242, 1997.
5. Bagley IJ et al: Magnetization transfer imaging of traumatic brain injury. J Magn Reson Imag, 11(1):1–8, 2000.
6. Bakay L, Glassauer FE: Head Injury. Boston, Little, Brown, 1980.
7. Benavidez DA, Fletcher JM, Hannay HJ, et al: Corpus callosum damage and interhemispheric transfer of information following closed head injury in children. Cortex 35(3):315–336, 1999.
8. Birbamer G et al: Post-traumatic segmental myoclonus associated with bilateral olivary hypertrophy. Acta Neurol Scand 87(6):505–509, 1993.
9. Blumbergs PC et al: Staining of amyloid precursor protein to study axonal damage in mild head injury. Lancet 344:1055–1056, 1994.
10. Brooks WM et al: Magnetic resonance spectroscopy in traumatic brain injury. J Head Trauma Rehabil 16(2):149–164, 2001.
11. Caveness WF: Incidence of cranio-cerebral trauma in 1976 with trend from 1970 to 1975. In: Thompson RA, Green JRG (eds): Advances in Neurology, vol 22. New York, Raven Press, pp. 1–3, 1979.
12. Condon B et al: Early ^{1}H magnetic resonance spectroscopy of acute head injury: Four cases. J Neurotrauma 15:563–571, 1998.
13. Cooper PR, Maravilla K, Kirkpatrick J, et al: Traumatically-induced brain stem hemorrhage and the computerized tomographic scan: Clinical, pathological, and experimental observations. Neurosurgery 4:115–124, 1979.
14. Cordobes F, Lobato RD, Rivas JJ, et al: Post-traumatic diffuse axonal brain injury: Análysis of 78 patients studied with computed tomography. Acta Neurochir 81:27–35, 1986.
15. Dawson SL, Hirsch CS, Lucas FV, et al: The contrecoup phenomenon: Reappraisal of a classic problem. Hum Pathol 11:155–166, 1980.
16. Friede RL, Roessman U: The pathogenesis of secondary midbrain hemorrhages. Neurology 16:1210–1216, 1968.
17. Gean AD: Imaging of Head Trauma. New York, Raven Press, 1994.

18. Gennarelli TA: Emergency department management of head injuries. Emerg Med Clin North Am 2:749–760, 1985.
19. Gennarelli TA, Thibault LE: Biomechanics of acute subdural hematoma. J Trauma 22:680–686, 1982.
20. Gentry LR et al: Prospective comparative study of intermediate field MR and CT in the evaluation of closed head trauma. AJNR 9:91–100, 1988.
21. Gentry LR, Godersky JC, Thompson BH: MR imaging of head trauma: Review of the distribution and radiopathologic features of traumatic lesions. AJR 150(3):663–672, 1988.
22. Gentry LR, Godersky JC, Thompson BH: Traumatic brain stem injury: MR imaging. Radiology 171:177–178, 1989.
23. Hammound DA, Wasserman BA: Diffuse axonal injuries: Pathophysiology and imaging. Neuroimag Clin North Am 12:205–216, 2002.
24. Hans JS, Kaufman B, Alfidi RJ, et al: Head trauma evaluated by magnetic resonance and computed tomography: A comparison. Radiology 150:71–77, 1984.
25. Hanstock C et al: Diffusion weighted imaging differentiates ischemic tissue from traumatic tissue. Stroke 25:843–848, 1994.
26. Hardman JM, Manoukian A: Pathology of head trauma. Neuroimag Clin North Am 12:175–187, 2002.
27. Hofman P et al: MR imaging, single photon emission CT, and neurocognitive performance after mild traumatic brain injury. AJNR 22:441–449, 2001.
28. Ito J et al: Characterization of edema by diffusion weighted imaging in experimental traumatic brain injury. J Neurosurg 84:97–103, 1996.
29. Jeret JS, Mandell M, Anziska B, et al: Clinical predictors of abnormality disclosed by computed tomography after mild head trauma. Neurosurgery 32(1):9–15, 1993.
30. Johnson MH, Lee SH: Computed tomography of acute cerebral trauma. Radiol Clin North Am 30(2):325–352, 1992.
31. Kelly AB, Zimmerman RD, Snow RB, et al: Head trauma: Comparison of MR and CT—experience in 100 patients. AJNR 9(4):699–708, 1988.
32. Kim PE, Zee CS: The radiologic evaluation of craniocerebral missile injuries. Neurosurg Clin North Am 6(4): 669–687, 1995.
33. LeRoux PD, Haglund MM, Newell DW, et al: Intraventricular hemorrhage in blunt head trauma: An analysis of 43 cases. Neurosurgery 31:678–684, 1992.
34. Liu AY et al: Traumatic brain injury: Diffusion weighted MR imaging findings. AJNR 20(9):1636–1641, 1999.
35. Lobato RD, Sarabia R, Cordobes F, et al: Posttraumatic cerebral hemispheric swelling. J Neurosurg 68:417–423, 1980.
36. McGowen J et al: Magnetization transfer imaging in the detection of injury associated with mild head trauma. AJNR 21:875–880, 2000.
37. Miller JD, Tocher JL, Jones PA: Extradural hematoma—earlier detection, better results [editorial] Brain Inj 2:83–86, 1988.
38. Mittl RL et al: Prevalence of MR evidence of diffuse axonal injury in patients with mild head injury and normal CT findings. AJNR 15:1583–1589, 1994.
39. Sasiadek M, Marciniak R, Bem Z: CT appearance of shearing injuries of the brain. Bildgebung 58(3):148–149, 1991.
40. Schynoll W, Overton D, Krome R, et al: A prospective study to identify high-yield criteria associated with acute intracranial computed tomography findings in head injury patients. Am J Emerg Med 11(4):321–326, 1993.
41. Segall HD, McComb JG, Tsai FY, Miller JH: Neuroradiology in head trauma. In: Gwinn JL, Stanley P (eds): Diagnostic Imaging in Pediatric Trauma. Berlin, Springer International, 1980, Chap. 3.
42. Servadei F, Piazzi G, Seracchioli A, et al: (1988) Extradural hematomas: An analysis of the changing characteristics of patients admitted from 1980 to 1986. Diagnostic and therapeutic implication in 158 cases. Brain Injury 2:87–100, 1988.
43. Sinson G et al: Magnetization transfer imaging and proton MR spectroscopy in the evaluation of axonal injury: Correlation with clinical outcome after traumatic brain injury. AJNR 22:143–151, 2001.
44. Sosin DM et al: Head injury–associated deaths in the United States from 1979 to 1986. JAMA 262(16):2251–2255, 1989.
45. Strich SJ: Shearing of nerve fibers as a cause of brain damage due to head injury, a pathological study of twenty cases. Lancet 1:2443–2448, 1961.
46. Tate DF, Bigler ED: Fornix and hippocampal atrophy in traumatic brain injury. Learn Mem 7(6):442–446, 2000.
47. Tsai FY, Huprich JE, Gardner FC, et al: Diagnostic and prognostic implications of computed tomography of head trauma. J Comput Assist Tomogr 2:323–331, 1978.
48. Udstuen GJ, Claar JM: Imaging of acute head injury in the adult. Neuroimag Clin North Am 11(3):433–445, 2001.
49. Yanagawa Y et al: A quantitative analysis of head injury using T2-weighted gradient-echo imaging. J Trauma 49:272–277, 1978.
50. Yoshino E, Yamaki T, Higuchi T, et al: Acute brain edema in fatal head injury: Analysis by dynamic CT scanning. J Neurosurg 63:830–839, 1985.
51. Zee CS et al: Imaging of sequelae of head trauma. Neuroimag Clin North Am 12:325–338, 2002.
52. Zee CS, Go JL: CT of head trauma. Neuroimag Clin North Am 8(3):525–539, 1998.
53. Zee CS, Segall HD, Destian S, Ahmadi J: Radiologic evaluation of head trauma. In: Wilkins R, Rengachary S (eds): Neurosurgery. New York: McGraw-Hill, pp 2675–2687, 1996.
54. Zimmerman RA, Bilaniuk LT, Gennarelli T: Computed tomography of shearing injuries of the cerebral white matter. Radiology 127:393–396, 1978.

Chapter 4
The Neuropathology of Trauma

DAVID I. GRAHAM,
KATHRYN E. SAATMAN,
NIKLAS MARKLUND, VALERIA CONTE,
DIEGO MORALES, NICOLAS ROYO,
AND TRACY K. McINTOSH

The epidemiology of head injury has been detailed in Chapter 1, where it can be readily seen that trauma to the central nervous system (CNS) is a major cause of death and persisting disability throughout the world. For example, in the United Kingdom, as in most industrialized countries, about 1800 per 100,000 persons present to accident and emergency departments with head injury, and between 200 and 300 per 100,000 are admitted for observation. Fortunately, the majority of the injuries are mild, but head injuries account for between 25% and 35% of all deaths from trauma.[280] A survey of head injuries by the European Brain Injury Consortium found that 3% of patients with head injury remained vegetative and 10% were severely disabled, 20% were moderately disabled, and 37% made a good recovery 6 months after their injury.[369] The cost to families and society is particularly high when it is remembered that trauma to the CNS is especially common in young adult males, many of whom have dependents.

Any classification of brain damage after injury to the head must take into account the full spectrum of clinical presentation and outcome, from the patient who remains in coma from the moment of injury until death to the patient who is apparently normal after the initial injury but who, as a result of a complication, subsequently lapses into a fatal coma. Clinical, neuroradiological, and neuropathological studies have shown that brain damage after head injury may be attributed to many different types of processes, with increasing evidence that what separates mild, moderate, and severe traumatic brain injury is not so much the nature of the lesion but its amount and distribution. Nevertheless, uncertainties remain as to whether or not there really is a continuum from mild to severe injury, and to what extent the changes seen postmortem in fatal cases can be extrapolated to the clinical and neuroradiological features that have been identified in those who survive head injury.

For any given level of injury, a good recovery is more likely in a healthy individual whose brain is normal than in an individual who, because of either a preexisting developmental or acquired disorder, has an abnormal brain. For example, the outcome even after a relatively minor head injury in a patient who has already experienced a stroke is likely to be worse than if such a premorbid condition is not present.[156,180]

Classification and Mechanisms of Brain Damage

There have been many studies on the neuropathological classification of brain damage in patients who die from a head injury (see Graham et al.[181]). In an attempt to provide clinico-pathological correlation, the existence of primary and secondary damage has been emphasized. This approach has helped to identify potentially preventable complications in patients with a head injury who "talk and die"[428] or "talk and deteriorate,"[330] as it is well recognized that an apparently trivial head injury can set in motion a progressive sequence of events leading to secondary brain damage with a fatal outcome or severe, persistent disability.[79,251] The merit of this classification is that from a neuropathological point of view, it recognizes that there are two main stages in the development of brain damage after injury to the head, namely, *primary damage*, which occurs at the moment of injury and takes the form of lacerations of the scalp, fracture of the skull, surface contusions and lacerations, diffuse traumatic axonal injury, and intracranial hemorrhage, and *secondary damage*, which is produced by complicating processes that are initiated at the moment of injury but do not present clinically for a period of time after injury, including brain damage due to ischemia, swelling, infection, and raised intracranial pressure.

A major contribution to the classification of brain injury after trauma has been provided by neuroradiology, including computed tomography (CT) and magnetic resonance imaging (MRI).[329,518] More recently, the use of positron emission tomography (PET) and single proton emission tomography (SPECT) have begun to provide functional correlates of the structural damage identified.[1,143,150,483] Such techniques have provided the alternative classification of *focal* damage, which includes lacerations of the scalp, fractures of the skull, surface contusions and lacerations, intracranial hematomas and raised intracranial pressure, and damage including ischemic brain damage, diffuse traumatic axonal injury, and diffuse brain swelling. Whereas the nature of focal lesions can be determined by imaging with a good degree of certainty, it is more difficult to be confident about the nature of diffuse brain damage in those patients who are in coma without evidence of intracranial hematoma.

The past decade or so has provided a wealth of clinical and laboratory information that has now established that the principal mechanisms of brain damage after head injury are due to either *contact* or *acceleration/deceleration*.[155,181] Lesions due to contact result from either something striking the head or vice versa and consist of local effects such as laceration of the scalp, fracture of the skull with or without an associated extradural hematoma, surface contusions and lacerations, and intracerebral hemorrhage. In contrast, acceleration/deceleration results from head movement in the instant after injury and leads to intracranial and intracerebral pressure gradients as well as shear, tensile, and compressive strains. Such inertial forces are responsible for two of the most important types of damage encountered in nonmissile head injury, namely, acute subdural hematoma resulting from the tearing of subdural bridging veins and widespread damage to axons.[157] Analysis of various datasets have shown that the focal pathologies associated with contact are more likely to result from a fall than from the diffuse pathologies that are most commonly associated with acceleration/deceleration after road traffic accidents.

Much of our knowledge about the pathology of brain damage after trauma is based on postmortem studies, a prerequisite of which is that the proper evaluation of specimens can only be undertaken if the brain is appropriately fixed prior to dissection and histological studies are carried out.[8] This applies both to *blunt* injuries, which are by far the most common in civilian practice and of which an account will follow, and to *missile* injuries, which will not be considered further in this chapter.

A comprehensive database of brain damage in fatal head injuries has been established in Glasgow that consists of a consecutive series of over 1500 documented blunt head injuries. The frequency of the observations will depend on the source of the material, namely, medico-legal, accident and emergency, or primary surgical or neurosurgical (Table 4.1).

Table 4.1. Data from a Consecutive Series of Fatal Blunt Head Injuries

Gender	Males	78%
	Females	22%
Cause of injury	Road traffic accidents	53%
	Falls	35%
	Assaults	5%
	Others	7%
Focal damage	Fracture of skull	75%
	Surface contusions and lacerations	95%
	Intracranial hematoma	60%
	Associated with raised intracranial pressure	75%
Diffuse damage	Diffuse traumatic axonal injury	95%
	Ischemic brain damage	55%
	Brain swelling	53%
	Intracranial infection	4%

Note: For definitions of types of damage, see the text.

Brain Damage in Fatal Blunt Head Injury in Adults

Although of considerable clinical importance, lesions of the scalp and fracture of the skull will not be considered further. The following is an account of the pathology of traumatic brain injury.

Focal Lesions

Scalp Injury and Skull Fracture

The scalp is often lacerated, and such lesions are the best indication of the site of contact. Further, they may bleed copiously.

The more severe the head injury, the greater the frequency of skull fracture. For example, the frequency is 3% in those who present to accident and emergency departments, 65% in patients admitted to a neurosurgical unit, and up to 80% in fatal cases.

A fracture of the skull is strongly associated with the development of an intracranial hematoma, particularly in a patient with a reduced level of consciousness. For example, one study determined that only 1 in 6000 patients who did not have any of these features while in the accident and emergency department subsequently developed an intracranial hematoma, whereas the risk became 1 in 4 if these clinical features were present.[355]

Surface Contusions and Lacerations

By definition, the pia-arachnoid is intact over surface contusions but torn in lacerations. Traditionally, contusions and lacerations have been considered the hallmark of brain damage due to head injury, and yet they may be absent in some 6% of fatal cases. They are most severe on the crests of gyri and have a very characteristic distribution affecting the frontal poles, the under aspects of the frontal lobes including the orbital gyri, the cortex above and below the sylvian fissures, the temporal poles, and the lateral and inferior aspects of the temporal lobes; less frequently, the under aspects of the cerebellar hemispheres are affected. In the acute stages they are hemorrhagic and swollen and may extend to involve related white matter. Over time they present as golden-brown shrunken scars and may be incidental findings in some 2.5% of autopsies in general hospitals.

Various types of contusions have been described: for example, *fracture contusions*, which occur at the site of a fracture; *coup contusions*, which occur at the site of impact in the absence of a fracture; *contrecoup contusions*, which occur in the brain diametrically opposite the point of impact; and *herniation contusions*, which occur where the medial parts of the temporal lobe make contact with the free edge of the tentorium or the cerebellar tonsils make contact with the foramen magnum at the time of injury. These various types of contusions occur on the surface of the brain, but reference is also made to *gliding contusions*, which are hemorrhagic lesions in the cerebral cortex and subjacent white matter at the dorsomedial margins of the cerebral hemispheres and which are now considered to be part of the vascular damage associated with diffuse injuries.

A contusion index has been developed that allows the depth and extent of contusions in various parts of the brain to be expressed quantitatively (see Graham et al.[181]). Using this index, it has been found, perhaps not surprisingly, that contusions are more severe in patients with a fracture of the skull than those without it; that they are significantly less severe in patients with diffuse traumatic axonal injury (see below) than in those without this type of brain damage; and that they are more severe in patients who do not experience a lucid interval than in those who do. The index has also shown that severe contusions are present in about 10% of fatalities, moderately severe contusions in 78%, and mild contusions in 6%. More recently, a *hemorrhagic lesion score* has been derived, which provides a finer discrimination of the distribution and severity of injury by including lesions involving corpus callosum, deep white matter, and deep gray matter.[446]

Lacerations are often associated with acute subdural and intracerebral and/or intracerebeller hemorrhage. The term *burst lobe* is then appropriate.

Intracranial Hemorrhage

This is the most common cause of clinical deterioration and death in patients who experience a lucid interval after their injury.[63] Traumatic intracranial hemorrhage is classified into *extradural* and *intradural* hematomas.

Clinical experience has shown that the effects of an intracranial hematoma are often delayed because it is the associated swelling of the brain that is largely responsible for subsequent events. The importance of intracranial hematoma as a source of secondary brain damage is emphasized by the study of patients who died although they were able to talk following a head injury.[330,428] The fact that the patients had talked shows that they did not have severe diffuse primary brain damage, subsequent deterioration being a consequence of the mass effect of an expanding intracranial lesion. This sequence of events is particularly characteristic of extradural hematoma, and some patients with an acute subdural hematoma also pursue a similar clinical course. An intracranial hematoma was present in about 60% of the cases in the Glasgow database.

EXTRADURAL HEMATOMA. This hematoma was present in some 4% of cases in the Glasgow database, and there was a fracture of the skull in some 85% of the adult patients. However, it is well recognized that extradural hematoma may occur in the absence of a fracture. This type of hematoma occurs most commonly in the temporal region, but in some 20% to 30% of cases the hematoma occurs elsewhere,[62,63,96] such as the frontal and parietal regions or within the posterior fossa; occasionally, the hematomas are multiple. Bleeding from the meningeal blood vessels causes the hematoma to enlarge and strip the dura from the skull to form a circumscribed oval mass that progressively indents and flattens the adjacent brain. Many extradural hematomas are associated with only minimal evidence of other types of brain damage. Over time, small hematomas become completely organized but larger hematomas may undergo partial organization, the centers of which become filled with dark viscous fluid.

INTRADURAL HEMATOMA. These hematomas are subdivided into *subarachnoid hematoma, subdural hematoma, discrete intracerebral* or *intracerebellar hematoma* not in continuity with the surface of the brain, and a *burst* lobe that is an intracerebral or intracerebellar hematoma in continuity with a related subdural hematoma.

Bilateral films showing blood in the subdural space are common in fatal head injury. Because the blood can spread freely throughout the subdural space, it tends to cover the entire hemisphere, with the result that a subdural hematoma is more extensive than an extradural hematoma. Large subdural hematomas were present in some 18% of the Glasgow database, the majority being due to rupture of veins that bridge the subdural space where they connect the superior surfaces of the cerebral hemispheres to the sagittal sinus. However, some subdural hematomas are arterial in origin. Most cases of acute subdural hematoma are associated with considerable brain damage. This is particularly true in cases with a burst lobe. This was present in some 23% of the cases in the Glasgow database and occurred most commonly in the frontal and temporal lobes.

Attempts to age hematomas on the basis of histological studies have not proved very satisfactory. The current opinion is moving toward classifying subdural hematoma as *acute* when it is composed of clot and blood (usually within the first 48 hours after injury), *subacute* when there is a mixture of clotted and fluid blood (developing between 2 and 14 days after injury), and *chronic* when the hematoma is fluid (developing more than 14 days after injury).[63]

Chronic subdural hematoma occurs weeks or months after what may appear to have been a trivial head injury. The hematoma becomes encapsulated and slowly increases in size, occasionally becoming large enough to produce distortion and herniation of the brain. Chronic subdural hematoma is more common in the older age group, in whom there is already some cerebral atrophy, than in younger patients.

Intracerebral hematomas were present in some 16% of the cases in the Glasgow database. They are often multiple and occur most commonly in the frontal and temporal lobes,[63] although they may also occur deep within the hemispheres. Less commonly, they occur in the cerebellum, although sometimes traumatic intracerebral hematomas are delayed for several days and a correct interpretation may have important medico-legal implications.

If a solitary hematoma is found in the brain of a patient who has experienced a head injury, the possibility that it is due to nontraumatic causes such as hypertension or rupture of a saccular aneurysm should be considered. Even when all the possibilities have been taken into consideration, it may still be difficult to reach a final conclusion.

Brain Damage Secondary to Raised Intracranial Pressure

This is a common complication in patients who sustain nonmissile head injury, being present in 75% of the cases in the Glasgow database.[185] The usual causes are mass lesions due to hematomas and associated brain swelling. As space occupation progresses, there is deformation of brain tissue, a reduction of the volume of cerebrospinal fluid (CSF), shift and distortion of the brain, and in the closed skull the formation of internal hernias. A space-occupying mass in one cerebral hemisphere may result in herniation of the cingulate gyrus beneath the free edge of the falx or herniation of the parahippocampal gyrus through the opening of the tentorium cerebelli. Within the posterior fossa, herniation of the cerebellar tonsil through the foramen magnum occurs. As internal hernias form, the basal cisterns are obliterated and pressure gradients develop between the various intracranial compartments. Eventually, these changes result in secondary damage to the brain stem, and they form midline hemorrhages and/or infarctions. At the same time, additional vascular lesions may develop, especially infarction within the distribution of one or both posterior cerebral arteries, the anterior choroidal arteries, and the superior cerebellar arteries.

Using the structural criterion of pressure necrosis in one or both parahippocampal gyri,[4] it has been possible to confirm that brain damage secondary to raised intracranial pressure is a common cause of deterioration and coma in patients who die within weeks of a severe head injury. While it might be anticipated that such brain damage is a common structural basis for severe disability or the vegetative state after head injury, this appears not to be the case, as the two most common findings are diffuse traumatic axonal injury and diffuse ischemic brain damage.[5,249] However, brain damage may occur in the absence of high intracranial pressure.[186]

Diffuse Lesions

Diffuse Traumatic Axonal Injury

Characterization in Humans

Using conventional histological techniques for the identification of axonal bulbs, diffuse traumatic axonal injury (TAI) has been found in most fatal cases and is the most common cause of the vegetative state and severe disability after injury.[5,249]

This type of brain damage was first called *diffuse degeneration of white matter*.[504] Since then, a variety of descriptive terms have been used, including *shearing injury*, [405,505] *diffuse damage of immediate impact type*,[9] *diffuse white matter shearing injury*,[575] *inner cerebral trauma*,[189] *diffuse axonal injury*,[7,158] and, more recently, *diffuse traumatic axonal injury*.[151,152]

In the original description of severe cases of diffuse axonal injury (DAI; now TAI) there were three distinctive features: (1) a focal lesion in the corpus callosum often involving the interventricular septum and associated with some intraventricular hemorrhage, (2) a focal lesion in one or both dorsolateral sectors of the rostral brain stem, and (3) microscopic evidence of widespread damage to axons.

The first two of these abnormalities can usually be seen at the time of brain cutting as long as the specimen has been properly fixed and dissected. Thus, if the patient survives for only a few days, the lesions in the corpus callosum and in the brain stem are usually hemorrhagic, but with survival the tissue becomes soft and granular and ultimately is represented by a shrunken, often cystic, scar. The third, and in many respects most important feature, can only be identified histologically, the appearances again depending on the length of survival. Thus, if survival is short (days), there are numerous axonal swellings that may be seen as eosinophilic masses on nerve fibers in sections stained by hematoxylin and eosin or as argyrophilic swellings in silver-stained preparations. They can also be demonstrated immunohistochemically.[160b,173,295b] These axonal swellings occur particularly in the parasagittal white matter, corpus callosum, internal capsule, thalami, and in the various ascending and descending tracts of the brain stem. If the patient survives for several weeks, axonal bulbs persist but the most characteristic lesion is the formation of large numbers of small clusters of microglia throughout the white matter of the cerebral and cerebellar hemispheres and in the brain stem; these are associated with an astrocytosis and lipid-filled macrophages. The principal neuropathology in those patients who survive for several months or longer is the identification of the breakdown products of myelin in those fiber tracts in which axonal bulbs and microglia were most frequently seen. Bulbs may persist for up to 6 weeks, although they are most easily seen within the first 2 weeks of injury, and clusters of microglia are most prominent between 4 and 6 weeks. In patients who survive in a vegetative state for many months or years, abnormalities in the brain may be limited to small, healed superficial contusions and Wallerian degeneration in deep white matter. On coronal section, the ventricles are enlarged because of the reduction in white matter, and in most cases it is possible to identify the telltale focal lesions in the corpus callosum and rostral brain stem.

Continuing experience confirms that patients with TAI form a distinct clinicopathological group that at the severe end of the spectrum is characterized by a statistically significant lower incidence of a lucid interval, a fracture of the skull, surface contusions, intracerebral hematomas, and evidence of raised intracranial pressure compared with patients without this type of brain damage. This pattern of damage is particularly associated with road traffic accidents[7] and assaults.[177] Cases have also been described following assault,[177,244] and there is a small number of patients who have fallen from a height greater than their own in whom this pattern of damage is also seen.[3]

It was originally considered that TAI is an all-or-none phenomenon, but the identification of less severe degrees of it now provides strong evidence that it is part of a continuum of diffuse brain injury that ranges clinically from concussion up to and including persistent posttraumatic coma.[48,153] Evidence for such a continuum has also been obtained from postmortem studies. For example, Pilz[414] described the occurrence of axonal swellings in human head injuries of varying severity, and as early as 1968, Oppenheimer[394] had shown that occasional clusters of microglia can be found in patients dying from some unrelated cause soon after a minor head injury. These findings were confirmed by Clark,[83] who also drew attention to the frequent occurrence of such clusters in the white matter in patients dying as a result of a head injury. More recently, Blumbergs et al.,[49] staining with an antibody against β-amyloid precursor protein, has shown evidence of axonal damage in a small series of patients who died from causes other than those associated with the previously sustained mild head injury.

Further support for the concept of varying degrees of TAI has been provided by a review of 122 cases in the Glasgow database,[2] as a result of which a new grading system was proposed. In grade 1, abnormalities were limited to histological evidence of axonal damage throughout the white matter, there being no focal accentuation in either the corpus callosum or the brain stem. Cases were designated grade 2 if, in addition to widely distributed axonal injury, there was a focal lesion in the corpus callosum. Grade 3 TAI, which represented the most severe end of the spectrum, was characterized by diffuse damage to axons in the presence of focal lesions in both the corpus callosum and brain stem. Concomitant with the appreciation that varying degrees of axonal injury may occur, it is now recognized that the lesser degrees of it may be associated with either a complete or partial lucid interval.[2] Indeed, of the 122 cases studied by Adams et al.,[2] there were 2 patients with a completely lucid interval who had grade 1 injury, and 15 with grade 2 axonal injury who had had a partially lucid interval. In contrast, none of the patients with grade 3 talked.

Given that it takes between 18 and 24 hours for classic axonal bulbs to be identified with certainty by silver impregnation techniques in the human brain after head injury, it is likely that, as revealed by the more sensitive technique of immunohistochemistry, the incidence of TAI is higher than the published figures suggest.[160,470] Indeed, in a recent study,[160b] we have shown that axonal injury of varying amounts is almost a universal finding in cases of fatal head injury. In spite of these advances, a definitive diagnosis of TAI cannot be made in patients who survive for only a short time (1–2 hours) after their injury, although it may be strongly suspected, particularly if there are focal lesions in the corpus callosum and in the brain stem, and if hemorrhages are present in the form of either gliding contusions or hematomas in the basal ganglia.[160b,295b]

Relevant Experimental Models

The term *diffuse axonal injury* arose as a clinicopathological entity that occurred in types of diffuse brain injury in which there was insufficient macroscopic evidence to account adequately for the clinical features of the patient. Diffuse brain injury is thought to occur primarily from tissue distortion and shear, caused by inertial forces present at injury.[154,339,407] As this concept has developed further, it has become apparent that there exists a wide spectrum of injuries, all of which are due to the same axonal pathology but differing in amount, location, and severity.[154]

In a recent overview of models of experimental traumatic brain injury (TBI), Laurer et al.[292] describes the exisiting experimental models of diffuse brain injury, displaying both the pros and cons of each, as well as the expectations beforehand and the consequences (both morphological and functional). Laurer et al. follow the earlier review by Gennarelli,[155] dividing their review of the models by percussion concussion and acceleration concussion. In fluid percussion, a small volume of liquid is injected into the subdural space or infused very rapidly by means of a percussion device. Many species have been used for studies of fluid percussion, including dog, rabbit, cat,[507] rat,[122,345,349,526] mouse,[68] and swine. In rigid percussion, a solid indentor is applied rapidly to the dura at varying velocities and depths of indentation; such studies have been performed in ferrets,[305] rats,[120,510] mice,[488] and pigs.[188]

The rotational acceleration forces needed to induce damage increase exponentially with respect to the animal's brain size; hence, few injury devices exist with the ability to meet all the parameters needed to reliably produce a purely diffuse traumatic brain injury.[327] Acceleration/concussion injury exists in various models of inertial injury and impact acceleration. Inertial injury models involve the acceleration of the head by distributing loading widely to minimize the effects of impact. Such studies have been carried out on nonhuman primates,[392,529] cats,[375] monkeys,[158,317] and, more recently, swine.[438] In the impact acceleration models, a piston or a weight is dropped either directly on the skull or onto a steel plate attached to the unrestrained skull, which serves to minimize localized skull loading and fracture.[327] These models have been developed in nonhuman primates,[393,465] cats,[287,525] and rats.[135,167,327,378,391]

Both experimental acceleration and fluid percussion appear to model adequately many different aspects of the clinical condition of TAI. However, in terms of the underlying structural pathology of diffuse brain damage as a cause of either severe disability or the vegetative state, models of inertial acceleration reproduce these changes better than fluid percussion at the severe end of the spectrum where extensive diffuse axonal injury occurs.[155] However, no single animal model is entirely successful in reproducing the complete spectrum of pathological changes observed after clinical TBI. Both Gennarelli[155] and Laurer et al.[292] make the important observation that many of the models are characterized by their ability to produce a common type of brain injury, that is, axonal damage. However, its distribution lacks the characteristic pattern found in humans, with the exception of the structural abnormalities induced in nonhuman primates using the inertial acceleration/rotation model, where focal lesions in the corpus callosum and in the dorsolateral sectors of the rostral brain stem, as well as microscopic evidence of diffuse damage to axons, are prevalent.[7,158]

Inherent in the term *diffuse axonal injury* is the premise that the morbidity associated with this type of TBI is due to damage to axons. The initial studies in humans suggested that axons are torn at the moment of injury. However, such immediate disruption of axons has not been identified following midline fluid percussion in the cat[127] or after stretch-induced injury to the optic nerve of the guinea pig.[159,337] These studies suggest that axotomy is delayed and does not occur until some time after the original injury, although primary axotomy or white matter tears may occur with more severe injuries.[187,452] This primary axotomy, which encompasses axonal shearing and resealing of the fragmented axonal membranes occurring at the moment of injury, appears to be irreversible.[176] A second mechanism, however, exists in which changes occur within the axon to disrupt axoplasmic transport.[340,418] With survival, there is an accumulation of transported axoplasm and organelles and local axonal swelling; ultimately, the axolemma is disrupted, resulting in secondary axotomy. There are two main theories concerning the mechanisms of secondary axotomy. The first one hypothesizes that an influx of calcium could activate proteases that degrade membrane proteins and neurofilaments. [347,449,454] This calcium hypothesis has received morphological support in studies that have combined the pyroantimonate reaction for free calcium and altered calcium ATPase activity[338] from studies demonstrating activation of calcium-dependent proteases. The second hypothesis concerning the genesis of injury is that the disruption of axonal transport possibly results from mechanical disturbance to the microtubular and neurofilamentous cytoskeleton.[559]

Many morphological studies have been carried out in the past decade using different types of TBI models. Some of these studies include cardiovascular and electrophysiological changes,[111,349] changes in regional cerebral blood flow,[29,111,140,271,562] the development and time course of cerebral edema,[29,271,386,492] changes in the blood–brain barrier (BBB),[30,99,540] changes in regional brain metabolism,[281,300,543] oxidative metabolism using 2-deoxy-D-glucose (2DG) autoradiography,[235] the development of neurological motor deficits,[301,332,349] and deficits in both cognitive memory and learning.[412,485]

Vascular Brain Damage

Characterization in Humans

It was not until the 1970s that there was full recognition of the frequency and distribution of ischemic brain damage after fatal blunt head injury, and that much of this damage could be attributed to a critical reduction in regional blood flow.[175,179] In this study,[175] ischemic damage was identified in 91% (138 of 151) of the cases. Ischemic damage was assessed as severe in 27%, moderately severe in 43%, and mild in 30%, and in the 138 cases it was found more frequently in the hippocampus (81%) and in the basal ganglia (79%) than in the cerebral cortex (46%) and the cerebellum (44%). There were statistically significant correlations between the ischemic brain damage and either an episode of hypoxia or raised intracranial pressure. As much of this damage was considered to be avoidable or preventable, it led to reappraisal of management and organization of patient care, with increased attention to the recognition that treatment of hypoxia and hypotension at the scene of the accident, during interhospital transfer, and in critical care units, and to the detection and release of cerebral compression by traumatic intracranial hematoma. An audit of the amount and distribution of ischemic damage in a second cohort of patients with fatal nonmissile head injuries was carried out some 10 years later[179] and showed that although it was still common (occurring in 88% of cases, with no statistical difference in the amount of moderately severe and severe ischemic damage—55% and 54%, respectively), there was an increase in the proportion of cases with diffuse damage in the cortex of the type seen after cardiac arrest or status epilepticus. This was rather surprising, as it was expected that the greater use of resuscitative measures would have reduced at least to some extent this type of brain damage. On the other hand, the events responsible may have occurred almost immediately after the injury, before first admission to the hospital and even before the arrival of any skilled personnel at the scene of the accident. Part of the explanation also lay in the fact that there was an increase in the number of severely head-injured patients transferred to the Department of Neurosurgery here at the Institute of Neurological Sciences, some of whom would have previously have died either in accident and emergency departments or in primary surgical wards.

There is now considerable clinical evidence that primary traumatic brain damage may be compounded by secondary insults that occur soon after trauma, during transfer to the hospital, and during the subsequent treatment of the head-injured patient. Such secondary insults are likely to be responsible for ischemic and other forms of secondary brain damage, may be of either intracranial or systemic origin, and may actually arise during initial management or later in the intensive care unit. In a series of papers between 1970 and 1985, a number of authors reported that in comatose head-injured patients, hypoxia was found in 30% and arterial hypotension in 15% of patients on arrival in the accident and emergency room. Probably because of better on-site resuscitation and transport arrangements, there has been a reduction in the frequency of these early insults. Of increasing importance is the awareness that secondary insults after head injury may actually occur within hours of injury,[51,463] including in the intensive care unit.[19] This awareness has largely been occasioned by continuous monitoring during intensive care and the correlations that exist between the adverse influences of the secondary insults and the outcome. Increasing experience suggests that secondary insults occur more frequently and last longer than had previously been thought, and that the duration of the insults matters as much as their severity.[79] Even the lowest grade of insult severity has been shown to adversely affect the outcome. Apparently, the most important predictors of mortality at 12 months postinjury were found to be the durations of hypotension, pyrexia, and hypoxemia.[251]

Relevant Experimental Models

The nature and distribution of diffuse ischemic brain damage after head injury is very similar, if not identical, to that described after cardiac arrest or status epilepticus. Because of the brain's extensive protective collateral circulation, attempts to arrest it in normothermic experimental animals has proven rather difficult. The principal methods used to arrest cerebral blood flow have been reviewed (see Graham, 1992).[174] In general, these studies endorsed the traditional view that complete recovery without neurological or histological damage was unlikely to occur after a complete arrest of the cerebral circulation for more than 4 or 5 minutes. It is now clear, however, that ischemic injury to selectively vulnerable areas such as CA1 of the hippocampus is compatible with survival and minimal neurological deficit. Newer experimental models of TBI have been shown to reproducibly mimic vascular dysfunction and ischemic injury associated with traumatic CNS injury.[110] The frequency and distribution of hypoxic hippocampal lesions in an acceleration model of brain injury has been undertaken,[279] in which lesions in the CA1 hippocampal subfield were present in 32/54 (59%) of the animals. Hippocampal CA1 damage has also been observed with other injury models, such as controlled cortical impact (CCI).[123] This hippocampal involvement was not associated with any marked elevation of the intracranial pressure or depression of cerebral perfusion pressure, but there was a correlation between what was termed *traumatically-induced neuronal necrosis of the hippocampus* and the length of time of unconsciousness and residual neurological deficit.

Hippocampal damage has been produced in fluid percussion injury in the rat[99,172,304] and has been attributed to various metabolic changes[117,130,166] or regional changes in cerebral blood flow.[165,562] Trauma-induced vasospasm has also been invoked with the suggestion that the blood vessels of the hippocampus are particularly susceptible to injury. Additional mechanisms include pathological neuronal excitation involving glutamate or other excitatory amino acid transmitters.[131,257,260,353,380,400,477] It is known, for example, that extracellular glutamate increases in the rat hippocampus after fluid percussion brain injury,[130,257] increasing the likelihood that excitotoxicity represents a mechanism involved in traumatic hippocampal damage.

The increasing awareness of the adverse affect of pyrexia has been reproduced experimentally. It has been shown than maintaining brain temperature at normothermia rather than at the lower levels induced spontaneously during brain ischemia may have a deleterious effect on the outcome.[65] The same principle appears to apply in TBI, namely, that hypothermia protects[54,336,399,506] and hyperthermia worsens the diffuse damage associated with fluid percussion.[89]

Brain Swelling

Brain swelling is common and may be localized or generalized. The cause of the swelling is not always clear, but it is generally due to an increase in either the cerebral blood volume (congestive brain swelling) or the water content of the brain (cerebral edema). There are three main types of brain swelling[246]:

Swelling adjacent to surface contusions or an intracranial hematoma. The physical disruption of tissue at sites of contusion damages the BBB, with leakage of water, electrolytes, and macromolecules into adjacent white matter to form vasogenic edema. The rate at which fluid accumulates is determined by a combination of tissue compliance and the amount of protein that accumulates in the fluid.

Diffuse swelling of one cerebral hemisphere. This is most often seen in association with an ipsilateral acute subdural hematoma. When the hematoma is evacuated, the brain expands to fill the space due to engorgement of a nonreactive vascular bed secondary to cerebral ischemia produced by high intracranial pressure.

Diffuse swelling of both cerebral hemispheres. This tends to develop most commonly in young patients,[178a,423c] and it seems likely that loss of vasomotor tone and consequent vasodilation contribute to the swelling. If vasodilation persists, the BBB may become defective, leading to vasogenic edema.

Outcome after Head Injury

Dementia Pugilistica

It is well recognized that large numbers of concussive or subconcussive blows, such as may be incurred by various sportsmen and in particular by boxers and horse riders, sometimes induce neurological signs and progressive dementia that may develop years after the last injury. This condition affects amateur as well as professional boxers, and it is most likely to develop in boxers with long careers who have been dazed, if not knocked out, on many occasions. Studies have revealed a characteristic pattern of damage, the principal features of which are abnormalities in the septum pellucidum and fenestration of its leaves and enlargement of the ventricles.[98] In some cases, there is thinning of the adjacent fornices of the corpus callosum, scarring with neuronal loss in the cerebellum, degeneration in the substantia nigra with a loss of pigmented neurons, the presence of numerous neurofibrillary tangles diffusely throughout the cerebral cortex and in the brain stem, and the demonstration of variable amounts of diffuse beta-amyloid staining plaques.[434] In contrast, neurofibrillary tangles are not more prevalent after a single episode of acute brain injury.[484] There is increasing evidence that head injury may be a risk factor for the subsequent development of Alzheimer's disease in genetically predisposed individuals.[183,184,192,377]

A major genetic risk factor for Alzheimer's disease is ApoE, the ϵ4 allele of which is overrepresented in groups of patients with Alzheimer's disease in comparison with age-matched controls, whereas Apoϵ2 is underrepresented.[466] In a group of fatally head-injured patients, a substantial difference was found in the ApoE genotype of patients with Alzheimer's disease without beta-amyloid deposits.[377] The Apoϵ4 allele frequency in the beta-amyloid-positive cases was 0.52 compared with 0.16 in the beta-amyloid-negative cases ($p < .0001$). The data linking the ApoE phenotype and findings in the brains of fatally injured patients stimulated investigation of the role of the Apoϵ4 genotype in the outcome of clinical cases. The results of a preliminary study of 100 patients admitted for neurosurgical care after head injury showed a highly significant association between possession of the Apoϵ4 gene subtype and an unfavorable outcome. This relationship held even when other prognostic factors such as age, coma score, and CT findings were taken into account. The rate of unfavorable outcomes (death or severe injury) was doubled for these patients with Apoϵ4 compared with control Apoϵ4–negative patients.

After the recognition that possession of the ϵ4 allele of the ApoE gene is a major risk factor for sporadic Alzheimer's disease, the relation of the polymorphism of the ApoE gene to the beta-amyloid deposits in fatal head injury was studied.[183,377] Subsequent studies have shown that patients with Apoe4 have a worse outcome after head injury[493] and are unlikely to have a good functional outcome.[142,517] The ApoE genotype influences the outcome of brain injury associated with boxing.[252] Recent demonstration of the accommodation of beta-amyloid in axons after TBI has suggested a mechanism that may contribute to long-term degeneration after trauma.[484]

Structural Basis of the Glasgow Outcome Scale

The Glasgow Outcome Scale has been widely adopted as a means of classifying the outcome after head injury[523]—death, vegetative state, severe disability, moderate disability, and good recovery.[250] Outcome has been shown to be associated with the cause and severity of injury: many more of the severe disability cases have sustained a head injury as a result of a traffic accident than as a result of a fall or an assault, with the cause of injury being similar in the vegetative state.[5] Most of the moderate disabilities resulted from a fall.[6,249] Fewer cases of severe disability and vegetative state had a fracture of the skull than the moderate disability cases, in which it was common; a similar association was found with intracranial hematoma. Contusions were most common in the moderate disability cases, being a particular feature of contact after a fall. In contrast, the principal trauma-related pathologies in the vegetative state and severe disability cases were the more severe grades of TAI, a pattern of damage that is well recognized with traffic accidents. It was concluded from these studies that the degree of disability after head injury, as measured by the Glasgow Outcome Scale, reflects both the type and amount of diffuse and focal pathologies sustained as a result of trauma. Quantitative studies are beginning to provide evidence for loss of neurons in different cell populations.[335]

Pathology of Cell Death and Axonal Injury

Progressive cell death after mechanical injury is one of the hallmark features of the pathophysiology of TBI. Both passive and active cell death mechanisms have been documented in the clinical setting and in experimental models of TBI developed to understand the mechanisms of this progressive and diffuse cell loss. Traditionally, treatment strategies for TBI have focused on the prevention of cell death using acute pharmacological therapy, but these strategies remain only partially effective. In addition to the prevention of cell death, a more novel therapeutic approach may be to use transplanted cells to replace lost cells and/or deliver neuroprotective molecules and/or pharmaceuticals.

Necrotic Cell Death after Experimental Traumatic Brain Injury

Degenerating cells exhibiting well-known features of necrosis under light and electron microscopy are observed within the first hour after lateral fluid-percussion (FP) brain injury in rats.[226,227] Morphologically, necrotic cell death associated with TBI can be differentiated from apoptosis and is generally characterized by a loss of membrane integrity, early organelle damage, cellular swelling, mitochondrial swelling, and uncontrolled cell lysis. Necrosis also induces an inflammatory response in brain tissue resulting in secondary damage. This type of necrotic cell death of neurons has been demonstrated in a variety of experimental models of TBI using Nissl,[99,226] acid fuchsin,[99,226] silver staining,[226] TUNEL,[424] and Fluoro-Jade staining[459] after TBI.

Following lateral FP brain injury in rats, Cortez et al.[99] observed necrotic neurons in the injured cortex, CA1, CA2, and CA3 regions of the hippocampus, granule cells in the dentate gyrus (DG) using acid fuchsin staining at acute time points (between 10 minutes and 24 hours), followed by a significant reduction in neurons in the injured pyramidal cell layer of the hippocampus and in the ventral and lateral posterior thalamus in the more chronic postinjury phase (between 1 and 4 weeks).[99,226] Intensely shrunken and acidophilic neurons were observed and reported to be undergoing necrosis. Others have observed dystrophic neurons after CCI injury in the rat localized to the DG, hippocampal CA1 and CA3 regions, amygdala, entorhinal and piriform cortices, and thalamic and hypothalamic regions.[92] Following FP brain injury in rats, neuronal cell body and dendrites are also often stained by silver stains and appear as dark or argyrophilic neurons.[147] Although necrotic neurons detected by silver staining appeared in a similar spatial pattern to the neurons detected by acid fuchsin, silver staining also stained microglia, astrocytes, and cellular debris. The acidic dye Fluoro-Jade, which is thought to stain the same substrates as acid fuchsin, has been used as a marker of degenerating neuronal cell bodies and their processes. Following lateral FP brain injury in rat, the regional distribution of Fluoro-Jade-labeled neurons corresponded to a similar pattern of silver and TUNEL staining.[423b,459] Severely injured neurons appeared in the cortex and hippocampus within 3 hours after injury and were most evident at 24 hours postinjury. In the thalamus, a delayed peak of necrotic neurons was observed at 7 days after injury and remained until 28 days.[554b] At later time points, the neuronal cell bodies and processes of these Fluoro-Jade-positive cells had degraded.

Although necrosis has been reported to be the primary cause of cell death following TBI, recent studies have also implicated programmed cell death, or apoptosis, as one mechanism of progressive cell death following TBI. However, distinguishing between apoptosis and necrosis within a particular group of cells at a particular time point after injury is often difficult, since cells appear to move freely between the two morphologies over the continuum of the death processes and may, in the process, assume biochemical characteristics inconsistent with the morphology they exhibit at a given time point (it is well known that dying cells can exibit DNA laddering patterns suggestive of apoptosis while having ultrastructural features consistent with a necrotic phenotype). It has been suggested that when sufficient sources of cellular energy are available, cell death will occur via a process consistent with the apoptotic morphology, but when energy is lacking, necrotic cell death will occur.[443] Thus, the constant balance between energy supply and consumption during the death continuum is a critical factor in determining whether cell death ultimately becomes an active (apoptotic) or passive (necrotic) process.

Apoptotic Cell Death after Experimental Traumatic Brain Injury

Apoptosis is the morphological manifestation of cells that die by programmed cell death (PCD) during CNS development. The classic pathological hallmarks of apoptosis include condensation and margination of the chromatin, activation of an endonuclease that degrades nuclear DNA, and formation of cellular fragments containing intact organelles. Using combined in situ DNA nick end labeling and DNA gel electrophoresis, numerous studies have detected internucleosomal DNA fragmentation following experimental TBI. Using the lateral FP brain injury model in rats, Rink and colleagues[433] first identified TUNEL-positive cells at acute time points (12–72 hours) and classified both type I (necrotic) and type II (apoptotic) populations of TUNEL(+) cells localized to the subcortical white matter, DG, and hippocampal CA3 region, in addition to the cortical site of injury. Consistent with these results, an apoptotic-like internucleosomal DNA gel electrophoresis fragmentation pattern (185–200 bp) was observed within tissue isolated from the injured cortex and hippocampus, and this degree of fragmentation directly correlated with the severity of the injury.[433] Colicos et al.[92] subsequently observed that at 24 hours following CCI injury in rats, a subpopulation of cells within the DG, CA1, and CA3 subfields exhibited apoptotic-like morphology. Conti et al.[95] also reported a biphasic increase of apoptotic cells in the injured cortex with an initial peak at 24 hours that colabeled with markers for neurons and oligodendrocytes and a secondary peak at 1 week following injury. Increased numbers of apoptotic cells were observed up to 8 weeks postinjury. Within the hippocampus, apoptotic neurons were significantly increased as early as 12 hours, with a peak at 48 hours, returning to control levels by 4 weeks. By 1 week following injury, apoptotic neurons were observed in the thalamus, with a significant peak at 2 weeks postinjury. Additional biochemical evidence exists to support the observation that DNA fragmentation is a result of the activation of endonucleases.

The molecular mechanisms underlying apoptotic cell death are multifactorial and too complex to be reviewed in their entirety in this chapter. One current area of critical investigation surrounds the stress-activated kinases, including the p38 mitogen-activated protein kinase (MAPK) and Jun N-terminal kinase (JNK), which are known to be activated in response to DNA damage.[163] However, the question of whether JNK or p38 plays a role in cell death following TBI remains highly controversial. Following lateral FP injury in rats, immunoreactivity for phospho-JNK, but not phospho-p38, has been observed to increase significantly within intact pyramidal cells of the injured hippocampus as early as 5 minutes and return to baseline expression levels at 1 hour, while phospho extracellular signal-regulated protein kinase (ERK) was also significantly increased in hippocampal regions vulnerable to TBI.[396] Recently, a more prolonged activation (up to 72 hours) of ERK1/2 and JNK has been reported in a similar model (Raghupathi et al., personal communication). In contrast, following CCI injury, phospho-ERK and p-p38, but not p-JNK, were transiently increased within the injured cortex at acute time points, and administration of an ERK kinase inhibitor, but not a p38/JNK kinase inhibitor, resulted in decreased traumatic lesion volume.[425] However, Dash et al.[103] reported a significant enhancement of loss of MAP-2 immunoreactivity within the CA3 subfield of the hippocampus upon administration of an ERK kinase inhibitor.

Axonal Injury after Experimental Traumatic Injury

Traumatic axonal injury is one of the most important types of brain damage that can occur as a result of nonmissile head injury.[254] The biomechanical pathogenesis of axonal injury involves acceleration and deceleration of the brain. This type of injury has been shown to produce coma in the absence of impact to the brain.[255] Initially, it was believed that axons were torn at the moment of injury, but subsequent observations have led to the conclusion that primary axotomy (occurring at the moment of injury) occurs only in the most severe cases and that the majority of axons undergo a secondary, progressive axotomy associated with intra-axonal perturbations, cytoskeletal alterations (e.g., neurofilament compaction and microtubule loss/misalignment), impaired axoplasmic transport, and ultimately axonal disconnection (for review, see Katayama et al.[257]). More recent studies suggest that there may be multiple phenotypes or distinct pathways resulting in traumatic secondary axotomy.[261] Whereas some axons appear to undergo progressive swelling over time, others seem to maintain their caliber despite compaction of the neurofilament cytoskeleton.[261] In the first scenario, mild injury results in subtle alterations in axolemma permeability, not detectable using a tracer such as horseradish peroxidase (HRP), and a submicromolar increase in axonal Ca^{2+} concentration. This is followed by activation of Ca^{2+}-calmodulin targets such as calcineurin, contributing to cytoskeletal misalignment, which in turn causes impaired axonal transport and accumulation of organelles.[263,273,289,291,294] In the second scenario, Povlishock and colleagues[419] hypothesized that moderate or severe injury produces an increase in axolemma permeability (observed by 5 minutes postinjury using the tracers HRP)[419] and allows a massive Ca^{2+} influx, followed by calpain activation, which is shown by the presence of spectrin breakdown products in injured axons by 15 minutes after injury.[298] In these axons, neurofilament compaction occurs by 5–15 minutes postinjury, perhaps due to dephosphorylation or calpain-mediated proteolysis of neurofilament sidearms, because spectrin breakdown products and neurofilament compaction have been shown to colocalize in the same injured axons.[298] Increased axonal Ca^{2+} is also followed by mitochondrial swelling, release of cytochrome c, and activation of caspase-3, which may further contribute to the cytoskeletal derangements observed in experimental models of TAI.[291] The final result in these pathways is axonal disconnection, followed by the downstream degeneration of axonal segments. The finding that the majority of traumatically injured axons appear to undergo a secondary, delayed axotomy means that there may be a therapeutic window for interfering in the progression of damage.

Pathophysiology of Traumatic Brain Injury

Glutamate

The excitatory amino acid (EAA) neurotransmitter glutamate is ubiquitous in the CNS, although only a fraction is present within the extracellular (EC) space or cerebrospinal fluid (CSF; 3–4 μM and 10 μM, respectively).[207] The gradient of glutamate across the plasma membrane is several thousand-fold, with the highest concentrations (100 mM) localized within the synaptic vesicles in nerve terminals.[499] In general, intracellular glutamate concentrations are considered nontoxic, but it is crucial that the EC glutamate concentration is kept low. This is achieved by rapid removal of glutamate by glial and neuronal glutamate transporters (GLT and GLAST), abundantly distributed within the mammalian brain (for review Danbolt[101]). Released glutamate acts on three major classes of glutamate receptors characterized by their genetic profile and classified according to the binding of various pharmacological compounds: *N*-methyl-D-aspartate (NMDA; the subunits NR1, NR2A, NR2B, NR2C, and NR2D), α-amino-3-hydroxy-5-methyl-4-isoxazole propionic acid (AMPA), kainate (GluR5-9, KA1 and KA2), and the metabotropic receptors, which again are subdivided into groups I (mGluR1 and mGluR5), II (mGluR2 and mGluR3), and III (mGluR4, mGluR6, mGluR7, and mGluR8). Regional distribution of both NMDA and AMPA/KA receptors has been directly related to the selective vulnerability of specific brain regions caused by CNS injury (for review see Choi[81]), and functional glutamate receptors and transporters are expressed in both gray and white matter tracts (for recent reviews, see Danbolt[101] and Matute et al.[334]).

After experimental TBI, EC glutamate levels are reversibly increased in the postinjury period, showing a strong dependency on the underlying injury severity and the models employed. Clinical studies have reported that glutamate concentrations are significantly elevated in the CSF of brain-injured patients for several days or perhaps weeks,[23,398] and the microdialysis technique has revealed significant and persisting increases in extracellular glutamate lasting for up to 9 days following the injury.[64,318,542] The pathological release of glutamate and subsequent activation of the glutamate receptors observed in TBI[101] results in a massive influx of Na^+ and efflux of K^+, allowing a large Ca^{2+} influx into the cell. This ionic influx can cause swelling, damage, or destruction of the cells (excitotoxicity) through direct or indirect pathways.[389] Mitochondrial depolarization, increased production of oxygen free radicals, and apoptotic and necrotic cell death have all been reported to result from excitotoxic stimuli and are factors known to occur in TBI.[80,139,303,321,436,520] Cortical injection of NMDA or AMPA produced remarkably similar histological lesions (cavitation and glial fibrillary acidic protein [GFAP] immunoreactions), as seen after CCI,[400] and cortical administration of glutamate through a microdialysis probe exacerbates lateral FP–induced histological damage,[114] support the notion that this increase in glutamate contributes to the pathology observed in TBI. Finally, the cognitive deficits observed following TBI have been linked to a high density of glutamate receptors and to the three- to fourfold elevation of EC glutamate levels seen in the hippocampus following CCI in the rat.

Reactive Oxygen and Nitrogen Species

An excess of tissue oxygen may be toxic to cells, mainly due to the formation of oxygen radicals (reactive oxygen species, ROS).[161] The definition of a radical is any atom or group of atoms that has an unpaired electron in the outer orbital, making the radical highly reactive. Upon subsequent addition of electrons to oxygen, the superoxide anion ($O_2^{\bullet-}$) hydroperoxyl radical ($HO_2^{\bullet-}$), hydrogen peroxide (H_2O_2), and the hydroxyl radical ($OH^\bullet$) are formed (Fig. 4.1). With normal cell metabolism, superoxide anion radicals are generated during mitochondrial electron transport reactions, reaching 1% to 2% of the total oxygen consumption,[52] and the superoxide radical may also be produced by the metabolism of arachidonic acid and activation of xanthine oxidase.[71,409] Superoxide does not react significantly with DNA, proteins, or phospholipids but rapidly reacts with nitric oxide (NO) to cause the formation of peroxynitrite ($ONOO^-$). Peroxynitrite, an increasingly recognized mediator of TBI-induced pathology, may damage and kill cells by inducing lipid peroxidation and protein tyrosine nitration.[33,198,202]

Hydrogen peroxide easily penetrates lipid bilayers but may not be cytotoxic in vivo except in

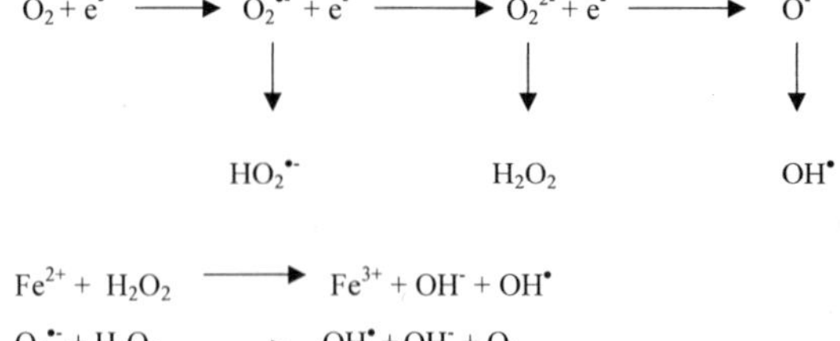

Figure 4.1. Production of reactice oxygen species. This reaction is extremely slow unless catalyzed by a transitional metal such as Fe^{2+} or copper (Cu^{2+}) ions (Fenton reaction). (Modified from Gamaley IA, Klyubin IV: Roles of reactive oxygen species: signaling and regulation of cellular functions. Int Rev Cytol. 188:203–255, 1999)

high and unphysiological concentrations.[109,554] Its probable role in the pathophysiology of TBI may be as a precursor of hydroxyl radicals (vide infra). Hydroxyl radicals ($OH^\bullet$) are extremely reactive, can react with practically any molecule present in cells, and may cause most of the TBI-induced pathology induced by ROS.[302] $OH^\bullet$ are formed when superoxide anion and hydroperoxide react according to the Haber-Weiss reaction,[199] catalyzed by a transitional metal such as iron (Fe^{2+}) or copper (Cu^{2+}) ions (Fenton reaction).

Oxidative damage in the CNS commonly manifests as lipid peroxidation, as the brain has a high content of peroxidable fatty acids and possesses a relatively poor antioxidant defense system,[473] as well as regions with high levels of iron and copper.[242] Brain tissue is highly vulnerable to oxidative damage because of its high rate of oxidative metabolic activity, intense production of reactive oxygen metabolites, relatively low antioxidant activity, low repair mechanism activity, and the high membrane surface to cytoplasm ratio (reviewed by Shohami et al.[473]).

The pathophysiology of ROS formation following TBI is complex, although there are several potential sites for ROS production that include mitochondrial leakage, increased free iron resulting from breakdown of extravasated hemoglobin, oxidation of catecholamines, breakdown of membrane phospholipids, and infiltrating neutrophils.[206,324,331] In addition, intracellular influx of calcium with resulting mitochondrial damage and phospholipase activation may cause ROS formation. Importantly, posttraumatic mitochondrial dysfunction may be caused by ROS overproduction,[229] implying that the mitochondria may be both an important source of ROS and a target for ROS-mediated damage.[139] Finally, increases in glutamate following TBI may generate ROS[464] and ROS may, in turn, further increase the release of glutamate and adversely affect glutamate uptake.[406,494] Detection of ROS formation following TBI is difficult due to their high reactivity and short half-life, but using various methods of radical trapping or indirect markers of oxidative damage, increased generation of ROS in TBI has commonly been observed.[201,321,421,473,534] Using microdialysis and the 4-hydroxybenzoic acid technique, maximally increased ROS formation was observed in the immediate postinjury phase following weight-drop injury in rats,[325] although isoprostanes, markers for lipid peroxidation, were sustained for longer periods postinjury.[421]

Nitric oxide, often referred to as a reactive nitrogen species (RNS), has important physiological functions in the brain, including maintenance of the BBB and regulation of resting cerebral blood flow (CBF).[420,513] Nitric oxide is synthesized from L-arginine by at least three isoforms of nitric oxide synthases (NOS); neuronal NOS (nNOS; type I), inducible NOS (iNOS; type II), and endothelial NOS (eNOS; type III). Evidence suggests that eNOS activity is neuroprotective after acute brain injury, whereas iNOS and nNOS activity may be detrimental.[241] The expression of the isoforms of NOS is markedly altered after TBI, where the most marked changes occur in the expression of iNOS in inflammatory cells invading brain tissue in both human and rat TBI.[145,146] Nitric oxide produced by eNOS has also been suggested to preserve rCBF following CCI in mice.[231]

Potassium

Widespread depolarization of neurons immediately after TBI is believed to result in a massive efflux of potassium. Such an acute, marked release of potassium could then trigger electrophysiological alterations, stimulate neurotransmitter release through disturbances in neuronal membrane and synaptic function, disrupt energy homeostasis, induce cerebral vasoconstriction, and alter cerebral glycolysis. In clinical studies, decreased plasma [K^+] has been reported in severely head-injured adults[415] and may be a predictor of injury severity.[32] However, in children with mild TBI, transient decreases in serum [K^+] were not correlated with Glasgow Coma Scale scores.[295] A number of clinical studies using cerebral microdialysis have shown that [K^+]e is increased for several hours after trauma in a subset of severely injured adults, and these increases correlate with increased extracellular glutamate levels and decreased regional CBF.[125,170,429] Furthermore, increased [K^+]e is associated with increased intracranial pressure and a poor outcome, and patients with a contusion have higher [K^+]e than those without contusions.[125,429]

Experimental models of TBI have confirmed these clinical findings. Following contusion brain injury in rats, [K^+]e increases rapidly but transiently,[257,379] with increases related to injury severity.[512] Total tissue levels of potassium decrease after either weight drop or lateral FP brain injury in rats[197,492] and may be attenuated by administration of NMDA receptor antagonists.[197,311] In hippocampal slices taken from rats subjected to lateral FP brain injury, electrophysiological recordings demonstrated reductions in K^+ currents and an accumulation of extracellular K^+ at 2 days following trauma in the CA3 region, a region selectively vulnerable to traumatic injury.[100]

Magnesium

In the CNS, magnesium is involved in a number of critical cellular processes, including glycolysis, oxidative phosphorylation, cellular respiration, and synthesis of DNA, RNA, and protein. Magnesium is mandatory for all enzyme reactions involving adenosine triphosphate (ATP) and is essential for mitochondrial and plasma membrane integrity.[12] In addition, magnesium is involved in the maintenance of normal cellular sodium and potassium gradients, the function of the NMDA subtype glutamate receptor, and cerebrovascular contractibility. Dysregulation of magnesium, therefore, may have multiple effects in the context of TBI. Phosphorus magnetic resonance spectroscopy has revealed significant increases in intracellular [Mg^{2+}] in head-injured patients,[149] although microdialysis techniques failed to detect a change in magnesium levels.[170] Early decreases in either serum or plasma [Mg^{2+}] have been described in patients admitted with mild to severe head injury.[18,72,253,354,415] Levels of serum [Mg^{2+}], but not total serum [Mg], have been shown to correlate with injury severity in humans.[354]

In rat models of both diffuse and focal brain injury, ionized magnesium levels in the blood significantly decrease in the acute posttraumatic period; injury-induced decreases persist for 1 to 4 days after trauma and correlate with the severity of motor dysfunction.[25,216] Early work by Vink and colleagues[545] established that lateral FP brain injury in the rat resulted in a profound, acute decrease in both total tissue magnesium and [Mg^{2+}] in the brain. Subsequent work has demonstrated similar declines in brain [Mg^{2+}] after focal brain injury in the rat[511] and after diffuse brain injury in the rat[217] and pig.[483] Decreases in brain [Mg^{2+}] may persist for 4 to 5 days after focal or diffuse TBI in rodents[217,544] and correlates with the magnitude of motor deficits.[217] Brain tissue total magnesium levels have also been shown to decrease after focal TBI and to be partially restored by posttraumatic administration of NMDA receptor antagonists.[311,467]

Calcium

Alterations in calcium homeostasis have been hypothesized to play a major role in neurodegeneration after traumatic CNS injury,[478,533] influencing necrosis, apoptosis, and axonal injury.[346,576] While some clinical studies have reported reductions in serum ionized calcium after acute head injury,[18] others suggest that plasma calcium levels are not significantly altered in patients with severe head injury.[415] However, using animal models of TBI, in which brain levels of calcium can be more readily measured, numerous investigators have documented significant acute, and sometimes persistent, disruption of calcium homeostasis. Total tissue calcium increased within 1 to 2 days following closed head trauma in rats,[311,467] while cortical extracellular [Ca^{2+}] levels decreased after cortical contusion in the rat, with more persistent decreases corresponding to regions of neuronal injury.[379] These findings are consistent with studies using $^{45}Ca^{2+}$ autoradiography that demonstrate acute increases in calcium flux following weight drop or FP brain injury in rats.[137,371] Interestingly, in regions of delayed cell damage such as the thalamus, calcium accumulation was delayed for several days following trauma. Furthermore, both cortical and thalamic regions that exhibited morphological damage showed persistent calcium accumulation, suggesting a link between continued calcium dysregulation and delayed cell death.[137,371,395]

Increases in total tissue calcium and calcium flux could be attenuated by treatment with NMDA receptor antagonists.[311,371,467] In vitro models of neuronal and axonal traumatic injury have confirmed that rapid deformation leads to increased intracellular [Ca^{2+}], which may be dependent on an influx of extracellular calcium and related to glutamate-mediated signaling.[290,306,556] Ultrastructural studies have revealed evidence of decreased Ca^{2+}-ATPase activity in injured axons and mitochondrial calcium accumulation after trauma.[338,557]

Calpains

Calpains are calcium-activated neutral cysteine proteases that are found in all cells of the CNS. The two major isoforms of calpains, calpain I (or μ-calpain) and calpain II (or m-calpain), require different calcium concentrations for activation.[168] Activation of calpain I may occur at free calcium levels on the order of 1 μM, while calpain II may require closer to 1 mM [Ca^{2+}]. Calpains have been shown to cleave numerous types of intracellular proteins, including cytoskeletal proteins, membrane-associated proteins (channels and receptors), enzymes (phosphatases, kinases), cell death–associated proteins, transcription factors, and more. Therefore, sustained calpain activation may initiate degradation of critical cell signaling molecules and compromise cell structure and membrane integrity, leading to cell death or dysfunction.[236,539] Postmortem examination of brain tissue from patients who died after blunt head injury has revealed evidence of calpain activation in the corpus callosum, a white matter region in which axonal injury is typically found in cases of diffuse head injury.[342] Degradation of neurofilament proteins was also found in these patients, suggesting that calpain activation may be involved in axonal cytoskeletal damage after trauma.

Activation of calpain and subsequent degradation of the cytoskeletal protein spectrin by calpains have been shown to occur within minutes after TBI in rats.[254,449] Activation of calpain I peaked at 6 hours after CCI brain injury in rats,[254] but accumulation of calpain-mediated spectrin breakdown products (BDPs) in neurons continued for up to 1 day.[254,417,449] Regions exhibiting extensive calpain-mediated proteolysis later showed widespread cell death, suggestive of a causative role for calpains in posttraumatic neuronal death. Nonetheless, under certain conditions, calpain activation has also been observed with sublethal tissue damage.[376] Interestingly, calpain activation appears to be an acute event in TAI, initiated within minutes after trauma.[61,447,449] In models of focal TBI, axonal calpain activation has been reported to be delayed.[376] Axonal degeneration following secondary axotomy may be associated with a delayed wave of calpain-mediated proteolysis.[447] A recent study by Kupina and colleagues[283] showed that calpain activation is substantially delayed in female compared to male mice after diffuse weight drop injury. The presence of calpain-mediated spectrin BDPs in the CSF has been demonstrated after experimental focal TBI, and has been proposed as a potential marker of TBI with clinical utility for diagnosis or evaluation of treatment efficacy.[413]

Caspases

The caspase family of proteins are interleukin-1β-converting enzyme (ICE)-like, aspartate-specific proteases, synthesized as procaspsases that are cleaved at active Asp-X sites, generating a large and a small subunit which together constitute the active protease. Caspases are known to be associated primarily with apoptotic cell death and can be categorized broadly into two groups: initiator caspases, which generally contain large prodomains, autoactivate, and are thought to be involved in the initiation of the apoptotic response, and executioner caspases, which generally contain short prodomains and are activated by initiator caspases. The activation of effector caspases, including caspase-3, appears to represent the cell's commitment to die and the convergence of numerous signaling pathways. Activation of caspase-3 has been observed after TBI, and central administration of the caspase-3 inhibitor z-DEVD-fmk was shown to reduce DNA cleavage and TUNEL staining and to improve the neurological outcome after FP injury.[103] Cytochrome c–mediated pathways as cytochrome c and activated caspase-3 are readily detected in damaged axons following the impact acceleration model of TBI in rats.[560] Following experimental TBI, caspase-8 mRNA and protein rapidly increase within neurons, astrocytes, and oligodendrocytes in the cortex and hippocampus.[34]

It is now clear that the homeostatic mechanisms involved in the activation of caspases are far more complex that the simple regulation of their cleavage. The Bcl-2 family of proteins plays a critical role in the intracellular apoptotic signaling transduction cascade. Following CCI injury with induced hypoxia in rats, bcl-2 expression has been shown to increase within primarily TUNEL(-) neurons, and to a lesser extend in the glia, the ipsilateral cortex, DG, and the CA3 region, beginning at 8 hours and continuing for 7 days.[60] Increased expression of Bcl-2 protein, but not Bcl-X_L or Bax, within neurons was also observed in the cortical regions of excised tissue from patients sustaining severe TBI.[85] Recent evidence has suggested the existence of a caspase-independent pathway of apoptosis involving the release of apoptosis-inducing factor (AIF) from the mitochondria. In dying cells, AIF relocates from the mitochondria to the nucleus, where its DNA binding activity is thought to mediate chromatin condensation and large-scale DNA fragmentation.[84]

Inflammation and Cytokines

The secondary injury factors believed to exacerbate the injury following TBI include an acute inflammatory response with breakdown of the BBB, edema formation, infiltration of peripheral blood cells, activation of resident immunocompetent cells, and intrathecal release of immune mediators such as cytokines.[232,297,361,475,489,497,553] Central nervous system inflammation has long been believed to be detrimental, causing sustained functional impairment and cell death, although there is increasing evidence that the activation of more chronic inflammatory pathways may be important for regenerative responses, while early inflammation is believed to be detrimental but may contribute to restoration and repair in the later postinjury phase.[297,361,461]

Infiltration and accumulation of polymorphonuclear leukocytes (PMNs) in brain parenchyma have been documented to occur in the acute posttraumatic period, reaching a peak by 24 hours postinjury,[489] and a relationship between cortical PMN accumulation and secondary brain injury, including lowered CBF, increased edema, and elevated intracranial pressure has been suggested.[574] The migration of PMNs requires adhesion to the cerebrovascular endothelium by expression of intercellular adhesion molecule (ICAM) –1, which is up-regulated in several models of experimental TBI.[69,248,426,471] Macrophages, natural killer (NK) cells, helper T cells, and T-cytotoxic suppressor cells are observed filling the cortical lesion and surrounding the hippocampal CA3 region as early as 2 days following weight drop, CCI, and lateral FP brain injury,[86,233,262,361,489,497] findings confirmed in human contusions.[232] The cellular inflammatory response also includes activation of astrocytes[228] and microglia postinjury.[313] In particular, microglia have been reported to up-regulate surface antigens involved in the inflammatory response, including the major histocompatibility complex (MHC) class II antigens.[313]

In addition, the cyclooxygenase enzyme may contribute to the pathophysiology of TBI,[282] and a number of studies have reported elevated COX-2 levels in injured cortex and in the ipsilateral hippocampus following experimental TBI in rats,[102] with increased synthesis of reactive prostaglandins.[282] While COX-2 induction following TBI may be beneficial, chronic COX-2 production may potentiate free radical–mediated cellular damage, vascular dysfunction, and alterations in cellular metabolism.[503]

Cytokines are polypeptides mediating inflammation and regulation of cell growth and differentiation, and include tumor necrosis factor (TNF), interleukins (IL), interferons, and growth factors including nerve growth factor (NGF) and transforming growth factor-β (TGF-β).[211,360,397,439] Tumor necrosis factor-α, IL-6, IL-1, and IL-18 are important mediators of neuroinflammation and are produced in response to acute brain injury by astrocytes, macrophage/microglial cells, neurons, and endothelial cells in the CNS.[133,134,171,267,423,457,475,514,566] Interleukin-10 is an anti-inflammatory cytokine that inhibits a variety of macrophage responses and is also a potent suppressor of T-cell proliferation and cytokine response by blocking expression of TNF and IL-1.[41,74]

Maximal increase of IL-6 mRNA and protein has been demonstrated at 6–8 hours following closed head injury,[212,432,475] and clinical studies have documented elevated levels of IL-6, soluble IL-6 receptor, and TNF- α in the CSF, plasma, or parenchyma of TBI patients up to several weeks following injury.[39,211,276,357,360,555] Following experimental TBI, increased levels of TNF-α protein and mRNA are also found in injured brain parenchyma within the first hours[134,267,475,514] that appear to remain elevated up to 3–6 days postinjury.[234,578] Tumor necrosis factor-α been reported to be increased in the CSF up to 48 hours postinjury following CCI in rats,[502] and increased hippocampal uptake of TNF-α from the bloodstream following weight drop injury in the mouse have been demonstrated.[401]

Chronic overexpression of either TNF-α or IL-6 has been shown to induce a neurodegenerative inflammatory encephalopathy, and IL-6 alone may promote demyelination, thrombosis, leukocyte infiltration, and BBB disruption and interfere with adult neurogenesis.[66,67,538] However, IL-6 has often been regarded as neuroprotective, as it has been suggested to promote survival, differentiation, and growth of neurons and to induce neurotrophin expression in response to CNS injury.[126,275,368] In vivo studies have suggested detrimental effects of TNF-α, demonstrating neuronal, endothelial, and glial cell damage and induction of apoptosis following exposure to TNF-α.[230,423,521,552] In vivo, intracerebroventricular (i.c.v) or intracisternal infusion of TNF-α induces apoptosis, intracranial inflammation, and BBB breakdown.[45,352,437] However, an anti-inflammatory and a neuroprotective role for TNF-α has also been demonstrated, showing prevention of excitotoxic and ischemic cell death,[28,56,307,374,422] and TNF-α may modulate tissue remodeling, gliosis, and scar formation.[76,286] Also, mice deficient in TNF receptors subjected to CCI brain injury developed larger lesions and more extensive BBB breakdown at 7 days postinjury, suggesting a neuroprotective effect of endogenous TNF-α.[508] Finally, in a study of TNF-α-deficient (TNF -/-) mice, attenuation of cognitive and neurological motor deficits was observed during the first week following TBI. However, up to 4 weeks postinjury, TNF -/- mice were significantly worse in cognitive and neurological motor function compared to wild-type controls, suggesting that early, but not late, inhibition of TNF-α may positively influence the outcome following TBI[461] and that TNF-α may be involved in recovery postinjury. Finally, using TNF/lymphotoxin-α-/- and IL-6 -/- mice,[496] increased mortality was observed following CCI, but the overall pathophysiological sequelae such as neurological motor performance, cell death, and polymorphonuclear cell infiltration were unaltered compared to those of their wild-type littermates,[496] suggesting that TNF and IL-6 do not influence the infiltration of neutrophils that may release ROS and hydrolytic enzymes, and are associated with increased secondary brain damage and a poor neurological outcome in experimental models of TBI.[69,86,331,495] The role of IL-6 and TNF-α up-regulation in the acute brain pathology following TBI remains elusive, as these cytokines may have both neuroprotective and neurotoxic properties.

Interleukin-1 includes three molecules (IL-1 α, IL-1β, and IL-1 receptor antagonist [IL-1ra]).[442]

Endogenous IL-1 has been associated with cognitive deficits and may mediate neurodegeneration in TBI.[441] Interleukin-1 up-regulates β-APP expression in vitro and in vivo (in nonneuronal cells), implicating IL-1 in the pathogenesis of Alzheimer's disease.[182,191] Interleukin-1 may also stimulate other inflammatory mediators, such as phospholipase A2, COX-2, prostaglandins, NO, and matrix metalloproteinases.[31,440] Interleukin-1 β mRNAs are elevated for up to 48 hours following injury by transient focal ischemia[558] and up to 24 hours following lateral FP brain injury in the rat.[133] Since IL-1 is also known to play a role in the induction of various types of apoptosis,[141] antagonism of IL-1 with the Il-1 receptor antagonists (IL-1ra) may exert an antiapoptotic neuroprotective effect in the injured brain.

Novel Therapeutic Strategies for Brain Injury

Excitatory Amino Acid Antagonists

Examples of NMDA channel blockers evaluated in experimental TBI include dextromethorphan and dextrorphan, ketamine, MK-801, magnesium, HU-211, and remacemide hydrochloride, all of which have been shown to decrease neuronal death, edema, and/or neurological dysfunction following experimental TBI and acute subdural hematoma.[326,535] However, compounds such as MK-801, phencyclidine (PCP), and ketamine have strong psychomimetic effects and cause vacuolization in neurons,[390,468] thus preventing their introduction into clinical practice. Newer noncompetitive NMDA receptor antagonists designed to have low toxicity but maintained efficacy include NPS 1506 and its analog NPS 846, and have been shown to improve neurological and cognitive deficits and delay edema following experimental TBI.[197,299] Of particular interest is the novel nonpsychotropic cannabinoid HU-211 (Dexanabinol), which was found to improve neuromotor and cognitive outcomes following brain trauma with a therapeutic window of 2–3 hours postinjury.[474,476] HU-211, a weak NMDA receptor antagonist with multiple mechanisms of action, including TNF-α inhibition, is currently being investigated in a Phase III clinical trial. In addition, the open-channel, noncompetitive NMDA blocker memantine can easily cross the BBB and shows minimal adverse effects on neuronal ultrastructure, learning, long-term potentiation (LTP), and synaptic transmission.[403] Following CCI in the rat, postinjury treatment with memantine decreased CA2 and CA3 cell death at 7 days postinjury.[427] NMDA-mediated receptor activation has a slow onset and a long decay phase relative to AMPA/ KA receptors, which is thought to result from the voltage-sensitive block within the NMDA receptor by Mg^{2+}.[341,381] Additionally, endogenous amines, including spermidine and spermine, enhance NMDA receptor activation, while the synthetic competitive antagonists of the polyamine site (eliprodil and ifenprodil) reduce NMDA receptor activation, and may have potential advantages over other noncompetitive antagonists due to less potential psychomimetic and neurotoxic side effects.[107] When administered immediately following CCI in the rat, ifenprodil attenuated brain edema, decreased BBB breakdown, and reduced cortical injury volume.[107] Eliprodil attenuated cortical tissue loss when delivered up to 18 hours after lateral FP injury, making this compound clinically interesting.[528]

Activation of the glycine site potentiates NMDA receptor binding, and inhibition of the glycine site has been shown to block the current evoked by NMDA.[237] When administered 15 minutes after injury, the glycine site antagonists kynurenate and I2CA both reduced cognitive and neurological motor deficits and reduced CA3 cell death at 2 weeks postinjury following lateral FP in the rat[224,487] and kynurenate reduced free fatty acid and diacylglycerol accumulation after lateral FP.[113] In addition, the compound ACEA1021 reduced ischemic damage in a model of acute subdural hematoma in the rat.[530]

Zn^{2+} is present at high concentrations in mammalian brain and is released in chelatable form after excitation of certain glutamatergic neurons. Zinc deficiency was associated with increased cell death following a cortical stab wound in the rat.[567] Recently, the zinc chelator calcium EDTA, administered i.c.v. prior to FP brain injury in rats, was shown to increase the expression of several neuroprotective genes, including heat shock proteins, and reduce the number of TUNEL-positive neurons.[222] To date, however, the role and importance of Zn^{2+} in the functional and behavioral deficits in TBI has yet to be investigated.

While NMDA receptors have a high affinity to glutamate and slowly inactivate, the low-affinity

AMPA/ KA receptors desensitize rather quickly. AMPA is thought to mediate the fast component, while NDMA receptors mediate the slow component of fast excitatory neurotransmission.[119] To date, only a few studies employing AMPA/ KA receptor antagonists in TBI have been published. However, postinjury treatment with the AMPA antagonist RPR117824 was recently shown to attenuate cortical lesion volume following lateral FP in the rat.[356] In addition, the AMPA antagonist Talampanel reduced CA1 damage and cortical lesion volume when administered 30 minutes after lateral FP.[37] Interestingly, the AMPA antagonist NBQX attenuated hippocampal damage when administered up to 7 hours following a weight drop injury in the rat.[43] Finally, YM872 was found to attenuate cerebral edema and lesion volume and improve neurological motor function following lateral FP brain injury in rats.

Abundant pre- and postsynaptically located metabotropic glutamate receptors (mGluRs) are thought to be important in modulating neurotransmission. Activation of group I receptors potentiates neuronal excitation and exacerbates excitotoxic cell death in vitro.[367] In contrast, group II and III agonists reduce excitation, perhaps through presynaptic inhibition of glutamate release[132,372] or modulation of adenylate cyclase activity.[57] Thus, mGluR activation may contribute to both neurotoxic and neuroprotective processes, depending on the activated receptor. In vivo, intracerebral or intraventricular administration of the group 1 inhibitors MCPG, AIDA, or MPEP has been used, starting pre-injury or up to 15 minutes following lateral FP, and consistent finding are improvements in neurological motor deficits, cortical lesion volume, and cognitive outcome.[132,169,316,364,367] In addition, i.v. administration of the $mGluR_1$ antagonist BAY 36-7620 attenuated ischemic damage in a model of acute subdural hematoma in the rat.[106]

The activation of group II and III mGlu receptors is expected to attenuate neuronal degeneration without hampering the efficiency of fast excitatory synaptic transmission. In vivo studies examining the role of groups II and III mGluR in brain injury are rare, but administration of the group II mGluR agonist LY 354740 after lateral FP injury in rats significantly improved neurological motor recovery.[16] When the compounds DCG-IV (group II) or (R,S)-4-phosphonophenylglycine (group III agonist) were injected into the CA2 and CA3 areas of the hippocampus immediately following lateral FP in the rat, only DCG-IV injections reduced the number of degenerating neurons in these regions.[579] Finally, the specific group II mGluR agonist LY379268 decreased cortical contusion volume at 7 days following CCI but did not attenuate edema at 24 hours.[501] Finally, animals injected i.c.v. with the specific mGluR4 agonist L-2-amino-4-phosphonobutyric acid (L-AP4) at 1 and 12 hours postinjury showed decreased neuronal loss and attenuated motor and cognitive deficits following diffuse head injury in rats.[573]

Modulation of EAA receptor activity may also be accomplished by inhibition of EAA release. BW1003C87 blocked glutamate release induced by the sodium channel agonist veratrine without blocking potassium-induced glutamate release and, when administered at 15 minutes after lateral FP in the rat, reduced edema in the ipsilateral cortex and hippocampus was found at 48 hours postinjury.[384] In addition, postinjury treatment with the sodium channel blocker and glutamate release inhibitor riluzole was found to attenuate neurological motor deficits, cognitive deficits, and cortical lesion volume after FP injury in the rat[24,27,550] and to reduce edema after CCI.[500] Finally, pretreatment with 619C89 attenuated neurological deficits and reduced CA1 and CA3 cell loss following FP injury.[509] It should be noted that these compounds may all have other mechanisms of action besides inhibiting glutamate release contributing to their neuroprotective properties, including a primary effect on inactive sodium channels (riluzole and 619C89).

The impressive reductions in functional and structural impairment following experimental TBI upon attenuating glutamate excitotoxicity have raised high expectations for neurological improvement following clinical TBI. Unfortunately, all clinical trials completed to date have failed to show any significant improvements in outcome.[373,516] Several new compounds with interesting profiles are currently being evaluated in various models of acute or chronic brain injuries in humans; these include memantine, HU-211 (Dexanabinol), currently in a Phase III trial for TBI, and [1-(2-thienyl) cyclohexyl]piperidine (TCP) and its derivative gacyclidine, a potent noncompetitive NMDA receptor antagonist that has been suggested to be devoid of adverse side effects.[358]

However, several reports have addressed the potentially beneficial actions of glutamate and glutamate receptor activation, findings that may explain part of the lack of clinical efficacy. NMDA antagonists such as MK-801 and PCP may inhibit LTP and cognitive processes,[105] and MK-801 produced a profound amnesia in a passive avoidance task following lateral FP.[209] Also, the NMDA agonist D-cycloserine improved cognitive outcome when administered 24 hours following lateral FP.[44,519] In addition, pretreatment with the NMDA receptor antagonist 4-(3-phospitonoproyl) piperazine-2-carboxylic acid (CPP) reduced but posttreatment *increased* apoptosis in the hippocampus following weight drop injury.[243] Administration of NMDA at 24 hours following a closed head injury in mice improved cognitive performance, blocked by coadministration with MK-801.[44] Although attenuation of excitotoxicity continues to be a potentially promising treatment strategy, these beneficial functions of glutamate receptor activation must be carefully considered.

Reactive Oxygen Species Scavengers

Increased ROS formation postinjury is believed to be detrimental, and inhibition of ROS with attenuation of ROS-mediated damage has been the topic of many studies (see below). The nonglucocorticoid 21-aminosteroid U74006F (tirilazad mesylate, TM) has no glucocorticoid activities, was found to attenuate ROS formation in concussive head injury in mice,[17] and was evaluated in a subsequent series of TBI studies. Tirilazad mesylate was found to improve grip strength and 1-week survival in mice with closed head injury,[205] attenuate posttraumatic cerebral edema in rats following lateral FP brain injury,[344,348,456] weight drop injury in rats[270] and closed head injury in cats,[118] and improve neurological motor function following lateral FP brain injury in rats.[456] In addition, the tirilazad-like 21-aminosteriod U74389G, was shown to reduce the extent of axonal injury following CCI in rats.[319] Tiriliazad has a very limited penetration into brain parenchyma of the BBB, and its action appears to be related to its ability to protect the microvascular endothelium and maintain normal BBB permeability. Unfortunately, Phase III clinical trials for ischemia, spinal cord injury, TBI[328] (1120 patients were enrolled), and subarachnoid hemorrhage all failed to show a positive outcome (see Hukkelhoven et al.[239]and Kavanagh and Kam[258]).

Vitamin E (α-tocopherol) is a naturally occurring antioxidant primarily acting as an inhibitor of lipid peroxidation. Administration of vitamin E prior to a weight drop injury in guinea pigs attenuated posttraumatic lipid peroxidation,[245] and postinjury treatment following central FP brain injury improved beam walk and reduced mortality in rats.[90] In addition, intracerebral infusion of D-α-tocopherol-enriched liposomes, delivered continuously for 7 days to the damaged cortex following bilateral lesioning of the frontal cortex, attenuated posttraumatic cognitive deficits.[498] In other reports, α-tocopherol analogues related to Trolox® were evaluated and showed reduction of paraplegia following concussive head injury in the mouse,[193] and MDL 74,180 attenuated cerebral edema following lateral FP.[408] More recently, in a study of TBI in Tg2576 mice, a mouse strain used in experimental models of Alzheimer's disease, vitamin E pretreatment attenuated lipid peroxidation and reduced cognitive deficits following TBI.[94]

The metal chelator deferoxamine may attenuate production of the hydroxyl radicals. Administration of dextran-deferoxamine reduced intracellular superoxide levels and attenuated the neurological impairment following closed head injury in mice,[402] and attenuated neurological motor deficits following a weight drop injury in rats.[572] Also, pretreatment with deferoxamine improved Morris water maze (MWM) performance following CCI in rats without reducing cortical lesion volume,[309] and a potent antioxidant and inhibitor of lipid peroxidation, LY341122, significantly reduced lesion volume and the number of necrotic neurons when administered both pre- and postinjury following lateral FP in the rat.[548]

Cytidine 5'-diphosphocholine (CDPC), or citicoline, is a naturally occurring endogenous compound that may attenuate the activation of phospholipase A_2 (PLA_2), and has been reported to provide neuroprotective effects after experimental cerebral ischemia[10] and in various neurological disorders associated with memory deficits (see Adibhatla et al.[11]). Citicoline was reported to attenuate BBB disturbance and reduce brain edema following CCI in rats,[30] improve MWM performance, and increase acetylcholine levels in the cortex and hippocampus following CCI.[124] It prevented hippocampal neuronal loss, decreased cortical contusion volume, and improved neurological recovery when given immediately following CCI in the rat.[108] Citicoline improved the outcome in a Phase III clinical trial of stroke[104] but provided inconclusive results in recent clinical trials of stroke and vascular dementia.[87,91] Its use in clinical TBI has yet to be investigated.

The spin-trapping agent α-phenyl-*tert*-*N*-butyl nitrone (PBN) was suggested to be neuroprotective due to its ability to form stable adducts with ROS.[388] The sulfonated derivatives of PBN, sodium 2-sulfophenyl-*N*-*tert*-butyl nitrone (S-PBN), were found to have similar or even superior neuroprotective properties in ischemia,[565] despite very poor penetration through the BBB. In a series of experiments, the effects of PBN and S-PBN were evaluated in TBI, and pretreatment with PBN was shown to improved MWM performance and reduce cortical lesion volume following weight drop injury in rats.[320] Furthermore, i.v. administration of PBN and S-PBN 30 minutes following lateral FP in rats was reported to improve cognitive and neurological motor outcomes and reduce lesion volume.[321] Both PBN and S-PBN also improved posttraumatic regional CBF (rCBF) attenuated the posttraumatic increase in glucose metabolism, and reduced ROS formation.[323,325] Currently, the related compound NXY-059 is in Phase III clinical trial for stroke.[190]

Nitroxides are stable free radicals that may serve as cell-permeable antioxidants. The neuroprotective properties of three nitroxides (2,2,6,6-tetramethylpiperidine-1-*N*-oxyl [TPO], the hydrophilic analog TPL, and its reduced form TPH) were evaluated in a model of closed head injury in the rat, and they all improved neurological recovery. Additionally, TPL was found to significantly reduce edema formation and to ameliorate BBB disruption with a therapeutic window of 4 hours after closed head injury.[36] The nitroxide 4-hydroxide-2,2,6,6-tetramethylpiperidine-1-oxyl (Tempol) attenuated ROS production and ischemic lesions after subdural hematoma formation in the rat when administered 10 minutes later i.v.[285] Finally, the highly lipophilic stilbazulenyl nitrone (STAZN), a novel second-generation azulenyl nitrone, has an antioxidant profile superior to that of PBN, and improved neurological motor function and reduced lesion volume up to 7 days following lateral FP brain injury in rats.[38]

Administration of the antioxidant enzyme superoxide dismutase (SOD) was reported to have beneficial effects on survival and neurological recovery.[473] The conjugation of polyethylene glycol to SOD (PEG-SOD, Dismutec), thereby improving BBB penetration and increasing its plasma half-life, has been shown to reduce motor deficits and reverse cerebral hypoperfusion after TBI in rats,[112,210] while administration of lecithinized SOD (PC-SOD) reduced brain edema following weight drop brain injury in rats.[569] In addition, SOD improved neurological recovery following CHI in the rat but did not affect brain edema.[569] Despite promising preclinical documentation,[366] PEG-SOD failed in the randomized Phase III multicenter trial including 463 patients. However, more PEG-SOD-treated patients had a favorable outcome and less disability 3 months postinjury compared to vehicle-treated controls, but this difference did not reach statistical significance.[568]

The antioxidant and the superoxide radical scavenger OPC-14117 were shown to reduce the contusion necrosis volume, attenuate neuronal cell death in the CA3 region of the hippocampus, and improve the Morris water maze performance following CCI in the rat.[21,259,362] Additionally, melatonin, the pineal hormone, may also have antioxidant properties following TBI.[82] When administered following CCI, a significantly reduced contusion volume was observed, but there was no effect on cerebral edema.[458]

Treatment with the selective inhibitors of neuronal NOS showed an improved neurological outcome in mice subjected to a weight drop injury (BN 80933)[73] and significantly decreased the contusion volume when given prior to lateral FP brain injury in the rat (3-bromo-7-nitroindazolem 7-NI),[549] although treatment postinjury with 3-bromo-7-nitroindazole (7-NI) or pre- or postinjury treatment with nitro-L-arginine-methyl ester (L-NAME) did not.[549] However, postinjury treatment with L-arginine significantly reduced the contusion volume following lateral FP brain injury in rats.[549] L-NAME and 7-NI, as well as pretreatment with 7-NI but not L-NAME, significantly reduced forelimb placing sensorimotor deficits 1 day after lateral FP brain injury in rats.[548] However, L-NAME increased mortality and failed to improve cognitive or neurological motor deficits following lateral FP brain injury in rats.[315] Finally, L-arginine reduced the cortical lesion volume following CCI in rats and mice.[78,231]

The (iNOS) inhibitor aminoguanidine showed a marked reduction in lesion volume and neuronal cell loss with a concomitant improvement in neurological motor performance and grip strength following lateral FP brain injury in rats[314] but failed to reduce contusion volume following CCI in rats.[549] Conflicting results have been reported following CCI with secondary hypoxemia in rats, where the iNOS inhibitors aminoguanidine and L-*N*-iminoethyllysine both worsened cognitive performance and increased CA1 and CA3 cell loss in the hippocampus.[482] The exact role of iNOS in TBI, therefore, remains to be determined. The NO donor (Z)-1-[*N*-(2–aminoethyl)-*N*-(2-ammonioethyl)amino]diazen-1-ium-1,2-diolate (DETA/NONOate) was shown to up-regulate neurogenesis and improve neurological motor outcome, but it did not reduce lesion volume when administered 24 hours following CCI in the rat.[312] Finally, the peroxynitrite scavenger penicillamine (or penicillamine methyl ester [PenME]), administered i.v. 5 minutes following closed head injury in the mouse, improved acute grip scores[203] and support work using nonpenetrating nitrones,[320,323,325] suggesting the microvasculature and endothelium as crucial pharmacological targets post-TBI.

Potassium Channel Antagonists

In comparison to preclinical studies of calcium channel antagonists and magnesium supplementation, less is known about the potential efficacy of modulating potassium channels. Intraventricular administration of tetrodotoxin (TTX) was shown to reduce potassium flux after trauma, but resulted in no improvement in either motor or memory function.[115] A recent study using BMS-204352, an opener of large-conductance calcium-activated potassium channels, reported that administration after lateral FP brain injury in rats resulted in decreased regional cerebral edema and improved motor function.[75] However, no cortical neuroprotection or improvement in cognitive function was observed.

Magnesium Supplementation

Numerous preclinical studies have documented the beneficial effects of posttraumatic magnesium supplementation in several animal species. Studies in the late 1980s established that pretreatment with magnesium sulfate attenuated posttraumatic declines in brain [Mg^{2+}] and improved cerebral metabolism and neuromotor function.[350,546] Subsequently, the behavioral efficacy of posttraumatic administration of magnesium salts was well established. For example, i.v. administration of MgC_{l2} after lateral FP brain injury in the rat was shown to improve motor function and memory but not learning, ability.[25,351,486] Using a model of severe diffuse brain injury in rats, Vink and colleagues reported that either MgC_{l2} or $MgSO_4$ given i.v. or i.m. attenuates posttraumatic motor deficits and learning impairment,[215,218,547] with improvement of motor function evident with as much as a 24-hour delay in initiating magnesium therapy.[218] Interestingly, improvements in motor function were not observed in a subset of brain-injured animals with subdural hematoma[220] or when MgC_{l2} treatment was followed by infusion of basic fibroblast factor (bFGF).[196]

Both $MgCl_2$ and $MgSO_4$, administered either i.v. or i.m, have been shown to penetrate the BBB and increase brain [Mg^{2+}].[219] Accordingly, posttraumatic magnesium supplementation has resulted in improvements in a wide range of neurochemical, physiological, and histological parameters in preclinical evaluations. Trauma-induced cerebral edema, BBB breakdown, decreases in endogenous antioxidant molecules, and increases in tissue lactate and malondialdehyde levels are attenuated by posttraumatic magnesium administration in several different models of contusion injury.[129,136,384,536,537] In addition, administration of $MgCl_2$ in the acute period following lateral FP brain injury in rats reduced cell loss, disruption of microtubule-associated protein-2, calpain-mediated proteolysis of spectrin, apoptosis, and expression of p53-related protein and mRNA, with more pronounced effects being observed in the cortex compared with the hippocampus.[26,296,365,448] An in vitro study of cortical neurons revealed that mechanical (stretch) injury reduced the Mg^{2+} blockade of the NMDA receptor, resulting in larger increases in intracellular free calcium.[571] These data suggest that one potential mechanism for the neuroprotective effects of magnesium supplementation may be the restoration of the magnesium-dependent blockade of the NMDA receptor. Currently, a National Institutes of Health–sponsored clinical trial of $MgSO_4$ in human TBI is underway.

Calcium Channel Antagonists

While glutamate receptor antagonists have been evaluated experimentally and clinically for efficacy, in part due to their potential for attenuating posttraumatic calcium influx, calcium channel blockers have also been tested in preclinical and clinical studies.[88,577] In rabbit models of TBI, the L-type calcium channel antagonist nimodipine produced beneficial effects on intracellular calcium levels, tissue lactate, malondialdehyde and endothelin levels, and cell damage[13,469,564] but had no effect on tissue antioxidant levels.[536] Posttraumatic administration of the N-type calcium channel antagonist, Ziconotide (SNX-11), reduced injury-induced accumulation of calcium in vulnerable tissue regions in a dose-dependent fashion,[455] enhanced mitochondrial function,[541] and improved both motor and cognitive functions[42] in rats subjected to either focal or diffuse brain injury. In rats receiving (S-)emopamil, a phenylalkylamine calcium channel blocker with serotonin receptor antagonist properties, significant attenuation of injury-induced rCBF decreases, brain edema, memory dysfunction, and motor deficits has been reported after lateral FP brain injury.[383,385] Calcium chelators have also been shown to limit axonal injury and cell damage after trauma.[222,419]

In the clinical setting, the efficacy of calcium channel antagonists has been far more disappointing. Early studies reported beneficial effects of nimodipine on cerebral vasospasm associated with severe head injury.[277,278] However, subsequent double-blind, placebo-controlled studies of nicardipine[93] and nimodipine[20,515] demonstrated no overall clinical benefit. Subgroup analysis in the HIT II clinical trial of nimodipine suggested a protective effect in patients with traumatic subarachnoid hemorrhage.[20] However, subsequent retrospective analyses failed to find support for these data.[288,370]

Calpain Inhibitors

Due to the relatively poor bioavailability of current-generation calpain inhibitors, this class of compounds has not yet been tested in clinical TBI. However, preclinical testing in animal models has shown encouraging results and should stimulate the development of inhibitors with improved pharmacological profiles. Postinjury administration of calpain inhibitors significantly attenuated behavioral dysfunction after lateral FP brain injury in rats[453] or diffuse weight drop brain injury in mice,[284] with a therapeutic window of up to 4 hours.[284] However, neither of the inhibitors used in these studies provided neuroprotection or reduction of spectrin proteolysis.[284,454] A calpain inhibitor that may also inhibit other cysteine proteases has been shown to inhibit degradation of neurofilament and spectrin proteins when administered 10 minutes after CCI brain injury in rats.[417] In a model of TAI, inhibition of calpain-mediated proteolysis, neurofilament alterations, and mitochondrial damage have been accomplished by pretreatment with a calpain inhibitor,[58] posttraumatic hypothermia,[59] or cyclosporin A administration.[59,387]

Caspase Inhibitors

Since activation of various pro-apoptotic caspases has been associated with cell death following experimental TBI,[24,35,84,268,561] one strategy to attenuate acute posttraumatic cell death is to inhibit these proteases, most notably, caspase-3. The most promising caspase inhibitors are ketones due to their ability to interact reversibly with the cysteine residue of the active site, as well as their stability in vivo. Problems with designing these compounds include their relative lack of ability to cross the BBB, their inability to penetrate cell membranes, and the lack of specificity for specific caspases while maintaining low affinity for other possible substrates. The pan-caspase inhibitor *N*-benzyloxycarbonyl-Val-Ala-Asp-fluoromethyl ketone (z-VAD-fmk), when administered i.c.v. following lateral FP brain injury in rats, has been shown to improve both motor and cognitive function (Knoblach et al.[268]; Yakovlev et al.[561]). In a mouse model of weight drop brain injury, z-VAD-fmk was reported to reduce lesion volume.[138] Since inhibition of apoptotic cell death may be either deleterious or protective in the period following TBI, and based on the difficult pharmacokinetics and lipophilicity of caspase inhibitors, further development of these molecules and testing in experimental models must be pursued before they are ready to enter clinical trials.

Anti-Inflammatory Strategies

The marked inflammatory response observed following TBI has generally been regarded as detrimental to the injured brain, and numerous anti-inflammatory drugs have been evaluated. High doses of anti-inflammatory glucocorticoids stabilize membranes and reduce ROS-induced lipid peroxidative injury.[55,204] Although many early clinical studies reported that high-dose steroid treatment has no effect in the treatment of TBI,[53,97,195] Giannotta et al.[162] reported that high-dose methylprednisolone significantly reduced mortality in severely head-injured patients, and the synthetic corticosteroid triamcinolone significantly reduced mortality and improved the long-term neurological outcome in severely head-injured patients.[194] The ongoing CRASH trial (Corticosteroid Randomization After Significant Head Injury) has been designed to determine the effects of short-term steroid treatment on death and disability following significant brain injury.[435] The nonselective COX inhibitors ibuprofen and indomethacin have been shown to improve neurological function and to decrease mortality following experimental TBI.[200,265] Administration of the selective COX-2 inhibitors 4-[5-(4-methylphenyl)-3-(trifluoromethyl)-1H-pyrazol-1-yl] benzenesulfonamide (Celecoxib) and nimesulide improved cognitive function after TBI, although their effect on motor function remains controversial.[240] In addition, neutralization of ICAM-1 may inhibit neutrophil accumulation and reduce release of neurotoxic mediators. However, treatment with the anti-ICAM-1 antibody 1A29 failed to significantly improve the learning deficits or histopathological damage following severe TBI in rats.[247] Finally, prostacyclin, known to inhibit leukocyte adherence and aggregation and platelet aggregation, was shown to reduce neocortical neuronal death following FP brain injury in rats.[40]

Intracerebroventricular administration of IL-1ra has been reported to reduce infarct volume in a variety of models of cerebral ischemia,[148,430,431,563] and i.c.v. administration of IL-1ra results in improved cognitive function, reduced lesion volume, and decreased CA3 cell counts without motor improvement.[457] Administration of recombinant IL1–ra resulted in reduced neuronal damage following lateral FP brain injury in rats.[527] These findings were supported by a report demonstrating reduction of cortical lesion volume induced by lateral FP brain injury by postinjury i.c.v. infusion of rhIL-1ra.[266] Finally, i.v. administration of the anti-inflammatory cytokine IL-18 binding protein given intraperitoneally 1 hour following closed head injury in the rat failed to attenuate cerebral edema but did improve the neurological outcome 1 week postinjury.[566] Interleukin-10 has been shown to improve neurological recovery and significantly reduce TNF expression in the traumatized cortex only when given both intravenously preinjury and subcutaneously 10 minutes following lateral FP brain injury, with no neuroprotective effects observed when i.c.v. infusion was started 15 minutes postinjury.[266]

Intracerebroventricular injection of IL-6 was shown to reduce infarct volume after permanent focal cerebral ischemia in vivo.[308] An improved outcome following experimental TBI with compounds (e.g., pentoxyfylline, HU-211, and soluble TNF-α receptor fusion protein) that block the action of TNF-α has been reported.[267,472,474] Pentoxyfylline, a compound known to prevent or attenuate the production of TNF-α,[570] and TNF-α binding protein (TNFBP) both reduced neurological motor deficits up to 4 days postinjury and decreased edema formation only when administered immediately in a single dose following closed head injury in the rat.[472] We have recently evaluated acute inhibition of TNF-α and IL-6 following lateral FP brain injury, where no significant change in the acute TBI-induced increase in brain water content or neurological and cognitive dysfunction was observed.[322] Finally, the nonpsychotropic cannabinoid HU-211 (Dexanabinol), a TNF-α inhibitor, was found to improve neuromotor and cognitive outcome following closed head injury with a short therapeutic window of 2–3 hours postinjury.[474,476]

Growth Factors

Nerve Growth Factor

Following TBI, deprivation of a target-derived survival signal such as nerve growth factor (NGF) may contribute to secondary cell death or cell dysfunction in remote areas containing neurons that project to the injury site. The administration of NGF directly in the target-deprived areas could rescue neurons from delayed death and/or dysfunction. In models of fimbria-fornix transection, basal forebrain cholinergic neurons are deprived of their source of NGF from their distal target (hippocampus). In rats, the subsequent massive cell loss can be significantly reduced by i.c.v. or intraparenchymal infusion of NGF[144,221,272,531] as well when cells are genetically transduced to overexpress NGF.[47] Following lateral FP brain injury in rats, intracerebral NGF infusion in the acute phase beginning 24 hours after injury and lasting until the time of sacrifice (72 hours, 1 week, 2 weeks) improved memory (when evaluated at 1 and 2 weeks after injury) but not motor function or hippocampal cell loss.[480] Intraparenchymal NGF infusion for 2 weeks after lateral FP brain injury in rats also reduced memory deficits up to 4 weeks after injury and concomitantly decreased cholinergic neuronal loss and apoptotic cell death in the medial septum,[479] suggesting that the behavioral improvements persist after cessation of NGF administration and that the beneficial effects of NGF may be related to its ability to attenuate traumatically induced apoptotic cell death. Dixon et al.[121] showed that i.c.v. NGF infusion improved memory and increased choline acetyltransferase (ChAT) immunoreactivity and release of acetylcholine (Ach) in the medial septum after CCI brain injury in the rat. Additionally, fetal cortical neural cell transplants were observed to survive and begin to differentiate in the host brain when engrafted into the traumatic lesion and supplemented with NGF infusions following FP brain injury in rats.[481] When transplanted 24 hours after FP brain injury in rats, neural stem cells genetically engineered to overexpress NGF have been shown to markedly improve cognitive function (both learning and memory) 1 week postinjury and to reduce hippocampal cell death.[410] Delivery of NGF via transplantation of genetically modified NT2N human neuronal cells in the medial septum has been recently shown to improve learning capacity in mice following CCI brain injury.[551] Therefore, NGF appears to be a potential candidate for therapeutic evaluation after TBI. However, the dose, timing (critical window), and route of delivery are critical parameters that should be further investigated. To date, the only studies of NGF administration in humans have been performed in patients with Alzheimer's disease and peripheral neuropathy. Nerve growth factor was infused i.c.v. in three patients with Alzheimer's disease for 3 months. Minimal cognitive improvement was observed, but significant dose-related side effects consisted of back pain, which occurred in all three patients, and weight loss, which occurred in the two patients who received higher doses,[128] suggesting that i.c.v. administration may not be the most efficacious route of NGF delivery. In addition, NGF has been administered subcutaneously in patients with diabetic and HIV-related neuropathy. Improvement in pain severity but not in neuropathy severity was observed.[22,462,522]

Brain-Derived Neurotrophic Factor

Brain-derived neurotrophic factor (BDNF) has important effects on anatomical plasticity and could potentially be very important for postinjury repair. After lateral FP and CCI brain injury in rats, alterations of dendritic morphology have been reported.[416,450] Overexpression of BDNF is shown to increase dendritic complexity in the hippocampal dentate gyrus, resulting in an increase in the number of dendrites, in total dendritic length, and in the number of branch points.[524] Long-term potentiation (LTP), a mechanism for synaptic learning, is impaired in BDNF-deficient mice and can be restored by supplying BDNF to the hippocampus via gene therapy.[274,404] Impairment in LTP, as well as learning and memory deficits related to hippocampal damage, have been shown after lateral FP injury in rats.[208,225,359] Intraseptal BDNF infusion beginning immediately after fimbria-fornix transection and lasting for 2 weeks showed greater efficacy than i.c.v. infusion, likely due to the low rate of diffusion of BDNF from the ventricle into the adjacent parenchyma.[363] To date, only one study in experimental TBI has examined the efficacy of BDNF administration, with rather disappointing results. Following intraparenchymal infusion of BDNF into either the cortex or the hippocampus after lateral FP brain injury in rats (beginning 4 hours postinjury and lasting for 2 weeks), no improvement in cognitive function or histological outcome was observed.[46]

Brain-derived neurotrophic factor administered subcutaneously in patients with amyotrophic lateral sclerosis (ALS) produced no significant beneficial effect but was well tolerated, with only minor side effects such as injection site reactions.[256] In a Phase I–II trial, when administered intrathecally in ALS patients by continuous infusion, BDNF caused paresthesias and sleep disturbances at higher doses.[522] Further studies are warranted to elucidate the role of endogenous BDNF in the injured brain and to evaluate the potential use of exogenous BDNF as a treatment for TBI.

Neurotrophin-4/5

There is a plethora of reports showing the neuroprotective effects of neurotrophin-4/5 (NT-4/5) both in vitro and in vivo, ranging from neuronal survival to activity-dependent neuronal plasticity. In vivo, NT-4/5 has been shown to protect basal forebrain cholinergic neurons following axotomy in rats.[15,238,532] Brain NT-4/5 infusion was demonstrated to stimulate the up-regulation expression of genes associated with axonal growth such as GAP-43 and Tα1-tubulin following cervical axotomy[269] and to promote axonal growth from regenerating retinal ganglion cells after optic nerve transection in rats.[460] Neurotrophin-4/5 protein has been shown to be transiently up-regulated in both the injured cortex and the underlying hippocampus.[445] Mice lacking NT-4/5 are more susceptible to selective cell loss in the CA3-CA2 subregion of the hippocampus following CCI, while no difference in brain lesion volume was observed. Similarly, prolonged intraparenchymal administration of NT-4/5 protects against the death of the selectively vulnerable pyramidal cells of the CA3-CA2 subfield of the hippocampus following lateral FP but has no effect on total brain lesion volume.[444]

Glial Cell–Derived Neurotrophic Factor

When glial cell–derived neurotrophic factor (GDNF) was infused i.c.v. for 7 days following TBI in rats, a significant decrease was observed in CA2 and CA3 cell loss.[264] Likewise, adenovirus-mediated GDNF expression into the sensorimotor cortex 24 hours prior to freeze injury in rats was shown to reduce the brain lesion volume, and the number of cells immunopositive for iNOS, activated capase-3, and TUNEL was observed.[223] Data gathered in animal models suggests that GDNF administration reduces neuronal damage after CNS insult. However, a recent clinical trial in which GDNF was injected i.c.v. into patients with advanced Parkinson's disease failed to show clinical benefit.[382] Severe side effects such as nausea, anorexia, and asymptomatic hyponatremia were noted. The result of this clinical trial suggests that improved methods of delivery and optimal dosing require further study, as the lack of efficacy may be related to a failure of GDNF to penetrate brain parenchyma following i.c.v administration. More recently, a Phase I clinical trial has showed good results when GDNF was injected directly into the putamen of patients with Parkinson's disease.[164] Improvement of motor deficits was observed without severe side effects; moreover, medication-induced dyskinesias were reduced. Based on these clinical data, direct infusion of GDNF may be a more attractive and promising means of delivery after CNS insults. Other possibilities for administration of GDNF include direct injection within the lesion or i.v. administration of OX-26–conjugated GDNF,[14] which allows GDNF to cross the BBB.

Insulin-like Growth Factor-I

Using in vivo models of peripheral nerve injury, local infusion of insulin-like growth factor-I (IGF-I) has been shown to stimulate axonal regeneration, enhance function recovery, and increase nerve sprouting.[70,213] Following FP brain injury in rats, subcutaneous injection of IGF-I 15 minutes post-injury, and every 12 hours for 14 days has been shown to improve learning and neuromotor function,[451] demonstrating that peripheral administration of IGF-I can result in therapeutic levels in the CNS following TBI.

A Phase II open label prospective randomized study to assess the safety and efficacy of i.v. administration of recombinant human IGF-I has been conducted on patients with moderate to severe head injury.[214] Continuous infusion of IGF for 14 days was given starting within 72 hours after injury. A trend toward improvement in neurological outcome scales and nutritional response was noted without serious side effects. Additional research will be needed to evaluate the potential of IGF-I as a therapeutic agent for patients with TBI, but to date it appears to be a promising candidate for the treatment of TBI.

Basic Fibroblast Growth Factor

Basic fibroblast growth factor (FGF) is believed to exert its protective effects by stabilizing calcium homeostasis[77] and by decreasing ROS formation and up-regulating levels of SOD, an antioxidant enzyme.[333] Following lateral FP brain injury in rats, i.v. administration of bFGF, beginning 30 minutes after injury and lasting for 3 hours, significantly reduces the volume of focal contusion and the number of posttraumatic necrotic cortical neurons.[116] Memory dysfunction associated with experimental FP brain injury can be also significantly attenuated by delayed infusion of exogenous bFGF directly in the injured cortex for 7 days starting 24 hours after injury, although no overt histological change has been associated with the observed cognitive improvement.[343] Immunohistochemical evaluation revealed a trend toward increased astrocytosis in the injured cortex of bFGF-treated animals compared to vehicle-treated animals. Interestingly, combined administration of bFGF and magnesium chloride over 24 hours beginning immediately after FP brain injury resulted in less neuromotor improvement than magnesium treatment alone.[196] Differences in the timing and length of exposure to bFGF administration or severity of injury may underlie the differences observed in these studies. Clinical studies designed to evaluate the administration of bFGF in head-injured patients have not been initiated, but studies of bFGF in stroke patients have been undertaken. Doses of 5–10 mg given i.v. over 24 hours were shown to be safe in a European clinical trial.[50] Although combinational pharmacotherapy should be used with caution, it is a potential strategy for the treatment of TBI and should be a focus of further research efforts.

Transplants to Deliver Protective Molecules

Cellular transplantation is one option to repair the injured CNS, aiming not only to replace the function of cells lost to injury but also chronically deliver trophic factors, pharmaceuticals, or neuroprotective molecules. Fetal cortical tissue, explants transplanted into the injured cortex of nonimmunosuppressed adult rats subjected to FP brain injury, survived best when transplanted between 2 days and 2 weeks postinjury[490] and were shown to ameliorate posttraumatic hippocampal cell death, suggesting that these grafts were producing a diffusible protective factor.[491] Transplantation at 4 weeks postinjury resulted in reduced graft integration, as measured by acetylcholinergic fibers crossing the graft–host interface, most likely due to increased glial scar formation at later postinjury time points. Recovery of both cognitive and motor function was observed after transplantation of fetal rat cortical tissue into the injured cortex in combination with NGF infusion after lateral FP TBI in nonimmunosuppressed adult rat.[491] Philips et al.[411] transplanted post mitotic human neurons (hNT) cells into the injured cortex of nonimmunosuppressed adult rats 24 hours after FP brain injury and observed viable hNT transplants up to 4 weeks, without attenuation of posttraumatic neuromotor deficits, while transplantation suggested a variable degree of graft rejection. More recently, transplantation of hNT cells transduced ex vivo to express NGF into the medial septum, following CCI injury in mice, attenuated long-term cognitive dysfunction and protected the NGF responsive cholinergic neurons of the septo-hippocampal pathway.[310,551] As other sources of cells for transplantation, multipotential immortalized stem and progenitor cell lines combine the advantages of cultured cells (unlimited expansion in cultures and the potential to be genetically manipulated in vitro) with the ability to give rise to multiple lineages.[551] The immortalized cell lines HiB5, MHP36, and C17.2 have been transplanted in experimental models of TBI. The HiB5 cells are conditionally immortalized progenitor cells derived from an embryonic (E16) rat hippocampus, and have been shown to differentiate into neurons and glia when transplanted into the neonatal hippocampus, cerebellum, and cortex or into the adult striatum. In rats subjected to FP brain injury, HiB5 cells transduced to secrete NGF (HiB5-NGF) were transplanted into three sites surrounding the injured cortex 24 hours after injury.[410] Brain-injured animals receiving either the HiB5-NGF cells or untransduced HiB5 cells showed similar improvement in neuromotor function and spatial learning. However, hippocampal cell death was significantly reduced only in the HiB5-NGF-engrafted group.[410] Although engrafted progenitor or stem cells are likely to secrete various trophic factors that can contribute to plasticity, regeneration, and neuroprotection, the transplantation of cells transduced to produce NGF, like the hNT cells and the HiB5 cells described above, or fetal tissue transplanted in combination with NGF infusion,[481] seem to have distinct advantages over cell engraftment alone. The use of transplanted migrating cells will allow long-term expression and diffuse delivery of neuroprotective factors and may have greater potential to integrate with the host tissue. In addition, autocrine and paracrine effects of the expressed neurotrophic factor might be important in increasing graft survival.

Despite improvements in the medical and surgical treatment of TBI, no neuroprotective agents are available to counteract secondary or delayed damage to the injured brain or to stimulate its repair and recovery. The development of cell replacement therapies, combined with delivery of neuroprotective molecules, may offer an alternative or a complementary strategy for the treatment of TBI. Recent advances both in the identification of a variety of cell lines with a potential for CNS transplantation and in the characterization of the neurogenic regions of the brain represent a new opportunity of great interest for delayed intervention in TBI patients.

REFERENCES

1. Abu-Judeh HH, Parker R, Singh M, el Zeftawy H, Atay S, Kumar M, Naddaf S, Aleksic S, Abdel-Dayem HM: SPECT brain perfusion imaging in mild traumatic brain injury without loss of consciousness and normal computed tomography. Nucl Med Commun 20:505–510, 1999.
2. Adams JH, Doyle D, Ford I, Gennarelli TA, Graham DI, McLellan DR: Diffuse axonal injury in head injury: Definition, diagnosis and grading. Histopathology 15:49–59, 1989.
3. Adams JH, Doyle D, Graham DI, et al: Diffuse axonal injury in head injuries caused by a fall. Lancet 2:1420–1422, 1984.
4. Adams JH, Graham DI: The relationship between ventricular fluid pressure and neuropathology of raised intracranial pressure. Neuropathol Appl Neurobiol 2:323–332, 1976.
5. Adams JH, Graham DI, Jennett B: The neuropathology of the vegetative state after an acute brain insult. Brain 123:1327–1338, 2000.
6. Adams JH, Graham DI, Jennett B: The structural basis of moderate disability after traumatic brain damage. J Neurol Neurosurg Psychiatry 71:521–524, 2001.
7. Adams JH, Graham DI, Murray LS, Scott G: Diffuse axonal injury due to nonmissile head injury in humans: An analysis of 45 cases. Ann Neurol 12:557–563, 1982.
8. Adams JH, Graham DI, Scott G, Parker LS, Doyle D: Brain damage in fatal non-missile head injury. J Clin Pathol 33:1132–1145, 1980.
9. Adams JH, Mitchell DE, Graham DI, Doyle D: Diffuse brain damage of immediate impact type. Brain 100:489–502, 1977.
10. Adibhatla RM, Hatcher JF, Dempsey RJ: Citicoline: Neuroprotective mechanisms in cerebral ischemia. J Neurochem 80:12–23, 2002.
11. Adibhatla RM, Hatcher JF, Dempsey RJ: Cytidine-5'-diphosphocholine affects CTP-phosphocholine cytidylyltransferase and lyso-phosphatidylcholine after transient brain ischemia. J Neurosci Res 76:390–396, 2004.
12. Aikawa JK: Magnesium: Its Biologic Significance. Boca Raton, FL, CRC Press, 1981.
13. Ak A, Ustun ME, Ogun CO, Duman A, Bor MA: Effects of nimodipine on tissue lactate and malondialdehyde levels in experimental head trauma. Anaesth Intens Care 29:484–488, 2001.
14. Albeck DS, Hoffer BJ, Quissell D, Sanders LS, Zerbe G, Granholm ACE: A noninvasive transport system for GDNF across the blood–brain barrier. NeuroReport 8:2293–2298, 1997.
15. Alderson RF, Wiegand SJ, Anderson KD, Cai N, Cho JY, Lindsay RM, Altar CA: Neurotrophin-4/5 maintains the cholinergic phenotype of axotomized septal neurons. Eur J Neurosci 8:282–290, 1996.
16. Allen JW, Ivanova SA, Fan L, Espey MG, Basile AS, Faden AI: Group II metabotropic glutamate receptor activation attenuates traumatic neuronal injury and improves neurological recovery after traumatic brain injury. J Pharmacol Exp Ther 290:112–120, 1999.
17. Althaus JS, Andrus PK, Williams CM, VonVoigtlander PF, Cazers AR, Hall ED: The use of salicylate hydroxylation to detect hydroxyl radical generation in ischemic and traumatic brain injury. Reversal by tirilazad mesylate (U-74006F). Mol Chem Neuropathol 20:147–162, 1993.
18. Altura BM, Memon ZS, Altura BT, Cracco RQ: Alcohol-associated acute head trauma in human subjects is associated with early deficits in serum ionized Mg and Ca. Alcohol 12:433–437, 1995.
19. Andrews PJD, Piper IR, Dearden NM, et al: Secondary insults during intrahospital transport of head-injured patients. Lancet 335:327, 1990.
20. Anonymous: A multicenter trial of the efficacy of nimodipine on outcome after severe head injury. The European Study Group on Nimodipine in Severe Head Injury. J Neurosurg 80:797–804, 1994.
21. Aoyama N, Katayama Y, Kawamata T, Maeda T, Mori T, Yamamoto T, Kikuchi T, Uwahodo Y: Effects of antioxidant, OPC-14117, on secondary cellular damage and behavioral deficits following cortical contusion in the rat. Brain Res 934:117–124, 2002.
22. Apfel SC, Schwartz S, Adornato BT, Freeman R, Biton V, Rendell M, Vinik A, Giuliani M, Stevens JC, Barbano R, Dyck PJ: Efficacy and safety of recombinant human nerve growth factor in patients with diabetic polyneuropathy: A randomized controlled trial. rhNGF Clinical Investigator Group. JAMA 284:2215–2221, 2000.
23. Baker AJ, Moulton RJ, MacMillan VH, Shedden PM: Excitatory amino acids in cerebrospinal fluid following traumatic brain injury in humans. J Neurosurg 79:369–372, 1993.
24. Bareyre FM, Raghupathi R, Saatman KE, McIntosh TK: DNase-I disinhibition is predominantly associated with actin hyperpolymerization after traumatic brain injury. J Neurochem 173–181, 2001.
25. Bareyre FM, Saatman KE, Helfaer MA, Sinson G, Weisser JD, Brown AL, McIntosh TK: Alterations in ionized and total blood magnesium after experimental traumatic brain injury: Relationship to neurobehavioral outcome and neuroprotective efficacy of magnesium chloride. J Neurochem 73:271–280, 1999.
26. Bareyre FM, Saatman KE, Raghupathi R, McIntosh TK: Post-injury treatment with magnesium chloride attenuates cortical damage after traumatic brain injury in rats. J Neurotrauma 17:1029–1039, 2000.
27. Bareyre FM, Wahl F, McIntosh TK, Stutzmann J-M: Time course of cerebral edema after traumatic brain injury in rats: Effects of riluzole and mannitol. J Neurotrauma 14:839–849, 1997.
28. Barger SW, Horster D, Mattson MP: Tumor necrosis factors a and b protect neurons against amyloid b-peptide

toxicity: Evidence for involvement of a kappa b–binding factor and attenuation of peroxide and Ca_{2+} accumulation. Proc Natl Acad Sci USA 92:9328–9332, 1995.

29. Barzo P, Marmarou A, Fatouros P, Corwin F, Dunbar J: Magnetic resonance imaging–monitored acute blood–brain barrier changes in experimental traumatic brain injury. J Neurosurg 85:1113–1121, 1996.
30. Baskaya MK, Dogan A, Rao AM, Dempsey RJ: Neuroprotective effects of citicoline on brain edema and blood–brain barrier breakdown after traumatic brain injury. J Neurosurg 92:448–452, 2000.
31. Basu A, Krady JK, O'Malley M, Styren SD, DeKosky ST, Levison SW: The type 1 interleukin-1 receptor is essential for the efficient activation of microglia and the induction of multiple proinflammatory mediators in response to brain injury. J Neurosci 22:6071–6082, 2002.
32. Beal AL, Scheltema KE, Beilman GJ, Deuser WE: Hypokalemia following trauma. Shock 18:107–110, 2002.
33. Beckman JS: Peroxynitrite versus hydroxyl radical: The role of nitric oxide in superoxide-dependent cerebral injury. Ann NY Acad Sci 738:69–75, 1994.
34. Beer R, Franz G, Krajewski S, Pike BR, Hayes RL, Reed JC, Wang KK, Klimmer C, Schmutzhard E, Poewe W, Kampfl A: Temporal and spatial profile of caspase 8 expression and proteolysis after experimental traumatic brain injury. J Neurochem 78:862–873, 2001.
35. Beer R, Franz G, Srinivasan A, Hayes RL, Pike BR, Newcomb JK, Zhao X, Schmutzhard E, Poewe W, Kampfl A: Temporal profile and cell subtype distribution of activated caspase-3 following experimental traumatic brain injury. J Neurochem 75:1264–1273, 2000.
36. Beit-Yannai E, Zhang R, Trembovler V, Samuni A, Shohami E: Cerebroprotective effect of stable nitroxide radicals in closed head injury in the rat. Brain Res 717:22–28, 1996.
37. Belayev L, Alonso OF, Liu Y, Chappell AS, Zhao W, Ginsberg MD, Busto R: Talampanel, a novel noncompetitive AMPA antagonist, is neuroprotective after traumatic brain injury in rats. J Neurotrauma 18:1031–1038, 2001.
38. Belayev L, Becker DA, Alonso OF, Liu Y, Busto R, Ley JJ, Ginsberg MD: Stilbazulenyl nitrone, a novel azulenyl nitrone antioxidant: Improved neurological deficit and reduced contusion size after traumatic brain injury in rats. J Neurosurg 96:1077–1083, 2002.
39. Bell MJ, Kochanek PM, Doughty LA, Carcillo JA, Adelson PD, Clark RS, Wisniewski SR, Whalen MJ, DeKosky ST: Interleukin-6 and interleukin-10 in cerebrospinal fluid after severe traumatic brain injury in children. J Neurotrauma 14:451–457, 1997.
40. Bentzer P, Mattiasson G, McIntosh TK, Wieloch T, Grande PO: Infusion of prostacyclin following experimental brain injury in the rat reduces cortical lesion volume. J Neurotrauma 18:275–285, 2001.
41. Benveniste EN, Tang LP, Law RM: Differential regulation of astrocyte TNF-alpha expression by the cytokines TGF-beta, IL-6 and IL-10. Int J Dev Neurosci 13:341–349, 1995.
42. Berman RF, Verweij BH, Muizelaar JP: Neurobehavioral protection by the neuronal calcium channel blocker Ziconotide in a model of traumatic diffuse brain injury in rats. J Neurosurg 93:821–828, 2000.
43. Bernert H, Turski L: Traumatic brain damage prevented by the non-*N*-methyl-D-aspartate antagonist 2,3-dihydroxy-6-nitro-7sulfamoylbenzo[f] quinoxaline. Proc Natl Acad Sci USA 93:5235–5240, 1996.
44. Biegon A, Fry PA, Paden CM, Alexandrovich A, Tsenter J, Shohami E: Dynamic changes in *N*-methyl-D-aspartate receptors after closed head injury in mice: Implications for treatment for neurological and cognitive deficits. Proc Natl Acad Sci USA 101:5117–5122, 2004.
45. Bjugstad KB, Flitter WD, Garland WA, Philpot RM, Kirstein CL, Arendash GW: CPI-1189 prevents apoptosis and reduces glial fibrillary acidic protein immunostaining in a TNF-alpha infusion model for AIDS dementia complex. J Neurovirol 6:478–491, 2000.
46. Blaha GR, Raghupathi R, Saatman KE, McIntosh TK: Brain-derived neurotrophic factor administration after traumatic brain injury in the rat does not protect against behavioral or histological deficits. Neuroscience 99:483–493, 2000.
47. Blomer U, Kafri T, Randolph-Moore L, Verma IM, Gage FH: Bcl-xL protects adult septal cholinergic neurons from axotomized cell death. Proc Natl Acad Sci USA 95:2603–2608, 1998.
48. Blumbergs PC, Jones NR, North JB: Diffuse axonal injury in head trauma. J Neurol Neurosurg Psychol 52:838–841, 1989.
49. Blumbergs PC, Scott G, Manavis J, Wainwright H, Simpson DA, McLean AJ: Staining of amyloid precursor protein to study axonal damage in mild head injury. Lancet 344:1055–1056, 1994.
50. Bogousslavsky J, Victor SJ, Salinas EO, Pallay A, Donnan GA, Fieschi C, Kaste M, Orgogozo JM, Chamorro A, Desmet A: Fiblast (trafermin) in acute stroke: Results of the European-Australian phase II/III safety and efficacy trial. Cerebrovasc Dis 14:239–251, 2002.
51. Bouma GJ, Muizelaar PJ, Stringer WA, Choi SC, Fatouros P, Young HF: Ultra-early evaluation of regional cerebral blood flow in severely head-injured patients using xenon-enhanced computerized tomography. J Neurosurg 77:360–368, 1992.
52. Boveris A: Determination of the production of superoxide radicals and hydrogen peroxide in mitochondria. Methods Enzymol 105:429–435, 1984.
53. Braakman R, Schouten HJ, Dishoeck MB, Minderhoud JM: Megadose steroids in severe head injury. J Neurosurg 58:326–330, 1983.
54. Bramlett HM, Dietrich WD, Green EJ, Busto R: Chronic histopathological consequences of fluid-percussion brain injury in rats: Effects of post-traumatic hypothermia. Acta Neuropathol 93:190–199, 1997.
55. Braughler JM, Hall ED, Means ED, Waters TR,

Anderson DK: Evaluation of an intensive methylprednisolone sodium succinate dosing regimen in experimental spinal cord injury. J Neurosurg 67:102–105, 1987.

56. Bruce AJ, Boling W, Kindy MS, Peschon J, Kraemer PJ, Carpenter MK, Holtsberg FW, Mattson MP: Altered neuronal and microglial responses to cerebrotoxic and ischemic brain injury in mice lacking TNF receptors. Nature Med 2:788–794, 1996.
57. Buisson A, Choi DW: The inhibitory mGluR agonist, S-4-carboxy-3-hydroxy-phenylglycine selectively attenuates NMDA neurotoxicity and oxygen-glucose deprivation-induced neuronal death. Neuropharmacology 34:1081–1087, 1995.
58. Buki A, Farkas O, Doczi T, Povlishock JT: Preinjury administration of the calpain inhibitor MDL-28170 attenuates traumatically induced axonal injury. J Neurotrauma 20:261–268, 2003.
59. Buki A, Koizumi H, Povlishock JT: Moderate posttraumatic hypothermia decreases early calpain-mediated proteolysis and concomitant cytoskeletal compromise in traumatic axonal injury. Exp Neurol 159:319–328, 1999.
60. Buki A, Okonkwo DO, Wang KK, Povlishock JT: Cytochrome c release and caspase activation in traumatic axonal injury. J Neurosci 20:2825–2834, 2000.
61. Buki A, Siman R, Trojanowski JQ, Povlishock JT: The role of calpain-mediated spectrin proteolysis in traumatically induced axonal injury. J Neuropathol Exp Neurol 58:365–375, 1999.
62. Bullock R, Graham DI: Non-penetrating injuries of the head. In: Cooper GJ, Dudley HAF, Gann DS (eds): Scientific Foundation of Trauma: Nonpenetrating Blunt Injury. Oxford, Buttwerworth Heinemann, 1997, pp 101–126.
63. Bullock R, Teasdale G: Surgical management of traumatic intracranial hematomas. In: Braakman R (ed): Handbook of Clinical Neurology, vol 15. Amsterdam, Elsevier, 1990, pp 249–298.
64. Bullock R, Zauner A, Woodward JJ, et al: Factors affecting excitatory amino acid release following severe human head injury. J Neurosurg 89:507–518, 1998.
65. Busto R, Dietrich W, Globus M, Ginsberg M: Small differences in intraischemic brain temperature critically determine the extent of ischemic neuronal injury. J Cereb Blood Flow Metab 7:729–738, 1987.
66. Campbell IL, Abraham CR, Masliah E, Kemper P, Inglis JD, Oldstone MB, Mucke L: Neurologic disease induced in transgenic mice by cerebral overexpression of interleukin 6. Proc Natl Acad Sci USA 90:10061–10065, 1993.
67. Campbell IL, Stalder AK, Akwa Y, Pagenstecher A, Asensio VC: Transgenic models to study the actions of cytokines in the central nervous system. Neuroimmunomodulation 5:126–135, 1998.
68. Carbonell WS, Maris DO, McCall T, Grady MS: Adaptation of the fluid percussion injury model to the mouse. J Neurotrauma 15:217–229, 1998.
69. Carlos TM, Clark RS, Franicola-Higgins D, Schiding JK, Kochanek PM: Expression of endothelial adhesion molecules and recruitment of neutrophils after traumatic brain injury in rats. J Leukoc Biol 61:279–285, 1997.
70. Caroni P, Grandes P: Nerve sprouting in innervated adult skeletal muscle induced by exposure to elevated levels of insulin-like growth factors. J Cell Biol 110:1307–1317, 1990.
71. Ceballos G, Tuttle JB, Rubio R: Differential distribution of purine metabolizing enzymes between glia and neurons. J Neurochem 62:1144–1153, 1994.
72. Cernak I, Savic VJ, Kotur J, Prokic V, Veljovic M, Grbovic D: Characterization of plasma magnesium concentration and oxidative stress following graded traumatic brain injury in humans. J Neurotrauma 17:53–68, 2000.
73. Chabrier PE, Auguet M, Spinnewyn B, Auvin S, Cornet S, Demerle-Pallardy C, Guilmard-Favre C, Marin JG, Pignol B, Gillard-Roubert V, Roussillot-Charnet C, Schulz J, Viossat I, Bigg D, Moncada S: BN 80933, a dual inhibitor of neuronal nitric oxide synthase and lipid peroxidation: A promising neuroprotective strategy [see comments.]. Proc Natl Acad Sci USA 96:10824–10829, 1999.
74. Chao CC, Hu S, Ehrlich L, Peterson PK: Interleukin-1 and tumor necrosis factor-α synergistically mediate neurotoxicity: Involvement of nitric oxide and of *N*-methyl-D-aspartate receptors. Brain Behav Immunol 9:355–365, 1995.
75. Cheney JA, Weisser JD, Bareyre FM, Laurer HL, Saatman KE, Raghupathi R, Gribkoff VK, Starrett JE, McIntosh TK: The Maxi-K potassium channel opener BMS-204352 attenuates regional cerebral edema and neurological motor impairment following experimental brain injury. J Cereb Blood Flow Metab 21:403, 2001.
76. Cheng B, Christakos S, Mattson MP: Tumor necrosis factors protect neurons against metabolic-excitotoxic insults and promote maintenance of calcium homeostasis. Neuron 12:139–153, 1994.
77. Cheng B, Mattson MP: NGF and bFGF protect rat hippocampal and human cortical neurons against hypoglycemic damage by stabilizing calcium homeostasis. Neuron 7:1031–1041, 1991.
78. Cherian L, Chacko G, Goodman C, Robertson CS: Neuroprotective effects of L-arginine administration after cortical impact injury in rats: Dose response and time window. J Pharmacol Exp Ther 304:617–623, 2003.
79. Chestnut RM, Marshall LF, Kauber MR, et al: The role of secondary brain injury in determing outcome from severe head injury. J Trauma 34:216–222, 1993.
80. Chihab R, Oillet J, Bossenmeyer C, Daval JL: Glutamate triggers cell death specifically in mature central neurons through a necrotic process. Mol Genet Metab 63:142–147, 1998.
81. Choi DW: Methods for antagonizing glutamate neurotoxicity. Cerebrovasc Brain Metab Rev 2:105–147, 1990.

82. Cirak B, Rousan N, Kocak A, Palaoglu O, Palaoglu S, Kilic K: Melatonin as a free radical scavenger in experimental head trauma. Pediatr Neurosurg 31:298–301, 1999.
83. Clark JM: Distribution of microglial clusters in the brain after head injury. J Neurol Neurosurg Psychiatry 37:463, 1974.
84. Clark RSB, Kochanek PM, Chen M, Watkins SC, Marion DW, Chen J, Hamilton RL, Loeffert JE, Graham SH: Increases in Bcl-2 and cleavage of caspase-1 and caspase-3 in human brain after head injury. FASEB J 13:813–821, 1999.
85. Clark RSB, Kochanek PM, Dixon CD, Chen M, Marion DW, Heinemann S, DeKosky ST, Graham SH: Early neuropathologic effects of mild or moderate hypoxemia after controlled cortical impact injury in rats. J Neurotrauma 14:179–189, 1997.
86. Clark RS, Schiding JK, Kaczorowski SL, Marion DW, Kochanek PM: Neutrophil accumulation after traumatic brain injury: Comparison of weight drop and controlled cortical impact models. J Neurotrauma 11:499–506, 1994.
87. Clark WM, Wechsler LR, Sabounjian LA, Schwiderski UE, Citicoline Stroke Study Group: A phase III randomized efficacy trial of 2000 mg citicoline in acute ischemic stroke patients. Neurology 57:1595–1602, 2001.
88. Clausen T, Bullock R: Medical treatment and neuroprotection in traumatic brain injury. Curr Pharm Des 7:1517–1532, 2001.
89. Clifton GL, Jiang JY, Lyeth BG, Jenkins LW, Hamm RJ, Hayes RL: Marked protection by moderate hypothermia after experimental traumatic brain injury. J Cereb Blood Flow Metab 11:114–121, 1991.
90. Clifton GL, Lyeth BG, Jenkins LW, Taft WC, DeLorenzo RJ, Hayes RL: Effect of D1 α-tocopheryl succinate and polyethylene glycol on performance tests after fluid percussion brain injury. J Neurotrauma 6:71–81, 1989.
91. Cohen RA, Browndyke JN, Moser DJ, Paul RH, Gordon N, Sweet L: Long-term citicoline (cytidine diphosphate choline) use in patients with vascular dementia: Neuroimaging and neuropsychological outcomes. Cerebrovasc Dis 16:199–204, 2003.
92. Colicos MA, Dixon CE, Dash PK: Delayed, selective neuronal death following experimental cortical impact injury in rats: Possible role in memory deficits. Brain Res 739:111–119, 1996.
93. Compton JS, Lee T, Jones NC, Waddell G, Teddy PJ: A double-blind placebo controlled trial of the calcium entry blocking drug nicardipine in the treatment of vasospasm following severe head injury. Br J Neurosurg 4:9–16, 1990.
94. Conte V, Uryu K, Fujimoto S, Yao Y, Longhi L, Trojanowski JQ, Lee VMY, McIntosh TK, Pratico D: Vitamin E reduces amyloidosis and improves cognitive function in Tg2576 mice folllowing repetitive concussive brain injury. J Neurochem 90:758–764, 2004.
95. Conti AC, Raghupathi R, Trojanowski JQ, McIntosh TK: Experimental brain injury induces regionally distinct apoptosis during the acute and delayed post-traumatic period. J Neurosci 18:5663–5672, 1998.
96. Cooper PR: Post-traumatic intracranial mass lesions. In: Cooper PR, Golfinos JF (eds): Head Injury. New York, McGraw-Hill, 2000, pp 293–340.
97. Cooper PR, Moody S, Clark WK, Kirkpatrick J, Maravilla K, Gould AL, Drane W: Dexamethasone and severe head injury. J Neurosurg 51:307–316, 1979.
98. Corsellis JA, Bruton CJ, Freeman-Browne D: The aftermath of boxing. Psychol Med 3:270–303, 1973.
99. Cortez SC, McIntosh TK, Noble L: Experimental fluid percussion brain injury: Vascular disruption and neuronal and glial alterations. Brain Res 482:271–282, 1989.
100. D'Ambrosio R, Maris DO, Grady MS, Winn HR, Janigro D: Impaired K(+) homeostasis and altered electrophysiological properties of post-traumatic hippocampal glia. J Neurosci 19:8152–8162, 1999.
101. Danbolt NC: Glutamate uptake. Prog Neurobiol 65:1–105, 2001.
102. Dash PK, Mach SA, Moore AN: Regional expression and role of cyclooxygenase-2 following experimental traumatic brain injury. J Neurotrauma 17:69–81, 2000.
103. Dash PK, Mach SA, Moore AN: The role of extracellular signal-regulated kinase in cognitive and motor deficits following experimental traumatic brain injury. Neuroscience 114:755–767, 2002.
104. Davalos A, Castillo J, Alvarez-Sabin J, Secades JJ, Mercadal J, Lopez S, Cobo E, Warach S, Sherman D, Clark WM, Lozano R: Oral citicoline in acute ischemic stroke: An individual patient data pooling analysis of clinical trials. Stroke 33:2850–2857, 2002.
105. Davis S, Butcher SP, Morris RGM: The NMDA receptor antagonist D-2-amino-5-phosphonopentanoate (DAP5) impairs spatial learning and LTP in vivo at intracerebral concentrations comparable to those that block LTP in vitro. J Neurosci 12:21–34, 1992.
106. De Vry J, Horvath E, Schreiber R: Neuroprotective and behavioral effects of the selective metabotropic glutamate mGlu(1) receptor antagonist BAY 36-7620. Eur J Pharmacol 428:203–214, 2001.
107. Dempsey RJ, Kaya MK, An A: Attenuation of brain edema, blood–brain barrier breakdown, and injury volume by ifenprodil, a polyamine-site *N*-methyl-D-aspartate receptor antagonist, after experimental traumatic brain injury in rats. Neurosurgery 47:399–404, 2000.
108. Dempsey RJ, Raghavendra R, V: Cytidinediphosphocholine treatment to decrease traumatic brain injury–induced hippocampal neuronal death, cortical contusion volume, and neurological dysfunction in rats. J Neurosurg 98:867–873, 2003.
109. Denu JM, Tanner KG: Specific and reversible inactivation of protein tyrosine phosphatases by hydrogen peroxide: Evidence for a sulfenic acid intermediate and implications for redox regulation. Biochemistry 37:5633–5642, 1998.

110. DeWitt DS, Prough DS: Traumatic cerebral vascular injury: The effects of concussive brain injury on the cerebral vasculature. J Neurotrauma 20:795–825, 2003.
111. DeWitt DS, Prough D, Taylor CL, Whitley J: Reduced cerebral blood flow oxygen delivery, and electroencephalographic activity after traumatic brain injury and mild hemorrhage in cats. J Neurosurg 76(5):812–821, 1992.
112. DeWitt DS, Smith TG, Deyo DJ, Miller KR, Uchida T, Prough DS: L-Arginine and superoxide dismutase prevent or reverse cerebral hypoperfusion after fluid-percussion traumatic brain injury. J Neurotrauma 14:223–233, 1997.
113. Dhillon HS, Prasad AS: Kynurenate attenuates the accumulation of diacylglycerol and free fatty acids after experimental brain injury in the rat. Brain Res 832:7–12, 1999.
114. Di X, Gordon J, Bullock R: Fluid percussion brain injury exacerbates glutamate-induced focal damage in the rat. J Neurotrauma 16:195–201, 1999.
115. Di X, Lyeth BG, Hamm RJ, Bullock MR: Voltage-dependent Na^+/K^+ ion channel blockade fails to ameliorate behavioral deficits after traumatic brain injury in the rat. J Neurotrauma 13:497–504, 1996.
116. Dietrich WD, Alonso O, Busto R, Finklestein SP: Posttreatment with intravenous basic fibroblast growth factor reduces histopathological damage following fluid-percussion brain injury in rats. J Neurotrauma 13:309–316, 1996.
117. Dietrich WD, Alonso O, Busto R, Ginsberg MD: Widespread metabolic depression and reduced somatosensory circuit activation following traumatic brain injury in rats. J Neurotrauma 11:629–640, 1994.
118. Dimlich RV, Tornheim PA, Kindel RM, Hall ED, Braughler JM, McCall JM: Effects of a 21-aminosteroid (U-74006F) on cerebral metabolites and edema after severe experimental head trauma. Adv Neurol 52:365–375, 1990.
119. Dingledine R, Borges K, Bowie D, Traynelis SF: The glutamate receptor ion channels. Pharmacol Rev 51:7–61, 1999.
120. Dixon CE, Clifton GL, Lighthall JW, Yaghmai A, Hayes RL: A controlled cortical impact model of traumatic brain injury in the rat. J Neurosci Meth 39:253–262, 1991.
121. Dixon CE, Flinn P, Bao J, Venya R, Hayes RL: Nerve growth factor attenuates cholinergic deficits following traumatic brain injury in rats. Exp Neurol 146:479–490, 1997.
122. Dixon CE, Lyeth BG, Povlishock JT, Findling R, Hamm R, Marmarou A, Young HF, Hayes RL: A fluid percussion model of experimental brain injury in the rat: Neurological, physiological, and histopathological characteristics. J Neurosurg 67:110–119, 1987.
123. Dixon CE, Ma X, Kline AE, Yan HQ, Ferimer H, Kochanek PM, Wisniewski SR, Jenkins LW, Marion DW: Acute etomidate treatment reduces cognitive deficits and histopathology in rats with traumatic brain injury. Crit Care Med 31:2222–2227, 2003.
124. Dixon CE, Ma X, Marion DW: Effects of CDP-choline treatment on neurobehavioral deficits after TBI and on hippocampal and neocortical acetylcholine release. J Neurotrauma 14:159–166, 1997.
125. Doppenberg EM, Reinert M, Zauner A, Massie TS, Bullock R: Determinants of cerebral extracellular potassium after severe human head injury. Acta Neurochir (Suppl) (Wien) 75:31–34, 1999.
126. Ebadi M, Bashir RM, Heidrick ML, Hamada FM, Refaey HE, Hamed A, Helal G, Baxi MD, Cerutis DR, Lassi NK: Neurotrophins and their receptors in nerve injury and repair. Neurochem Int 30:347–374, 1997.
127. Erb DE, Povlishock JT: Axonal damage in severe traumatic brain injury: An experimental study in the cat. Acta Neuropathol (Berl) 76:347–358, 1988.
128. Eriksdotter JM, Nordberg A, Amberla K, Backman L, Ebendal T, Meyerson B, Olson L, Seiger, Shigeta M, Theodorsson E, Viitanen M, Winblad B, Wahlund LO: Intracerebroventricular infusion of nerve growth factor in three patients with Alzheimer's disease. Dement Geriatr Cogn Disord 9:246–257, 1998.
129. Esen F, Erdem T, Aktan D, Kalayci R, Cakar N, Kaya M, Telci L: Effects of magnesium administration on brain edema and blood–brain barrier breakdown after experimental traumatic brain injury in rats. J Neurosurg Anesthesiol 15:119–125, 2003.
130. Faden AI, Demediuk P, Panter SS, Vink R: The role of excitatory amino acids and NMDA receptors in traumatic brain injury. Science 244:789–800, 1989.
131. Faden AI, Demediuk P, Panter SS, Vink R: The role of excitatory amino acids and NMDA receptors in traumatic brain injury. Science 244:798–800, 1989.
132. Faden AI, O'Leary DM, Fan L, Bao W, Mullins PG, Movsesyan VA: Selective blockade of the mGluR1 receptor reduces traumatic neuronal injury in vitro and improves outcome after brain trauma. Exp Neurol 167:435–444, 2001.
133. Fan L, Young PR, Barone FC, Feuerstein GZ, Smith DH, McIntosh TK: Experimental brain injury induces expression of interleukin-1b mRNA in the rat brain. Mol Brain Res 30:125–130, 1995.
134. Fan L, Young PR, Barone FC, Feuerstein GZ, Smith DH, McIntosh TK: Experimental brain injury induces differential expression of tumor necrosis factor-α mRNA in the CNS. Mol Brain Res 36:287–291, 1996.
135. Feeney DM, Boyeson MG, Linn RT, Murray HM, Dail WG: Responses to cortical injury. I. Methodology and local effects of contusions in the rat. Brain Res 211:67–77, 1981.
136. Feldman Z, Gurevitch B, Artru AA, Oppenheim A, Shohami E, Reichenthal E, Shapira Y: Effect of magnesium given 1 hour after head trauma on brain edema and neurological outcome. J Neurosurg 85:131–137, 1996.
137. Fineman I, Hovda DA, Smith M, Yoshino A, Becker DP: Concussive brain injury is associated with a prolonged accumulation of calcium: A ^{45}Ca autoradiographic study. Brain Res 624:94–102, 1993.

138. Fink KB, Andrews LJ, Butler WE, Ona VO, Li M, Bogdanov M, Endres M, Khan SQ, Namura S, Stieg PE, Beal MF, Moskowitz MA, Yuan J, Friedlander RM: Reduction of post-traumatic brain injury and free radical production by inhibition of the caspase-1 cascade. Neuroscience 94:1213–1218, 1999.
139. Fiskum G: Mitochondrial participation in ischemic and traumatic neural cell death. J Neurotrauma 17:843–855, 2000.
140. Forbes ML, Hendrich KS, Kochanek PM, Williams DS, Schiding JK, Wisniewski SR, Kelsey SF, DeKosky ST, Graham SH, Marion DW, Ho C: Assessment of cerebral blood flow and CO_2 reactivity after controlled cortical impact by perfusion magnetic resonance imaging using arterial spin-labeling in rats [erratum appears in J Cereb Blood Flow Metab 1997 Nov;17(11): 1263]. J Cereb Blood Flow Metab 17:865–874, 1997.
141. Friedlander RM, Gagliardini V, Rotello RJ, Yuan J: Functional role of interleukin 1 beta (IL-1 beta) in IL-1 beta-converting enzyme-mediated apoptosis. J Exp Med 184:717–724, 1996.
142. Friedman G, Froom P, Sazbon L, Grinblatt I, Shochina M, Tsenter J, Babaey S, Yehuda B, Groswasser Z: Apolipoprotein E-epsilon4 genotype predicts a poor outcome in survivors of traumatic brain injury. Neurology 52:244–248, 1999.
143. Friedman SD, Brooks WM, Jung RE, Hart BL, Yeo RA: Proton MR spectroscopic findings correspond to neuropsychological function in traumatic brain injury. Am J Neuroradiol 19:1879–1885, 1998.
144. Gage FH, Armstrong DM, Williams LR, Varon S: Morphological response of axotomized septal neurons to nerve growth factor. J Comp Neurol 269:147–155, 1988.
145. Gahm C, Holmin S, Mathiesen T: Temporal profiles and cellular sources of three nitric oxide synthase isoforms in the brain after experimental contusion. Neurosurgery 46:169–177, 2000.
146. Gahm C, Holmin S, Mathiesen T: Nitric oxide synthase expression after human brain contusion. Neurosurgery 50:1319–1326, 2002.
147. Gallyas F, Zoltay G, Balas I: An immediate light microscopic response of neuronal somata, dendrites and axons to contusing concussive head injury in the rat. Acta Neuropathol (Berl) 83:394–401, 1992.
148. Garcia JH, Liu KF, Relton JK: Interleukin-1 receptor antagonist decreases the number of necrotic neurons in rats with middle cerebral artery occlusion. Am J Pathol 147:1477–1486, 1995.
149. Garnett MR, Corkill RG, Blamire AM, Rajagopalan B, Manners DN, Young JD, Styles P, Cadoux-Hudson TA: Altered cellular metabolism following traumatic brain injury: A magnetic resonance spectroscopy study. J Neurotrauma 18:231–240, 2001.
150. Gean AD: Imaging of Head Trauma. New York, Raven Press, 1994.
151. Geddes JF, Vowles GH, Beer TW, Ellison DW: The diagnosis of diffuse axonal injury: Implications for forensic practice. Neuropathol Appl Neurobiol 23:339–347, 1997.
152. Geddes JF, Whitwell HL, Graham DI: Traumatic axonal injury: Practical issues for diagnosis in medicolegal cases. Neuropathol Appl Neurobiol 26:105–116, 2000.
153. Gennarelli TA: Cerebral concussion and diffuse brain injuries. In: Cooper PR (ed): Head Injury. Philadelphia, Williams & Wilkins, 1993, pp 137–158.
154. Gennarelli TA: Mechanisms of brain injury. J Emerg Med 11(suppl 1):5–11, 1993.
155. Gennarelli TA: Animate models of human head injury. J Neurotrauma 11:357–368, 1994.
156. Gennarelli TA: The pathobiology of traumatic brain injury. Neuroscientist 3:73–81, 1997.
157. Gennarelli TA, Thibault LE: Biomechanics of acute subdural hematoma. J Trauma: Inj Inf Crit Care 22:680–686, 1982.
158. Gennarelli TA, Thibault LE, Adams JH, Graham DI, Thompson C, Marcincin RP: Diffuse axonal injury and traumatic coma in the primate. Ann Neurol 12:564–574, 1982.
159. Gennarelli TA, Thibault LE, Tipperman R, Gennarelli LM, Duhaime AC, Boock R, Greenberg J: Axonal injury in the optic nerve: A model that simulates diffuse axonal injury in the brain. J Neurosurg 71:244–253, 1989.
160a. Gentleman SM, Nash MJ, Sweeting CJ, et al: β-Amyloid precursor protein (b-APP) as a marker for axonal injury after head injury. Neurosci Lett 160:134–144, 1993.
160b. Gentleman, SM, Graham DI, Roberts GW: Molecular pathology of head trauma: altered beta APP metabolism and the aetiology of Alzhemer's disease. Progress in Brain Research 96:237–246, 1993.
161. Gerschman R, Gilbert DL, Nye SW, Dwyer P, Fenn WO: Oxygen poisoning and x-irradiation: A mechanism in common. Science 119:623–626, 1954.
162. Gianotta SL, Weiss MH, Apuzzo ML, Martin E: High dose glucocorticoids in the management of severe head injury. Neurosurgery 15:497–501, 1984.
163. Gibson S, Widmann C, Johnson GL: Differential involvement of MEK kinase 1 (MEKK1) in the induction of apoptosis in response to microtubule-targeted drugs versus DNA damaging agents. J Biol Chem 274:10916–10922, 1999.
164. Gill SS, Patel NK, Hotton GR, O'Sullivan K, McCarter R, Bunnage M, Brooks DJ, Svendsen CN, Heywood P: Direct brain infusion of glial cell line–derived neurotrophic factor in Parkinson disease. Nature Med 9:589–595, 2003.
165. Ginsberg MD, Zhao W, Alonso OF, Loor-Estades JY, Dietrich WD, Busto R: Uncoupling of local cerebral glucose metabolism and blood flow after acute fluid-percussion injury in rats. Am J Physiol 272:H2859–H2868, 1997.
166. Ginsberg MD, Zhao W, Belayev L, Alonso OF, Liu Y, Loor JY, Busto R: Diminution of metabolism/blood flow uncoupling following traumatic brain injury in rats in response to high-dose human albumin treatment. J Neurosurg 94:499–509, 2001.

167. Goldman H, Hodgson V, Morehead M, Hazlett J, Murphy S: Cerebrovascular changes in a rat model of moderate closed-head injury. J Neurotrauma 8:129–144, 1991.
168. Goll DE, Thompson VF, Li H, Wei W, Cong J: The calpain system. Physiol Rev 83:731–801, 2003.
169. Gong QZ, Delahunty TM, Hamm RJ, Lyeth BG: Metabotropic glutamate antagonist MCPG in the treatment of traumatic brain injury in rats. Brain Res 700(1–2):299–302, 1995.
170. Goodman JC, Valadka AB, Gopinath SP, Uzura M, Grossman RG, Robertson CS: Simultaneous measurement of cortical potassium, calcium, and magnesium levels measured in head injured patients using microdialysis with ion chromatography. Acta Neurochir (Suppl) (Wien) 75:35–37, 1999.
171. Gourin CG, Shackford SR: Production of tumor necrosis factor-α and interleukin-1b by human cerebral microvascular endothelium after percussive trauma. J Trauma 42:1101–1107, 1997.
172. Grady MS, Charleston JS, Maris D, Witgen BM, Lifshitz J: Neuronal and glial cell number in the hippocampus after experimental traumatic brain injury: Analysis by stereological estimation. J Neurotrauma 20:929–941, 2003.
173. Grady MS, McLaughlin MR, Christman CW, Valadka AB, Fligner CL, Povlishock JT: The use of antibodies targeted against the neurofilament subunits for the detection of diffuse axonal injury in humans. J Neuropathol Exp Neurol 52:143–152, 1993.
174. Graham DI: Hypoxia and vascular disorders. In: Adams HJ, Duchen IW (eds): Greenfield's Neuropathology. New York, Oxford University Press, 1992, pp 153–268.
175. Graham DI, Adams JH, Doyle D: Ischaemic brain damage in fatal non-missle head injuries. J Neurol Sci 39:213–234, 1978.
176. Graham DI, Adams JH, Nicoll JA, Maxwell WL, Gennarelli TA: The nature, distribution and causes of traumatic brain injury. Brain Pathol 5:397–406, 1995.
177. Graham DI, Clark JC, Adams JH, Gennarelli TA: Diffuse axonal injury caused by assault. J Clin Pathol 45: 840–841, 1992.
178a. Graham DI, Ford I, Adams JH, Doyle D, Lawrence AE, McLellan DR, Ng HK: Fatal head injury in children. J Clin Pathol 42:18–22, 1989.
178b. Graham DI, Smith C, Reichard R, Leclercq PD, Gentleman SM. Trials and tribulations of using beta-amyloid precursor protein immunohistochemistry to evaluate traumatic brain injury in adults. Forensic Sci Int. 146: 89–96, 2004.
179. Graham DI, Ford I, Adams JH, Doyle D, Teasdale G, Lawrence A, McLellan DR: Ischaemic brain damage is still common in fatal nonmissile head injury. J Neurol Neurosurg Psychiatry 52:346–350, 1989.
180. Graham DI, Gennarelli TA, McIntosh TK: Cellular and molecular consequences of TBI. In: Graham DI, Luntus PL (eds): Greenfield's Neuropathology. London, Arnold, 2002, pp 823–898.
181. Graham DI, Gennarelli TA, McIntosh TK: Cellular and molecular consequences of TBI. In: Graham DI, Luntus PL (eds): Greenfield's Neuropathology. London, Arnold, 2002, pp 823–898.
182. Graham DI, Gentleman SM, Nicoll JAR, Royston MC, McKenzie JE, Roberts GW, Griffin WS: Altered beta-APP metabolism after head injury and its relationship to the aetology of Alzheimer's disease. Acta Neurochir (Suppl) (Wien) 66:96–102, 1996.
183. Graham DI, Gentleman SM, Nicoll JA, Royston MC, McKenzie JE, Roberts GW, Mrak RE, Griffin WS: Is there a genetic basis for the deposition of beta-amyloid after fatal head injury? Cell Mol Neurobiol 19:19–30, 1999.
184. Graham DI, Horsburgh K, Nicoll JA, Teasdale GM: Apolipoprotein E and the response of the brain to injury. Acta Neurochir (Suppl) (Wien) 73:89–92, 1999.
185. Graham DI, Lawrence AE, Adams JH, et al: Brain damage in non-missile head injury secondary to high intracranial pressure. Neuropathol Appl Neurobiol 13: 209–217, 1987.
186. Graham DI, Lawrence AE, Adams JH, et al: Brain damage in fatal non-missile head injury without high intracranial pressure. J Clin Pathol 41:34–37, 1988.
187. Graham DI, Raghupathi R, Saatman KE, Meaney DF, McIntosh TK: Tissue tears in the white matter after lateral fluid percussion brain injury in the rat: Relevance to human brain injury. Acta Neuropathol 99:117–124, 2000.
188. Grate LL, Golden JA, Hoopes PJ, Hunter JV, Duhaime AC: Traumatic brain injury in piglets of different ages: Techniques for lesion analysis using histology and magnetic resonance imaging. J Neurosci Methods 123:201–206, 2003.
189. Grcevic N: Topography and pathogenic mechanisms of lesions. In: Inner Cerebral Trauma. Nauke: Rad.Jun .Akad.ZNSM.UMJ.Od.Med., 1982, pp 265–331.
190. Green AR, Ashwood T, Odergren T, Jackson DM: Nitrones as neuroprotective agents in cerebral ischemia, with particular reference to NXY-059. Pharm Ther 100:195–214, 2003.
191. Griffin WS, Sheng JG, Gentleman SM, Graham DI, Mrak RE, Roberts GW: Microglial interleukin-1 alpha expression in human head injury: Correlations with neuronal and neuritic beta-amyloid precursor protein expression. Neurosci Lett 176:133–136, 1994.
192. Griffin WS, Sheng JG, Royston MC, Gentleman SM, McKenzie JE, Graham DI, Roberts GW, Mrak RE: Glial–neuronal interactions in Alzheimer's disease: The potential role of a "cytokine cycle" in disease progression. Brain Pathol 8:65–72, 1998.
193. Grisar JM, Bolkenius FN, Petty MA, Verne J: 2,3-Dihydro-1-benzofuran-5-ols as analogues of alpha-tocopherol that inhibit in vitro and ex vivo lipid autoxidation and protect mice against central nervous system trauma. J Med Chem 38:453–458, 1995.
194. Grumme T, Baethmann A, Kolodziejczyk D, Krimmer J, Fischer M, von Eisenhart Rothe B, Pelka R,

Bennefeld H, Pollauer E, Kostron H: Treatment of patients with severe head injury by triamcinolone: A prospective, controlled multicenter clinical trial of 396 cases. Res Exp Med 195:217–229, 1995.
195. Gudeman SK, Miller JD, Becker DP: Failure of high-dose steroid therapy to influence intracranial pressure in patients with severe head injury. J Neurosurg 51: 301–306, 1979.
196. Gulama K, Saatman KE, Brown A, Raghupathi R, McIntosh TK: Sequential pharmacotherapy with magnesium chloride and basic fibroblast factor (bFGF) after fluid percussion brain injury results in less neuromotor efficacy than that achieved with magnesium alone. J Neurotrauma 16:311–321, 1999.
197. Gurevich B, Artru AA, Lam AM, Mueller AL, Merkind V, Talmor D, Katchko L, Shapira Y: Neuroprotective effects of NPS 846, a novel *N*-methyl-D-aspartate receptor antagonist, after closed head trauma in rats. J Neurosurg 88:1066–1074, 1998.
198. Gutteridge JM, Halliwell B: Free radicals and antioxidants in the year 2000. A historical look to the future. Ann NY Acad Sci 899:136–147, 2000.
199. Haber F, Weiss J: The catalytic decomposition of hydrogen peroxide by iron salts. Proc R Soc Lond Ser A 147:351, 1934.
200. Hall ED: Beneficial effects of acute intravenous ibuprofen on neurologic recovery of head-injured mice: Comparison of cyclooxygenase inhibition with inhibition of thromboxane A2 synthetase or 5-lipoxygenase. Cent Nerv Syst Trauma 2:75–83, 1985.
201. Hall ED, Andrew PK, Yonker PA: Brain hydroxyl radical generation in acute experimental head injury. J Neurochem 60:588–594, 1993.
202. Hall ED, Detloff MR, Johnson K, Kupina NC: Peroxynitrite-mediated protein nitration and lipid peroxidation in a mouse model of traumatic brain injury. J Neurotrauma 21:9–20, 2004.
203. Hall ED, Kupina NC, Althaus JS: Peroxynitrite scavengers for the acute treatment of traumatic brain injury. Ann NY Acad Sci 890:462–468, 1999.
204. Hall ED, McCall JM, Chase RL, Yonkers PA, Braughler JM: A non-glucocorticoid steroid analog of methylprednisolone duplicates its high-dose pharmacology in models of central nervous system trauma and neuronal membrane damage. J Pharmacol Exp Ther 242:137–142, 1987.
205. Hall ED, Yonkers PA, McCall JM, Braughler JM: Effects of the 21-aminosteroid U74006F on experimental head injury in mice. J Neurosurg 68:456–461, 1988.
206. Halliwell B, Gutteridge JMC: Oxygen free radicals and iron in relation to biology and medicine: Some problems and concepts. Arch Biochem Biophys 246:501–514, 1986.
207. Hamberger A, Nystrom B: Extra- and intracellular amino acids in the hippocampus during development of hepatic encephalopathy. Neurochem Res 9:1181–1192, 1984.
208. Hamm RJ, Lyeth BG, Jenkins LW, O'Dell DM, Pike BR: Selective cognitive impairment following traumatic brain injury in rats. Behav Brain Res 59:169–173, 1993.
209. Hamm RJ, Pike BR, O'Dell DM, Lyeth BG: Traumatic brain injury enhances the amnesic effect of an NMDA antagonist in rats. J Neurosurg 81:267–271, 1994.
210. Hamm RJ, Temple MD, Pike BR, Ellis EF: The effect of postinjury administration of polyethylene glycol-conjugated superoxide dismutase (Pegorgotein Dismutec®) or lidocaine on behavioral function following fluid-percussion brain injury in rats. J Neurotrauma 13:325–332, 1996.
211. Hans VH, Kossmann T, Joller H, Otto V, Morganti-Kossmann MC: Interleukin-6 and its soluble receptor in serum and cerebrospinal fluid after cerebral trauma. NeuroReport 10:409–412, 1999.
212. Hans VH, Kossmann T, Lenzlinger PM, Probstmeier R, Imhof H, Trentz O, Morganti-Kossmann MC: Experimental axonal injury triggers interleukin-6 mRNA, protein synthesis and release into cerebrospinal fluid. J Cereb Blood Flow Metab 19:184–194, 1999.
213. Hansson H-A: Insulin-like growth factors and nerve regeneration. Ann NY Acad Sci 692:161–171, 1993.
214. Hatton J, Rapp RP, Kudsk KA, Brown RO, Luer MS, Bukar JG, Chen SA, McClain CJ, Gesundheit N, Dempsey RJ, Young B: Intravenous insulin-like growth factor-I (IGF-I) in moderate-to-severe head injury: A phase II safety and efficacy trial. J Neurosurg 86:779–786, 1997.
215. Heath DL, Vink R: Magnesium sulphate improves neurologic outcome following severe closed head injury in rats. Neurosci Lett 228:175–178, 1997.
216. Heath DL, Vink R: Blood-free magnesium concentration declines following graded experimental traumatic brain injury. Scand J Clin Lab Invest 58:161–166, 1998.
217. Heath DL, Vink R: Brain free magnesium concentration is predictive of motor outcome following traumatic axonal brain injury in rats. Magnes Res 12:269–277, 1999.
218. Heath DL, Vink R: Delayed therapy with magnesium up to 24 h following traumatic brain injury improves motor outcome. J Neurosurg 90:504–509, 1999.
219. Heath DL, Vink R: Optimization of magnesium therapy after severe diffuse axonal brain injury in rats. J Pharmacol Exp Ther 288:1311–1316, 1999.
220. Heath DL, Vink R: Subdural hematoma following traumatic brain injury causes a secondary decline in brain free magnesium concentration. J Neurotrauma 18:465–469, 2001.
221. Hefti F: Nerve growth factor promotes survival of septal cholinergic neurons after fimbrial transections. J Neurosci 6:2155–2162, 1986.
222. Hellmich HL, Frederickson CJ, DeWitt DS, Saban R, Parsley MO, Stephenson R, Velasco M, Uchida T, Shimamura M, Prough DS: Protective effects of zinc chelation in traumatic brain injury correlate with upregulation of neuroprotective genes in rat brain. Neurosci Lett 355:221–225, 2004.
223. Hermann DM, Kilic E, Kugler S, Isenmann S, Bahr M:

Adenovirus-mediated glial cell line–derived neurotrophic factor (GDNF) expression protects against subsequent cortical cold injury in rats. Neurobiol Dis 8:964–973, 2001.
224. Hicks RR, Gennarelli TA, McIntosh TK: Kynurenate is neuroprotective following experimental brain injury in the rat. Brain Res 655:91–96, 1994.
225. Hicks RR, Smith DH, Lowenstein DH, Saint Marie RL, McIntosh TK: Mild experimental brain injury in the rat induces cognitive deficits associated with regional neuronal loss in the hippocampus. J Neurotrauma 10:405–414, 1993.
226. Hicks RR, Smith DH, McIntosh TK: Temporal response and effects of excitatory amino acid antagonism on microtubule-associated protein 2 immunoreactivity following experimental brain injury in rats. Brain Res 678:151–160, 1995.
227. Hicks RR, Soares HD, Smith DH, McIntosh TK: Temporal and spatial characterization of neuronal injury following lateral fluid-percussion brain injury in the rat. Acta Neuropathol 91:236–246, 1996.
228. Hill-Felberg SJ, McIntosh TK, Oliver DL, Raghupathi R, Barbarese E: Concurrent loss and proliferation of astrocytes following lateral fluid percussion brain injury in the adult rat. J Neurosci Res 57:271–279, 1999.
229. Hillered L, Ernster L: Respiratory activity of isolated rat brain mitochondria following in vitro exposure to oxygen radicals. J Cereb Blood Flow Metab 3:207–214, 1983.
230. Hisahara S, Shoji S, Okano H, Miura M: ICE/CED-3 family executes oligodendrocyte apoptosis by tumor necrosis factor. J Neurochem 69:10–20, 1997.
231. Hlatky R, Lui H, Cherian L, Goodman JC, O'Brien WE, Contant CF, Robertson CS: The role of endothelial nitric oxide synthase in the cerebral hemodynamics after controlled cortical impact injury in mice. J Neurotrauma 20:995–1006, 2003.
232. Holmin S, Biberfeld P, Mathiesen T: Intracerebral inflammation after human brain contusion. Neurosurgery 42:291–299, 1998.
233. Holmin S, Mathiesen T, Shetye J, Biberfeld P: Intracerebral inflammatory response to experimental brain contusion. Acta Neurochir (Wien) 132:110–119, 1995.
234. Holmin S, Schalling M, Hojeberg B, Nordqvist AC, Skeftruna AK, Mathiesen T: Delayed cytokine expression in rat brain following experimental contusion. J Neurosurg 86:493–504, 1997.
235. Hovda DA, Yoshino A, Kawamata T, Katayama Y, Becker DP: Diffuse prolonged depression of cerebral oxidative metabolism following concussive brain injury in the rat: A cytochrome oxidase histochemistry study. Brain Res 567:1–10, 1991.
236. Huang Y, Wang KK: The calpain family and human disease. Trends Mol Med 7:355–362, 2001.
237. Huettner JE: Indole-2-carboxylic acid: A competitive antagonist of potentiation by glycine at the NMDA receptor. Science 243:1611–1613, 1989.
238. Hughes PE, Alexi T, Hefti F, Knusel B: Axotomized septal cholinergic neurons rescued by nerve growth factor or neurotrophin-4/5 fail to express the inducible transcription factor c-Jun. Neuroscience 78:1037–1049, 1997.
239. Hukkelhoven CW, Steyerberg EW, Farace E, Habbema JD, Marshall LF, Maas AI: Regional differences in patient characteristics, case management, and outcomes in traumatic brain injury: Experience from the tirilazad trials [see comment]. J Neurosurg 97:549–557, 2002.
240. Hurley SD, Olschowka JA, O'Banion MK: Cyclooxygenase inhibition as a strategy to ameliorate brain injury. J Neurotrauma 19:1–15, 2002.
241. Iadecola C: Bright and dark sides of nitric oxide in ischemic brain injury. Trends Neurosci 20:132–139, 1997.
242. Ikeda Y, Ikeda K, Long DM: Protective effect of the iron chelator deferoxamine on cold-induced brain edema. J Neurosurg 71:233–238, 1989.
243. Ikonomidou C, Stefovska V, Turski L: Neuronal death enhanced by *N*-methyl-D-aspartate antagonists. Proc Natl Acad Sci USA 97:12885–12890, 2000.
244. Imajo T, Challener RC, Roessman U: Diffuse axonal injury by assault. Am J Forensic Med Pathol 8:217–219, 1987.
245. Inci S, Ozcan OE, Kilinc K: Time-level relationship for lipid peroxidation and the protective effect of alpha-tocopherol in experimental mild and severe brain injury. Neurosurgery 43:330–335, 1998.
246. Ironside JW, Pickard JD: Raised intracranial pressure, oedema and hydrocephalus. In: Graham DI, Lantos PL (eds): Greenfield's Neuropathology. London, Arnold, 2002, pp 193–231.
247. Isaksson J, Hillered L, Olsson Y: Cognitive and histopathological outcome after weight-drop brain injury in the rat: Influence of systemic administration of monoclonal antibodies to ICAM-1. Acta Neuropathol 102:246–256, 2001.
248. Isaksson J, Lewen A, Hillered L, Olsson Y: Upregulation of intercellular adhesion molecule 1 in cerebral microvessels after cortical contusion trauma in a rat model. Acta Neuropathol 94:16–20, 1997.
249. Jennett B, Adams JH, Murray LS, Graham DI: Neuropathology in vegetative and severely disabled patients after head injury. Neurology 56:486–490, 2001.
250. Jennett B, Bond M: Assessment of outcome after severe brain injury: A practical scale. Lancet 1:480, 1975.
251. Jones PA, Andrews PJD, Midgley S: Measuring the burden of secondary insults in head-injured patients during intensive care. J Neurosurg Anesthesiol 6:4–14, 1994.
252. Jordan BD, Relkin NR, Ravdin LD, Jacobs AR, Bennett A, Gandy S: Apolipoprotein E epsilon4 associated with chronic traumatic brain injury in boxing. JAMA 278:136–140, 1997.
253. Kahraman S, Ozgurtas T, Kayali H, Atabey C, Kutluay T, Timurkaynak E: Monitoring of serum ionized magnesium in neurosurgical intensive care unit: Preliminary results. Clin Chim Acta 334:211–215, 2003.

254. Kampfl A, Posmantur R, Nixon R, Grynspan F, Zhao X, Liu SJ, Newcomb JK, Clifton GL, Hayes RL: M-calpain activation and calpain mediated cytoskeletal proteolysis following traumatic brain injury. J Neurochem 67:1575–1583, 1996.
255. Kantrow SP, Piantadosi CA: Release of cytochrome c from liver mitochondria during permeability transition. Biochem Biophys Res Commun 232:669–671, 1997.
256. Kasarskis EJ, Shefner JM, Miller R, Smith RA, Licht J, Mitsumoto H, Hopkins LC, Rosenfeld J, Pascuzzi R, Cornblath DR, Armon C, Strong MJ, Kula R, Windebank A, Bosch EP, Smith BE, Cashman N, Sivak M, Sergay S, Siddique T, Sufit RL, Johnston W, Brooke MB, Graves MC, Olney RK, Roos RP, Neville H, Ringel SP, Ross M, Bradley WG, Sharma KR, Parry G, Mandler R, Giuliani M, Thornton CA, Jackson C, Bryan W, Bromberg M, Tandan R, Fries T, Phillips L, Brooks BR, Fenichel G, Pestronk A, Bear M, Beatey R, Fuller C, Hill R, Malta E, Nakanishi A, Patel A, Thurmond B, Cedarbaum JM, Stambler N: A controlled trial of recombinant methionyl human BDNF in ALS. Neurology 52:1427–1433, 1999.
257. Katayama Y, Becker DP, Tamura T, Hovda DA: Massive increases in extracellular potassium and the indiscriminate release of glutamate following concussive brain injury. J Neurosurg 73:889–900, 1990.
258. Kavanagh RJ, Kam PC: Lazaroids: Efficacy and mechanism of action of the 21-aminosteroids in neuroprotection. Br J Anaesth 86:110–119, 2001.
259. Kawamata T, Dietrich WD, Schallert T, Gotts JE, Cocke RR, Benowitz LI, Finklestein SP: Intracisternal basic fibroblast growth factor enhances functional recovery and up-regulates the expression of a molecular marker of neuronal sprouting following focal cerebral infarction. Proc Natl Acad Sci USA 94:8179–8184, 1997.
260. Kawamata T, Katayama Y, Hovda DA, Yoshino A, Becker DP: Lactate accumulation following concussive brain injury: The role of ionic fluxes induced by excitatory amino acids. Brain Res 674:196–204, 1995.
261. Kaya SS, Mahmood A, Li Y, Yavuz E, Goksel M, Chopp M: Apoptosis and expression of p53 response proteins and cyclin D1 after cortical impact in rat brain. Brain Res 818:23–33, 1999.
262. Keeling KL, Hicks RR, Mahesh J, Billings BB, Kotwal GJ: Local neutrophil influx following lateral fluid-percussion brain injury in rats is associated with accumulation of complement activation fragments of the third component (C3) of the complement system. J Neuroimmunol 105:20–30, 2000.
263. Kempermann G, van Praag H, Gage FH: Activity-dependent regulation of neuronal plasticity and self repair. Prog Brain Res 127:35–48, 2000.
264. Kim BT, Rao VL, Sailor KA, Bowen KK, Dempsey RJ: Protective effects of glial cell line–derived neurotrophic factor on hippocampal neurons after traumatic brain injury in rats. J Neurosurg 95:674–679, 2001.
265. Kim HJ, Levasseur JE, Patterson JL, Jackson GF, Madge GE, Povlishock JT, Kontos HA: Effect of indomethacin pretreatment on acute mortality in experimental brain injury. J Neurosurg 71:565–572, 1989.
266. Knoblach SM, Faden AI: Interleukin-10 improves outcome and alters proinflammatory cytokine expression after experimental traumatic brain injury. Exp Neurol 153:143–151, 1998.
267. Knoblach SM, Fan L, Faden AI: Early neuronal expression of tumor necrosis factor-alpha after experimental brain injury contributes to neurological impairment. J Neuroimmunol 95:115–125, 1999.
268. Knoblach SM, Nikolaeva M, Huang X, Fan L, Krajewski S, Reed JC, Faden AI: Multiple caspases are activated after traumatic brain injury: Evidence for involvement in functional outcome. J Neurotrauma 19: 1155–1170, 2002.
269. Kobayashi NR, Fan DP, Giehl KM, Bedard AM, Wiegand SJ, Tetzlaff W: BDNF and NT-4/5 prevent atrophy of rat rubrospinal neurons after cervical axotomy, stimulate GAP-43 and T alpha 1-tubulin mRNA expression, and promote axonal regeneration. J Neurosci 17: 9583–9595, 1997.
270. Koc RK, Kurtsoy A, Pasaoglu H, Karakucuk EI, Oktem IS, Meral M: Lipid peroxidation and oedema in experimental brain injury: Comparison of treatment with methylprednisolone, tirilazad mesylate and vitamin E. Res Exp Med 199:21–28, 1999.
271. Kochanek PM, Marion DW, Zhang W, Schiding JK, White M, Palmer AM, Clark RS, O'Malley ME, Styren SD, Ho C: Severe controlled cortical impact in rats: Assessment of cerebral edema, blood flow, and contusion volume. J Neurotrauma 12:1015–1025, 1995.
272. Koliatsos VE, Applegate MD, Knusel B, Junard EO, Burton LE, Mobley WC, Hefti FF, Price DL: Recombinant human nerve growth factor prevents retrograde degeneration of axotomized basal forebrain cholinergic neurons in the rat. Exp Neurol 112:161–173, 1991.
273. Kontos HA: Oxygen radicals in cerebral vascular injury. Circ Res 57:508–516, 1985.
274. Korte M, Griesbeck O, Gravel C, Carroll P, Staiger V, Thoenen H, Bonhoeffer T: Virus-mediated gene transfer into hippocampal CA1 region restores long-term potentiation in brain-derived neurotrophic factor mutant mice. Proc Natl Acad Sci USA 93:12547–12552, 1996.
275. Kossmann T, Hans V, Imhof HG, Trentz O, Morganti-Kossmann MC: Interleukin-6 released in human cerebrospinal fluid following traumatic brain injury may trigger nerve growth factor production in astrocytes. Brain Res 713:143–152, 1996.
276. Kossmann T, Stahel PF, Lenzlinger PM, Redl H, Dubs RW, Trentz O, Schlag G, Morganti-Kossmann MC: Interleukin-8 released into the cerebrospinal fluid after brain injury is associated with blood-brain barrier dysfunction and nerve growth factor production. J Cereb Blood Flow Metab 17:280–289, 1997.
277. Kostron H, Rumpl E, Stampfl G, Russegger L, Grunert V: Treatment of cerebrovasospasm following severe head injury with the calcium channel influx blocker

nimodipine. Acta Neurochir (Wein) 28:103–109, 1985.

278. Kostron H, Twerdy K, Stampfl G, Mohsenipour I, Fischer J, Grunert V: Treatment of the traumatic cerebral vasospasm with the calcium channel blocker nimodipine. Neurol Res 6:29–32, 1984.

279. Kotapka MJ, Gennarelli TA, Graham DI, Adams JH, Thibault LE, Ross DT, Ford I: Selective vulnerability of hippocampal neurons in acceleration-induced experimental head injury. J Neurotrauma 8:247–258, 1991.

280. Kraus JF, McArthur DL: Epidemiology of head njury. In: Cooper PR, Golfinos JF (eds): Head Injury. New York, McGraw-Hill, 2000, pp 1–26.

281. Krishnappa IK, Contant CF, Robertson CS: Regional changes in cerebral extracellular glucose and lactate concentrations following severe cortical impact injury and secondary ischemia in rats. J Neurotrauma 16:213–224, 1999.

282. Kunz T, Marklund N, Hillered L, Oliw EH: Cyclooxygenase-2, prostaglandin synthases, and prostaglandin H2 metabolism in traumatic brain injury in the rat. J Neurotrauma 19:1051–1064, 2002.

283. Kupina NC, Detloff MR, Bobrowski WF, Snyder BJ, Hall ED: Cytoskeletal protein degradation and neurodegeneration evolves differently in males and females following experimental head injury. Exp Neurol 180:55–73, 2003.

284. Kupina NC, Nath R, Bernath EE, Inoue J, Mitsuyoshi A, Yuen PW, Wang KK, Hall ED: The novel calpain inhibitor SJA6017 improves functional outcome after delayed administration in a mouse model of diffuse brain injury. J Neurotrauma 18:1229–1240, 2001.

285. Kwon TH, Chao DL, Malloy K, Sun D, Alessandri B, Bullock MR: Tempol, a novel stable nitroxide, reduces brain damage and free radical production after acute subdural hematoma in the rat. J Neurotrauma 20:337–345, 2003.

286. La Fleur M, Underwood JL, Rappolee DA, Werb Z: Basement membrane and repair of injury to peripheral nerve: Defining a potential role of macrophages, matrix metalloproteinases, and tissue inhibitor of metalloproteinases-1. J Exp Med 184:2311–2326, 1996.

287. Langfitt TW, Tannanbaum HK, Kassell NF: The etiology of acute brain swelling following experimental head injury. J Neurosurg 24:172, 1966.

288. Langham J, Goldfrad C, Teasdale G, Shaw D, Rowan K: Calcium channel blockers for acute traumatic brain injury. Cochrane Database Syst Rev CD000565, 2003.

289. LaPlaca MC, Raghupathi R, Verma A, Pieper AA, Saatman KE, Snyder SH, McIntosh TK: Temporal patterns of poly(ADP-ribose) polymerase activation in the cortex following experimental brain injury in the rat. J Neurochem 73:205–213, 1999.

290. LaPlaca MC, Thibault LE: Dynamic mechanical deformation of neurons triggers an acute calcium response and cell injury involving the *N*-methyl-D-aspartate glutamate receptor. J Neurosci Res 52:220–229, 1998.

291. LaPlaca MC, Zhang J, Raghupathi R, Li JH, Smith F, Bareyre FM, Snyder SH, Graham DI, McIntosh TK: Pharmacologic inhibition of poly(ADP-ribose) polymerase is neuroprotective following traumatic brain injury in rats. J Neurotrauma 18:369–376, 2001.

292. Laurer HL, Lenzlinger PM, McIntosh TK: Models of traumatic brain injury. Eur J Trauma 26:95–110, 2000.

293. Laurer HL, McIntosh TK: Experimental models of brain trauma. Curr Opin Neurol 12:715–721, 1999.

294. Laurer HL, McIntosh TK: Pharmacologic therapy in traumatic brain injury: Update on experimental treatment strategies. Curr Pharm Design 7:1505–1516, 2001.

295a. Lazar L, Erez I, Gutermacher M, Katz S: Brain concussion produces transient hypokalemia in children. J Pediatr Surg 32:88–90, 1997.

295b. Leclercq PD, Stephenson MA, Graham DI, Gentleman SM. Morphological measurements of axonal swellings are not sufficient to date traumatic lesions. Neuropathol Appl Neurobiol 27:161 (Abstract), 2001.

296. Lee JS, Han YM, Yoo do S, Choi SJ, Choi BH, Kim JH, Kim YH, Huh PW, Ko YJ, Rh HK, Cho KS, Kim DS: A molecular basis for the efficacy of magnesium treatment following traumatic brain injury in rats. J Neurotrauma 21:549–561, 2004.

297. Lenzlinger PM, Morganti-Kossmann MC, Laurer HL, McIntosh TK: The duality of the inflammatory response to traumatic brain injury. Mol Neurobiol 24:169–181, 2001.

298. Leonard JR, Maris DO, Grady SM: Fluid percussion injury causes loss of forebrain choline acetyltransferase and nerve growth factor receptor immunoreactive cells in the rat. J Neurotrauma 11:379–392, 1994.

299. Leoni MJ, Chen X-H, Cheney JA, McIntosh TK, Smith DH: NPS-1506 attenuates cognitive dysfunction and hippocampal neuron death following brain trauma in the rat. Exp Neurol 166:442–449, 2000.

300. Levasseur JE, Alessandri B, Reinert M, Bullock R, Kontos HA: Fluid percussion injury transiently increases then decreases brain oxygen consumption in the rat. J Neurotrauma 17:101–112, 2000.

301. Lewen A, Fredriksson A, Li GL, Olsson Y, Hillered L: Behavioral and morphological outcome of mild cortical contusion trauma of the rat brain: Influence of NMDA-receptor blockade. Acta Neurochir (Suppl) (Wien) 141: 183–202, 1999.

302. Lewen A, Matz P, Chan PH: Free radical pathways in CNS injury. J Neurotrauma 17:871–890, 2000.

303. Lewen A, Skoglosa Y, Clausen F, Marklund N, Chan PH, Lindholm D, Hillered L: Paradoxical increase in neuronal DNA fragmentation after neuroprotective free radical scavenger treatment in experimental traumatic brain injury. J Cereb Blood Flow Metab 21:344–350, 2001.

304. Lifshitz J, Friberg H, Neumar RW, Raghupathi R, Welsh FA, Janmey P, Saatman KE, Wieloch T, Grady MS, McIntosh TK: Structural and functional damage sustained by mitochondria after traumatic brain injury in the rat: Evidence for differentially sensitive populations in the cortex and hippocampus. J Cereb Blood Flow Metab 23:219–231, 2003.

305. Lighthall JW: Controlled cortical impact: A new experimental brain injury model. J Neurotrauma 5:1–15, 1988.
306. Limbrick DD Jr, Sombati S, DeLorenzo RJ: Calcium influx constitutes the ionic basis for the maintenance of glutamate-induced extended neuronal depolarization associated with hippocampal neuronal death. Cell Calcium 33:69–81, 2003.
307. Liu J, Marino MW, Wong G, Grail D, Dunn A, Bettadapura J, Slavin AJ, Old L, Bernard CC: TNF is a potent anti-inflammatory cytokine in autoimmune-mediated demyelination. Nature Med 4:78–83, 1998.
308. Loddick SA, Turnbull AV, Rothwell NJ: Cerebral interleukin-6 is neuroprotective during permanent focal cerebral ishemia in the rat. J Cereb Blood Flow Metab 18:176–179, 1998.
309. Long DA, Ghosh K, Moore AN, Dixon CE, Dash PK: Deferoxamine improves spatial memory performance following experimental brain injury in rats. Brain Res 717:109–117, 1996.
310. Longhi L, Watson DJ, Saatman KE, Thompson HJ, Zhang C, Fujimoto S, Royo NC, Castelbuono D, Raghupathi R, Trojanowski JQ, Lee VMY, Wolfe JH, Stocchetti N, McIntosh TK: Ex vivo therapy using targeted engraftment of NGF-expressing human NT2N neurons attenuates cognitive deficits following traumatic brain injury in mice. J Neurotrauma 21:1723–1736, 2004.
311. Lorber A, Artru AA, Lam MA, Mueller LA, Karpas Z, Roytblat L, Shapira Y: NPS 1506: A novel NMDA receptor antagonist: Neuroprotective effects in a model of closed head trauma in rats. J Neurosurg Anesthesiol 12:345–355, 2000.
312. Lu D, Mahmood A, Zhang R, Copp M: Upregulation of neurogenesis and reduction in functional deficits following administration of DEtA/NONOate, a nitric oxide donor, after traumatic brain injury in rats. J Neurosurg 99:351–361, 2003.
313. Lu J, Moochhala S, Kaur C, Ling EA: Cellular inflammatory response associated with breakdown of the blood-brain barrier after closed head injury in rats. J Neurotrauma 18:399–408, 2001.
314. Lu J, Moochhala S, Shirhan M, Ng KC, Teo AL, Tan MH, Moore XL, Wong MC, Ling EA: Neuroprotection by aminoguanidine after lateral fluid-percussive brain injury in rats: A combined magnetic resonance imaging, histopathologic and functional study. Neuropharmacology 44:253–263, 2003.
315. Lu YC, Liu S, Gong QZ, Hamm RJ, Lyeth BG: Inhibition of nitric oxide synthase potentiates hypertension and increases mortality in traumatically brain-injured rats. Mol Chem Neuropathol 30:125–137, 1997.
316. Lyeth BG, Gong QZ, Shields S, Muizelaar JP, Berman RF: Group I metabotropic glutamate antagonist reduces acute neuronal degeneration and behavioral deficits after traumatic brain injury in rats. Exp Neurol 169:191–199, 2001.
317. Margulies SS, Gennarelli TA, Thibault LE: Physical model simulations of brain injury in the primate. J Biomechanics 23(8):823–836, 1990.
318. Marion DW, Puccio A, Wisniewski SR, Kochanek P, Dixon CE, Bullian L, Carlier P: Effect of hyperventilation on extracellular concentrations of glutamate, lactate, pyruvate, and local cerebral blood flow in patients with severe traumatic brain injury. Crit Care Med 30: 2619–2625, 2002.
319. Marion DW, White MJ: Treatment of experimental brain injury with moderate hypothermia and 21-aminosteroids. J Neurotrauma 13:139–147, 1996.
320. Marklund N, Clausen F, Lewen A, Hovda DA, Olsson Y, Hillered L: alpha-Phenyl-tert-*N*-butyl nitrone (PBN) improves functional and morphological outcome after cortical contusion injury in the rat. Acta Neurochir (Wien) 143:73–81, 2001.
321. Marklund N, Clausen F, McIntosh TK, Hillered L: Free radical scavenger posttreatment improves functional and morphological outcome after fluid percussion injury in the rat. J Neurotrauma 18:821–832, 2001.
322. Marklund N, Keck C, Hoover R, Soltesz K, Millard M, LeBold D, Spangler Z, Banning A, Benson J, McIntosh TK: Inhibition of the inflammatory mediators tumor necrosis factor alpha and interleukin-6 does not attenuate acute behavioral deficits following experimental traumatic brain injury in the rat. Rest Neurol Neurosci 23:31–42, 2005.
323. Marklund N, Lewander T, Clausen F, Hillered L: Effects of the nitrone radical scavengers PBN and S-PBN on in vivo trapping of reactive oxygen species after traumatic brain injury in rats. J Cereb Blood Flow Metab 21:1259–1267, 2001.
324. Marklund N, Salci K, Lewen A, Hillered L: Glycerol as a marker for post-traumatic membrane phospholipid degradation in rat brain. NeuroReport 8:1457–1461, 1997.
325. Marklund N, Sihver S, Langstrom B, Bergstrom M, Hillered L: Effect of traumatic brain injury and nitrone radical scavengers on relative changes in regional cerebral blood flow and glucose uptake in rats. J Neurotrauma 19:1139–1153, 2002.
326. Marklund N, Stover JF, McIntosh TK: Excitotoxicity and traumatic brain injury. Pathology, treatment approaches and controversies. In: Ferrarese C, Beal MF (eds): Excitotoxicity in Neurological Diseases. Boston, Kluwer Academic, 2004, pp .
327. Marmarou A, Foda MAA-E, van den Brink W, Campbell J, Kita H, Demetiadou K: A new model of diffuse brain injury in rats. Part I: Pathophysiology and biomechanics. J Neurosurg 80:291–300, 1994.
328. Marshall LF, Maas AI, Marshall SB, Bricolo A, Fearnside M, Iannotti F, Klauber MR, Lagarrigue J, Lobato R, Persson L, Pickard JD, Piek J, Servadei F, Wellis GN, Morris GF, Means ED, Musch B: A multicenter trial on the efficacy of using tirilazad mesylate in cases of head injury. J Neurosurg 89:519–525, 1998.
329. Marshall LF, Marshall SB, Klauber MR, et al: The diagnosis of head injury requires a classification based on

computed axial tomography. J Neurotrauma (Suppl 1) 9:S287, 1992.
330. Marshall LF, Toole BM, Bowers SA: The national traumatic coma data bank II. Patients who talk and deteriorate: Implications for treatment. J Neurosurg 59:285–288, 1983.
331. Matsuo Y, Kihara T, Ikeda M, Ninomiya M, Onodera H, Kogure K: Role of neutrophils in radical production during ischemia and reperfusion of the rat brain: Effect of neutrophil depletion on extracellular ascorbyl radical formation. J Cereb Blood Flow Metab 15:941–947, 1995.
332. Mattiasson GJ, Philips MF, Tomasevic G, Johansson BB, Wieloch T, McIntosh TK: The rotating pole test: Evaluation of its effectiveness in assessing functional motor deficits following experimental brain injury in the rat. J Neurosci Methods 95:75–82, 2000.
333. Mattson MP, Lovell MA, Furukawa K, Markesbery WR: Neurotrophic factors attenuate glutamate-induced accumulation of peroxides, elevation of intracellular Ca^{2+} concentration, and neurotoxicity and increase antioxidant enzyme activities in hippocampal neurons. J Neurochem 65:1740–1751, 1995.
334. Matute C, Alberdi E, Ibarretxe G, Sanchez-Gomez MV: Excitotoxicity in glial cells. Eur J Pharmacol 447:239–246, 2002.
335. Maxwell WL, Dhillon K, Harper L, Espin J, MacIntosh TK, Smith DH, Graham DI: There is differential loss of pyramidal cells from the human hippocampus with survival after blunt head injury. J Neuropathol Exp Neurol 62:272–279, 2003.
336. Maxwell WL, Domleo A, McColl G, Jafari SS, Graham DI: Post-acute alterations in the axonal cytoskeleton after traumatic axonal injury. J Neurotrauma 20:151–168, 2003.
337. Maxwell WL, Graham DI: Loss of axonal microtubules and neurofilaments after stretch-injury to guinea pig optic nerve fibers. J Neurotrauma 14:603–614, 1997.
338. Maxwell WL, McCreath BJ, Graham DI, Gennarelli TA: Cytochemical evidence for redistribution of membrane pump calcium-ATPase and ecto-Ca-ATPase activity, and calcium influx in myelinated nerve fibres of the optic nerve after stretch injury. J Neurocytol 24:925–942, 1995.
339. Maxwell WL, Povlishock JT, Graham DI: A mechanistic analysis of nondisruptive axonal injury: A review. J Neurotrauma 14:419–440, 1997.
340. Maxwell WL, Watt C, Graham DI, Gennarelli TA: Ultrastructural evidence of axonal shearing as a result of lateral acceleration of the head in non-human primates. Acta Neuropathol 86:136–144, 1993.
341. Mayer ML, Westbrook GL: The action of *N*-methyl-D-aspartic acid on mouse spinal neurones in culture. J Physiol (Lond) 361:65–90, 1985.
342. McCracken E, Hunter AJ, Patel S, Graham DI, Dewar D: Calpain activation and cytoskeletal protein breakdown in the corpus callosum of head-injured patients. J Neurotrauma 16:749–761, 1999.
343. McDermott KL, Raghupathi R, Fernandez SC, Saatman KE, Protter AA, Finkelstein SP, Smith DH, McIntosh TK: Delayed administration of basic fibroblast growth factor attenuates cognitive dysfunction following parasagittal fluid percussion brain injury in the rat. J Neurotrauma 14:191–200, 1997.
344. McIntosh TK, Banbury M, Smith DH, Thomas MJ: The novel 21-aminosteroid U-74006F attenuates cerebral edema and improves survival after brain injury in the rat. In: Reulen HJ, Baethmann A, Fenstermacker J, Marmarou A, Spatz M (eds): Brain Edema VIII. New York, Springer-Verlag, 1990, pp 329–330.
345. McIntosh TK, Noble L, Andrews B, Faden AI: Traumatic brain injury in the rat: Characterization of midline fluid-percussion model. Cent Nerv Syst Trauma 4:119–134, 1987.
346. McIntosh TK, Saatman KE, Raghupathi R: Calcium and the pathogenesis of traumatic CNS injury: Cellular and molecular mechanisms. Neuroscientist 3:169–175, 1997.
347. McIntosh TK, Saatman KE, Raghupathi R, Graham DI, Smith, DH, Lee VM, Trojanowski JQ: The Dorothy Russell Memorial Lecture. The molecular and cellular sequelae of experimental traumatic brain injury: pathogenetic mechanisms. Neuropathol Appl Neurobiol 24:251–267, 1998.
348. McIntosh TK, Thomas MJ, Smith DH, Banbury M: The novel 21-aminosteroid U74006F attenuates cerebral edema and improves survival after brain injury in the rat. J Neurotrauma 9:33–40, 1992.
349. McIntosh TK, Vink R, Noble L, Yamakami I, Fernyak S, Faden AI: Traumatic brain injury in the rat: Characterization of a lateral fluid percussion model. Neuroscience 28:233–244, 1989.
350. McIntosh TK, Vink R, Yamakami I, Faden AI: Magnesium deficiency exacerbates and pretreatment improves outcome following traumatic brain injury in rats. ^{31}P magnetic resonance spectroscopy and behavioral studies. J Neurotrauma 5:17–31, 1988.
351. McIntosh TK, Vink R, Yamakami I, Faden AI: Magnesium protects against neurological deficit after brain injury. Brain Res 482:252–260, 1989.
352. Megyeri P, Abraham CS, Temesvari P, Kovacs J, Vas T, Speer CP: Recombinant human tumor necrosis factor alpha constricts pial arterioles and increases blood–brain barrier permeability in newborn piglets. Neurosci Lett 148:137–140, 1992.
353. Meldrum B: Protection against ischemic neuronal damage by drugs acting on excitatory neurotransmission. Cerebrovasc Brain Metab Rev 2:27–57, 1990.
354. Memon ZI, Altura BT, Benjamin JL, Cracco RQ, Altura BM: Predictive value of serum ionized but not total magnesium levels in head injuries. Scand J Clin Lab Invest 55:671–677, 1995.
355. Mendelow AD, Teasdale G, Jennett B, Bryden J, Hessett C, Murray G: Risks of intracranial hematoma in head injured adults. Br Med J Clin Res Ed 287:1173–1176, 1983.

356. Mignani S, Bohme GA, Birraux G, Boireau A, Jimonet P, Damour D, Debono MW, Pratt J, Vuilhorgne M, Wahl F, Stutzmann J-M: 9-Carboxymethyl-5H,10H-imidazo[1,2-a]indeno[1,2-e]pyrazin-4-one-2-carbolic acid (RPR117824): Selective anticonvulsive and neuroprotective AMPA antagonist. Bioorg Med Chem 10: 1627–1637, 2002.
357. Minambres E, Cemborain A, Sanchez-Velasco P, Gandarillas M, Diaz-Reganon G, Sanchez-Gonzalez U, Leyva-Cobian F: Correlation between transcranial interleukin-6 gradient and outcome in patients with acute brain injury. Crit Care Med 31:933–938, 2003.
358. Mitha AP, Maynard KI: Gacyclidine (Beaufour-Ipsen). Curr Opin Invest Drugs 2:814–819, 2001.
359. Miyazaki S, Katayama Y, Lyeth BG, Jenkins LW, DeWitt DS, Goldberg SJ, Newlon PG, Hayes RL: Enduring suppression of hippocampal long-term potentiation following traumatic brain injury in rat. Brain Res 585:335–339, 1992.
360. Morganti-Kossmann MC, Lenzlinger PM, Stahel P, Csuka E, Ammann E, Stocker R, Trentz O, Kossmann T: Production of cytokines following brain injury: Beneficial and deleterious for the damaged tissue. Mol Psychol 2:133–136, 1997.
361. Morganti-Kossmann MC, Rancan M, Stahel PF, Kossmann T: Inflammatory response in acute traumatic brain injury: A double-edged sword. Curr Opin Crit Care 8:101–105, 2002.
362. Mori T, Kawamata T, Katayama Y, Maeda T, Aoyama N, Kikuchi T, Uwahodo Y: Antioxidant, OPC-14117, attenuates edema formation, and subsequent tissue damage following cortical contusion in rats. Acta Neurochir (Suppl) (Wien) 71:120–122, 1998.
363. Morse JK, Wiegand SJ, Anderson K, You Y, Cai N, Carnahan J, Miller J, DiStefano PS, Altar CA, Lindsay RM: Brain-derived neurotrophic factor (BDNF) prevents the degeneration of medial septal cholinergic neurons following fimbria transection. J Neurosci 13: 4146–4156, 1993.
364. Movsesyan VA, O'Leary DM, Fan L, Bao W, Mullins PG, Knoblach SM, Faden AI: mGluR5 antagonists 2-methyl-6-(phenylethynyl)-pyridine and (E)-2-methyl-6-(2-phenylethenyl)-pyridine reduce traumatic neuronal injury in vitro and in vivo by antagonizing *N*-methyl-D-aspartate receptors. J Pharmacol Exp Ther 296:41–47, 2001.
365. Muir JK, Raghupathi R, Emery DL, Bareyre F, McIntosh TK: Postinjury magnesium treatment attenuates traumatic brain injury–induced cortical induction of p53 mRNA in rats. Exp Neurol 159:584–593, 1999.
366. Muizelaar JP, Marmarou A, Young HF, Choi SC, Wolf A, Schneider RL, Kontos HA: Improving the outcome of severe head injury with the oxygen radical scavenger polyethylene glycol–conjugated superoxide dismutase: A phase II trial. J Neurosurg 78:375–382, 1993.
367. Mukhin A, Fan L, Faden AI: Activation of metabotropic glutamate receptor subtype mGluR1 contributes to post-traumatic neuronal injury. J Neurosci 16:6012–6020, 1996.
368. Munoz-Fernandez MA, Fresno M: The role of tumour necrosis factor, interleukin 6, interferon-gamma and inducible nitric oxide synthase in the development and pathology of the nervous system. Prog Neurobiol 56:307–340, 1998.
369. Murray GD, Teasdale GM, Braakman R, Cohadon F, Dearden M, Iannotti F, Karimi A, Lapierre F, Maas A, Ohman J, Persson L, Servadei F, Stocchetti N, Trojanowski T, Unterberg A: The European Brain Injury Consortium survey of head injuries. Acta Neurochir (Wien) 141:223–236, 1999.
370. Murray GD, Teasdale GM, Schmitz H: Nimodipine in traumatic subarachnoid haemorrhage: A re-analysis of the HIT I and HIT II trials. Acta Neurochir (Wien) 138:1163–1167, 1996.
371. Nadler V, Biegon A, Beit-Yannai E, Adamchik J, Shohami E: ^{45}Ca accumulation in rat brain after closed head injury; attenuation by the novel neuroprotective agent HU-211. Brain Res 685:1–11, 1995.
372. Nakanishi S: Metabotropic glutamate receptors: Synaptic transmission, modulation, and plasticity. Neuron 13:1031–1037, 1994.
373. Narayan RK, Michel ME, Ansell B, Baethmann A, Biegon A, Bracken MB, Bullock MR, Choi SC, Clifton GL, Contant CF, Coplin WM, Dietrich WD, Ghajar J, Grady SM, Grossman RG, Hall ED, Heetderks W, Hovda DA, Jallo J, Katz RL, Knoller N, Kochanek PM, Maas AI, Majde J, Marion DW, Marmarou A, Marshall LF, McIntosh TK, Miller E, Mohberg N, Muizelaar JP, Pitts LH, Quinn P, Riesenfeld G, Robertson CS, Strauss KI, Teasdale G, Temkin N, Tuma R, Wade C, Walker MD, Weinrich M, Whyte J, Wilberger J, Young AB, Yurkewicz L: Clinical trials in head injury. J Neurotrauma 19:503–557, 2002.
374. Nawashiro H, Tasaki K, Ruetzler CA, Hallenbeck JM: TNF-a pretreatment induces protective effects against focal cerebral ischemia in mice. J Cereb Blood Flow Metab 17:483–490, 1997.
375. Nelson LR, Auen EL, Bourke RS, et al: A new head injury model for evaluation of treatment modalities. Neurosci Abstr 5:516, 1979.
376. Newcomb JK, Kampfl A, Posmantur RM, Zhao X, Pike BR, Liu SJ, Clifton GL, Hayes RL: Immunohistochemical study of calpain-mediated breakdown products to α-spectrin following controlled cortical impact injury in the rat. J Neurotrauma 14:369–383, 1997.
377. Nicoll JAR, Roberts GW, Graham DI: Apolipoprotein E e4 allele is associated with deposition of amyloid b-protein following head injury. Nature Med 1(2):135–137, 1995.
378. Nilsson B, Ponten U, Voight G: Experimental head injury in the rat. Part I: Mechanics, pathophysiology, and morphology in an impact acceleration trauma model. J Neurosurg 47:241–251, 1977.
379. Nilsson P, Hillered L, Olsson Y, Sheardown M, Hansen A: Regional changes in interstitial K^+ and Ca^{2+} levels following cortical compression contusion trauma in rats. J Cereb Blood Flow Metab 13:183–192, 1993.

380. Nilsson P, Hillered L, Ponten U, Urgerstedt V: Changes in cortical extracellular levels of energy-related metabolites and amino acids following concussive brain injury in rats. J Cereb Blood Flow Metab 10:631–637, 1990.
381. Nowak L, Bregestovski P, Ascher P, Herbelt A, Prochiantz A: Magnesium gates glutamate-activated channels in mouse central neurons. Nature 307:462–465, 1984.
382. Nutt JG, Burchiel KJ, Comella CL, Jankovic J, Lang AE, Laws ER, Lozano AM, Penn RD, Simpson RK, Stacy M, Wooten GF: Randomized, double-blind trial of glial cell line–derived neurotrophic factor (GDNF) in PD. Neurology 60:69–73, 2003.
383. Okiyama K, Rosenkrantz TS, Smith DH, Gennarelli TA, McIntosh TK: (S)-Emopamil attenuates regional cerebral blood flow reduction following experimental brain injury. J Neurotrauma 11:83–95, 1994.
384. Okiyama K, Smith DH, Gennarelli TA, Simon RP, Leach M, McIntosh TK: The sodium channel blocker and glutamate release inhibitor BW1003C87 and magnesium attenuate regional cerebral edema following experimental brain injury in the rat. J Neurochem 64(2): 802–809, 1995.
385. Okiyama K, Smith DH, Thomas MJ, McIntosh TK: Evaluation of a novel calcium channel blocker (S)-emopamil on regional cerebral edema and neurobehavioral function after experimental brain injury. J Neurosurg 77:607–615, 1992.
386. Okiyama K, Smith DH, White WF, McIntosh TK: Effects of the NMDA antagonist CP-98,113 on regional cerebral edema and cardiovascular, cognitive, and neurobehavioral function following experimental brain injury in the rat. Brain Res 792:291–298, 1998.
387. Okonkwo DO, Buki A, Siman R, Povlishock JT: Cyclosporin A limits calcium-induced axonal damage following traumatic brain injury. NeuroReport 10:353–358, 1999.
388. Oliver CN, Starke-Reed PE, Stadtman ER, Liu GJ, Carney JM, Floyd RA: Oxidative damage to brain proteins, loss of glutamine synthetase activity, and production of free radicals during ischemia/reperfusion-induced injury to gerbil brain. Proc Natl Acad Sci USA 87:5144–5147, 1990.
389. Olney JW, Ho OL, Rhee V: Cytotoxic effects of acidic and sulphur-containing amino acid on the infant mouse central nervous system. Exp Brain Res 14:61–76, 1971.
390. Olney JW, Ikonomidou C, Mosinger JL, Frierdich G: MK-801 prevents hypobaric ischemic neuron degeneration in infant rat brain. J Neurosci 9:1701–1704, 1989.
391. Ommaya AK, Geller A, Parsons LC: The effect of experimental head injury on one-trial learning in rats. Int J Neurosci 1:371, 1971.
392. Ommaya AK, Gennarelli TA: Cerebral concussion and traumatic unconsciousness. Correlation of experimental and clinical observations on blunt head injuries in man. Brain 97:633–654, 1974.
393. Ommaya AK, Hirsch AE, Flamm ES, et al: Cerebral concussion in the monkey: An experimental model. Science 153:211, 1966.
394. Oppenheimer DR: Microscopic lesions of the brain following head injury. J Neurol Neurosurg Psychiatry 31: 299–306, 1968.
395. Osteen CL, Moore AH, Prins ML, Hovda DA: Age-dependency of ^{45}calcium accumulation following lateral fluid percussion: Acute and delayed patterns. J Neurotrauma 18:141–162, 2001.
396. Otani N, Nawashiro H, Fukui S, Nomura N, Shima K: Temporal and spatial profile of phosphorylated mitogen-activated protein kinase pathways after lateral fluid percussion in the cortex of the rat brain. J Neurotrauma 19:1587–1596, 2002.
397. Ott L, McClain CJ, Gillespie M, Young B: Cytokines and metabolic dysfunction after severe head injury. J Neurotrauma 11:447–472, 1994.
398. Palmer AM, Marion DW, Botscheller ML, Bowen DM, DeKosky ST: Increased transmitter amino acid concentration in human ventricular CSF after brain trauma. NeuroReport 6:153–156, 1994.
399. Palmer AM, Marion DW, Botscheller ML, Redd EE: Therapeutic hypothermia is cytoprotective without attenuating the traumatic brain injury–induced elevations in interstitial concentrations of aspartate and glutamate. J Neurotrauma 10:363–372, 1993.
400. Palmer AM, Marion DW, Botscheller ML, Swedlow PE, Styren SD, DeKosky ST: Traumatic brain injury–induced excitotoxicity assessed in a controlled cortical impact model. J Neurochem 61:2015–2024, 1993.
401. Pan W, Kastin AJ, Rigai T, McLay R, Pick CG: Increased hippocampal uptake of tumor necrosis factor alpha and behavioral changes in mice. Exp Brain Res 149:195–199, 2003.
402. Panter SS, Braughler JM, Hall E: Dextran-coupled deferoxamine improves outcome in a murine model of head injury. J Neurotrauma 9:47–53, 1992.
403. Parsons CG, Hartmann S, Spielmanns P: Budipine is a low affinity, *N*-methyl-D-aspartate receptor antagonist: Patch clamp studies in cultured striatal, hippocampal, cortical and superior colliculus neurones. Neuropharmacology 37:719–727, 1998.
404. Patterson SL, Abel T, Deuel TAS, Martin KC, Rose JC, Kandel ER: Recombinant BDNF rescues deficits in basal synaptic transmission and hippocampal LTP in BDNF knockout mice. Neuron 16:1137–1145, 1996.
405. Peerless SJ, Newcastle NB: Shear injuries of the brain. Can Med Assoc J 96:577–582, 1967.
406. Pellegrini-Giampietro DE, Cherici G, Alesiani M, Carla V, Moroni F: Excitatory amino acid release and free radical formation may cooperate in the genesis of ischemia-induced neuronal damage. J Neurosci 10:1035–1041, 1990.
407. Pettus EH, Christman CW, Giebel ML, Povlishock JT: Traumatically induced altered membrane permeability: Its relationship to traumatically induced reactive axonal change. J Neurotrauma 11:507–522, 1994.
408. Petty MA, Poulet P, Haas A, Namer IJ, Wagner J:

Reduction of traumatic brain injury–induced cerebral oedema by a free radical scavenger. Eur J Pharmacol 307:149–155, 1996.

409. Peuchen S, Bolanos JP, Heales SJ, Almeida A, Duchen MR, Clark JB: Interrelationships between astrocyte function, oxidative stress and antioxidant status within the central nervous system. Prog Neurobiol 52:261–281, 1997.

410. Philips MF, Mattiasson G, Wieloch T, Bjorklund A, Johansson BB, Tomasevic G, Martinez-Serrano A, Lenzlinger PM, Sinson G, Grady MS, McIntosh TK: Neuroprotective and behavioral efficacy of nerve growth factor–transfected hippocampal progenitor cell transplants after experimental traumatic brain injury. J Neurosurg 94:765–774, 2001.

411. Philips MF, Muir JK, Saatman KE, Raghupathi R, Lee VMY, Trojanowski JQ, McIntosh TK: Survival and integration of transplanted postmitotic human neurons following experimental brain injury in immunocompetent rats. J Neurosurg 90:116–124, 1999.

412. Pierce JES, Smith DH, Trojanowski JQ, McIntosh TK: Enduring cognitive, neurobehavioral, and histopathological changes persist for up to one year following severe experimental brain injury in rats. Neuroscience 87:359–369, 1998.

413. Pike BR, Flint J, Dutta S, Johnson E, Wang KK, Hayes RL: Accumulation of nonerythroid alpha II-spectrin and calpain-cleaved alpha II-spectrin breakdown products in cerebrospinal fluid after traumatic brain injury in rats. J Neurochem 78:1297–1306, 2001.

414. Pilz P: Survival after traumatic lesions of the pontomedullary junction: Report of 4 cases. Acta Neurochir (Suppl) (Wien) 32:77, 1983.

415. Polderman KH, Bloemers FW, Peerdeman SM, Girbes AR: Hypomagnesemia and hypophosphatemia at admission in patients with severe head injury. Crit Care Med 28:2022–2025, 2000.

416. Posmantur RM, Kampfl A, Liu SJ, Heck K, Taft WC, Clifton GL, Hayes RL: Cytoskeletal derangements of cortical neuronal processes three hours after traumatic brain injury in rats: An immunofluorescence study. J Neuropathol Exp Neurol 55:68–90, 1996.

417. Posmantur R, Kampfl A, Siman R, Liu SJ, Zhao X, Clifton GL, Hayes RL: A calpain inhibitor attenuates cortical cytoskeletal protein loss after experimental traumatic brain injury in the rat. Neuroscience 77:875–888, 1997.

418. Povlishock JT: Traumatically induced axonal injury: Pathogenesis and pathobiological implications. Brain Pathol 2:1–12, 1992.

419. Povlishock JT, Buki A, Koiziumi H, Stone J, Okonkwo DO: Initiating mechanisms involved in the pathobiology of traumatically induced axonal injury and interventions targeted at blunting their progression. Acta Neurochir (Suppl) (Wien) 73:15–20, 1999.

420. Prado R, Watson BD, Kuluz J, Dietrich WD: Endothelium-derived nitric oxide synthase inhibition. Effects on cerebral blood flow, pial artery diameter, and vascular morphology in rats. Stroke 23:1118–1123, 1992.

421. Pratico D: Alzheimer's disease and oxygen radicals: New insights. Biochem Pharmacol 63:563–567, 2002.

422. Probert L, Akassoglou K, Kassiotis G, Pasparakis M, Alexopoulou L, Kollias G: TNF-alpha transgenic and knockout models of CNS inflammation and degeneration. J Neuroimmunol 72:137–141, 1997.

423a. Pulliam L, Zhou M, Stubblebine M, Bitler CM: Differential modulation of cell death proteins in human brain cells by tumor necrosis factor alpha and platelet activating factor. J Neurosci Res 54:530–538, 1998.

423b. Raghupathi R, Conti AC, Graham DI, Krajewski S, Reed JC, Grady, MS, Trojanowsky JQ, McIntosh TK. Mild traumatic brain injury induces apoptotic cell death in the cortex that is preceded by decreases in cellular Bcl-2 immunoreactivity. Neuroscience 110:605–616, 2002.

423c. Quinn TJ, Smith C, Murray L, Stewart J, Nicoll JAR, Graham DI. There is no evidence of an association in children and teenagers between the apolipoprotein E ϵ4 allele and post-traumatic brain swelling. Neuropathol Appl Neurobiol 30:569-575, 2004.

424. Raghupathi R, Graham DI, McIntosh TK: Apoptosis after traumatic brain injury. J Neurotrauma 17:927–938, 2000.

425. Raghupathi R, Muir JK, Fulp CT, Pittman RN, McIntosh TK: Acute activation of mitogen-activated protein kinases following traumatic brain injury in the rat: Implications for post-traumatic cell death. Exp Neurol 183:438–448, 2003.

426. Rancan M, Otto VI, Hans VH, Gerlach I, Jork R, Trentz O, Kossmann T, Morganti-Kossmann MC: Upregulation of ICAM-1 and MCP-1 but not of MIP-2 and sensorimotor deficit in response to traumatic axonal injury in rats. J Neurosci Res 63:438–446, 2001.

427. Rao VL, Dogan A, Todd KG, Bowen KK, Dempsey RJ: Neuroprotection by memantine, a non-competitive NMDA receptor antagonist after traumatic brain injury in rats. Brain Res 911:96–100, 2001.

428. Reilly PL, Graham DI, Adams JH, et al: Patients with head injury who talk and die. Lancet 2:375–377, 1975.

429. Reinert M, Khaldi A, Zauner A, Doppenberg E, Choi S, Bullock R: High level of extracellular potassium and its correlates after severe head injury: Relationship to high intracranial pressure. J Neurosurg 93:800–807, 2000.

430. Relton JK, Martin D, Thompson RC, Russel DA: Peripheral administration of interleukin-1 receptor antagonist inhibits brain damage after focal cerebral ischemia in the rat. Exp Neurol 138:206–213, 1996.

431. Relton JK, Rothwell NJ: Interleukin-1 receptor antagonist inhibits ischaemic and excitotoxic neuronal damage in the rat. Brain Res Bull 29:243–246, 1992.

432. Rhodes JK, Andrews PJ, Holmes MC, Seckl JR: Expression of interleukin-6 messenger RNA in a rat model of diffuse axonal injury. Neurosci Lett 335:1–4, 2002.

433. Rink AD, Fung K-M, Trojanowski JQ, Lee V, Neuge-

bauer E, McIntosh TK: Evidence of apoptotic cell death after experimental traumatic brain injury in the rat. Am J Pathol 147:1575–1583, 1995.

434. Roberts GW, Allsop D, Bruton C: The occult aftermath of boxing. J Neurol Neurosurg Psychiatry 53:373–378, 1990.

435. Roberts I: The CRASH trial: The first large-scale, randomised, controlled trial in head injury. Crit Care (Lond) 5:292–293, 2001.

436. Rose ME, Huerbin MB, Melick J, Marion DW, Palmer AM, Schiding JK, Kochanek PM, Graham SH: Regulation of interstitial excitatory amino acid concentrations after cortical contusion injury. Brain Res 943:15–22, 2002.

437. Rosenberg GA, Estrada EY, Dencoff JE, Stetler-Stevenson WG: Tumor necrosis factor-α-induced gelatinase B causes delayed opening of the blood–brain barrier: An expanded therapeutic window. Brain Res 703:151–155, 1995.

438. Ross DT, Meaney DF, Sabol M, Smith DH, Thibault LE, Gennarelli TA: Distribution of forebrain diffuse axonal injury following inertial closed head injury in miniature swine. Exp Neurol 126:291–299, 1994.

439. Rothwell NJ, Hopkins SJ: Cytokines and the nervous system II: Actions and mechanisms of action. TINS 18:130–136, 1995.

440. Rothwell NJ, Luheshi GN: Interleukin 1 in the brain: Biology, pathology and therapeutic target. Trends Neurosci 23:618–625, 2000.

441. Rothwell NJ, Relton JK: Involvement of cytokines in acute neurodegeneration in the CNS. Neurosci Biobehav Rev 17:217–227, 1993.

442. Rothwell NJ, Strijbos PJ: Cytokines in neurodegeneration and repair. Int J Dev Neurosci 13:179–185, 1995.

443. Roy M, Sapolsky R: Neuronal apoptosis in acute necrotic insults: Why is this subject such a mess? Trends Neurosci 22:419–422, 1999.

444. Royo NC, Davis JE, Shimizu S, Conte V, Saatman KE, McIntosh TK: Neurotrophin-4/5 is a selective hippocampal neuroprotectant after experimental traumatic brain injury. Int Neurotrauma Symp, Adelaide, submitted (Poster), 2004.

445. Royo NC, Shimizu S, Saatman KE, McIntosh TK: Alterations in nerve growth factor (NGF) and neurotrophin-4/5 (NT-4/5) after traumatic brain injury in rats. J Neurotrauma 19(10):1362, 2002.

446. Ryan GA, McLean AJ, Vilenius AT, Kloeden CN, Simpson DA, Blumbergs PC, Scott G: Brain injury patterns in fatally injured pedestrians. J Trauma: Inj Inf Crit Care 36:469–476, 1994.

447. Saatman KE, Abai B, Grosvenor A, Vorwerk CK, Smith DH, Meaney DF: Traumatic axonal injury results in biphasic calpain activation and retrograde transport impairment in mice. J Cereb Blood Flow Metab 23:34–42, 2003.

448. Saatman KE, Bareyre FM, Grady MS, McIntosh TK: Acute cytoskeletal alterations and cell death induced by experimental brain injury are attenuated by magnesium treatment and exacerbated by magnesium deficiency. J Neuropathol Exp Neurol 60:183–194, 2001.

449. Saatman KE, Bozyczko-Coyne D, Marcy V, Siman R, McIntosh TK: Prolonged calpain-mediated spectrin breakdown occurs regionally following experimental brain injury in the rat. J Neuropathol Exp Neurol 55:850–860, 1996.

450. Saatman KE, Bozyczko-Coyne D, Marcy VR, Siman R, McIntosh TK: Prolonged calpain-mediated spectrin breakdown occurs regionally following experimental brain injury in the rat. J Neuropathol Exp Neurol 55:850–860, 1996.

451. Saatman KE, Contreras PC, Smith DH, Raghupathi R, McDermott KL, Fernandez SC, Sanderson KL, Voddi M, McIntosh TK: Insulin-like growth factor-1 (IGF-1) improves both neurological motor and cognitive outcome following experimental brain injury. Exp Neurol 147:418–427, 1997.

452. Saatman KE, Graham DI, McIntosh TK: The neuronal cytoskeleton is at risk after mild and moderate brain injury. J Neurotrauma 15:1047–1058, 1998.

453. Saatman KE, Murai H, Bartus RT, Smith DH, Hayward NJ, Perri BR, McIntosh TK: Calpain inhibitor AK295 attenuates motor and cognitive deficits following experimental brain injury in the rat. Proc Natl Acad Sci USA 93:3428–3433, 1996.

454. Saatman KE, Zhang C, Bartus RT, McIntosh TK: Behavioral efficacy of posttraumatic calpain inhibition is not accompanied by reduced spectrin proteolysis, cortical lesion, or apoptosis. J Cereb Blood Flow Metab 20:66–73, 2000.

455. Samii A, Badie H, Fu K, Luther RR, Hovda DA: Effects of an N-type calcium channel antagonist (SNX 111; Ziconotide) on calcium-45 accumulation following fluid-percussion injury. J Neurotrauma 16:879–892, 1999.

456. Sanada T, Nakamura T, Nishimura MC, Isayama K, Pitts LH: Effect of U74006F on neurologic function and brain edema after fluid percussion injury in rats. J Neurotrauma 10(1):65–71, 1993.

457. Sanderson KL, Raghupathi R, Martin D, Miller G, McIntosh TK: Systemic administration of interleukin-1 receptor antagonist (IL-1ra) attenuates neuronal death and cognitive dysfunction but not neurological motor deficits following lateral fluid-percussion brain injury in the rat. J Cereb Blood Flow Metab 19:1118–1125, 1999.

458. Sarrafzadeh AS, Thomale UW, Kroppenstedt SN, Unterberg AW: Neuroprotective effect of melatonin on cortical impact injury in the rat. Acta Neurochir 142:1293–1299, 2000.

459. Sato M, Chang E, Igarashi T, Noble LJ: Neuronal injury and loss after traumatic brain injury: Time course and regional variability. Brain Res 917:45–54, 2001.

460. Sawai H, Clarke DB, Kittlerova P, Bray GM, Aguayo AJ: Brain-derived neurotrophic factor and neurotrophin-4/5 stimulate growth of axonal branches from regenerating retinal ganglion cells. J Neurosci 16:3887–3894, 1996.

461. Scherbel U, Raghupathi R, Nakamura M, Saatman KE, Trojanowski JQ, Neugebauer E, Marino M, McIntosh TK: Differential acute and chronic responses of tumor necrosis factor–deficient mice to experimental brain injury. Proc Natl Acad Sci USA 96:8721–8726, 1999.
462. Schifitto G, Kieburtz K, McDermott MP, McArthur J, Marder K, Sacktor N, Palumbo D, Selnes O, Stern Y, Epstein L, Albert S: Clinical trials in HIV-associated cognitive impairment: Cognitive and functional outcomes. Neurology 56:415–418, 2001.
463. Schroder ML, Muizelaar JP, Bullock MR, Salvant JB, Povlishock JT: Focal ischemia due to traumatic contusions documented by stable xenon-CT and ultrastructural studies. J Neurosurg 82:966–971, 1995.
464. Schulz JB, Henshaw DR, Siwek D, Jenkins BG, Ferrante RJ, Cipolloni PB, Kowall NW, Rosen BR, Beal MF: Involvement of free radicals in excitotoxicity in vivo. J Neurochem 64:2239–2247, 1995.
465. Sekino H, Nakamura N, Kiruchi A, et al: Experimental head injury in monkeys using rotational acceleration impact. Neurol Med Chir 20:27, 1979.
466. Selkoe DJ: Alzheimer's disease: A central role for amyloid. J Neuropathol Exp Neurol 53:438–447, 1994.
467. Shapira Y, Lam AM, Artu AA, Eng C, Soltow L: Ketamine alters calcium and magnesium in brain tissue following experimental head trauma in rats. J Cereb Blood Flow Metab 13:962–968, 1993.
468. Sharp F, Jasper P, Hall J, Noble L, Sagar SM: MK-801 and ketamine induce heat shock protein HSP72 in injured neurons in posterior cingulate and retrosplenial cortex. Ann Neurol 30:801–809, 1991.
469. Shen G, Zhou Y, Xu M, Liu B, Xu Y: Effects of nimodipine on changes of endothelin after head injury in rabbits. Chin J Traumatol 4:172–174, 2001.
470. Sherriff FE, Bridges LR, Sivaloganathan S: Early detection of axonal injury after human head trauma using immunocytochemistry for β-amyloid precursor protein. Acta Neuropathol 87:55–62, 1994.
471. Shibayama M, Kuchiwaki H, Inao S, Yoshida K, Ito M: Intercellular adhesion molecule-1 expression on glia following brain injury: Participation of interleukin-1b. J Neurotrauma 13:801–808, 1996.
472. Shohami E, Bass R, Wallach D, Yamin A, Gallily R: Inhibition of tumor necrosis factor alpha (TNFα) activity in rat brain is associated with cerebroprotection after closed head injury. J Cereb Blood Flow Metab 16:378–384, 1996.
473. Shohami E, Beit-Yannai E, Horowitz M, Kohen R: Oxidative stress in closed-head injury: Brain antioxidant capacity as an indicator of functional outcome. J Cereb Blood Flow Metab 17:1007–1019, 1997.
474. Shohami E, Novikov M, Bass R: Long-term effect of HU-211, a novel noncompetitive NMDA antagonist, on motor and memory functions after closed head injury in the rat. Brain Res 674:55–62, 1995.
475. Shohami E, Novikov M, Bass R, Yamin A, Gallily R: Closed head injury triggers early production of TNFα and IL-6 by brain tissue. J Cereb Blood Flow Metab 14:615–619, 1994.
476. Shohami E, Novikov M, Mechoulam R: A nonpsychotropic cannabinoid, HU-211, has cerebroprotective effects after closed head injury in the rat. J Neurotrauma 10:109–119, 1993.
477. Siesjö BK: Calcium, ischemia, and death of brain cells. Ann NY Acad Sci 522:638, 1988.
478. Siesjo BK: Basic mechanisms of traumatic brain damage. Ann Emerg Med 22:959–969, 1993.
479. Sinson G, Perri BR, Trojanowski JQ, Flamm ES, McIntosh TK: Improvement of cognitive deficits and decreased cholinergic neuronal cell loss and apoptotic cell death following neurotrophin infusion after experimental traumatic brain injury. J Neurosurg 86:511–518, 1997.
480. Sinson G, Voddi M, McIntosh TK: Nerve growth factor administration attenuates cognitive but not neurobehavioral motor dysfunction or hippocampal cell loss following fluid-percussion brain injury in rats. J Neurochem 65:2209–2216, 1995.
481. Sinson G, Voddi M, McIntosh TK: Combined fetal neural transplantation and nerve growth factor infusion: Effects on neurological outcome following fluid-percussion brain injury in the rat. J Neurosurg 84:655–662, 1996.
482. Sinz EH, Kochanek PM, Dixon CE, Clark RS, Carcillo JA, Schiding JK, Chen M, Wisniewski SR, Carlos TM, Williams D, DeKosky ST, Watkins SC, Marion DW, Billiar TR: Inducible nitric oxide synthase is an endogenous neuroprotectant after traumatic brain injury in rats and mice. J Clin Invest 104:647–656, 1999.
483. Smith DH, Cecil KM, Meaney DF, Chen X-H, McIntosh TK, Gennarelli TA, Lenkinski RE: Magnetic resonance spectroscopy of diffuse brain trauma in the pig. J Neurotrauma 15:665–674, 1998.
484. Smith DH, Chen XH, Iwata A, Graham DI: Amyloid b accumulation in axons after traumatic brain injury in humans. J Neurosurg 98:1072–1077, 2003.
485. Smith DH, Lowenstein DH, Gennarelli TA, McIntosh TK: Persistent memory dysfunction is associated with bilateral hippocampal damage following experimental brain injury. Neurosci Lett 168:151–154, 1994.
486. Smith DH, Okiyama K, Gennarelli TA, McIntosh TK: Magnesium and ketamine attenuate cognitive dysfunction following experimental brain injury. Neurosci Lett 157:211–214, 1993.
487. Smith DH, Okiyama K, Thomas MJ, McIntosh TK: Effects of the excitatory amino acid receptor antagonists kynurenate and indole-2-carboxylic acid on behavioral and neurochemical outcome following experimental brain injury. J Neurosci 13:5383–5392, 1993.
488. Smith DH, Soares HD, Pierce JES, Perlman KG, Saatman KE, Meaney DF, Dixon CE, McIntosh TK: A model of parasagittal controlled cortical impact in the mouse: Cognitive and histopathologic effects. J Neurotrauma 12(2):169–178, 1995.

489. Soares HD, Hicks RR, Smith DH, McIntosh TK: Inflammatory leukocytic recruitment and diffuse neuronal degeneration are separate pathological processes resulting from traumatic brain injury. J Neurosci 15:8223–8233, 1995.
490. Soares HD, McIntosh TK: Fetal cortical transplants in adult rats subjected to experimental brain injury. J Neural Transplant Plast 2(3–4):207–220, 1991.
491. Soares HD, Sinson G, McIntosh TK: Fetal hippocampal transplants attenuate hippocampal CA_3 pyramidal cell death resulting from fluid percussion brain injury in the rat. J Neurotrauma 12:1059–1067, 1995.
492. Soares HD, Thomas M, Cloherty K, McIntosh TK: Development of prolonged focal cerebral edema and regional cation change following experimental brain injury in the rat. J Neurochem 58:1845–1852, 1992.
493. Sorbi S, Nacmias N, Piacentini S, Repice A, Latorraca S, Forleo P, Amaducci L: ApoE as a prognostic factor for post-traumatic coma. Nature Med 1:852, 1995.
494. Sorg O, Horn TF, Yu N, Gruol DL, Bloom FE: Inhibition of astrocyte glutamate uptake by reactive oxygen species: Role of antioxidant enzymes. Mol Med 3:431–440, 1997.
495. Stahel PF, Morganti-Kossmann MC, Kossmann T: The role of the complement system in traumatic brain injury. Brain Res Rev 27:243–256, 1998.
496. Stahel PF, Shohami E, Younis FM, Kariya K, Otto VI, Lenzlinger PM, Grosjean MB, Eugster HP, Trentz O, Kossmann T, Morganti-Kossmann MC: Experimental closed head injury: Analysis of neurological outcome, blood–brain barrier dysfunction, intracranial neutrophil infiltration, and neuronal cell death in mice deficient in genes for pro-inflammatory cytokines. J Cereb Blood Flow Metab 20:369–380, 2000.
497. Stahel PF, Shohami E, Younis FM, Kariya K, Otto VI, Lenzlinger PM, Grosjean MB, Eugster HP, Trentz O, Kossmann T, Morganti-Kossmann MC: Experimental closed head injury: Analysis of neurological outcome, blood–brain barrier dysfunction, intracranial neutrophil infiltration, and neuronal cell death in mice deficient in genes for pro-inflammatory cytokines. J Cereb Blood Flow Metab 20:369–380, 2002.
498. Stein DG, Halks-Miller M, Hoffman SW: Intracerebral administration of α-tocopherol-containing liposomes facilitates behavioral recovery in rats with bilateral lesions of the frontal cortex. J Neurotrauma 8:281–292, 1991.
499. Storm-Mathisen J, Danbolt NC, Rothe F, Torp R, Zhang N, Aas JE, Kanner BI, Langmoen I, Ottersen OP: Ultrastructural immunocytochemical observations on the localization, metabolism and transport of glutamate in normal and ischemic brain tissue. Prog Brain Res 94:225–241, 1992.
500. Stover JF, Beyer TF, Unterberg AW: Riluzole reduces brain swelling and contusion volume in rats following controlled cortical impact injury. J Neurotrauma 17:1171–1178, 2000.
501. Stover JF, Sakowitz OW, Beyer TF, Dohse NK, Kroppenstedt S-N, Thomale U-W, Schaser K-D, Unterberg AW: Effects of LY379268, a selective group II metabotropic glutamate receptor agonist, on EEG activity, cortical perfusion, tissue damage, and cortical glutamate, glucose, and lactate levels in brain-injured rats. J Neurotrauma 20:315–326, 2003.
502. Stover JF, Schoning B, Beyer TF, Woiciechowsky C, Unterberg AW: Temporal profile of cerebrospinal fluid glutamate, interleukin-6, and tumor necrosis factor-alpha in relation to brain edema and contusion following controlled cortical impact injury in rats. Neurosci Lett 288:25–28, 2000.
503. Strauss KI, Barbe MF, Marshall RM, Raghupathi R, Mehta S, Narayan RK: Prolonged cyclooxygenase-2 induction in neurons and glia following traumatic brain injury in the rat. J Neurotrauma 17:695–711, 2000.
504. Strich SJ: Diffuse degeneration of the cerebral white matter in severe dementia following head injury. J Neurol Neurosurg Psychiatry 19:163–185, 1956.
505. Strich SJ: Shearing of nerve fibers as a cause of brain damage due to head injury. A pathological study of twenty cases. Lancet 2:443–448, 1961.
506. Suehiro E, Ueda Y, Wei EP, Kontos HA, Povlishock JT: Posttraumatic hypothermia followed by slow rewarming protects the cerebral microcirculation. J Neurotrauma 20:381–390, 2003.
507. Sullivan HG, Martinez J, Becker DP, Miller JD, Griffin R, Wist AO: Fluid percussion model of mechanical brain injury in the cat. J Neurosurg 45:520–534, 1976.
508. Sullivan PG, Bruce-Keller AJ, Rabchevsky AG, Christakos S, Clair DK, Mattson MP, Scheff SW: Exacerbation of damage and altered NF-kappa B activation in mice lacking tumor necrosis factor receptors after traumatic brain injury. J Neurosci 19:6248–6256, 1999.
509. Sun F-Y, Faden AI: Neuroprotective effects of 619C89, a use-dependent sodium channel blocker, in rat traumatic brain injury. Brain Res 673:133–140, 1995.
510. Sutton RL, Lescaudron L, Stein DG: Unilateral cortical contusion injury in the rat: Vascular disruption and temporal development of cortical necrosis. J Neurotrauma 10:135–149, 1993.
511. Suzuki M, Nishina M, Endo M, Matsushita K, Tetsuka M, Shima K, Okuyama S: Decrease in cerebral free magnesium concentration following closed head injury and effects of VA-045 in rats. Gen Pharmacol 28:119–121, 1997.
512. Takahashi H, Tanaka S, Sano K: Changes in extracellular potassium concentration in cortex and brain stem during the acute phase of experimental closed head injury. J Neurosurg 55:708–717, 1981.
513. Tanaka K, Gotoh F, Gomi S, Takashima S, Mihara B, Shirai T, Nogawa S, Nagata E: Inhibition of nitric oxide synthesis induces a significant reduction in local cerebral blood flow in the rat. Neurosci Lett 127:129–132, 1991.

514. Taupin V, Toulmond S, Serrano A, Benavides J, Zavala F: Increase in IL-6, IL-1 and TNF levels in rat brain following traumatic lesion. Influence of pre- and post-traumatic treatment with Ro54864, a peripheral-type (*p* site) benzodiazepine ligand. J Neuroimmunol 42:177–186, 1993.
515. Teasdale G: A randomized trial of nimodipine in severe head injury: HIT 1. J Neurotrauma 37:S545–S550, 1992.
516. Teasdale GM, Bannan PE: Neuroprotection in head injury. In: Reilly P, Bullock R (eds): Head Injury. London, Chapman & Hall, 1997, pp 423–438.
517. Teasdale GM, Nicoll JA, Murray G, Fiddes M: Association of apolipoprotein E polymorphism with outcome after head injury. Lancet 350:1069–1071, 1997.
518. Teasdale G, Teasdale E, Hadley D: Computed tomographic and magnetic resonance imaging classification of head injury. In: Jane JA, Anderson DK, Torner JC, Young W (eds): Central Nervous System Trauma Status Report. J Neurotrauma (Suppl 1), 9:S249–S257, 1992.
519. Temple MD, Hamm RJ: Chronic, postinjury administration of D-cycloserine, an NMDA partial agonist, enhances cognitive performance following experimental brain injury. Brain Res 741:246–251, 1996.
520. Tenneti L, Lipton SA: Involvement of activated caspase-3-like proteases in *N*-methyl-D-aspartate–induced apoptosis in cerebrocortical neurons. J Neurochem 74:134–142, 2000.
521. Terada LS, Willingham IR, Guidot DM, Shibao GN, Kindt GW, Repine JE: Tungsten treatment prevents tumor necrosis factor–induced injury of brain endothelial cells. Inflammation 16:13–19, 1992.
522. Thoenen H, Sendtner M: Neurotrophins: From enthusiastic expectations through sobering experiences to rational therapeutic approaches. Nat Neurosci 5 (suppl): 1046–1050, 2002.
523. Thornhill S, Teasdale GM, Murray GD, McEwen J, Roy CW, Penny KI: Disability in young people and adults one year after head injury: Prospective cohort study. BMJ 320:1631–1635, 2000.
524. Tolwani RJ, Buckmaster PS, Varma S, Cosgaya JM, Wu Y, Suri C, Shooter EM: BDNF overexpression increases dendrite complexity in hippocampal dentate gyrus. Neuroscience 114:795–805, 2002.
525. Tornheim PA, Linwicz BH, Hirsch CS, Brown DL, McLaurin LR: Acute responses to blunt head trauma: Experimental model and gross pathology. J Neurosurg 59:431–438, 1983.
526. Toulmond S, Duval D, Serrano A, Scatton B, Benavides J: Biochemical and histological alterations induced by fluid percussion brain injury in the rat. Brain Res 620:24–31, 1993.
527. Toulmond S, Rothwell NJ: Interleukin-1 receptor antagonist inhibits neuronal damage caused by fluid percussion injury in the rat. Brain Res 671:261–266, 1995.
528. Toulmond S, Serrano A, Benavides J, Scatton B: Prevention by eliprodil (SL 82.0715) of traumatic brain damage in the rat. Existence of a large (18 h) therapeutic window. Brain Res 620:32–41, 1993.
529. Tsubokawa T, Yamamoto T, Miyazaki S, et al: Pathogenic mechanism of cerebral concussion due to rotational angular acceleration impact. Neurol Med Chir 21:657, 1981.
530. Tsuchida E, Bullock R: The effect of the glycine site-specific *N*-methyl-D-aspartate antagonist ACEA1021 on ischemic brain damage caused by acute subdural hematoma in the rat. J Neurotrauma 12:279–288, 1995.
531. Tuszynski MH: Intraparenchymal NGF infusions rescue degenerating cholinergic neurons. Cell Transplant 9:629–636, 2000.
532. Tuszynski MH, Mafong E, Meyer S: Central infusions of brain-derived neurotrophic factor and neurotrophin-4/5, but not nerve growth factor and neurotrophin-3, prevent loss of the cholinergic phenotype in injured adult motor neurons. Neuroscience 71:761–771, 1996.
533. Tymianski M, Tator CH: Normal and abnormal calcium homeostasis in neurons: A basis for the pathophysiology of traumatic and ischemic central nervous system injury. Neurosurgery 38:1176–1195, 1996.
534. Tyurin VA, Tyurina YY, Borisenko GG, Sokolova TV, Ritov VB, Quinn PJ, Rose M, Kochanek P, Graham SH, Kagan VE: Oxidative stress following traumatic brain injury in rats: Quantitation of biomarkers and detection of free radical intermediates. J Neurochem 75:2178–2189, 2000.
535. Uchida K, Nakakimura K, Kuroda Y, Haranishi Y, Matsumoto M, Sakabe T: Dizocilpine but not ketamine reduces the volume of ischaemic damage after acute subdural hematoma in the rat. Eur J Anaesthesiol 18:295–302, 2001.
536. Ustun ME, Duman A, Ogun CO, Vatansev H, Ak A: Effects of nimodipine and magnesium sulfate on endogenous antioxidant levels in brain tissue after experimental head trauma. J Neurosurg Anesthesiol 13: 227–232, 2001.
537. Ustun ME, Gurbilek M, Ak A, Vatansev H, Duman A: Effects of magnesium sulfate on tissue lactate and malondialdehyde levels in experimental head trauma. Intens Care Med 27:264–268, 2001.
538. Vallieres L, Campbell IL, Gage FH, Sawchenko PE: Reduced hippocampal neurogenesis in adult transgenic mice with chronic astrocytic production of interleukin-6. J Neurosci 22:486–492, 2002.
539. Vanderklish PW, Bahr BA: The pathogenic activation of calpain: A marker and mediator of cellular toxicity and disease states. Int J Exp Pathol 81:323–339, 2000.
540. Vaz R, Sarmento A, Borges N, Cruz C, Azevedo I: Effect of mechanogated membrane ion channel blockers on experimental traumatic brain oedema. Acta Neurochir (Wien) 140:371–374, 1998.
541. Verweij BH, Muizelaar JP, Vinas FC, Peterson PL, Xiong Y, Lee CP: Improvement in mitochondrial dysfunction as a new surrogate efficiency measure for preclinical trials: Dose-response and time-window profiles for administration of the calcium channel blocker Ziconotide in experimental brain injury. J Neurosurg 93:829–834, 2000.

542. Vespa P, Prins M, Ronne-Engstrom E, Caron M, Shalmon E, Hovda DA, Martin NA, Becker DP: Increase in extracellular glutamate caused by reduced cerebral perfusion pressure and seizures after human traumatic brain injury: A microdialysis study. J Neurosurg 89:971–982, 1998.
543. Vink R, Faden AI, McIntosh TK: Changes in cellular bioenergetic state following graded traumatic brain injury in rats: Determination by phosphorus 31 magnetic resonance spectroscopy. J Neurotrauma 5:315–330, 1988.
544. Vink R, Heath DL, McIntosh TK: Acute and prolonged alterations in brain free magnesium following fluid-percussion induced brain trauma in rats. J Neurochem 66:2477–2483, 1996.
545. Vink R, McIntosh TK, Demediuk P, Faden AI: Decrease in total and free magnesium concentration following traumatic brain injury in rats. Biochem Biophys Res Commun 149:594–599, 1987.
546. Vink R, McIntosh TK, Demediuk P, Weiner MW, Faden AI: Decline in intracellular free Mg^{2+} is associated with irreversible tissue injury following brain trauma. J Biol Chem 263:757–761, 1988.
547. Vink R, O'Connor CA, Nimmo AJ, Heath DL: Magnesium attenuates persistent functional deficits following diffuse traumatic brain injury in rats. Neurosci Lett 336:41–44, 2003.
548. Wada K, Alonso OF, Busto R, Panetta J, Clemens JA, Ginsberg MD, Dietrich WD: Early treatment with a novel inhibitor of lipid peroxidation (LY341122) improves histopathological outcome after moderate fluid percussion brain injury in rats. Neurosurgery 45:601–608, 1999.
549. Wada K, Chatzipanteli K, Busto R, Dietrich WD: Role of nitric oxide in traumatic brain injury in the rat. J Neurosurg 89:807–818, 1998.
550. Wahl F, Renou E, Mary V, Stutzmann J-M: Riluzole reduces brain lesions and improves neurological function in rats after a traumatic brain injury. Brain Res 756:247–255, 1997.
551. Watson DJ, Longhi L, Lee EB, Fulp CT, Fujimoto S, Royo NC, Passini MA, Trojanowski JQ, Lee VMY, Wolfe JH: Genetically modified NT2N human neuronal cells mediate long-term gene expression as CNS grafts in vivo and improve functional cognitive outcome following experimental traumatic brain injury. J Neuropathol Exp Neurol 62:368–380, 2003.
552. Westmoreland SV, Kolson D, Gonzalez-Scarano F: Toxcity of TNF-α and platelet activating factor for human NT2N neurons: A tissue culture model for human immunodeficiency virus dementia. J Neurovirol 2:118–226, 1996.
553. Whalen MJ, Carlos TM, Kochanek PM, Clark RS, Heineman S, Schiding JK, Franicola D, Memarzadeh F, Lo W, Marion DW, DeKosky ST: Neutrophils do not mediate blood–brain barrier permeability early after controlled cortical impact in rats. J Neurotrauma 16: 583–594, 1999.
554a. Whisler RL, Goyette MA, Grants IS, Newhouse YG: Sublethal levels of oxidant stress stimulate multiple serine/threonine kinases and suppress protein phosphatases in Jurkat T cells. Arch Biochem Biophys 319: 23–35, 1995.
554b. Wilson S, Raghupathi R, Saatman KE, MacKinnon M-A, McIntosh TK, Graham DI. Continued *in situ* DNA fragmentation of microglial/macrophages in white matter weeks and months after traumatic brain injury. J Neurotrauma 21:239–250, 2004.
555. Winter CD, Pringle AK, Clough GF, Church MK: Raised parenchymal interleukin-6 levels correlate with improved outcome after traumatic brain injury. Brain 127:315–320, 2004.
556. Wolf JA, Stys PK, Lusardi T, Meaney D, Smith DH: Traumatic axonal injury induces calcium influx modulated by tetrodotoxin-sensitive sodium channels. J Neurosci 21:1923–1930, 2001.
557. Xiong Y, Peterson PL, Muizelaar JP, Lee CP: Mitochondrial dysfunction and calcium perturbation induced by traumatic brain injury. J Neurotrauma 14:23–34, 1997.
558. Yabuuchi K, Minami M, Katsumata S, Yamazaki A, Satoh M: An in situ hybridization study on interleukin-1 beta mRNA induced by transient forebrain ischemia in the rat. brain. Brain Res 26:135–142, 1994.
559. Yaghmai A, Povlishock JT: Traumatically induced reactive change as visualized through the use of monoclonal antibodies targeted to neurofilament subunits. J Neuropathol Exp Neurol 51:158–176, 1992.
560. Yakovlev AG, Knoblach S, Fan L, Fox GB, Goodnight R, Faden AI: Activation of CPP32–like caspases contributes to neuronal apoptosis and neurological dysfunction after traumatic brain injury. J Neurosci 17: 7415–7424, 1997.
561. Yakovlev AG, Wang G, Stoica BA, Simbulan-Rosenthal CM, Yoshihara K, Smulson ME: Role of DNAS1L3 in Ca^{2+}- and Mg^{2+}-dependent cleavage of DNA into oligonucleosomal and high molecular mass fragments. Nucl Acids Res 27:1999–2005, 1999.
562. Yamakami I, McIntosh TK: Alterations in regional cerebral blood flow following brain injury in the rat. J Cereb Blood Flow Metab 11:655–660, 1991.
563. Yamasaki Y, Matsuura N, Shozuhara H, Onodera H, Itoyama Y, Kogure K: Interleukin-1 as a pathogenic mediator of ischemic brain damage in rats. Stroke 26: 676–680, 1995.
564. Yang SY, Wang ZG: Therapeutic effect of nimodipine on experimental brain injury. Chin J Traumatol 6:326–331, 2003.
565. Yang Y, Li Q, Shuaib A: Neuroprotection by 2-h postischemia administration of two free radical scavengers, alpha-phenyl-*n*-tert-butyl-nitrone (PBN) and *N*-tert-butyl-(2-sulfophenyl)-nitrone (S-PBN), in rats subjected to focal embolic cerebral ischemia. Exp Neurol 163:39–45, 2000.
566. Yatsiv I, Morganti-Kossmann MC, Perez D, Dinarello CA, Novick D, Rubinstein M, Otto VI, Rancan M, Kossmann T, Redaelli CA, Trentz O, Shohami E, Stahel

PF: Elevated intracranial IL-18 in humans and mice after traumatic brain injury and evidence of neuroprotective effects of IL-18-binding protein after experimental closed head injury. J Cereb Blood Flow Metab 22:971–978, 2002.

567. Yeiser EC, Vanlandingham JW, Levenson CW: Moderate zinc deficiency increases cell death after brain injury in the rat. Nutr Neurosci 5:345–352, 2002.

568. Young B, Runge JW, Harrington T, Wilberger J, Muizelaar JP, Boddy A, Kupiec JW: Effects of perorgotein on neurologic outcome of patients with severe head. A multicenter, randomized controlled trial. JAMA 276:638–543, 1996.

569. Yunoki M, Kawauchi M, Ukita N, Noguchi Y, Nishio S, Ono Y, Asari S, Ohmoto T, Asanuma M, Ogawa N: Effects of lecithinized superoxide dismutase on traumatic brain injury in rats. J Neurotrauma 14:739–746, 1997.

570. Zabel P, Wolter DT, Schonharting MM, Schade UF: Oxpentifylline in endotoxaemia. Lancet 2:1474–1477, 1989.

571. Zhang L, Rzigalinski BA, Ellis EF, Satin LS: Reduction of voltage-dependent Mg^{2+} blockade of NMDA current in mechanically injured neurons. Science 274:1921–1923, 1996.

572. Zhang RL, Shohami E, Beit-Yannai E, Bass R, Trembovler V, Samuni A: Mechanism of brain protection by nitroxide radicals in experimental model of closed-head injury. Free Rad Biol Med 24:332–340, 1998.

573. Zhou F, Hongmin B, Xiang Z, Enyu L: Changes of mGluR4 and the effects of its specific agonist L-AP4 in a rodent model of diffuse brain injury. J Clin Neurosci 10:684–688, 2003.

574. Zhuang J, Shackford SR, Schmoker JD, Anderson ML: The association of leukocytes with secondary brain injury. J Trauma 35:415–422, 1993.

575. Zimmerman RA, Bilaniuk LT, Gennarelli TA: Computed tomography of shearing injuries of the cerebral white matter. Radiology 127:393–396, 1978.

576. Zipfel GJ, Babcock DJ, Lee JM, Choi DW: Neuronal apoptosis after CNS injury: The roles of glutamate and calcium. J Neurotrauma 17:857–869, 2000.

577. Zornow MH, Prough DS: Neuroprotective properties of calcium-channel blockers. New Horiz 4:107–114, 1996.

578. Zou L, Yotnda P, Zhao T, Yuan X, Long Y, Zhou H, Yang K: Reduced inflammatory reactions to the inoculation of helper-dependent adenoviral vectors in traumatically injured rat brain. J Cereb Blood Flow Metab 22:959–970, 2002.

579. Zwienenberg M, Gong QZ, Berman RF, Muizelaar JP, Lyeth BG: The effect of groups II and III metabotropic glutamate receptor activation on neuronal injury in a rodent model of traumatic brain injury. Neurosurgery 48:1119–1126, 2001.

Chapter 5

The Postconcussion Syndrome and the Sequelae of Mild Head Injury

RANDOLPH W. EVANS

Although neurologists frequently evaluate and treat patients with mild head injury, the persistent sequelae are controversial.[80] The following two cases illustrate some elements of this controversy, including the credibility of the patient with subjective complaints and the effect of secondary gain and litigation on persistent symptoms. The chapter will then review the Hollywood head injury myth, definitions, epidemiology, historical aspects, neuropathology, nonorganic explanations, sequelae, diagnostic testing, prognosis, and treatment.

Case 1. Neurosurgeon as Victim

"This 42-year-old moderately coordinated neurological surgeon was in Vail, Colorado in 1984, for a meeting of the National Traumatic Coma Data Bank. Following the morning meeting, he spent the afternoon touring the mountains of Vail, and while descending one that had only a modest incline, he lost his balance and fell, striking his head. He was rendered immediately unconscious for a period of a few seconds—certainly no more than 10–15. Upon awakening, the world appeared upside down, with the sky below and terra firma above. This condition cleared, but a very modest vertigo persisted. This did not interfere in any way with descent from the mountain, and in fact did not interfere with further skiing activities. Neuropsychological testing was soon recommended by the neuropsychologists at the meeting, but was respectfully declined.

Upon returning home, the neurosurgeon noted that he was a bit more distractible than was his norm and that he had a great deal of difficulty remembering recent events, including particularly the location of objects necessary for work, such as a dictaphone, briefcase, and keys. List making in order to recall meetings scheduled and tasks to be performed became necessary, whereas they were not necessary before. Referencing articles from memory storage was difficult; authors were frequently transposed and dates incorrectly recalled. Information processing did not appear to be affected, but the ability to attend to a task required a higher level of energy expenditure than previously. These symptoms persisted, but they improved gradually over a period of approximately 18 months and by the fall of 1985, they appeared to have reached their asymptote. Modest improvement in information storage retrieval has continued, indicating that neither Alzheimer's nor a presenile dementia was revealed by the head injury. Function, as judged by others remains good, but is not optimal."[184]

Case 2. Unforseen Misfortune

Penny Pellito, age 52, was a customer in a Home Depot store in Fort Lauderdale, Florida, in April 1987. Vertically stacked lumber fell, striking her on the top of her head (Larry Keller, personal communication, 1991). She had a small scalp laceration, but there was no loss of consciousness. She sued Home Depot, Inc., for at least $100,000 for alleged brain damage and an unspecified amount for paranormal injury. She claimed that the mild head injury had robbed her of a supernatural power: her ability to go on "automatic"—to undergo pain-free surgery without anesthesia.

On February 8, 1991, the Broward Circuit Court jury of three men and three women awarded Penny Pellito $5000 for physical injuries but found that she was 80% negligent. They also awarded her husband, James, $1000 for loss of her services.

"The jurors are 'in the majority of the way people feel,' Pellito said after the verdict. 'Welcome to the real world. They don't look beyond, to what can be.' Her husband was less sanguine.'They are still in the caveman stage,' he said. Home Depot's attorney, James Zloch, was elated with the verdict. In the immortal words of [singer] James Brown, 'I feel good,' he said.

"Pellito also says she is a psychic but had she foreseen the outcome of her lawsuit, she may not have proceeded to trial. She and her husband rejected a pretrial settlement offer of $17,000 from Home Depot, insisting on more than $1 million, Zloch said.

"Judge Paul M. Marko III agonized for two days before letting the jury even consider awarding Pellito money for paranormal damages.'There's no legal precedent for either allowing it or denying it,' he said after the verdict."[149]

The Hollywood Head Injury Myth

Although extensive data of the past three decades strongly support an organic basis for sequelae from mild head injury, much doubt exists among some physicians[82,150] and authors of population-based prevalence studies,[200] as well as laypersons,[12] defense attorneys, and agents of insurance companies. One explanation is that for many people, their knowledge of the sequelae of head injuries is entirely the product of "movie magic." What I have termed the *Hollywood head injury myth*[81] and what Robertson has called the *Three Stooges Model*[233] has been an extreme source of misinformation. The reader can easily reference many different movies and television programs and bring to mind examples.

In western movie barroom brawls, the cowboy may be punched in the face and hit repeatedly over the head with chairs without much effect before one of the showgirls comes up from behind, striking the cowboy over the head with a liquor bottle. The cowboy collapses, unconscious, only to be fully recovered in the next scene. In detective, boxing, Kung Fu, and other action stories, kicks, punches, and blows (which in reality would be fatal or near-fatal) delivered to the face and head in rapid succession are brushed off by the combatants after eliciting only a grimace and a grunt. The infliction of head trauma is one of the funniest routines in cartoons and slapstick movies of any vintage. Our actual experience is minuscule compared to the thousands of simulated head injuries the average person witnesses in the movies and on television. Therefore, the neurologist has a difficult job educating a public reared on this mythology.

To help make the opposite point, the neurologist can conjure up the image of the havoc wreaked by the powerful fists of professional boxers, even with the ample padding of 8- or 10- ounce gloves. Most people are familiar with the meaning of the abbreviations TKO and KO. The punch-drunk syndrome of cumulative head trauma in boxers[231] (well described by Martland in 1928[185]) and the examples of two of the most successful boxers, Joe Louis and Muhammad Ali, are also quite familiar to most persons. In other sports, there is growing awareness of the effects of cumulative concussions—for example, in professional football (quarterbacks Steve Young, Troy Aikman, and Stan Humphries) and hockey (Pat Lafontaine). Starting with examples from sports, the public may then be more receptive to the presentation of general factual information. This chapter will review definitions, epidemiology, historical aspects, neuropathology, sequelae, testing, prognosis, medico-legal aspects, and treatment.

Definitions of Mild Head Injury, Concussion, and Postconcussion Syndrome

The terms *mild* and *minor head injury* are frequently used. The term *mild head injury*, however, is preferred to delineate the continuum of mild, moderate, and severe. In addition, *minor* can denote an injury of little consequence, which can be misleading. Mild head injury is typically defined by the following criteria: loss of consciousness lasting for 30 minutes or less or being dazed without loss of consciousness, an initial Glasgow Coma Scale (GCS) score of 13 to 15 without subsequent deterioration, and absence of focal neurological deficits without evidence of depressed skull fractures, intracranial hematoma, or other neurosurgical pathology.

Since this definition includes a heterogeneous population, there may be merit in segregating those with GCS scores of 15 from those with scores of 13 and 14. Computed tomography (CT) scans are more likely to be abnormal and the need for neurosurgical intervention is greater with scores of 13 and 14 than 15.[53] The Neurotraumatology Committee of the World Federation of Neurosurgical Societies has further suggested stratification based upon risk factors for neurosurgical pathology for those with GCS scores of 14 and 15.[250] In addition, because the risk of intracranial lesions is similar, the Committee recommends reclassifying patients with a GCS score of 13 in the group with moderate head injury (GCS scores of 9–12). Patients classified as low-risk mild are those with an admission GCS score of 15 without a history of loss of consciousness, amnesia, vomiting, or diffuse headache where the risk of intracranial hematoma requiring surgical evaluation is less than 0.1:100. Those considered medium risk mild have a GCS score of 15 with one or more of the following symptoms: loss of consciousness, amnesia, vomiting, or diffuse headache. The risk of intracranial hematoma requiring surgical evacuation is in the range of 1–3:100, and a CT scan should be obtained. High-risk mild head injury patients have an admission GCS score of 14 or 15 with a skull fracture and/or neurological deficits. The risk of intracranial hematoma requiring surgical evacuation is in the range of 6–10:100, and a CT scan must be obtained. Patients with risk factors including coagulopathy, drug or alcohol consumption, previous neurosurgical procedures, pretraumatic epilepsy, or age over 60 years are included in the high-risk group independent of the clinical presentation.

The Quality Standards Subcommittee of the American Academy of Neurology defines concussion as a trauma-induced alteration in mental status that may or may not involve loss of consciousness.[224] The postconcussion syndrome usually follows mild head injury and comprises one or more of the following symptoms and signs: headaches, dizziness, vertigo, tinnitus, hearing loss, blurred vision, diplopia, convergence insufficiency, light and noise sensitivity, diminished taste and smell, irritability, anxiety, depression, personality change, fatigue, sleep disturbance, decreased libido, decreased appetite, memory dysfunction, impaired concentration and attention, slowing of reaction time, and slowing of information-processing speed. Rare sequelae of mild head injury include subdural and epidural hematomas, seizures, transient global amnesia, tremor, and dystonia (Table 5.1). The most common complaints are headaches, dizziness, fatigue, irritability, anxiety, insomnia, loss of concentration and memory, and noise sensitivity.[65,73,74,204,241] Loss of consciousness does not have to occur for the postconcussion syndrome to develop. Over 50% of patients with mild head injury will develop the postconcussion syndrome.[16]

Many physicians are appropriately concerned with the use of a grab bag diagnosis with many vague subjective symptoms, which can easily be overused and used improperly. The symptoms are also common in the general population. The term *grab bag diagnosis* refers to a heterogeneous patient population with varying degrees of injury to the head and brain. Individual patient characteristics may alter the expression of the injury. When evaluating individual patients, the physician should give each symptom and sign a cause or a classification, when that is appropriate, as specifically as possible (for example, posttraumatic migraine, convergence insufficiency, benign positional vertigo).

A subdivision into an early postconcussion syndrome and a late or persistent postconcussion syndrome when symptoms and signs persist for more than 6 months can be useful.[5] In the late group, psychological factors and compensation issues may contribute to persisting symptoms.[44] These patients are very similar to those with chronic pain syndromes and may have an interaction of chronic headaches and depression.[4,279]

Table 5.1. Sequelae of Mild Head Injury

Headaches
Muscle contraction or tension type
Cranial myofascial injury
Secondary to neck injury (cervicogenic)
Myofascial injury
Intervertebral discs
Cervical spondylosis
C2-3 facet joint (third occipital headache)
Secondary to temporomandibular joint injury
Greater and lesser occipital neuralgia
Migraine with and without aura
Footballer's migraine
Medication rebound
Cluster
Supraorbital and infraorbital neuralgia
Resulting from scalp lacerations or local trauma
Dysautonomic cephalgia
Carotid or vertebral artery dissection
Subdural or epidural hematomas
Hemorrhagic cortical contusions
Low cerebrospinal fluid pressure syndrome
Hemicrania continua
Chronic paroxysmal hemicranial
SUNCT
Mixed
Cranial Nerve Symptoms and Signs
Dizziness
Vertigo
Tinnitus
Hearing loss
Blurred vision
Diplopia
Convergence insufficiency
Light and noise sensitivity
Diminished taste and smell
Psychologic and Somatic Complaints
Irritability
Anxiety
Depression
Personality change
Post-traumatic stress disorder
Fatigue
Sleep disturbance
Decreased libido
Decreased appetite
Initial nausea or vomiting
Cognitive Impairment
Memory dysfunction
Impaired concentration and attention
Slowing of reaction time
Slowing of information processing speed
Rare Sequelae
Subdural and epidural hematomas
Cerebral venous thrombosis
Second impact syndrome
Seizures
Nonepileptic post-traumatic seizures
Transient global amnesia
Tremor
Dystonia

Source: Evans RW. Post-concussion syndrome. In: Evans RW, Baskin DS, Yatsu FM (eds): Prognosis of Neurological Disorders. 2nd ed. New York, Oxford University Press, 2000. pp. 366–380, with permission.

SUNCT, short-lasting unilateral neuralgiform headache attacks with conjunctival injection, tearing, sweating, and rhinorrhea.

Epidemiology

Head trauma of all degrees is one of the most important public health problems. Mild head injury accounts for 75% or more of all brain injuries.[158] The annual incidence of mild head injury per 100,000 population has been estimated to be 131 for San Diego County, California,[156] 149 for Olmsted County, Minnesota,[9] and 511 for Auckland, New Zealand.[289] However, the incidence of mild head injury may be as high as 640 per 100,000 population, as many cases go unreported.[20] In addition, some patients may have hidden traumatic brain injury in which they develop a postconcussion syndrome but do not make the causal connection between the injury and its consequences.[104] For an industrialized country such as the United States, estimates of the relative causes of head trauma are as follows: motor vehicle accidents 45%, falls 30%, occupational accidents 10%, recreational accidents 10%, and assaults 5%.[144] In the elderly, falls are more likely the cause, and motor vehicle accidents are more common in the young.[234] Males are injured twice as often as females. About one-half of all patients are between the ages of 15 and 34. It has been estimated that 20% to 40% of all patients with mild head injuries in the United States do not seek medical care.[96]

Historical Aspects

The postconcussion syndrome has been recognized for at least the past few hundred years.[80,260,273] One interesting historical case involved a 26-year-old maid servant who had been hit over the head with a stick and complained of retrograde amnesia. Six months later, she was still complaining of headaches, dizziness, tinnitus, and fatigue. A judge requested the opinion of the Swiss physician J.J. Wepfer and two other surgeons, who stated, "We can't say anything definite, but it is certain that this will leave its mark in the form of an impediment." Although similar prognostic opinions are still given, this particular statement was made in 1694.[60] Boyer in 1822, Astley Cooper in 1827, and Duputren in 1839 all described the clinical picture of cerebral concussion with persistent symptoms.

In 1879, Rigler[229] raised the important issue of compensation neurosis when he described the increased incidence of posttraumatic invalidism after a system for financial compensation was established for accidental injuries on the Prussian railways in 1871. Countering this view, Erichsen,[77] a London surgeon, felt that minor injuries to the head and spine could result in severe disability due to "molecular disarrangement" or anemia of the spinal cord. His 1882 book, *On Concussion of the Spine: Nervous Shock and Other Obscure Injuries of the Nervous System in Their Clinical and Medico-Legal Aspects*, was the medico-legal authority of the time and was frequently cited in court cases.

In 1888, Strumpell discussed how the desire for compensation could lead to exaggeration. In 1889, Oppenheim popularized the concept of traumatic neurosis, in which a strong afferent stimulus resulted in impairment of function of the central nervous system. Charcot countered Oppenheim's work and suggested that the impairment described was actually due to hysteria and neurasthenia. The *Boston Medical and Surgical Journal in 1883*[35] published several articles covering these different points of view. The leading article drew the following conclusions:

> In this iconoclastic age when we are not allowed to believe in a personal devil, or good honest ghosts, or even to coddle our own pet superstitions and hobbies without a suspicicion of mental degeneration, it is natural that the medical "bugaboo" raised by Mr. Erichsen some years ago, and christened spinal concussion, should meet with little quarter at the hands of the modern scientific observer. It is possible, however, that in this, as in other things, the skeptic may have gone too far, and that although it was no ghost that has alarmed us there may actually have been some phosphorescent light which we do not understand, and the nature of which we cannot fully explain. . . . A rose, however, under any other name, will remain as fragrant to the sufferer, and whether the ailment be termed railway spine or traumatic neurasthenia, the condition is equally distressing."

Another landmark work was the 1934 paper by Strauss and Savitsky.[260] They argued that concussion can occur without loss of consciousness and cited examples of significant intracranial trauma such as subdural hematomas, which can be caused by injuries not resulting in loss of consciousness. Strauss and Savitsky discussed the interrelationships of the head injury, premorbid personality, and the stress resulting from dealing with the aftermaths of the injury:

> There can be no denying that the present mode of handling these unfortunate persons in compensation bureaus multiplies the psychic stresses and strains and complicates an already almost intolerable situation of life. The harshness, injustice and brutal disregard of complaints show by the physicians and representatives of the insurance companies and their ready assumption of intent to swindle do not foster wholesome patterns of reaction in injured persons. The frequent expression of unjustifiable skepticism on the part of examiners engenders resentment, discouragement and hopelessness and too often forces these people to resort to more primitive modes of response (hysterical). The repeated psychic traumas bring out the worst that there is in them and makes manifest all their frailties and constitutional insufficiencies. This is especially true in view of the fact that the blow itself is known to give rise to defects in personality integratation. In addition, the premorbid make-up of the injured persons varies considerably and undoubtedly contributes much to the manner in which they handle their problems. The trauma, moreover, lowers resistances and thresholds and brings prominently into consciousness repressed conflicts and difficulties.

They concluded:

> In our opinion, the subjective posttraumatic syndrome, characterized by headache, dizziness, inordinate fatigue on effort, intolerance to intoxicants and vasomotor instability, is organic and is dependent on a disturbance in intracranial equilibrium due directly to the blow on the head. We suggest the term "postconcussion syndrome" for this symptom complex.

The use of the term *postconcussion syndrome* in this article and in Grinker's textbook,[108] also published in 1934, are the earliest uses of the term that I could find.

In 1961, Miller summarized the viewpoint of those who believe that the postconcussion syndrome is really a compensation neurosis: "The most consistent clinical feature is the subject's unshakable conviction of unfitness for work. . . ."[202] Symonds[266] took an equally strong opposing position in 1962 when he wrote, "It is questionable whether the effects of concussion, however slight, are ever completely reversible."

Neuropathology

In 1835, Gama[97] wrote, "Fibers as delicate as those of which the organ of mind is composed are liable to break as a result of violence to the head." For the next 120 years, neuropathologists described more obvious focal contusions due to coup and contrecoup injuries and hematomas.

In 1956, and with more cases in 1961,[261,262] Strich observed diffuse axonal injury resulting from shear and tensile strain damage. Microscopically, these injuries have the appearance of retraction balls, which were first described and named by Cajal.[42] Strich[262] explained that "when a nerve-fibre in the peripheral or central nervous system is cut, axoplasm flows out of both cut ends and is visible as a large blob." In 1968, Oppenheimer[214] extended this observation to five cases of mild head injury in which the patients died from fat embolism or pneumonia.

The observation of diffuse axonal injury in cases of mild head injury has been further confirmed.[2,25,103,170,223] A neurochemical substrate for mild head injury with release of the putative excitatory neurotransmitters acetylcholine, glutamate, and aspartate has been suggested.[121,122] Axonal rupture can occur at the time of injury. However, a gradient of axonal damage can occur, ranging from disruption of axoplasmic transport to delayed rupture due to release of putative neurotransmitters and other mechanisms.[223] Animal studies, including studies of monkeys and cats subjected to mild head injury, have demonstrated similar diffuse axonal injury.[140,223] Abnormalities in cerebral hemodynamics have been demonstrated in animals and humans after mild head injury.[68,227,267,271] Neuroimaging abnormalities are discussed later in this chapter, including serial magnetic resonance imaging (MRI) studies showing the development of generalized atrophy perhaps due to apoptotic processes.[182] Neuropathological and chemical abnormalities are discussed further in Chapter 4.

Nonorganic Explanations of Persistent Postconcussion Symptoms

For the minority of patients with persistent postconcussion symptoms, a variety of nonorganic explanations have been advanced that will be further discussed later in the chapter, including the following: psychogenic disorders (stress and premorbid neurosis, depression, and other types of personality and psychiatric disorders); psychosocial problems; chronic pain; posttraumatic stress disorder; expectation of chronic symptoms; the base rate phenomenon; malingering; and secondary gain due to litigation. Since many of the postconcussion symptoms are common in the general population, the base rate phenonomen is misattribution of symptoms to the injury.

Headache Types

Headaches are variably estimated as occurring in 30% to 90% of persons who are symptomatic following mild head injury.[204] Paradoxically, headache prevalence and lifetime duration are greater in those with mild head injury compared to those with more severe trauma.[50,51,291] Posttraumatic headaches are more common in those with a history of headache.[237]

Interestingly, patients who sustain iatrogenic trauma when undergoing a craniotomy for brain tumor (other than acoustic neuroma) or intractable epilepsy often have a self-limited combination of tension-type and site-of-injury headache, if they have any headache at all.[99] However, 3 months following removal of a vestibular schwannoma via the retrosigmoid approach, 34% of patients still complain of severe headaches.

According to the International Headache Society's criteria in the second edition of its *International Classification of Headache Disorders*, the onset of the headache should be less than 7 days after the injury.[123] This time period is arbitrary, particularly since the etiology of posttraumatic migraine is not understood. For example, posttraumatic epilepsy may have a latency of months or years. Similarly, it would not be surprising if there was a latency of weeks or months for posttraumatic migraine to develop. Conversely, since migraine is a rather common disorder, the longer the latency between the trauma and migraine onset, the more likely that the trauma may not have been causative. Consider the hypothetical case of a 27-year-old male who develops new-onset migraine 2 months after a mild head injury in a motor vehicle accident. The incidence of migraine in males under the age of 30 is 0.25% per year or, in this case, 0.042% per 2 months. Was the new-onset migraine due to the mild head injury or coincidence? Three months seems a more reasonable latency for onset than 7 days.[115]

Many patients have more than one type of headache or have headaches with tension and migraine features.[70,71,215] Neck injuries commonly accompany head trauma and can produce headaches. Headaches are also commonly associated with whiplash injuries (see Chapter 22). Although not part of postconcussion syndrome, headaches associated with subdural and epidural hematomas are also described.

Tension Type

About 85% of posttraumatic headaches are of the tension type. The headaches can occur in a variety of distributions including generalized, nuchal-occipital, bifrontal, bitemporal, cap-like, or headband. The headache, which may be constant or intermittent, with variable duration, is usually described as a pressure, tight, or dull aching. The headache may be present daily. Temporomandibular joint injury can be caused either by direct trauma or by jarring associated with the head injury.[37] Patients may complain of jaw pain and hemicranial or ipsilateral frontotemporal aching or pressure headaches.

Occipital Neuralgia and Third Occipital Headache

The term *occipital neuralgia* is in some ways a misnomer because the pain is not necessarily from the occipital nerve and does not usually have a neuralgic quality. Greater occipital neuralgia is a common type of posttraumatic headache but frequently is seen without injury as well.[52,124] The aching, pressure, stabbing, or throbbing pain may be in a nuchal-occipital and/or parietal, temporal, frontal, periorbital, or retro-orbital distribution. Occasionally, a true neuralgia may be present with paroxysmal shooting-type pain. The headache may last for minutes to hours to days and can be unilateral or bilateral. Lesser occipital neuralgia can similarly occur, with pain generally referred more laterally over the head.

The headache may be due to an entrapment of the greater occipital nerve in the aponeurosis of the superior trapezius or semispinalis capitis muscle or instead may be referred pain without nerve compression from trigger points in these or other suboccipital muscles. Digital pressure over the greater occipital nerve at the mid-superior nuchal line (halfway between the posterior mastoid and the occipital protuberance) reproduces the headache.

The C2-3 facet joint is innervated by the third occipital nerve. Pain referred from an injured C2–3 facet joint, third occipital headache[28,179] may produce a headache similar to occipital neuralgia. Tenderness over the C2–3 facet joint is suggestive of the diagnosis, which can be established by an anesthetic block.

Migraine[254]

Recurring attacks of migraine with and without aura can result from mild head injury.[17,286] Impact can also cause acute migraine episodes, often in adolescents with a family history of migraine. This condition was originally termed *footballer's migraine* to describe young men playing soccer who had multiple migraine with aura attacks triggered only by impact.[188] Similar attacks can be triggered by mild head injury in any sport.[11,18] The most famous example involved the running back of the Denver Broncos and was witnessed by hundreds of millions of people around the world during the 1998 Super Bowl. Terrell Davis, who had preexisting migraine, developed a migraine with aura after a ding on the helmet at the end of the first quarter. After successfully using DHE nasal spray, he was able to return for the third quarter, scored the winning touchdown, set a Super Bowl rushing record, and was voted Most Valuable Player.

Following minor head trauma, children, adolescents, and young adults can develop a variety of transient neurological sequelae that are not always associated with headache and are perhaps due to vasospasm.[116] Five clinical types can cause the following: hemiparesis; somnolence, irritability, and vomiting; a confusional state;[256] transient blindness, often precipitated by occipital impacts; and brain stem signs.[285]

Cluster, Hemicrania Continu (HC); Short-Lasting Unilateral Neuralgiform Headache Attacks with Conjunctival Injection, Tearing, Sweating, and Rhinorrhea. (SUNCT); and Chronic Paroyxmal Hemicrani (CPH)

Rare case reports have attributed trauma to the onset of cluster headaches,[275] HC,[83] SUNCT,[219] and CPH.[186]

Supraorbital and Infraorbital Neuralgia

Injury of the supraorbital branch of the first trigeminal division as it passes through the supraorbital foramen just inferior to the medial eyebrow can cause supraorbital neuralgia. Similarly, infraorbital neuralgia can result from trauma to the inferior orbit. Shooting, tingling, aching, or burning pain, along with decreased or altered sensation and sometimes decreased sweating in the appropriate nerve distribution, may be present. The pain can be paroxysmal or fairly constant. A dull aching or throbbing pain may also occur around the area of injury.

Scalp Lacerations and Local Trauma

Dysesthesias over scalp lacerations occur frequently. In the presence or absence of a laceration, an aching, soreness, tingling, or shooting pain over the site of the original trauma can develop.[282] The symptoms may persist for weeks or months but rarely for more than 1 year.

Subdural Hematoma

In one series, headaches occurred in 11% of patients with acute, 53% with subacute, and 81% with chronic subdural hematomas.[197] Since many of the patients with acute subdural hematomas had alteration of consciousness, headaches may have been underreported. The headaches associated with subdurals are nonspecific, ranging from mild to severe and from paroxysmal to constant. Unilateral headaches are usually due to ipsilateral subdural hematomas. Headaches associated with chronic subdural hematomas have at least one of the following features present in 75% of cases: sudden onset; severe pain; exacerbation with coughing, straining, or exercise; and vomiting and/or nausea.

One rare cause of subdural hematomas causing headaches is "roller-coaster headache."[26,90] Acceleration-deceleration forces of riding on a roller coaster without direct head trauma can tear bridging veins leading to a subdural hematoma. Roller coaster rides can also cause headaches due to internal carotid artery dissection;[24b] middle fossa arachnoid cyst as a risk factor for bilateral subdural hygromas;[130b] posttraumatic migraine;[193b] and cerebrospinal fluid leak.[243b]

Epidural Hematomas

The headaches of acute and chronic epidural hematomas may be unilateral or bilateral and can be nonspecific. Up to 30% of epidural hematomas are of the chronic type. The patient is often a child or young adult who sustains what appears to be a trivial injury, often without loss of consciousness. A persistent headache then develops, often associated with nausea, vomiting, and memory impairment, which might seem consistent with a postconcussion syndrome. After the passage of days to weeks, focal findings develop.

Low Cerebrospinal Fluid Pressure Headache

Trauma can cause a cerebrospinal fluid (CSF) leak through a dural root sleeve tear or a cribiform plate fracture and result in a low CSF pressure headache with the same features as a postlumbar puncture headache.[206]

Dysautonomic Cephalgia

This is a rare headache due to injury of the anterior triangle of the neck or carotid sheath.[281] Acute local pain and tenderness in the anterior triangle can be followed weeks or months later by severe unilateral frontotemporal headache, ipsilateral increased sweating of the face, dilation of the ipsilateral pupil, blurred vision, ipsilateral photophobia, and nausea. The headache can occur a few times per month and last for hours to days.

Other Types

Hemorrhagic cortical contusions can cause a headache due to subarachnoid hemorrhage. Rarely, posttraumatic headaches can be due to to carotid and vertebral artery dissections.

Cranial Nerve Symptoms and Signs

Dizziness and Hearing Loss

Dizziness is a common complaint following mild head injury, occurring in 53% of patients within 1 week of the injury[173] and persisting in 18% after 2 years.[44] Various types of peripheral and central pathology can cause the dizziness. Mild head injury without a temporal bone fracture can result in a labyrinthine concussion with vertigo, hearing loss, and tinnitus. Spontaneous or positional nystagmus and occasionally hypoactive calorics can be recorded with electronystagmography (ENG). Peripheral vestibular disturbances with canal paresis have been described in 17.1% of patients after mild head injury.[274] Positional nystagmus has been noted in 30% of patients with dizziness on discharge from the hospital after mild head injury.[44]

Mild head injury can also cause benign paroxysmal positional vertigo owing to dislodged otoconia from the utricular macule settling onto the cupula of the posterior semicircular canal.[13] The resulting dizziness can recur over a period of 1 to 10 years.[13] Occasionally, mild head injury without a skull fracture can result in a perilymph fistula, with the sudden onset of vertigo, hearing loss, or both. Prolonged I-V latencies on auditory brain stem evoked potential recordings are consistent with brain stem injury as the cause of dizziness in some cases.[208] Postural imbalance caused by disturbances of postural tonic activity can be demonstrated by abnormal statokinesimetry studies.[14]

In a prospective study of 58 patients with dizziness after a mild head injury referred to a vestibular clinic, the diagnoses were as follows: 41%, posttraumatic vestibular migraine; 28%, posttraumatic positional vertigo; 19%, posttraumatic spatial disorientation; and 12% could not be characterized.[129] The spatial disorientation group had distinct abnormalities of the vestibulo-ocular reflex and the vestibulo-spinal reflex and the following history: a constant feeling of unsteadiness worsened when standing still but present even when sitting or lying down, drifting to one side while walking, and shifting weight when standing still. At 1 year, 4% of the 58 patients were no better.

Conductive-type hearing loss can occur following mild head injury due to blood in the middle ear or disruption of the ossicular chain. Occasionally, sensorineural hearing loss can occur due to an unsuspected temporal bone fracture with normal skull radiographs.[39] Routine otoscopic examination is essential to detect hemotympanum. Bilateral sensorineural hearing loss without a fracture can also occur.[274]

Visual Symptoms

Blurred vision following mild head injury is reported by 14% of patients.[204] Convergence insufficiency is the most common cause. Although the anatomical localization is not known, lesions of the occipital lobe and upper midbrain are possibilities.[159] The diagnosis can be made by measurements of convergence fusional reserves. The near point of convergence alone is an unreliable measure.[159] Diplopia due to third, fourth, and sixth cranial nerve palsies can be caused by mild head injury. Trauma is the most common cause of fourth nerve palsy and may follow apparently trivial head trauma.[160] Bilateral internuclear ophthalmoplegia can very rarely result from mild head injury.[284] Optic nerve contusions can result in diminished visual acuity and hue discrimination.

Other Symptoms

Head trauma is the most common cause of anosmia.[61,125] Decreased smell and taste is reported by more than 5% of patients after mild head injury.[204] In a prospective study of 111 patients tested 2 weeks after a mild traumatic brain injury, 22% had hyposmia and 4% had anosmia.[59] Damage to the olfactory filaments can be caused by mild head trauma. Light and noise sensitivity were reported by 7.2% and 15% of patients, respectively, 14 days following mild head injury.[111] This sensitivity has been documented in two studies comparing patients after mild head injury to controls.[30,283]

Psychological and Somatic Complaints

Nonspecific psychological symptoms are common following mild head injury and include personality change, irritability, anxiety, and depression.[226,253a] Within 3 months of injury, up to 51% to 84% of patients have posttraumatic symptoms.[230,240] The symptoms can be quite persistent, with an incidence estimated at 15% to 33% at 1 year[62,241] and 15% after 3 years.[62] Lishman[177] has suggested interpreting these complaints in the context of pre-, peri-, and posttraumatic factors (Table 5.2). There is an increased risk of developing depression in patients after mild head injury compared to controls,[244] with a point prevalence of 14% to 29%.[226] Acute psychosis,[191] mania,[153] and Ganser syndrome[56] have been reported as rare sequelae of mild head trauma.

Posttraumatic stress disorder may also occur following mild closed head injury and has some symptoms similar to those of the postconcussion syndrome (see Chapter 34). In a study of patients with posttraumatic headache present for more than 3 months, nearly 30% were diagnosed with posttraumatic stress disorder.[48] In a prospective study with an initial cohort of 79 patients who sustained a mild traumatic brain injury in a motor vehicle accident, acute stress disorder was diagnosed in 14% at 1 month and posttraumatic stress disorder was diagnosed in 22% and 24% at 6 months and 2 years, respectively.[120a]

Table 5.2. Factors Relevant to Psychiatric Disability

1. Pre-traumatic
    - Age
    - Alcoholism
    - Mental constitution
        - Genetic vulnerability
        - Previous psychiatric illness
        - Personality (including being prone to accidents)
    - Pre-existing psychosocial difficulties
        - Domestic
        - Financial
        - Occupational
    - Recent life events
2. Peri-traumatic
    - Brain damage
        - Transient
        - Permanent
    - Other physical damage (skull, scalp, vestibular apparatus)
    - Emotional impact and meaning
        - Fear of accident
        - Fear of early symptoms
    - Circumstances of accident
        - Setting
        - Significance
        - Type (road traffic accident, industrial, domestic, sport)
    - Iatrogenic (early information, management, investigations)
3. Post-traumatic
    - Intellectual impairment
    - Other impairments (physical disabilities, deformity, scars)
    - Epilepsy
    - Emotional repercussions of accident (including depression)
    - Ensuring psychosocial difficulties
        - Domestic
        - Financial
        - Occupational
    - Compensation and litigation

Source: Lishman WA: Physiogenesis and psychogenesis in the "post-concussional syndrome." Br J Psychiatry 153:460–469, 1988, with permission.

Fatigue is a common complaint reported by 29% of patients at 4 weeks after the trauma and by 23% at 6 months.[204] Possible explanations include sleep deprivation; frustration with persisting symptoms such as headaches, dizziness, and blurred vision; the increased effort necessary to compensate for cognitive deficits;[110] and stress brought on by extra-injury factors such as impaired school and work performance, financial and family problems, interaction with health care providers, and pending litigation. These factors can also contribute to the decrease in appetite and libido reported by some patients.

Disruption of sleep patterns after mild head injury has been described.[218] Difficulty with falling asleep and arousal are the most common problems and are reported by 15% of patients 6 weeks post-injury.[240] Less often, increased sleep duration and daytime naps are reported. There has been a suggestion that chronic excessive daytime drowsiness can be triggered by mild head injury, but the data are inconclusive.[113]

Cognitive Impairment

In a study 4 weeks following mild head injury, 19% of patients complained of loss of memory, and 21% complained of difficulty with concentration.[204] Consistent with these complaints, deficits in cognitive functioning have been documented, including a reduction in information processing speed,[111] attention,[100] reaction time,[208,264] and memory for new information.[66,173] Neuropsychological testing needs to be tailored to detect these specific types of nonlocalizing deficits. Cognitive impairment is further discussed in Chapter 11.

Rare Sequelae

Subdural and Epidural Hematomas

Jennett et al.[145] estimated that a subdural hematoma occurs in fewer than 1 in 5000 patients who are seen in the hospital after mild head injury. For adults with mild head injury and an initial GCS score of 13 to 15, three other studies in the United States have variably reported the incidence of subdural hematomas as 0.5%,[54] 0.8%,[258] and 1.0%[147] and that of epidural hematomas as 0.2%,[54] 0.3%,[147] and 1%.[258] Mild head injuries without loss of consciousness or superficial cranial trauma can result in intracranial hematomas.[251] The incidence of neurosurgical complications after mild head injury has been estimated to be between 1% and 3%.[54]

Bollinger[32] first introduced the concept of delayed traumatic intracranial hematoma in 1891. Both subdural and epidural hematomas can later appear after an initial CT scan is normal.[64,168,203] After an apparently mild head injury, an epidural hematoma can have a delayed evolution of symptoms and mimic postconcussion syndrome.[19] The clinician needs to be vigilant to recognize these rare complications.[64]

Second Impact Syndrome

Diffuse cerebral swelling is a rare complication of mild head injury, usually occurring in children and adolescents and resulting in death or a persistent vegetative state.[40] When diffuse cerebral swelling occurs after a second concussion when an athlete is still symptomatic from an earlier concussion, the term *second impact syndrome* is used. This syndrome is a rare and somewhat controversial complication[195] (also see Chapter 26).

Seizures

The relative risk within 5 years of a posttraumatic seizure after a mild head injury with loss of consciousness or posttraumatic amnesia of less than 30 minutes and without a skull fracture in one population study was 1.5.[8] Another study in Taiwan of 4232 adult patients with mild head injuries and a normal neurological examination reported that 2.36% of these patients developed seizures within 1 week.[165] Posttraumatic seizures are discussed further in Chapter 7.

Transient Global Amnesia

Transient global amnesia has been described after mild head injury. Haas and Ross[118] described nine patients, ages 11 to 28, who had episodes of transient global amnesia lasting for 2 to 24 hours following mild head injury, probably without loss of consciousness. Five of the patients had a headache associated with the amnestic episode. During the episode, almost all of the patients voiced repetitive queries or comments. A 12-year-old boy had a second similar episode subsequently triggered by a second mild head injury at the age of 14. He had a paternal grandmother with an episode of transient global amnesia at the age of 73. A 16-year-old subject of the study had a 15-year-old brother who had had two similar episodes of transient global amnesia after mild head injury. Based on the generally young age of the patients, associated headaches in some, and a positive family history in others, Haas and Ross suggested that these episodes were due to posttraumatic confusional migraine. Additional patients with similar episodes have been described.[93,162]

Movement Disorders

Movement disorders have been described as sequelae of mild head injury142.[141,155] Biary et al.[22] described a posttraumatic tremor similar to essential tremor, although myoclonic-like jerking was frequently present. Six of their seven patients had a postural and kinetic tremor, and the seventh had a resting , postural, and kinetic tremor. The tremor could involve the head, hands, legs, trunk, and tongue. The onset of the tremor occurred anywhere from immediately after the head injury to 4 weeks later. All of the patients had normal CT or MRI scans of the brain. Clonazepam reduced the tremor in three patients and propranolol decreased it in another. Primidone was not of benefit. The tremor did not resolve in any of the patients studied. I have treated two similar patients, one with nadolol and the other with alprazalom, with modest improvement.

Parkinson's syndrome can follow severe head trauma or multiple episodes of mild head injury.[210] Stern et al.,[259a] however, have suggested that head trauma should be reassessed as a potential risk factor for Parkinson's disease based on their study of various environmental exposures, early life experiences, and head injuries in 149 patients. Head injury or stress caused by motor vehicle accidents may transiently increase the dysfunction of Parkinson's disease without altering the long-term prognosis.[101]

Mild head injury associated with a whiplash injury has been reported as causing torticollis.[142,248] Mild head injury has also been associated with hemidystonia.[155,157] Dysfunction of the lenticulothalamic neuronal circuit may be related to the development of dystonia following head trauma.[164] Posttraumatic movement disorders are discussed further in Chapter 33.

Mild Head Injury as a Risk Factor for Alzheimer's Disease

Neuropathological studies suggest that brain injury can lead to Alzheimer's disease. The brains of boxers with dementia pugilistica demonstrate β amyloid protein containing diffuse plaques and neurofibrillary tangles, pathological features similar to those of Alzheimer's disease.[231] In a study of 152 patients after a severe head injury with a survival time of between 4 hours and 2.5 years, 30% demonstrated β amyloid protein deposits in one or more cortical areas.[232] The plaques occurred more frequently than in neurologically normal controls. This suggests "that increased expression of β amyloid precursor protein (β APP) is part of an acute phase response to neuronal injury in the human brain, that extensive overexpression of β APP can lead to deposition of β amyloid protein and the initiation of an Alzheimer disease–type process within days, and that head injury may be an important aetiological factor in Alzheimer's disease."[232]

Epidemiological studies have also investigated this issue. Head injury with loss of consciousness may[189,190,280] or may not[45] be a risk factor for the development of Alzheimer's disease. A meta-analysis found that head injury was a risk factor with an odds ratio of 2.29 only in males.[95] Mild head injury is not a proven risk factor for the development of Alzheimer's disease. Studies showing a causal relationship should be interpreted with caution because early Alzheimer's disease may cause falls with a head injury and the possibility of recall bias in retrospective studies.[280] Prospective population-based case-controlled studies could provide additional information.

Testing

The judicious use of testing needs to be individualized for each patient.[295] Routine imaging studies available include CT scan and MRI studies of the brain. Neurophysiological studies include electroencephalography (EEG) and auditory brain stem responses (ABRs). For some patients with prominent complaints of dizziness, hearing loss, or tinnitus, referral to an otorhinolaryngologist and ENG, audiometric, and posturography testing may be worthwhile to assess for the presence of peripheral and central pathology, as discussed in the prior section. Patients with persisting blurred vision, diplopia, acuity changes, or field cuts may require referral to an ophthalmologist and formal assessment of visual fields.

When performed by a knowledgeable and experienced psychologist, neuropsychological evaluation can be quite helpful for evaluating patients with prominent cognitive complaints or psychological problems. The referring physician, however, should be aware that the findings are easily subject to mis- and overinterpretation for a variety of reasons,[94,225] especially in medico-legal cases.[194] Neuropsychological testing is discussed further in Chapters 11 and 12.

Imaging Studies

Computed Tomography Scan

Patients with a GCS score of less than 15, an abnormal mental status, or hemispheric neurological deficits should have a CT scan.[92,258] In a study by Feuerman et al.,[92] 3 of 137 adults with GCS scores of 13 or 14 had operative hematomas and another 3 had significant deterioration while in the hospital under observation. Stein and Ross[258] reported CT abnormalities in 37.5% of adults with a GCS score of 13 and in 24.2% with a score of 14.

For patients with a GCS score of 15, the indications for CT are less certain. Feuerman et al.,[92] based upon a retrospective review of 236 adults, 68% with loss of consciousness, recommended that patients with a GCS score of 15, normal mental status, and no hemispheric neurological deficit be discharged for observation without a CT scan. Stein and Ross,[258] however, reported a 13% risk of an abnormal CT scan in 1117 patients with a GCS score of 15 and no focal neurological deficits. The number of these patients who required neurosurgical intervention was not reported. The authors recommended a routine CT scan in all head injury patients who have lost consciousness or are amnesic, even if all other physical findings are normal. Jeret et al.,[147] in a prospective study of 712 adults with a GCS score of 15, found significant CT abnormalities in 9.4%, including 2 with epidural, 9 with subdural, and 7 with intracerebral hematomas. Only two (0.3%) required neurosurgical intervention, and one died. Risk factors for an abnormal CT scan included older age, white race, signs of basilar skull fracture, and being either a pedestrian hit by a motor vehicle or a victim of an assault. Based upon a meta-analysis of 73 studies, the estimated prevalence of intracranial CT scan abnormalities is 5% in patients presenting to the hospital with a GCS score of 15 and 30% or higher in patients presenting with a score of 13.[34] About 1% of all treated patients with mild traumatic brain injury require neurosurgical intervention.

Two clinical decision instruments have been proposed to identify criteria to guide in CT use in patients with mild head injury. Haydel et al.[120c] performed CT scans on 1429 patients age more than 3 years with minor head injuries with loss of consciousness seen in the emergency room within 24 hours of the injury with a GCS score of 15 and a normal neurological examination. Ninety-three patients had positive CT scans and 6 (.4%) underwent neurosurgery for the lesions. They suggested that CT is only indicated in patients with minor head injury with one of seven risk factors or criteria with a sensitivity of 100% and specificity of 24.5%. The New Orleans Criteria (NOC) are the following: headache, vomiting, an age over 60 years, drug or alcohol intoxication, deficits in short-term memory, physical evidence of trauma above the clavicles, and seizure.

Stiell et al.[259c] performed a prospective emergency department study on 3121 persons over 16 years of age with GCS scores of 13–15. They derived the Canadian CT head rule (CCHR) that consists of five high-risk factors (failure to reach GCS of 15 within 2 hours, suspected open skull fracture, any sign of basal skull fracture, vomiting >two episodes, or age >65 years) and two additional medium-risk factors (amnesia before impact >30 minutes and dangerous mechanism of injury). The high-risk factors were 100% sensitive for predicting need for neurological intervention and would require only 32% of patients to undergo CT. The medium-risk factors were 98.4% sensitive and 49.6% specific for predicting clinically important brain injury and would require only 54% of patients to undergo CT.

Two studies provide external validation for these instruments. Stiell et al.[259b] performed a prospective study of 2707 adults who presented with blunt head trauma resulting in witnessed loss of consciousness, disorientation, or definite amnesia and a GCS score of 13 to 15 and underwent CT scans in Canadian emergency departments. Of 1822 patients with GCS score of 15, eight (.4%) required neurosurgical intervention and 97 (5.3%) had clinically important brain injury. The NOC and the CCHR both had 100% sensitivity but the CCHR was more specific (76.3% vs. 12.1%) for predicting need for neurosurgical intervention. For clinically important brain injury, the CCHR and the NOC were both 100% sensitive but the CCHR was more specific (50.6% vs. 12.7%), and would result in lower CT rates (52.1% vs. 88.0%). The kappa values for physician interpretation of the rules, CCHR vs. NOC, were 0.85 vs. 0.47. Physicians misinterpreted the rules as not requiring imaging for 4.0% of patients according to CCHR and 5.5% according to NOC (P = .04). Among all 2707 patients with a GCS score of 13 to 15, the CCHR had a sensitivity of 100% for 41 patients requiring neurosurgical intervention and 100% for 231 patients with clinically important brain injury.

Smits et al.[253b] performed a prospective study of 3181 patients with a GCS score of 13–15 who presented to four university hospitals in The Netherlands with GCS score of 13–14 or with 15 and at least one risk factor (including the 7 NOC). Of 3181 patients with a GCS score of 13–15, neurosurgical intervention was performed in 17 patients (0.5%). Traumatic CT findings were present in 312 patients (9.8%). Sensitivity for neurosurgical intervention was 100% for both the CCHR and the NOC. The NOC had a higher sensitivity for traumatic findings and for clinically important findings (97.7%–99.4%) than did the CCHR (83.4%–87.2%). Specificities were very low for the NOC (3.0%–5.6%) and higher for the CCHR (37.2%–39.7%). The estimated potential reduction in CT scans for patients with minor head injury would be 3.0% for the adapted NOC and 37.3% for the adapted CCHR.

There are some caveats in using these two clinical decision instruments.[120b] The instrument may not be optimal for the patient population or setting. Both studies exclude patients without loss of consciousness. However, Smits et al.[253b] found that almost 30% of patients who required neurosurgical intervention had not lost consciousness. Due to inclusion criteria in the original studies, neither instrument can be applied to patients with anticoagulation and the CCHR cannot be applied to those with posttraumatic seizures. Finally, patient and family anxiety and medicolegal concerns may also enter the decision making.

Magnetic Resonance Imaging

Magnetic resonance imaging is more sensitive than CT scan in evaluating head injury. Hesselink et al.,[128] in a comparative study of MRI and CT scans, reported that MRI detected 98% of brain contusions compared with only 56% detected by CT scan. Magnetic resonance imaging was superior in demonstrating brain contusions during the subacute and chronic stages after head trauma. Yokota et al.[293] performed another comparative study of 177 patients with mild to severe head injury. They found that MRI was superior to CT scan in diagnosing acute nonhemorrhagic contusions. In addition, MRI provided some information allowing clinicians to evaluate the severity of diffuse axonal injury and to predict delayed traumatic intracerebral hematoma.

Levin et al.[175] performed a comparative study of CT and MRI on 50 consecutive patients admitted with mild to moderate nonmissile head injuries. Magnetic resonance imaging detected parenchymal lesions, primarily in the frontotemporal region, in 80% of patients, including 26% of those with a normal CT scan and in 52% in whom MRI showed more lesions than were seen on CT. Eighteen percent had lesions on CT not detected on MRI. Follow-up scans at 1 and 3 months showed marked reduction in the size of lesions.

The prevalence of MRI abnormalities in patients with mild head injury alone is not clear from these studies. In a study of 20 patients with mild head injury using a 1.5 T magnet, MRI abnormalities compatible with diffuse axonal injury were reported in 30% of cases with normal CT findings.[205] This study also demonstrated the additional sensitivity of a high-field-strength magnetic and gradient-echo imaging.

Hughes et al.[132] performed MRI studies on a 1.0 T scanner and neuropsychological assessment on 80 consecutive patients with a mean age of 31 years within 24 to 72 hours of presentation to the emergency department with a mild traumatic brain injury (94% had a GCS score of 15). Abnormalities were detected on 32.5% of the scans, but only 6.3% were definitely posttraumatic. The rest were foci of high signal in white matter detected on fluid attenuated inversion recovery (FLAIR) sequences; it is not possible to be certain whether these represented incidental findings or were subtle evidence of axonal injury. (The FLAIR sequence is particularly sensitive to diffuse axonal injury, cortical contusion, and subdural hematomas, as well as to incidental high-signal foci.) However, 81% of the abnormalities were in the frontal lobes, consistent with a traumatic etiology. Follow-up scans were attempted at 3 months, but attendance was poor. There was weak correlation of abnormal MRI findings with abnormal neuropsychological tests for attention in the acute period. There was no significant correlation of abnormal MRI findings with a questionnaire for postconcussion syndrome and return-to-work status.

MacKenzie et al.[182] performed a retrospective longitudinal quantitative analysis of the volume of brain parenchyma (VBP) on serial MRI scans of 11 patients with mild head injury and 3 with moderate head injury. At an average of 11 months after trauma, whole-brain atrophy was present, with a loss of brain parenchyma 2.8 times greater (4.2% versus 1.5% change in %VBP) and a rate of %VBP loss greater for the group with traumatic brain injury than for the control subjects. The authors suggest that the etiology is a neurodegenerative or apoptotic process. In another serial MRI study, Hofman et al.[130a] also reported whole-brain atrophy in 57% of subjects with a mild traumatic brain injury and an initial GCS score of 14 or 15.

Mild head injury might result in an increase in dilated perivascular or Virchow-Robin spaces. Inglese et al. obtained MRI scans in 24 consecutive adult patients with a mean age of 33.6 years with mild head injuries and compared them to normal controls.[136b] Fifteen patients underwent MR imaging within a mean interval of 3.6 days and nine patients after an average of 3.7 years. The mean number of high-convexity Virchow-Robin spaces was significantly higher in the injured than controls. Although the number of spaces correlated with age in controls, the number did not correlate with age or elapsed time from injury in injured subjects. They suggest that the findings reflect early and permanent brain changes that may result from the accumulation of inflammatory cells and/or changes of vascular permeability. This intriguing finding is being explored in a larger study with serial MRI, clinical, and neuropsychological evaluations.

Functional Magnetic Resonance Imaging

A few studies have investigated the utility of functional MRI in the evaluation of mild traumatic brain injury. McAllister et al.[192] evaluated the brain activation patterns of 18 patients with mild traumatic brain injury within 1 month of their injury compared to 12 controls in response to a task involving an increasing working memory load. The patients showed a different pattern of allocation of processing resources associated with a high processing load condition compared to the healthy controls despite similar task performance.

Jantzen et al.[143] acquired preseason baseline levels of blood oxygen level–dependent (BOLD) activity during a test battery on eight college football players.[143] Four players who sustained a concussion were retested within 1 week of the injury. Compared with control subjects, concussed players had a marked within-subject increase in the amplitude and extent of BOLD activity during a finger sequencing task, primarily in the parietal and lateral frontal and cerebellar regions.

Chen et al.[46] compared the results of BOLD functional MRI studies of 16 elite athletes (15/16 still symptomatic) 1–16 months after a concussion to 8 matched controls on a task of working memory. The athletes had weaker BOLD changes within the right mid-dorsolateral prefrontal cortex. In addition, almost all of the symptomatic athletes had additional atypical activations that deviated from the control group in at least one region, suggesting use of compensatory mechanisms through alternative cognitive resources.

Single Photon Emission Computed Tomography Scans

Technetium-99m-hexamethylpropyleneamine (HMPAO) single photon emission computed tomography (SPECT) may have application in the evaluation of mild head injury. Ichise et al.[134] evaluated 15 patients with a history of mild head injury who were still symptomatic at least 6 months after the injury. SPECT detected abnormalities in 53% compared with 31% on MRI and 11% on CT. The SPECT abnormalities, areas of decreased gray matter perfusion, were predominantly in the frontal and temporal lobes.

Jacobs et al.[138] evaluated 25 patients with minor neurological complaints after mild head injury with no history of loss of consciousness or retrograde amnesia and no CT abnormalities. HMPAO SPECT scans performed within 4 weeks of the injury were abnormal in nine patients (36%). A repeat scan of these nine patients after a mean interval of 3 months showed persistent abnormalities in seven. The SPECT scan results were highly significant predictors of the clinical outcome. All the patients with normal initial scans had resolution of postconcussion symptoms and a normal neurological examination, memory, and concentration tests (termed *clinically negative*) when reevaluated at a mean time of 3 months. In the group with abnormal initial scans, at follow-up, one of seven patients with an abnormal scan and two of two with a normal scan were clinically negative.

Abu-Judeh et al.[1] retrospectively performed SPECT scans on 228 symptomatic patients within 3 years of a mild or moderate traumatic head injury (28% unknown and 18% had no loss of consciousness). Seventy-seven percent had abnormal findings, most commonly basal ganglia followed by frontal lobe and temporal lobe hypoperfusion. There was no control group.

Hofman et al.[130a] performed MRI scans and neurocognitive assessment on 21 consecutive patients and SPECT scans (on 18/21) who sustained a mild traumatic brain injury. Fifty-seven percent had abnormal MRI findings and 61% had abnormal SPECT findings with areas of hypoperfusion. Three patients had normal SPECT scans with abnormal MRI studies, and four patients had normal MRI studies with abnormal SPECT scans. The mean neurocognitive performance of all subjects was within the normal range. There was no difference in neurocognitive performance between patients with normal and abnormal MRI findings. Patients with abnormal MRI findings only showed significantly slower reaction times during a reaction-time task. Seven patients had persistent neurocognitive complaints, and one patient met the criteria for a postconcussion syndrome.

Bonne et al.[33] compared the results of SPECT scans of 28 symptomatic patients (with abnormal neuropsychological test results but normal structural brain imaging studies) who had sustained mild traumatic brain injuries a mean of 5.2 years previously to those of 20 matched controls. Patients demonstrated regions of hypoperfusion in frontal, prefrontal, and temporal cortices and subcortical structures. Hypoperfusion in frontal, left posterior, and, to a lesser extent, subcortical subgroups was concordant with neuropsychological localization.

The authors concluded, "Although group analysis is appropriate for the generation of statistically significant differences, the clinical application of brain SPECT imaging in MTBI calls for a capability to associate clinical examination, neuropsychological assessment and cerebral perfusion at the individual subject level. Such competence is still to be attained."

Despite these interesting studies, the clinical use of SPECT scans in evaluating the sequelae of mild head injury in individual patients is questionable. SPECT scan abnormalities are not specific. For example, depression and polydrug abuse can produce perfusion deficits similar to those described after head injury.[147a,169] Because of these questions of sensitivity and specificity, the use of SPECT scans in medico-legal cases is difficult to justify.[228]

Positron Emission Tomography and Magnetic Source Imaging

Although positron emission tomography (PET) has been reported to show widespread abnormalities in cerebral glucose metabolism after severe head injury,[3] little information is available about the findings after mild head injury. One study of three patients with cognitive impairment after mild head injury demonstrated decreased glucose metabolism.[133]

Chen et al.[47] compared the results of PET scans of five symptomatic patients who had sustained mild head injuries with persistent symptoms a mean of 16.6 months previously to five matched controls. During the spatial working memory task, patients had a smaller increase in regional cerebral blood flow than controls in the right prefrontal cortex. Positron emission tomography studies are limited by their cost, limited resolution, and limited availability.[217]

Magnetic source imaging (MSI) combines magnetoencephelography and MRI information into a merged graphic dataset.[176] Studies of abnormal low-frequency magnetic activity (ALFMA) involve analyses of spontaneous neuromagnetic signals that correspond to focal delta or theta frequency EEG slowing. In a study of 30 patients after mild head injury, MRI abnormalities were found in only 6, while ALFMA was identified in 18.[176] Of the original group of patients, six underwent two or more sequential examinations. The persistence or resolution of ALFMA correlated with the persistence or resolution of symptoms.

Lewine et al.[176] compared the results of MRI, EEG, and MSI in 20 control subjects, 10 subjects with complete recovery from mild head injuries, and 20 subjects with persistent postconcussion symptoms. The percentage of MRI, EEG, and MSI abnormalities, respectively, were as follows: controls, 0%, 5%, 5%; recovered injured, 0%, 10%, 10%; and persistent symptoms, 20%, 20%, 65%. Magnetic source imaging indicated brain dysfunction in significantly more patients with postconcussive symptoms than either EEG or MRI. While these studies provide additional confirmation of pathology caused by mild head injury, clinical application depends upon confirmation in additional studies and more widespread availability of the technology.

Neurophysiological Assessment

Electroencephalography

During the past 50 years, EEG studies have frequently been done to evaluate mild head injury. Dow et al.[69] reported an interesting patient series in 1944. They equipped a room of the first aid station at Kaiser's Oregon Ship Building Corporation with an EEG machine. During the study at this site, where 33,000 people were employed, 197 employees underwent EEG studies shortly after sustaining mild head injuries and were compared to 211 coworker controls. Sixty-two percent of the control group and 57% of the head-injured group had normal EEGs. Thirty percent of the control group and 33% of the head-injured groups had borderline records with increased theta activity. Eight percent of the control group and 10% of the head-injured group had abnormal EEGs. The EEGs performed within 30 minutes of the injury showed a greater percentage of abnormalities than those taken after 30 minutes. Clinical judgment was more predictive of time lost from work than the EEG results.

As this shipyard study demonstrates, abnormal studies in patients after mild head injury are not specific because of the high frequency of abnormal EEG studies in controls. Lorenzoni[180] further confirmed this poor specificity in an EEG study of 72 patients with head injuries in whom an EEG had been obtained before the injury. The pretraumatic EEG studies were obtained between 2 and 8 years before the accident, with 33 normal and 39 abnormal results. The posttraumatic EEG studies were obtained within 4 weeks of the injury. Fifty-seven percent of the pretraumatic normal records were still normal, and 43% showed focal or generalized slow wave activity after the injury. Thirty-one percent of the studies that were abnormal before the injury were normal after the injury, 23% were unchanged, and 46% were worse. Spike and wave complexes were not present following the head injury unless they had been present before.

Although it is difficult to determine with certainty in the individual whether abnormalities were caused by the mild head injury, as a group athletes with prior mild head injuries do have an increased incidence of abnormal EEG recordings. Tysvaer et al.[277] studied 37 former soccer players of the Norwegian National Team. Sixteen of them had chronic symptoms such as headache, irritability, dizziness, lack of concentration, and loss of memory. A significantly increased incidence of EEG abnormalities was found in former players compared with matched controls. The number of cumulative mild head injuries may be reflected in an EEG study of a group. In a study of 40 ex-boxers, Ross et al.[235] found a significant correlation between EEG abnormalities and the number of bouts fought.

Electroencephalographic studies after mild head injury may be abnormal in only a minority of patients, showing diffuse or asynchronous theta and delta activity and a decrease of alpha amplitude and frequency. These abnormalities may resolve with time. An EEG study may be very helpful when a posttraumatic seizure disorder is suspected. The utility of EEG studies following mild head injuries is restricted due to their limited sensitivity and specificity.[213b]

Brain Mapping

Abnormalities in EEG power spectral analyses have been reported following mild head injury.[208,269,270] These studies provide additional information suggesting cerebral cortical dysfunction following mild head injury. However, EEG discriminant analysis is subject to misdiagnosis.[213a,213b] When presented in courtrooms in the United States, computerized EEG studies contain a high frequency of serious errors.[76] The Therapeutics and Technology Assessment Subcommittee of the American Academy of Neurology does not recommend routine use of EEG brain mapping for evaluation of mild head injury.[212]

Auditory Brain Stem Response

Auditory brain stem responses (ABRs) have been reported as being abnormal following mild head injury, providing additional evidence of a disturbance of brain stem function.[245] Montgomery et al.[207,208] reported an abnormal I-V interval in one-half of a group of patients following mild head injury. The abnormality persisted in most for at least 6 weeks. In a similar study, Schoenhuber et al.[247] found abnormal ABR results in about 10% of patients after mild head injury. No specific pattern of abnormality was detected, although interpeak latency I–III was most often affected.

Schoenhuber et al.[246] reported a prospective study of 103 patients in whom ABRs were recorded within 48 hours of mild head injury. At 1-year follow-up, 80% of the patients had at least one persisting complaint, with irritability reported by 54%, memory loss by 47%, and depression by 39%. Auditory brain stem response abnormalities, however, were found with the same prevalence in patients with and without a postconcussion syndrome. The data suggest that ABRs not be used for medico-legal evaluation of patients with a postconcussion syndrome.

Event Related Potentials

Event related potential abnormalities provide additional evidence of impaired brain functioning after mild head injury. When an infrequent or oddball visual stimulus is presented to a subject, a positive wave is elicited after 300 ms (the P300) and recorded using an averaged time-locked EEG. The P300 amplitude was reduced in 20 college athletes with postconcussion syndrome compared to controls.[72] The amplitude was also attenuated in 10 college athletes who were still symptomatic compared to 10 who had recovered from mild concussions.[163] Abnormal findings have also been reported in symptomatic patients after mild head injury using event related potentials in an auditory oddball task.[222] In another interesting study, as a group, 10 asymptomatic college students who had sustained mild head injuries an average of 6.4 years previously had significantly reduced P300 amplitude on auditory oddball tasks compared to controls.[249]

Biochemical Markers

Neuron specific enolase (NSE) and S-100B are markers of cell damage of the central nervous system. Neuron specific enolase is an isoenzyme of enolase and is located mainly in neurons but also in smooth muscle fibers and adipose tissue. S-100 (soluble in 100% ammonium sulfate) is an acidic calcium binding protein found in the brain as the isoforms S-100B (95%) and S-100A1 (5%). S-100B is found in high concentrations in glial cells and Schwann cells and is highly specific for lesions of the central nervous system. S-100A1 is found in neurons. S-100A1 and S-100B form the heterodimer S100A1B. After brain injury, increased concentrations of NSE and S-100B can be measured in peripheral blood serum, with peak concentrations occurring within 6 hours and half-lives of about 20 and 2 hours, respectively.

In a 6-month study of 29 patients evaluated within 1 day of a mild head injury, elevated serum S-100B protein levels and, to a lesser degree, NSE levels, were significantly associated with disorders of attentional performance on neuropsychological testing.[126] Elevated serum S-100B protein levels were also predictive of abnormalities in another study that evaluated neuropsychological test results at 3 months in patients who had sustained mild head injuries.[136a]

Ingebrigtsen et al.[135] prospectively evaluated 182 patients with mild head injuries within 24 hours. Undetectable serum levels of S-100 protein predicted a normal CT scan of the brain. Of the 38% of patients with an elevated level, 5% had intracranial pathology on CT (mostly brain contusions). On 3-month follow-up, there was a trend toward an increased frequency of postconcussion symptoms among patients with detectable levels.

De Kruijk et al.[58] prospectively evaluated parameters that may be predictive of the severity of posttraumatic complaints 6 months after mild traumatic brain injury in a series of 79 patients presenting to the emergency room within 6 hours of the injury. After 6 months, 28% of the patients were still symptomatic. An elevated S-100B level was correlated with the severity of forgetfulness after 6 months. Increased NSE concentrations were positively associated with the severity of dizziness and headache after 6 months. The presence of headache, dizziness, or nausea in the emergency room was strongly associated with the severity of most posttraumatic complaints after 6 months.

Savola and Hillborn[242] evaluated 172 consecutive patients with mild head injury seen in the emergency room within 6 hours of the injury. At 1-month follow-up, 22% reported postconcussion symptoms. An elevated serum protein S-100B level had a specificity for postconcussion symptoms at 1 month of 93% but a sensitivity of only 27%. Other significant predictors of postconcussion symptoms were skull or facial fractures, dizziness, and headache. These abnormal biochemical markers are additional objective evidence of an organic basic for the postconcussion syndrome.

De Boussard[56a] and colleagues found S100 proteins not to be predictive of cognitive impairment. In a prospective study of 97 patients with mild traumatic brain injuries and GCS scores of 14 and 15 compared to controls, concentrations of S100B and S100A1B were above cutoff in 31% and 48%, respectively, but were not significantly associated with abnormal symptoms or signs of cognitive impairment 3 months after injury. In another study of subjects with mild traumatic brain injuries, Stapert et al.[256a] found that elevation of the S100B protein concentration was not predictive of abnormal neuropsychological performance assessed at a median of 13 days after injury.

Prognosis

During the past 60 years, many prognostic studies have been performed. Comparison among the studies, however, is difficult due to significant differences, including the definition of mild head injury, testing employed, study design, and subject characteristics (Table 5.3).[38,81,171]

Loss of Consciousness and Posttraumatic Amnesia

The probability of having persistent symptoms and neuropsychological deficits is the same whether a patient is only dazed or if loss of consciousness of varying duration of less than 1 hour occurs.[62,167] The duration of posttraumatic amnesia has been reported as being predictive[204] and not predictive[74] of postconcussion sequelae. There is no correlation between duration of posttraumatic amnesia and time off from work following the injury.[290]

Subject Characteristics

Many subject characteristics may affect the prognosis, including age,[102] sex, occupation, socioeco-

Table 5.3. Variables in Prognostic Studies

Definition of Mild Head Injury
Loss of consciousness and if so, duration
Duration, if present, of post-traumatic amnesia
Glasgow Coma Scale score
Inclusion of skull fractures/or cerebral contusions.
Radiological
Neurophysiological
Neuropsychological
Use of Testing
Study Design
Prospective vs. retrospective
Length of follow-up
Spontaneous volunteering of symptoms vs. responding to a checklist
Face to face interview vs. a mailed questionnaire
Use of matched controls
Number of subjects
Symptoms assessed
Subject Variables
Cause of head injury
Hospital vs. outpatient presentation
Geographic and cultural differences
Age and gender
Socioeconomic and educational level
Pre-morbid personality and psychopathology
Prior head trauma
Use of alcohol and drugs
Multiple trauma
Pending or completed litigation
Attrition rate of subjects

Source: Evans RW. Post-concussion syndrome. In: Evans RW, Baskin DS, Yatsu FM (eds): Prognosis of Neurological Disorders, 2nd ed. New York, Oxford University Press, 2000, pp. 366–380, with permission.

nomic status, personality, intelligence, social adversity, history of prior head injuries, prior use of alcohol or illicit drugs, and multiple trauma. Age over 40 years is a risk factor for increased duration and number of postconcussion symptoms[62,74,127] and slower recovery from cognitive deficits.[15,110] Late symptoms occur more often in women than in men.[74,239] Ferrari et al.[91] and others have also stated that expectation of chronic symptoms after mild head injury may be a significant factor in producing chronic complaints.

Symonds[265] observed, "The symptom picture depends not only upon the kind of injury, but upon the kind of brain." Preexisting psychopathology and premorbid personality are important factors.[152] Patients with high IQ recover more rapidly than low-IQ patients, even though the degree of initial impairment of information processing speed is not related to intelligence.[109] The greater motivation of high achievers may be responsible. Patients with adverse life events in the year preceding injury may be at increased risk for the emergence and persistence of a postconcussion syndrome.[89]

Cumulative diffuse axonal injuries and contusions may explain why prior head injury is a risk factor for persistence and for the number of postconcussion symptoms.[43,112,137] An increased number of posttraumatic sequelae and additional slowing of reaction time are associated with a history of prior alcohol abuse.[43] Alcohol intoxication makes the initial assessment of patients with head injury more difficult[36] and is a risk factor for neurosurgical sequelae. Finally, multiple trauma with associated orthopedic or soft tissue injuries contributes to the persistence and frequency of postconcussion symptoms[66] and can cause additional functional impairment, depression, anxiety, and stress.[21,43]

Postconcussion Symptoms

The percentage of patients reported with various symptoms following mild head injury varies (Table 5.4). The percentage of patients with headaches at 1 month is variably reported as 31.3%[204] and 90%[62] and at 3 months as 47%[173] and 78%.[230] At 4 years, 24% of the patients had persisting headaches.[74] The frequency of dizziness at 1 week varies from 19%[44] to 53%.[173] Dizziness is reported in 25% of patients at 1 year[201] and in 18% at 2 years[44,62] and at 4 years.[74] Memory problems are reported in 18.8% of patients at 1 month,[204] 59% at 3 months,[230] 15.3% at 6 months,[204] variably as 3.8%,[241] 4.2%,[6] and 25% at 1 year,[201] and 19% at 4 years.[74] At 1 month, 24.7% of patients reported irritability,[204] and variably at 1 year, so did 5.3%[241] and 21%.[201]

Comparison to controls is important because the symptoms of postconcussion syndrome are so common in the general population. Dikmen et al.[66] compared 20 patients with mild head injuries to carefully matched controls 1 month after the injury. The subjects and controls endorsed the following symptoms: headaches 51%, 38%; memory difficulties 52%, 6%; difficulty concentrating 42%, 21%; irritability 68%, 42%; dizziness 41%, 11%; fatigue 68%, 41%; noise sensitivity 52%, 10%; and light sensitivity 32%, 28%.

Table 5.4. Percentage of Patients with Persistence of Symptoms After Mild Head Injury

	1 Week	1 Month	6 Weeks	2 Months	3 Months	6 Months	1 Year	2 Years	3 Years	4 Years	5 Years
Headache	71[173] 36[44]	90[62] 31.3[204] 56.0[173]	24.8[241]	31.5[62]	78[230] 47[173]	21.6[204] 27[44]	35[62] 8.4[241] 18[44]	22[62] 24[44]	20[62]	24[74]	12[257] (headaches and/or dizziness)
Dizziness	53[173] 19[44]	12[62] 21.9[204] 35[173]	14.5[241]	23[62]	22[173]	13.1[204] 22[44]	26[62] 4.6[241] 14[44]	18[62] 18[44]	16[62]	18[74]	
Memory problem		18.8[204]	8.3[241]		59[230]	15.3[204]	3.8[241]			19[74]	
Irritability		24.7[204]	9[241]			19.6[204]	5.3[241]				

Note: Superscript numbers refer to references.

Source: Evans RW: The post-concussion syndrome. In: Evans RW, Baskin DS, Yatsu FM (eds): Prognosis of Neurological Disorders, 2nd ed. New York, Oxford University Press, 2000, pp. 366–380, with permission.

Neuropsychological Deficits

Deficits in cognitive functioning owing to mild head injury include a reduction in information processing speed, attention, reaction time, and memory for new information. Recovery of information processing speed occurs within 3 months in most patients.[111,131,173] Persisting impairment of attention deficits is still present at 3 months.[100] Reaction time is abnormal at 6 weeks[181] and 3 months,[131] with recovery occurring by about 6 months.[181] Memory for new information recovers over 1 to 3 months,[66,173] although persisting impairment in visual memory and performance of digit span has been noted in one subgroup.[173]

Subjective symptoms may persist even after testing demonstrates resolution of cognitive impairment. In the study of Levin et al.,[173] although testing demonstrated almost complete cognitive recovery 3 months after the injury, 47% of subjects reported headaches, 22% dizziness, and 22% decreased energy.

Residual brain impairment may be present even after resolution of cognitive impairment and symptoms. As discussed earlier, the sequelae of mild head injury are cumulative even in persons who have clinically recovered. Physical, psychosocial, and environmental stress may reveal asymptomatic brain damage. Ewing et al.[85] compared university students who had made a full recovery from mild head injury 1 to 3 years previously with matched controls. The two groups were tested at ground level and at a simulated altitude of 12,500 feet. The mild head injury group showed significant impairment compared with the controls in tests of memory and vigilance performed with the mild hypoxia, although both groups performed similarly at ground level.

A minority of patients have persistent postconcussion difficulties and cognitive deficits after 3 months.[29,66,167] Leininger et al.[167] compared 53 patients with mild head injury who had persisting symptoms after 1 or more months to matched controls. Thirty-two percent of the patients were dazed, without loss of consciousness, and 58% were unconscious for 20 minutes or less. Testing was performed 1 to 22 months after injury. Deficits were documented on tests of reasoning, information processing, and verbal learning. Test results were similar in patients assessed within 3 months of the injury compared to the others tested after 3 months. Bohnen et al.[29] found that patients with postconcussion symptoms demonstrated deficits on tests of attention and information processing 6 months after the injury compared with patients without postconcussion symptoms and healthy controls. Patients who had recovered from an uncomplicated mild head injury did not differ in cognitive functioning from healthy control subjects. Vanderploeg et al.[279a] administered a neuropsychological test battery to three groups matched on premorbid cognitive ability: 254 nonreferred subjects with a history of mild traumatic brain injury an average of 8 years previously, a second group with no history of head injury or a motor vehicle accident, and a third group with a history of non-head injuries in a motor vehicle accident. Compared to the other two groups, the group with a history of mild brain injury was found to have deficits in subtle aspects of complex attention and working memory.

Return to Work

Four prospective studies of hospitalized patients have found variable percentages returning to work after different intervals. These findings may not necessarily be similar in patients who are not hospitalized after mild head injury. Rimel et al.[230] in Charlottesville, Virginia, reported that the following variables were significant predictors for return to work by 3 months: older age; higher level of education, employment, and socioeconomic status; and greater income. By 3 months, 100% of executives and business managers had returned to work compared to 68% of skilled laborers and 57% of unskilled laborers.

Englander et al.,[75] in San Jose, California, performed a prospective study of insured patients hospitalized after mild head injury. An average of 55 days postdischarge, follow-up was obtained with 62% of the subjects, who had a mean age of 26 years. Seventy-four percent of the patients reported no problems from the head injury. Eighty-eight percent had returned to their former level of employment or school.

Dikmen et al.,[67] in Seattle, Washington, performed a prospective study of 366 hospitalized patients with all degrees of head injury. The following variables were predictive of those less likely to return to work or to take a longer time to return to work: a more severe head injury; injuries to other body systems and their severity; age over 50; less than a high school education; and an unstable preinjury work history. Of the 213 patients who sustained a mild head injury with an initial GCS score of 13 to 15, the percentage who returned to work at various times after the injury was as follows: 25%, 1 month; 63%, 6 months; 80%, 12 months; and 83%, 24 months.

Van der Naalt et al.[279] performed a prospective study of 43 patients hospitalized in Groningen, the Netherlands, after mild head injuries with GCS scores of 13 to 14.[279] On 1-year follow-up, 79% had returned to previous work, school, or other activities completely. With multiple regression analysis, the duration of posttraumatic amnesia and the number of complaints at 3 months were important for outcome and return to work.

Litigation and Compensation Claims

Physician as Expert Witness

As previously discussed in the "Historical Aspects" section, the possible effects of pending litigation or compensation claims have been controversial for the past century. In 1888, Everts[84] discussed the problems with using the physician as an expert witness:

> What, then, is the real value of medical expert testimony? And who should be considered as medical experts? . . . Does that aggregration of knowledge known as "medicine" furnish the necessary principles for their qualifications as experts in all such cases? . . .
>
> . . . the more important qualification of the medical expert to determine questions of mental manifestations, and human actions, whether or not influenced by pathological conditions of brains, or other organs, remains to be accounted for. What has medicine in its widest range of instruction to offer on this subject? After all, how little! . . .
>
> Physiology, as taught in our schools, is indeed, still in doubt respecting the relation of mind to body. . . .
>
> . . . The natural tendency of experts, however, is to invalidate their opinions more or less, by the admission of color derived, imperceptibly, it may be, from the interest taken in behalf of the parties employing them. Instigated, also, by professional pride, experts, like detectives, are more zealous in finding what they are supposed to be peculiarly qualified to find, than otherwise. . . .

Compensation Neurosis and Malingering

As a matter of routine, defense attorneys still cite Miller's 1961 study[202] of 200 consecutive cases of mild head injury seen for medico-legal examination in Newcastle upon Tyne, England, and invariably raise questions of secondary gain and malingering. Forty-seven of the 200 patients were reported to have gross and unequivocally psychoneurotic complaints. They exhibited characteristic behaviors during the consultation and displayed an attitude of "martyred gloom." The patients frequently arrived late and were accompanied by a family member who took an active part in the interview process. In more than half of the patients, an obvious dramatization of symptoms was perceived to be present.

> The most consistent feature is the subject's unshakable conviction of unfitness for work, a conviction quite unrelated to overt disability, even if his symptomatology is accepted at its face value. At a later stage, the patient will declare his fitness for light work, which is often not available. . . . Another cardinal feature is an absolute refusal to admit any degree of symptomatic improvement.

Miller makes behavioral observations of a biased sample, which may have some validity, although they are by necessity quite subjective and judgmental. Symptoms are dismissed as being minor without substantiation, and information is not provided on the percentage of patients with various complaints such as headaches, dizziness, and memory problems. Investigations such as MRI scans of the brain and current neuropsychological testing techniques were, of course, not available. Miller did not totally reject the concept of a postconcussion syndrome. He stated in the same paper, "The consistency of the post-concussional syndrome of headache, postural dizziness, irritability, failure of concentration, and intolerance of noise, argues a structural or at least a pathophysiological basis." Miller's study has stimulated many other investigators to further explore issues of compensation.

Guthkelch[114] reported on 398 consecutive head injury patients he had examined in connection with a claim for compensation. Accident neurosis was defined by bizarre and inconsistent complaints, exaggeration of the length of the initial unconsciousness, and attention-seeking behaviors. For example, two of the patients claimed to be unable to stand or take a single step without support and then were observed walking normally in the street within a few minutes after the examination. Three patients claimed compensation from disability while surreptitiously working full-time. Headaches were blinding or terrible and did not improve with time. In several cases, the patients gave an unsolicited and histrionic assertion of complete indifference to money, which was at variance with their dealings with their attorney. Some patients claimed that they wanted to return to work but were forbidden by their attending physician, when in actuality this was not the case.

All of the patients were employed at the time of the injury. About one-half of the patients returned to work but left within a few days complaining of headaches and noise intolerance. About one-half of the patients did not return to work until their compensation claim had been settled or they were turned down for disability. Accident neurosis was more common in manual workers sustaining accidents at work than in nonmanual workers. Psychiatric treatment was not found to be helpful. Guthkelch concluded, "Accident neurosis is not particularly common; even in this series, which was exclusively composed of patients with a compensation problem, it was identified in only 6.8% of patients."

Potential indicators of malingering following mild head injury include the following: premorbid factors (antisocial and borderline personality traits, poor work record, and prior claims for injury); behavioral characteristics (uncooperative, evasive, or suspicious); neuropsychological test performance (missing random items, giving up easily, inconsistent test profile, or frequently stating, "I don't know"); postmorbid complaints (describing events surrounding the accident in great detail or reporting an unusually large number of symptoms); and miscellaneous items (engaging in general activities not consistent with reported deficits, having significant financial stressors, showing resistance, and exhibiting a lack of reasonable follow-through on treatments).[24a,236]

In evaluating the sequelae of mild head injury, the physician should always consider a patient's motivation and to what degree secondary gain may be playing a part.[263] Patients with premorbid neuroticism, inadequate or histrionic personalities, and psychosocial problems can certainly exaggerate or fabricate complaints.[23,177] Comprehensive multidisciplinary evaluations may be required to detect malingering.[86,236] Subjective criteria for making a diagnosis of postconcussion syndrome should be clearly delineated from objective findings. Evaluation can be done in a nonthreatening manner; the physician does not have to be a district attorney. The diagnosis of accident neurosis, malingering, or conversion neurosis should be made with a great deal of caution because some patients with seemingly hysterical signs and symptoms may actually have underlying organic disease.[105]

Are Litigants Different from Nonlitigants?

Patients with litigation and compensation claims are quite similar to those without them. Similar symptoms improving with time[167,196,199] and similar cognitive test results[167,196] are present in both groups. Patients applying for compensation do not have increased symptoms compared to those without applications.[209] A study of posttraumatic migraine suggests that both groups respond similarly to appropriate treatment.[287]

However, Andrikopoulos[7] compared 72 mildly head-injured litigants with headaches without improvement or worsening to 39 with improving headache. Those who had no improvement or worsening performed more poorly on cognitive tests and had greater psychopathology on the Minnesota Multiphasic Personality Inventory–Version 2 than those who had improving headaches, suggesting the possibility of malingering. In addition, Feinstein et al.[88] found an increased level of psychological distress in litigants compared to nonlitigants attending an outpatient hospital clinic when assessed an average of 42.2 days after a mild head injury. There were no cognitive differences between the two groups. They concluded that the pursuit of compensation may influence the subjective expression of symptoms following mild traumatic brain injury.

Just having litigation pending, however, may increase the level of stress for some claimants,[119] may increase the number of subjective complaints,[166] and may result in an increased frequency of symptoms after settlement.[87,198] The skepticism of treating physicians and insurance companies about persistent symptoms may accentuate this level of stress.

Not Cured by a Verdict

The end of litigation does not mean the end of symptoms or return to work for many claimants: they are not cured by a verdict.[198] Fee and Rutherford[87] reported that 39% of patients were symptomatic at the time of settlement, and 34% were still symptomatic 1 year after the settlement of claims. Patients who are older or employed in more dangerous occupations often do not return to work after settlement.[151] Packard[215] interviewed 50 patients who had persistent posttraumatic headaches when litigation was settled. At the time of follow-up, an average of 23 months after settlement, all 50 patients continued to report persistent headache symptoms, with an improvement in the headache pattern reported by only 4 patients.

Mild Head Injury in Lithuania: Outside the Medico-Legal Context

Lithuania has been selected to evaluate postconcussion syndrome outside the medico-legal context because there are minimal possibilities for economic gain, as that nation's fledgling insurance companies do not recognize postconcussion syndrome and because there seem to be fewer expectations of persisting symptoms than in a Western society.[91] Mickevičiene et al.[200] prospectively evaluated 300 subjects with a mild head injury for 1 year in Kaunas, Lithuania, with questionaires. The prevalence, frequency, and visual analogue scale scores of headaches both after 3 months and after 1 year did not differ significantly between the injured and the controls. After 1 year, most symptoms did not differ between the injured and the controls with the exceptions of slightly significant findings of more sporadic memory problems, concentration problem, and dizziness in the injured. The authors conclude that "our results cast doubts on the validity of PCS as a useful clinical entity, at least for head injuries with loss of consciousness for <15 minutes." Thus, no litigation, no expectation of symptoms, no postconcussion syndrome.

However, the results of this study may not be generalizable for the following reasons: other studies have variably defined mild head injury as including loss of consciousness for up to 30 minutes; 66% of the cohort and controls were male (late symptoms occur more often in women); and 66% of the injuries were due to assaults. In addition, the prevalence of headaches for more than 14 days in the controls (6% at 3 months and 8% at 1 year) was higher than that reported in other countries. Although I am not aware of any prevalence studies in Lithuania, compare this to population-based studies revealing the prevalence of chronic daily headache in 2.98% (4.18% in females and 1.62% in males) in France[161] and 4.1% in the United States (5% in females and 2.8% in males).[243a] The prevalence of headaches in controls in this study is especially high when you consider that 66% of both head-injured patients and controls were males. While litigation and, to a much lesser extent, the expectation of chronic symptoms may certainly be factors to consider in the persistence of symptoms in some cases, they clearly do not suffice to explain away persistent postconcussion syndrome.

Treatment

Treatment for the postconcussion syndrome is individualized after the patient's particular problems are diagnosed. Simple reassurance is often the major treatment since most patients will improve within 3 months.

Headaches

Amitriptyline has been widely used for posttraumatic tension-type headaches,[276] as well as for nonspecific symptoms such as irritability, dizziness, depression, fatigue, and insomnia. Nortriptyline may be better tolerated than amitriptyline and perhaps maybe as effective. Tension-type headaches may also respond to nonsteroidal anti-inflammatory drugs (NSAIDs) and muscle relaxant-type medications including baclofen and tiazanidine. An inpatient program of repetitive intravenous dihydroergotamine and metoclopramide may provide relief of refractory chronic posttraumatic headaches.[193a,294]

Greater occipital neuralgia frequently responds to greater occipital nerve block[124] with a local anesthetic,[252] which can also be combined with an injectable corticosteroid.[10] Muscle relaxant-type medications and NSAIDs, transcutaneous electrical nerve stimulation (TENS) units,[255] physical therapy, and manipulation[146] may also be beneficial. Paroxysms of shooting pain may respond to carbamazepine, baclofen, gabapentin, or tiazanidine. Greater occipital nerve section or decompression is rarely indicated.[55,107,220]

A diagnosis of headache due to third occipital headache, similar to greater occipital neuralgia but much less common, can be established with an anesthetic nerve block of the C2-3 facet.[28] Percutaneous radiofrequency neurotomy of the third occipital nerve can result in complete relief of the headache for 88% of patients for a median duration of 297 days.[106] A repeat neurotomy may result in even longer relief.

Traumatically induced migraine headaches may respond to the usual migraine medications. For prevention, a 70% response to propranolol or amitriptyline used alone or in combination has been reported.[287] Topirimate and valproic acid[187] are also effective migraine preventatives. The usual symptomatic medications for migraine, including triptans, may be effective.[98] Barbiturates such as butalbital and narcotics[296] should be used infrequently for posttraumatic headaches to avoid habituation and rebound headaches. Rebound headaches can also result from frequent use of over-the-counter medications including acetaminophen, acetaminophen/aspirin/caffeine combinations, and ibuprofen.

A short course of biofeedback training may be worthwhile for patients with persistent headaches of all types. Acupuncture[49] and naltrexone[268] have been reported to be helpful for relieving headaches in single reports. Botulinum toxin injections may also be effective for intractable headaches.[178]

Psychological and Cognitive Complaints

Treatment with oxiracetam has been described as being helpful for postconcussion symptoms in a single report.[238] CDP-choline has been reported as useful for memory impairment in a single preliminary report.[174] Six patients with chronic symptoms after mild head injury reported subjective cognitive improvement in an open label study of donepezil.[148] The vasopressin analogue desglycinamide-arginine-vasopressin does not have a positive effect on cognitive recovery after mild head injury.[31]

The use of cognitive retraining for cognitive difficulties after mild head injury is controversial. Because cognitive rehabilitation can be quite costly, additional prospective studies are needed to demonstrate its efficacy before widespread application can be recommended. Training in the use of a notebook and visual imagery may be helpful. This topic is discussed further in Chapter 13, When the psychological symptoms are particularly prominent, supportive psychotherapy and use of antidepressant and antianxiety-type medications may be helpful.

Education

One of the most important roles for the physician is education of the patient and family members, other physicians, and, as appropriate, employers, attorneys, and representatives of insurance companies.[27] Many patients are greatly reassured to discover that their symptoms are not unique or crazy but are instead part of a well-described syndrome. The treatment program of education, short-term bed rest, and timely follow-up may hasten recovery in some patients.[204,211] Provision of an information booklet has been reported as reducing anxiety and reporting of ongoing postconcussion symptoms at 3 months[221] and as having no effect.[6] Disbelieving family members may become more supportive with education. Perhaps third parties such as some employers and insurance companies could also become less hostile to injured patients if provided with education.

Bed Rest

De Kruijk et al.[57] randomized 107 patients presenting to the emergency room after a mild head injury to either no bed rest (mobile from the first day after the trauma, with at most a little bed rest and return to work on the fifth day) or bed rest (for the first 6 days following the trauma and then progressive mobilization and return to work like the no-bed-rest group). Although bed rest reduced complaints of dizziness in the first week after injury, there was no difference in the severity of posttraumatic complaints at 3 months or 6 months.

Summary

The postconcussion syndrome refers to a large number of symptoms and signs that may occur alone or in combination following usually mild head injury. The most common complaints are headaches, dizziness, fatigue, irritability, anxiety, insomnia, loss of concentration and memory, and noise sensitivity. Mild head injury is a major public health concern since its annual incidence is about 150 per 100,000 population, accounting for 75% or more of all head injuries.

The postconcussion syndrome has been recognized for at least the past few hundred years and has been the subject of intense controversy for over 100 years. The Hollywood head injury myth has been an important contributor to persisting skepticism and might be countered by educational efforts and counterexamples from boxing.

The organicity of the postconcussion syndrome has now been well documented. Abnormalities following mild head injury have been reported in neuropathological, neurophysiological, neuroimaging, biochemical, and neuropsychological studies.

There are multiple sequelae of mild head injury, including headaches of multiple types, cranial nerve symptoms and signs, psychological and somatic complaints, and cognitive impairment. Rare sequelae include hematomas, second impact syndrome, seizures, transient global amnesia, tremor, and dystonia. Neuroimaging, physiological, and psychological testing should be used judiciously based upon the problems of the particular patient rather than in a cookbook fashion.

Prognostic studies clearly substantiate the existence of a postconcussion syndrome. Manifestations of the syndrome are common, with resolution in most patients by 3 to 6 months after the injury. Persistent symptoms and cognitive deficits are present in a distinct minority of patients for additional months or years. Risk factors for persisting sequelae include age over 40 years; lower educational, intellectual, and socioeconomic levels; female gender; alcohol abuse; prior head injury; and multiple trauma. Although a small minority are malingerers or frauds or have compensation neurosis, most patients have genuine complaints. Contrary to the popular perception, most patients with litigation or compensation claims are not cured by a verdict.

Treatment is individualized, depending upon the specific complaints of the patient. Although a variety of medication and psychological treatments are currently available, ongoing basic and clinical research of all aspects of mild head injury is crucial to provide more efficacious treatment in the future.

REFERENCES

1. Abu-Judeh HH, Parker R, Aleksic S, et al: SPECT brain perfusion findings in mild or moderate traumatic brain injury. Nucl Med Rev Cent East Eur 3(1):5–11, 2000.
2. Adams JH, Graham DI, Murray LS, et al: Diffuse axonal injury due to non-missile head injury in humans: An analysis of 45 cases. Ann Neurol 12:557–563, 1982.
3. Alavia A, Fezekas T, Alves W, et al: Positron emission tomography in the evaluation of head injury. J Cereb Blood Flow Metab 7(suppl 1):S646, 1986.
4. Alexander MP: Neuropsychiatric correlates of persistent postconcussive syndrome. J Head Trauma Rehabil 7:60–69, 1992.
5. Alexander MP: Mild traumatic brain injury: Pathophysiology, natural history, and clinical management. Neurology 45:1253–1260, 1995.
6. Alves W, Macciocchi SN, Barth JT: Postconcussive symptoms after uncomplicated mild head injury. J Head Trauma Rehabil 8:48–59, 1993.

7. Andrikopoulos J. Post-traumatic headache in mild head injured litigants. Headache 43:553, 2003.
8. Annegers JF, Coan SP: The risks of epilepsy after traumatic brain injury. Seizure 9:453–457, 2000.
9. Annegers JF, Grabow JD, Kurland LT, et al: The incidence, causes, and secular trends of head trauma in Olmsted County, Minnesota, 1935–1974. Neurology 30:912–919, 1980.
10. Anthony M: Headache and the greater occipital nerve. Clin Neurol Neurosurg 94:297–301, 1992.
11. Ashworth B: Migraine, head trauma and sport. Scott Med J 30:240–242, 1985.
12. Aubrey J, Dobbs AR, Rule BG: Laypersons' knowledge about the sequelae of minor head injury and whiplash. J Neurol Neurosurg Psychiatry 52:842–846, 1989.
13. Baloh RW, Honrubia V, Jacobson K: Benign positional vertigo: Clinical and oculographic features in 240 cases. Neurology 37:371–378, 1987.
14. Baron JB: Postural aspects of the post-concussional syndrome. Chin Otolaryngol 5:215–219, 1980.
15. Barth JT, Macciocchi SN, Giordani B, et al: Neuropsychological sequelae of minor head injury. Neurosurgery 13:529–533, 1983.
16. Bazarian JJ, Wong T, Harris M: Epidemiology and predictors of post-concussive syndrome after minor head injury in an emergency population. Brain Injury 13:173–189, 1999.
17. Behrman S: Migraine as a sequela of blunt head injury. Injury 9:74–76, 1977.
18. Bennett DR, Fuenning SI, Sullivan G, et al: Migraine precipitated by head trauma in athletes. Am J Sports Med 8(3):202–205, 1980.
19. Benoit BG, Russell NA, Richard MT, et al: Epidural hematoma: Report of seven cases with delayed evolution of symptoms. Can J Neurol Sci 9:321–324, 1982.
20. Bernstein DM: Recovery from mild head injury. Brain Inj 13:151–172, 1999.
21. Berrol S: Other factors: Age, alcohol, and multiple injuries. In: Hoff JT, Anderson TE, Cole TM (eds): Mild to Moderate Head Injury. Boston, Blackwell Scientific, 1989, pp 135–142.
22. Biary N, Cleeyes L, Findley L, et al: Post-traumatic tremor. Neurology 39:103–106, 1989.
23. Binder LM: Persisting symptoms after mild head injury: A review of the postconcussive syndrome. J Clin Exp Neuropsychol 8:323–346, 1986.
24a. Binder LM, Rohling ML: Money matters: A meta-analytic review of the effects of financial incentives on recovery after closed-head injury. Am J Psychiatry 153:7–10, 1996.
24b. Blacker DJ, Wijdicks EF: A ripping roller coaster ride. Neurology 61:1255, 2003.
25. Blumbergs PC, Jones NR, North JB: Diffuse axonal injury in head trauma. J Neurol Neurosurg Psychiatry 52:838–841, 1989.
26. Bo-Abbas Y, Bolton CF: Roller-coaster headache. N Engl J Med 332:1585, 1995.
27. Boake C, Bobetic KM, Bontke CF: Rehabilitation of the patient with mild traumatic brain injury. Neurorehabilitation 1:70–78, 1991.
28. Bogduk N: The neck and headaches. Neurol Clin 22(1): 151–171, 2004.
29. Bohnen N, Jones J, Twijnstra A: Neuropsychological deficits in patients with persistent symptoms six months after mild head injury. Neurosurgery 30:692–696, 1992.
30. Bohnen N, Twijnstra A, Wijnen G, et al: Tolerance for light and sound of patients with persistent postconcussional symptoms six months after mild head injury. J Neurol 238:443–446, 1991.
31. Bohnen NI, Twijnstra A, Jones J: A controlled trial with vasopressin analogue (DGAVP) on cognitive recovery immediately after head trauma. Neurology 43: 103–106, 1993.
32. Bollinger O: Uber traumatische Spat-Apoplexie ein Beitrag zur Lehre yon der Hirnerschutterung. Internationale Beitrage zur wissenschaftlichen Medizin, Festschrift, Virchow, R Berlin, A Hirschwald. Vol 2. 1891, pp 457–470.
33. Bonne O, Gilboa A, Louzoun Y, et al: Cerebral blood flow in chronic symptomatic mild traumatic brain injury. Psychiatry Res 124(3):141–152, 2003.
34. Borg J, Holm L, Cassidy JD, et al: Diagnostic procedures in mild traumatic brain injury: Results of the WHO Collaborating Centre Task Force on Mild Traumatic Brain Injury. J Rehabil Med 43(suppl):61–75, 2004.
35. Boston Med Surg J: Leading article 109:400, 1883.
36. Brismar B, Engstrom A, Rydberg U: Head injury and intoxication: A diagnostic and therapeutic dilemma. Acta Chir Scand 149:11–14, 1983.
37. Brooke RI, Lapointe IIJ: Temporomandibular joint disorders following whiplash. Spine: State Art Rev 7:443–454, 1993.
38. Brown SJ, Farm JR, Grant I: Postconcussional disorder: Time to acknowledge a common source of neurobehavioral morbidity. J Neuropsychiatry Clin Neurosci 6:15–22, 1994.
39. Browning GC, Swan IRC, Gatehouse S: Hearing loss in minor head injury. Arch Otolaryngol 108:474–477, 1982.
40. Bruce DA: Delayed deterioration of consciousness after trivial head injury in childhood. Br Med J 289:715–716, 1984.
41. Cabral RJ: Simulation and malingering after injuries to the brain and spinal cord. Lancet 2:953, 1972.
42. Cajal SR: Degeneration and Regeneration of the Nervous System. Oxford, Oxford University Press, 1928.
43. Carlsson GS, Svardsudd K, Welin L: Long-term effects of head injuries sustained during life in three male populations. J Neurosurg 67:197–205, 1987
44. Cartlidge NEF: Postconcussional syndrome. Scott Med J 23:103, 1978.
45. Chandra V, Kokmen E, Schoenberg BS, Beard CM: Head trauma with loss of consciousness as a risk factor for Alzheimer's disease. Neurology 39:1576–1578, 1989.

46. Chen JK, Johnston KM, Frey S, et al: Functional abnormalities in symptomatic concussed athletes: An fMRI study. Neuroimage 22(1):68–82, 2004.
47. Chen SH, Kareken DA, Fastenau PS, et al: A study of persistent post-concussion symptoms in mild head trauma using positron emission tomography. J Neurol Neurosurg Psychiatry 74(3):326–332, 2003.
48. Chibnall JT, Duckro PN: Post-traumatic stress disorder in chronic post-traumatic headache patients. Headache 34:3.57–361, 1994.
49. Chilvers CD: Acupuncture in the post-concussional syndrome. NZ Med J 98:658, 1985.
50. Couch JR, Bearss C: Chronic daily headache in the post-head injury syndrome (PHIS). Headache 34:296, 1994.
51. Couch JR, Bearss C: Chronic daily headache in the posttrauma syndrome: Relation to extent of head injury. Headache 41:559–564, 2001.
52. Cox CL, Cocks GR: Occipital neuralgia. J Med Assoc State Al 48:23–32, 1979.
53. Culotta VP, Sementilli ME, Gerold K, Watts CC: Clinicopathological heterogeneity in the classification of mild head injury. Neurosurgery 38(2):245–250, 1996.
54. Dacey RG, Alves WM, Rimel RW, et al: Neurosurgical complications after apparently minor head injury. J Neurosurg 65:203–210, 1986.
55. Dalessio DJ: Occipital neuralgia. Headache 20:107, 1980.
56. Dalfen AK, Anthony F. Head injury, dissociation, and the Ganser syndrome. Brain Inj 14(12):1101–1105, 2000.
56a. de Boussard CN, Lundin A, Karlstedt D, et al: S100 and cognitive impairment after mild traumatic brain injury. J Rehabil Med. 37:53–57, 2005.
57. de Kruijk JR, Leffers P, Meerhoff S, et al: Effectiveness of bed rest after mild traumatic brain injury: A randomised trial of no versus six days of bed rest. J Neurol Neurosurg Psychiatry 73(2):167–172, 2002.
58. de Kruijk JR, Leffers P, Menheere PP, et al: Prediction of post-traumatic complaints after mild traumatic brain injury: Early symptoms and biochemical markers. J Neurol Neurosurg Psychiatry 73(6):727–732, 2003.
59. de Kruijk JR, Leffers P, Menheere PP, et al: Olfactory function after mild traumatic brain injury. Brain Inj 17:73–78, 2003.
60. de Morsier G: Les encephalopathies traumatiques. Etude neurologique. Schweiz Arch Neurol Neurochir Psychiatry 50:161, 1943.
61. Deems DA, Doty RL, Settle RG, et al: Smell and taste disorders, a study of 750 patients from the University of Pennsylvania smell and taste center. Arch Otolaryngol Head Neck Surg 117:519–528, 1991.
62. Denker PG: The postconcussion syndrome: Prognosis and evaluation of the organic factors. NY State J Med 44:379–384, 1944.
63. Dennv-Brown D: Disability arising from closed head injury. JAMA 127:429–436, 1945.
64. Diaz FG, Yoch DEI, Larson D, et al: Early diagnosis of delayed post-traumatic intracerebral hematomas. J Neurosurg 50:217–223, 1979.
65. Dikmen SS, Levin HS: Methodological issues in the study of mild head injury. J Head Trauma Rehabil 8:30–37, 1993.
66. Dikmen SS, McLean A, Temkin N: Neuropsychological and psychosocial consequences of minor head injury. J Neurol Neurosurg Psychiatry 49:1227–1232, 1986.
67. Dikmen SS, Temkin NR, Machamer JE, et al: Employment following traumatic head injuries. Arch Neurol 51:177–186, 1994.
68. Dila C, Bouchard L, Myer E, et al: Microvascular response to minimal brain trauma. In: McLaurin RL (ed): Head Injuries, Second Chicago Symposium on Neural Trauma. New York, Grune & Stratton, 1976, pp 213–215.
69. Dow RS, Ulett G, Raaf J: Electroencephalographic studies immediately following head injury. Am J Psychiatry 101:174–183, 1944.
70. Duckro PN, Chibnall JT, Greenberg M, Schultz KT: Muscle factors in chronic post-traumatic headache. Headache 34:304–305, 1994.
71. Duckro PN, Greenberg M, Schultz KT, et al: Clinical features of chronic post-traumatic headache. Headache Q 3:295–308, 1992.
72. Dupuis F, Johnston KM, Lavoie M, et al: Concussions in athletes produce brain dysfunction as revealed by event-related potentials. NeuroReport 11(18):4087–4092, 2000.
73. Edna T-H: Disability 3–5 years after minor head injury. J Oslo City Hosp 37:41–48, 1987.
74. Edna T-H, Cappelen J: Late postconcussional symptoms in traumatic head injury. An analysis of frequency and risk factors. Acta Neurochir (Wien) 86:12–17, 1987.
75. Englander J, Hall K, Stimpson T, Chaffin S: Mild traumatic brain injury in an insured population: Subjective complaints and return to employment. Brain Inj 6:161–166, 1992.
76. Epstein CM: Computerized EEG in the courtroom. Neurology 44:1566–1569, 1994.
77. Erichsen JE: On Concussion of the Spine: Nervous Shock and Other Obscure Injuries of the Nervous System in Their Clinical and Medico-Legal Aspects. London, Longmans Green, 1882.
78. Evans RW: Postconcussive syndrome: An overview. Texas Med 83:49–53, 1987.
79. Evans RW: The postconcussion syndrome and the sequelae of mild head injury. Neurol Clin 10:815–847, 1992.
80. Evans RW: The postconcussion syndrome: 130 years of controversy. Semin Neurol 14:32–39, 1994.
81. Evans RW: The post-concussion syndrome. In: Evans RW, Baskin DS, Yatsu FM (eds): Prognosis of Neurological Disorders, 2nd ed. New York, Oxford University Press, 2000, pp 366–380.

82. Evans RW, Evans RI, Sharp MJ: The physician survey on the postconcussion and whiplash syndromes. Headache 34:268–274, 1994.
83. Evans RW, Lay CL. Posttraumatic hemicrania continua? Headache 40:761–762, 2000.
84. Everts O: Expert testimony and medical experts. JAMA 11:873–876, 1888.
85. Ewing R, McCarthy D, Gronwall D, et al: Persisting effects of minor head injury observable during hypoxic stress. J Clin Neuropsychol 2:147–155, 1980.
86. Faust D: The detection of deception. Neurol Clin 13: 255–265, 1995.
87. Fee CRA, Rutherford WH: A study of the effect of legal settlement on postconcussion symptoms. Arch Emerg Med 5:12–17, 1988.
88. Feinstein A, Ouchterlony D, Somerville J, Jardine A: The effects of litigation on symptom expression: A prospective study following mild traumatic brain injury. Med Sci Law 41(2):116–121, 2001.
89. Fenton G, McClelland R, Montgomery A, MacFlynn G, Rutherford W: The postconcussional syndrome: Social antecedents and psychological sequelae. Br J Psychiatry 162:493–497, 1993.
90. Fernandes CMB, D'aya MR: A roller coaster headache: Case report. J Trauma 37:1007–1010, 1994.
91. Ferrari R, Obelieniene D, Russell AS, et al: Symptom expectation after minor head injury. A comparative study between Canada and Lithuania. Clin Neurol Neurosurg 103(3):184–190, 2001.
92. Feuerman T, Wackym PA, Gade GF, et al: Value of skull radiography, head computed tomographic scanning, and admission for observation in cases of minor head injury. Neurosurgery 22:440–453, 1988.
93. Fisher CM: Concussion amnesia. Neurology 16:826–830, 1966.
94. Fisher JM, Williams AD: Neuropsychologic investigation of mild head injury: Ensuring diagnostic accuracy in the assessment process. Semin Neurol 14:53–59, 1994.
95. Fleminger S, Oliver DL, Lovestone S, et al: Head injury as a risk factor for Alzheimer's disease: The evidence 10 years on; a partial replication. J Neurol Neurosurg Psychiatry 74:857–862, 2003.
96. Frankowski RE, Annegers JF, Whitman S: The descriptive epidemiology of head trauma in the United States. In: Becker DP, Povlishock JT (eds): Central Nervous System Trauma Status Report. Bethesda, MD, NINCDS, National Institutes of Health, 1985.
97. Gama JHP: Traité des plaies de tete et de l'encéphalite. Paris, 1835.
98. Gawel MJ, Rothbart P, Jacobs H: Subcutaneous sumatriptan in the treatment of acute episodes of posttraumaHc headache. Headache 33:96–97, 1993.
99. Gee JR, Ishaq Y, Vijayan N: Postcraniotomy headache. Headache 43:276–278, 2003.
100. Gentilini M, Nichelli P, Schoenhuber R: Assessment of attention in mild head injury. In: Levin HS, Eisenberg HM, Benton AL (eds): Mild Head Injury. New York, Oxford University Press, 1989, pp 163–175.
101. Goetz CG, Stebbins GT: Effects of head trauma from motor vehicle accidents on Parkinson's disease. Ann Neurol 29:191–193, 1991.
102. Goldstein FC, Levin HS: Neurobehavioral outcome of traumatic brain injury in older adults: Initial findings. J Head Trauma Rehabil 10:57–73, 1995.
103. Goodman JC: Pathologic changes in mild head injury. Semin Neurol 14:19–24, 1994.
104. Gordon WA, Brown M, Sliwinksi M: The enigma of "hidden" traumatic brain injury. J Head Trauma Rehabil 13:39–56, 1998.
105. Gould R, Miller BL, Goldberg MA, et al: The validity of hysterical signs and symptoms. J Nerv Ment Dis 174:593–597, 1986.
106. Govind J, King W, Bailey B, Bogduk N: Radiofrequency neurotomy for the treatment of third occipital headache. J Neurol Neurosurg Psychiatry 74:88–93, 2003
107. Graff-Radford SB, Jaeger BJ, Reeves JL: Myofascial pain may present clinically as occipital neuralgia. Neurosurgery 19:610–613, 1986.
108. Grinker RR: Neurology. Springfield, IL, Charles C Thomas, 1934, p 790.
109. Gronwall D: Concussion: Does intelligence help? NZ Psychol 5:72–78, 1976.
110. Gronwall D: Cumulative and persisting effects of concussion on attention and cognition. In: Levin HS, Eisenberg HM, Benton AL (eds): Mild Head Injury. New York, Oxford University Press, 1989, pp 153–162.
111. Gronwall D, Wrightson P: Delayed recovery of intellectual function after minor head injury. Lancet 2:605–609, 1974.
112. Gronwall D, Wrightson P: Cumulative effects of concussion. Lancet 2:995–997, 1975.
113. Guilleminault C, Faull KF, Miles L, van der Hoed J: Posttraumatic excessive daytime sleepiness: A review of 20 patients. Neurology 33:1584–1589, 1983.
114. Guthkelch AN: Posttraumatic amnesia, post-concussional symptoms and accident neurosis. Eur Neurol 19:91–102. 1980.
115. Haas DC: Chronic post-traumatic headaches classified and compared with natural headaches. Cephalalgia 16:486–493, 1996.
116. Haas DC, Lourie H: Trauma-triggered migraine: An explanation for common neurological attacks after mild head injury. J Neurosurg 68:181–188, 1988.
117. Haas DC, Pineda GS, Lourie H: Juvenile head trauma syndromes and their relationship to migraine. Arch Neurol 32:721–730, 1975.
118. Haas DC, Ross GS: Transient global amnesia triggered by mild head trauma. Brain 109:251–257, 1986.
119. Ham LP, Andrasik F, Packard RC, Bundrick CM: Psychopathology in individuals with post-traumatic headaches and other pain types. Cephalagia 14:118–126, 1994.
120a. Harvey AG, Bryant RA: Two-year prospective evaluation of the relationship between acute stress disorder

and posttraumatic stress disorder following mild traumatic brain injury. Am J Psychiatry 157:626–628, 2000.

120b. Haydel MJ: Clinical decision instruments for CT scanning in minor head injury. JAMA 28; 294(12):1551–1553, 2005.

120c. Haydel MJ, Preston CA, Mills TJ,et al. Indications for computed tomography in patients with minor head injury. N Engl J Med 13:343(2):100–105, 2000.

121. Hayes RL, Dixon CE: Neurochemical changes in mild head injury. Semin Neurol 14:25–31, 1994.

122. Hayes RL, Lyeth BG, Jenkins LW: Neurochemical mechanisms of mild and moderate head injury: Implications for treatment. In: Levin HS, Eisenberg HM, Benton AL (eds): Mild Head Injury. New York, Oxford University Press, 1989, pp 37–53.

123. Headache Classification Subcommittee of the International Headache Society: The International Classification of Headache Disorders, second edition. Cephalalgia 24(suppl 1):59, 2004.

124. Hecht JS. Occipital nerve blocks in postconcussive headaches: A retrospective review and report of ten patients. J Head Trauma Rehabil 19(1):58–71, 2004.

125. Hendriks APJ: Olfactory dysfunction. Rhinology 26:229–251, 1988.

126. Herrmann M, Curio N, Jost S, et al: Release of biochemical markers of damage to neuronal and glial brain tissue is associated with short and long term neuropsychological outcome after traumatic brain injury. J Neurol Neurosurg Psychiatry 70(1):95–100, 2001.

127. Hernesniemi J: Outcome following head injuries in the aged. Acta Neurochir (Wien) 49:67–79, 1979.

128. Hesselink JR, Dowd CF, Healy ME, et al: MR imaging of brain contusions: A comparative study with CT. AJR 150:1133–1142, 1988.

129. Hoffer ME, Gottshall KR, Moore R, et al: Characterizing and treating dizziness after mild head trauma. Otol Neurotol 25:135–138, 2004.

130a. Hofman PA, Stapert SZ, van Kroonenburgh MJ, et al: MR imaging, single-photon emission CT, and neurocognitive performance after mild traumatic brain injury. Am J Neuroradiol 22(3):441–449, 2001.

130b. Huang PP: Roller coaster headaches revisited. Surg Neurol 60:398–401, 2003.

131. Hugenholtz H, Stuss DT, Stetbem LL, et al: How long does it take to recover from a mild concussion? Neurosurgery 22:853–858, 1988.

132. Hughes DG, Jackson A, Mason DL, et al: Abnormalities on magnetic resonance imaging seen acutely following mild traumatic brain injury: Correlation with neuropsychological tests and delayed recovery. Neuroradiology 46:550–558, 2004.

133. Humayun MS, Presty SK, Lafrance ND, et al: Local cerebral glucose abnormalities in mild closed head injured patients with cognitive impairments. Nucl Med Commun 10:355–344, 1989.

134. Ichise M, Chung DG, Wang P, et al: Technetium-99m-HMPAO SPECT, CT and MRI in the evaluation of patients with chronic traumatic brain injury: A correlation with neuropsychological performance. J Nucl Med 35: 211–226, 1994.

135. Ingebrigtsen T, Romner B, Marup-Jensen S, et al: The clinical value of serum S-100 protein measurements in minor head injury: A Scandinavian multicentre study. Brain Inj 14(12):1047–1055, 2000.

136a. Ingebrigtsen T, Waterloo K, Jacobsen EA, et al: Traumatic brain damage in minor head injury: Relation of serum S-100 protein measurements to magnetic resonance imaging and neurobehavioral outcome. Neurosurgery 45(3):468–475, 1999.

136b. Inglese M, Bomsztyk E, Gonen O, et al: Dilated perivascular spaces: Hallmarks of mild traumatic brain injury. Am J Neuroradiol 26:719–724, 2005.

137. Iverson GL, Gaetz M, Lovell MR, Collins MW: Cumulative effects of concussion in amateur athletes. Brain Inj 18(5):433–443, 2004.

138. Jacobs A, Put E, Ingels M, Bossuvt A: Prospective evaluation of technetium-99m-HMPAO SPECT in mild and moderate traumatic brain injury. J Nucl Med 35:942–947, 1994.

139. Jacobsen J, Baadsgaard SE, Thompsen S, et al: Prediction of post-concussional sequelae by reaction time test. Acta Neurol Scand 75:341–345, 1987.

140. Jane JA, Steward O, Genarelli T: Axonal degeneration induced by experimental noninvasive minor head injury. J Neurosurg 62:96–100, 1985.

141. Jankovic J: Post-traumatic movement disorders: Central and peripheral mechanisms. Neurology 44:2006–2014, 1994.

142. Jankovic J, van der Linden C: Dystonia and tremor induced by peripheral trauma: Predisposing factors. J Neurol Neurosurg Psvchiatry 51:1512–1519, 1988.

143. Jantzen KJ, Anderson B, Steinberg FL, Kelso JA: A prospective functional MR imaging study of mild traumatic brain injury in college football players. Am J Neuroradiol 25(5):738–745, 2004.

144. Jennett B, Frankovyski RF: The epidemiology of head injury. In: Braakman R (ed): Handbook of Clinical Neurology, Vol 13. New York, Elsevier, 1990, pp 1–16.

145. Jennett B, Teasdale G, Murray G, et al: Head injury. In: Evans RW, Baskin DS, Yatsu FM (eds): Prognosis of Neurological Disorders. Oxford, Oxford University Press, 1992, pp 85–96.

146. Jensen OK, Nielsen FF, Vosmar L: An open study comparing manual therapy with the use of cold packs in the treatment of post-traumatic headache. Cephalagia 10: 241–250, 1990.

147. Jeret JS, Mandell M, Anziska B, et al: Clinical predictors of abnormality disclosed by computed tomography after mild head trauma. Neurosurgery 32:9–16, 1993.

147a. Juni JE: Taking brain SPECT seriously: Reflections on recent clinical reports in The Journal of Nuclear Medicine. J Nucl Med 35:1891–1895, 1994.

148. Kaye NS, Townsend JB 3rd, Ivins R: An open-label trial of donepezil (Aricept) in the treatment of persons with mild traumatic brain injury. J Neuropsychiatry Clin Neurosci 15(3):383–384, 2003.

149. Keller L: Unforeseen misfortune: Florida psychic's "power loss" met by skeptical jury. Houston Chronicle, February 9:9A 1991.
150. Kelly R: The post-traumatic syndrome: An iatrogenic disease. Forensic Sci 6:17, 1975.
151. Kelly R, Smith BN: Post-traumatic syndrome: Another myth discredited. J R Soc Med 74:275–277, 1981.
152. Keshavan MS, Channabasavanna SM, Reddy GN: Post-traumatic psychiatric disturbances: Patterns and predictors of outcome. Br J Psychiatry 138:157–160, 1981.
153. Khanna S, Srinath S: Symptomatic mania after minor head injury. Can J Psychiatry 30:236–237, 1985.
154. Kirsch NL: The implications of prognostic uncertainty for rehabilitation after mild head injury. In: Hoff JT Anderson TE, Cole TM (eds): Mild to Moderate Head Injury. Boston, Blackwell Scientific, 1989, pp 145–151.
155. Koller WC, Wong GF, Lang A: Posttraumatic movement disorders: A review. Mov Disord 4(1):20–36, 1989.
156. Kraus JF, Black MA, Hessol N, et al: The incidence of acute brain injury and serious impairment in a defined population. Am J Epidemiol 119:186–201, 1984.
157. Krauss JK, Mohadjer M, Braus DF, et al: Dystonia following head trauma: A report on nine patients and review of the literature. Mov Disord 7:263–272, 1992.
158. Kraus JF, Nourjah P: The epidemiology of mild uncomplicated brain injury. J Trauma 28:1637–1643, 1988.
159. Krohel GB, Kristan RYA, Simon JW, et al: Posttraumatic convergence insufficiency. Ann Ophthalmol 18: 101–104, 1986.
160. Kwartz J, Leatherbarrow B, Davis H: Diplopia following head injury. Injury 21:351–352, 1990.
161. Lanteri-Minet M, Auray JP, El Hasnaoui A, et al: Prevalence and description of chronic daily headache in the general population in France. Pain 102(1–2):143–149, 2003.
162. Laplane D, Trlrelle JL: Le mechanisme de l'ictus amnesique: A propos de quelques formes inhabituelles. Nouv Presse Med 3:721–725, 1974.
163. Lavoie ME, Dupuis F, Johnston KM, et al: Visual p300 effects beyond symptoms in concussed college athletes. J Clin Exp Neuropsychol 26(1):55–73, 2004.
164. Lee MS, Rinne JO, Ceballos-Baumann A, Thompson PD, Marsden CD: Dystonia after head trauma. Neurology 44:1374–1378, 1994.
165. Lee ST, Lui TN: Early seizures after mild closed head injury. J Neurosurg 76:435–439, 1992.
166. Lees-Haley PR, Brown RS: Neuropsychological complaint basis rates of 170 personal injury claimants. Arch Clin Neuropsychiatry 8:203–209, 1993.
167. Leininger BE, Gramling SE, Farrel AD, et al: Neuropsychological deficits in symptomatic minor head injury patients after concussion and mild concussion. J Neurol Neurosurg Psychiatry 53:293–296, 1990.
168. Lesoin F, Viaud C, Pruvo J, et al: Traumatic and alternating delayed intracranial hematomas. Neuroradiology 26:515–516, 1984.
169. Lesser IM, Mena I, Boone KB, et al: Reduction of cerebral blood flow in older depressed patients. Arch Gen Psychiatry 51:677–686, 1994.
170. Levi L, Guilburd JN, Lemberger A, et al: Diffuse axonal injury: Analysis of 100 patients with radii logical signs. Neurosurgery 27:429–432, 1990.
171. Levin HS: Neurobehavioral outcome of mild to moderate head injury. In: Hoff JT, Anderson TE, Cole TM (eds): Mild to Moderate Head Injury. Boston, Blackwell Scientific, 1989, pp 153–183.
172. Levin HS, Gary HE, High WM, et al: Minor head injury and the postconcussional syndrome: Methodological issues in outcome studies. In: Levin HS, Grafman J, Eisenberg HM (eds): Neurobehavioral Recovery from Head Injury. New York, Oxford University Press, 1987, pp 262–275.
173. Levin HS, Mattis S, Ruff RM, et al: Neurobehavioral outcome following minor head injury. A three-center study. J Neurosurg 66:234–243, 1987.
174. Levin HS, Williams D, Eisenberg HM: Treatment of postconcussional symptoms with CDP-choline. Neurology 40(suppl 1):326, 1990.
175. Levin HS, Williams DH, Eisenberg HM, High WM, Guinto FC: Serial MRI and neurobehavioral findings after mild to moderate closed head injury. J Neurol Neurosurg Psychiatry 5:255–262, 1992.
176. Lewine JD, Davis JT, Sloan JH, et al: Neuromagnetic assessment of pathophysiologic brain activity induced by minor head trauma. Am J Neuroradiol 20(5):857–866, 1999.
177. Lishman WA: Physiogenesis and psychogenesis in the "post-concussional syndrome." Br J Psychiatry 153:460–469, 1988.
178. Loder E, Biondi D: Use of botulinum toxin for chronic headaches: A focused review. Clin J Pain 18(6 suppl): S169–S176, 2002.
179. Lord SM, Barnsley L, Wallis BJ, Bogduk N: Third occipital headache: A prevalence study. J Neurol Neurosurg Psvchiatry 57:1187–1190, 1994.
180. Lorenzoni E: Electroencephalographic studies before and after head injuries. Electroencephalogr Clin Neurophysiol 28:216, 1970.
181. MacFlvnn G, Montgomery EA, Fenton GW, et al: Measurement of reaction time following minor head injury. J Neurol Neurosurg Psychiatry 47:1326–1331, 1984.
182. MacKenzie JD, Siddiqi F, Babb JS, et al: Brain atrophy in mild or moderate traumatic brain injury: A longitudinal quantitative analysis. AJNR 23(9):1509–1515, 2002.
183. Mandel S: Minor head injury may not be "minor." Postgrad Med 85(6):213–225, 1989.
184. Marshall LF, Ruff RN: Neurosurgeon as victim. In: Levin HS, Eisenberg HM, Benton Al (eds): Mild Head Injury. Oxford, Oxford University Press, 1989, pp 276–280.
185. Martland HS: Punch-drunk. JAMA 19:1103–1107, 1928.
186. Matharu MS, Goadsby PJ: Post-traumatic chronic paroxysmal hemicrania with aura. Neurology 56:273–275, 2001.

187. Mathew N, Saper JR, Silberstein SD, et al: Migraine prophylaxis with divalproex. Arch Neurol 52:281–286, 1995.
188. Matthews WB: Footballer's migraine. Br Med J 2:326–327, 1972.
189. Mayeux R, Ottman R, Maestre G, et al: Synergistic effects of traumatic head injury and apolipoprotein-e4 in patients with Alzheimer's disease. Neurology 45:555–557, 1995.
190. Mayeux R, Ottman R, Tang MX, et al: Genetic susceptibility and head injury as risk factors for Alzheimer's disease among community-dwelling elderly persons and their first-degree relatives. Ann Neurol 33:494–501, 1993.
191. McAllister TW: Neuropsychiatric sequelae of head injuries. Psychiatr Clin 15:395–413, 1992.
192. McAllister TW, Sparling MB, Flashman LA, et al: Differential working memory load effects after mild traumatic brain injury. Neuroimage 14(5):1004–1012, 2001.
193a. McBeath JG, Nanda A: Use of dihydroergotamine in patients with postconcussion syndrome. Headache 34: 148–151, 1994.
193b. McBeath JG, Nanda A: Roller coaster migraine: An underreported injury? Headache 40:745–747, 2000.
194. McCaffrey RJ, Williams AD, Fisher JM, Laing LC: Forensic issues in mild head injury. J Head Trauma Rehabil 8:38–47, 1993.
195. McCrory P: Does second impact syndrome exist? Clin J Sport Med 11(3):144–149, 2001.
196. McKinlay WW, Brooks DN, Bond MR: Postconcussional symptoms, financial compensation and outcome of severe blunt head injury. J Neurol Neurosurg Psychiatry 46:1084–1091, 1983.
197. McKissock W: Subdural hematoma. A review of 389 cases. Lancet 1:1365–1370, 1960.
198. Mendelson G: Not "cured by a verdict": Effect of legal settlement on compensation claimants. Med J Aust 2: 132–134, 1982.
199. Merskey H, Woodforde JM: Psychiatric sequelae of minor head injury. Brain 95:521–528, 1972.
200. Mickevičiene D, Schrader H, Obelieniene D, et al: A controlled prospective inception cohort study on the post-concussion syndrome outside the medicolegal context. Eur J Neurol 11(6):411–419, 2004.
201. Middelboe T, Andersen HS, Birket-Smith M, Friis ML: Minor head injury: Impact on general health after 1 year. A prospective follow-up study. Acta Neurol Scand 85:5–9, 1992.
202. Miller H: Accident neurosis. Br Med J 1:919, 1961.
203. Milo R, Razon N, Schiffer J: Delayed epidural hematoma. A review. Acta Neurochir 84:13–23, 1987.
204. Minderhoud JM, Boelens MEM, Huizenga J, et al: Treatment of minor head injuries. Clin Neurol Neurosurg 82:127–140, 1980.
205. Mittl RL, Grossman RI, Hiehle JF, et al: Prevalence of MR evidence of diffuse axonal injury in patients with mild head injury and normal head CT findings. Am J Neuroradiol 15:1583–1589, 1994.
206. Mokri B: Low cerebrospinal fluid pressure syndrome. Neurol Clin 22:55–74, 2004.
207. Montgomery EA, Fenton GW, McClelland RJ: Delayed brainstem conduction time in post-concussional syndrome. Lancet 1:1011, 1984.
208. Montgomery EA, Fenton GW, McClelland RJ, et al: The psychobiology of minor head injury. Psychol Med 21:375–384, 1990.
209. Mureriwa J: Head injury and compensation: A preliminary investigation of the postconcussional syndrome in Harare. Cent Afr J Med 36:315–318, 1990.
210. Nayernouri T: Post-traumatic parkinsonism. Surg Neurol 24:263–264, 1985.
211. Newcombe F, Babbitt P, Briggs M: Minor head injury: Pathophysiologic or iatrogenic sequelae? J Neurol Neurosurg Psychiatry 57:709–716, 1994.
212. Nuwer MR: Assessment of digital EEG, quantitative EEG, and EEG brain mapping: Report of the American Academy of Neurology and the American Clinical Neurophysiology Society. Neurology 49(1):277–292, 1997.
213a. Nuwer MR, Hauser HKI: Erroneous diagnosis using EEG discriminant analysis. Neurology 44:1998–2000, 1994.
213b. Nuwer MR, Hovda DA, Schrader LM, Vespa PM: Routine and quantitative EEG in mild traumatic brain injury. Clin Neurophysiol 116(9):2001–2025, 2005.
214. Oppenheimer DR: Microscopic lesions in the brain following head injury. J Neurol Neurosurg Psychiatry 31: 299–306, 1968.
215. Packard RC: Posttraumatic headache: Permanency and relationship of legal settlement. Headache 32:496–500, 1992.
216. Packard RC: Posttraumatic headache. Semin Neurol 14:40–45, 1994.
217. Packard RC, Ham LP: Promising techniques in the assessment of mild head injury. Semin Neurol 14:74–83, 1994.
218. Parsons LC, *Ver Beek D*: Sleep-awake patterns following cerebral concussion. Nurs Res 31:260–264, 1982.
219. Piovesan EJ, Kowacs PA, Werneck LC: S.U.N.C.T. syndrome: Report of a case preceded by ocular trauma. Arq Neuropsiquiatr 54:494–497, 1996.
220. Poletti CE: Proposed operation for occipital neuralgia: C-2 and C-3 root decompression. Neurosurgery 12: 221–224, 1983.
221. Ponsford J, Willmott C, Rothwell A, et al: Impact of early intervention on outcome following mild head injury in adults. J Neurol Neurosurg Psychiatry 73:330–332, 2002.
222. Potter DD, Bassett MR, Jory SH, Barrett K: Changes in event-related potentials in a three-stimulus auditory oddball task after mild head injury. Neuropsychologia 39(13):1464–1472, 2001.
223. Povlishock JT, Coburn TH: Morphopathological change associated with mild head injury. In: Levin HS, Eisenberg HM, Benton AL (eds): Mild Head Injury. New York, Oxford University Press, 1989, pp 37–53.

224. Practice parameter: The management of concussion in sports (summary statement). Report of the Quality Standards Subcommittee of the American Academy of Neurology. Neurology 48:581–585, 1997.
225. Prigatano GP, Redner JE: Uses and abuses of neuropsychological testing in behavioral neurology. Neurol Clin 11:219–231, 1993.
226. Rapoport MJ, McCullagh S, Streiner D, et al: The clinical significance of major depression following mild traumatic brain injury. Psychosomatics 44:31–37, 2003.
227. Reid RH, Gulenchyn KY, Ballinger JR, et al: Cerebral perfusion imaging with technetium-99m HMPAO following cerebral trauma. Initial experience. Clin Nucl Med 15:383–388, 1990.
228. Ricker JH, Zafonte RD: Functional neuroimaging and quantitative electroencephalography in adult traumatic head injury: Clinical applications and interpretive cautions. J Head Trauma Rehabil 15(2):859–868, 2000.
229. Rigler J: Ueber die Verletzungen auf Eisenbahnen Insbesondere der Verletzungen des Rueckenmarks. Berlin, Reimer, 1879.
230. Rimel RW, Giordani B, Barth JT, et al: Disability caused by minor head injury. Neurosurgery 9:221–228, 1981.
231. Roberts GW, Allsop D, Bruton C: The occult aftermath of boxing. J Neurol Neurosurg Psychiatry 53:373–378, 1990.
232. Roberts GW, Gentleman SM, Lynch A, et al: β amyloid protein deposition in the brain after severe head injury: Implications for the pathogenesis of Alzheimer's disease. J Neurol Neurosurg Psychiatry 57:419–425, 1994.
233. Robertson A: The post-concussional syndrome then and now. Aust NZ J Psychiatry 22:396–403, 1988.
234. Roy CW, Pentland B, Miller JD: The causes and consequences of minor head injury in the elderly. Injury 17:220–223, 1986.
235. Ross RJ, Cole M, Thompson JS, et al: Boxers—computer tomography, EEG, and neurological evaluation. JAMA 249:211–213, 1983.
236. Ruff RM, Wylie T, Tennant W: Malingering and malingering-like aspects of mild closed head injury. J Head Trauma Rehabil 8:60–73, 1993.
237. Russell MB, Olesen J: Migraine associated with head trauma. Eur J Neurol 3:424–428, 1996.
238. Russello D, Randazzo G, Favetta A, et al: Oxiracetam treatment of exogenous postconcussion syndrome. Statistical evaluation of results. Minerva Chir 45:1309–1314, 1990.
239. Rutherford WH: Postconcussion symptoms: Relationship to acute neurological indices, individual differences, and circumstances of injury. In: Levin HS, Eisenberg HM, Benton AL (eds): Mild Head Injury. Oxford, Oxford University Press, 1989, pp 217–228.
240. Rutherford WH, Merrett JD, McDonald JR: Sequelae of concussion caused by minor head injuries. Lancet 1:1–4, 1977.
241. Rutherford WH, Merrett JD, McDonald JR: Symptoms at one year following concussion from minor head injuries. Injury 10:225–230, 1978.
242. Savola O, Hillborn M. Early predictors of post-concussion symptoms in patients with mild head injury. Eur J Neurol 10:175–181, 2003.
243a. Scher AI, Stewart WF, Lieberman J, Lipton RB: Prevalence of frequent headache in a population sample. Headache 38:497–506, 1998.
243b. Schievink WI, Ebersold MJ, Atkinson JL: Roller-coaster headache due to spinal cerebrospinal fluid leak. Lancet 18;347(9012):1409, 1996.
244. Schoenhuber R, Gentilini M: Anxiety and depression after mild head injury: A case control study. J Neurol Neurosurg Psychiatry 51:722–724, 1988.
245. Schoenhuber R, Gentilini M: Neurophysiological assessment of mild head injury. In: Levin HS, Eisenberg HM, Benton AL (eds): Mild Head Injury. Oxford, Oxford University Press, 1989, pp 142–150.
246. Schoenhuber R, Gentilini M, Orlando A: Prognostic value of auditory brainstem responses for late postconcussion symptoms following minor head injury. J Neurosurg 68:742–744, 1988.
247. Schoenhuber R, Gentilini M, Scarano M, et al: Longitudinal study of auditory brainstem response in patients with minor head injuries. Arch Neurol 144:1181–1182, 1987.
248. Schott GD: Induction of involuntary movements by peripheral trauma: An analogy with causalgia. Lancet 2:712–716, 1986.
249. Segalowitz SJ, Bernstein DM, Lawson S: P300 event-related potential decrements in well-functioning university students with mild head injury. Brain Cogn 45(3):342–356, 2001.
250. Servadei F, Teasdale G, Merry G, Neurotraumatology Committee of the World Federation of Neurosurgical Societies: Defining acute mild head injury in adults: A proposal based on prognostic factors, diagnosis, and management. J Neurotrauma 18(7):657–664, 2001.
251. Shah AK, Guyot AM, Ham SD, et al: "CT or not to CT": ER evaluation of head trauma. Neurology 41(suppl 1):308, 1991.
252. Sjaastad O: The headache of challenge in our time: Cervicogenic headache. Fund Neurol 5:155–158, 1990.
253a. Slagle DA: Psychiatric disorders following closed head injury: An overview of biopsychological factors in their etiology and management. Int J Psychiatr Med 20:1–35, 1990.
253b. Smits M, Dippel DW, de Haan GG,et al: External validation of the Canadian CT Head Rule and the New Orleans Criteria for CT scanning in patients with minor head injury. JAMA 28;294(12):1519–1525, 2005.
254. Solomon S: Posttraumatic migraine. Headache 38:772–778, 1998.
255. Solomon S, Guglielmo KM: Treatment of headache by transcutaneous electrical stimulation. Headache 25:12–15, 1985.
256. Soriani S, Cavaliere B, Faggioli R, et al: Confusional

migraine precipitated by mild head trauma. Arch Pediatr Adolesc Med 154:90–91, 2000.

256a. Stapert S, de Kruijk J, Houx P, et al: S-100B concentration is not related to neurocognitive performance in the first month after mild traumatic brain injury. Eur Neurol 53:22–26, 2005.

257. Steadman JH, Graham JG: Rehabilitation of the brain-injured. Proc R Soc Med 63:23–28, 1969.

258. Stein SC, Ross SE: Mild head injury: A plea for routine early CT scanning. J Trauma 33:11–13, 1992.

259a. Stern M, Dulaney E, Gruber SB, et al: The epidemiology of Parkinson's disease. Arch Neurol 48:903–907, 1991.

259b. Stiell IG, Clement CM, Rowe BH, et al: Comparison of the Canadian CT Head Rule and the New Orleans Criteria in patients with minor head injury. JAMA 28; 294(12):1511–1518, 2005.

259c. Stiell IG, Wells GA, Vandemheen K, et al: The Canadian CT Head Rule for patients with minor head injury. Lancet 5;357(9266):1391–1396, 2001.

260. Strauss I, Savitsky N: Head injury: Neurologic and psychiatric aspects. Arch Neurol Psychiatry 31:893–955, 1934.

261. Strich SJ: Diffuse degeneration of the cerebral white matter in severe dementia following head injury. J Neurol Neurosurg Psychiatry 19:163–185, 1956.

262. Strich SJ: Shearing of nerve fibers as a cause of brain damage due to head injury. Lancet 2:443–448, 1961.

263. Stuss DT: A sensible approach to mild traumatic brain injury. Neurology 45:1251–1252, 1995.

264. Stuss DT, Stethem LL, Hugenholtz H, et al: Reaction time after head injury: Fatigue, divided and focused attention, and consistency of performance. J Neurol Neurosurg Psychiatry 52:742–748, 1989.

265. Symonds C: The assessment of symptoms following head injury. Guys Hospital Gazette 51:4641, 1937.

266. Symonds C: Concussion and its sequelae. Lancet l:1–5, 1962.

267. Tenjin H, Ueda S, Mizukawa N, et al: Positron emission tomographic studies on cerebral hemodynamics in patients with cerebral contusion. Neurosurgery 26:971–979, 1990.

268. Tennant FS, Wild J: Naltrexone treatment for postconcussional syndrome. Am J Psychiatry 144:813–814, 1987.

269. Thatcher RW, Walker RA, Gerson I, et al: EEG discriminant analyses of mild head injury. Electroencephalogr Clin Neurophysiol 73:94–1061, 1989.

270. Thornton K: The electrophysiological effects of a brain injury on auditory memory functioning. The QEEG correlates of impaired memory. Arch Clin Neuropsychol 18(4):363–378,2003.

271. Tikofsky RS: Predicting outcome in traumatic brain injury: What role for rCBF/SPECT? J Nucl Med 35:947–948, 1994.

272. Travell JG, Simons DG: Myofascial Pain and Dysfunction. The Trigger Point Manual. Baltimore, Williams & Wilkins, 1983.

273. Trimble M: Post-traumatic Neurosis: From Railway Spine to the Whiplash. Chichester, Wiley, 1981.

274. Tuohimaa P: Vestibular disturbances after acute mild head injury. Acta Otolaryngol 359(suppl):1–59, 1978.

275. Turkewitz LJ, Wirth O, Dawson GA, Casaly JS: Cluster headache following head injury: A case report and review of the literature. Headache 32:504–.506, 1992.

276. Tyler GS, McNeely HE, Dick ML: Treatment of post-traumatic headache with amitriptyline. Headache 20: 213–216, 1980.

277. Tysvaer AT, Storli OV, Bachen NI: Soccer injuries to the brain. A neurologic and electroencephalographic study of former players. Acta Neurol Scand 80:1.51–156, 1989.

278. Uomoto JM, Esselman PC, Cardenas DD: Treatment of postconcussion syndrome. West J Med 157:665, 1992.

279. van der Naalt J, van Zomeren AH, Sluiter WJ, Minderhoud JM: One year outcome in mild to moderate head injury: The predictive value of acute injury characteristics related to complaints and return to work. J Neurol Neurosurg Psychiatry 66(2):207–213, 1999.

279a. Vanderploeg RD, Curtiss G, Belanger HG: Long-term neuropsychological outcomes following mild traumatic brain injury. J Int Neuropsychol Soc 11:228–236, 2005.

280. Van Duijn CM, Tanja TA, Haaxma R, et al: Head trauma and the risk of Alzheimer's disease. Am J Epidemiol 135:775–782, 1992.

281. Vijayan N: A new post-traumatic headache syndrome: Clinical and therapeutic observations. Headache 17(1): 19–22, 1977.

282. Vijayan N, Watson C: Site of injury headache. Headache 28:297, 1988.

283. Waddell PA, Gronwall DMA: Sensitivity to light and sound following minor head injury. Acta Neurol Scand 69:270–276, 1984.

284. Walsh WP, Hafner JW Jr, Kattah JC: Bilateral internuclear ophthalmoplegia following minor head trauma. J Emerg Med 24:19–22, 2003.

285. Weinstock A, Rothner AD: Trauma-triggered migraine: A cause of transient neurologic deficit following minor head injury in children. Neurology 45 (suppl 4):A347–A348, 1995.

286. Weiss HD, Stern BJ, Goldberg J: Post-traumatic migraine: Chronic migraine precipitated by minor head or neck trauma. Headache 31:451–456, 1991.

287. Wilkinson MN, Gilchrist E: Post-traumatic headache. Ups J Med Sci 31:48–51, 1980.

288. Williams DH, Levin HS, Eisenberg HM: Mild head injury classification. Neurosurgery 27:422–428, 1990.

289. Wrightson P: Management of disability and rehabilitation services after mild head injury. In: Levin HS, Eisenberg HM, Benton AL (eds): Mild Head Injury. New York, Oxford University Press, 1989, pp 245–256.

290. Wrightson P, Gronwall D: Time off work and symptoms after minor head injury. Injury 12:445–454, 1981.

291. Yamaguchi M: Incidence of headache and severity of head injury. Headache 32:427–431, 1992.

292. Yatham LN, Benbow JC, Jeffers AM: Mania following head injury. Acta Psychiatr Scand 77:359–360, 1988.
293. Yokota H, Kurokawa A, Otsuka T, et al: Significance of magnetic resonance imaging in acute head injury. J Trauma 31:351–357, 1991.
294. Young WB, Hopkins MM, Janyszek B, Primavera JP: Repetitive intravenous DHE in the treatment of refractory post-traumatic headache. Headache 34:297, 1994.
295. Young WB, Silberstein SD: Imaging and electrophysiologic testing in mild head injury. Semin Neurol 14:46–52, 1994.
296. Ziegler DK: Opiate and opioid use in patients with refractory headache. Cephalagia 14:5–10, 1994.

Chapter 6

Posttraumatic Cranial Neuropathies

JAMES R. KEANE AND
ROBERT W. BALOH

Diagnostic Difficulties

Perseverance is required to diagnose cranial nerve injury in the presence of severe head trauma.[49] Coma may obscure all but cranial nerve III, VI, and VII damage.[59] Diagnosis of trochlear nerve injury in particular requires a high level of patient cooperation.[54] Injury to the orbital muscles may be impossible to distinguish from ocular motor nerve damage. Loss of smell from nasal obstruction may be confused with olfactory nerve damage, and blockage of the auditory canal or damage to the middle ear may be difficult to distinguish from nerve VIII interruption. Craniofacial and skull base fracture can be overlooked while treating more life-threatening injuries.[42]

Head trauma is a recurrent event. As with strokes, the greatest risk factor is a similar previous experience. Memory falters with successive blows to the head, alcohol further dulls recollection, and the possibility of previous unacknowledged injuries must be kept in mind. Cranial nerve signs may be old, the frozen eye may be prosthetic rather than paralyzed, and even the bullet seen on head scans may be old and incidental. With motorcyclists in particular, only death or multiple dismemberment dampens the ardor for repeat encounters with large objects.[55]

Neurological disabilities are often linked in patients' minds to recent episodes of trauma. If the connection seems unlikely, it probably is. Even when head injury is the immediate cause of cranial neuropathy, an underlying problem may be present. Trivial blows resulting in surprising palsies to cranial nerves III or IV or lower cranial nerves may be acting on nerves already compromised by tumor.[22]

Which Nerves Are Injured Most Commonly?

The exact incidence of damage to each cranial nerve varies with patient selection and length of follow-up (Table 6.1)[18,24a,24b,25,30,39,87,91,103] There is general agreement that the olfactory and facial nerves and audiovestibular function are damaged most often by blunt head injury. Trauma to the optic nerve and each of the ocular motor nerves is intermediate in frequency, whereas the trigeminal nerve trunk and the lower cranial nerves are rarely injured.

Table 6.1. Percentage of Patients with Traumatic Damage to Each Cranial Nerve

Reference No.	No. of Patients	I	II	III	IV	V	VI	VII	IX, X
22	430	2.6	—	—	0.1	0.2	0.4	1.6	—
27	1285	3.0	—	0.5	—	—	0.4	2.9	0.16
35	1800	0.5	4.0	4.0	1.4	3.6	4.1	4.7	0.05
75*	291	14.0	2.7	6.6	—	—	2.7	3.0	—
91	1550	7.7	1.8	1.0	1.0	1.0	1.0	3.0	0.06

*Limited to severe head injury.

Delayed Signs

The facial nerve may appear normal initially and then develop weakness several days after head injury. Delayed nerve VI palsies are usually due to increased intracranial pressure or hemorrhagic meningitis. Late appearance of oculomotor nerve paresis, even without pupillary involvement,[45] is a more ominous sign indicating transtentorial herniation. Tentorial herniation is not a cause of trochlear or abducens damage. Rarely, damage to intracranial arteries can result in delayed cranial neuropathies owing to aneurysm formation.[37] Serial follow-up evaluations are necessary therefore to fully evaluate cranial nerve trauma (Fig. 6.1).

Type of Injury

Cranial nerve findings can predict the type of head injury. Gunshot trajectories among survivors showing cranial nerve damage follow two general paths: In many suicide and some homicide attempts, an entry wound in front of the ear takes a transverse path that results in blindness. Eye movement limitation is common, but brain damage may be minimal.[50] Such cases have been reported regularly since the introduction of radiographs; Cushing published one of the more dramatic illustrations (Fig. 6.2).[13] More common in homicide attempts is an infraorbital entry with a downward path to either side of the neck, sparing the brain but damaging the lower cranial nerves and frequently the carotid artery and the sympathetic trunk. Facial paralysis and deafness are more common with missile injury to the temporal bone than following blunt trauma.[84]

With blunt head injuries, many middle and lower traumatic cranial neuropathies are accompanied by basilar fractures. All cranial nerves (except IX to XII) are at risk, but the olfactory nerve and the facial nerve are most commonly injured.[69] Symmetric middle cranial neuropathies often result from skull-crushing injuries,[99] such as happens when an automobile slips off the jack onto the mechanic's head. This pressure cracks the skull like an egg, stretching the nerves but sparing the brain (Fig. 6.3). Hyperextension neck injuries may selectively interrupt cranial nerves VI and XII bilaterally, but associated direct damage to the pontomedullary junction or indirect brain stem infarction following vertebral artery injury may obscure cranial nerve damage.[51]

Stretching injuries tend to damage nerves at fixed attachments or at points of sharp angulation. Autopsy reports come largely from coroners' offices and emphasize rapidly fatal injuries. The high frequency with which nerves are pulled loose from the brain stem in these reports reflects the severe forces involved and provides an explanation for failure of recovery in more than half of traumatic cranial neuropathies.[34] The optic nerve is a somewhat special case. It is tethered within the optic canal—the usual site of injury—and is subject to stretching with brain shifts. In addition, however, the bony architecture of the orbit directly transfers force from the superolateral orbital rim to the optic nerve canal.[28]

Terrorist bomb attacks are an increasingly common cause of cranial nerve injuries in civilians.[67] Cranial nerves VII and VIII are particularly vulnerable to shrapnel penetrating the temporal bone. The examining physician must be alert to small skin imperfections around the ear canal to identify penetrating wounds.

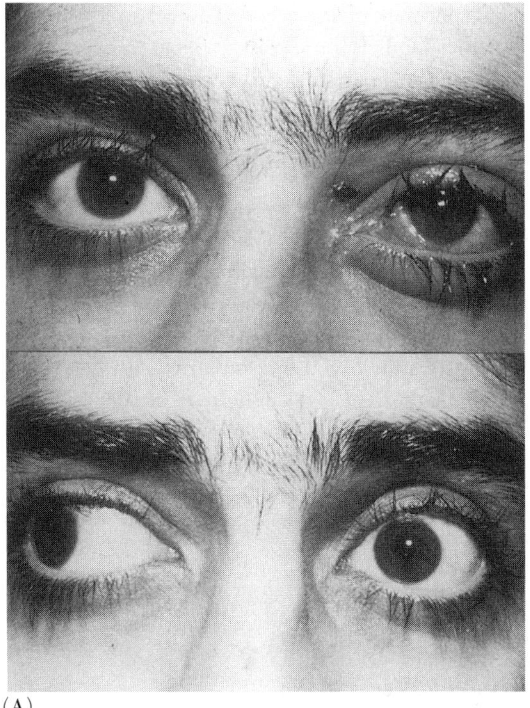

(A)

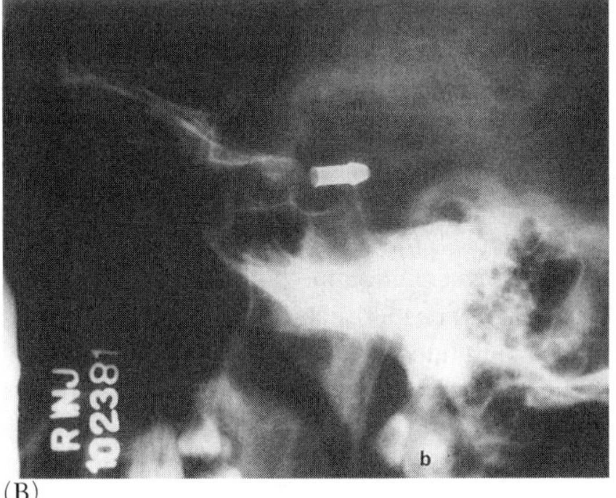

(B)

Figure 6.1. Vagaries of trauma are illustrated by a patient who was stabbed at the inner canthus of the left eye (*A*—top) by a ballpoint pen that penetrated the skull (*B*) but spared the medial rectus muscle, cranial nerves, and carotid artery. Left medial rectus weakness (*A*—bottom) was seen 2 years later when he returned with internuclear ophthalmoplegia as the presenting sign of multiple sclerosis.

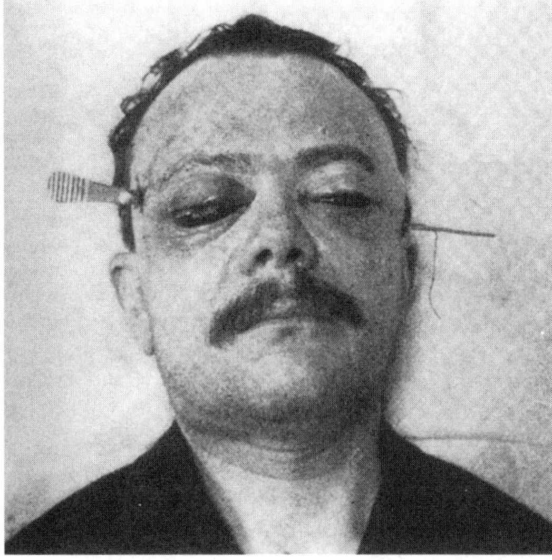

Figure 6.2. An awake patient with blindness following gunshot wound in a suicide attempt. *Source*: Cushing.[13]

Recovery

It is uncertain how often, how soon, and how well patients recover from traumatic cranial neuropathies. Follow-ups are notoriously poor in this group. When patients do return, the average physician will skip the olfactory nerve, be casual about testing vision and hearing, and record aberrant regeneration of nerve III as recovery. Chances of return of function vary with the nerve involved: The facial nerve usually recovers, the ocular motor nerves return to normal about 40% of the time,[90] and the first two cranial nerves show significant improvement in less than one-third of cases.[38,101] Lesions of the audiovestibular nerve are usually permanent.

Treatment

There are few situations in which any therapy is of unequivocal benefit in restoring cranial nerve function after traumatic injury. In particular, strong opinions concerning treatment of optic nerve damage generate heat rather than light. Various measures have been advocated after injury to cranial nerves II through VIII and are discussed in those sections.

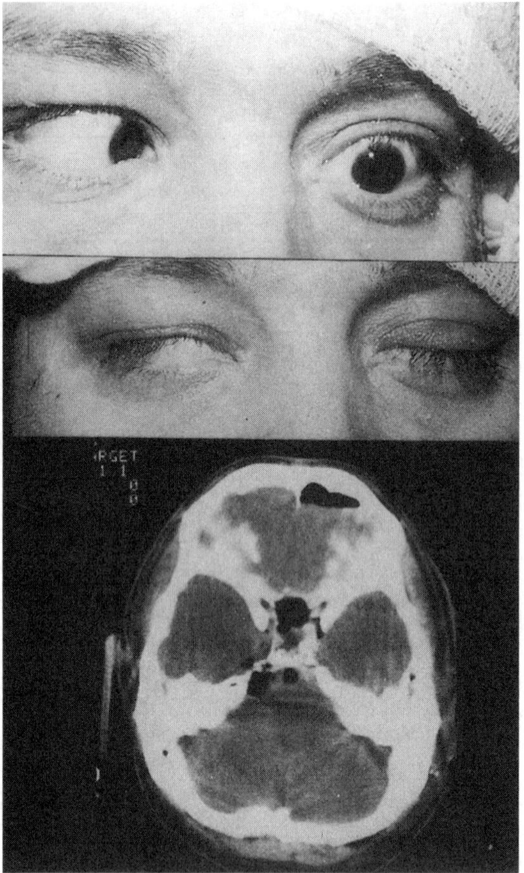

Figure 6.3. Patient following crush injury to the skull looking left (top) and showing one (of two) nerve VI palsies: closing the eyes (center), showing bilateral nerve VII pareses; and computed tomography (bottom) illustrating pneumocephalus accompanied by a subjective splashing sound with head movement.

Olfactory Nerve

Medical students and house officers increasingly begin their cranial nerve examination with vision, as in "cranial nerves II through XII intact." This neglect in testing the sense of smell transfers to the patient the burden of detecting a loss of taste and smell.[16] Of all patient complaints of loss of smell at a "nasal dysfunction clinic," 10% were related to trauma, and two-thirds had inflammatory/viral causes.[15]

Anosmia is more common with occipital than with frontal blows and can result from trauma to any part of the head. Recovery occurs in more than one-third of cases, usually during the first 3 months. Some patients, however, are reported to show improvement as late as 5 years after injury. Trivial blows can cause permanent loss of smell, but the incidence of anosmia parallels the severity of head trauma. A high percentage of patients with posttraumatic olfactory dysfunction (88%) show abnormalities in the olfactory bulbs and tracts and the inferior frontal lobes on magnetic resonance imaging (MRI).[104]

Sumner extensively reviewed previous studies[100] and credited Hughlings Jackson with the first report of posttraumatic anosmia in 1864. Most studies agree that the olfactory nerve is the cranial nerve most often damaged by blunt head trauma. Leigh[71] found anosmia in 5.0% of patients with head injuries, Turner[103a] in 7.7%, Hughes[39] in 10.5%, Friedman and Merritt[25] in 2.5%, Sumner[100] in 7.1%, and Zusho[105] in 4.2%. Sumner suggests an overall incidence of 7%, rising to 30% with severe head injuries or anterior fossa fractures.[101]

Optic Nerve

Clinical Presentation

Type of Injury

About one-fourth of civilian optic nerve trauma is due to penetrating injury (Table 6.2). Gunshot wounds are the usual cause, with orbital perforating injuries and surgical complications being less common. American men strongly prefer handguns for suicide. The usual technique of holding the muzzle to the temple frequently destroys both optic nerves, but even less common methods such as positioning the muzzle beneath the chin or "swallowing the barrel" may produce blindness in one or both eyes.[50]

Indirect optic nerve injury results from trauma to the ipsilateral outer eyebrow with astonishing regularity. Forces exerted there are transmitted

Table 6.2. Traumatic Optic Nerve Injuries*

Blunt injury	191	
Unilateral	150	(78%)
Bilateral	22	(12%)
Chiasmal	19	(10%)
Penetrating injury	53	
Unilateral	44	(83%)
Bilateral	8	(15%)
Chiasmal	1	(2%)

*Inpatients seen at the Los Angeles County/University of Southern California Medical Center over 24 years.

directly to the optic nerve canal,[6b,28] the usual site of traumatic optic neuropathy.[12,75] Occasionally, temporal-parietal blows will damage the optic nerve, but occipital trauma rarely produces optic neuropathy. In a few patients, injuries to the globe result in avulsion of the optic nerve, with associated fundus hemorrhage and disruption.[3a] Rarer still are the psychotic individuals who heed the advice given by the apostle Matthew: "If thy right eye offend thee, pluck it out."[68] Removal of an eye and the attached optic nerve is a relatively simple procedure for the motivated, and unfortunately, many self-enucleations are bilateral.

The optic nerves, like the olfactory and trochlear nerves, can be damaged by trivial blows, but most traumatic optic neuropathies are associated with severe head injury with unconsciousness. (In the horse, unconsciousness rarely accompanies such injuries.[78]) On a neurosurgery service, optic nerve damage tends to be severe and the diagnosis delayed. Restoration of vision is unlikely, and precedence is naturally given to protecting life and brain function. Emergency room patients in whom monocular visual loss is the chief complaint have injuries that are milder and often isolated. In such cases, diagnosis and treatment should be prompt.

Visual Loss

The most common result of optic nerve injury is complete blindness in one eye, but any degree of impairment of visual acuity may occur.[15,63,66,72] Similarly with partial damage, any type of visual field loss may occur, but inferior altitudinal defects are relatively frequent. About 10% of patients will show signs of bilateral optic nerve or chiasmal damage (Fig. 6.4),[93] usually in association with severe head injuries. Many chiasmal lesions are asymmetric, with unilateral severe optic neuropathy associated with contralateral temporal hemianopia.

Occasionally, a patient will present with spurious visual loss after head trauma. If that possibility is kept in mind, the diagnosis is not difficult.[51] The usual picture is that of monocular blindness or severe monocular visual loss accompanied by a tunnel field or spurious hemianopia.[60] Lack of an afferent pupillary defect confirms the diagnosis of functional visual loss, and a firm, optimistic prognosis should be rendered.

Indirect optic nerve trauma usually produces immediate visual loss. Spontaneous improvement is rarely documented in an inpatient neurosurgical setting but may occur in more than one-third of patients in more favorable situations.[37,63,93] The presence of blood within the posterior ethmoid cells, age over 40 years, loss of consciousness with the traumatic optic neuropathy, and absence of recovery after 48 hours of steroid treatment are all poor prognostic factors for recovery of vision.[11]

Delayed visual loss is potentially reversible. A small percentage of patients develop progressive

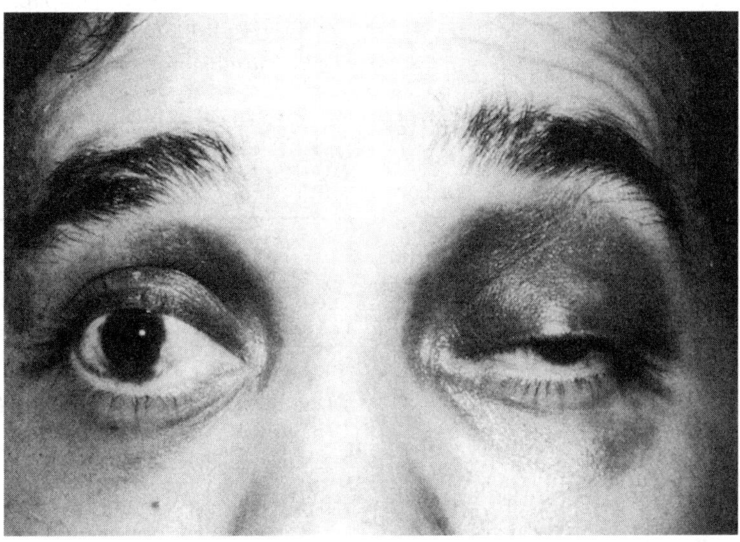

Figure 6.4. Patient with damage to the chiasm, left nerve III, and bilateral nerves VI following blunt head injury.

visual loss several hours to several days after injury, presumably owing to edema or ischemia within the canal or compression from an evolving orbital subperiosteal hematoma.[24c] Rarer still is a delay of days to weeks resulting from enlargement of traumatic mucoceles[70] or posttraumatic aneurysms.[44]

Evaluation

Clinical evaluation of the conscious patient consists of prompt testing of visual acuity and fields and using the swinging flashlight test to search for an afferent pupillary defect. In the unresponsive patient, evaluation depends on afferent pupillary function, and the frequent association of efferent pupillary damage may make this a difficult task. Although early optic disk pallor does not appear until 1 month after injury, funduscopy is necessary to rule out vitreous or retinal hemorrhage as the cause of visual loss.

Radiographic and laboratory testing are of limited value in the presence of immediate visual loss. Fractures through the optic canal can be demonstrated in about one-half of such patients, but this finding is of limited practical concern. Small optic nerve sheath hematomas occasionally accompany optic nerve injuries. Similar sheath hemorrhages are frequently seen with subarachnoid hemorrhage and other acute intracranial bleeding,[46] where they do not interfere with vision. Their presence after head trauma is expected, will rarely be a factor in visual loss, and should not overly excite the surgeon.

Treatment

There is agreement that prompt treatment is imperative in cases of delayed visual loss. The effectiveness of treating immediate injuries remains unproven. The optic nerve and the spinal cord are similar in being central nervous system tracts contained within bony canals, and effective therapy for one may well benefit the other. Evidence that immediate high-dose steroid therapy results in an improved outcome after spinal cord injuries[7] is a strong recommendation for its prompt use in nearly all cases of traumatic optic neuropathy. The dangers of fluid rhinorrhea must be weighed against potential benefit to the optic nerve.

Continuing the analogy to the spinal cord in the case of surgery, which has proven of little benefit in stable spinal cord injuries, is not encouraging for the role of surgical decompression of the traumatized canicular optic nerve. In practice, however, favorable results of decompression have been reported with increasing frequency and enthusiasm.[26,74,76,81,98,102] (These reports should be tempered by recalling the decade of perfervid testimonial to the efficacy of decompression in Bell's palsy.) Unfortunately, definitive studies do not exist. The International Optic Nerve Trauma Study was inconclusive because of the limited number of eligible patients.[73] A recent prospective nonrandom study of steroids and endoscopic optic nerve decompression showed visual improvement in 70% of patients treated within 7 days of injury compared to only 24% of patients treated after 7 days.[86a] However, in patients who are not completely blind, improvement can occur even when surgery is undertaken a few months after injury.[62]

Ocular Motor Nerves (III, IV, AND VI)

Clinical Presentation

Nerve III

The dilated pupil and turned-out eye of a patient with a major nerve III palsy provide a distinctive appearance even in the unconscious patient.[58] The principal temptation is overdiagnosis of oculomotor nerve paresis in the face of concomitant orbital trauma. A fixed, dilated pupil after face and head trauma commonly represents traumatic mydriasis owing to iris injury or orbital parasympathetic damage. Distinguishing nerve III damage from diffuse orbital muscle limitation depends on relative spar-

Table 6.3. Ocular Motor Nerve Palsies*

Nerve Affected Trauma	Number as a Result of All Causes	Number as a Result of Trauma	Percent Due to Trauma
Nerve III			
Direct trauma	197	843	23
Herniation	128		—
Nerve IV (bilateral 35)	116	185	63
Nerve VI (bilateral 65)	181	889	20
Total III-IV-VI palsies	494	1917	26

*Inpatients seen at the Los Angeles County/University of Southern California Medical Center over 24 years.

ing of lateral movement and may need to await reduction in orbital swelling. Infraorbital numbness suggests an orbital blowout fracture and argues against a nerve III palsy.

A fracture through the orbital roof is much less common than a floor fracture and is even more important to diagnose promptly[57]; the accompanying subfrontal hematomas may require emergency neurosurgery.[86b] Roof fracture often mimics superior division palsies of nerve III (Fig. 6.5). The levator and superior rectus muscles are paralyzed, but in these cases, damage is due to direct muscle injury by "blow-in" bone fragments or hemorrhage.

Recovery of oculomotor nerve function more than 6 weeks after trauma, with disproportionate improvement in adduction and highly variable ptosis, suggests aberrant regeneration. Demonstration that the lid elevates when the eye is turned in and down confirms the diagnosis.

Nerve IV

Traumatic trochlear nerve palsies are rarely diagnosed on acute neurosurgical services.[52,56] As the patient slowly awakens from coma in a convalescent setting, he or she inadvertently closes one eye to focus. As lethargy declines, the patient complains of vertical double vision on looking downward. Examination shows one eye to be slightly higher, especially on gaze down and in. Contralateral head tilt will improve diplopia, whereas tilting the head to the ipsilateral side will increase the separation of images and confirm the diagnosis.

The most common mistake in diagnosing a trochlear nerve palsy is overlooking lesser paresis of the opposite nerve IV. Using a red glass to demonstrate reversal of hypertropia on down gaze to alternate sides will confirm bilateral involvement. Orbital muscle injury, minor nerve III paresis, and skew deviation enter the differential diagnosis, but if the pattern of diplopia fits, nerve IV palsy is more likely. Magnetic resonance imaging (fluid attenuated inversion recovery—FLAIR) may show a high-intensity lesion of the trochlear nerve in the ambient cistern consistent with subarachnoid blood.[32]

Nerve VI

Minor degrees of lateral rectus limitation are ambiguous after head injury, and patient cooperation is necessary to establish a diagnosis of nerve VI palsy. Although bilateral nerve III palsies are rare, bilateral nerve IV and VI pareses are common and may even be confused with each other in a stuporous patient who exhibits esotropia on downward gaze.

Rarely, apparent bilateral nerve VI palsies will vary dramatically from moment to moment. This inconsistency raises the possibility of voluntary convergence spasm. Observing that miosis occurs in proportion to esotropia will establish the diagnosis.[48]

Diagnostic Tests

Recorded diplopia fields (Lancaster or others) are useful for diagnosis and follow-up of cooperative patients with minimal diplopia. A computed tomography (CT) scan is automatic after any significant head trauma. The formerly paramount question concerning whether a nerve III palsy was immediate and due to direct trauma or delayed and due to tentorial herniation is now answered before it arises. One surprise with scanning has been the unexpectedly high incidence of dorsolateral midbrain contusion with trochlear palsy.[26] Computed tomography and MRI scans are highly useful in sorting out the cause of delayed diplopia. Slowly evolving tentorial herniation may be subtle and carries high mortality and morbidity even in the scan era.[45,47,53,60]

Treatment

Initial treatment of diplopia consists of patching for comfort. Most patients will choose to patch the more limited eye, and it is not necessary for adults to alternate the patch. Some patients with trochlear palsies will prefer to achieve single vision by tilting the head and tucking the chin down. Overall, about one patient in five will find a patch more nuisance than help. Like hospital gowns, eye patches of unusual cheapness seem to appeal to hospital administrators. A decent patch should be comfortably convex, with sufficient elastic to avoid secondary glaucoma. Patients who experience diplopia only in a small field of vision can apply semitransparent tape to the appropriate portion of one lens of their glasses for a better cosmetic and functional result.

Paste-on prisms, combined with considerable patience by both physician and patient, may occasionally improve the area of binocular single vision. Injection of botulinum toxin into the antagonists of paralyzed muscles is a technique that promises

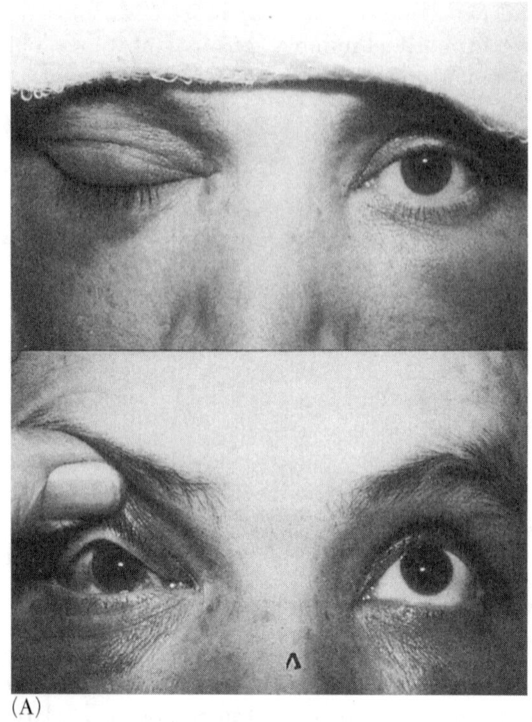

(A)

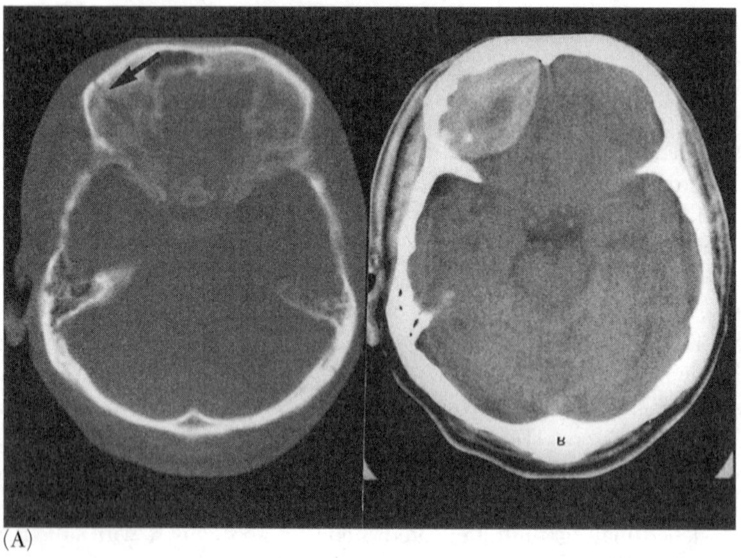

(A)

Figure 6.5. Right ptosis (*A*—top) and paralysis of elevation (*A*—bottom) simulate superior division nerve III palsy. However, these signs are due to local muscle damage from an orbital roof fracture (arrow) (*B*—left). A commonly associated frontal bone fracture (*B*—left) and a subfrontal epidural hematoma (*B*—right) are evident.

to reduce contractures. Surgery of the extraocular muscles is usually delayed 9 to 12 months or until diplopia has been stable for 6 months. Surgery aims to eliminate diplopia in the forward and the downward reading positions[92] and can be very helpful for persisting trochlear palsies, less so for abducens pareses, sometimes of benefit with nerve III damage, and only occasionally of use in the presence of aberrant regeneration of nerve III.

Trigeminal Nerve

Branches of the trigeminal nerve are frequently injured by facial lacerations and fractures. One of the most common causes of maxillary nerve injury is an orbital floor blowout fracture.[27] Mandibular nerve injury is common after dental procedures.[86c] When head and face trauma result in infraorbital (V2) numbness and limitation of ocular elevation, sometimes accompanied by a sluggish pupil, the temptation to diagnose nerve V and III pareses should be restrained, as this is a common pattern with orbital floor fractures.

The gasserian ganglion and the trigeminal trunk are rarely involved in closed head injuries. Jefferson and Schorstein reviewed the literature in 1955 and found five cases of traumatic complete trigeminal neuropathy after gunshot wounds and seven resulting from blunt trauma.[41] They added seven personal examples resulting from penetrating wounds and nine from blunt trauma. Of 11 cases at Los Angeles County Hospital involving injury to the entire trigeminal nerve, 5 resulted from intracranial gunshot wounds and 6 from blunt trauma. Patients with closed head injuries had basilar fractures and concomitant involvement of nerves VI and VII and often other cranial nerves.

Facial Nerve

Clinical Presentation

Because of its long, tortuous course through the temporal bone, the facial nerve is especially vulnerable to penetrating or blunt trauma to the head (Fig. 6.6).[4,103b] Objects entering the middle ear damage the relatively exposed horizontal segment of the facial nerve. The most common penetrating injuries to the middle ear result from self-instrumentation of the ear canal (usually with Q-tips) or accidental entry of the ear canal by foreign objects, such as the branch of a tree. A common industrial injury is penetration of the middle ear by hot sparks produced by a welding torch. Major blunt trauma to the skull often leads to fractures at the base.[64] Laceration of the facial nerve within the internal auditory canal occurs in about 50% of patients with transverse fractures of the temporal bone.[10] The more common longitudinal fractures of the temporal bone do not cross the internal auditory canal but may involve a portion of the fallopian canal, particularly the tympanic or mastoid portion. In these cases, facial paralysis is often delayed in onset because the injury is due to edema rather than to a direct interruption of the nerve. Some cases of severe blunt head injury may result in tearing of the facial nerve at the root entry zone into the brain stem. Patients with this injury invariably have a prolonged period of unconsciousness at the time of the accident, and there are nearly always associated symptoms and signs of brain stem injury.

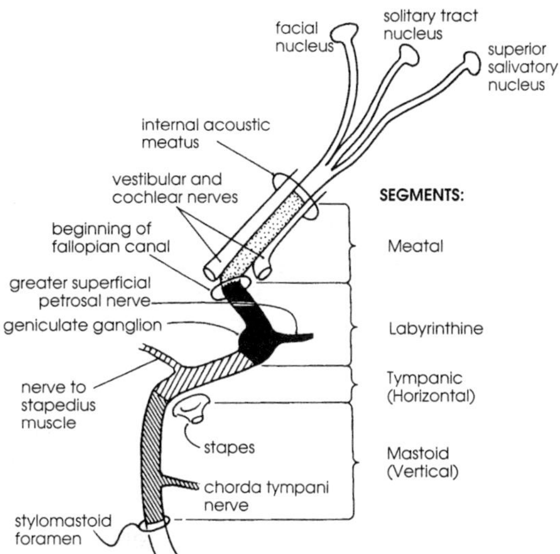

Figure 6.6. The branches of the facial nerve as it passes through the temporal bone. (From Baloh RW, Honrubia V: Clinical Neurophysiology of the Vestibular System, 2nd ed. Philadelphia, FA Davis, 1990, p 24, with permission.)

Diagnostic Tests

Topographic Testing of the Facial Nerve
Knowledge of the three major branches of the facial nerve within the temporal bone allows one to localize the site of the lesion within the fallopian canal (see Fig. 6.6).[17] Lesions of the vertical mastoid segment result in loss of taste on the ipsilateral anterior two-thirds of the tongue. Lesions involving the horizontal segment within the middle ear produce a loss of both the stapedius reflex and ipsilateral taste. The former is manifested by hypersensitivity to loud sounds. Finally, a lesion of the most proximal labyrinthine segment of the facial nerve results in impaired ipsilateral lacrimation in addition to the loss of the stapedius reflex and ipsilateral taste. Lesions within the internal auditory canal commonly involve both cranial nerves VII and VIII, so facial symptoms are combined with hearing loss and vertigo.

Electrical Stimulation of the Facial Nerve
The Hilger stimulator is the most commonly used device for percutaneous electrical stimulation of the facial nerve. Typically, thresholds are determined for minimal and maximal movement of the facial musculature on the involved side and on the normal side. Absence of response on the involved side immediately after an accident may be evidence of a complete interruption of the facial nerve. Even if the facial nerve is interrupted, however, it may continue to stimulate for up to 4 days because the distal segment remains intact. After a 4-day waiting period, repeat percutaneous stimulation should provide a good estimate of the level of facial nerve function. If the involved side stimulates as well as the normal side, the prognosis is excellent for return of function. Absence of stimulation on the involved side after 4 days is a poor prognostic indicator, and surgical exploration may be needed to evaluate the status of the facial nerve.[20]

Imaging Studies
High-resolution CT scanning with bone windows is the radiological procedure of choice for evaluating trauma to the temporal bone and skull base.[64] Over one-third of temporal bone fractures are missed by clinical diagnosis alone.[21] The clinician must work closely with the radiologist so that appropriate cuts are made of all the potentially involved areas. Computed tomography with contrast can be helpful when there is suspected intracranial involvement. Magnetic resonance imaging is most sensitive for identifying soft tissue lesions but is of little use for identifying fractures. Angiography with digital subtraction may be necessary if the fracture line runs through one of the vascular structures within the temporal bone.

Treatment

Surgery
Decisions regarding surgery for facial nerve injury after trauma can be very difficult.[23,6c] As suggested earlier, if there is only partial paresis and the facial nerve stimulates after 4 days, the prognosis is good and surgical intervention is unlikely. Often the history of the onset and progression of the facial nerve injury is less clear, however, particularly when the surgeon first sees the patient several months after the accident. The most clear-cut indication for surgery is a transverse fracture of the temporal bone, in which case the facial paralysis is usually associated with severe loss of auditory and vestibular function as well. In this case, the surgeon performs a mastoidectomy and decompresses the facial nerve, informing the patient that the loss of auditory and vestibular function is permanent. Because temporal bone fractures often involve the facial nerve in more than one location, the entire length of the facial canal must be explored. The most frequent location of involvement is in the area of the geniculate ganglion. Success of reconstructive surgery rests on the extent of the injury, availability of the proximal stump, the time since injury, and the duration of muscle denervation.[85]

Eye Care
Prophylactic eye care using artificial tears should be instituted in all patients with facial paralysis, regardless of whether they have adequate or inadequate tear production.[97] The artificial tears should be used several times a day and a sterile ointment instilled at night. Further, the patient should tape the eye closed at night using paper tape. If the patient develops any pain or redness, a referral to an ophthalmologist is indicated. Partial or complete tarsorrhaphy is often required in patients with permanent facial paralysis. A simple marginal lid adhesion tarsorrhaphy can easily be reversed if facial nerve function returns.

Physiotherapy
With prolonged facial paralysis, electrical stimulation of the denervated muscles can help maintain tone and prevent contractures. The patient also can massage the muscles to relieve spasms and avoid contractures. As nerve function recovers, exercises can be performed in front of a mirror to aid recovery of muscle function.

Audiovestibular Nerve

Clinical Presentation

Fractures of the Skull Base
Fractures of the temporal bone most commonly result from direct lateral blunt trauma to the skull in the parietal region of the head.[10] Because the otic capsule surrounding the inner ear is very dense bone, the fracture usually courses around it to involve the major foramina in the skull base, the most common being that of the carotid artery and the jugular bulb. Fractures commonly occur near the root of the external auditory canal and run parallel along the petrous apex, extending anteriorly to the foramen lacerum and the carotid artery. They may extend into the temporomandibular joint region.

Longitudinal fractures account for between 70% and 90% of temporal bone fractures. They pass parallel to the anterior margin of the petrous pyramid and usually extend medially from the region of the gasserian ganglion to the middle ear and laterally to the mastoid air cells (Fig. 6.7). Typically, the fracture line transverses the tympanic annulus, lacerating the tympanic membrane and producing a step-like deformity in the external auditory canal. Sensorineural hearing loss and vertigo, characteristic of inner ear concussion, frequently accompany a longitudinal temporal bone fracture, but the bony labyrinth is rarely fractured.[95] Damage to the VIII cranial nerve is infrequent.

Transverse fractures of the temporal bone account for less than 20% of fractures in this region, but they are commonly associated with damage to both cranial nerves VII and VIII. They usually pass through the vestibule of the inner ear, tearing the membranous labyrinth and lacerating the vestibular and cochlear nerve, thus producing complete loss of vestibular and cochlear function. Because the tympanic membrane remains intact, bleeding is usually confined to the middle ear, where it can be seen through the intact membrane. Spinal fluid leakage is common with these injuries, often first detected as clear fluid drains from the eustachian tube into the throat. Meningitis is a late complication of both types of temporal bone fractures.[2]

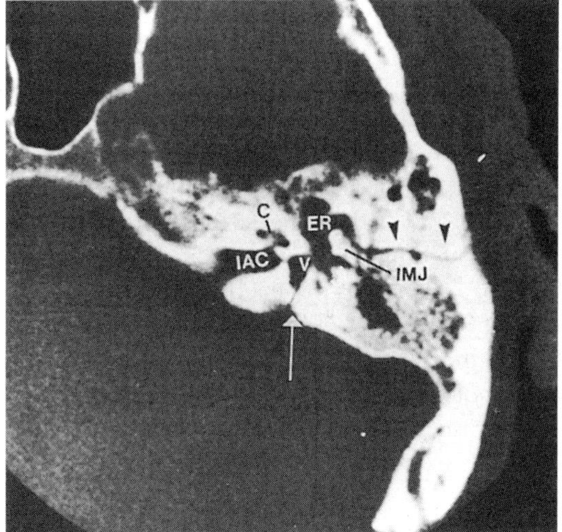

Figure 6.7. Computed tomography scan of the temporal bone showing longitudinal and transverse fractures in the same patient. The longitudinal fracture (black arrowheads) crosses the middle ear, disrupting the ossicular chain, and the transverse fracture (white arrow) enters the vestibule, damaging the membranous labyrinth. C = cochlea, ER = epitympanic recess, IMJ = incudomalleal joint, V = vestibule, IAC = internal auditory canal. (From Baloh RW, Honrubia V: Clinical Neurophysiology of the Vestibular System, 2nd ed. Philadelphia, FA Davis, 1990, p 246, with permission.)

It should be kept in mind that fracture lines can extend in almost any direction across the base of the skull and that multiple fractures are not uncommon (e.g., see Fig. 6.7). A detailed clinical evaluation of all of the structures at the skull base therefore should be conducted to determine the extent of injury.

Labyrinthine Concussion
Auditory and vestibular symptoms (either isolated or in combination) frequently follow blows to the head that do not result in temporal bone fracture. The absence of associated brain stem symptoms and signs and the usual rapid improvement in symptoms following injury support a peripheral localization of the lesion. Although protected by a bony capsule, the delicate labyrinthine membranes

are susceptible to blunt trauma.[96] In most cases, the blow is severe enough to result in associated loss of consciousness.[14]

Sudden deafness following a blow to the head without associated vestibular symptoms is often partially or completely reversible. It is likely caused by intense acoustic stimulation from pressure waves created by the blow, which are transmitted through the bone to the cochlea just as pressure waves are transmitted from air through the conduction mechanism.[40] Supporting this possibility, the pathological changes in the cochlea produced by experimental head blows in animals are similar to those produced by intense airborne sound stimuli.[96] These changes consist of degeneration of hair cells and cochlear neurons in the middle turns of the cochlea. Pure tone hearing loss is usually most pronounced at 4000 to 8000 Hz.

Posttraumatic Positional Vertigo

The most common neurotological sequela of head injury is so-called benign positional vertigo. The patient develops sudden brief attacks of vertigo and nystagmus precipitated by changing the head position such as turning over in bed, getting into and out of bed, bending over and straightening up, and reaching for an object on a high shelf.[5] The attacks of vertigo last for less than a minute, but the patient is left with a more nonspecific dizziness along with nausea and imbalance. Barber[6a] reported positional vertigo with 47% of head injuries associated with longitudinal temporal bone fractures and with 21% of head injuries of comparable severity without skull fracture. Posttraumatic benign positional vertigo is thought to result when calcium carbonate crystals, dislodged from the macula of the utricle, enter the posterior semicircular canal.[9,19,31] The blow to the head dislodges the crystals, which enter the long arm of the posterior semicircular canal when the head is held backward (Fig. 6.8*B*). When the patient sits upright, a clot of the calcium carbonate crystals forms at the most dependent portion of the posterior semicircular canal (Fig. 6.8*A*). Movement of the head back and to the side in the plane of the posterior canal (such as with the standard Dix-Hallpike positional test) will cause the clot to move away from the cupula, producing an ampullofugal displacement of the cupula due to the *plunger* effect of the clot moving within the narrow canal. Fatigability with repeated positional testing is explained by dispersion of the particles from the clot, making the plunger effect less effective. The induced attacks of vertigo and nystagmus are brief in duration since, once the clot reaches its lowest position in the canal with respect to gravity, the cupula returns to its primary position due to its elasticity. The latency before the onset of nystagmus is explained by the delay in setting the clot into motion.

Once the diagnosis of benign positional vertigo is made, a simple explanation of the nature of this disorder and its favorable prognosis can relieve the patient's anxiety. It is important to be aware, however, that although it is a benign disorder, recurrences are common. In our study[5] the episodes of positional vertigo typically occurred in flurries, and more than half of the patients had one exacerbation after an initial remission. The likelihood of a recurrence should be explained to patients so that they are not unduly frightened if it occurs.

Traumatic Perilymph Fistula

With this disorder, limiting membranes of the labyrinth are disrupted, usually at the oval or round windows. A perilymph fistula should be considered in any patient who has an abrupt onset of hearing loss, vertigo, or tinnitus immediately after a blow to the head, particularly if the symptoms fluctuate with time.[80]

The classic presentation of a perilymph fistula is a sudden audible pop in the ear immediately followed by hearing loss, tinnitus, and vertigo. Symptoms may be aggravated by coughing, sneezing, or straining.

Diagnostic Tests

The first step in evaluating a patient who develops dizziness or hearing loss immediately after head trauma is a careful examination of the external auditory canal and the tympanic membrane. Laceration of the tympanic membrane with blood in the external auditory canal is common with a longitudinal fracture of the temporal bone, whereas hemotympanum is often seen with a transverse fracture. With the former, the fracture line traverses the tympanic annulus, producing a step-like deformity in the external auditory canal. Audiometric examination can help document the magnitude of hearing loss and the site of the lesion. Similarly, electronystagmography testing can identify uni-

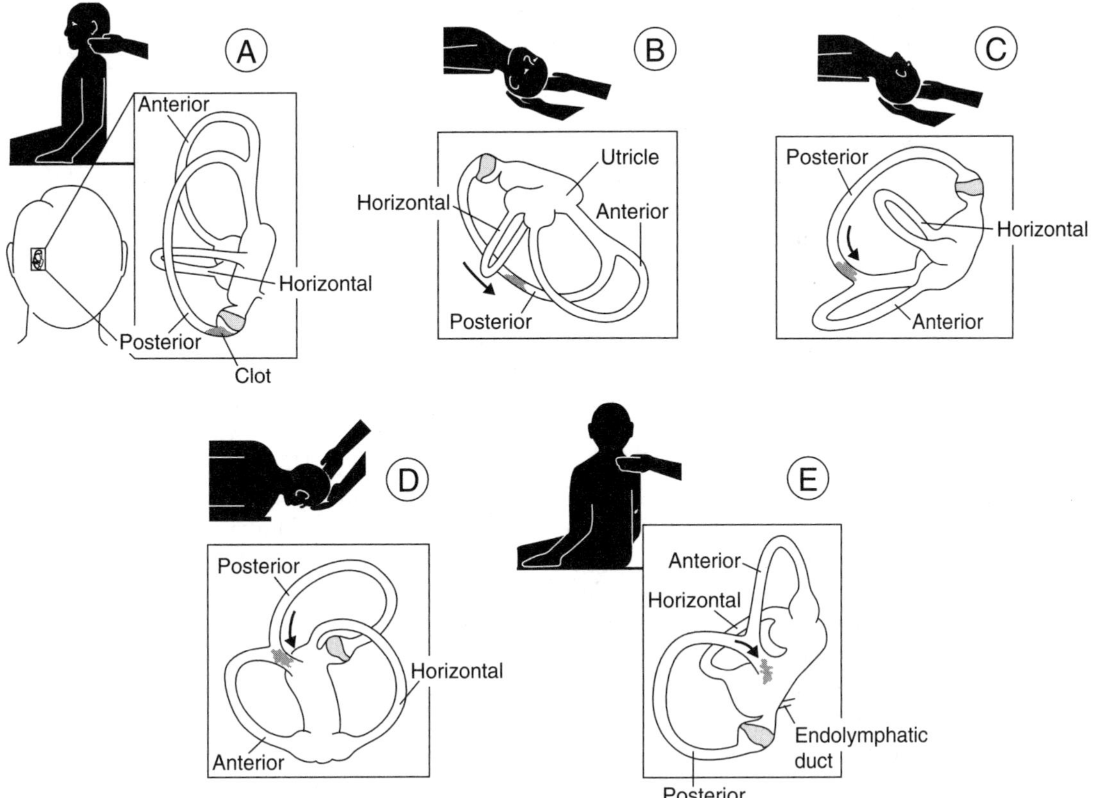

Figure 6.8. Positional maneuver for treating benign positional vertigo. (*A*) The patient is seated, and the clot of calcium carbonate crystals is at the lowermost position in the posterior semicircular canal. (*B*) The patient is moved to the head-hanging position with the abnormal ear down, and the clot begins to move around the posterior canal (arrows). (*C*) The head is then moved across to the opposite head-hanging position, and the clot moves farther along the posterior canal. (*D*) The patient rolls onto his side and the head is rotated toward the ground, and the clot enters the common crus of the posterior and anterior semicircular canals. (*E*) Finally, the patient returns to the sitting position, and the clot falls into the utricle.

lateral peripheral vestibular loss and associated central signs when present.

As with the facial nerve, the radiological procedure of choice for evaluating trauma to the temporal bone and skull base is CT scanning. One often can identify multiple fracture lines spreading throughout the base of the skull.

Treatment

There is no specific treatment for sensorineural hearing loss due to temporal bone trauma unless there is evidence of a perilymph fistula. If conductive hearing loss is identified, surgical intervention may lead to restoration of normal hearing. Separation of the incudostapedial joint, with or without dislocation of the body of the incus from the articulation with the malleus head, is the most common type of ossicular dislocation occurring with temporal bone injury.[36] The surgeon can usually deal with these problems through a transcanal route under local anesthesia using a tympanomeatal flap.

Damage to the vestibular apparatus results in acute symptoms, with gradual improvement as central compensation occurs. Symptomatic treatment of vertigo is helpful initially, and the patient is encouraged to begin vestibular exercises as soon as possible to accelerate the compensation process.[4] Persistent fluctuating vestibular symptoms may indicate the presence of a perilymph fistula and necessitate exploration of the middle ear.

Posttraumatic benign positional vertigo can usually be treated and cured at the bedside by a simple positioning maneuver (see Fig. 6.8).[19,32,35] The maneuver was designed to liberate the calcium carbonate clot from the posterior semicircular canal. The patient is moved around the plane of the posterior semicircular canal so that the clot moves around the canal and out into the utricle (see Fig. 6.8). Once the clot enters the utricle, it presumably becomes attached to the membrane or is cleared through the endolymphatic duct and sac so that it can no longer interfere with the semicircular canal dynamics. The patient is instructed to avoid lying flat for at least 2 days after the maneuver is performed to prevent the clot from reentering the posterior canal orifice. Positioning exercises in which the patient repeatedly moves from a sitting to a head-hanging position and repeatedly induces the positional vertigo and nystagmus also lead to remissions in a large percentage of patients.[8] However, these positional exercises designed to disperse the calcium carbonate crystals are less well tolerated by patients than the single positioning maneuver described above. Occasionally the otolith debris can become trapped in the horizontal or anterior semicircular canals or become attached to the cupula of any of the canals requiring different treatment maneuvers in each case.[3b]

Vagus Nerve

The lower cranial nerves are only occasionally affected by head trauma. In the few reported cases, penetrating neck wounds from bullets or stab wounds are the usual cause.[83] One early study, however, was concerned with the bullfight neck wounds of toreadors.[94] Vagus nerve injuries from blunt trauma are usually associated with occipital condyle or jugular foramen fractures.[33,89] Two patients with unilateral vocal cord and soft palate paralysis were apparent exceptions, without skull base abnormalities.[65] On rare occasions, whiplash hyperextension neck injuries may selectively affect the vagus nerve.[88]

Hypoglossal Nerve

Surgical trauma is a common cause of injury to all of the cranial nerves and may be the most frequent cause of hypoglossal nerve trauma because of the popularity of carotid endarterectomy. In one large study,[77] 16 of 336 (4.8%) endarterectomies were followed by tongue weakness—usually transient. Injuries to the vocal cord (6%) and the facial nerve (2.4%) were also common.

Mitchell[82] reported one of the earliest cases of damage to the hypoglossal nerve caused by a Civil War gunshot wound. World War I provided many examples of unilateral and bilateral tongue paralysis from bullet wounds, and gunshot and knife wounds have continued to be common causes of hypoglossal injury.[1a] At Los Angeles County Hospital, 6 of 45 examples (13%) of extramedullary hypoglossal nerve palsy were the result of gunshot wounds of the neck. Of 78 examples of nerve XII palsy at the Los Angeles County/University of Southern California Medical Center, 11 were due to nonsurgical trauma: 10 from gunshot wounds and 1 associated with blunt trauma in an automobile accident.

Blunt injury of the hypoglossal nerve is rare and usually caused by hyperextension neck injuries, with or without hypoglossal tubercle separation[61] or cervical spine fractures. Bilateral abducens nerve injury is a frequent concomitant of such severe whiplash injuries, and other lower cranial nerves are occasionally involved.[29,79] When the anterior pons is torn or infarcted in hyperextension injuries, a locked-in syndrome may obscure damage to the lower cranial nerves.[51]

Summary

Injury to cranial nerves is a common sequela of blunt head trauma. The olfactory, facial, and audiovestibular nerves are damaged most often, followed by the optic and ocular motor nerves. The trigeminal and lower cranial nerves are rarely involved. Chances of recovery are greatest for the facial nerve, intermediate for the ocular motor nerves, and least likely for the olfactory, optic, and audiovestibular nerves. Treatment is usually symptomatic, although steroids or surgical decompression of the optic and facial nerves can lead to dramatic results in selected patients.

REFERENCES

1a. Alrich EM, Baker GS: Injuries of the hypoglossal nerve: Report of ten cases. Mil Surg 103:20, 1948.
1b. Alberio N, Cultrera F, Antonelli V, Servadei F: Isolated glossopharyngeal and vagus nerves palsy due to frac-

ture involving the left jugular foramen. Acta Neurochir (Wien) 147:791–794, 2005.

2. Applebaum E: Meningitis following trauma to the head and face. JAMA 173:1818, 1960.

3a. Archer DB, Canavan YM: Contusional injuries of the distal optic nerve. Trans Ophthalmol Soc NZ 35:14, 1983.

3b. Aw ST, Todd MJ, Aw GE, et al: Benign positional nystagmus: A study of its three-dimensional spatio-temporal characteristics. Neurology 64:1897–1905, 2005.

4. Baloh RW, Honrubia V: Clinical Neurophysiology of the Vestibular System, 3rd ed. Philadelphia, FA Davis, 2001.

5. Baloh RW, Honrubia V, Jacobson K: Benign positional vertigo: Clinical and oculographic features in 240 cases. Neurology 37:371–378, 1987.

6a. Barber H: Positional nystagmus especially after head injury. Laryngoscope 74:891, 1964.

6b. Bento RF, Pirana S, Sweet R, et al: The role of the middle fossa approach in the management of traumatic facial paralysis. Ear Nose Throat J 83:817–823, 2004.

6c. Borruat FX, Kawasaki A: Optic nerve massaging: an extremely rare cause of self inflicted blindness. Am J Ophthalmol 139:715–716, 2005.

7. Bracken MB, Shepard MJ, Collins WF, et al: A randomized, controlled trial of methylprednisolone or nalozone in the treatment of acute spinal-cord injury. N Engl J Med 322:1405–1411, 1990.

8. Brandt T, Daroff RB: Physical therapy for benign paroxysmal positional vertigo. Arch Otolaryngol 106:484–485, 1980.

9. Brandt T, Steddin S: Current view of the mechanism of benign paroxysmal positional vertigo: Cupulolithiasis or canalithiasis? J Vest Res 3:373–382, 1993.

10. Cannon CR, Jahrsdorfer RA: Temporal bone fractures: Review of 90 cases. Arch Otolaryngol 109:285–288, 1983.

11. Carta A, Ferigno L, Salvo M, et al: Visual prognosis after indirect traumatic optic neuropathy. J Neurol Neurosurg Psychiatry 74:246–248, 2003.

12. Crompton MR: Visual lesions in closed head injury. Brain 93:785, 1970.

13. Cushing H: Surgery of the head. In: Keen WW (ed): Surgery: Its Principles and Practice by Various Authors, Vol 3. Philadelphia, WB Saunders Co, 1908, p 17.

14. Davey LM: Labyrinthine trauma in head injury. Conn Med 29:250, 1965.

15. Davidson M: The indirect traumatic optic atrophies. Am J Ophthalmol 21:7, 1938.

16. Davidson TM, Jalowayski A, Murphy C, et al: Evaluation and treatment of smell dysfunction. West J Med 146:434, 1987.

17. Dobie RA: Tests of facial nerve function. In: Cummings CW et al (eds): Otolaryngology—Head and Neck Surgery. 3rd ed. Vol. 4. St. Louis, CV Mosby, 1998, pp 2757–2766.

18. Edmund J, Godtfredsen E: Unilateral optic atrophy following head injury. Acta Ophthalmol 41:693, 1963.

19. Epley JM: The canalith repositioning procedure: For treatment of benign paroxysmal positional vertigo. Otolaryngol Head Neck Surg 107:399–404, 1992.

20. Exadaktylos AK, Sclabas GM, Muyens M, et al: The clinical correlation of temporal bone fractures and spiral computed tomographic scan: A prospective and consecutive study at a level I trauma center. J Trauma 55:704–706, 2003.

21. Eyster EF, Hoyt WF, Wilson CB: Oculomotor palsy from minor head trauma. JAMA 220:1083, 1972.

22. Fisch U: Facial paralysis in fracture of the petrous bone. Laryngoscope 84:214, 1974.

23. Foerster O: As cited in ref. 25.

24a. Friedman AP, Merritt HH: Damage to cranial nerves resulting from head injury. Bull LA Neurol Soc 9:135, 1944.

24b. Garcia TA, McGetrick BA, Janik JS: Spectrum of ocular injuries in children with major trauma. J Trauma 59:169–174, 2005.

24c. Gerbino R, Ramieri GA, Nasi A: Diagnosis and treatment of retrobulbar hematomas following blunt orbital trauma: a description of eight cases. Int J. Oral Maxillofac Surg 34:172–131, 2005.

25. Gilden DH: Clinical practice. Bell's Palsy. N Engl J Med 351:1323–1331, 2004.

26. Girard BCH, Bouzas EA, Lamas G, Soudant J: Visual improvement after transethmoid-sphenoid decompression in optic nerve injuries. J Clin Neuro-ophthalmol 12:142–148, 1992.

27. Greenwald HS Jr, Keeney AH, Shannon GM: A review of 128 patients with orbital fractures. Am J Ophthalmol 78:655, 1974.

28. Gross CE, DeKock JR, Panje WR, et al: Evidence for orbital deformation that may contribute to monocular blindness following minor frontal head trauma. J Neurosurg 55:963–986, 1981.

29. Grundy DJ, McSweeney T, Jones HWF: Cranial nerve palsies in cervical injuries. Spine 9:339–343, 1984.

30. Gurdjian ES, Webster JE: Head Injuries: Mechanisms, Diagnosis and Management. Toronto, Little, Brown, 1958.

31. Hall SF, Ruby SRF, McClure JA: The mechanics of benign paroxysmal vertigo. J Otolaryngol 8:151–158, 1979.

32. Hara N, Kan S, Simizu K: Localization of post-traumatic trochlear nerve palsy associated with hemorrhage at the subarachnoid space by magnetic resonance imaging. Am J Ophthalmol 32:443–445, 2001.

33. Hashimoto T, Watanabe O, Takase M, et al: Collet-Sicard syndrome after minor head trauma. Neurosurgery 23:367–370, 1988.

34. Heinze J: Cranial nerve avulsion and other neural injuries in road accidents. Med J Aust 2:1246, 1969.

35. Herdman SJ, Tusa RJ, Zee DS, et al: Single treatment approaches to benign paroxysmal positional vertigo. Arch Otolaryngol Head Neck Surg 119:450–454, 1992.

36. Hongli J, Stuart W: Middle ear injuries in skull trauma. Laryngoscope 78:899, 1968.

37. Hooper RS: Orbital complications of head injury. Br J Surg 39:126, 1951.
38. Hughes B: Indirect injuries of the optic nerves and chiasma. Bull Johns Hopkins Hosp 111:98, 1962.
39. Hughes B: The results of injury to special parts of the brain and skull: The cranial nerves. In: Rowbotham GR (ed): Acute Injuries of the Head, Edinburgh, Livingston, 1964, p 410.
40. Igarashi M, Schuknecht H, Myers E: Cochlear pathology in humans with stimulation deafness. J Laryngol 78:115, 1964.
41. Jefferson G, Schorstein J: Injuries of the trigeminal nerve, its ganglion and its divisions. Br J Surg 42:561, 1955.
42. Katzen JT, Jarrahy R, Mathiasen RA, et al: Craniofacial and skull base trauma. J Trauma 54:1026–1034, 2003.
43. Keane JR: Hysterical hemianopia: The 'missing half' field defect. Arch Ophthalmol 97:865, 1979.
44. Keane JR: Posttraumatic intracavernous aneurysm: Epistaxis with monocular blindness preceded by chromatopsia. Arch Ophthalmol 87:701, 1972.
45. Keane JR: Oculomotor palsy with pupillary sparing in subdural hematoma: Two cases with documented tentorial herniation. Mount Sinai J Med 41:161, 1974.
46. Keane JR: Retinal hemorrhage: Its significance in 100 patients with acute encephalopathy of unknown cause. Arch Neurol 36:691, 1979.
47. Keane JR: Blindness following tentorial herniation. Ann Neurol 8:186–190, 1980.
48. Keane JR: Neuro-ophthalmic signs and symptoms of hysteria. Neurology 32:757–762, 1982.
49. Keane JR: Eye signs of head trauma. In: Rose FC (ed): The Eye in General Medicine. London, Chapman and Hall, 1983, pp 276–290.
50. Keane JR: Blindness from self-inflicted gunshot wounds. J Clin Neuro-ophthalmol 6:247–249, 1986.
51. Keane JR: Locked-in syndrome after head and neck trauma. Neurology 36:80–82, 1986.
52. Keane JR: Trochlear nerve pareses with brainstem lesions. J Clin Neuro-ophthalmol 6:242–246, 1986.
53. Keane JR: Bilateral ocular motor signs after tentorial herniation in 25 patients. Arch Neurol 43:806–807, 1986.
54. Keane JR: Traumatic internuclear ophthalmoplegia. J Clin Neuro-ophthalmol 7:165–166, 1987.
55. Keane JR: Neurologic eye signs following motorcycle accidents. Arch Neurol 46:761, 1989.
56. Keane JR: Fourth nerve palsy: Historical review and study of 215 inpatients. Neurology 43:2439–2443, 1993.
57. Keane JR: Ptosis and levator paralysis caused by orbital roof fractures: Three cases with subfrontal epidural hematomas. J Clin Neuro-ophthalmol 13:225–228, 1993.
58. Keane JR: Third-nerve palsy due to penetrating trauma. Neurology 43:1523–1527, 1993.
59. Keane JR: Eye movements in coma. In: Albert DM, Jakobiec W (eds): Principles and Practice of Ophthalmology. Philadelphia, WB Saunders, 1994, pp 2499–2507.
60. Keane JR, Itabashi HH: Locked-in syndrome due to tentorial herniation. Neurology 35:1647–1649, 1985.
61. Kendrick MM, Bredfeldt RC, Sheridan CD: Bilateral injury to the hypoglossal nerve. Arch Phys Med Rehabil 58:578, 1977.
62. Kern RC, Quinn B, Rosseau G, Farbman AI: Post-traumatic olfactory dysfunction. Laryngoscope 110:2106–2109, 2000.
63. King AB, Walsh FB: Trauma to the head with particular reference to the ocular signs. Part 1. Injuries involving the cranial nerves. Am J Ophthalmol 32:191, 1949.
64. Kinney SE: Trauma. In: Cummings CW et al (eds): Otolaryngology—Head and Neck Surgery, vol 4. St. Louis, CV Mosby, 1986, p 3033.
65. Kitanaka C, Sugaya M, Yamada H: Avellis syndrome after minor head trauma: Report of two cases. Surg Neurol 37:236–239, 1992.
66. Kline LB, Morawetz RB, Swaid SN: Indirect injury of the optic nerve. Neurosurgery 14:756–764, 1984.
67. Koren I, Shimonove M, Shvero Y, Feinmesser R: Unusual primary and secondary facial blast injuries. Am J Otolaryngol 24:75–77, 2003.
68. Krauss HR, Yee RD, Foos RY: Autoenucleation. Surv Ophthalmol 29:179, 1984.
69. Kruse JJ, Awasthi D: Skull-base trauma: Neurosurgical perspective. J Craniomaxillofac Trauma 4:8–14, 1998.
70. Larson CH, Adkins WY, Osguthorpe JD: Posttraumatic frontal and frontoethmoid mucoceles causing reversible visual loss. Otolaryngol Head Neck Surg 91:691–694, 1983.
71. Leigh AD: Defects of smell after head injuries. Lancet 1:38, 1943.
72. Lessell S: Indirect optic nerve injury. Arch Ophthalmol 107:382–386, 1989.
73. Levin LA, Beck RW, Jospeh MP, et al: The treatment of traumatic optic neuropathy: The International Optic Nerve Trauma Study. Ophthalmology 106:1268–1277, 1999.
74. Levin LA, Joseph MP, Rizzo JF 3rd, Lessel S: Optic canal decompression in indirect optic nerve trauma. Ophthalmology 101:566–569, 1994.
75. Lindenberg R, Walsh FB, Sacks JG: Neuropathology of Vision: An Atlas. Philadelphia, Lea & Febiger, 1973.
76. Mahapatra AK, Tandon DA: Traumatic optic neuropathy in children: A prospective study. Pediatr Neurosurg 19:34–39, 1993.
77. Maniglia AJ, Han DP: Cranial nerve injuries following carotid endarterectomy: An analysis of 336 procedures. Head Neck 13:121–124, 1991.
78. Martin L, Kaswan R, Chapman W: Four cases of traumatic optic nerve blindness in the horse. Equine Vet J 18:133, 1986.
79. Matthia P, Coudray C, Cornec J, et al: Traumatisme cervical indirect et paralysie des deux dernieres paires craniennes, a propos de deux observations. Rev Otoneuro-ophthalmol 52:43–51, 1980.
80. Mattox DE: Perilymph fistulas. In: Cummings CW et al

(eds): Otolaryngology—Head and Neck Surgery, vol 4. St. Louis, CV Mosby, 1986, p 3113.

81. Mauriello JA, DeLuca J, Krieger A, et al: Management of traumatic optic neuropathy—a study of 23 patients. Br J Ophthalmol 76:349–352, 1992.
82. Mitchell SW: Injuries of the Nerves and Their Consequences. Philadelphia, Lippincott, 1872, p 335.
83. Mohanty SK, Barrios M, Fishbone H, et al: Irreversible injury to cranial nerves 9 though 12 (Collet-Sicard syndrome), case report. J Neurosurg 38:86, 1973.
84. Moore PL, Selby G, Irving RM: Gunshot injuries to the temporal bone. J Laryngol Otol 117:71–74, 2003.
85. Myckatyn TM, Mackinnon SE: The surgical management of facial nerve injury. Clin Plast Surg 30:307–318, 2003.
86a. Rajiniganth MG, Gupta AK, Gupta A, Bapuraj JR: Traumatic optic neuropathy. Arch Otolaryngol Head Neck Surg 129:1203–1206, 2003.
86b. Ratilal BO, Galo SM, Luiz CA: Intrinsic hematoma of the oculomotor nerve: case report and review of the literature. Neurosurgery 57:E370; discussion E370, 2005.
86c. Robert RC, Bacchetti P, Pogrel MA: Frequency of trigeminal nerve injuries following third molar removal. J Oral Maxillofac Surg 63:732–735; discussion 736, 2005.
87. Roberts AH: Severe Accidental Head Injury. London, Macmillan, 1979.
88. Robertson JC, Todd GB, Lobb M: Bilateral vocal cord paralysis due to whiplash injury. Br Med J 288:1876, 1984.
89. Rosa L, Carol M, Bellegarrigue R: Multiple cranial nerve palsies due to a hyperextension injury to the cervical spine. J Neurosurg 61:172–173, 1984.
90. Rush JA, Younge BR: Paralysis of cranial nerves III, IV, and VI; cause and prognosis in 1000 cases. Arch Ophthalmol 99:76–79, 1981.
91. Russell WR: Injury to cranial nerves including the optic nerves and chiasma. In Brock S (ed): Injuries of the Skull, Brain and Spinal Cord, 2nd ed. Baltimore, Williams & Wilkins, 1943, p 104.
92. Sabates NR, Gonce MA, Farris BK: Neuro-ophthalmological findings in closed head trauma. J Clin Neuro-ophthalmol 11:273–277, 1991.
93. Savino PJ, Glaser JS, Schatz NJ: Traumatic chiasmal syndrome. Neurology 30:963–970, 1980.
94. Schoenberg BS, Massey EW: Tapia's syndrome: The erratic evolution of an eponym. Arch Neurol 36:257, 1979.
95. Schuknecht H, Davison R: Deafness and vertigo from head injury. Arch Otolaryngol 63:513, 1956.
96. Schuknecht H, Neff W, Perlman H: An experimental study of auditory damage following blows to the head. Ann Otol Rhinol Laryngol 60:273, 1951.
97. Smith MFW, Goode RL: Eye protection in the paralyzed face. Laryngoscope 89:435, 1979.
98. Steinsapir KD, Goldberg RA: Traumatic optic neuropathy. Surv Ophthalmol 38:487–518, 1994.
99. Summers CG, Wirtshafter JD: Bilateral trigeminal and abducens neuropathies following low-velocity, crushing head injury. J Neurosurg 50:508, 1979.
100. Sumner C: Post-traumatic anosmia. Brain 87:107, 1964.
101. Sumner D: Disturbances of the senses of smell and taste after head injuries. In: Vinken PJ, Bruyn BW (eds): Injuries of the Brain and Skull, part 2 (Handbook of Clinical Neurology, vol 24). Amsterdam, Elsevier, 1976, p 1.
102. Tandon DA, Thakar A, Mahapatra AK, et al: Transethmoidal optic nerve decompression. Clin Otolaryngol 19:98–104, 1944.
103a. Turner JWR: Indirect injuries of the optic nerve. Brain 66:140, 1943.
103b. Ulug T, Ulubil SA: Bilateral traumatic facial paralysis associated with unilateral abducens palsy: a case report. J Laryngol Otol 119144–147, 2005.
104. Yousem DM, Geckle RJ, Bilker WB, et al: Posttraumatic olfactory dysfunction: MR and clinical evaluation. AJNR 17:1171–1179, 1996.
105. Zusho H: Posttraumatic anosmia. Arch Otolaryngol 108:90, 1982.

Chapter 7
Posttraumatic Epilepsy

L. JAMES WILLMORE

Severe head injury results in a sequence of pathophysiological changes in brain that tend to correlate with the severity of injury.[12] Acute traumatic brain injury causes changes in brain metabolism, blood flow, and homeostasis that are a threat to survival. Seizures occur because of the acute injury and are liable to complicate management. Such immediate seizures[50] that occur either acutely or within the first 24 hours of injury may require initiation of treatment at the injury scene or may occur later in the course of treating the injured patient. Phenytoin is an anticonvulsant that is effective in preventing seizures that occur in the period following an acute injury.[93] However, occurrence of a seizure in a head-injured patient requires immediate brain imaging to define a possible cause, including the accumulation of blood within the cranium.

Risks for Development of Epilepsy

The risk of developing of posttraumatic epilepsy (PTE) is related to the severity of injury.[17,106,107] Within the first year after severe head injury, the incidence of seizures exceeds 12 times the population risk for the development of epilepsy.[17,38] Patients with severe head trauma and cortical injury with neurological deficits on physical examination, but with the dura mater remaining intact, have an incidence of epilepsy ranging from 7% to 39%. However, increased severity of trauma, with dural penetration and neurological abnormalities, yields an incidence range of epilepsy of 20% to 57%[4,17] Guidelines identifying patients at risk for late epilepsy (Table 7.1) include factors associated with the severity of neocortical contusion, including the presence of an intracerebral hematoma and the need for surgical repair of a depressed skull fracture.[50]

To improve the prediction of who might be liable to develop PTE,[34] refinement of risk factors was attempted by using a formula with weighted trauma categories. Variables included brain loca-

Table 7.1. Factors Associated with Increased Incidence of Late Epilepsy

Factor	*n*	%
No early epilepsy	29/868	3%
Early epilepsy	59/238	25%*
No hematoma	27/854	3%
Hematoma	45/128	35%*
No depressed fracture	27/832	3%
Depressed fracture	76/447	17%*

*$p < .001$.

Source: Modified from Jennett and Teasdale,[50] with permission.

tion, the agent of injury, severity, complications, and the presence of focal neurological deficits.[34] The highest numeric values of risk were associated with missile wound with dural penetration, central-parietal location, occurrence of an early seizure, and the presence of an intracerebral hematoma. Predictive factors for the risk of epilepsy in the Vietnam Head Injury Survey included cortical involvement, moderate volume of brain tissue loss, intracerebral hematoma, and retained metal fragments.[81] Other studies of patients with PTE showed prolonged posttraumatic amnesia, the presence of a cortical laceration from a depressed skull fracture with dural laceration, and intracerebral hematoma to be predictive.[48,52,91] The risk of developing seizures is increased following hemorrhagic cerebral infarction[24,77] and spontaneous intracerebral hematoma.[33] These facts resulted in the development of a hypothesis by Willmore et al. suggesting that trauma-induced hemorrhage with blood in contact with the neuropil is an important etiological factor in the development of PTE.[1,56,114]

Latency from injury to the development of epilepsy varies, although 57% of patients have onset of seizures within the first year after injury.[81] Whether a seizure occurs immediately after injury, within the first week, or beyond the first week may have prognostic significance for the development of epilepsy.[50] Immediate seizures, occurring within hours after trauma, or a sequence of seizures with development of posttraumatic status epilepticus will complicate management of an injured patient by causing hypoxia, hypertension, and metabolic changes. Although an immediate seizure may be a nonspecific reaction to head trauma, an intracranial hematoma may present this way and must be excluded. An early seizure, occurring during the first week after injury, is associated with increased incidence of late epilepsy.[50]

Closed head injury in the civilian population of such severity to cause hospitalization results in an overincidence of PTE of 4% to 7%.[3,38,50] The incidence of PTE is considerably higher among patients undergoing rehabilitation for head injury.[10,51,82] Patients with penetrating head injury have an epilepsy incidence of 35% to 50%.[5,17–19,81] However, not all factors are understood since trivial head injury has been associated with the development of PTE.[25]

Occurrence of a seizure after head injury is not always predictive for the development of epilepsy, nor does such a complication predict an eventual enduring problem with chronic epilepsy. Between 50% and 65% of patients with a seizure will have that event within 12 months of injury.[19,23,81] Approximately 80% who seize will have done so by 2 years after injury.[102,103] Of interest, approximately 50% of all patients will have a single seizure, without recurrence, while another 25% will have only two or three seizures. Although the risk of recurrence following a single seizure without trauma as the etiology is 30% at 5 years,[46] at least 80% of those with a single seizure will have a second seizure by 2 years after injury, supporting the practice of labeling a patient as having PTE after only one seizure.[38]

Timing of a seizure in relation to head injury provides some predictive information. From 20% to 30% of patients with a seizure within 1 week of injury will have late seizures, that is, beyond 1 week of injury.[49,81,102,105] Such later seizure recurrence seems better correlated with seizure frequency during the first year. While these observations suggest that the overall prognosis is good,[104] intractability becomes a major clinical problem for some patients.

A history of febrile seizures is found as part of the patterns of risk for development of typical mesial temporal sclerosis (MTS) and the clinical problem of complex partial seizures. However head injury, particularly during childhood, is a factor in some cases.[32] The UCLA series[9,61] found head trauma associated in 16% of their cases with MTS. Such an occurrence is not typically dual pathology[16,57] but may represent the consequences of transmitted forces with selective vulnerability of the hippocampus, as has been observed in animals.[59]

Patients with PTE may develop intractable epilepsy. Since such patients are unresponsive to antiepileptic drug therapy, the usual strategy is to evaluate the patient for consideration for resective surgery. The challenge of the monitoring process, and of the accompanying planning for potential resective surgery, is the unpredictable nature of the process of lesion formation following head injury. Head trauma of sufficient intensity to result in the development of PTE causes spatial dispersion of injured cortex in temporal and extratemporal regions.[58] Location of the clinically important regions of injury causing epilepsy may require an intracranial electrode array. Knowledge observers, including family members, must review taped seizures to be sure that the clinical events reflect patient's typical seizures. The patient must understand the success rate of resective surgery and the potential need to pursue further assessment should the initial surgical effort fail.

Prevention and Prophylaxis

Prophylaxis is the process of guarding against the development of a specific disease by an action or treatment that affects its pathogenesis. Prevention renders a process impossible by an advanced provision.[109] One example of prevention is administration of anticonvulsants to patients with severe head trauma to prevent seizures that could cause the complications of hypertension and hypoxia. Such use of antiepileptic medications for patients who are thought to be at risk for tonic-clonic seizures is intended to prevent the complications that are associated with convulsive seizures. Prophylactic use of antiepileptic drugs in patients with head trauma, or for patients undergoing neurosurgical procedures requiring incision of the neocortex, has the intention of interfering with epileptogenesis.[73] Although prevention of acute seizures following head injury is a practical goal,[93] such treatment has not had a prophylactic effect against later development of epilepsy.[8]

Clinical observations indicating the efficacy of antiepileptic drugs as prophylactic against the development of posttraumatic epilepsy appeared within a few years of the availability of phenytoin.[73] Young et al.[117] compared the observed 6% epilepsy occurrence in their treated head-injured patients to historical controls developing posttraumatic seizures. They concluded that early administration of antiepileptic drugs prevented the development of posttraumatic epilepsy, and recommended prophylactic administration of phenytoin to patients with a 15% or greater risk of developing posttraumatic epilepsy.

Rish and Caveness[78] did not detect a difference in early seizure occurrence between phenytoin-treated and untreated patients. However, Wohns and Wyler[116] reviewed patients selected with critical trauma indicators that included depressed skull fracture, dural or cortical laceration, or a prolonged period of posttraumatic amnesia. Although the authors acknowledged selection bias they introduced in their study, they concluded that antiepileptic drug administration prevented the development of posttraumatic epilepsy.

Because the uncontrolled studies suggested that antiepileptic drugs might have a prophylactic effect, prospective, placebo-controlled studies were undertaken (Table 7.2). Penry et al.[70] administered phenytoin and phenobarbital to head-injured patients in a double-blind fashion, with a phenytoin vehicle as the initial placebo control. Seizure probability was 21% in the treated group and 13% in the controls. The lack of significant difference between the treatment and control groups supported the conclusion that anticonvulsant administration had no effect on the development of posttraumatic epilepsy in the treated patients.

Young et al.[118] used a double-blind, prospective study of 179 head-injured patients treated with phenytoin or placebo for 18 months. Eighty-five patients were included in the treated group, and 74 patients were enrolled as placebo controls. Seizures occurred in 12.9% of the treated patients and in 10.8% of the control patients. Temkin et al.[93] reported their experience with 404 patients treated in a prospective fashion. Patients with severe head trauma were assigned to receive an intravenous loading dose of either phenytoin or placebo. Serum levels were measured at regular intervals, blood levels of drug were maintained in the therapeutic range, and efforts were made to ensure that evaluations were blinded. At 1 year, no difference in the incidence of PTE was found between the treatment and control groups. However, the authors did observe that phenytoin was effective in preventing seizures during the acute period immediately after injury. By 2 years, PTE

Table 7.2. Summary of Double-Blind, Placebo-Controlled Prospective Studies of the Efficacy of Antiepileptic Drugs as Prophylaxis of Posttraumatic Epilepsy

		Percent Developing Epilepsy	
Reference	**Drug**	**Control**	**Treated**
Penry et al.[70]	Phenytoin Phenobarbital[118]	13%	23%
Young et al.	Phenytoin	10.8%	12.9%
Temkin et al.[93]	Phenytoin	21.1%	27.5%
Temkin et al.[92]	Valproic acid	15%	24%

Source: From L.J. Willmore: Head trauma and the development of posttraumatic epilepsy. In: Ettinger and Devinsky: Managing epilepsy and co-existing disorders. Butterworth-Heinemann 2002, with permission.

had occurred in 27.5% of phenytoin-treated patients and in 21.1% of controls. Thus, early posttraumatic seizures can be prevented with administration of phenytoin for 1 or 2 weeks, but reduction in seizure occurrence is not associated with reduction of mortality.[45]

Valproic acid had an effect on kindling in animals[83] and was evaluated in humans as well.[92] It was given for 1 month or 6 months, or patients were treated for 1 week with phenytoin as controls; 379 patients were enrolled in this study. Patients were followed for 2 years. Both phenytoin and valproic acid were effective in preventing early seizures, with 1.5% in the phenytoin group and 4.5% in the valproic acid group developing seizures within the first week of injury. Valproic acid failed to prevent the development of posttraumatic seizures, with late seizures developing in 15% of the phenytoin group, 16% in the 1-month valproic acid group, and 24% in the 6-month valproic acid group. A trend toward higher mortality in the long-term valproic acid treatment group was noted; no specific cause was reported.[92]

Mechanisms of Brain Injury

Blunt impact to the head with deformation of the skull causes transmission of a pressure wave through the brain that results in abrupt, and transient cavitation in brain tissue. Mechanical forces propagate a pressure wave through the brain.[58,72] Mechanical forces of head injury cause the brain to accelerate, with induction of rotation and shearing injury to fiber tracts and blood vessels and contusion.[41] Contusion results in hemorrhage that is an admixture of red blood cells, coagulation necrosis, and edema caused by mechanical disruption of blood vessels or by cellular diapedesis. Histopathological studies of material obtained from traumatized brain show formation of axonal retraction balls, reactive gliosis, Wallerian degeneration, and microglial star formation within cystic white matter lesions.[54,94,100] Mechanical effects cause bulk displacement of tissue, with secondary responses that include alterations in cerebral vasomotor regulation, vasospasm, altered cerebral blood flow, changes in intracranial pressure, and altered vascular permeability.[108] Immediate effects include increased extracellular calcium and glutamate from transporter failure and free radical formation. Delayed effects of acute head trauma include focal or diffuse brain edema, ischemia, necrosis, gliosis, and neuronal loss.

Biochemical Effects of Brain Injury

Contusion or cortical laceration causes bleeding followed by hemolysis of red blood cells and deposition of hemoglobin within the neuropil. Iron liberated from hemoglobin and transferrin and deposited as hemosiderin is found within the brains of patients with PTE.[69] Iron is critical to biological functions, but the two stable oxidation states and the redox properties of iron pose a biological hazard. Although oxidation of ferrous iron to ferric iron is a simple reaction yielding insoluble hydroxide complexes, autoxidation reactions in aqueous solution or biological fluids, with or without chelators, causes a complicated series of one-electron transfer reactions yielding free radical intermediates.[1] Addition of iron salts or heme compounds to solutions containing polyunsaturated fatty acids (PUFA) or to suspensions of subcellular organelles results in the formation of highly reactive free radical oxidants, including perferryl ions, superoxide radicals, singlet oxygen, and hydroxyl radicals.[1,36,37,86,111] Although free radical species may form by iron-catalyzed Haber-Weiss reactions,[22,53] these oxidants are also actively generated by iron in biologically chelated forms in heme or with ADP.[6,37]

Free radicals react with methylene groups adjacent to double bonds of PUFA and lipids within cellular membranes, causing hydrogen abstraction and subsequent propagation of peroxidation reactions.[37] This nonenzymatic initiation and propagation of lipid peroxidation causes disruption of membranes of subcellular organelles, degrades deoxyribose and amino acids, and yields diene conjugates and fluorescent chromophores.[7,65,95] Inorganic iron salts, hematin, and hemoproteins stimulate peroxidation of lipids of microsomes and mitochondria, as well as changing cellular thiodisulfide function.[84] Alkyl hydroxyl and peroxyl species of fatty acids propagate until a termination reaction occurs with a membrane constituent capable of electron donation without formation of a free radical. Such constituents include tocopherol, cholesterol, proteins, and the sulfhydryl group of glutathione.[2,6,96,113] Histopathological alterations following injection of aqueous iron into neural tissue can be prevented by pretreatment of animals with alpha-tocopherol and selenium, further supporting the contention that peroxidative reactions are important in trauma-induced brain injury responses.[2,96,112,113]

Cellular Mechanisms of Epileptogenesis

Interictal epileptiform discharges reflect stereotyped cellular patterns of depolarization shift (PDS).[71] Transition from interictal to ictal discharge is characterized by loss of hyperpolarization and by synchronization of neurons in the focus. Amplification of excitatory postsynaptic potentials (EPSP) that underlie the PDS may be produced by mechanisms that include withdrawal of inhibition, frequency potentiation of EPSPs, change in the space constant of the dendrites of the postsynaptic neuron, activation of *N*-methyl-D-aspartate (NMDA) receptors, and potentiation by neuromodulators.[26]

Biochemical injury to neurons may cause a sequence of changes ranging from cellular loss with replacement gliosis to subtle alterations in the neuronal plasma membrane. Membrane changes initiated by biochemical effects of injury may alter the densities and distribution of ion channels on the neuronal membrane. Alteration of membrane ionotophores could affect Na^+ and Ca^{2+} currents, alter thresholds, and lead to progressive depolarization. Intrinsic cellular bursting may also develop with an increase in extracellular K^+ or a reduction of extracellular Ca^{2+}. Development or recruitment of a critical mass of neurons sufficient to cause clinical manifestations requires synchronization of a critical mass of cells.[26,71]

The mechanism or critical physiological changes causing posttraumatic epileptogenesis remains unknown. However, several processes may provide useful areas for investigation. Trauma may cause mechanical shearing of fiber tracts with loss of inhibitory interneurons following anterograde transsynaptic neuronal degeneration.[80] Trauma-induced release of aspartate or glutamate, with attendant activation of NMDA receptors,[31] elaboration of nerve growth factor,[40] or enhancement of reactive gliosis may be operant as well.[66] Assessment of hippocampal tissue obtained during surgical resection for temporal lobe seizures and stained for identification of acetylcholine esterase shows enhancement of staining in the outer portion of the molecular layer of the dentate gyrus.[42] Histochemical staining of rodent kindled hippocampus shows abundant mossy fiber synaptic terminals in the supragranular region and the inner molecular layer of the dentate gyrus.[85] Expression of the immediate early gene proteins c-Fos, c-Jun, and Zif/268 does not appear to be critical to the development of mossy fiber sprouting.[64] Although speculative, synaptic reorganization may increase recurrent excitation in granule cells, favoring epileptogenesis. Experimental foci experience the loss of axosomatic GABAergic terminals, as represented by asymmetric synapses. The GABAergic pericellular basket plexus that provides tonic inhibition was thought to be sensitive to hypoxia, given the implied dependence on aerobic metabolism evidenced by the presence of increased numbers of mitochondria within the altered synapses.[75] Intrinsic membrane changes with enhanced NMDA synaptic conductances suggest a potential mechanism as well.[13]

Genetic and Molecular Factors

Cellular responses to the generation of free radical oxidants following decompartmentalization of hemoglobin- or iron-containing heme compounds may depend upon the induction of protective mechanisms. For example, strains of *Escherichia coli* may be differentiated observing responses to peroxide. Induction of enzymes to repair DNA damage induced by Fenton-derived free radicals appears to be critical for cellular survival.[15,47] Although speculative, sustained membrane changes that are associated with continuing alterations causing focal epileptiform discharges may result from free radical injury to neuronal nuclear or mitochondrial DNA. Differentiation of the susceptibility to develop epilepsy after a given trauma dose may be related to the ability of repair response induction following initiation of lipid peroxidation.

Specific brain genetic factors that cause a liability to the development of PTE remain unknown. A possible genetic predisposition has been observed with the detection of decreased levels of serum haptoglobin in familial epilepsy.[68] Haptoglobins are acute phase glycoproteins in the alpha-1-globulin fraction of serum that form stable complexes with hemoglobin.[43] Since antioxidants such as superoxide dismutase and peroxidases are not found in high concentration in extracellular fluid, containment of factors that initiate oxidation must depend upon binding of reactive metals to carrier proteins, including transferrin, lactoferrin, ceruloplasmin, and haptoglobins.[43] Since one mechanism of protection against induction of oxidant stress is sequestration of free hemoglobin with haptoglobins, identification of impairment in the synthesis of these glycoproteins may identify an inherent susceptibility to the development of epilepsy after head trauma.

Regulation of glutamate may be critical in the process of epileptogenesis. Microdialysis measurements from humans with spontaneous seizures from the hippocampus show transient release of glutamate.[29] Most glutamate is cleared from the extrasynaptic space by the action of high-affinity transporters called *glutamate transporter* (GLAST) and *glial transporter-1* (GLT-1). These proteins are found predominantly in glia.[55,79] Decreasing GLAST and GLT-1 expression would be the result of down-regulation, since the mRNAs of these protein are decreased even though progressive gliosis is a characteristic of the hippocampus from rats who spontaneously seize.[87,88] Down-regulation of GLASTs, with a resultant increase in tissue glutamate concentration, contributes to excitatory synaptic transmission, occurrence of seizures, and neurodegeneration in the hippocampus. Animals with chronic and spontaneous iron-induced amygdalar seizures[99] have been found to have down-regulation of GLAST production as a marker of epileptogenesis.[28,98]

Molecular changes appear to correlate with depolarization-induced elevation of extracellular glutamate levels in the hippocampus, as determined by in vivo microdialysis. A protein called GAT-1 transports GABA. This transporter protein is reported to be responsible for approximately 85% of GABA reuptake.[11] GAT-1 is widely distributed in neurons and astrocytes in hippocampal and limbic regions.[30,63,76] Alterations in GABA uptake may be important to the process of chronic epileptogenesis following head trauma.[97]

Alteration of Brain Injury Responses

Since antiepileptic drugs administered prophylactically fail to inhibit the process of epileptogenesis, are there biochemical strategies that could disrupt brain injury responses associated with the development of epilepsy?

Antiperoxidants may be of value in modulating brain injury responses. Hydroxyl radicals, superoxide radicals, and peroxides generated in biological systems by oxidative chemistry or by actions of heme-containing compounds liberated within lipid systems are quenched by the action of enzymes such as catalase, peroxidase, and superoxide dismutase.[39] Glutathione peroxidase, using glutathione as a cosubstrate and selenium as a metallic cofactor, reduces intracellular formation of hydrogen peroxide and free radicals. Oxidative stress increases the activity of glutathione reductase, glucose-6-phosphate dehydrogenase, and glutathione peroxidase.[67,90] Selenium, a metallic cofactor of glutathione peroxidase, also seems to act synergistically with alpha-tocopherol in preventing peroxidation of structural membrane components.

Alpha-tocopherol prevents peroxidative injury of sulfhydryl groups of glycolipids and glycoproteins, apparently augmenting the antioxidant effects of enzyme systems such as glutathione peroxidase. Tocopherol also prevents peroxidation of unsaturated fatty acids and lipids by reaction of phenolic hydroxyl groups with propagating lipid radicals that were initiated by oxidative carbonyl hydrogen abstraction.[62,74,89,115] Further, the phytyl side chain of tocopherol may intercalate within the acyl chains of polyunsaturated phospholipids, causing lipid membrane stabilization and reduction of membrane permeability.[27,60] Tocopherol may also act as a free radical scavenger and a singlet oxygen quenching agent.[115] A novel nonglucocorticoid 21-aminosteroid with properties inhibiting iron-dependent lipid peroxidation had a salutary effect on concussive injury to mice.[44,110]

Superoxide radicals induce cellular and vasogenic edema.[21,35,101] Initiation of focal edema by cold-induced injury to the cerebral cortex of rodents increases the levels of superoxide radicals.[21] Administration of liposome-entrapped copper-zinc superoxide dismutase interferes with the development of cold-induced edema, suggesting that superoxide dismutase interruption of oxygen free radical–induced fatty acid injury may have potential for interruption of trauma-induced brain injury.[21]

Decisions about how to manage head-injured patients with regard to the development of epilepsy are confounded by the lack of specific information upon which to base recommendations. Using an antiepileptic drug as a prophylactic treatment must be accompanied by informed consent by patients and members of families. Misunderstanding about the intent of treatment with antiepileptic drugs may cause problems with compliance or may leave the impression that discontinuation of such medication

Box 7.1. Rational Guide for Managing Antiepileptic Drug Administration in Patients with Head Injury

1. *High-risk patients*: Patients with severe head injury and a high risk of occurrence of seizures, and in whom the physiological consequences would complicate management, should receive preventive phenytoin treatment. They should be given a loading dose of 18 mg/kg by peripheral vein at a rate not to exceed 25 mg/min. A maintenance dose of 5 mg/kg/day should be given intravenously until oral intake of phenytoin is possible. Avoid simultaneous nasogastric feeding and phenytoin administration. Blood levels should be maintained within the recognized therapeutic range of 10–20 μg/ml. Because an allergic rash may develop in as many as 10% of patients treated in this fashion, regular skin inspection must be performed. If an allergic reaction occurs, then discontinue phenytoin and use parenteral administration of an anticonvulsant drug such as phenobarbital.

2. *Maintenance of preventive treatment*: Phenytoin is effective in preventing seizures for at least 1 month after injury. Maintain therapeutic plasma levels of phenytoin for at least 1 month after injury. At that time, the drug should be tapered over the following 4 weeks. Obtain an electroencephalogram (EEG) prior to drug tapering. Although the EEG is not predictive of the potential for development of epilepsy immediately after injury, the observation of epileptiform patterns on the EEG after injury may be of value in making a decision about whether to continue administration of an anticonvulsant drug.

3. *Discontinuation of treatment*: Patients occasionally are maintained on antiepileptic drugs for 6 months or more after injury. Since long-term treatment is not effective as prophylaxis, early tapering is preferred. If a patient ends up on long-term prophylaxis even without having a seizure, then the patient and the physician face a clinically challenging problem. The patient may be anxious about long-term treatment and may not be willing to risk discontinuing the drug. If the patient agrees to discontinue antiepileptic drug treatment, then special cautions regarding prohibition of driving during the time of drug tapering must be individualized. Realistic discussion of the risk along with EEG assessment, followed by discontinuation over 6 weeks, may be best.

4. *Natural history of PTE*: As with other forms of epilepsy, those patients with few seizures that are easily controlled tend to have the best prognosis. Walker and Erculei[104] observed that 50% of patients identified as having PTE would be in complete remission by 15 years after injury. Assessment and decisions about discontinuation of medication after a long seizure-free interval should be governed by guidelines that apply to any patient who is a candidate for a trial off medication.[14,20]

will render the patient vulnerable to the development of epilepsy. Because long-term prophylaxis with currently available antiepileptic drugs has not been shown to be effective in preventing PTE, the algorithm in Box 7.1 provides a rational guide for the management of these patients.

REFERENCES

1. Aisen P: Some physicochemical aspects of iron metabolism. In: Ciba Foundation Symposium. #51 New York, Elsevier, 1977, pp 1–14.
2. Anderson DK, Means ED: Lipid peroxidation in spinal cord. FeCl2 induction and protection with antioxidants. Neurochem Pathol 1:249–264, 1983.
3. Annegers JF, Grabow JD, Grover RV, Laws ER, Elveback LR, Kurland LT: Seizures after head trauma: A population study. Neurology 30:683–689, 1980.
4. Annegers JF, Hauser WA, Coan SP, Rocca WA: A population-based study of seizures after traumatic brain injuries. N Engl J Med 338:20–24, 1998.
5. Ascroft PB: Traumatic epilepsy after gunshot wounds of the head. Br Med J 1:739–744, 1941.
6. Aust SD, Svingen BA: The role of iron in enzymatic lipid peroxidation. In: Pryor WA (ed): Free Radicals in Biology. New York, Academic Press, 1982, pp 1–28.
7. Baker N, Wilson L: Water-soluble products of UV-irradiated, autoxidized linoleic and linolenic acids. J Lipid Res 7:341–348, 1966.
8. Beghi E: Overview of studies to prevent posttraumatic epilepsy. Epilepsia 44:s21–s26, 2003.
9. Betz P, Eisenmenger W: Traumatic origin of a meningioma? Int J Legal Med 107:326–328, 1995.
10. Bontke CF, Lehmkuhl LD, Englander J, et al: Medical complications and associated injures of patients treated in TBI Model System programs. J Head Trauma Rehabil 8:34–46, 1993.
11. Borden LA, Smith KE, Hartig PR, Branchek TA, Weinshank RL: Molecular heterogeneity of gamma-

aminobutyric acid (GABA) transport system. J Biol Chem 267:21098–21104, 1992.
12. Bruns J, Hauser WA: The epidemiology of traumatic brain injury: A review. Epilepsia 44:s2–s10, 2003.
13. Bush PC, Prince DA, Miller KD: Increased pyramidal excitability and NMDA conductance can explain posttraumatic epileptogenesis without disinhibition: A model. J Neurophysiol 82:1748–1758, 1999.
14. Callaghan N, Garrett A, Goggin T: Withdrawal of anticonvulsant drugs in patients free of seizures for two years. N Engl J Med 318:942–946, 1988.
15. Carlsson J, Carpenter VS: The *recA*[+] gene product is more important than catalase and superoxide dismutase in protecting *Escherichia coli* against hydrogen peroxide toxicity. J Bacteriol 142:319–321, 1980.
16. Cascino GD, Jack CR, Parisi JE, Sharbrough FW, Schreiber CP, Kelly PJ, Trenerry MR: Operative strategy in patients with MRI-identified dual pathology and temporal lobe epilepsy. Epilepsy Res 33:639–644, 1993.
17. Caveness WF: Epilepsy, a product of trauma in our time. Epilepsia 17:207–215, 1976.
18. Caveness WF, Liss HR: Incidence of post-traumatic epilepsy. Epilepsia 2:123–129, 1961.
19. Caveness WF, Meirowsky AM, Rish BL, Mohr JP, Kistler JP, Dillon JD, Weiss GH: The nature of posttraumatic epilepsy. J Neurosurg 50:545–553, 1979.
20. Chadwick D, Reynolds EH: When do epileptic patients need treatment? Starting and stopping medication. Br Med J 290:1885–1888, 1985.
21. Chan PH, Fishman RA: Transient formation of superoxide radicals in polyunsaturated fatty acid–induced brain swelling. J Neurochem 35:1004–1007, 1980.
22. Czapski G, Ilan YA: On the generation of the hydroxylation agent from superoxide radical. Can the Haber-Weiss reaction be the source of OH radicals? Photochem Photobiol 28:651–653, 1978.
23. da Silva AM, Vaz AR, Riberiro I, Melo AR, Nune B, Correia M: Controversies in posttraumatic epilepsy. Acta Neurochir (Wien) 50:48–51, 1990.
24. DeCarolis P, D'Alessandro R, Ferrara R, Andreoli A, Sacquegna T, Lugaresi E: Late seizures in patients with internal carotid and middle cerebral artery occlusive disease following ischaemic events. J Neurol Neurosurg Psychiatry 47:1345–1347, 1984.
25. Devinsky O: Epilepsy after minor head trauma. J Epilepsy 9:94–97, 1996.
26. Dichter MA, Ayala GF: Cellular mechanisms of epilepsy: A status report. Science 237:157–164, 1987.
27. Diplock AT, Lucy JA: The biochemical modes of action of vitamin E and selenium: A hypothesis. FEBS Lett 29:205–210, 1973.
28. Doi T, Ueda Y, Tokumaru J, Mitsuyama Y, Willmore LJ: Sequential changes in glutamate transporter mRNA during Fe^{+++} induced epileptogenesis. Mol Brain Res 75: 105–112, 2000.
29. During MJ, Spencer DD: Extracellular hippocampal glutamate and spontaneous seizure in the conscious human brain. Lancet 341:1607–1610, 1993.
30. Durkin MM, Smith KE, Borden LA, Weinshank RL, Branchek TA, Gustafson EL: Localization of messenger RNAs encoding three GABA transporters in rat brain: An in situ hybridization study. Mol Brain Res 33:7–21, 1995.
31. Faden AI, Demediuk P, Panter SS, Vink R: The role of excitatory amino acids and NMDA receptors in traumatic brain injury. Science 244:798–800, 1989.
32. Falconer MA, Serafetinides EA, Corsellis JAN: Etiology and pathogenesis of temporal lobe epilepsy. Arch Neurol 10:233–248, 1964.
33. Faught E, Peters D, Bartolucci A, Moore L, Miller PC: Seizures after primary intracerebral hemorrhage. Neurology 39:1089–1093, 1989.
34. Feeney DM, Walker AE: The prediction of posttraumatic epilepsy. A mathematical approach. Arch Neurol 36:8–12, 1979.
35. Fishman RA, Chan PH, Lee J, Quan S: Effects of superoxide free radicals on the induction of brain edema. Neurology 29:546, 1979.
36. Fong KL, McCay BP, Poyer JL, Keele BB, Misra H: Evidence that peroxidation of lysosomal membranes is initiated by hydroxyl free radicals produced during flavin enzyme activity. J Biol Chem 248:7792–7797, 1973.
37. Fong KL, McCay PB, Poyer JL, Misra HP, Keele BB: Evidence of superoxide-dependent reduction of Fe^{3+} and its role in enzyme-generated hydroxyl radical formation. Chem-Biol Interactions 15:77–89, 1976.
38. Frey LC: Epidemiology of posttraumatic epilepsy: A critical review. Epilepsia 44:s11–s17, 2003.
39. Fridovich I: Superoxide dismutase. Adv Enzymol 41:35–97, 1974.
40. Gall CM, Isackson PJ: Limbic seizures increase neuronal production of messenger RNA for nerve growth factor. Science 245:758–761, 1989.
41. Gennarelli TA, Thibaulat LE, Adams JH, Graham DI, Thompson CJ, Marcincin RP: Diffuse axonal injury and traumatic coma in the primate. Ann Neurol 12:564–574, 1982.
42. Green RC, Blume HW, Kupferschmid SB, Mesulam M-M: Alterations of hippocampal acetylcholinesterase in human temporal lobe epilepsy. Ann Neurol 26:347–351, 1989.
43. Gutteridge JMC: The antioxidant activity of haptoglobin towards haemoglobin-stimulated lipid peroxidation. Biochim Biophys Acta 917:219–223, 1987.
44. Hall ED, Yonkers PA, McCall JM, Braughler JM: Effects of the 21-aminosteroid U74006F on experimental head injury in mice. J Neurosurg 68:456–461, 1988.
45. Haltiner AM, Newell DW, Temkin NR, Dikmen SS, Winn HR: Side effects and mortality associated with use of phenytoin for early posttraumatic seizure prophylaxis. J Neurosurg 91:588–592, 2000.
46. Hauser WA, Anderson VE, Loewenson RB, McRoberts SM: Seizure recurrence after a first unprovoked seizure. N Engl J Med 307:522–528, 1982.
47. Imlay JA, Linn S: DNA damage and oxygen radical toxicity. Science 240:1302–1309, 1988.

48. Jennett B: Epilepsy and acute traumatic intracranial haematoma. J Neurol Neurosurg Psychiatry 38:378–381, 1975.
49. Jennett WB, Lewin W: Traumatic epilepsy after closed head injuries. J Neurol Neurosurg Psychiatry 23:295–301, 1960.
50. Jennett B, Teasdale G: Management of Head Injuries, Philadelphia, FA Davis, 1981, pp 271–288.
51. Kalisky Z, Morrison P, Meyers CA, Von Laufen AV: Medical problems encountered during rehabilitation of patients with head injury. Arch Phys Med Rehabil 66:25–29, 1985.
52. Kaplan HA: Management of craniocerebral trauma and its relation to subsequent seizures. Epilepsia 2:111–116, 1961.
53. Koppenol WH, Butler J, van Leeuwen JW: The Haber-Weiss cycle. Photochem Photobiol 28:655–660, 1978.
54. Langfitt TW, Weinstein JD, Kassell NF: Vascular factors in head injury. Contribution to brain-swelling and intracranial hypertension. In: Caveness WE, Walker AE (eds): Head Injury. Philadelphia, Lippincott, 1966, pp 172–194.
55. Lehre KP, Levy LM, Ottersen OP, Storm-Mathisen J, Danbolt NC: Differential expression of two glial glutamate transporters in the rat brain: Quantitative and immunocytochemcial observations. J Neurosci 15:1835–1853, 1995.
56. Levitt P, Wilson WP, Wilkins RH: The effects of subarachnoid blood on the electrocorticogram of the cat. J Neurosurg 35:185–191, 1971.
57. Li LM, Cendes F, Watson C, Andermann F, Fish DR, Dubeau F, Free S, Olivier A, Harkness W, Thomas DGT, Duncan JS, Sander JWAS, Shorvon SD, Cook MJ, Arnold DL: Surgical treatment of patients with single and dual pathology: Relevance of lesion and of hippocampal atrophy to seizure outcome. Neurology 48:437–444, 1997.
58. Lingren SO: Experimental studies of mechanical effects in head injury. Acta Chir Scand 132(suppl 360):1–32, 1966.
59. Lowenstein DH, Thomas MJ, Smith DH, McIntosh TK: Selective vulnerability of dentate hilar neurons following traumatic brain injury: A potential mechanistic link between head trauma and disorders of the hippocampus. J Neurosci 12:4846–4853, 1992.
60. Lucy JA: Functional and structural aspects of biological membranes: A suggested structural role for vitamin E in the control of membrane permeability and stability. Ann NY Acad Sci 203:4–11, 1972.
61. Mathern GW, Babb TL, Armstrong DL: Hippocampal sclerosis. In: Engel J Jr, Pedley TA (eds): Epilepsy: A Comprehensive Textbook. Philadelphia, Lippincott-Raven, 1997, pp 133–155.
62. McCay PB, King MM: Vitamin E: Its role as a biological free radical scavenger and its relationship to the microsomal mixed-function oxidase system. In: Machlin LJ (ed): Vitamin E. New York, Marcel Dekker, 1980, pp 289–317.
63. Minelli A, Brecha NC, Karschin C, DeBiasi S, Conti F: GAT-1, a high affinity GABA plasma membrane transporter, is localized to neurons and astroglia in the cerebral cortex. J Neurosci 15:7734–7746, 1995.
64. Nahm WK, Noebels JL: Nonobligate role of early or sustained expression of immediate-early gene proteins c-Fos, c-Jun, and Zif/268 in hippocampal mossy fiber sprouting. J Neurosci 18:9245–9255, 1998.
65. Niehaus WG, Samuelsson B: Formation of malonaldehyde from phospholipid arachidonate during microsomal lipid peroxidation. Eur J Biochem 6:126–130, 1968.
66. Nieto-Sampedro M: Astrocyte mitogen inhibitor related to epidermal growth factor receptor. Science 240:1784–1786, 1988.
67. Orlowski M, Karkowsky A: Glutathione metabolism and some possible functions of glutathione in the nervous system. Int Rev Neurobiol 19:75–121, 1976.
68. Panter SS, Sadrzadeh SM, Hallaway PE, Haines J, Anderson VE, Eaton JW: Hypohaptoglobinemia associated with familial epilepsy. J Exp Med 161:748–754, 1985.
69. Payan H, Toga M, Berard-Badier M: The pathology of post-traumatic epilepsies. Epilepsia 11:81–94, 1970.
70. Penry JK, White BG, Brackett CE: A controlled prospective study of the pharmacologic prophylaxis of posttraumatic epilepsy. Neurology 29:600–601, 1979.
71. Prince DA, Connors BW: Mechanisms of epileptogenesis in cortical structures. Ann Neurol 16(suppl):s59–s64, 1984.
72. Pudenz RH, Shelden CH: The lucite calvarium-a method for direct observation of the brain. J Neurosurg 3:487–505, 1946.
73. Rapport RL, Penry JK: Pharmacologic prophylaxis of post-traumatic epilepsy: A review. Epilepsia 13:295–304, 1972.
74. Rehncrona S, Smith DS, Akesson B, Westerberg E, Siesjo BK: Peroxidative changes in brain cortical fatty acids and phospholipids, as characterized during Fe^{2+}- and ascorbic acid–stimulated lipid peroxidation in vitro. J Neurochem 34:1630–1638, 1980.
75. Ribak CE, Harris AB, Vaughn JE, Roberts E: Inhibitory GABAergic nerve terminals decrease at sites of focal epilepsy. Science 205:211–214, 1979.
76. Ribak CE, Tong WMY, Brecha NC: GABA plasma membrane transporters, GAT-1 and GAT-2, display different distributions in the rat hippocampus. J Comp Neurol 367:595–606, 1996.
77. Richardson EP, Dodge PR: Epilepsy in cerebrovascular disease. Epilepsia 3(series 3):49–74, 1954.
78. Rish BL, Caveness WF: Relation of prophylactic medication to the occurrrence of early seizures following craniocerebral trauma. J Neurosurg 38:155–158, 1973.
79. Rothstein JD, Dykes-Hoberg M, Pardo CA, Bristol LA, Jin L, Kuncl RW, Kanai Y, Hediger MA, Wang Y, Schielke JP, Welty DF: Knockout of glutamate transporters reveals a major role for astroglial transport in excitotoxicity and clearance of glutamate. Neuron 16:675–686, 1996.
80. Saji M, Reis DJ: Delayed transneuronal death of substantia nigra neurons prevented by gamma-aminobutyric acid agonist. Science 235:66–69, 1987.

81. Salazar AM, Jabbari B, Vance SC, Grafman J, Amin D, Dillon JD: Epilepsy after penetrating head injury. I. Clinical correlates: A report of the Vietnam Head Injury Study. Neurology 35:1406–1414, 1985.
82. Sazbon L, Groswasser Z: Outcome in 134 patients with prolonged posttraumatic unawareness. Part 1: Parameters determining late recovery of consciousness. J Neurosurg 72:75–80, 1990.
83. Silver JM, Shin C, McNamara JO: Antiepileptogenic effects of conventional anticonvulsants in the kindling model of epilespy. Ann Neurol 29:356–363, 1991.
84. Smith GJ, Dunkley WL: Initiation of lipid peroxidation by a reduced metal ion. Arch Biochem Biophys 98:46–48, 1962.
85. Sutula T, Cascino G, Cavazos J, Parada I, Ramirez L: Mossy fiber synaptic reorganization in the epileptic human temporal lobe. Ann Neurol 26:321–330, 1989.
86. Svingen BA, O'Neal FO, Aust SD: The role of superoxide and singlet oxygen in lipid peroxidation. Photochem Photobiol 28:803–809, 1978.
87. Tanaka S, Kondo S, Tanaka T, Yonemasu Y: Long-term observation of rats after unilateral intra-amygdaloid injection of kainic acid. Brain Res 463:163–167, 1988.
88. Tanaka T, Tanaka S, Fujita T, Takano K, Fukida H, Sako K, Yonemasu Y: Experimental complex partial seizures induced by a microinjection of kainic acid into limbic structures. Prog Neurobiol 38:317–334, 1992.
89. Tappel AL: Vitamin E and free radical peroxidation of lipids. Ann NY Acad Sci 203:12–28, 1972.
90. Tappel AL: Lipid peroxidation damage to cell components. Fed Proc 32:1870–1874, 1973.
91. Temkin NR: Risk factors for posttraumatic seizures in adults. Epilepsia 44:s18–s20, 2003.
92. Temkin NR, Dikmen SS, Anderson GD, Wilensky AJ, Holmes MD, Cohen W, Newell DW, Nelson P, Awan A, Winn HR: Valproate therapy for prevention of posttraumatic seizures: A randomized trial. J Neurosurg 91: 593–600, 1999.
93. Temkin NR, Dikmen SS, Wilensky AJ, Keihm J, Chabal S, Winn HR: A randomized, double-blind study of phenytoin for the prevention of post-traumatic seizures. N Engl J Med 323:497–502, 1990.
94. Tornheim PA, Liwnicz BH, Hirsch CS, Brown DL, McLaurin RL: Acute responses to blunt head trauma. J Neurosurg 59:431–438, 1983.
95. Triggs WJ, Willmore LJ: In vivo lipid peroxidation in rat brain following intracortical Fe^{2++} injection. J Neurochem 42:976–980, 1984.
96. Triggs WJ, Willmore LJ: Effect of [dl]-a-tocopherol on $FeCl_2$-induced lipid peroxidation in rat amygdala. Neurosci Lett 180:33–36, 1994.
97. Ueda Y, Willmore LJ: Hippocampal gamma-aminobutyric acid transporter alterations following focal epileptogenesis induced in rat amygdala. Brain Research Bulletin 52:357–361, 2000.
98. Ueda Y, Willmore LJ: Sequential changes in glutamate transporter protein levels during Fe^{+++} induced epileptogenesis. Epilepsy Res 39:201–219, 2000.
99. Ueda Y, Willmore LJ, Triggs WJ: Amygdalar injection of $FeCl_3$ causes spontaneous recurrent seizures. Exp Neurol 153:123–127, 1998.
100. Unterharnscheidt F, Sellier K: Mechanisms and pathomorphology of closed head injuries. In: Caveness WF, Walker AE (eds): Head Injury. Philadelphia, Lippincott, 1966, pp 321–341.
101. Wagner FC, Stewart WB: Effect of trauma dose on spinal cord edema. J Neurosurg 54:8802–8806, 1981.
102. Walker AE: Posttraumatic epilepsy in World War II veterans. Surg Neurol 32:235–236, 1989.
103. Walker AE, Blumer D: The fate of World War II veterans with posttraumatic seizures. Arch Neurol 46:23–26, 1989.
104. Walker AE, Erculei F: Posttraumatic epilepsy 15 years later. Epilepsia 11:17–26, 1970.
105. Walker AE, Jablon S: A follow-up of head injured men of World War II. J Neurosurg 16:600–610, 1959.
106. Weiss GH, Feeney DM, Caveness WF, Dillon D, Kistler JP, Mohr JP: Prognostic factors for the occurrence of posttraumatic epilepsy. Arch Neurol 40:7–10, 1983.
107. Weiss GH, Salazar AM, Vance SC, Grafman JH, Jabbari B: Predicting posttraumatic epilepsy in penetrating head injury. Arch Neurol 43:771–773, 1986.
108. Willmore LJ: Posttraumatic epilepsy: Cellular mechanisms and implications for treatment. Epilepsia 31(suppl. 3):s67–s73, 1990.
109. Willmore LJ: Prophylactic use of anticonvulsant drugs. In: Resor SR, Kutt H (eds): Medical Treatment of Epilepsy. New York, Marcel Dekker, 1992, pp 73–77.
110. Willmore LJ: Post-traumatic epilepsy: Mechanisms and prevention [review]. Psychiatry Clin Neurosci 49:s171–s173, 1995.
111. Willmore LJ, Hiramatsu M, Kochi H, Mori A: Formation of superoxide radicals, lipid peroxides and edema after $FeCl_3$ injection into rat isocortex. Brain Res 277: 393–396, 1983.
112. Willmore LJ, Rubin JJ: Antiperoxidant pretreatment and iron-induced epileptiform discharge in the rat: EEG and histopathologic study. Neurology 31:63–69, 1981.
113. Willmore LJ, Rubin JJ: Effects of antiperoxidants on $FeCl_2$-induced lipid peroxidation and focal edema in rat brain. Exp Neurol 83:62–70, 1984.
114. Willmore LJ, Sypert GW, Munson JB: Recurrent seizures induced by cortical iron injection: A model of posttraumatic epilepsy. Ann Neurol 4:329–336, 1978.
115. Witting LA: Vitamin E and lipid antioxidants in free-radical-initiated reactions. In: Pryor WA (ed): Free Radicals in Biology, vol. 4. New York, Academic Press, 1980, pp 295–319.
116. Wohns RNW, Wyler AR: Prophylactic phenytoin in severe head injuries. J Neurosurg 51:507–509, 1979.
117. Young B, Rapp R, Brooks WH, Madauss W, Norton JA: Post-traumatic epilepsy prophylaxis. Epilepsia 20:671–681, 1979.
118. Young B, Rapp RP, Norton JA, Haack D, Tibbs PA, Bean JR: Failure of prophylactically administered phenytoin to prevent late post-traumatic seizures. J Neurosurg 58:236–241, 1983.

Chapter 8
Traumatic Intracranial Hemorrhage

JOSHUA M. AMMERMAN,
S. TAYLOR JARELL, AND
RICHARD S. POLIN

In the United States, the direct and indirect costs of care for individuals suffering a traumatic brain injury (TBI) are estimated at more than $56 billion annually.[49] The overall impact is even more substantial when one considers that the majority of severe head injuries occur in adolescents and young adults.

Following head trauma, the spectrum of TBI ranges from concussion to diffuse axonal injury with irreversible coma. Within this spectrum lie the patients with traumatic intracranial hemorrhages (TIH).

When the results from the Traumatic Coma Data Bank are reviewed, it becomes apparent that intracranial mass lesions represent the predominant diagnosis. Twenty percent of mass lesions evacuated were acute subdural hematomas, 14% were traumatic intracerebral hemorrhages or contusions, and 5% were epidural hematomas. Of note, the overall mortality rate for trauma craniotomies approached 40%.[30,31]

In this chapter, five varieties of TIH are discussed based on their location within the intracranial compartment: traumatic subarachnoid hemorrhage, acute subdural hematoma, chronic subdural hematoma, acute epidural hematoma, and traumatic intracerebral hemorrhage or contusion. The clinical presentation, pathophysiology, radiographic characteristics, management, and outcome will be discussed for each, as well as the general medical management of TIH.

Traumatic Subarachnoid Hemorrhage

Head trauma is by far the most common etiology for subarachnoid hemorrhage (SAH). These hemorrhages result from the disruption of small pia-arachnoid vessels within the subarachnoid space that are sheared at the time of impact.[9] The anatomic distribution of these hemorrhages is primarily within the basal cisterns and over the convexity of the brain. When patients with severe TBI are screened with computed tomographic (CT) scanning, 50% to 60% demonstrate traumatic SAH at initial assessment.[28]

In isolation, traumatic SAH generally follows a benign course. Patients usually complain of headache and other mild postconcussive symptoms. Deterioration in neurological status is exceedingly rare in this patient population. General medical management for this condition is based on that of associated intracranial mass lesions, which frequently accompany severe closed head injury.

Radiographic assessment for traumatic SAH is best performed via noncontrast CT scanning. Subarachnoid hemorrhage appears as a hyperdensity filling normal cerebrospinal fluid (CSF) spaces. Contrast administration should be avoided, as it tends to highlight the intracranial vasculature, making the detection of the hyperdense acute SAH difficult. Repeated CT scanning for patients with isolated traumatic SAH is rarely indicated.

An important issue to be considered when caring for patients with traumatic SAH is whether or not the SAH resulted from head trauma or the head trauma resulted from loss of consciousness secondary to a spontaneous SAH. In patients with a questionable history for primary head injury or SAH in an atypical location, cerebrovascular imaging is indicated to rule out a primary vascular lesion. With the recent advent of high-quality CT angiography, this screening can be performed without the added morbidity of a conventional cerebral angiogram.[5]

Much like sufferers of aneurysmal SAH, up to 20% of patients with severe TBI and traumatic SAH may develop symptomatic cerebral vasospasm.[22,47] Treatment of this vasospasm following traumatic SAH is similar to that for aneurysmal SAH, including hypertensive, hypervolemic therapy, papaverine, and possibly calcium channel blocking medications.[3]

In addition to inducing vasospasm, traumatic SAH may occasionally lead to the development of hydrocephalus. This results from clogging of the arachnoid villi with blood degradation products and a subsequent reduction in CSF absorption. In the majority of cases, this hydrocephalus is transient; however, a small number of patients may require either temporary ventriculostomy or permanent CSF diversion via shunting.[4]

Aside from its roles in posttraumatic vasospasm and hydrocephalus, traumatic SAH is felt to serve as a prognostic marker for a poorer patient outcome and more severe CT findings.[32] In a large head injury series, up to 41% of patients without traumatic SAH achieved a good recovery compared to only 15% of patients with traumatic SAH. This poor overall outcome is likely a feature of the associated intracranial mass lesions and brain stem shear injury seen in patients with severe TBI.[43]

Acute Subdural Hematoma

Hematoma formation within the subdural space, a potential space, is generally the result of rupture of the veins bridging the cortical surface and the sagittal sinus following significant craniocerebral trauma. Other sites for the origin of acute subdural hematoma (aSDH) have been reported, including cortical arterial hemorrhage and venous sinus laceration.[10,14] Additional risk factors for the development of aSDH include alcohol use, liver disease, pharmacological anticoagulation, and increasing age. Of note, hemorrhage within the subdural space can travel freely and may frequently cover an entire hemisphere. This is in contrast to extradural hematomas, which are generally bounded by dural-calvarial attachments.

Acute subdural hematomas are often large enough to act as mass lesions and occur at rates as high at 63% in nonmissile cranial injuries.[13] Given the significant kinetic energy required to generate an aSDH, an underlying parenchymal injury is a frequent associated finding.[15] These injuries may include contusion, venous infarction, and/or diffuse axonal injury and carry mortality rates ranging from 50% to 90%.[18] In trauma victims suffering an aSDH, over 50% are rendered unconscious at the time of injury and up to 75% lose consciousness at some point during their initial evaluation.[45]

Computed tomography scanning is the optimal modality for assessing an aSDH. The classical appearance of an aSDH is a crescent-shaped hyperdensity between the inner table of the skull and the brain parenchyma (Fig. 8.1). These hematomas are most commonly found on the surface of the brain but may also form in the interhemispheric space or along the tentorium.[24]

In deciding whether surgical evacuation of an aSDH is indicated, the critical factors are the patient's neurological status, the radiographic appearance, and the extent of parenchymal injury. There is little debate regarding surgical intervention for a rapidly deteriorating patient harboring an expanding intracranial hematoma with significant mass effect. As a rule, all acute traumatic extra-axial hematomas 10 mm thick or more should undergo exploration and evacuation. For less clear situations controversy remains, but several reasonable guidelines exist. An extra-axial hematoma over 5 mm thick with an equivalent midline shift in a patient with a Glasgow Coma Scale (GCS) score

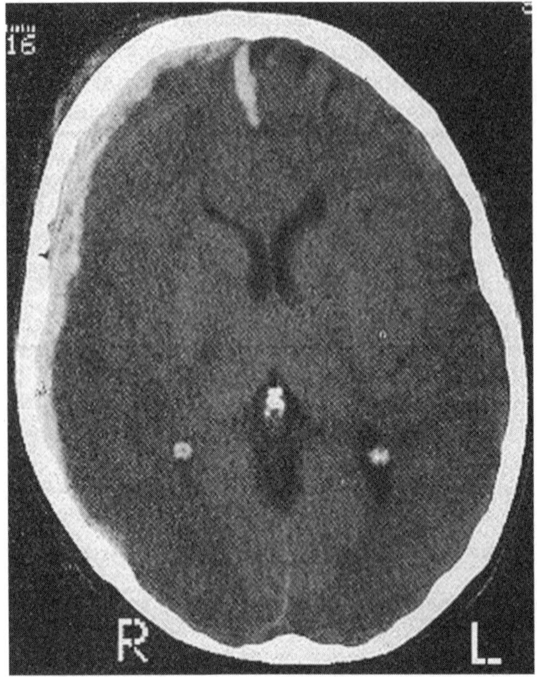

Figure 8.1. Noncontrast computed tomography scan demonstrating a right acute subdural hematoma with interhemispheric extension.

of 8 or less should undergo urgent evacuation. However, operative decompression of a thin rim SDH, associated with significant brain swelling and midline shift, is unlikely to improve the patient's condition.[33] For these patients, medical management alone or, alternatively, more aggressive decompressive procedures should be considered.

Another somewhat controversial group of patients are those with an aSDH 5 to 10 mm thick with a GCS of 9 to 13. Urgent surgical management is warranted in all patients with a deteriorating level of consciousness, pupillary abnormalities, or hemiparesis or when CT scanning reveals a hematoma in the temporal fossa exerting mass effect. Patients who can be managed in the intensive care unit (ICU) include those who have a stable or improving level of consciousness, absence of focal neurological findings, and normal basilar cisterns on CT without an appreciable midline shift. Any deterioration warrants an urgent repeat CT scan.[1]

Another subset of patients who should be considered for conservative management are those with an interhemispheric aSDH without a significant neurological deficit. A conservative course may be warranted given the risks of operating on a potentially bleeding sagittal venous sinus.

The outcome following traumatic aSDH has been carefully studied over time. Among the prognostic variables, the time to definitive therapy remains a strong predictive marker. In a series of 82 patients with aSDH, those who underwent hematoma evacuation within 4 hours of injury had a 30% mortality rate versus a 90% mortality rate if evacuation was delayed beyond 4 hours.[42] Age also appears to play a significant role in the outcome following aSDH. Approximately 40% of patients under age 35 remain persistently vegetative or die following a traumatic aSDH compared to 80% of those aged 55 or more.[19]

Mortality in patients sustaining a traumatic aSDH with evidence of brain stem herniation has also been evaluated. Functional recovery to a moderate level of disability was seen in only 25% of patients, with a 64% mortality at 1 year. The mortality of patients with bilateral loss of pupillary reactivity for 6 hours or more approached 100%.[41]

Chronic Subdural Hematoma

Chronic subdural hematoma (cSDH) is primarily a disease of the elderly. As individuals age, their brains undergo normal atrophy and shrinkage. This shrinkage causes the brain to move away from the inner surface of the dura and places the veins bridging the cortical surface and sagittal sinus on stretch. Thus, even minor head trauma may cause rupture of these vessels.

Slow bleeding from this low-pressure venous system can enable large hematomas to form before clinical signs become apparent. In patients who have sustained a head injury, 25% become symptomatic within 1–4 weeks. Another 25% experience symptoms between 5 and 12 weeks before coming to medical attention. Only 33% of patients fail to have an asymptomatic period.

Small SDHs may resorb spontaneously. Larger cSDHs can organize and form vascularized membranes. Repeated bleeding from small, friable vessels in these membranes may account for the slow expansion of CSDHs.[37]

In patients with cSDH, blood flow to the deep gray structures appears to be particularly affected compared to that to the rest of the brain. Tanaka et al.[46] suggested that impaired thalamic function might lead to a spreading depression that impairs cortical activity. They found that a 7% decrease in cerebral blood flow (CBF) was associated with headache, whereas a 35% decrease was associated with focal deficits such as hemiparesis.

Given that the pathophysiology of cSDH is often associated directly with cerebral volume loss, it is not surprising that cSDH is seen in association with conditions that cause cerebral atrophy such as alcoholism and dementia. In a single series, alcoholics constituted over 50% of the patient population with cSDH.[12] Other associated factors include coagulopathy, seizure disorder, and CSF shunts. Thus, careful attention must be paid to coagulation profiles and platelet studies when managing patients with cSDH. Rapid correction of deficiencies in blood clotting in this patient population is mandatory.

The radiographic diagnosis of cSDH is best made on noncontrast CT scans. As has been previously stated, acute blood appears hyperdense on CT scan, progressing to isodense and then hypodense over a few weeks (Fig. 8.2). Chronic subdural hematomas are thus arbitrarily defined as hematomas presenting 21 days or more after injury. In the pre-CT era, failure to diagnosis was frequent in the setting of cSDH. A history of antecedent head injury was absent in 25% to 50% of patients in most series. Common misdiagnoses include dementia, stroke, transient ischemic attack, tumor, and meningoencephalitis. Of note, cSDHs may occur bilaterally in up to 20% of patients.[40]

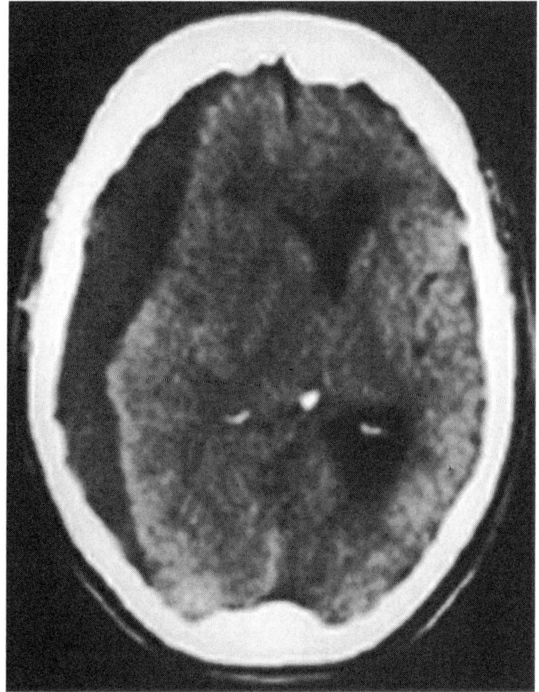

Figure 8.2. Noncontrast computed tomography scan demonstrating a right chronic subdural hematoma with midline shift.

Headache is the most common presenting feature, occurring in up to 90% of cases. Other common symptoms include confusion, weakness, seizures, and incontinence. Hemiparesis and a decreased level of consciousness are the most common neurological signs, occurring in approximately 58% and 40%, respectively. Gait dysfunction is another common finding. When the signs of cSDH are compared across age groups, somnolence, confusion, and memory loss are significantly more common in elderly patients. Signs of increased intracranial pressure, such as headache and vomiting, are more likely to be seen in the younger patient population.

Symptomatic cSDH should be evacuated. However, the optimal surgical approach remains in debate. Williams et al.[50] examined the outcome of 62 patients with cSDH treated with either burr hole drainage or twist drill craniostomy. They found that 64% of twist drill patients required repeated evacuations compared with 11% of those with burr holes only and 7% of those with burr-holes plus drainage. Formal craniotomy is another valid option. However, burr hole drainage and twist drill craniostomy can be performed under local anesthesia. Removal of the hematoma, by whichever means, classically reveals a thin liquid resembling old motor oil.

Many physicians treating patients with cSDH feel that patients should be kept flat in bed for a period of time to help promote brain reexpansion. However, a prospective, randomized study of 46 patients with cSDH failed to show a statistically significant difference in patients kept flat for 3 days postoperatively versus those assuming a sitting position on the day of operation.[38] A lower rate of repeat surgery has also been observed in patients who underwent subdural drain placement, regardless of whether there was visible evidence of brain reexpansion on CT scan.[23] Postoperative CT scans often show a residual subdural fluid collection that may be left alone unless it continues to exert significant mass effect.

The functional outcome following treatment for cSDH is fairly good. In a review of 500 consecutive patients treated for cSDH, 89% had good recovery, 8% showed no change, and 2% worsened. Hematoma recurrence was noted in 10% of patients at 1 to 8 weeks after the first operation. Advanced age, preexisting cerebral infarction, and persistence of subdural air after surgery were significantly correlated with poor brain reexpansion postoperatively.[34]

Acute Epidural Hematoma

Acute epidural hematomas (aEDH) are not infrequent sequelae of severe closed head injury. While potentially devastating, aEDHs remain among the most treatable traumatic intracranial mass lesions.

Acute epidural hematomas result from stripping of the periosteal dural layer away from the inner table of the skull by an expanding collection of blood. The source of these hematomas may be bleeding bone edges or lacerated venous sinuses, but most of them usually result from a torn meningeal vessel.[2] The middle meningeal artery runs in a groove within the squamous portion of the temporal bone. Fractures across this thin bone result in laceration of this vessel and formation of a hematoma adjacent to the temporal fossa.

The clinical presentation of traumatic aEDHs has been subject to much debate. The classic description is that of a patient initially rendered unconscious by a blow, followed by neurological recovery and then rapid deterioration with signs of brain stem herniation. In reality, this *lucid interval* likely occurs in only a small percentage of cases and should not be considered the hallmark of traumatic aEDH.[25]

The imaging study of choice for the diagnosis of aEDH, like that of most traumatic intracranial lesions, is noncontrast CT scanning. The classic appearance of an aEDH is a lenticular or biconvex hyperdense lesion bounded by dural margins (Fig. 8.3). It should be noted that following an initially negative CT scan, up to 12% of patients can develop a delayed aEDH.[21]

The management of traumatic aEDH demands an aggressive surgical approach given the potential for rapid neurological decline and the excellent results of surgical intervention. Any patient with a depressed level of consciousness or signs of impending brain stem herniation should undergo emergent craniotomy and hematoma evacuation. Observation should be reserved for patients with small hematomas and good neurological function. They should be screened with serial CT scans at regular intervals, and any change in neurological exam or hematoma enlargement should prompt surgical evacuation.[6]

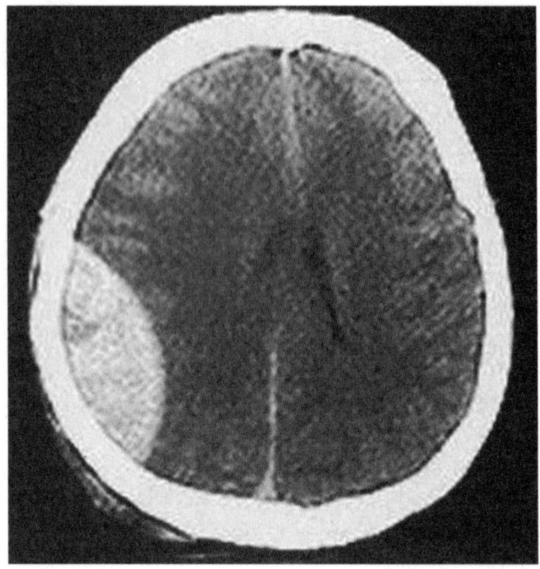

Figure 8.3. Noncontrast computed tomography scan demonstrating a right acute epidural hematoma.

Acute epidural hematomas of the posterior fossa is quite rare but nonetheless merits discussion. Given the small, already crowded posterior fossa, addition of even a small amount of hematoma can have disastrous consequences. Compression of the posterior fossa contents and collapse of the fourth ventricle may lead to obstructive hydrocephalus in severe cases. Not surprisingly, the morbidity and mortality due to this entity are potentially greater than those resulting from the supratentorial variety, and urgent surgical evacuation should receive strong consideration.

The outcome following traumatic aEDH is good for those patients receiving definitive care in a timely fashion. A favorable outcome is seen in up to 89% of patients.[39] The most important prognostic factors appear to be the preoperative level of consciousness and the degree of associated intracranial injuries seen on CT scanning. Patients who are conscious before surgery, a favorable outcome has been achieved in up to 90%, while mortality has ranged from 0% to 5%. Patients presenting with a GCS score of 8 or less achieved favorable outcomes in 38% to 73% of cases and had a mortality rate of up to 41%.[17]

Traumatic Intracerebral Hemorrhage/Contusion

The distinction between *traumatic intracerebral hemorrhage* (ICH) and *contusion* is arbitrary, and thus these terms will be used interchangeably. These lesions generally result from parenchymal impact against the bony prominences of the skull base and subsequent rupture of small subpial vessels. Therefore, these hematomas are most often seen at the frontal and temporal poles where the cortical surface comes in contact with the frontal fossa floor and the sphenoid wing. Coup contusions occur beneath the site of impact, and contrecoup contusions are classically located opposite the site of impact. Gliding contusions consist of an area of focal hemorrhage along the superior medial margins of the cerebral hemispheres. They are often symmetrical and involve mainly white matter adjacent to the cortex.

The acute presentation of cerebral contusions is much like that of the other traumatic intracranial hematomas, and traumatic ICH is frequently seen in association with extra-axial hematomas. Up to 7% of patients suffering a severe closed head injury may develop a traumatic ICH in a delayed fashion.[7] Delayed traumatic ICH may develop in areas of previously demonstrated contusion but more often occur in the presence of a completely normal initial CT scan. Patients with this diagnosis typically meet the following criteria: a clear history of trauma and an asymptomatic interval followed by acute deterioration.

Once again, noncontrast CT scanning is the imaging modality of choice for the diagnosis of a traumatic ICH. An area of hyperdensity within the substance of the brain, most frequently on gyral crests, is the hallmark of this lesion. As time passes, approximately one-third of patients develop a halo of surrounding edema that may exert greater mass effect than the ICH itself.

Management of traumatic ICH should begin with standard medical management, discussed elsewhere in this chapter. Intracerebral hemorrhages with clinical evidence of herniation or significant mass effect should be evacuated. Smaller lesions should be followed cautiously with serial imaging and neurological exams. Contusions of the temporal lobe should receive special attention. Given the proximity of the temporal lobe to the tentorial notch, expanding hematomas can rapidly precipitate uncal herniation.

The outcome in patients with an ICH, whether evacuated or managed conservatively, is favorable in approximately 25%, with a mortality rate of 27% to 50%.[30,31] A low initial GCS score and associated intracranial injuries are also predictive of a poor outcome.

Medical Management of Traumatic Intracranial Hemorrhage

The primary goal of medical management of TIH is minimization of secondary brain injury. This is best accomplished by tight control of blood pressure, oxygenation, and ventilation, and aggressive stepwise management of intracranial hypertension. As a reminder, all surgically treatable lesions should be addressed simultaneously with medical management.

Hypotension and hypoxia remain two of the most powerful predictors of a poor outcome following severe closed head injury. As illustrated by the Traumatic Coma Data Bank literature, a single episode of hypotension (systolic blood pressure <90 mm Hg) doubles the expected mortality following severe closed head injury. Patients who experience an episode of hypoxia ($PaO_2 < 60$ mm Hg) carry a 28% mortality rate, and those suffering both hypoxic and hypotensive episodes carry a mortality rate of 57%. As well, Manley et al.[27] showed a threefold increase in mortality in patients suffering a hypotensive episode in the emergency department. These poor outcomes following hypotension and hypoxia underscore the need for aggressive airway and circulatory support both in the field and in the emergency department for this patient population.

Once the critical issues of hypoxia and hypotension have been addressed, the remainder of medical management centers on tight control of intracranial pressure (ICP). It should be remembered that ICP greater than 20–25 mm Hg is pathological and requires intervention. Failure to control significant ICP elevations results in a nearly

100% mortality rate. Of note, the proposed algorithm for management of elevated ICP (Fig. 8.4) is based primarily on Class II and III data and should serve only as a guideline.

The initial step in the management of intracranial hypertension is placement of an ICP monitor. The primary indication for ICP monitoring is a head-injured patient with a GCS score of 8 or less and an abnormal CT scan. As well, older patients and those suffering an episode of hypotension may benefit from ICP monitoring despite initially unimpressive CT scans. The decision to use parenchymal, subarachnoid, or subdural monitors versus ventriculostomy depends on the physician's preference. However, ventriculostomy offers the potential benefit of CSF diversion, which will be discussed later in this section.

Once the decision to monitor ICP has been made, a few initial simple steps can result in dramatic improvement in ICP. Neutral alignment of the neck and elevation of the head of the bed 15 to 30 degrees can dramatically improve venous return and lower ICP. In patients with potential spine injuries, the bed can be placed in the reverse Trendelenberg position to elevate the head while keeping the spine straight. Pain and agitation lead to increases in ICP. Therefore, patients should receive adequate sedation, analgesia, and pharmacological paralysis if necessary. Given that the vast majority of patients with severe CHI are intubated, ventilator settings employing high levels of positive end-expiratory pressure should be avoided, as elevated intrathoracic pressure reduces central venous return.

When ICP remains elevated despite the above measures, the first tier of therapeutic options—osmotic diuresis, ventricular drainage, and mild hyperventilation—is instituted. Osmotic diuresis with intravenous mannitol (0.25–1 g/kg), administered on an intermittent basis, can result in rapid, significant reduction in ICP. Patients receiving mannitol must be carefully monitored for hypovolemia. Serum osmolarity should be followed on a regular basis and kept below 320 mOsm/kg to prevent renal dysfunction. Mannitol is felt to act by drawing interstitial fluid out of the brain and also by improving the rheological properties of erythrocytes.[36] With extended usage, small amounts of mannitol can cross the blood–brain barrier and lead to rebound intracranial hypertension.[20] In severely refractory cases, small amounts of furosemide can be used to augment diuresis.

Ventricular drainage is another highly effective means to lower ICP. If a patient has previously had a ventriculostomy placed for ICP measurement, either continuous or intermittent CSF diversion is generally successful in bring ICP into an acceptable range. However, there is no Class I or Class II evidence to support the establishment of CSF diversion if this is not already in place for monitoring purposes. The primary complications of ventriculostomy placement are iatrogenic intracranial hemorrhage (1% incidence) and infection. Ventricular catheters carry up to a 10% risk of infection in general, and this risk quadruples in the face of an open skull fracture.[26] Posttraumatic hydrocephalus is an entirely different entity and should be treated accordingly.

As the final option in first-tier ICP management, mild hyperventilation is a rapidly effective method of reducing elevated ICP. Carbon dioxide (CO_2) is a potent cerebrovasodilator; thus, hyperventilation leads to a reduction in CO_2 levels and a subsequent drop in ICP. As a rule, every 1 mm Hg reduction in CO_2 leads to a 3% reduction in CBF. However, during the first few days following injury, CBF is generally lower than normal, and hyperventilation may lead to or exacerbate cerebral ischemia.[29] Therefore, when used as a first-line agent for ICP control, hyperventilation should be brief and should not reduce the $PaCO_2$ below 30–35 mm Hg.

In patients with ICP elevations refractory to first-line measures, pharmacologically induced coma, hypothermia, and aggressive hyperventilation are second-tier options for ICP control. Decompressive craniectomy is also considered among second-tier measures, but its discussion is beyond the scope of this chapter. Many neurointensivists consider barbiturates, specifically pentobarbital, the drug of choice for inducing coma. These agents work to suppress cerebral metabolic activity and therefore uncouple CBF. This can lead to a significant reduction in ICP. Other anesthetic agents, such as propofol and etomidate, have proved useful for cerebral protection in the operating room but have not been used as extensively for ICP control. Patients placed in barbiturate coma should be monitored for burst suppression via continuous bedside electroencephalography, with a target suppression pattern of 15–20 seconds. Dosing for pentobarbital is as follows: a 10 mg/kg loading dose over 30 minutes, followed by 5 mg/kg/hr for 3 hours and then a 1 mg/kg/hr maintenance infusion. The

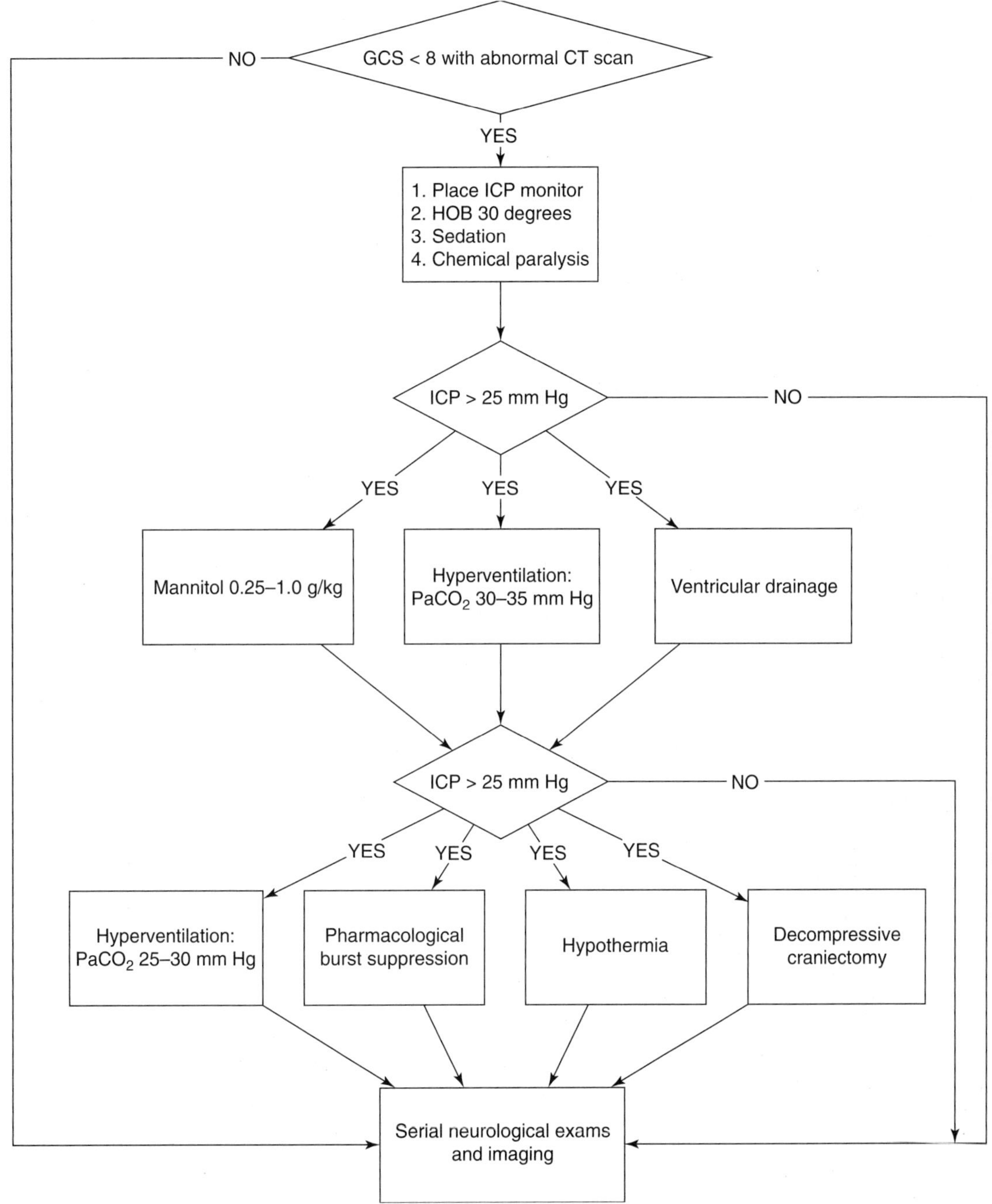

Figure 8.4. Algorithm for the medical management of elevated intracranial pressure.

use of barbiturate-induced coma is not without risks. Barbiturates are known cardiodepressants and appear to suppress the immunological system, increasing the risk of nosocomial infection. Barbiturates should be tapered slowly over 24–48 hours to prevent rebound ICP elevation.[11]

Hypothermia also acts to lower ICP by cerebral metabolic suppression. For every 1°C drop in core body temperature, the cerebral metabolic rate drops by 5%.[8] Cooling blankets, cold gastric lavage, and cold saline infusion have been used to reduce body temperature to 32–33°C. The available data on the use of hypothermia to control refractory ICP are conflicting regarding the functional outcome, and in head-injured patients it should be used on a case-by-case basis.[16] In addition, hypothermia, to levels used in cerebral protection, may lead to arrhythmias, sepsis, and coagulopathy. All patients receiving induced hypothermia must undergo constant core temperature monitoring in addition to the standard ICU monitoring for CHI.

Aggressive hyperventilation takes advantage of the previously stated effect of cerebral CO_2 reduction on ICP. Reduction of $PaCO_2$ to 25–30 mm Hg can lead to a 30% reduction in ICP. The profound cerebral vasoconstriction seen at these CO_2 concentrations and the potential for lethal cerebral ischemia suggest that invasive brain oxygen saturation and extraction monitoring be considered for patients receiving this therapy. Once again, no compelling data exist to suggest that the ICP reductions achieved with this manuver translate into an improved neurological outcome.[35,44]

The role of corticosteroids in head injury has remained a topic of controversy in recent years. A 1996 survey of UK neuroscience intensive-care units showed that corticosteroids were used in 14% of units to treat traumatic brain injury (TBI), and a similar study in the United States demonstrated steroid administration to be a component of TBI therapy in nearly two-thirds of US trauma centers.[15b,19b] Results of a systematic review conducted in 1997 suggested that steroid therapy for patients with closed head-injuries decreased the absolute risk for death by 1%–2% compared with no steroid treatment.[1a] However, an evidence-based review of the available literature, conducted by the Cochrane Group in 2000, failed to demonstrate any conclusive benefit of corticosteroids administration in TBI patients.[1b]

Recently a large multi-center, randomized clinical trial (CRASH) has been completed to address the question of steroid therapy in closed head injury. Ten thousand eight patients were enrolled at 239 hospitals in 49 countries. Inclusion criteria required a Glasgow coma scale scores of 14 or less and initiation of treatment within 8 hours of injury. Patients were randomized to receive either methylprednisolone or placebo for 48 hours. Primary outcomes were mortality within 2 weeks and death and disability at 6 months. At 2 weeks, 21.1% of patients treated with corticosteroids and 17.9% of those treated with placebo had died (relative risk, 1.18; $P = 0.0001$). At 6 months, 25.7% of the corticosteroid group had died vs. 22.3% of the placebo group (relative risk 1.15, $p = 0.0001$). Subset analysis showed that the mortality difference was not affected by injury severity score, time from injury to initiation of steroids, or degree of extra-cranial trauma.[11a,40a]

Based on the class I data now available from the CRASH trial, and supported by recent Cochrane Group analysis, it does not appear that the routine administration of corticosteroids has a role in the management of TBI.[1c]

An additional topic that deserves discussion is posttraumatic epilepsy. Seizures following head injury are often divided into early (less than 1 week after injury) and late (more than 1 week after injury) events. Patients suffering a severe CHI have a 30% risk of developing early posttraumatic seizures and a 13% risk of developing late seizures. Prophylactic antiepileptic medications, specifically phenytoin, have been shown to decrease the risk of early posttraumatic seizures but not that of late seizures. Therefore, all patients with severe CHI should receive phenytoin for only 1 week, maintained at therapeutic levels.[48] Subsequent development of a seizure disorder should be treated in the standard fashion.

Summary

As should now be apparent, traumatic intracranial hemorrhages are frequent sequelae of severe closed head injuries. A clear understanding of the pathophysiology, presentation, radiology, and treatment of these lesions is paramount to the care of brain-injured patients. Maintenance of a high level of suspicion for TIH and aggressive therapy, both surgical and medical, can lead to a reduction in mortality and an improvement in functional outcome for this patient population.

REFERENCES

1a. Alderson P, Roberts I: Corticosteroids in acute traumatic brain injury: a systematic review of randomized trials. BMJ 314:1855–1859, 1997.

1b. Alderson P, Roberts I: Corticosteroids for acute traumatic brain injury. Cochrane Database Syst Rev 2:CD000196, 2000.

1c. Alderson P, Roberts I: Corticosteroids for acute traumatic brain injury. Cochrane Database Syst Rev 1:CD000196, 2005.

1d. Aldrich EF, Eisenberg HM: Acute subdural hematoma. In: Apuzzo MJ (ed): Brain Surgery Complication Avoidance and Management. New York, Churchill Livingstone, 1993, pp 1283–1293.

2. Baykaner K, Alp H, Ceviker N, et al: Observation of 95 patients with extradural hematomas and review of the literature. Surg Neurol 30:339–341, 1988.

3. Cairns CJ, Finfer SR, Harrington TJ, Cook R: Papaverine angioplasty to treat cerebral vasospasm following traumatic subarachnoid haemorrhage. Anaesth Intens Care 31(1):87–91, 2003.

4. Cardoso ER, Galbraith S: Posttraumatic hydrocephalus —a retrospective review. Surg Neurol 23:261–264, 1985.

5. Chappell ET, Moure, FC, Good MC: Comparison of computed tomographic angiography with digital subtraction angiography in the diagnosis of cerebral aneurysms: A meta-analysis. Neurosurgery 52:624–631, 2003.

6. Chen TY, Wong CW, Chang CN, et al: The expectant treatment of "asymptomatic" supratentorial epidural hematomas. Neurosurgery 32:176–179, 1993.

7. Clifton Gl, McCormick WF, Grossman RG: Neuropathology of early and late deaths after head injury. Neurosurgery 8:309–314, 1981.

8. Cormino M, Claudia SR, Narayan RK: Secondary insults to the injured brain. J Clin Neurosci 2:132–148, 1997.

9. Crooks DA: Pathogenesis and biomechanics of traumatic intracranial hemorrhages. Virchows Arch 418:479, 1991.

10. Delfini R, Santoro A, Innocenzi G, et al: Interhemispheric subdural hematoma. Case report. J Neurosurg Sci 35:217–220, 1991.

11a. Edward P et al: Final results of MRC CRASH, a randomised placebo-controlled trial of intravenous corticosteroid in adults with head injury-outcomes at 6 months. Lancet 365:1957–1959, 2005.

11b. Eisenberg HM, Frankowski RF, Contant CF, et al: High-dose barbiturate control of elevated intracranial pressure in patients with severe head injury. J Neurosurg 68:15–23, 1988.

12. Foelholm R, Waltimo O: Epidemiology of chronic subdural haematoma. Acta Neurochir 32:247–250, 1975.

13. Freytag E: Autopsy findings in head injury from blunt forces. Arch Pathol 75:402, 1963.

14. Gartman JJ, Atstupenas EA, Vollmer DG, et al: Traumatic laceration of pericallosal artery resulting in interhemispheric subdural hematoma: Case report. Neurol Med Chir 36:377–379, 1996.

15a. Gennarelli TA, Thibault LE: Biomechanics of acute subdural hematoma. J Trauma 22:680–686, 1982.

15b. Ghajar J, Hariri R, Narayan R, Lacono L, Firlik K, Patterson R: Survey of critical care management of comatose head injured patients in the United States. Crit Care Med 23:560–567, 1995.

16. Harris OA, Colford JM, Good MC, Matz PG: The role of hypothermia in the management of severe brain injury: A meta-analysis. Arch Neurol 59:1007–1083, 2002.

17. Haselsberger K, Pucher R, Auer LM: Prognosis after acute subdural or epidural hemorrhage. Acta Neurochir 90:111–116, 1988.

18. Hatashita S, Koga N, Hosaka Y, et al: Acute subdural hematoma: Severity of injury, surgical intervention and mortality. Neurol Med Chir 33:13–18, 1993.

19a. Jane JA, Francel PC: Age and outcome of head injury. In: Narayan RK (ed): Neurotrauma. New York, McGraw-Hill, 1996, pp 793–804.

19b. Jeevaratnum DR, Menon DK: Survey of intensive care of severely head injured patients in the United Kingdom. BMJ 312:944–947, 1996.

20. Kaufmann AM, Cardoso ER: Aggravation of vasogenic cerebral edema by multiple-dose mannitol. J Neurosurg 77:584–589, 1992.

21. Korinth M, Weinzierl M, Gilsbach, JM: Treatment options in traumatic epidural hematomas. Unfallchirurgie 105:224–230, 2002.

22. Lee JH, Martin NA, Alsina G, et al: Hemodynamically significant cerebral vasospasm and outcome after head injury: A prospective study. J Neurosurg 87:221–223, 1997.

23. Lind CR, Lind CJ, Mee EW: Reduction in the number of repeated operations for the treatment of subacute and chronic subdural hematomas by placement of subdural drains. J Neurosurg 99:44–46, 2003.

24. Llamas L, Ramos-Zuniga R, Sandoval L: Acute interhemispheric subdural hematoma: Two case reports and analysis of the literature. Minim Invasive Neurosurg. 45:55–58, 2002.

25. Lobato RD, Rivas JJ, Gomez PA, et al: Head-injured patients who talk and deteriorate into coma. Analysis of 211 cases studied with computerized tomography. J Neurosurg 75:256–261, 1991.

26. Lozier AP, Sciacca RR, Romagnoli MF, Connolly ES: Ventriculostomy-related infections: A critical review of the literature. Neurosurgery 51:170–178, 2002.

27. Manley G, Knudson MM, Morabito D, Damron S, et al: Hypotension, hypoxia, and head injury: Frequency, duration, and consequences. Arch Surg 136:118–1123, 2001.

28. Marion D: Pathophysiology of cranial trauma. In: Batjer HH, Loftus CM (eds): Textbook of Neurosurgery: Principles and Practices. Philadelphia, Lippincott Williams & Wilkins, 2003, pp 2798–2803.

29. Marmarou A, Maset AL, Ward JD, et al: Contribution of CSF and vascular factors to elevation of ICP in severely head-injured patients. J Neurosurg 66:883–890, 1987.

30. Marshall LF et al: The outcome of severe closed head injury from report on Traumatic Coma Data Bank. J Neurosurg 75(suppl):536–538, 1991.

31. Marshall LF, Gautille T, Klauber MR, et al: The outcome of severe closed head injury. J Neurosurg 75:S28–S36, 1991.

32. Mattioli C, Beretta L, Gerevini S, Veglia F, et al: Traumatic subarachnoid hemorrhage on the computerized tomography scan obtained at admission: A multicenter assessment of the accuracy of diagnosis and the potential

impact on patient outcome. J Neurosurg 98(1):37–42, 2003.
33. Miller JD: Evaluation and treatment of head injury in adults. Neurosurgery 2:28–43, 1992.
34. Mori K, Maeda M: Surgical treatment of chronic subdural hematoma in 500 consecutive cases: Clinical characteristics, surgical outcome, complications, and recurrence rate. Neurol Med-Chir 41:371–381, 2001.
35. Muizelaar JP, Marmarou A, Ward JD, et al: Adverse effects of prolonged hyperventilation in patients with severe head injury: A randomized clinical trial. J Neurosurg 75:731–739, 1991.
36. Muizellar JP, Wei EP, Kontos HA, et al: Mannitol causes a compensatory cerebral vasoconstriction and vasodilatation in response to blood viscosity changes. J Neurosurg 59:822–828, 1983.
37. Murakami H, Hirose Y, Sagoh M, et al: Why do chronic subdural hematomas continue to grow slowly and not coagulate? Role of thrombomodulin in the mechanism. J Neurosurg 96:877–884, 2002.
38. Nakajima H, Yasui T, Nishikawa M, et al: The role of postoperative patient posture in the recurrence of chronic subdural hematoma: A prospective randomized trial. Surg Neurol 58:385–387, 2002.
39. Phonprasert C, Suwanwela C, Hongsaprabhas C, et al: Extradural hematoma: Analysis of 138 cases. J Trauma 20:679–683, 1980.
40a. Roberts I et al: Effect of intravenous corticosteroids on death within 14 days in 10008 adults with clinically significant head injury (MRC CRASH trial): Randomised placebo-controlled trial. Lancet 364:1321–1328, 2004.
40b. Robinson RG: Chronic subdural hematoma: Surgical management in 133 patients. J Neurosurg. 61:263–268, 1984.
41. Sakas DE, Bullock MR, Teasdale GM: One-year outcome following craniotomy for traumatic hematoma in patients with fixed dilated pupils. J Neurosurg 82:961–965, 1995.
42. Seelig JM, Becker DP, Miller JD, et al: Traumatic acute subdural hematoma: Major mortality reduction in comatose patients treated within four hours. N Engl J Med 304:1511–1518, 1981.
43. Servadei F, Murray GD, Teasdale GM, Dearden M, et al: Traumatic subarachnoid hemorrhage: Demographic and clinical study of 750 patients from the European Brain Injury Consortium survey of head injuries. Neurosurgery 50(2):261–267, 2002.
44. Sheinberg M, Kanter MJ, Robertson CS, Contant CF, Narayan RK, Grossman RG: Continuous monitoring of jugular venous oxygen saturation in head-injured patients. J Neurosurg 76:212–217, 1992.
45. Stone JL, Rifai MH, Sugar O, et al: Subdural hematomas: I. Acute subdural hematoma: Progress in definition, clinical pathology and therapy. Surg Neurol 19:216–231, 1983.
46. Tanaka A, Yoshinaga S, Kimura M: Xenon-enhanced computed tomographic measurement of cerebral blood flow in patients with chronic subdural hematomas. Neurosurgery 27:554–561, 1990.
47. Taneda M, Kataoka K, Akai F, Asai T, Sakata I: Traumatic subarachnoid haemorrhage: Analysis of 89 cases. Acta Neurochir (Wien) 122:45–48, 1993.
48. Temken NR, Dikmen SS, Wilensky AJ, et al: A randomized double-blind study of phenytoin for the prevention of post-traumatic seizures. N Engl J Med 323:497–502, 1990.
49. Thurman D: The epidemiology and economics of head trauma. In: Miller L, Hayes R (eds): Head Trauma: Basic, Preclinical, and Clinical Directions. New York, Wiley 2001, pp
50. Williams GR, Baskaya MK, Menendez J, Polin R, et al: Burr-hole versus twist-drill drainage for the evacuation of chronic subdural haematoma: A comparison of clinical results. J Clin Neurosci 8:551–554, 2001.

Chapter 9
Neurovascular Trauma

ANIL NANDA, SATISH RUDRAPPA, HAKAN TUNA, AND PRASAD VANNEMREDDY

Historical Note and Nomenclature

Ambroise Paré, who had the distinct privilege of operating on King Henry II of France, was the first to describe the successful treatment of a carotid injury when, in 1552, he repaired a penetrating injury to the left carotid artery caused by a sword using a cotton pack and suture.[5] The next mention of this form of injury appeared at sea, on the *HMS Tonnant* in 1803, where a carotid laceration was repaired with no neurological deficit.[23] In 1872, Verneuil presented the first case of nonpenetrating trauma to the carotid artery with thrombus and intimal tear at autopsy.[68] The first reported case of a traumatic intracranial aneurysm was by Guibert, who, in 1895, described a traumatic internal carotid artery aneurysm found at autopsy. Neurovascular trauma had a colorful and rich history in the glorious times of sword fights and gallantry. Unfortunately, the chivalry of the sixteenth century has been replaced by the staccato of urban gunfire and accelerating motor vehicles, making cerebrovascular system trauma a common occurrence today.

Traumatic vascular lesions can occur after severe or even the mildest form of head and cervical trauma. These injuries must be strongly suspected based on the mechanism of trauma, which might be penetrating (obvious) or blunt (concealed); the former might obviate the need for exploration of the injured artery, while the latter may make it more difficult to diagnose the extent of injury. The scenario is further complicated in the setting of polytrauma, where shock, sensorium, and sedation confound the diagnosis.[52]

Injury to the cerebrovascular tree can result in disruption, contusion, laceration, thrombosis, dissection, stenosis, pseudoaneurysm formation, and occlusion of carotid and vertebrobasilar systems. The true incidence of these entities remains uncertain because of the subtle nature of injuries in blunt trauma and the infrequent use of invasive angiography in head and neck trauma at present. The cost effectiveness of noninvasive studies in such instances is also questionable given the long latency and probably infrequent occurrence of clinical presentation with stroke.[44]

Carotid Artery Injury

Injury to the carotid arteries is divided into two distinct entities; penetrating and nonpenetrating or blunt carotid artery injury. They have entirely different presentations and management options.

Based on anatomical facts and injury mechanisms, the carotid and vertebrobasilar arterial systems present with different pathologies. The long, mobile segments of both of these arteries also predispose them to trauma more often than is the case with other large arteries. The osseous structures through which these vessels pass to enter the cranial cavity along with the dural and other soft tissue elements produce a tethering effect contributing to damage to the vessels wall, especially at the point of contact with bony structures such as the carotid tubercle and styloid process. Clinical presentation of such an etiology would take a fairly long time. Diagnosis of this kind of delayed presentation requires clinical suspicion and prompt investigation. Nanda et al.[52] found an almost equal incidence of blunt and penetrating trauma to the carotids.

Penetrating Carotid Artery Injury

Etiopathology

Penetrating trauma is more obvious and often gets attention due to the extent of the injury. The common carotid artery is injured in 75% of cases, with penetrating trauma in a report of 25 years' experience by Rubio et al.[59] In spite of its posterior location in the carotid sheath, the internal carotid artery was injured in 58% of cases with penetrating injuries in our series,[52] probably because of the head turning to the opposite side and/or assaults from the lateral aspect of the neck.

Epidemiology

The incidence of extracranial carotid artery injury during trauma is difficult to determine. In a series of 2000 cases from Egypt that encompassed both civilian and wartime experience, there were only 6 cases (0.3%) of extracranial carotid injury.[20] However, penetrating injuries of the carotid artery tend to be far more common than blunt injuries, and almost 80% of penetrating wounds to the carotid artery are caused by gunshot wounds, the rest being secondary to stab wounds.[59]

The incidence of cervical vessel involvement in head and neck trauma is 25%, and carotid artery injury makes up 5% to 10% of all arterial injuries.[34] Injuries to the cervical vessels can be subdivided into those resulting from penetrating trauma and those due to blunt trauma. Penetrating injuries are the major cause of cervical vessel injuries. Nonpenetrating injuries to the cervical vessels are rare, accounting for less than 10% of all cervical vessel injuries.[34]

Clinical Manifestations

Open injury to the carotids in the neck present with self-explanatory features like massive bleeding, altered sensorium, shock, neurological deficits, and airway obstruction. In closed head injury, signs of carotid artery injury are a cervical bruit, a quickly growing cervical hematoma, and absence of a carotid artery pulse. Pulse deficits in the superficial temporal artery, signs of air embolism, oropharyngeal bleeding, widened mediastinum, and so on are subtle signs. A review of the cumulative data suggests that almost a third of patients present with neurological deficits.[25,59] In a series of more than 128 patients, 46 (36%) presented with hypotension and shock and 42 (33%) with airway compromise.[60] Shock is always secondary to massive hemorrhage, which can cause compromise of the airway in the neck. In the presence of hypotension and shock, it is sometimes difficult to rule out a coexisting head injury. Penetrating injury can also lead to complete or partial thrombosis of the carotid artery and possible pseudoaneurysm formation. Some individuals can tolerate a complete occlusion of the carotid artery, but up to 30% are unable to do so and present with symptoms of cerebral ischemia from decreased blood flow or emboli from the site of injury.[59]

Diagnostic Workup

The extent of the diagnostic workup depends upon the extent of injury in polytrauma and the severity of shock in penetrating injuries. Most of the discrepancy in the incidence of the different types of injuries is due to the time frame dictated by the injury severity score and the central nervous system status. The trauma protocol in a given center might still be followed until the cost effectiveness of a given diagnostic workup is established, especially for invasive angiographic studies.

The site of injury should be examined and, most importantly, a complete neurological evaluation should be performed and documented. A routine lateral cervical spine exam is important to rule out any cervical subluxation with possible associated vertebral artery injury, and a chest x-ray should always be performed to rule out a pneumo- or hemothorax. If the platysma been violated surgical exploration is required. A preoperative angiogram is necessary, but is not mandatory in life-threatening hemorrhage. In our series,[52] 6 of the 12 patients with penetrating trauma had exploration without angiographic evaluation; 4 of them survived after arterial reconstruction. Radiological findings and physical examination are good predictors of arterial injuries in patients with penetrating neck wounds and can exclude injury in the majority of patients. Although arteriography is a sensitive test, it tends to have a lower yield. As arteriography is an invasive procedure and has certain complications, it is reserved for Zone I and III injuries. According to du Toit et al.,[19] preoperative angiography does not influence mortality or stroke rates in hemodynamically stable patients. Duplex examination is the preferred diagnostic method for Zone II injuries.[26,35] In patients with high-velocity penetrating neck injury, a computed tomography, (CT) scan is useful to assess possible associated head trauma. The roles of CT angiography (CTA) and magnetic resonance angiography (MRA) as diagnostic tools are being evaluated.

Management

In patients with hypotension and airway obstruction, stabilization of cardiorespiratory functions is essential. Most patients respond to crystalloid intravenous solution rapidly, but those with concomitant head injury and agitation may require elective intubation. Patients with active pulsatile hemorrhage or a growing cervical hematoma may require urgent surgical exploration. Treatment paradigms are directed at preventing cerebral ischemia and potentially hemorrhagic lesions such as pseudoaneurysms. Diffusion and perfusion magnetic resonance imaging (MRI) may be useful to determine the presence of any ischemic lesion that might require urgent revascularization. Transcranial Doppler sonography may be indicated in cases of suspected intimal flaps, pseudoaneurysms, or dissections that are actively generating emboli.[64]

Conservative management is aimed at preventing embolic events, especially when patients tolerate a blocked carotid without any evidence of ischemia. Many authors[47] have reported favorable results with anticoagulation as a primary therapeutic modality for these patients. Systemic anticoagulation (1) minimizes clot formation at the site of intimal injury, (2) decreases propagation of the clot by allowing the fibrinolytic system to dissolve the clot, and (3) prevents embolization from the clot within the sac of the pseudoaneurysm. Fabian et al.[22] reported that over a period of time, 62% of nonocclusive dissections resolve with anticoagulation. However, 29% of initial dissections develop pseudoaneurysms on follow-up angiography, which are unlikely to resolve once formed. Mokri et al.[48] thus advocated surgical repair of posttraumatic pseudoaneurysms when they were producing symptoms.

Operative management consists of restoration of flow through the injured carotid artery, whether by primary repair of the lacerated carotid or with a patch graft. If a segment of the carotid artery has been lost, the saphenous vein from the thigh can be harvested and an interposition graft placed. These methods are defined as repair, as opposed to ligation, which is defined as deliberate surgical interruption of flow through the injured vessel. In patients who are neurologically intact, the balloon occlusion test and blood flow studies may be done to review the possibility of carotid sacrifice. While mortality after arterial repair was 17.6%, procedural mortality associated with arterial ligation was reported as 45%, and no surviving patient experienced a change in the preligation neurological state.[19] Arterial ligation should be considered only for distal arterial occlusion, for impossible distal control, and in the patient with multiple trauma in whom instability precludes extensive surgery. In patients with severe neurological deficits and coma, there is reason to view aggressive intervention with some trepidation, as these patients have a dismal prognosis; the rate of mortality resulting from carotid artery injury ranges from 7% to 33%, with the average at about 20%. The majority of the deaths seem to occur in patients who present in refractory hemorrhagic shock, in coma, or with severe neurological deficits.[52] Endovascular stents or stent-grafts can be helpful in providing urgent revascularization at the time of diagnostic angiography, though no large series or long-term data are available on the safety and efficacy of these devices.[37]

Blunt Carotid Artery Injury

Etiopathology

The carotid artery is relatively fixed at the base of the skull in the petrous canal. Therefore, sudden hyperextension with rotation causes the internal carotid artery to pull against the lateral mass of either C1 or C2. This area, as well as the area just above the bifurcation of the carotid artery, is a frequent site for intimal dissection and disruption. Intracranially, the most common site is above the supraclinoid process, and dissections at this site can involve the middle cerebral artery. Careful neurological assessment is required even in blunt injuries since a dissection can present with rapid deterioration secondary to ischemia and can result in death.[53] Chiropractic maneuvers for neck pain have also been implicated in injury to the carotids and vertebral arteries, mostly producing dissections.[2] The role of this type of minor trauma producing blunt carotid artery injury (BCI) has received much attention, especially for the cost effectiveness of the screening procedures adopted by different trauma centers and stroke protocols.[44]

Fleming and Petrie[24] described four types of BCI. Type I involves the cervical carotid artery and occurs in older patients with atherosclerotic vessels, injuring the intima and portions of the media. This is seen in 50% of dissection cases. Type II injuries produce stretching of the internal carotid artery, with injury to the intima and media while preserving the adventitia. This type of BCI is seen in hyperextension of the neck. Type III injuries involve intraoral trauma and are commonly seen in children. Type IV injuries are skull base fractures and can result in transection of the carotid cartery at the petrous bone. In all of these instances, the initiating point is a breach in the intimal layer resulting in pooling of blood in the subintimal space and dissecting intima into the lumen of the blood vessel. This can lead to complete obstruction of the blood vessel or to stenosis of the artery following thrombus formation, which could become the source of embolization of intracranial vasculature. A dissection or tear in the adventitial layer results in pseudoaneurysm formation.

Epidemiology

Blunt cerebrovascular artery injury is being recognized with increasing frequency after motor vehicle collisions. Davis et al.[17] reported the characteristics of blunt cerebrovascular injuries in motor vehicle collisions. Among the 940 individuals with blunt cerebrovascular injury, half were belted (57.4%) and 82.3% had airbag deployment; 16.2% were partially or completely ejected from the vehicle. Head and thoracic injuries were common (44.4% and 40.8%, respectively); 27.8% sustained a cervical spine fracture, and 21.0% sustained a soft tissue injury to the neck. The case fatality rate was 44.5%. The majority of BCI patients were drivers (76.0%). Among belted patients, the lap/shoulder belt was most commonly considered the injury source (61.4%). Davis et al.[15] demonstrated an 0.08% incidence of BCI over a 4-year period in their trauma population. Laitt et al.[36] reported an incidence of 0.4% from 2024 blunt trauma patients over a 3-year period. Almost 70% of all BCIs are caused by motor vehicle accidents and 12% all caused by sporting events, with the rest being secondary to fights and falls.[55] A 10-year medical record review by Mayberry et al.[44] found that 17 (0.05%) of 35,212 blunt trauma admissions had a BCI, 11 of whom had a stroke within 12 hours. Spontaneous dissection of the carotid artery has an annual incidence of 2.5 per 100,000 in community-based studies and may account for nearly 2% of all ischemic strokes (predominantly in young and middle-aged patients, with a 10% to 25% occurrence.[61,63]

Clinical Manifestations

Nonpenetrating Injuries of the Carotid Artery

Vascular injury after head trauma must be suspected especially in the presence of a neurological deficit or a progressive neurological deficit in the absence of a mass lesion.[29] Headaches are the most common presenting symptom of BCI. However, the lack of clear etiology and the delay in presenting symptoms make the initial clinical symptoms hard to determine. Most patients present with focal ischemic features; typical signs are unilateral neurological deficits including hemiparesis, aphasia, or transient visual loss. The third most common sign is ipsilateral Horner's syndrome and, less frequently, a bruit with neck swelling or focal tenderness. Epistaxis, cranial nerve deficits, and different forms of stroke may also herald the presentation.[52] Bruising from a seat belt following a motor vehicle crash might be indicative of silent injury to the carotids. Massive cerebral infarcts secondary to acute dissection of the middle cerebral artery following BCI were also reported at autopsy.[53] At this point, it is important to not a report from two level 1 trauma centers, where a retrospective analysis of 10 years' experience revealed that BCI and stroke due to BCI occur too rarely to justify, according to the authors, routine use of aggressive angiographic screening protocols at their trauma centers.[44]

Diagnostic Workup

Angiography remains the gold standard in the diagnosis of blunt injury to the internal carotid artery in the neck and head.[41] Computed tomography scanning is normally unremarkable unless there is associated infarction, which would only be present at a later stage. Angiography may reveal a *string sign* (a tapered occlusion beginning just after the cervical bifurcation), a stenosis, a pseudoaneurysm, or even a complete thrombosis. Magnetic resonance imaging is an advance over routine angiography and is a noninvasive means of diagnosing dissections. It can provide sensitive information regarding infarction in the brain parenchyma. Axial MRI may also reveal subintimal hematomas in the petrous and supraclinoid sections of the carotid with some sensitivity. Laster et al.[38] reported that MRA was a fairly accurate screening method that compared well with routine angiography in the evaluation of the carotid bifurcation. In a recent study, the sensitivity, specificity, positive predictive value, and negative predictive value of CTA were reported as 68%, 67%, 65%, and 70%, respectively. In the same study, the authors found the sensitivity, specificity, positive predictive value, and negative predictive value of MRA to be 75%, 67%, 43%, and 89%.[10] Both CTA and MRA have been cited to have controversial results. Duplex ultrasonography, though cost effective for imaging neck vessels, has not been evaluated as an alternative because of its inability to visualize the intracranial vasculature.[44,47]

The important end point in the management of BCI is the development of stroke and the diagnosis. Some of the risk factors for the development of stroke in BCI are basilar skull factures and midfacial factures, hanging, neck seat-belt contusion, cervical spine injury, and severe blow to the head with poor Glasgow Coma Scale scores. In such instances, angiographic evaluation of the extra- and intracranial vasculature is indicated.

Management

The mainstay of treatment for nonpenetrating injuries to the carotid artery that result in dissection or thrombosis is anticoagulation.[14,71] Current studies suggest that early anticoagulation in patients with nonpenetrating carotid artery injury reduces the stroke rate and the resultant neurological morbidity. Miller et al.[46] reported that the stroke rate for patients treated with heparin and antiplatelet therapy was 6.8% compared with 64% in untreated patients ($p < .01$). To prevent propagation of thrombosis or embolic events, the patient is heparinized for 7 days and treated with Coumadin for approximately 3 months. At this stage, a repeat angiogram is taken; in most cases, there is complete resolution of radiological abnormalities. If the patient develops symptoms despite anticoagulation treatment, then the surgical options include trapping of the vessel with or without an extracranial-intracranial bypass procedure and possible proximal ligation. In some cases, if the lesion is fairly low in the cervical carotid, an endarterectomy is also an option. The extracranial-intracranial bypass study did not show any benefit for transient ischemic attacks, but this procedure may be used in cases of dissection refractory to medical management. Although the blood flow in these extracranial-intracranial bypasses is low (approximately 30 ml/min), with a saphenous vein bypass graft from the internal carotid to middle cerebral artery, the flow is nearly tripled, to almost 100 ml/min. This method has been fairly successful with skull base tumors and has recently been used in the treatment of carotid artery dissections as well.[50] Recently, some authors have proposed the use of antiplatelet therapy as an alternative to anticoagulant therapy for blunt carotid injury.[70] Antiplatelet agents can be used in patients at high risk of bleeding complications from either intracranial or other major injuries. Although there are some series, the role of carotid stents in the treatment of nonpenetrating carotid artery injury remains undetermined.[11,13,18]

Traumatic dissections tend to have a high incidence of associated aneurysms and progress more easily to occlusion than do spontaneous dissections. With spontaneous dissections, resolution of stenosis occurs in 80% to 90% of cases compared to approximately 50% of those with traumatic dissections. A study by Mokri and colleagues[48] showed that the risk of recurrent dissection was almost 8% within the first month. A prolonged follow-up showed that the rate of recurrent dissection was only about 1% per year. Furthermore, younger patients were more likely to have recurrent dissections, and most recurrences were symptomatic. Revascularization for persistently symptomatic traumatic internal carotid artery dissection was recently shown to eliminate ischemic complications.[69] In summary, the risk of neurological morbidity with the chance of a repeat dissection is fairly low with long-term follow-up.[62]

Vertebrobasilar Injury

Etiopathology

Injuries to the vertebral artery tend to be blunt rather than penetrating in origin since they are difficult to reach inside the foramina of cervical vertebrae. Interestingly, they occur without fractures or dislocations. Many of these lesions go undetected because they are compensated for by the contralateral vertebral artery and thus are not symptomatic. The vertebral artery is most susceptible to injury at the point of entrance at the foramen transversarium at C6 because it is relatively fixed to the bony orifice of the foramen, and the increased mobility at C5-6 makes it vulnerable. The next most common site is C1-2, with rotation of the atlanto-occipital and atlanto-axial joints. Even in patients without any symptoms referable to the vertebrobasilar system, the vertebral artery may be occluded by mere extension of the neck with rotation during routine angiography.[16]

Injuries to the vertebral system can result in thrombosis, dissection, aneurysm, and arteriovenous fistula formation. Furthermore, spontaneous vertebral dissections can occur without any obvious underlying etiology; incriminating factors like fibromuscular dysplasia, autosomal dominant polycystic kidney, migraine headaches, oral contraceptive use, and Marfan's syndrome are described in the literature.[49] In instances where dissections of the vertebral artery have been described as caused by activities ranging from the sublime to the ridiculous, the predisposing factors may play a significant role and a detailed history would be helpful. The basilar artery, due to its location deep within the cranium, is rarely injured even in penetrating trauma due to gunshots.

Epidemiology

Vertebrobasilar injuries are far less frequent than carotid artery injuries. In a series including 7000 arterial injuries, only 15 cases of vertebral artery injury were documented.[57] Vertebral artery injuries tend to be secondary to blunt rather than penetrating injury. The cause of the blunt trauma to the vertebrobasilar system is most commonly motor vehicle accidents.[7] The anatomical location of the vertebral artery, rather deep in the neck and protected by the vertebral column, makes it less vulnerable to injury. The incidence of vertebral artery injury with cervical spine trauma is higher than is generally thought because most patients with cervical spine injuries do not undergo routine angiography. Moreover, symptoms of vertebral artery injury are neither forthcoming nor dramatic. Willis et al.[72] reported vertebral artery injury in 46% of 26 patients with blunt trauma of the cervical spine, producing a subluxation from a *locked* or *perched* facet, facet destruction with evidence of instability, or a fracture involving the foramen transversarium. Kral et al.[33] reported that the incidence of vertebral artery injury was 4% in all types of blunt cervical spinal injury but increased to 16% in cases suspicious for vertebral artery injury, that is, cases with mono- or bifacet dislocation and/or cases with fractures extending into the transverse foramen.

Clinical Manifestations

Most injuries to the vertebrobasilar system remain silent because a unilateral vertebral thrombosis is usually well compensated for by the other vertebral artery unless one vertebral is congenitally hypoplastic. The most common symptom of extracranial vertebral dissection is headache associated with neck pain. However, symptoms of ischemia in the brain stem, cerebellum, and occipital lobes can present with a wide spectrum of clinical findings. These include lateral medullary infarction (Wallenberg's syndrome), hemiatrophy, ataxia, dysmetria, tremor associated with nystagmus, tinnitus, deafness, dysphasia, cortical blindness, and, in the most morbid manifestation, with basilar artery thrombosis involving coma with decerebrate rigidity. Extracranial lesions may remain asymptomatic, present as a painful pulsatile mass, and may elicit a thrill upon palpation. Dissections that extend up to the fourth part of the vertebral artery may rupture intracranially, leading to a subarachnoid hemorrhage. These patients present with severe headaches, photophobia, and signs of meningismus and, in severe cases, can be moribund. Even after minor whiplash injuries, fatal basilar thrombosis may occur. Thrombotic disease of the vertebrobasilar circulation is associated with a poor prognosis. It may occur in trauma patients, especially those with neck injuries, even several months after the initial insult.

Diagnostic Workup

For carotid injuries, angiography, MRI, and MRA are diagnostic tools. As a screening procedure, a Doppler study of the vertebral arteries is noninvasive and less expensive.

Management

In cases where there is a complete thrombosis of the vertebral artery and adequate compensation from the contralateral side, there may be no need for any treatment at all. Currently, anticoagulation is the mainstay of treatment for symptomatic dissections and usually consists of heparinization for 7 days, followed by Coumadin for 3 months. Most dissections resolve with this treatment; however, those that are refractory to medical management will require neuroradiological and surgical intervention.

Neuroradiological intervention techniques include the placement of coils or latex balloons, which are effective for pseudoaneurysms and arteriovenous fistulas. This is a relatively low-risk procedure with a high rate of success.[8] Other modalities include thrombolytic therapy for acute vertebrobasilar embolism and the use of intra-arterial streptokinase and recombinant tissue plasma activator; however, these are still in the clinical trial phase, and only anecdotal reports exist.[31]

Surgical treatment consists of proximal ligation of the vertebral artery to prevent propagation of clots in cases in which medical therapy has failed. The vertebral artery can be trapped if there is adequate collateral circulation, and in some cases, retromastoid craniotomy may be required to clip the vessel intracranially proximal to the posterior inferior cerebellar artery. In patients with subarachnoid hemorrhage due to an intracranial vertebral artery dissection, clipping or trapping may be required and anticoagulation is contraindicated. In intracranial dissections, hematomas exist between the internal elastic lamina and the media, as opposed to their location in the extracranial vessels, where they are located between the media and the adventitia.[9] Innovative bypass procedures have been recommended for some types of vertebrobasilar insufficiencies secondary to dissection, but their use in the clinical setting has not been widespread.[4] Since the extracranial-intracranial study showed little benefit from these low-flow bypasses, there is some doubt about their ultimate value. In summary, most cases of extracranial dissection respond well to anticoagulation, and rarely is neuroradiological or surgical intervention required. The vast majority of occult penetrating and blunt cervical vascular injuries remain asymptomatic, and a significant percentage of symptomatic arterial injuries thoughout the body are known to heal without causing clinical abnormalities.[10,27]

Traumatic Aneurysms

Etiopathology

Traumatic aneurysms can occur after penetrating injury or, more commonly, after closed head trauma. Blunt head injury can result in traumatic aneurysms because of the different velocities of the brain and the skull. A traumatic aneurysm of the internal carotid artery following closed head trauma may be due to one of the following mechanisms: a basal skull fracture may directly injure the internal carotid artery, the impact of the head trauma may cause overstretching or torsion of the internal carotid artery, or nearby prominent bony structures such as the anterior or posterior clinoid processes may tear the internal carotid artery. These aneurysms are more often located at the cranial base in the presence of a skull fracture or peripherally in the distal branches of the anterior cerebral or cortical arteries. Levy et al.,[40] in a retrospective study, found that 3.2% of the patients who presented with subarachnoid hemorrhage after a gunshot wound to the head harbored an aneurysm. A history of trauma may be easily forthcoming in patients with aneurysm rupture where the cause and effect are actually unrelated.

Epidemiology

Traumatic intracranial aneurysms comprise less than 1% of intracranial aneurysms. Laun's[39] study of 73 traumatic aneurysms showed that 27% were located on the meningeal, 40% on the middle cerebral, and 135 on the anterior cerebral arteries. The time between trauma and diagnosis of aneurysm ranges from a few hours to as long as 10 years, with a mean time of 2 to 3 weeks.

Clinical Manifestations

Most traumatic aneurysms are false aneurysms and become symptomatic several weeks after trauma.[1,12] In aneurysms of the skull base, cranial nerve involvement is not uncommon, with the optic nerve being most frequently involved. Furthermore, carotid injury of the skull base can present with a triad of unilateral blindness, basal skull fracture, and recurrent epistaxis.[43] In children, traumatic aneurysms can present with enlarging skull fractures and tend to be more frequent.[12]

Diagnostic Workup

Since routine angiography is no longer performed for head injuries, a high index of suspicion must exist to warrant a study of the blood vessels. Normally, patients with penetrating injuries and moderate amounts of blood in the brain associated with delayed deterioration should have angiography performed. Patients with sphenoid sinus fractures and massive epistaxis should undergo angiography soon after stabilization. However, angiography performed within hours after the injury may occasionally show no abnormality because the lesions may take time to develop. The literature suggests that angiography should be performed as quickly as possible in cases with both sphenoid sinus lateral wall fractures and massive epistaxis, but screening angiography should be deferred until the third week after trauma in cases with fractures without epistaxis. With the introduction of MRA, this entity may be diagnosed more frequently. In patients who present after several years of progressive headaches and visual loss, angiography can confirm the diagnosis. In current clinical practice, delayed subarachnoid hemorrhage, unexplained neurological deterioration, massive epistaxis, cranial nerve palsy, and unexplained cortical bleeding in patients with head injuries heralds the presence of traumatic aneurysms.

Management

The mortality rate for patients operated on for traumatic aneurysms is between 18% and 22%; patients treated nonsurgically have a higher mortality rate ranging from 41% to 50%.[12] Most traumatic aneurysms require neuroradiological or surgical intervention. The treatment of traumatic aneurysms can be hazardous. If the aneurysm is located in a safe, accessible area, surgical resection is recommended due to the disastrous nature and frequency of the hemorrhage. However, in the case of false aneurysms located deep in the brain or near an eloquent area, more conservative measures have been advocated.[3] Certain skull base aneurysms, particularly those in the cavernous sinus, may be treated with balloon occlusion, but if the carotid cannot be sacrificed, a saphenous vein bypass may be needed. Surgically, these aneurysms tend to be technically more demanding since they are false aneurysms and do not have well-formed necks. Therefore, innovative clipping is required and tandem clips are often used. Another treatment option is endovascular occlusion of the traumatic aneurysm or parent artery.[32] Current treatment of traumatic aneurysms involves occlusion of the main artery using either endovascular or surgical techniques.[67] In patients in whom test occlusion is not tolerated, extracranial to intracranial bypass surgery is the treatment of choice. Literature reviews consistently find that patients fare better with surgical treatment of traumatic aneurysms.

Gomez et al.[28] proposed endovascular treatment for the following subpopulations: (1) patients who cannot be anticoagulated for symptomatic dissection, (2) patients receiving anticoagulation therapy for symptomatic dissection with surgically inaccessible locations (like skull base), and (3) patients with asymptomatic dissection and poor neurological reserve/cerebral collateral circulation.

Endovascular stents, stent-assisted coiling, and covered-stent graft treatment of these posttraumatic lesions have recently been reported.[37]

Traumatic Arteriovenous Fistula

Etiopathology

Anatomically, the cavernous sinus is a plexus of veins through which the carotid artery runs. The arterial branches of the intracavernous carotid artery are the meningohypophyseal trunk, the artery of the inferior cavernous sinus, and the capsular arteries of McConnel. Carotid-cavernous sinus fistulas (CCFs) are anomalous connections between the intracavernous carotid artery, or one of its branches, and the cavernous sinus. When associated with trauma, CCF is usually a high-flow lesion that produces a distinctive clinical syndrome characterized by pulsating exophthalmos and a bruit.[30] Tears at the origin of any of these small vessels can lead to a CCF known as an *indirect* or *low-flow* CCF. The mechanisms include direct injury as a result of skull base fracture, injury due to torsion or stretching of the carotid siphon on impact, or impingement of the vessel on bony prominences. Hemodynamically, direct CCF is differentiated from indirect (low-flow) CCF by a high flow. The cavernous sinus is invested with dura, and any rupture there rarely extends into the subarachnoid space; thus, the likelihood of a catastrophic intracranial hemorrhage is rare. Arteriovenous fistulas in the neck are rare even with close proximity of the great vessels inside the carotid sheath; they seldom result from penetrating injuries.[52]

Epidemiology

The incidence of traumatic arteriovenous fistulas is extremely low. They are usually formed secondary to a depressed skull fracture or penetrating trauma and may be associated with intracranial hematomas. Most commonly, they involve the meningeal vessels, and the middle meningeal artery communicates with one of the meningeal veins.[51]

Clinical Manifestations

The traumatic CCF occurs in younger men and presents mainly with ipsilateral and sometimes bilateral symptoms. Commonly, these include pulsatile headaches, chemosis, hyperlacrimation, proptosis, exophthalmos, and even complete ophthalmoplegia in high-flow fistula. The patient may present with a subjective bruit and decreased vision in the affected eye. Prominent veins on the forehead in the drainage area of the corresponding cavernous sinus are evident. Advanced cases may show corneal ulcerations with painful ophthalmoplegia and progression to secondary glaucoma and phthisis bulbi. A low-flow fistula presents with chronic features of arterialized veins and oculomotor paralysis. Subarachnoid hemorrhage is a rare occurrence, and most CCFs do not cause major neurological deficits or endanger life. Most traumatic CCFs present almost a month after the initial trauma. Posttraumatic vertebral arteriovenous fistulas normally occur in the extradural portion of the vertebral artery and present with tinnitus, vertigo and other features of vertebrobasilar insufficiency.

Diagnostic Workup

As with other cerebrovascular injuries, the diagnosis is confirmed with an arteriogram. Both CT and MRA offer useful diagnostic information and are noninvasive. However, dynamic visualization of the fistulous tract and its topography requires a standard arteriogram. A routine invasive angiogram is both diagnostic and therapeutic in most cases. Retrograde venography via the superior ophthalmic vein for CCF is less invasive than arteriography and is equally effective for therapeutic options.

Management

Traditionally, the management of CCF was surgical and included ligating of the carotid artery or exposing the cavernous sinus and packing the fistula with thrombogenic material. The introduction of endovascular management using balloons revolutionized the treatment of these fistulas, with drastic reductions in morbidity and mortality. The first use of endovascular treatment with balloon catheter to occlude CCF was reported by Prolo and Hanberry.[56] At present, endovascular detachable balloon placement is the standard of care with arterial or venous routes to reach the fistula. Retrograde venography was first reported by Tress et al.[65] Subsequently, several reports described the safety and optimal results of the venous route via the superior ophthalmic vein.[6,45] An occasional case might require open placement of the catheters and balloons with an incision on the upper eyelid to reach the ophthalmic vein.

Prognosis

The natural history of dissections of the intracranial arteries is much more dismal than that of dissections of the cervical carotid and vertebral arteries, which usually resolve spontaneously. Traumatic intracranial aneurysms also carry a high mortality rate. Parkinson and West[54] reported that the mortality is 50% in untreated cases. The prognosis for vertebrobasilar artery injury has come a long way from the time of Matas' description in 1893, when the overall mortality among 20 patients with traumatic vertebral aneurysms was 70%. Mortality from BCI ranges from 12% to 40%.[21,58] A literature review by Unger et al.[66] reported an overall mortality of about 21% in patients with penetrating carotid artery injury. Patients who had arterial repair showed greater improvement than those who had carotid artery ligation (34% versus 14%). Patients presenting with coma, shock, and severe neurological deficits had higher mortality.[42,55,66]

REFERENCES

1. Acosta C, Williams PE Jr, Clark K: Traumatic aneurysms of the cerebral vessels. J Neurosurg 36(5):531–536, 1972.
2. Ahl B, Bokemeyer M, Ennen JC, Kohlmetz C, Becker H, Weissenborn K: Dissection of the brain supplying arteries over the life span. J Neurol Neurosurg Psychiatry 75: 1194–1196, 2004.
3. Amirjamshidi A, Rahmat H, Abbassioun K: Traumatic aneurysms and arteriovenous fistulas of intracranial vessels associated with penetrating head injuries occurring during war: Principles and pitfalls in diagnosis and management. A survey of 31 cases and review of the literature. J Neurosurg 84(5):769–780, 1996.
4. Ausman JI, Diaz FG, Vacca DF, Sadasivan B: Superficial temporal and occipital artery bypass pedicles to superior, anterior inferior, and posterior inferior cerebellar arteries for vertebrobasilar insufficiency. J Neurosurg 72(4): 554–558, 1990.
5. Bagwell CE: Ambroise Paré and the renaissance of surgery. Surg Gynecol Obstet 152(3):350–354, 1981.
6. Baldauf J, Spuler A, Hoch HH, Molsen HP, Kiwit JC, Synowitz M: Embolization of indirect carotid-cavernous sinus fistulas using the superior ophthalmic vein approach. Acta Neurol Scand 110:200–204, 2004.
7. Beaudry M, Spence JD: Motor vehicle accidents: The most common cause of traumatic vertebrobasilar ischemia. Can J Neurol Sci 30(4):320–325, 2003.
8. Beaujeux RL, Reizine DC, Casasco A, Aymard A, Rufenacht D, Khayata MH, Riche MC, Merland JJ: Endovascular treatment of vertebral arteriovenous fistula. Radiology 183(2):361–367, 1992.
9. Berger MS, Wilson CB: Intracranial dissecting aneurysms of the posterior circulation. Report of six cases and review of the literature. J Neurosurg 61(5):882–894, 1984.
10. Biffl WL, Ray CE Jr, Moore EE, Mestek M, Johnson JL, Burch JM: Noninvasive diagnosis of blunt cerebrovascular injuries: A preliminary report. J Trauma 53(5):850–856, 2002.
11. Brandt MM, Kazanjian S, Wahl WL: The utility of endovascular stents in the treatment of blunt arterial injuries. J Trauma 51(5):901–905, 2001.
12. Buckingham MJ, Crone KR, Ball WS, Tomsick TA, Berger TS, Tew JM Jr: Traumatic intracranial aneurysms in childhood: Two cases and a review of the literature. Neurosurgery 22(2):398–408, 1988.
13. Coldwell DM, Novak Z, Ryu RK, Brega KE, Biffl WL, Offner PJ, Franciose RJ, Burch JM, Moore EE: Treatment of posttraumatic internal carotid arterial pseudoaneurysms with endovascular stents. J Trauma 48(3): 470–472, 2000.
14. Cothren CC, Moore EE, Biffl WL, Ciesla DJ, Ray CE Jr, Johnson JL, Moore JB, Burch JM: Anticoagulation is the gold standard therapy for blunt carotid injuries to reduce stroke rate. Arch Surg. 139(5):540–545, 2004.
15. Davis J, Holbrook T, Hoyt D, et al: Blunt carotid artery dissection: Incidence, associated injuries, screening, and treatment. J Trauma 30:1514–1517, 1990.
16. Davis JM, Zimmerman RA: Injury of the carotid and vertebral arteries. Neuroradiology 25(2):55–69, 1983.
17. Davis RP, McGwin G Jr, Melton SM, Reiff DA, Whitley D, Rue LW 3rd: Specific occupant and collision characteristics are associated with motor vehicle collision-related blunt cerebrovascular artery injury. J Trauma 56:64–67, 2004.
18. Duke BJ, Ryu RK, Coldwell DM, Brega KE: Treatment of blunt injury to the carotid artery by using endovascular stents: An early experience. J Neurosurg 87(6):825–829, 1997.
19. du Toit DF, van Schalkwyk GD, Wadee SA, Warren BL: Neurologic outcome after penetrating extracranial arterial trauma. J Vasc Surg 38(2):257–262, 2003.
20. El Gindi S, Salama M, Tawfik E, Aboul Nasr H, El Nadi F: A review of 2,000 patients with craniocerebral injuries with regard to intracranial haematomas and other vascular complications. Acta Neurochir (Wien) 48(3–4):237–244, 1979.
21. Fabian TC, George TC, Croce MA, Mangiante EC, Voeller G, Kudska KA: Carotid artery trauma: Management based on mechanism of injury. J Trauma 30:953–963, 1990.
22. Fabian TC, Patton JH Jr, Croce MA: Blunt carotid injury. Importance of early diagnosis and anticoagulant therapy. Ann Surg 223:513–522, 1996.
23. Fleming D: Case of rupture of the carotid artery and wounds of several of its branches, successfully treated by

tying the common trunk of the carotid itself. Med Chir J Rev 3:2–4, 1817.

24. Fleming JFR, Petrie D: Traumatic thrombosis of the internal carotid artery with delayed hemiplegia. Can J Surg 11:166–172, 1968.
25. Flint LM, Snyder WH, Perry MO, Shires GT: Management of major vascular injuries in the base of the neck. An 11-year experience with 146 cases. Arch Surg 106(4): 407–413, 1973.
26. Fry WR, Dort JA, Smith RS, Sayers DV, Morabito DJ: Duplex scanning replaces arteriography and operative exploration in the diagnosis of potential cervical vascular injury. Am J Surg 168(6):693–695, 1994.
27. Frykberg ER: Advances in the diagnosis and treatment of extremity vascular trauma. Surg Clin North Am 75:207–223, 1995.
28. Gomez CR, May AK, Terry JB: Endovascular therapy of traumatic injuries of the extracranial cerebral arteries. Crit Care Clin 15:789–809, 1999.
29. Guyot LL, Kazmierczak CD, Diaz FG: Vascular injury in neurotrauma. Neurol Res 23(2–3):291–296, 2001.
30. Harris AE, McMenamin PG: Carotid artery–cavernous sinus fistula. Arch Otolaryngol 110(9):618–623, 1984.
31. Herderschee D, Limburg M, Hijdra A, Koster PA: Recombinant tissue plasminogen activator in two patients with basilar artery occlusion. J Neurol Neurosurg Psychiatry 54(1):71–73, 1991.
32. Komiyama M, Nakajima H, Nishikawa M, Yasui T: Endovascular treatment of traumatic aneurysms of the superficial temporal artery. J Trauma 43(3):545–548, 1997.
33. Kral T, Schaller C, Urbach H, Schramm J: Vertebral artery injury after cervical spine trauma: A prospective study. Zentralbl Neurochir 63(4):153–158, 2002.
34. Kumar SR, Weaver FA, Yellin AE: Cervical vascular injuries. Surg Clin North Am 81(6):1331–1356, 2001.
35. Kuzniec S, Kauffman P, Molnar LJ, Aun R, Puech-Leao P: Diagnosis of limbs and neck arterial trauma using duplex ultrasonography. Cardiovasc Surg 6(4):358–366, 1998.
36. Laitt RD, Lewis TT, Bradshaw JR: Blunt carotid arterial trauma. Clin Radiol 51(2):117–122, 1996.
37. Larsen DW: Traumatic vascular injuries and their management. Neurosurg Clin North Am 12:249–269, 2002.
38. Laster RE Jr, Acker JD, Halford HH 3rd, Nauert TC: Assessment of MR angiography versus arteriography for evaluation of cervical carotid bifurcation disease. AJNR 14(3):681–688, 1993.
39. Laun A: Intracranial traumatic aneurysms. Unfallheilkunde 81(7):482–491, 1978.
40. Levy ML, Rezai A, Masri LS, Litofsky SN, Giannotta SL, Apuzzo ML, Weiss MH: The significance of subarachnoid hemorrhage after penetrating craniocerebral injury: Correlations with angiography and outcome in a civilian population. Neurosurgery 32(4):532–540, 1993.
41. Li MS, Smith BM, Espinosa J: Nonpenetrating trauma to the carotid artery. Seven cases and a literature review. J Truama–Inj Infec Crit Care 36: 265–272, 1994.
42. Liekweg WG Jr, Greenfield LJ: Management of penetrating carotid arterial injury. Ann Surg 188:587–592, 1978.
43. Maurer JJ, Mills M, German WJ: Triad of unilateral blindness, orbital fractures and massive epistaxis after head injury. J Neurosurg 18:837–840, 1961.
44. Mayberry JC, Brown CV, Mullins RJ, Velmahos GC: Blunt carotid artery injury. Arch Surg 139: 609–613, 2004.
45. Miller NR, Monsein H, Debrun GM, Tamargo RJ, Nauta HJ: Treatment of carotid-cavernous sinus fistulas using a superior ophthalmic vein approach. J Neurosurg 84:838–842, 1995.
46. Miller PR, Fabian TC, Bee TK, et al: Blunt cerebrovascular injuries: Diagnosis and treatment. J Trauma 51:279–285, 2001.
47. Miller PR, Fabian TC, Croce MA, et al: Prospective screening for blunt cerebrovascular injuries: Analysis of diagnostic modalities and outcomes. Ann Surg 236:386–395, 2002.
48. Mokri B, Piepgras DG, Houser OW: Traumatic dissections of the extracranial internal carotid artery. J Neurosurg 68:189–197, 1988.
49. Mokri B, Sundt TM Jr, Houser OW, Piepgras DG: Spontaneous dissection of the cervical internal carotid artery. Ann Neurol 19(2):126–138, 1986.
50. Morgan MK, Sekhon LH: Extracranial-intracranial saphenous vein bypass for carotid or vertebral artery dissections: A report of six cases. J Neurosurg 80(2):237–246, 1994.
51. Nakamura K, Tsugane R, Ito H, Obata H, Narita H: Traumatic arterio-venous fistula of the middle meningeal vessels. J Neurosurg 25(4):424–429, 1966.
52. Nanda A, Vannemreddy PSSV, Willis BK, Baskaya MK, Jawahar AJ: Management of carotid artery injuries: Louisiana State University Shreveport experience. Surg Neurol 59:184–190, 2003.
53. Pampin BJ, Tamayo MN, Fonseca HR, Payne-James JJ, Jerreat P: Delayed presentation of carotid dissection, cerebral ischemia and infarction following blunt trauma: Two cases. J Clin Forensic Med 9:136–140, 2002.
54. Parkinson D, West M: Traumatic intracranial aneurysms. J Neurosurg 52(1):11–20, 1980.
55. Perry M, Snyder W, Thal E: Carotid artery injuries caused by blunt trauma. Ann Surg 192:74–77, 1980.
56. Prolo DJ, Hanberry JW: Intraluminal occlusion of the carotid-cavernous sinus fistula with a balloon catheter. Technical note. J Neurosurg 35:237–242, 1971.
57. Rich N et al: Vascular Trauma. Philadelphia, WB Saunders, 1978.
58. Rossenwasser R, Delgado T, Bucheit W: Cerebral vascular complications of closed neck and head trauma: Injuries to the carotid artery. Surg Rounds 56–65, 1993.
59. Rubio PA, Reul GJ Jr, Beall AC Jr, Jordan GL Jr, DeBakey ME: Acute carotid artery injury: 25 years' experience. J Trauma 14(11):967–973, 1974.
60. Sampson DS: Cervical carotid injuries. Clin Neurosurg 29:647–656, 1995.
61. Schievink WI: Spontaneous dissection of the carotid and vertebral arteries. N Engl J Med 344: 898–906, 2001.
62. Schievink WI, Limburg M: Dissection of cervical arteries as a cause of cerebral ischemia or cranial nerve dysfunction. Ned Tijdschr Geneeskd 134(38):1843–1848, 1990.

63. Schievink WI, Mokri B, O'Fallon WM: Recurrent spontaneous cervical-artery dissection. N Engl J Med 330(6): 393–397, 1994.
64. Srinivasan J, Newell DW, Sturzenegger M: Transcranial Doppler in the evaluation of internal carotid artery dissection. Stroke 27:1226–1230, 1996.
65. Tress BM, Thomson KR, Klug GL, Mee RR, Crawford B: Management of carotid-cavernous sinus fistulas by surgery combined with interventional radiology. Report of two cases. J Neurosurg 59:1076–1081, 1983.
66. Unger SW, Tucker WS Jr, Mrdeza MA, Wellons HA Jr, Chandler JG: Carotid arterial trauma. Surgery 87: 477–487, 1980.
67. Uzan M, Cantasdemir M, Seckin MS, Hanci M, Kocer N, Sarioglu AC, Islak C: Traumatic intracranial carotid tree aneurysms. Neurosurgery 43(6):1314–1320, 1998.
68. Verneuil M: Contusions multiples: délire violent; hémiplégie á droite, signes de compression cérébrale. Bull Acad Nat Med (Paris) 1:46–56, 1872.
69. Vishteh AG, Marciano FF, David CA, Schievink WI, Zabramski JM, Spetzler RF: Long-term graft patency rates and clinical outcomes after revascularization for symptomatic traumatic internal carotid artery dissection. Neurosurgery 43(4):761–767, 1998.
70. Wahl WL, Brandt MM, Thompson BG, Taheri PA, Greenfield LJ: Antiplatelet therapy: An alternative to heparin for blunt carotid injury. J Trauma 52(5):896–901, 2002.
71. Watridge CB, Muhlbauer MS, Lowery RD: Traumatic carotid artery dissection: Diagnosis and treatment. J Neurosurg 71:854–857, 1989.
72. Willis BK, Greiner F, Orrison WW, Benzel EC: The incidence of vertebral artery injury after midcervical spine fracture or subluxation. Neurosurgery 34(3):435–441, 1994.

Chapter 10
Medical Complications of Head Injury

JOSEPH L. VOELKER
AND ALISON M. WILSON

A significant part of the morbidity produced by cerebral injury comes in the form of medical complications. The brain, through autonomic, hormonal, and biochemical mechanisms, influences most of the body's organ systems. This finely tuned control may be markedly disrupted by trauma to the central regulatory areas. In caring for head-injured patients, it is important that the resulting derangements in organ system function be recognized and treated. This chapter presents an overview of several medical complications that may develop following head injury.

Cardiovascular Effects of Head Injury

Following severe head trauma, patients exhibit signs of sympathetic hyperactivity. The resulting cardiovascular changes include hypertension, tachycardia, increased cardiac index, and decreased peripheral vascular resistance. Unlike essential hypertension, the blood pressure may be quite labile, with varying cardiac output and vascular resistance. Elevated levels of plasma norepinephrine (NE) have been found in this group.[13,14,53,81] The degree of NE elevation is proportional to the severity of head injury as measured by the Glasgow Coma Scale (GCS) score.[14]

The elevated sympathetic neuronal activity can result in a variety of electrocardiographic (ECG) abnormalities following head injury, especially if there is raised intracranial pressure (ICP). These include prominent U waves, ST-T segment changes, notched T waves, inverted T waves, and shortening and prolongation of Q-T intervals.[14,34] Supraventricular tachycardia is the most common arrhythmia associated with trauma to the brain and is also related to sympathetic overactivity.[18,90]

Subendocardial hemorrhages are found in up to 50% of severely head-injured patients undergoing autopsy, again related to a sympathetically mediated hyperdynamic state.[13,18,53] The myocardial injury can occur in the absence of coronary artery disease and produces typical ischemic ECG changes and elevation of cardiac enzymes. Some patients do not survive the cardiac ischemia.[53] Reversible myocardial contractile dysfunction (stunned myocardium) has also been seen after head trauma.[82]

Beta-adrenergic receptor blockage can prevent or ameliorate myocardial injury in this setting. Treating brain trauma patients with the $beta_1$-selective agent atenolol was shown to prevent myocardial necrosis and reduced the incidence of supraventricular tachycardia.[18] Propranolol has been successfully used to treat hypertension in this group.[74] Sedation or analgesia may control mild, transient blood pressure elevation. Vasodilating drugs such as hydralazine and nitroprusside should be used with caution, as they may increase the ICP.[16,74]

Before manipulating the blood pressure in these patients, it is important to remember that a disturbance in cerebral autoregulation has been demonstrated to occur after head injury.[19,74] As a result, the cerebral blood flow (CBF) will vary directly with the mean arterial pressure (MAP), and a drop in cerebral perfusion pressure (CPP)—where CPP = MAP − ICP—can produce cerebral ischemia. The current recommendation calls for maintaining the CPP > 70 mm Hg.[64,78] Elevated ICP should be treated before blood pressure control is begun, and control of arterial hypertension is generally necessary only when the systolic pressure approaches 180 to 200 torr or signs of cardiac ischemia occur. In addition, recent studies have shown that elevated blood pressure may exacerbate intracranial hypertension and worsen the outcome.[19,64]

Systemic hypotension is frequently found in victims of multiple trauma with concurrent cerebral injury. This is most commonly due to blood loss and hypovolemia. In a small percentage of patients the hypotension may have a neurogenic cause.[10] Hypotension is the single most important cause of secondary brain insult in this group, and an episode of hypotension doubles the mortality of a patient with severe head injury.[11] Hypotension should be prevented or rapidly corrected with fluids and, if necessary, inotropic agents. The patient should be kept euvolemic and seen by the trauma surgeon to rule out ongoing hemorrhage as a cause for the hypotension.

Respiratory System Complications of Head Injury

Respiratory dysfunction is common after head injury. Potential problems include neurogenic pulmonary edema (NPE), hypoxemia, hypocarbia, nosocomial pneumonia, pulmonary embolism, and aspiration. Additionally, the head-injured patient may have sustained direct chest trauma. Although pulmonary complications are not independent predictors of worsened outcomes, patients with these disorders do tend to have poorer clinical outcomes.[25]

Neurogenic pulmonary edema is a variant of the adult respiratory distress syndrome (ARDS). It has been reported to occur in 32% of those who die at the scene of an accident and in up to 50% of those who die in the first 96 hours.[75] Neurogenic pulmonary edema most often presents in the initial 4 hours following injury[24] but may be delayed for 12 hours to several days. Typical clinical findings include dyspnea and tachypnea, hypoxemia, decreased pulmonary compliance, and an ARDS-like pattern of *fluffy* infiltrates on chest roentgenograms. Usually NPE is self-limited and resolves over hours to days.

Neurogenic pulmonary edema has also been seen in many other pathological central nervous system conditions. The common anatomical locus of damage is the brain stem. The areas most likely associated with NPE include the A1 and A5 areas in the medulla, the nucleus tractus solitarius, the area postrema, the vagal nuclei, and the hypothalamus.[15]

Multiple mechanisms may cause NPE after brain injury. Catecholamines released due to hypothalamic stress result in myocardial depression and dysfunction, adding to the hydrostatic pressure injury in the pulmonary capillaries.[50] Use of inotropes such as dobutamine can improve cardiac function and decrease pulmonary vascular resistance.[20]

Early hypoxemia may occur in a significant number of severely head-injured patients. Although hypoxemia is dangerous at any time, its presence in the prehospital setting has been found to be associated with increased mortality and poorer recovery in survivors.[11] In many head-injured patients, concurrent chest trauma is responsible for the hypoxia.

Treatment of these pulmonary complications is mainly supportive. Adequacy of the airway must be ensured; any head-injured patient with a GCS score ≤8 should be endotracheally intubated as soon as possible. Supplemental oxygen should be administered early to combat the hypoxemia and prevent secondary brain insult. If hypoxemia persists, positive-pressure mechanical ventilation must be instituted. Positive end-expiratory pressure (PEEP) may be used as necessary. Although it is unclear whether levels of PEEP ≤20 cm H_2O in mechanically ventilated head-injured patients deleteriously affect ICP, ICP monitoring is generally recommended if the level of PEEP exceeds 10 cm H_2O.

Other pulmonary complications of head trauma include aspiration and pneumonia. Pulmonary infections are a major source of morbidity and the most common infectious complication in cerebral injury. In the severely head-injured patient requiring long-term mechanical ventilation, the incidence of pneumonia has been reported to be 35% to 70%, with up to 50% mortality. In addition to the usual risk factors for pneumonia in intensive care unit (ICU) patients, such as impaired airway reflexes, aspiration, and more than 24 hours of ventilatory support, head-injured patients having ICP monitoring or receiving barbiturates or steroid therapy for intracranial hypertension are at additional risk.[46,92] Treatment still relies upon early diagnosis, prompt identification of the pathogen, and vigorous treatment.

Deep Vein Thrombosis and Pulmonary Embolus

Deep vein thrombosis (DVT) and pulmonary embolus (PE) can be devastating complications in head-injured patients. This population often has risk factors such as coagulation abnormalities, immobility, trauma to the pelvis or legs, age over 40 years, and obesity.[30] As a result, those sustaining brain trauma are considered to be at high risk for DVT and PE.[76] The incidence of DVT is estimated to be approximately 15%, with a 1% to 3% rate of fatal PE.[94] The majority of DVTs develop within the first 2 weeks following injury; however, they may continue to occur during periods of prolonged immobility.[94]

Preventative Therapy

The best strategy in treating such patients is immediate prophylaxis, either mechanical or pharmacological. The most efficacious mechanical method seems to be intermittent external pneumatic compression (IPC) of the calf, which is thought to work via local and systemic fibrinolysis.[30,89] For patients with extremity fractures in whom IPC cannot be used, foot pumps may be an alternative for mechanical prophylaxis.[84]

Pharmacological prophylaxis involves the use of anticoagulants to stop the propagation of clots, but it has been thought to be problematic in this group because of the risk of intracranial hemorrhage. The use of prophylactic low-dose subcutaneous heparin after craniotomy has been shown to produce no increase in postoperative complications or bleeding.[49] In another report, the use of unfractionated heparin within the first 72 hours following traumatic brain injury did not cause an increase in intracranial bleeding or deterioration on the neurological exam.[40] Early results from a study evaluating enoxaparin, a low molecular weight heparin, after intracranial injuries suggest that it is safe if employed 24 hours after admission or craniotomy.[63] Although it appears that low molecular weight heparin may be effective and safe,[30] it must be noted that further data are required since large, prospective studies are not yet available.

There is still controversy about when to start anticoagulation after traumatic brain injury, and practices vary from 24 hours to 14 days. In very-high-risk situations or when anticoagulation is contraindicated, an inferior vena cava (IVC) filter may be employed.[76] Prophylactic IVC filters have been shown to have a low complication rate and offer up to 99% protection from fatal PE.[45] Failure has been associated with filter tilt of 14 degrees or more or the presence of strut malfunction.[77]

Deep Vein Thrombosis

Unfortunately, even with prophylaxis, DVT may develop. It is important to remember that the chance of developing PE is 40% to 50% if the thrombus arises in or proximal to the popliteal vein. In addition, DVT is often clinically silent.[61] A high index of suspicion is mandatory. Some institutions use periodic screening for DVT in the ICU. Unfortunately, the use of the D-dimer assay has not been found to be predictive in the setting of head injury.[56] The most common test currently used to detect proximal thrombosis is Doppler ultrasonography with B-mode imaging.

If DVT arises early after head trauma while anticoagulation is contraindicated, an IVC filter should be placed. Although associated with risks related to insertion, failure, and thrombosis,[2] these devices have been used with success.[47] Anticoagulants should be added as soon as it is safe in order to minimize thrombosis. If the DVT occurs after 10 to 14 days, the usual anticoagulation treatment with heparin and warfarin can be started and continued for 3 months.

Pulmonary Embolus

The main problem with DVT is that it leads to PE, many cases of which may be silent.[61] Sudden hypoxia or cardiovascular collapse may be the only sign. If there is any question that a PE has occurred, a vigorous attempt should be made to confirm the diagnosis. The ventilation/perfusion scan is difficult to perform in the ICU and is inaccurate in the presence of other lung pathologies such as atelectasis or pneumonia, which a majority of these patients will have. The gold standard has been pulmonary arteriography, but computed tomography (CT) of the chest with PE protocol is being used increasingly. As this technology is becoming more advanced, even small emboli in the tertiary, pulmonary vasculature can be detected. If the scan shows a PE, the patient should be treated with an IVC filter or with anticoagulation.[67]

Coagulopathy

Hemostasis

Hemostasis consists of the local control of bleeding resulting from three interacting systems—the vessel wall, the clotting factors, and the platelets. Injury to tissue releases into the bloodstream phospholipoproteins that activate clotting factors. Clotting mechanisms and platelets can also be activated by exposure to vessel walls damaged by hypoxia, acidosis, or shock and denuded of endothelium. There is a parallel set of mechanisms to limit the process and preserve the patency of the general circulation. The result is a dynamic balance between coagulation and anticoagulation.[26,35,38]

Disseminated Intravascular Coagulation

A variety of disease processes can produce such marked activation of the coagulation system that the normal feedback control mechanisms are overwhelmed, and disseminated intravascular coagulation (DIC) results.[6] Excessive fibrin clot is formed systemically in affected patients, leading to thrombosis of large and small vessels, ischemia, and end-organ damage. Platelets are trapped in the partially occluded microcirculation, causing thrombocytopenia, and erythrocytes are damaged, producing a microangiopathic hemolytic anemia. Bleeding results from thrombocytopenia, depletion of clotting factors, and the formation of fibrin(ogen) degradation products (FDP) that interfere with both clot formation and platelet function. In addition, complement activation and kinin generation increase vascular permeability, leading to hypotension and shock.

Approximately 10% to 35% of head-injured patients develop a coagulopathy, and there is evidence of DIC in 8% of all brain trauma victims and in up to 40% of those severely injured.[8b,68,80,85] The brain is a rich source of tissue thromboplastin, and its release into the general circulation following trauma incites the coagulation disorder.[26,38,90] There is evidence of systemic coagulation and platelet activation in most patients after cerebral trauma.[35,38,80] Also, petechial hemorrhages due to thrombosis followed by clot lysis and hemorrhage are often present in the brains and spinal cords of these patients.[68] When searched for, intravascular fibrin microthrombi are a frequent finding in injured brain tissue.[38,85] The increase in circulating catecholamines following head injury further enhances platelet reactivity. The severity of abnormal hemostasis correlates with the extent of brain injury, as well as with survivability and outcome.[65,68] The peak occurrence of coagulopathy is during the first 2 to 4 days following injury.[68] Delayed traumatic intracranial hematomas occur in 8% or more of severely head-injured patients, and coagulopathy is a primary cause.[37]

Diagnosis

The symptoms and signs of DIC are variable but include petechiae, purpura, wound bleeding, oozing from venipuncture sites or intra-arterial lines, and subcutaneous hematomas.[6] Fever, hypotension, acidosis, proteinuria, and hypoxia may be seen. The laboratory criteria are evidence of procoagulant activity, fibrinolytic activation, inhibitor consumption, and end-organ damage or failure.[6] The prothrombin time, activated partial thromboplastin time, and thrombin time are nonspecific and not consistently altered in DIC. Of the commonly available tests, the D-dimer assay is the most reliable, being abnormal in 93% of DIC patients.[6] Other reliable tests include prothrombin fragment 1+2, antithrombin III level, fibrinogen A level, and FDP titer. The platelet count may be decreased in DIC, but the range is quite variable. Tests of platelet function are more commonly abnormal due to

FDP coating of platelet membranes.[6] End-organ damage can be inferred from an elevated lactate dehydrogenase (LDH) or creatinine level or from a decreased pH or PaO_2. Various DIC scores can be calculated to aid in diagnosis.[6,65]

Treatment

It is uncertain if treating DIC can improve the patient's outcome since the coagulopathy may be a reflection of the severity of injury, which is irreversible. Since patients who develop DIC are at risk for hemorrhagic and ischemic complications and have poorer outcomes, however, it seems reasonable to treat the condition aggressively. General supportive care with correction of acidosis, hypotension, and hypovolemia is important.[90] Clotting factors are replaced with fresh frozen plasma and cryoprecipitate. Platelet transfusions may be necessary. Heparin has been used in cases of protracted DIC but probably has no role in head trauma. Low molecular weight heparin has been shown to lessen the pathological effects of brain injury in experimental animals.[85] Activated protein C reduced the mortality rate in a study of sepsis-related DIC.[91]

Water and Electrolyte Balance

Over one-half of the total body weight in normal adults is made up of water. In young men, total body water accounts for 60% of body weight, and in young women 52%.[1b,57] In the elderly, the amount of body water is about 6% lower. Two-thirds of the water is intracellular and the remainder is extracellular. The extracellular fluid can be subdivided into the interstitial fluid and the plasma volume, which is about 3 l for a 70-kg man. Approximately 98% of the body's potassium is intracellular, where it is the principal cation. The main intracellular anions are organic acids, phosphate, and sulfate. Ninety-five percent of sodium, however, is extracellular, and it is the predominant extracellular cation. Chloride is the main extracellular anion.

Syndrome of Inappropriate Antidiuretic Hormone Secretion

Electrolyte abnormalities occur in nearly 60% of those with severe head injury.[68] Hyponatremia is the most common electrolyte derangement in these patients, and is often caused by the syndrome of inappropriate antidiuretic hormone secretion (SIADH) with an incidence of 5% to 12%.[1b] Trauma-related stress leads to the release of antidiuretic hormone (ADH) and aldosterone. Elevated ICP and positive-pressure ventilation can also stimulate ADH release.[57,90] Antidiuretic hormone increases the urine concentration by augmenting the reabsorption of water in the renal distal tubules and collecting ducts. In patients with SIADH, a dilutional hyponatremia develops due to an expanded extracellular fluid volume.

The occurrence of symptoms is related both to the level of hyponatremia and to the rate at which it develops.[57] Mild hyponatremia may produce lethargy, confusion, fatigue, anorexia, nausea, vomiting, muscle cramps, and loss of muscle stretch reflexes. A more marked drop in serum sodium can result in hypothermia, seizures, Cheyne-Stokes respiration, stupor, and coma, leading ultimately to death in the most severe cases.

The diagnosis is made by identifying a low serum sodium (<135 mmol/l), a low serum osmolarity (<280 mOsm/l), inappropriately high urine sodium (>20 mmol/l), urine osmolarity greater than serum osmolarity, and normal renal, adrenal, and thyroid function, as well as by the absence of cirrhosis, congestive heart failure, peripheral edema, or dehydration.[32,57]

Mild to moderate hyponatremia can be successfully treated with fluid restriction to 800–1000 ml/day. More severely depressed sodium values below 115 mmol/l may require 3% saline infusion. The hyponatremia must not be corrected too rapidly, however, as this may result in the osmotic demyelination syndrome with central pontine myelinolysis. This occurs more commonly in cases of chronic hyponatremia, and a sudden rise in serum osmolarity may be more important than changes in the sodium level.[72] The serum sodium should not be increased by more than 12 mmol/l per 24 hours.[87] Chronic or refractory cases of SIADH may occasionally be seen. Oral demeclocycline blocks the effect of ADH on the kidney tubule, producing a reversible partial nephrogenic diabetes insipidus.[9,27] It can be effective in the chronic management of SIADH at doses of 600–1200 mg/day. Mineralocorticoids such as fludrocortisone can also be used to treat this condition.[1b,90]

Cerebral Salt Wasting

Cerebral salt wasting (CSW) is another important cause of hyponatremia in the head trauma population. In fact, it may occur as frequently as or even more frequently than SIADH.[33,62] The principal features are a renal loss of sodium with a decreased extracellular fluid volume and hypovolemia. These patients may exhibit orthostatic hypotension, tachycardia, dry mucous membranes, skin tenting, and flat neck veins. The pathophysiological mechanism of CSW is unknown. The brain injury may result in decreased sympathetic output to the kidneys.[32] Alternatively, faulty cerebral regulation of atrial natriuretic peptide or brain natriuretic peptide may play a role.[32] Treatment involves correcting the hypovolemia with intravenous fluids and replenishing the body's sodium stores. Depending on the severity of hyponatremia, this can be accomplished with intravenous 0.9% saline, 3% saline, or enteral salt.

The differential diagnosis between these two causes of hyponatremia is important because the treatment of SIADH (fluid restriction) is the opposite of the treatment of CSW (rehydration with normal saline). Both conditions may result in similar changes in serum sodium level, serum osmolarity, urine osmolarity, and urine sodium levels. The main distinguishing feature is the patient's volume status: euvolemia to slight hypervolemia in SIADH and hypovolemia in CSW. Evidence in favor of CSW includes weight loss, a negative fluid balance, a low central venous pressure, or a low pulmonary capillary wedge pressure. Elevations of the hematocrit, the blood urea nitrogen:creatinine ratio, and the serum protein concentration suggest dehydration related to CSW. The serum uric acid is usually normal in CSW but is decreased in SIADH. Isotope-dilution studies of plasma volume can be performed at the bedside.[33]

Other Electrolyte Abnormalities

Hypernatremia may develop in persons sustaining head trauma. Treatment of increased ICP with mannitol or furosemide promotes diuresis and may iatrogenically elevate the serum sodium level. There may be excessive insensible water loss in patients who are mechanically ventilated, have a tracheostomy, or are febrile. Hypernatremia may also result from traumatic diabetes insipidus (DI) or from the use of high-calorie, hyperosmolar, or high-salt enteral tube feedings. Phenytoin is often given to this group of patients as seizure prophylaxis. It inhibits ADH release but may worsen hypernatremia. Correcting the free water deficit with intravenous 5% dextrose in water or increased oral intake will lower the sodium level.

Hypokalemia is frequently seen in patients with cerebral injury. In a group of 18 severely head-injured patients, moderate hypokalemia developed in 8 and severe hypokalemia (<3.0 mmol/l) in 4.[69] The stress-related aldosterone release promotes renal potassium excretion, as can therapeutic use of corticosteroids, diuretics, or mannitol. The large catecholamine discharge produced by severe head injury can lead to hypokalemia.[70] Treatment of increased ICP with hyperventilation results in respiratory alkalosis with movement of potassium ions into cells and decreased plasma levels. Excessive gastrointestinal losses, insulin therapy, hypomagnesemia, and certain antibiotics (amphotericin B, gentamicin, and penicillin derivatives) may also lower serum potassium.[83] Symptoms may occur when the potassium level falls below 3 mmol/l and include fatigue, muscle weakness, ECG changes, and arrhythmias. Treatment is performed with small intravenous boluses of potassium chloride or oral replacement. Hyperkalemia occurs less often but may be associated with renal failure or metabolic acidosis.

Extensive blood transfusion can result in hypocalcemia due to citrate chelation. Alkalosis, hypomagnesemia, pancreatitis, and sepsis are other possible etiologies.[1b] Correction can be accomplished with intravenous calcium chloride or calcium gluconate, or with oral supplementation in less severe cases. Hypercalcemia is less common but may occur secondary to prolonged immobilization in a comatose patient, renal failure, or excessive calcium replacement.

Hypomagnesemia is frequently associated with both hypokalemia and hypocalcemia.[69] Increased renal excretion from traumatic DI, mannitol, or diuretics can lead to hypomagnesemia.[1b] Other causes include sepsis, alkalosis, and aminoglycoside antibiotics. It is more common in malnourished or alcoholic individuals. Normal levels can be restored with intravenous magnesium sulfate or oral replacement. Associated hypokalemia or hypocalcemia should be corrected simultaneously.

Increased urinary loss of phosphate due to diuretics or hypomagnesemia can produce hypophosphatemia.[1b] Prolonged hyperventilation to treat elevated ICP leads to respiratory alkalosis, intracellular shifts of phosphate, and lowered serum levels. Corticosteroids and phosphate-binding antacids are also associated with hypophosphatemia. Phosphate can be replaced intravenously or orally.

Hypothalamic and Pituitary Dysfunction

Pathophysiology

Head trauma results in physiological stress and provokes an increase in serum cortisol due to an elevated adrenocorticotropic hormone (ACTH) release. Most patients with a significant head injury have an abnormal diurnal cortisol pattern.[42,86] There is diminished or absent feedback regulation of cortisol upon ACTH release. The resulting elevation in steroid levels contributes to the negative nitrogen balance in these patients.[42,71]

Traumatic injury to the hypothalamus and pituitary is seen in up to 60% of severe, fatal head injuries.[17,44,71] Areas of petechial hemorrhage are found in the anterior hypothalamic nuclei and the mammillary bodies. They are due to transmitted forces from the impact to the head, the effects of increased ICP, or traumatic vasospasm. Pathological examination of the pituitary reveals areas of hemorrhage in the neurohypophysis and anterior lobe infarction caused by shearing stresses that compress or disrupt the pituitary stalk and interrupt the hypothalamic-hypophyseal portal vessels.[31] These injuries can be demonstrated clinically with magnetic resonance imaging.[52]

Diabetes Insipidus

Posttraumatic DI is seen in less than 2% of severely head-injured patients, probably because a brain injury sufficiently severe to damage the hypothalamus and pituitary is usually fatal.[1b,44] It results from injury to the hypothalamus, pituitary stalk, or neurohypophysis and is more likely to be found if there are fractures adjacent to the sella turcica.[90] The hallmarks of this condition are polyuria and polydipsia. In the adult, the urine output increases to over 200 ml/hr up to 10–15 l/day, and hypernatremia can quickly occur.[1b] The urine is hypo-osmolar with respect to plasma, and the specific gravity is below 1.005. Such a rapid volume loss can lead to hypotension with an adverse effect on the cerebral perfusion pressure (CPP).[71]

Diabetes insipidus may be partial or transient, and the alert patient with an intact thirst mechanism can increase oral free water intake and maintain normal hydration.[1a] In the stuporous or comatose patient, urinary losses should be replaced intravenously with 5% dextrose in water, with careful attention to the overall fluid balance. Aqueous pitressin is a short-acting agent that may be used early in the course of treatment when it is unclear if the DI is transient or will be prolonged. Permanent DI is controlled more effectively by intravenous or intranasal administration of desmopressin acetate (DDAVP). Patients sustaining a mild closed head injury can develop subclinical, partial DI that may be related to the postconcussion syndrome.[7]

Hypopituitarism

Complete panhypopituitarism occurs less frequently than DI because a large proportion of the adenohypophysis must be destroyed to produce clinical symptoms.[31,44] Although hemorrhagic or ischemic pituitary infarction is found in up to 45% of fatal head injuries, a significant part of the anterior gland may remain intact.[31,41] A portion of the gland can survive even complete transaction of the pituitary stalk.[44] In some cases, hypothalamic injury may be responsible for the hypopituitarism due to an insufficiency of releasing factors.[71]

Partial hypopituitarism occurs more frequently than was previously realized and may develop in 30% to 80% of head trauma survivors.[21] The gonadotrophic and somatotrophic cells are the most sensitive to trauma, and hypogonadism and growth hormone deficiency are the most common abnormalities.[5,39] Any of the anterior pituitary hormones can be affected, but may produce only subtle symptoms that evade detection for months or years.[5,39,48] Thyroid-stimulating hormone and ACTH insufficiency may conceal coexistent DI, which then manifests itself when glucocorticoid replacement is begun.[71]

Metabolic Physiology, Pathophysiology, and Management

The outcome from trauma is dependent upon the ability of the body to sustain itself and recover from the damage of the injury. To accomplish this, a variety of protective responses occur in its metabolic physiology to facilitate an optimal milieu for cellular and organ reconstitution and function. When reviewing general metabolism, the most important aspects to consider are energy and protein metabolism, although fats, minerals, and vitamins are also relevant. Normal metabolism, metabolic changes due to trauma and specifically head injury, evaluation of nutritional status, and nutritional support will be discussed.

Normal Metabolism

The human body is made up of organic material, minerals, and water. There is a large reserve of fat, a minimal reserve of carbohydrate, and a modest reserve of protein. There is also a modest reserve of potassium but only a limited reserve of sodium. The brain uses 25% of the energy of basal metabolism. Some tissues, especially nervous tissue and red blood cells, rely on glucose as their main source of energy, whereas the rest use nonesterified fatty acids or their oxidation products—acetoacetate or hydroxybutyrate (ketone bodies). Energy is produced by oxidation, and if there is insufficient oxygen, the process stops with the production of lactate, which is inefficient.[79]

Metabolic Homeostasis in Injury

Following trauma, the local injury initially stimulates an inflammatory reaction that causes edema and depression of local metabolism. However, this reaction is soon replaced by a generalized increase in metabolism resulting from elevated sympathetic activity with mobilization of carbohydrate and fat stores. After a short period, muscle protein catabolism begins. The purpose of these metabolic responses is to promote survival and healing. It is an obligatory process that cannot be suppressed by even large intakes of calories and protein. In extreme cases, depletion of protein can lead to muscle wasting and poor wound healing. If the injury is not overwhelming and sufficient nutrients are supplied, however, adaptation will occur. A reduction in protein catabolism and glucose utilization are subsequently seen. There is increased lipolysis, and the liver forms more ketone bodies. The brain also adjusts and can obtain as much as half of its energy requirements from ketone bodies.

Concomitant problems and complications may exacerbate the situation. Fever raises the energy expenditure 13% for each 1°C increase. Hypoxia, shock, or infection may occur, and surgery may be required.

Metabolic Pathophysiology in Head Injury

It is evident that brain injury stimulates tremendous changes in metabolism that are inversely related to the GCS score and may persist throughout the duration of the coma. Autonomic and endocrine alterations occur, producing an increase in circulating catecholamines, steroids, insulin, and glucagon. Elevated cardiac output, hyperventilation, fever, restlessness, posturing, seizures, and secondary infections can cause additional metabolic demands. Head-injured patients may have a 120% to 200% rise in resting energy expenditure and twice the normal oxygen consumption. Catabolism of endogenous protein leads to depletion of lean body mass and excretion of large amounts of nitrogen.[79,97]

Nutritional Support and Assessment

Adequate nutrition is commonly recognized as a crucial aspect of critical care. Appropriate nutritional support has been shown clinically and experimentally to improve the outcome and decrease complications, particularly infections.[88] Nutritional support may be delivered enterally or parenterally. Much debate continues over the preferred route and timing. Enteral feeding is less expensive and is associated with decreased infectious complications, improved gastric protection, and a better clinical outcome.[43,93] Additionally, since the gut may be important in the development of multiple organ failure syndrome, early institution of enteral feeding may decrease infectious complications in these patients, particularly pneumonia.[60] There are concerns about delayed gastric emptying following head trauma,[36] and pro-kinetic agents have failed to show a benefit in the brain-injured patient.[51] The optimal delivery systems—intragastric versus postpyloric—continue to be debated, but both appear to be equally efficacious.[43,88] To help decrease the risk of aspiration, appropriate patient positioning is important in all cases of enteral feeding. If enteral feeding cannot be tolerated, then total parenteral nutrition should be considered, although it carries a risk and is expensive.[28] There are significant data to support early nutritional support, whether enteral or parenteral, and all victims of head injury should receive full nutrition within the first 7 days.[58,88] Some nutrients, such as zinc, copper, and glutamine, may be particularly important.[66,96]

Calories should be delivered in sufficient quantities to obtain efficient utilization of the protein and should equal the daily metabolic expenditure, as calculated or measured by indirect calorimetry. Another method of estimating caloric requirements involves giving them in a fixed ratio to the protein intake using a calorie:nitrogen ratio of approximately 150:1. The goal of the nutritional regimen should be to provide nutrients in sufficient quantities to minimize losses, rather than to achieve positive nitrogen balance, for in the acute phase after injury this may be neither possible nor desirable.[79]

Protein requirements can be calculated by a ratio to the estimated caloric intake (1 g nitrogen/150 kcal), by using established tables (for adults, 1.3 to 3.0 g protein/kg), or by monitoring the excretion of nitrogen or urea.[54] Because of glucose intolerance, perhaps more than half of these calories should be from fat initially, with the proportion decreasing over time.[79] Overfeeding can cause hyperglycemia, uremia, and increased production of CO_2, which can compromise respiratory function, often already a problem in the head-injured patient. Additional research is needed to define the optimum protein and calorie needs for these patients.

Nutritional assessment may be carried out using a standard battery of biochemical, immunological, and hematological tests. Various plasma proteins can help determine the visceral protein status. Proteins with long half-lives, such as albumin (20 days), may help reveal the baseline nutritional and visceral protein status, whereas shorter half-life proteins, such as transferrin (8 days), thyroxine-binding prealbumin (24 hours), and retinol-binding protein (12 hours), can help define acute changes. The 24-hour urine nitrogen excretion and urea can demonstrate the nitrogen balance. The presence of anergy can be disclosed by skin antigen testing or a total lymphocyte count.

Despite the provision of energy, amino acids, and other essential nutrients, it may not be possible to compensate for hypermetabolism and endogenous protein breakdown. Therefore, other strategies such as alteration of the stress response, provision of specific fuels, and administration of growth factors are being studied as methods of treating adverse metabolic responses to trauma.[95,97]

Gastrointestinal Complications of Head Injury

A primary concern in evaluating any severely head-injured patient is the determination of trauma to other systems, particularly the intra-abdominal organs. Early in the resuscitation and management process, a trauma surgeon should evaluate the patient and, as indicated, perform a diagnostic peritoneal lavage or CT scan of the abdomen to evaluate for intra-abdominal bleeding or organ injury. Identification and management of these injuries are important, as they can be responsible for continued blood loss and hypotension.

Gastrointestinal bleeding can be a devastating complication of critical illness. Prior to the advent and widespread use of prophylaxis, upper gastrointestinal bleeding in the ICU had an incidence of up to 75%.[29] Administration of prophylactic agents and the provision of adequate nutrition have decreased the incidence to approximately 2% to 4%.[99] Head injury has been shown to be an independent risk factor for gastric stress erosions.[8a] Other prominent risk factors include the presence of hypotension or septicemia.[59] Endoscopic methods of treatment and aggressive medical therapy can treat the majority of these episodes. Despite aggressive prophylaxis, some patients will require surgical intervention, for which both brain and spinal cord injury are risk factors.[98] Many of these patients will have had a herald bleed approximately 1 week previously.[99]

The optimal type of prophylaxis has been debated. Since these lesions have been associated with hyperacidity, preventative treatment with antacids or H_2 blockers is often instituted. H_2 blockers are effective in decreasing the incidence of upper gastrointestinal bleeding.[55,73] There is also evidence that ranitidine, an H_2 blocker, improves lymphocyte function.[73] However, there are data to suggest that neutralization of gastric pH allows bacterial overgrowth to occur and may be a causative factor in the development of pneumonia. For this reason, some institutions prefer sucralfate, a topically active agent that does not alter the gastric pH.[22] Although many studies exist, none show any medication to be superior when rate of bleeding, pneumonia, additional risk factors, and cost are evaluated. Proton pump inhibitors are becoming increasingly used and appear to be superior to H_2 blockers. However, large prospective studies comparing them to other forms of prophylaxis are not yet available.

Another recently recognized but important entity is abdominal compartment syndrome (ACS). This has been shown clinically and experimentally to be associated with multisystem organ failure and increased mortality.[4] An intra-abdominal pressure greater than 20 mm Hg is considered significant, and a pressure greater than 30 mm Hg requires intervention. Intra-abdominal pressures are determined by measuring the bladder pressure. Abdominal compartment syndrome can result from intra-abdominal injury but can also occur secondary to resuscitation. In trauma patients, the requirement of 10 l or more of fluid in the first 24 hours is an independent risk factor.[3] Elevated intra-abdominal pressure and ACS have been shown to increase the ICP.[12,23] The mechanism is thought to be transmission of pressure through the central venous system to the cerebrospinal fluid. Abdominal compartment syndrome has been proven to be an important entity in the critically ill but is probably still underrecognized.

REFERENCES

1a. Agha A. Thornton E, O'Kelly P, et al: Posterior pituitary dysfunction after traumatic brain injury. J Clin Endocrinol Metab 89:5987–5992, 2004.

1b. Andrews BT: Fluid and electrolyte disorders in neurosurgical intensive care. Neurosurg Clin North Am 5:707–723, 1994.

2. Athanasoulis CA: Complications of vena cava filters. Radiology 188:614–615, 1993.

3. Balogh Z, McKinley BA, Cocanour CS, et al: Supranormal trauma resuscitation causes more cases of abdominal compartment syndrome. Arch Surg 138:637–642, 2003.

4. Balogh Z, McKinley BA, Holcomb JB, et al: Both primary and secondary abdominal compartment syndrome can be predicted early and are harbingers of multiple organ failure. J Trauma 54:848–859, 2003.

5. Benvenga S, Campenni A, Ruggeri RM, et al: Clinical review 113: Hypopituitarism secondary to head trauma. J Clin Endocrinol Metab 85:1353–1361, 2000.

6. Bick RL: Disseminated intravascular coagulation: Current concepts of etiology, pathophysiology, diagnosis, and treatment. Hematol Oncol Clin North Am 17:149–176, 2003.

7. Bohnen N, Twijnstra A, Jolles J: Water metabolism and postconcussional symptoms 5 weeks after mild head injury. Eur Neurol 33:77–79, 1993.

8a. Brown TH, Davidson PF, Larson GM: Acute gastritis occurring within 24 hours of severe head injury. Gastrointest Endosc 35:37–40, 1989.

8b. Carrick MM, Tyroch AH, Youens CA et al: Subsequent development of thrombocytopenia and coagulopathy in moderate and severe head injury: support for serial laboratory examination. J Trauma 58:725–730, 2005.

9. Cherrill DA, Stote RM, Birge JR, et al: Demeclocycline treatment in the syndrome of inappropriate antidiuretic hormone secretion. Ann Intern Med 83:654–656, 1975.

10. Chesnut RM, Gautille T, Blunt BA, et al: Neurogenic hypotension in patients with severe head injuries. J Trauma 44:958–964, 1998.

11. Chesnut RM, Marshall LF, Klauber MR, et al: The role of secondary brain injury in determining outcome from severe head injury. J Trauma 34:216–222, 1993.

12. Citerio G, Vascotto E, Villa F, et al: Induced abdominal compartment syndrome increases intracranial pressure in neurotrauma patients: A prospective study. Crit Care Med 29:1466–1471, 2001.

13. Clifton GL, Robertson CS, Kyper K, et al: Cardiovascular response to severe head injury. J Neurosurg 59:447–454, 1983.

14. Clifton GL, Ziegler MG, Grossman RG: Circulating catecholamines and sympathetic activity after head injury. Neurosurgery 8:10–14, 1981.

15. Colice GL: Neurogenic pulmonary edema. Clin Chest Med 6:473–489, 1985.

16. Cottrell JE, Patel K, Turndorf J, et al: Intracranial pressure changes induced by sodium nitroprusside in patients with intracranial mass lesions. J Neurosurg 48:329–331, 1978.

17. Crompton MR: Hypothalamic lesions following closed head injury. Brain 94:165–172, 1971.

18. Cruickshank JM, Neil-Dwyer G, Hayes Y, et al: Stress/catecholamine-induced cardiac necrosis: Reduction by $beta_1$-selective blockade. Postgrad Med 83:140–147, 1988.

19. Czosnyka M, Smielewski P, Piechnik S, et al. Cerebral autoregulation following head injury. J Neurosurg 95:756–763, 2001.

20. Deehan SC, Grant IS: Haemodynamic changes in neurogenic pulmonary oedema: Effect of dobutamine. Intens Care Med 22:672–676, 1996.

21. Dimopoulou I, Tsagarakis S, Kouyialis AT, et al: Hypothalamic-pituitary-adrenal axis dysfunction in critically ill patients with traumatic brain injury: Incidence, pathophysiology, and relationship to vasopressor dependence and peripheral interleukin-6 levels. Crit Care Med 32: 404–408, 2004.

22. Driks MR, Craven DE, Celli BR, et al: Nosocomial pneumonia in intubated patients given sucralfate as compared with antacids or histamine type 2 blockers. The role of gastric colonization. N Engl J Med 317:1376–1382, 1987.
23. Ertel W, Oberholzer A, Platz A, et al: Incidence and clinical pattern of the abdominal compartment syndrome after "damage control" laparotomy in 311 patients with severe abdominal and/or pelvic trauma. Crit Care Med 28:1747–1753, 2000.
24. Fontes RB, Aguiar PH, Aznetti MV, et al: Acute neurogenic pulmonary edema: Case reports and literature review. J Neurosurg Anesthesiol 15:144–150, 2003.
25. Friedman JA, Pichelmann MA, Piepgras DG, et al: Pulmonary complications of aneurysmal subarachnoid hemorrhage. Neurosurgery 52:1025–1031, 2003.
26. Fujii Y, Tanaka R, Takeuchi S, et al: Serial changes in hemostasis after intracranial surgery. Neurosurgery 35: 26–33, 1994.
27. Graze K, Molitch ME, Post K: Chronic demeclocycline therapy in the syndrome of inappropriate ADH secretion due to brain tumor: Case report. J Neurosurg 47:933–936, 1977.
28. Hadley MN: Hypermetabolism following head trauma: Nutritional considerations. In: Barrow DL (ed): Complications and Sequelae of Head Injury. Park Ridge, IL, American Association of Neurological Surgeons, 1992, pp 161–168.
29. Halloran LG, Zfass AM, Gayle WE, et al: Prevention of acute gastrointestinal complications after severe head injury: A controlled trial of cimetidine prophylaxis. Am J Surg 139:44–48, 1980.
30. Hamilton MG, Hull RD, Pineo GF: Venous thromboembolism in neurosurgery and neurology patients. A review. Neurosurgery 34:280–296, 1994.
31. Harper CG, Doyle D, Adams JH, et al: Analysis of abnormalities in pituitary gland in non-missile head injury: Study of 100 consecutive cases. J Clin Pathol 39:769–773, 1986.
32. Harrigan MR: Cerebral salt wasting syndrome: A review. Neurosurgery 38:152–160, 1996.
33. Harrigan MR: Cerebral salt wasting syndrome. Crit Care Clin 17:125–138, 2001.
34. Jachuck SJ, Ramani PS, Clark F, et al: Electrocardiographic abnormalities associated with raised intracranial pressure. Br Med J 1:242–244, 1975.
35. Jacoby RC, Owings JT, Holmes J, et al: Platelet activation and function after trauma. J Trauma 51:639–647, 2001.
36. Kao CH, ChangLai SP, Chieng PU, et al: Gastric emptying in head-injured patients. Am J Gastroenterol 93:1108–1112, 1998.
37. Kaufman HH: Delayed posttraumatic intracerebral hematoma. In: Kaufman HH (ed): Intracerebral Hematomas. New York, Raven Press, 1992, pp 173–179.
38. Kaufman HH, Hui K-S, Mattson JC, et al: Clinicopathological correlations of disseminated intravascular coagulation in patients with head injury. Neurosurgery 15:34–42, 1984.
39. Kelly DF, Gaw Ganzalo IT, Cohan P, et al: Hypopituitarism following traumatic brain injury and aneurysmal subarachnoid hemorrhage: A preliminary report. J Neurosurg 93:743–752, 2000.
40. Kim J, Gearhart MM, Zurick A, et al: Preliminary report on the safety of heparin for deep venous thrombosis prophylaxis after severe head injury. J Trauma 53:38–43, 2002.
41. King LR, Knowles HC, McLaurin RL, et al: Pituitary hormone response to head injury. Neurosurgery 9:229–235, 1981.
42. King LR, McLaurin RL, Lewis HP, et al: Plasma cortisol levels after head injury. Ann Surg 172:975–984, 1970.
43. Klodell CT, Carroll M, Carrillo HE, et al: Routine intragastric feeding following traumatic brain injury is safe and well tolerated. Am J Surg 179:168–171, 2000.
44. Kornblum RN, Fisher RS: Pituitary lesions in craniocerebral injuries. Arch Pathol Lab Med 88:242–248, 1969.
45. Langan EM, Miller RS, Casey WJ, et al: Prophylactic inferior vena cava filters in trauma patients at high risk: Follow-up examination and risk/benefit assessment. J Vasc Surg 30:484–488, 1999.
46. Langer M, Cigada M, Mandelli M, et al: Early onset pneumonia: A multicenter study in intensive care units. Intens Care Med 13:342–346, 1987.
47. Leach TA, Pastena JA, Swan KG, et al: Surgical prophylaxis for pulmonary embolism. Am Surg 60:292–295, 1994.
48. Lieberman SA, Oberoi AL, Gilkison CR, et al: Prevalence of neuroendocrine dysfunction in patients recovering from traumatic brain injury. J Clin Endocrinol Metab 86:2752–2756, 2001.
49. Macdonald RL, Amidei C, Lin G, et al: Safety of perioperative subcutaneous heparin for prophylaxis of venous thromboembolism in patients undergoing craniotomy. Neurosurgery 45:245–251, 1999.
50. Macmillan CS, Grant IS, Andrews PJ: Pulmonary and cardiac sequelae of subarachnoid haemorrhage: Time for active management? Intens Care Med 28:1012–1023, 2002.
51. Marino LV, Kiratu EM, French S, et al: To determine the effect of metoclopramide on gastric emptying in severe head injuries: A prospective, randomized, controlled clinical trial. Br J Neurosurg 17:24–28, 2003.
52. Mark AS, Phister SH, Jackson DE, et al: Traumatic lesions of the suprasellar region: MR imaging. Radiology 182:49–52, 1992.
53. McLeod AA, Neil-Dwyer G, Meyer CHA, et al: Cardiac sequelae of acute head injury. Br Heart J 47:221–226, 1982.
54. McMahon MM, Farnell MB, Murray MJ: Nutritional support of critically ill patients. Mayo Clin Proc 68:911–920, 1993.
55. Metz CA, Livingston DH, Smith JS, et al: Impact of multiple risk factors and ranitidine prophylaxis on the development of stress-related upper gastrointestinal bleeding: A prospective, multicenter, double-blind, randomized trial. Crit Care Med 21:1844–1849, 1993.
56. Meythaler JM, Fisher WS, Rue LW, et al: Screening for venous thromboembolism in traumatic brain injury:

Limitations of D-dimer assay. Arch Phys Med Rehabil 84:285–290, 2003.
57. Miller M: Syndromes of excess antidiuretic hormone release. Crit Care Clin 17:11–23, 2001.
58. Minard G, Kudsk KA, Melton S, et al: Early versus delayed feeding with an immune-enhancing diet in patients with severe head injuries. JPEN 24:145–149, 2000.
59. Misra UK, Kalita J, Pandey S, et al: Predictors of gastrointestinal bleeding in acute intracerebral haemorrhage. J Neurol Sci 208:25–29, 2003.
60. Moore EE, Jones TN: Benefits of immediate jejunostomy feeding after major abdominal trauma—a prospective, randomized study. J Trauma 26:874–881, 1986.
61. Neilsen HK, Husted SE, Krusell LR, et al: Silent pulmonary embolism in patients with deep venous thrombosis. Incidence and fate in a randomized, controlled trial of anticoagulation versus no anticoagulation. J Intern Med 235:457–461, 1994.
62. Nelson PB, Seif SM, Maroon JC, et al. Hyponatremia in intracranial disease: Perhaps not the syndrome of inappropriate secretion of antidiuretic hormone (SIADH). J Neurosurg 55:938–941, 1981.
63. Norwood SH, McAuley CE, Berne JD, et al: Prospective evaluation of the safety of enoxaparin prophylaxis for venous thromboembolism in patients with intracranial hemorrhagic injuries. Arch Surg 137:696–701, 2002.
64. Oertel M, Kelly DF, Lee JH, et al: Efficacy of hyperventilation, blood pressure elevation, and metabolic suppression therapy in controlling intracranial pressure after head injury. J Neurosurg 97:1045–1053, 2002.
65. Olson JD, Kaufman HH, Moake J, et al: The incidence and significance of hemostatic abnormalities in patients with head injuries. Neurosurgery 24:825–832, 1989.
66. Penkowa M, Giralt M, Thomsen PS, et al: Zinc or copper deficiency–induced impaired inflammatory response to brain trauma may be caused by the concomitant metallothionein changes. J Neurotrauma 18:447–463, 2001.
67. Persson AV, Davis RJ, Villavicencio JL: Deep vein thrombosis and pulmonary embolism. Surg Clin North Am 71: 1195–1209, 1991.
68. Piek J, Chestnut RM, Marshall LF, et al: Extracranial complications of severe head injury. J Neurosurg 77:901–907, 1992.
69. Polderman KH, Bloemers FW, Peerdeman SM, et al: Hypomagnesemia and hypophosphatemia at admission in patients with severe head injury. Crit Care Med 28:2022–2025, 2000.
70. Pomeranz S, Constantini S, Rappaport ZH: Hypokalaemia in severe head trauma. Acta Neurochir (Wien) 97:62–66, 1989.
71. Popp AJ, Feustel PJ, Kimelberg HK: Pathophysiology of traumatic brain injury. In: Wilkins RH, Rengachary SS (eds): Neurosurgery, 2nd ed. New York, McGraw-Hill, 1996, pp 2623–2637.
72. Riggs JE, Schochet SS: Osmotic stress, osmotic myelinolysis, and oligodendrocyte topography. Arch Pathol Lab Med 113:1386–1388, 1989.
73. Rixen D, Livingston DH, Loder P, et al: Ranitidine improves lymphocyte function after severe head injury: Results of a randomized, double-blind study. Crit Care Med 24:1787–1792, 1996.
74. Robertson CS, Clifton GL, Taylor AA, et al: Treatment of hypertension associated with head injury. J Neurosurg 59:455–460, 1983.
75. Rogers FB, Shackford SR, Trevisani GT, et al: Neurogenic pulmonary edema in fatal and nonfatal head injuries. J Trauma 39:860–866, 1995.
76. Rogers FB, Shackford SR, Wilson J, et al: Prophylactic vena cava filter insertion in severely injured trauma patients. Indications and preliminary results. J Trauma 35: 637–642, 1993.
77. Rogers FB, Strindberg G, Shackford SR, et al: Five-year follow-up of prophylactic vena cava filters in high-risk trauma patients. Arch Surg 133:406–411, 1998.
78. Rosner MJ, Daughton S: Cerebral perfusion pressure management in head injury. J Trauma 30:933–941, 1990.
79. Rowlands BJ, Litofsky NS, Kaufman HH: Metabolic physiology, pathophysiology and management. In: Wirth FP, Ratcheson RA (eds): Neurosurgical Critical Care. Baltimore, Williams & Wilkins, 1987, pp 81–108.
80. Scherer RU, Spangenberg P: Procoagulant activity in patients with isolated severe head trauma. Crit Care Med 26:149–156, 1998.
81. Schulte am Esch J, Murday H, Pfeifer G: Haemodynamic changes in patients with severe head injury. Acta Neurochir (Wien) 54:243–250, 1980.
82. Sharkey SW, Shear W, Hodges M, et al: Reversible myocardial contraction abnormalities in patients with an acute noncardiac illness. Chest 114:98–105, 1998.
83. Singer GG, Brenner BM: Fluid and electrolyte disturbances. In: Braunwald E, Fauci AS, Kasper DL, Hauser SL, Longo DL, Jameson JL (eds): Harrison's Principles of Internal Medicine, 15th ed. New York, McGraw-Hill, 2001, pp 271–283.
84. Spain DA, Bergamini TM, Foffmann JF, et al: Comparison of sequential compression devices and foot pumps for prophylaxis of deep venous thrombosis in high-risk trauma patients. Am Surg 64:522–525, 1998.
85. Stein SC, Chen X-H, Sinson GP, et al: Intravascular coagulation: A major secondary insult in nonfatal traumatic brain injury. J Neurosurg 97:1373–1377, 2002.
86. Steinbok P, Thompson G: Serum cortisol abnormalities after craniocerebral trauma. Neurosurgery 5:559–565, 1979.
87. Sterns RH, Riggs JE, Schochet SS: Osmotic demyelination syndrome following correction of hyponatremia. N Engl J Med 314:1535–1542, 1986.
88. Taylor SJ, Fettes SB, Jewkes C, et al: Prospective, randomized, controlled trial to determine the effect of early enhanced enteral nutrition on clinical outcome in mechanically ventilated patients suffering head injury. Crit Care Med 27:2525–2531, 1999.
89. Thromboembolic Risk Factors (THRIFT) Consensus Group: Risk of and prophylaxis for venous thromboembolism in hospital patients. BMJ 305:567–574, 1992.
90. Tien R, Chestnut RM: Medical management of the trau-

matic brain-injured patient. In: Cooper PR, Golfinos JG (eds): Head Injury, 4th ed. New York, McGraw-Hill, 2000, pp 457–482.

91. Toh CH, Dennis M: Disseminated intravascular coagulation: Old disease, new hope. BMJ 327:974–977, 2003.
92. Torres A, Aznar R, Gatell JM, et al: Incidence, risk and prognosis factors of nosocomial pneumonia in mechanically ventilated patients. Am Rev Respir Dis 142:523–528, 1990.
93. Ulusoy H, Usul H, Aydin S, et al: Effects of immunonutrition on intestinal mucosal apoptosis, mucosal atrophy, and bacterial translocation in head injured rats. J Clin Neurosci 10:596–601, 2003.
94. Velmahos GC, Nigro J, Tatevossian R, et al: Inability of an aggressive policy of thromboprophylaxis to prevent deep venous thrombosis (DVT) in critically injured patients: Are current methods of DVT prophylaxis insufficient? J Am Coll Surg 187:529–533, 1998.
95. Wilmore DW: Catabolic illness. Strategies for enhancing recovery. N Engl J Med 325:695–702, 1991.
96. Yeiser EC, Vanlandingham JW, Levenson CW: Moderate zinc deficiency increases cell death after brain injury in the rat. Nutr Neurosci 5:345–352, 2002.
97. Young B, Ott L, Norton J, et al: Nutrition and brain injury. J Neurotrauma 9:S375–S383, 1992.
98. Zarazur BL, Kudsk KA, Carter K, et al: Stress ulceration requiring definitive surgery after severe trauma. Am Surg 67:875–879, 2001.
99. Zeltsman D, Rowland M, Shanavas Z: Is the incidence of hemorrhagic stress ulceration in surgical critically ill patients affected by modern antacid prophylaxis? Am Surg 62:1010–1013, 1996.

Chapter 11
Neurobehavioral Outcome of Head Trauma

DANIEL X. CAPRUSO AND
HARVEY S. LEVIN

Neurobehavioral outcome in survivors of head trauma ranges from rapid recovery of cognition with no discernible sequelae to survival without recovery of consciousness. For those patients whose outcome falls between these two extremes, cognitive deficits and personality change frequently result in marked impairments of social and occupational functioning. These deficits in thought and behavior contribute more to disability than do physical (motor and sensory) sequelae in 72% of severe head trauma survivors.[97]

Classification of Initial Severity

The Glasgow Coma Scale (GCS)[98,236] is used to grade the initial severity of head trauma into the categories of mild, moderate, and severe based on the sum score of the patient's eye opening, motor, and verbal responses, which are typically the first scores recorded after resuscitation. To describe these categories in simplified terms: The acute presentation of patients with *mild head trauma* ranges from fully alert to mildly confused. Patients with *moderate head trauma* present with some impairment of consciousness, but they can be awakened and show signs of cognitive activity or at least localize the site of tactile stimulation by the examiner and display some eye opening. Patients with *severe head trauma* are initially comatose or deteriorate to coma (Table 11.1). *Coma* is defined as no eye opening, no motor response to command, and no comprehensible speech. There is some range in the depth of coma that is largely secondary to variation in the motor response.

Sequence of Neurobehavioral Recovery

Head trauma arising from acceleration/deceleration of the head typically induces an acute alteration of consciousness that may range from a mild dazing to a deep coma. From this initial disturbance of consciousness, patients usually pass through a sequence of neurobehavioral syndromes until alertness and orientation are restored (Fig. 11.1). At the mild end of the spectrum, a person who has sustained a concussion may suffer a shallow, transient confusion that clears within a few minutes, leaving either no permanent residual interval of memory loss or a loss of memory for those seconds or minutes that followed the impact.

Table 11.1. Head Injury Classification

Category	Acute GCS	Clinical Features
Mild	13–15	Loss of consciousness for <20 minutes, no deterioration of GCS, no focal neurological deficit or complication (e.g., hypotension), no intracranial mass lesion or intracranial surgery.
Moderate	9–12	Includes GCS >12, with complication or focal brain lesion seen on computed tomography scan, and may include patients rapidly recovered from coma.
Severe	3–8	No eye opening, no motor response to command, no verbal response or speech. Coma duration must be ≥ 6 hours.

GCS, Glasgow Coma Scale.

Among survivors at the most severe end of the spectrum, long-term survival may occur without recovery of consciousness, as in the persistent vegetative state described below.

The recovery of full consciousness following severe head trauma is typically a gradual and evolving process, as emergence from an initial period of coma is followed by an interval of posttraumatic amnesia.[217,220] The hallmarks of this transitional period are disorientation and failure to register and recall ongoing events. The term *posttraumatic amnesia* is a partial misnomer, because the memory loss of the recovering patient often occurs either in the context of a reduction in the level of consciousness (i.e., *hypokinetic confusion*) or in the context of excessive arousal (i.e., *hyperkinetic confusion* or *delirium*).[80,189] This period is also characterized by marked attentional disturbance.[232b]

There is a higher frequency of restlessness, agitation, and other socially inappropriate behaviors during posttraumatic amnesia when lesions are present that overlap the frontal and temporal lobes.[240] The period of posttraumatic amnesia is considered to have ended when patients regain normal orientation and when they are able to store and retrieve ongoing events. *Islands* of intact memory amid ongoing posttraumatic amnesia may be observed.[219] The resolution of posttraumatic amnesia may be reliably measured in objective and standardized fashion using the Galveston Orientation and Amnesia Test.[151]

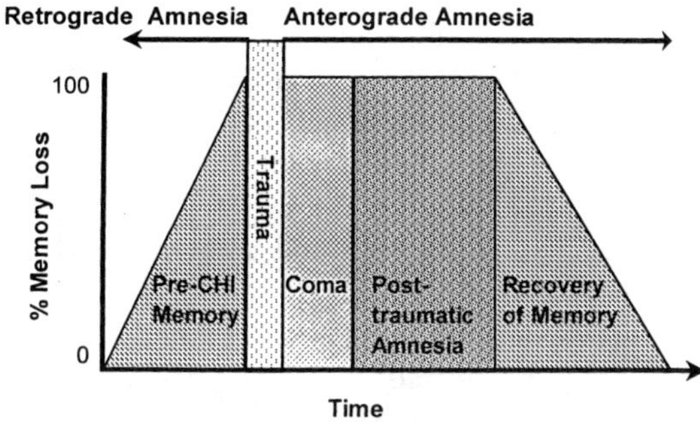

Figure 11.1. Sequence of acute alterations in memory following closed head injury (CHI). (Created from KdeS Hamsher, adaptation of reference 119, p 74, with permission.)

Classification of Outcome

The five categories of the original Glasgow Outcome Scale (GOS)[96–98] include death and four levels of survival:

1. *Death*
2. *Vegetative State* The hallmark of the vegetative state is an apparent absence of cognitive function, as reflected by the total abolition of psychologically meaningful behavior. Unlike persons in coma, patients in a vegetative state may have eye-opening, visual tracking, and sleep/wake cycles. Although these patients may be *awake*, they are not *aware*. Patients in a vegetative state may demonstrate a variety of spontaneous or reflexive motor actions, but these motoric responses are not indicative of consciousness unless they communicate clearly and reliably or imply some type of cognitive activity.
3. *Severe Disability* Conscious but dependent patients are included in this category. Although the degree of dependence may vary, these patients must rely on a caregiver for some activities throughout the day. In some patients, physical functioning may remain relatively intact, but they may be so disinhibited or apathetic that they cannot manage their own behavior. Patients who cannot be trusted

to care for themselves over a 24-hour interval are included here.

4. *Moderate Disability* Independent but disabled patients are included in this category. Although they may live alone, these patients have a degree of cognitive or physical handicap that limits them in comparison to premorbid functioning. Many patients in this category continue to work, although they are unable to assume their previous level of occupational responsibility.
5. *Good Recovery* Independent patients who are capable of returning to their work or other premorbid activities without major limitations are included in this category. These patients may have mild persisting neurological or cognitive deficits, but these deficits are not severe enough to interfere substantially with their general functioning. These patients are socially competent and capable of comporting themselves adequately and without a suggestion of marked personality change. For relatives and friends who know these patients well, subtle reductions in cognitive and social acumen may be apparent, despite an otherwise near-complete recovery.

Jennett et al.[97] found that the three categories of conscious survivorship in the original GOS were too broad, and were therefore insensitive to gradations of improvement during recovery. They introduced the extended GOS (GOSE), in which each conscious survival category is subdivided into an upper and a lower category, producing a 6-point scale for conscious survivors. When used with a structured interview and compared against the original GOS, the GOSE is more reflective of the functional outcome, neuropsychological status, and affective functioning of patients 3 to 12 months postinjury.[121,200]

Course of Global Recovery

Prediction of outcome based exclusively on the initial hospitalization is not as accurate as prediction based on the level of recovery at 3 months.[34] The greatest rate of recovery in survivors of severe head trauma typically occurs within the first 6 months and then begins to level off, with smaller incremental gains thereafter.[98] Among survivors of severe head trauma reaching the GOS category of good recovery at 12 months, 90% have already attained good recovery by 6 months.[97]

Interaction of Trauma, Brain Structure, and Neurobehavioral Outcome

In a typical closed head injury of the acceleration/deceleration type, such as those caused by motor vehicle accidents and falls, the destructive force is not equally distributed in all areas of the brain. Rather, the maximum concentration of force and neuronal shear strain occur in the orbitofrontal and anterior temporal lobes due to the relative structural (gyral and sulcal) irregularity of these areas, their distance from the brain's center of gravity, and the arc of rotation induced in the brain by the force imparted.[61,90] As a result, a high concentration of extraparenchymal and parenchymal lesions are apparent in the frontal and anterior temporal lobes, regardless of the site of exterior impact.[61,117] The orbitofrontal and anterior temporal areas not only sustain the most diffuse axonal injury in the parenchyma wrought by shear strain, but are also the most susceptible to contusion.[54] Again, regardless of the external site of impact, the protrusions of the sphenoid ridges and frontal fossa underlying these areas bruise and lacerate the cortical surface as the brain is displaced over these bony ridges by the force of the trauma (see Fig.11.2).[2,61,77]

Following head trauma, focal areas of contusion or mass lesions such as hematoma may produce classic neurobehavioral syndromes that have a strong correlation with the locus and extent of the lesion. More common is a syndrome produced by the underlying diffuse effects of head trauma on cerebral functioning. In correlation with the known neuropathological distribution of macroscopic and microscopic lesions in the orbitofrontal and anterior temporal areas, head injury frequently produces a predictable syndrome of deficit in which memory, self-regulation, and appropriate social functioning are the areas of thought and behavior most severely affected. Thus, even when a classic neurobehavioral syndrome with implications for focal brain functioning is present, it is typically superimposed on underlying and more global deficits produced by the diffuse insult.

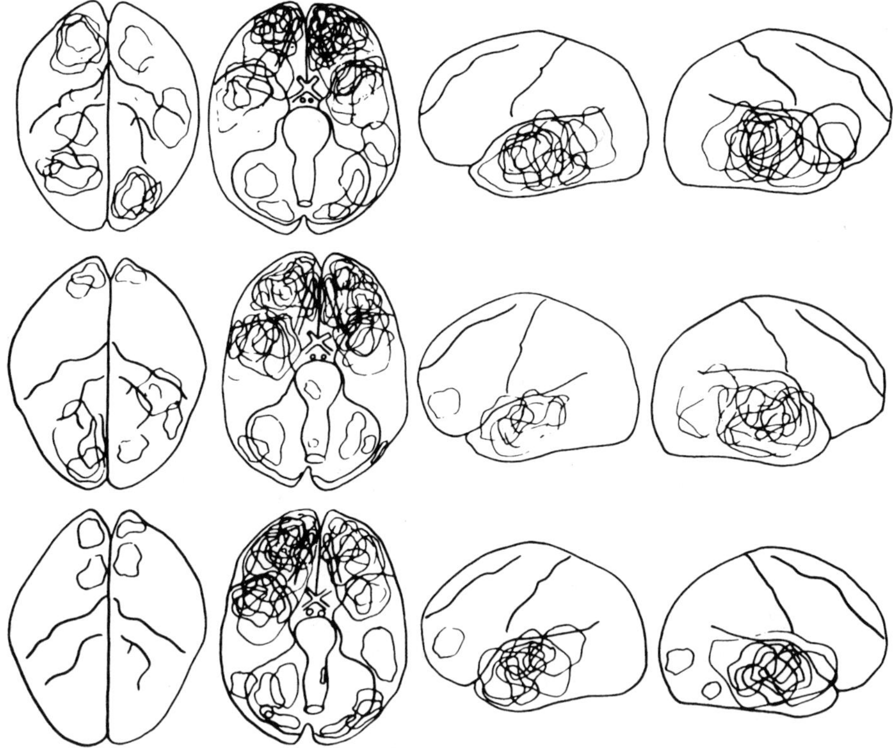

Figure 11.2. Composite of cerebral contusions in autopsies following craniocerebral trauma, showing concentration of contusions in the frontal and temporal lobes, with relative sparing of the parietal and occipital lobes. (From reference 77, p 46, with permission.)

Neurobehavioral Outcome of Head Injury in Adults

Cognitive Effects

The effects of head injury on functioning in various cognitive domains are described below.

Memory

In most cases of head injury, memory is the cognitive domain that is most severely affected.[134,138,195] As described above, the neuropathological effects of parenchymal shear strain and surface contusion concentrated in the anterior temporal lobes affect the hippocampus and its related neuronal structures, which normally perform storage and retrieval of new memories.[184,231] The hippocampus is particularly susceptible to hypoxic and ischemic complications,[71] and it may also be damaged by the release of excitotoxic amino acids following head injury.[112]

Posttraumatic and Retrograde Amnesia

During the early stages of recovery, there are both *retrograde* and *anterograde* components of posttraumatic memory deficit. As illustrated in Figure 11.1, retrograde amnesia extends *backward in time* from the moment of trauma, whereas anterograde amnesia extends *forward in time* from the moment of trauma.[219,220] Thus, the retrograde component of amnesia refers to memory loss for events that occurred before the injury, whereas the anterograde component of amnesia refers to an inability to recall events occurring after the injury. Russell and Nathan[220] found that in recovered patients, the duration of retrograde amnesia is correlated with and almost always much briefer than the duration of anterograde amnesia. The majority of patients recovered from mild to moderate head injury have a residual retrograde amnesia that is limited to seconds or minutes.

Modern understanding of retrograde memory loss began in 1882 with Ribot,[211] who surveyed cases of amnesia stemming from head trauma and a variety of other pathologies. As a result of his observations, Ribot proposed his *Law of Regression*, which stated that the memories formed most recently are most susceptible to disruption by neurological disease. Ribot's proposed temporal gradient of retrograde memory loss for head injury patients was confirmed by Levin et al.[145] for autobiographical materials. The extent of retrograde memory loss observed may be dependent on the stage of the patient's recovery. During posttraumatic amnesia, retrograde memory loss may be seen to *shrink* in time toward the point of trauma as the patient recovers normal mental status, such that a retrograde amnesia that initially extended backward by several years may resolve to a permanent retrograde amnesia that encompasses only the last minutes before the trauma.[218] High et al.[89] found that the pattern of recovery of orientation in head trauma patients is consistent with the concept of shrinking retrograde amnesia. Their head trauma patients typically misstated the date backwards in time, and then, as they recovered, their orientation errors typically receded forward in time to approximate the current date. Also consistent with the concept of shrinking retrograde amnesia, Levin et al.[145] found that the proportion of recall of autobiographical events from recent years recovered from a mean of under 35% in patients still in posttraumatic amnesia to a mean of over 75% in patients who had recovered from posttraumatic amnesia.

Levin et al.[151] found that prolonged posttraumatic amnesia was related to computed tomography (CT) findings of bilateral mass lesioning and diffuse injury. Wilson et al.[255] reported similar findings; a prolonged duration of posttraumatic amnesia was associated with increased numbers of both central (basal ganglia, callosal, brain stem, or cerebellum) and hemispheric lesions on magnetic resonance imaging (MRI), whereas variables such as GCS and coma duration were only associated with more central lesions.

Residual Memory Deficit

Although recovery from posttraumatic amnesia indicates that a patient has regained a relatively intact level of orientation and awareness of ongoing events, this improved mental status does not imply that the patient's memory has returned to normal premorbid levels. Levin et al.[134] found that among patients who recovered normal intellectual functioning (IQ of 85 or higher), a disproportionately severe memory deficit was found in 16% of patients recovered from moderate head trauma and in 25% of patients recovered from severe head trauma. Levin et al.[138] found verbal learning deficits in 10% of patients with good recovery, in 44% of patients with moderate disability, and in 100% of patients with severe disability. These psychometric findings are validated by the ecological observations of Oddy et al.,[195] who found that 7 years after severe head trauma, memory deficit was the single most frequent symptom reported by both patients (53%) and their relatives (79%). The lower rate of memory complaints by the patients likely reflects the lack of insight into the deficit that is common following head trauma.[206]

Intelligence

Intelligence is the sum of a person's knowledge and problem-solving skills. The Wechsler Adult Intelligence Scale (WAIS)-III[247] is most commonly used and yields an omnibus Full Scale IQ as well as a Verbal IQ (VIQ) and a Performance IQ (PIQ). The IQ scores are themselves multifactorial in that the VIQ contains tests of both Verbal Comprehension (declarative knowledge) and Working Memory (attention-concentration), whereas the PIQ contains measures of both Perceptual Organization (sequencing, pattern recognition, spatial reasoning, and constructional ability) and Processing Speed.

When IQ scores are below expectation following head trauma, it is typically the tests of Perceptual Organization and Processing Speed that are relatively impaired.[138,164] These tasks are more sensitive to head trauma because of their complexity and the demands they make on rapid, efficient performance. In contrast to the Verbal Comprehension subtests, which generally demand response with rote and overlearned knowledge, several of the Perceptual Organization subtests are novel tasks that demand active problem solving. The ability to find solutions to novel tasks is often inordinately affected by head trauma, presumably in correlation with the relatively high concentration of neuropathology in the frontal lobes,[1,61,117] where functions such as cognitive flexibility are traditionally localized. Relative impairments on the Verbal Conceptual subtests are associated with recovery from left hemisphere mass lesions such as hematoma or hemorrhagic contusion, although equivalent impairments in Perceptual Organization are found with mass lesion of either hemisphere.[239]

Consistent with the Wechsler IQ's validated ability to predict adaptive behavior,[167] the IQ score in survivors of head trauma has a significant relationship to the GOS category attained. In a study of 27 patients followed after severe head trauma, Levin et al.[138] found that all patients with good recovery showed IQs >85; IQ scores of patients with moderate disability ranged from 73 to 114; and IQ scores of patients with severe disability ranged from 39 to 69.

Substantial improvements in intellectual functioning can be expected as patient recovery continues. Dikmen et al.[42] tested median IQ scores at 1, 12, and 24 months following moderate to severe head trauma. Compared with the postinjury baseline, they found a +17 point improvement in VIQ and a +25 point improvement in PIQ at 12 months. There were additional improvements of +4 points in VIQ and +7 points in PIQ at 24 months. It should be noted that in controls, *practice effects* from repeated testing produced a +7 improvement on PIQ, with no practice effect apparent on VIQ.

Language

Only about 2% of patients admitted consecutively to neurosurgery services after head trauma are aphasic.[85] However, Sarno et al.[227] found classic aphasia syndromes in approximately one-third of severe head injury patients referred for subsequent rehabilitation. Of these aphasic patients, 51% had fluent aphasias, 35% had nonfluent aphasias, and 14% had global aphasias. Approximately one-third of the nonaphasic head injury patients referred for rehabilitation were dysarthric, and all patients in the series demonstrated language deficits on psychometric testing. Sarno et al. described many of these patients as having *subclinical aphasia*, in that they had adequate conversational language but showed a clear language deficit under the increased challenge of psychometric testing. The most commonly seen language disturbance following head injury is anomia,[123,136] with sparing of fluency, repetition, and comprehension, although circumlocution and semantic paraphasia may be present. The psychometric profiles of aphasic patients show the highest rate of deficit in confrontation naming, with lower frequencies of deficit in comprehension, writing, and verbal associative fluency, and with repetition relatively preserved.[136]

Language deficits in the acute phase of recovery typically occur in the context of a mass lesion in the left hemisphere, whereas chronic language deficits are related to coma duration and left lateral ventricular enlargement.[139] As with other etiologies, right hemiplegia is associated with aphasia after head injury.[227] There is a fairly optimistic prognosis for the resolution of acute aphasic deficits following head injury. Levin et al.[139] found that of 21 patients suffering acute aphasia following head trauma, 43% had full recovery of language functioning, 29% remained globally aphasic, and 29% had resolution to specific language deficits, predominately anomia. Posttraumatic mutism is present in approximately 3% of head injury patients despite recovery of consciousness and the ability to communicate through a nonspeech channel.[146] These mute patients typically have lesions in the putamen and internal capsule, or they have cortical lesions of the left hemisphere.

Even with recovery of basic language abilities, the conversational discourse of patients with head injury may be impaired secondary to deficits that go beyond the standard language dimensions of fluency, naming, repetition, and comprehension. Several investigators[4,193] have demonstrated that the communication of patients with left prefrontal lesions is characterized by disorganization and impoverished narrative. In contrast, the communication of patients with right prefrontal lesions tends to be tangential and socially inappropriate.[4] Galski et al.[59] found that the discourse of nonaphasic persons recovered from head trauma tended to contain more irrelevant statements, was more disorganized, and contained an increased number of paraphasic errors compared to the discourse of normal controls.

Visual Perception

Visuoperceptual ability is relatively preserved in the majority of patients recovered from head trauma.[137] Of patients with intracranial mass lesions, visuoperceptual deficit was generally confined to those with right hemisphere hematoma. Visuospatial judgment is relatively preserved in patients surviving severe head injury,[135] as is constructional praxis.[132] These findings of relative preservation of complex perception following head trauma are consistent with the rostrocaudal gradient of tissue destruction induced by head injury. The relative sparing of the perceptual processing systems localized in the posterior cortices is also secondary to the lesser degree of structural irregularity in these areas, which are surrounded by relatively smooth and convex skull surfaces.[1,117,179]

Attention-Concentration

Profound deficit in attention-concentration is often a prominent clinical feature of posttraumatic amnesia, and is a part of the residual disturbance of consciousness and arousal apparent during the early stage of recovery from head injury. After the resolution of posttraumatic amnesia, performance on simple tests of attentional capacity, such as Digit Span, often recovers to relatively normal levels.[180] However, prominent deficits may be seen in these same patients when more sophisticated measures are used, as attentional processing is now recognized to subsume multiple dimensions such as vigilance (sustained attention), freedom from distraction (focused attention), and capacity for divided attention. Risser and Hamsher[213] found that whereas only 9% of consecutively referred patients recovering from severe head injury had impairments in vigilance, 77% showed increased distractability in the context of normal vigilance.

Levin et al.[144] found an interaction between severe head injury and sustained attention over the time taken to perform a task. Although normal subjects were generally able to sustain attention over successive time blocks on a cognitive task, persons recovered from head trauma showed worsening performance over time, again suggesting that simple and brief measures of attentional capacity will not truly capture the attentional deficits apparent when more rigorous testing is performed. Whyte et al.[252] found that compared to controls, patients with head trauma had lower rates of on-task performance in both quiet and distracting environments, although the head trauma patients were also more susceptible to distraction when it was introduced. An analysis of fidgeting behavior indicated that the attention-concentration of head injury patients could not be attributed to hyperactivity.

Processing Speed

Slowed processing speed is a common result of head trauma.[73,144] As the complexity of a choice reaction time task is increased, patients recovering from head trauma tend to show disproportionate slowing in mental speed.[183,241] The Paced Auditory Serial Addition Task (PASAT)[74] has been used to study divided attention (multitasking) under progressively accelerating rates of information processing speed. Patients recovering even from mild head injury tend to show deficits on this task,[74,76,144] although the information processing deficits of these patients with mild head injury tend to be restricted to the first 1 to 3 months of recovery.

Executive Functioning

The executive, or frontal lobe system, functions are those cognitive abilities involved in the planning, initiation, execution, and regulation of behavior.[158] Executive functioning represents the process by which behavior is motivated, and then checked for the efficiency and appropriateness of task performance. Like memory, executive functions are highly susceptible to the destructive effects of head injury. Because executive functions involve frontally guided, distributed networks,[135] the prominence of executive deficit in head injury patients is likely related to diffuse axonal injury and to the high concentration of parenchymal and extraparenchymal lesions induced in the frontal lobes by accelerative/decelerative trauma.[1,117,157,179]

Standard clinical interviews and basic psychological testing will often fail to detect the presence of executive deficits. In the standard interview, the clinician frequently guides and structures the interview while the patient passively provides what may well be habitual answers. Likewise, during the standard psychometric examination, the patient is usually given explicit instructions on performing a series of highly structured tasks, with correction provided by the examiner when rules are violated. These situations provide samples of behavior that do not adequately reflect real-world requirements of self-structuring the solutions to complex problems, nor do they measure the active self-monitoring of performance necessary to ensure that appropriate progress toward a relevant goal is being achieved. Despite a satisfactory performance in the psychology laboratory, persons recovered from head trauma with executive dysfunction may lack the initiative to perform necessary tasks once they leave the professional's office, or they may lack the judgment, insight, and critical capacity necessary to monitor and evaluate whether their actions are accomplishing anything. Adaptive functioning of persons recovered from head trauma is often impaired because they lack the flexibility of reasoning and problem solving to respond to an environment where each day may bring completely new problems demanding novel and creative solutions.

An illustration of the dissociations by executive deficits can be discerned when the language performance of head trauma patients is evaluated by neuropsychological testing. Although measured vocabulary levels are relatively resistant to head trauma, when patients are given 1 minute to generate as many words as they can that start with a specific letter, their performance is often impoverished.[157] In these cases, the patients' lexicon may be well preserved, but they lack the mental flexibility necessary to access the breadth of words potentially available to them. As a nonverbal analogue, patients may demonstrate above-average constructional ability when copying models, but when asked to generate their own designs independently, they often have surprising difficulties.[135,159]

The Wisconsin Card Sorting Test[83] is a test of executive functioning that provides little explicit instruction, and which demands that patients discover the rules of the task by themselves, eliminate alternative hypotheses through logic, make continuous use of feedback, and shift their problem-solving strategies when necessary. Severe head trauma patients with both frontal and nonfrontal lesions on MRI frequently perform below normal levels on this task.[135]

Goldstein and Levin[65] used a "Twenty Questions" procedure in which the patient was shown an array of objects and given the task of guessing which object had been secretly selected by the examiner. A logical and efficient strategy is to ask *constraint* questions that will narrow the item down to a specific quality or category, for example by asking "Is it a tool?" Patients with severe head trauma required significantly more questions to guess the correct object, while asking more narrow questions which suggest an inefficient and concrete stategy. Instead of narrowing the possible solutions, they had a greater tendency to ask repeated specific and concrete questions like "Is it a fish?," "Is it a jacket?," "Is it a hammer?" and so on.

The Tower of London task demands that the patient rearrange three colored beads on three pegs of varying height to match a particular configuration. To perform the task efficiently, the patient must think several steps ahead instead of considering each move by itself. Despite its status as a purported test of frontal lobe functioning, the Tower of London test of planning ability did not discriminate between controls and a small sample of head-injured adults with frontal or nonfrontal MRI lesions.[135] This negative finding was replicated by Cockburn.[37]

Perseveration is a feature of executive dysfunction that may appear prominently across a number of tests.[135] Patients with head trauma will often persist in attempting an incorrect solution despite repeated feedback that they are performing the task in the wrong way. They may also repeatedly give a previously correct response, despite instructions that they provide a novel and alternate solution on each trial.

That deficits in executive functioning account for a significant proportion of the disability suffered by head injury patients was demonstrated by Mazaux et al.[172] In a study of impairments on various ecological activities in patients 5 years after head injury, they found that the performance of administrative tasks and successful management of finances, two tasks requiring intact organizational and executive skills, were most difficult for patients. Also prominently impaired were the activities of writing letters, planning the week, and using public transportation, all complex tasks drawing on executive functions such as initiative, organization, and prospective thought.

Neurobehavioral Sequelae of Mild Head Injury

Studies of individuals with mild head injury[41,60,74,75,127,147] generally indicate that impairments on sensitive tasks of memory, attention, information processing, and psychomotor speed are present within the first week of recovery, but that rapid improvement to a normal level of neurobehavioral functioning is apparent within 1 to 3 months of injury. Newcombe et al.[192] could find essentially no cognitive deficit within 48 hours of mild head injury. Although the early (and eventually resolving) cognitive impairment seen following mild head trauma is likely to be of neurogenic origin, chronic cognitive complaints attributed to head injury may reflect the precipitation of a somatoform or depressive reaction by an initial neurogenic event. There are dissenting views to this interpretation.[27,114]

Williams et al.[253] found that among patients with initial (and lowest) GCS scores of 13 to 15, those patients having a parenchymal contusion or hematoma on CT had worse memory performances and slower information processing capacity than patients who had initially presented with mild impairment of consciousness and negative CT scans. The presence of a subdural or epidural hematoma, irrespective of the presence of an intracerebral lesion, was associated with lowered verbal fluency. At 6 months, 97% of patients with uncomplicated mild head injury had obtained good recovery compared with 83% of those with extraparenchymal lesions and 75% of those with parenchymal lesions. Patients with moderate head injury had a good recovery rate of 73%. Depressed skull fracture was associated with a 94% rate of good recovery at 6 months. The necessity of intracranial surgery had no effect on the outcome. These findings led Williams et al. to propose that patients with GCS scores of 13–15, but with lesions visible on CT, would be more accurately categorized as having moderate head trauma.

Dikmen et al.[41] progressively subdivided 157 patients with mild head trauma to create four subgroups based on severity of complications. Thus, in addition to their total group, there was a group that also followed commands within 1 hour, a group that also had normal CT scans, and a group that also had less than 24 hours of posttraumatic amnesia. The total mild head trauma sample had a high (37%) rate of preexisting conditions including treatment for alcoholism, prior head trauma, previous brain disease, psychiatric conditions, and learning disability, so a control group was created matched on the prevalence of those factors. Neuropsychological testing at 1 month indicated that all patients with mild head trauma differed from controls only on verbal learning and only at 1 month postinjury, not at 1 year. The PIQ and a test of speeded executive functioning (Trail Making Test —Part B) did not differ from controls. The subgroups of patients who did not suffer the various complications described above did not differ from controls at 1 month or 1 year. Regression analysis for the total mild head trauma sample at 1 month indicated that neuropsychological performance was predicted not only by head trauma, but also by the pre-existing psychiatric and neurological conditions, age at or over 50 years, and educational level. At 1 year, these various preexisting conditions and demographic variables were much more powerful predictors of performance than was the mild head injury. The results suggest that a relatively limited degree of early cognitive dysfunction may be seen in mild head injury cases at 1 month, but that at 1 year any residual effects are probably due to other factors. Continuing morbidity after the acute phase of recovery is likely due to social, psychiatric, and illness factors that are separable from the current mild head trauma.

Teasdale and Engberg[235] studied 1220 men who had undergone cognitive testing by the Danish Draft Board. Where the population rate for dysfunctional performance on the draft cognitive testing was 20%, they found that an increased rate of cognitive dysfunction (50%) was apparent only when the men were tested within 1 week of head trauma. Furthermore, the men who were injured *after* the cognitive testing had a significantly higher rate of cognitive dysfunction (30%) than the men who were injured more than 1 week before testing (24%). At first, these results make little sense, as performance in an injury group should only be worse after the injury, not before. But the results are logical when it is considered that, as explained below, the group of persons sustaining head trauma contains an overrepresentation of those with characterological and other psychopathology that negatively impacts cognitive functioning even before the trauma. These results confirm not only that the effects of mild head trauma are typically transient, but also that there is a higher rate of preexisting cognitive dysfunction in the mild head trauma population.

The experience of multiple concussions over time may have subtle deleterious effects on cognitive functioning. Patients suffering multiple mild head injuries have slower recovery of information processing speed than is observed following a single mild head trauma, suggesting that some degree of cumulative cognitive impairment may follow multiple concussive episodes.[75] Furthermore, when athletes who had suffered three or more previous concussions again sustain mild head trauma, they are more likely to experience loss of consciousness, confusion, and anterograde amnesia than athletes with no history of concussion.[38] Of course, there may also be a bias toward an increased base rate of pathology for those who sustain multiple concussive events.

A *postconcussion syndrome* of headache, fatigue,

dizziness, sleep disturbance, memory loss, depression, anxiety, and other vague and specific cognitive, emotional, and somatic complaints is apparent in the acute phase of recovery from mild head injury.[3,204,221,222] The validity of this syndrome has been questioned, as there is a high base rate of these nonspecific complaints in the general population.[127,259] Also, persons recovering from mild head injury have been shown to significantly underestimate the premorbid frequency of the symptoms that comprise the postconcussion syndrome.[185] Although the subjective complaints of most patients resolve within weeks of a mild head injury, approximately 15% of patients are left with persisting and chronic postconcussive complaints. The presence of these complaints cannot be explained solely on the basis of a preexisting psychiatric disorder.[186] It is possible that for this minority of chronic patients following mild head injury, concussion acts as a catalyst for the emergence of somatoform pathology.

Capruso et al.[28] investigated 30 patients whose postconcussive symptoms continued beyond the 3-month period during which recovery typically occurs in the majority of patients with mild head injury. Time since injury in these patients ranged from 3 to 88 months. There was no relationship between recovery time and cognitive performance, although there was a significant correlation (r = –.55) between attentional disturbance in these patients and severity of real or simulated psychopathology as measured by the Minnesota Multiphasic Personality Inventory (MMPI)-2 F Scale. Memory functioning in these chronic postconcussive patients was correlated with extent of psychological denial or lying (MMPI-2 L Scale) or with excessive endorsement of both vague and specific somatic complaints (MMPI-2 Scales 1 and 3).

Psychosocial Outcome of Head Injury in Adults

Behavioral Profile of Head Trauma Patients

Levin et al.[143] interviewed 101 mildly, moderately, and severely head-injured patients and rated their behavior by the objective criteria of the Neurobehavioral Rating Scale. The following types of behavioral disturbance were most characteristic of patients and were also related to the severity of trauma:

- *Conceptual disorganization*: Confused, disconnected, and disorganized thought processes were apparent. Social communication tended to be tangential and perseverative.
- *Poor planning*: Unrealistic goals and poorly formulated plans for the future were apparent, with a failure to take the degree of disability into account.
- *Inaccurate insight and self-appraisal*: Also apparent were poor insight, exaggerated self-opinion, and a tendency to overrate the current ability level while underrating the personality change.

Memory loss and depression were other symptoms that were rated as occurring with high frequency in the head injury patients. Patients with detectable frontal lobe lesions did not differ in symptom severity from patients without detectable frontal lobe lesions, although the relative proportion of *metacognitive* deficit was greater in the frontal group. That is, patients with clear frontal lobe lesions had diminished self-awareness of their deficit.

Vanier et al.[242] revised the Neurobehavioral Rating Scale and applied it to 286 patients in France 1 to 3 months after mild, moderate, or severe head trauma. Memory difficulties, conceptual disorganization, planning difficulties, anxiety, inattention, decreased initiative, or decreased motivation were most frequently observed. Nearly identical results were found by McCauley et al.[175] in a study of 210 head trauma patients in the United States and Canada. The extent of cognitive deficits observed was related to the severity of the injury, whereas emotional difficulties were observed with equal frequency across mild, moderate, and severe head trauma groups, which suggests that extraneural psychosocial factors contribute to the irritability, anxiety, and depression that occur during recovery.[208]

Spatt et al.[230] evaluated the psychosocial outcome in 33 persons approximately 8 years after moderate to severe closed head injury. Both the recovered patients and their relatives rated the patients as less socially competent and less socially resonant, and as more depressive and introverted. Whereas relatives rated the patients as more impulsive and less controlled, the patients saw themselves as adequately controlled. Only 20% of the patients had returned to jobs that were equivalent to the positions that they had held premorbidly.

Psychiatric Disorder Following Head Trauma

Premorbid Psychopathology in Head Injury Patients. There is a disproportionate incidence of premorbid psychiatric illness and personality disorder in persons sustaining head injury. In a review of the literature on the influence of psychopathology on motor vehicle accidents, Tsuang et al.[238] found that head-injured drivers had high premorbid rates of hostile, immature, antisocial, and impulsive personality characteristics. Haselkorn et al.[81] found that in the year prior to head injury, 29% of head-injured patients had received a citation for a moving violation compared to 4% of controls hospitalized for stroke, isolated extremity fractures, or appendicitis. For many persons sustaining head trauma, the automobile presents an opportunity to express risk-taking and aggressive behaviors.

Greve et al.[72] studied head trauma patients demonstrating significant problems with impulsive aggression during rehabilitation. They found that 74% of these patients had substantial preinjury histories of impulsive and aggressive behaviors compared to 26% of the patients who displayed a less volatile demeanor. In contrast to premorbid personality, neither coma duration nor neuropsychological functioning was predictive of impulsive aggression.

Among consecutive admissions to a trauma center for head injury, Whetsell et al.[250] found that alcohol intoxication was involved in 49% of cases, and that 47% of patients with blunt trauma and 88% of patients with penetrating trauma had a substantial degree of premorbid psychopathology. Pettigrew et al.[200] found that in a series of 80 head injury patients, 65% had been drinking alcohol at the time of injury, 15% had been treated for alcoholism, 10% used illegal drugs on a regular basis, and 34% had previously sought psychiatric intervention. Kelly et al.[107] found that 56% of head trauma patients given toxicology screens on admission tested positive for alcohol or illicit drugs. When tested an average of 1 month postinjury, the patients with negative alcohol and drug screens had significantly better performances on tests of intellect, memory, and attention than those with a positive alcohol or drug screen. MacMillan et al.[163] found that preinjury psychiatric and substance abuse histories predicted employment status after recovery from head trauma. Substance abuse history also predicted subsequent independent living status. These studies demonstrate that it can be difficult to separate the effect of head trauma from the neurotoxic and psychosocial effects of previous substance abuse.

Psychosis

Levin et al.[119] isolated 10 patients displaying bizarre and agitated behavior during subacute recovery from a series of 800 admissions for head trauma. Only 1 of these 10 patients had a previous psychiatric history, consisting of hyperactivity and truancy. The chief psychotic symptoms observed in these patients were confabulations and fragmented delusions. Of these 10 patients, visual hallucinations were present in 4, auditory hallucinations were present in 1, and 1 patient had hallucinations in both modalities. Diffuse cerebral swelling and mass effect associated with hematoma were common neurological findings in these psychotic patients. Nakase-Thompson et al.[189] found a 20% rate of delusions and a 16% rate of hallucinations in the acute phase of recovery from head trauma.

Mood and Anxiety Disorders

The development of depression secondary to head injury is more common in patients with premorbid histories of psychiatric disorder or substance abuse.[101] Jorge et al.[100] found a 26% rate of major depression among consecutive admissions to a trauma center for acute head injury. Of those patients who were not initially depressed, 27% went on to develop major depressive episodes within 1 year of injury. In the acute phase of recovery, depression was associated with left dorsolateral frontal or left basal ganglia lesions or with subcortical lesions. Both neurovegetative and psychological symptoms of depression were frequent among recovering patients, with lack of energy being the most chronic neurovegetative symptom. The presence of a comorbid generalized anxiety disorder was associated with the presence of a right hemisphere lesion and indicated a longer clinical course of depression.[103] Manic episodes occurred in 9% of one series,[102] and these episodes were associated with basal lesions in the temporal poles. Levin et al.[122] found a 17% rate of depression in patients sustaining mild to moderate head trauma compared to 6% in patients suffering from other (extracranial) trauma. Although 42% of the head trauma patients had a resulting intracranial lesion, there was no relationship between presence or locus of lesion and depression.

Hibbard et al.[87] found that the rates of preinjury mood, anxiety, and substance abuse disorders in head trauma patients exceeded those of the general population. The rates of major depression, obsessive-compulsive disorder, panic disorder, and generalized anxiety disorder tripled in patients once they had sustained head trauma. For most of these disorders, about half of the patients experienced resolution of psychiatric illness in the 8 years that followed injury. Deb et al.[40] also found dramatic increases in the rates of major depression and panic disorder following head trauma.

Personality Disorder

The 1848 case of Phineas Gage stands as the classic description of personality change induced by head trauma.[162,232a] Before his head trauma, Gage had been described as well balanced, honest, efficient, reliable, and capable. Parts of his left frontal lobe and temporal pole were blasted away when an explosion propelled an iron rod through his skull. In contrast to his premorbid good character, after his recovery Gage was described as childish, capricious, inconsiderate and profane, and as having poor judgment. It was said that the balance between his intellectual abilities and his animal propensities had been destroyed, and friends described him as "No longer Gage." Benton[10] has cited similar descriptions in a series of pathological personality changes reported by Welt in 1888, some from traumatic etiologies and all involving lesions of the orbital gyri.

Blumer and Benson[14] have suggested a neuroanatomical and behavioral dichotomy of personality disorder following head trauma. Lesions of the dorsomedial aspects of the frontal lobes or the frontal poles are thought to induce a *pseudodepressed personality syndrome* characterized by apathy and limited emotional reactivity. Lesions of the orbital frontal cortex are thought to induce a *pseudopsychopathic personality syndrome* characterized by disinhibition, egocentricity, and sexual inappropriateness. The validity of this distinction has not been thoroughly investigated.

The Relative's Perspective

Brooks and McKinlay[22] found that 1 year after severe head trauma, relatives described patients as having a poor temper, social withdrawal, irritability, depression, emotional lability, childishness, and unreasonableness. In other studies, caregivers described patients as fatigued, slow, and socially withdrawn in the first year of recovery,[78,176] with caregivers becoming increasingly concerned about their self-centeredness and aggressiveness after the second year of recovery. Thomsen[237] followed 31 patients with posttraumatic amnesia of at least 1 month for 20 years following head injury. Of these patients, 48% lived alone, 13% were married, 13% lived with their parents, and 26% were in nursing homes. For the 32% of patients with chronic and severely disturbed behavior, the most characteristic problems were aggressiveness, violent tendencies, and inappropriate sexual behavior. A complete lack of friendships was apparent in 61% of patients, and 42% of patients had no interests. On the positive side, 23% of Thomsen's patients had a relatively good outcome. The lack of social activity found by Thomsen was also reported by Oddy et al.[195] in patients 7 years after head injury, with insight regarding their deficits as the crucial variable distinguishing the good and poor outcome groups. Following head injury, patients often have diminished awareness and understanding of their deficits, especially in the context of bilateral and multifocal lesions.[206] A substantial social and emotional toll may be also be exacted on the families of patients with head injury.[21]

Return to Work after Head Injury

Mclean et al.[178] found that 0% of patients with severe head injury had returned to work by 1 month but that 46% had returned to work by 1 year. Among patients with mild head injury, 29% returned to work at 1 month, and 79% returned to work by 1 year. Brooks et al.[23] followed up survivors of severe head injury within 2 to 7 years of injury. Before injury 86% were working, whereas 29% were working 7 years after injury. Younger patients were more likely to return to work, as were patients with technical and managerial positions, although relatives sometimes suggested that in patients with more advanced positions, their coworkers "carried" them by providing them with additional assistance or assuming some of their responsibilities. Among cognitive variables, positive predictors of return to employment were adequate verbal learning and information processing capacity (PASAT). Deficits in social discourse (conversational skills) or personal hygiene were negative predictors. Patients who were unable to assume responsibility for running a household or patients who had poor control of mood and anger were much less likely to be employed following severe head injury.

Boake et al.[15] found that normal performance on most neuropsychological tests increased the probability of an ultimate return to productive employment or academic work by 40% to 130%. Similar findings were reported by Cattelani et al.,[29] who found that approximately half of the patients recovered from head trauma were able to return to work, and that the employed patients had VIQs and PIQs approximately one standard deviation (+15 IQ points) greater than those of patients who were unable to resume employment. The employed patients also had significantly higher performance on tests of memory, attention, and executive functioning.

Neurobehavioral Outcome of Head Trauma in the Elderly

Rothweiler et al.[216] followed the outcome in cross sections of patients with closed head injury across the adult life span. They found that even when injury severity was controlled for, persons of advanced age had significantly worse global outcomes as measured by the GOS, and significantly fewer older adults returned to their former living status. Older patients required significantly more time to reach a level of alertness in which they could follow commands, and they were more likely to suffer from medical complications than were younger patients. Even for patients with mild head injury who were following commands within 24 hours, GOS scores at 1 year were lower for patients over age 60 years.

Kilaru et al.[108] reviewed the outcome 3 years after severe head trauma in 40 elderly patients ages 65 to 95 years. A history of premorbid coexisting disease was present in 87% of the sample. None of the elderly patients with GCS scores of 3 to 5 survived in a conscious state. Of the elderly patients with GCS scores of 6 to 7, 55% survived in a conscious state but all were disabled. Of the elderly patients with GCS scores of 8, 60% survived as disabled but independent and 20% had a good recovery.

Goldstein and Levin[66] and Goldstein et al.[68] evaluated patients 50 to 79 years old 1 month following mild to moderate head trauma. Patients recovering from mild head injury performed equivalently to controls, but those sustaining moderate head trauma had deficits in verbal memory, naming, executive functioning, and psychomotor speed. Approximately one-third of the head trauma patients suffered from subjective symptoms of depression, but the frequency of depression did not differ in the mild versus moderate severity groups. Elderly persons recovering from moderate head trauma were rated as having disturbances in cognition, energy level, and metacognition, whereas both mild and moderate groups had worsened somatic concerns and anxiety. The results of these studies indicated that, like their younger counterparts, elderly persons sustaining mild head trauma do not suffer from persistent, clinically significant cognitive deficits, a finding that has been replicated.[188] However, lowered GCS scores and intracranial pathology in a person suffering from moderate head trauma was associated with a poorer outcome, even in the absence of loss of consciousness or an interval of posttraumatic amnesia.[66,68] When these elderly patients were followed up at 1 year, Goldstein et al.[67] found that their relatives rated them as having only slight worsening in cognition and mood. Less satisfactory recovery may be seen if even a mild or moderate head trauma is superimposed on a preexisting or nascent dementia process.

Head Injury as a Risk Factor for Alzheimer's Disease and the APOE-e4 Genotype

A number of studies have found that the presence of the apolipoprotein E-epsilon 4 (APOE-e4) genotype is associated with a worsened outcome after both mild and severe head trauma compared to patients possessing one of the other three APOE alleles.[58,160,233] In contrast, Millar et al.[182] evaluated 396 patients 15 to 25 years after surviving mild, moderate, or severe head traumas and could find no effect for APOE-e4 either on GOS score (extended) or on a battery of neuropsychological tests.

A number of studies have proposed that head injury is a significant risk factor for the subsequent development of Alzheimer's disease,[45,133,187,209] whereas others[57] have failed to replicate the association between history of head injury and Alzheimer's disease. Mayeux et al.[171] suggested a synergistic relationship between head injury and the presence of the APOE-e4 genotype for the development of Alzheimer's disease. O'Meara et al.[197] replicated the increased risk, but found the presence of the APOE-e4 allele to be an independent or additive risk factor for the development of Alzheimer's disease not related to a history of head injury. Salib and Hillier[226] found that an increased risk for dementia after head trauma was not specific to Alzheimer's disease, but was also found for vascular dementia and dementias due to other etiologies as well.

The concept of reduced *cerebral reserve* has also been invoked to explain the association of head injury and Alzheimer's disease. Because severe head injury is known to reduce the neuronal population in the brain, a head injury survivor may have a lower threshold for the development of dementia, as the neuropathology of Alzheimer's disease pushes the cerebral neuronal population below the critical mass necessary for adequate functioning of memory and intellect, with resulting social incompetence. In view of the conflicting findings, head injury continues to be considered a putative risk factor for Alzheimer's disease, especially in the context of APOE-e4 gene penetrance.

Vegetative Survivors of Head Injury

Among persons suffering severe head injury, approximately 10% are discharged in a vegetative state.[120] According to the guidelines of the American Neurological Association, a *persistent* vegetative state is present if the patient has not recovered consciousness within 30 days of eye opening.[6] The diagnosis of vegetative state implies that the patient does not have the critical mass of functioning or connected neuronal tissue necessary to sustain psychologically meaningful behavior.[95] The neuropathology underlying the vegetative state is widespread diffuse axonal injury and associated degeneration of ascending and descending subcortical white matter. This pattern of neuropathology was confirmed in vivo using MRI by Kampfl et al.[104] in 42 patients with persistent vegetative state. The most common common type of traumatic lesion detected by MRI was diffuse white matter injury sparing the overlying cortex. In descending order, the corpus callosum (splenium and body), corona radiata, and frontal and temporal lobe white matter were the areas most frequently lesioned.

Levin et al.[152] found that factors associated with development of the vegetative state were older age, lower GCS score, bilateral pupillary abnormality, CT scan showing diffuse injury with swelling, and hypotension or hypoxia on admission. With regard to recovery, of 84 patients vegetative at the time of hospital discharge (median duration of stay = 59 days), 52% regained consciousness within 1 year, but only a further 6% of the remaining vegetative patients regained consciousness in the following 2 years. Although development of the vegetative state in survivors could be predicted as described above, analysis of the same prognostic factors did not predict the outcome once a patient had entered the vegetative state. Neither age, nor acute neurological indices, nor CT findings determined which patients would recover consciousness, persist in a vegetative state, or die within 3 years of discharge.

Braakman et al.[18] found that of 140 patients vegetative 1 month after injury, by 1 year 51% had died, 11% persisted as vegetative, 26% had severe disability, and 10% were independent. All patients regaining independence were under 40 years old. Of 49 patients still vegetative 3 months after injury, by 1 year 49% had died, 31% persisted as vegetative, 20% were severely disabled, and 0% regained independence. More optimistic findings were reported by Choi et al.,[34] who found that of an initial 73 patients discharged as vegetative, rates of recovered consciousness were 45% at 3 months, 69% at 6 months, and 72% at 12 months. Of the conscious patients, 44% were severely disabled, 17% were moderately disabled, and 11% had a good recovery.

Consistent with the findings of Levin et al.,[152] Choi et al.[34] found no variables that could significantly predict the outcome from the vegetative state. In a review of the literature, Higashi[88] concluded that the probability of recovery from a persistent vegetative state depends mainly on the chronicity of the patient's condition, with a conscious outcome much less likely if the duration of the vegetative state is greater than 1 month. Kampfl et al.[105] also found that age, GCS score, and pupillary reactivity could not predict recovery from the persistent vegetative state in 80 patients, but they also found that the frequency of lesions in the corpus callosum, corona radiata, and dorsolateral upper brain stem significantly differentiated patients who remained in a persistent vegetative state 1 year after injury from those who recovered consciousness.

Quigley et al.[207] have proposed the *3-4-5* rule using a simple combination of age and admission/postresuscitation GCS score to predict a conscious versus dead/vegetative outcome in persons suffering catastrophically severe head injuries. Their data show that conscious survival is essentially zero for persons beyond their 30s with a GCS score of 3; persons beyond their 40s with a GCS score of 4; and persons beyond their 50s with a GCS score of 5. Although their initial sample size was large ($n = 375$), small sample sizes in some age/GCS cohorts make the validity of the 3-4-5 rule questionable. For example, their prediction of essentially no conscious survivorship for patients over age 50 with a GCS score of 5 is based on only eight patients in that particular age/GCS cohort. With relevance to this point, Quigley et al. state that an "extensive" review of the literature did not disclose a single patient outcome that would violate their 3-4-5 rule. Consistent with Quigley et al.'s claim, similar findings by Kilaru et al.[108] are described above in the section on elderly survivors of head injury.

Penetrating Missile Wounds

The neuropathology generated by penetrating missiles, such as bullets or shrapnel, is markedly different from that induced by accelerative/decelerative or blunt trauma.[245] The extent of damage with missile wound depends on the path, velocity, and tumbling action of the projectile within the cranium, with further damage possible from shock waves and expansion of hot gases in the wake of the missile. Wounds that cross the midsagittal or midcoronal planes are associated with a poor outcome.[202] Survival is rare for patients in deep coma. Retention of consciousness in the acute phase of injury by many patients suffering missile wounds[225] demonstrates that penetrating injuries may remain focal in nature, in contrast with the diffuse neuropathological consequences of accelerative/decelerative trauma. As with closed head trauma, the GCS score is related to the outcome. Zafonte et al.[262] found that of 442 penetrating head trauma patients with initial GCS scores of 3–8, 75% died, 3% were discharged to a skilled nursing facility, 17% were discharged to rehabilitation or long-term care, and 4% were discharged to a private residence. In contrast, 26% of patients with initial GCS scores of 9–12 were discharged to private residences, as were 79% of patients with intial GCS scores of 13–15.

Newcombe's[191] classic work demonstrated that there is a clinical correlation between the path of damage caused by a penetrating missile wound and the resulting cognitive deficit. Focal penetrating missile wounds did not cause generalized intellectual deficit in her patients, and there were clear dissociations in the deficits seen in unilateral lesion groups. Left hemisphere wounds produced dysphasia and verbal deficits, whereas right hemisphere wounds produced deficits in complex visual perception.

Schwab et al.[229] found that of 520 Vietnam War veterans with penetrating missile wounds (mostly shrapnel), 56% were eventually employed, in comparison with an 82% employment rate for uninjured Vietnam veteran controls. Posttraumatic epilepsy, paresis, visual field defects, memory loss, psychological disturbance, and violent behavior each contributed to employment status, with a cumulative relationship among the presence of these variables and the likelihood of employment. These investigators[70] also found more frequent aggressive verbal confrontations in patients who had sustained frontal ventromedial lesions as compared to controls and patients with lesions in other brain areas. The presence of aggressive behavior was not associated with lesion volume. Virkkunen et al.[244] followed up 1830 Finnish veterans 32 to 37 years after they had suffered penetrating missile wounds in World War II and found that the incidence of criminal behavior in these veterans was comparable to that of controls.

Predictors of Neurobehavioral Outcome in Adults

Age

In an analysis of 5600 patients who sustained severe head trauma, Hukkelhoven et al.[91] determined that there is an essentially linear relationship between age and outcome as measured by the GOS (Fig. 11.3). Despite the fact that older persons tend to suffer more frequently from low-velocity (e.g. falls) than high-velocity (e.g., motor vehicle) accidents, increasing age is still associated with deeper coma (GCS score of 3–5) and increased numbers

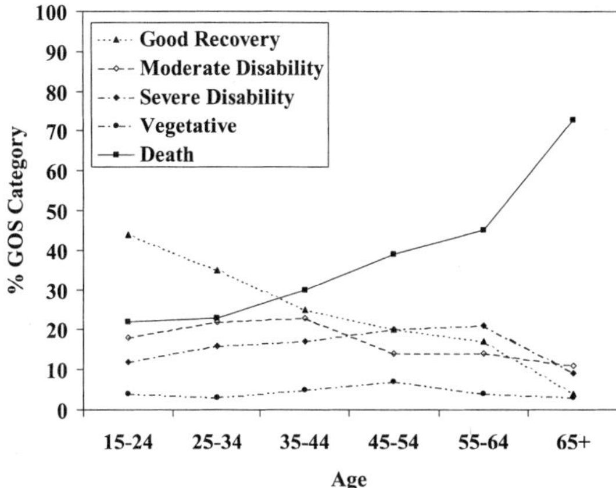

Figure 11.3. The relationship of age at injury to Glasgow Outcome Scale (GOS) category for adults with severe head trauma. (Adapted from reference 910).

of lesions visualized on CT. After age 65, the incidence of nonreactivity in both pupils doubles. These factors suggest that advancing age renders the brain more vulnerable to the effects of impacts of equal or even lesser severity than those experienced by younger persons. As discussed above, Rothweiler et al.[216] found that even with initial GCS scores controlled across age cohorts, advanced age is associated with more severe neurobehavioral consequences, which again suggests that the aged brain is more vulnerable to the deleterious primary or secondary effects of head injury than to the young adult brain.

Glasgow Coma Scale

The acute GCS score is a predictor of coma duration[255] and of neurobehavioral outcome as categorized by the GOS. Levin et al.[132] found that among survivors of severe head injury at 1 year, vegetative patients typically had a worst postresuscitation GCS score of 3–4, those with severe disability typically had GCS scores of 4–6, those with moderate disability typically had GCS scores of 4–7, and those with good recovery typically had GCS scores of 6–7. However, within each range of GCS score, there was variation in outcome. Cognitive outcome, as gauged by the ability to participate meaningfully in neuropsychological testing, was also related to acute GCS score. Alexandre et al.[5] found that GCS scores at admission predicted the cognitive outcome, as measured by psychometric testing 2 years after injury (Table 11.2), and that improved prediction was obtained using the GCS score at 24 hours. Patients with a very brief coma

Table 11.2. Cognitive Outcome in Conscious Survivors of Head Injury at 2 Years in Relation to Acute Neurologic Indices*

	Initial GCS† Score			**Neurological Syndrome‡**		
	8–15	*5–7*	*3–4*	*Hemisph.*	*Dienceph.*	*Mesenceph.*
No/minimal deficit§	84%	34%	11%	91%	25%	—
Mild deficit‖	16%	40%	25%	9%	56%	23%
Severe deficit¶	—	26%	64%	—	19%	77%
Posttraumatic Coma Duration (days)				***Amnesia Duration (Days)***		
	<1	*1–3*	*≥4*	*≤7*	*8–14*	*>14*
No/minimal deficit	50%	36%	38%	56%	38%	29%
Mild deficit	30%	21%	35%	19%	31%	38%
Severe deficit	20%	43%	27%	25%	31%	33%

*Subjects were 100 survivors of closed head injury.

†Glasgow Coma Scale.

‡Level of neurological syndrome as diagnosed by a neurologist based on evaluation of pyramidal and extrapyramidal systems, intrinsic and extrinsic ocolumotor systems, respiration, and reactivity to stimulation. Hemisph, hemispheric; Dienceph., diencephalic; Mesenceph., mesencephalic.

§No/minimal deficit: No/minimal reduction in memory, Full Scale Intelligence Quotient (FSIQ) >90, no significant difference between Verbal IQ (VIQ) and Performance IQ (PIQ).

‖Mild deficit: Memory deficit and either FSIQ 70–90 or VIQ-PIQ difference ≥ 20 points.

¶Severe deficit: Memory deficit and FSIQ <70.

Source: Adapted from reference 12.

duration have a greater probability of achieving a good recovery, but the relationship between longer coma duration and cognitive outcome is unreliable.[5,138]

Brain Stem Reflexes

According to the centripetal model of head injury proposed by Ommaya and Gennarelli,[198] diffuse shear strain is maximal at the neocortex, which is the most peripheral aspect of the brain, less severe in the subcortical structures and their diencephalic connections, and least severe at the level of the mesencephalon. Consistent with this model, the finding of abnormal brain stem reflexes strongly suggests that substantial force has been imparted to the deepest, core areas of the brain, implying that even more severe shear strain has also been generated throughout the cerebrum, with a resulting massive, diffuse insult. Brain stem reflex findings, as described below, are associated with a poor prognosis. As a caveat, deficits in these reflexes can also be caused by damage outside the brain stem.[98]

Pupillary Reactivity

Jennett et al.[99] found that in severely injured patients with nonreactive pupils during the first 24 hours of coma, 91% have dead or vegetative outcomes and 4% have moderate disability or good recovery. In contrast, there is a 50% rate of moderate disability or good recovery among patients with reactive pupils. As shown in Table 11.3, a similar relationship between favorable GOS score at 1 year and intact pupillary reactivity after severe head injury was found by Levin et al.[132] As shown in Table 11.4, residual deficits in memory and intellect are also predicted by pupillary reactivity.[134] Levin et al.[132] found an interaction between the ability of GCS scores and pupillary reactivity to predict the cognitive outcome, such that a low GCS score was only predictive of severe neurobehavioral sequelae in the context of nonreactive pupils. A low GCS score occurring with intact pupillary reactivity may reflect transient effects of raised intracranial pressure, medication, or other acute variables, rather than the depth and extent of diffuse shear strain imparted throughout the brain. Thus, the finding of a low GCS score concomitant with nonreactive pupils provides a less equivocal indication of the depth and extent of structural injury.

Table 11.3. Glasgow Outcome Scale Findings by Pupillary Reactivity 1 Year After Survival of Severe Head Injury*

	Pupils	
Glasgow Outcome Scale	**Both Reactive**	**One or Both Nonreactive**
Good recovery	57%	22%
Moderate disability	22%	20%
Severe disability	16%	42%
Vegetative	5%	16%

*Subjects were 259 survivors of severe head injury admitted to trauma centers with coma or who deteriorated to coma (Glasgow Coma Scale score ≤ 8).

Source: Adapted from reference 132.

Oculovestibular Reflex

Levin et al.[138] found that coma accompanied by a deficit in the oculovestibular reflex predicted a probable outcome at 1 year of moderate to severe disability, marked memory deficit, and intellect in the borderline to deficit range. Consistent with this report, Heiden et al.[84] found that only 4% of patients with abnormal oculovestibular reflexes had good recoveries.

Intracranial Pressure

Levin et al.[152] found that maximum levels of intracranial pressure, or the total time during which intracranial pressure exceeded 20 mg Hg, did not differentiate severely injured patients who recovered consciousness from those persisting in a vegetative state. Among survivors of severe head injury, intracranial pressure exceeding 20 mm Hg had a modest relationship with impaired memory functioning at 6 months after head injury, but this effect could not be replicated at 12 months after head injury.[128] Likewise, Levin et al.[132] found negligible effects of intracranial pressure on cognitive outcome 1 year following severe head injury. Resnick et al.[210] have also failed to find a relationship between outcome, mean or peak intracranial pressure, duration of time with raised intracranial pressure, or lowest recorded cerebral perfusion pressure. More recently, Clifton et al.[36] found that intracranial pressure, greater than 25 mm Hg was associated with poor outcome, as measured by the GOS.

Table 11.4. Cognitive Outcome as Related to Acute Neurological Indices 15 to 42 Months After Head Injury*

	Median Time		Pupils	
	Lowest to Median GCS	Follow Commands (Days)	Reactive	Nonreactive
Normal	8	1	69%	19%
Memory deficit (IQ ≥85)	7	10	12%	31%
Global deficit (IQ <85)	6	18	19%	50%

*Subjects were 42 patients with moderate to severe closed head injury.
Source: Adapted from reference 134.

Ventricular Enlargement

Considered irrespective of time of onset, ventricular enlargement is correlated with length of coma, but shows only a modest relationship with the outcome on tests of memory and intellect.[150] In fact, striking dissociations between extent of ventricular enlargement and outcome were apparent in 13% of patients studied. Meyers et al.[181] studied the correlates of ventricular enlargement with consideration of the time of onset. Patients with "early" ventricular enlargement (occurring 0 to 28 days after injury), largely secondary to subarachnoid or intraventricular hemorrhage, were contrasted with patients showing "late" (presumably ex-vacuo) ventricular enlargement (occurring 40 or more days after injury), which purportedly reflected degeneration of the periventricular white matter. The GCS score and coma duration were related only to late ventricular enlargement. The relationship between early ventricular enlargement and cognitive outcome was not significant. There was a modest relationship between late ventricular enlargement and intellectual performance.

Neurological Syndrome

Bricolo et al.[19] found worsening GOS scores after 1 year of recovery for vegetative patients as the classification of acute neurological syndrome progressed in depth from hemispheric to diencephalic, mesencephalic, and finally pontomedullary. Similar findings were reported by Alexandre et al.[5] and are shown in Table 11.2. These findings are again consistent with Ommaya and Genarelli's centripetal model of brain injury.[198]

Duration of Unconsciousness

The length of unconsciousness, as measured until the time a patient is able to consistently follow commands, provides moderate to low prediction of functional independence ($r = -.40$) and level of cognitive functioning ($r = -.35$) on discharge from rehabilitation.[251]

Duration of Posttraumatic Amnesia

Russell[217] and Russell and Nathan [220]established that the duration of posttraumatic amnesia is related to the degree of residual memory deficit, Dikmen et al.[42] found that it is related to the degree of disability following head trauma. Levin et al.[151] found that a duration of posttraumatic amnesia of less than 14 days is predictive of good recovery, whereas a duration greater than 14 days is predictive of moderate to severe disability (see Table 11.2). This finding is also apparent in the observations of Jennett et al.,[97] Alexandre et al.,[5] and more recently in the study of van der Naalt, and Sluiter.[240] Zafonte et al.[261] found that the duration of posttraumatic amnesia predicted both functional independence and degree of disability on discharge from a rehabilitation center.

Psychosocial outcome is also predicted by the duration of posttraumatic amnesia. Brooks and McKinlay[22] found that longer periods of posttraumatic amnesia were associated with a higher probability of personality change following head injury. Oddy et al.[196] found that 6 months after head injury, those patients with posttraumatic amnesia of less than 7 days had a 71% rate of return to work compared to a 27% return rate for those with more than 7 days of posttraumatic amnesia. Ellenberg et al.[46] found that the duration of posttraumatic amnesia predicts the GOS score at 6 months even when the interval of conscious disorientation is separated from the period of coma. Cattelani et al.[29] found that length of posttraumatic amnesia, but not admission GCS score, predicted eventual return to employment.

Neuroimaging

Computed Tomography

Although of great diagnostic value in acute treatment, CT contributes only modestly to prediction of the neurobehavioral outcome of severe head injury.[29,61,132,211] Uzzell et al.[239] found that when considered alone, CT findings of diffuse axonal injury (midline hemorrhages or multiple small hemorrhages at the gray–white matter junction) predicted a poorer GOS category at 6 months compared to CT findings of diffuse swelling or focal lesions. The relationship with more specific cognitive measures was not impressive. IQ and language scores did not differ among the CT groups at 8 months, although differences in gradients of recovery in memory and mental speed were apparent. Levin et al.[132] found that the type of injury imaged on CT scan (diffuse swelling, mass effect, other abnormality) was unrelated to cognitive performance at 1 year. More recently, Mataro et al.[168] found that the presence of a mass lesion on CT predicted performance at 6 months on tests of motor or psychomotor speed but not on other neuropsychological tests.

Magnetic Resonance Imaging

Among patients with GCS scores of 9 to 15, MRI will detect 80% to 85% more intracranial lesions than CT.[117,157] The correlations between the site of lesions seen on MRI and performance in specific neuropsychological domains remains modest at best in group comparisons, although striking clinical correlations may be seen in individual cases.[7,117,135,140,157]

Levin et al.[156] examined the relationship between depth of brain lesion on MRI and various clinical variables in 94 patients with head injuries of varying severity. Consistent with Ommaya and Gennarelli's[198] centripetal model of diffuse neuronal damage following head injury, deep central gray matter or brain stem lesions were associated with lower levels of consciousness, longer durations of impaired consciousness, increased ventricular enlargement, and more severe disability at 6 months (Fig. 11.4). The duration of posttraumatic amnesia was not predicted by depth of lesion. Although Kampfl et al.[105] have shown that MRI can predict recovery from the persistent vegetative state, other outcome studies have indicated that MRI does not consistently provide incremental information over more basic variables such as age, GCS score, and pupillary reactivity. In a similar vein, Pierallini et al.[201] found that at 1 year, the total volume of lesions imaged on MRI could predict the level of cognitive functioning, but it is not clear that MRI added predictive power over other clinical variables gauging injury severity.

Posttraumatic Epilepsy

Mazzini et al.[173] found that 19% of 143 patients admitted consecutively after severe head trauma developed posttraumatic epilepsy, with some patients developing seizures more than 3 years postinjury. Posttraumatic epilepsy was predicted neither by GCS score nor by the number and size of le-

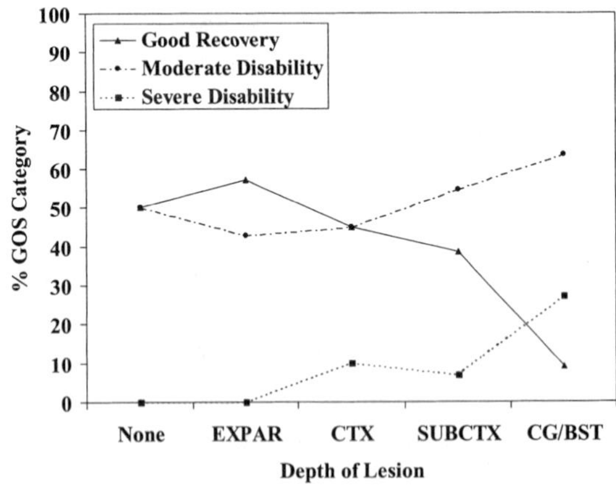

Figure 11.4. Relationship between maximum depth of lesion on magnetic resonance imaging and probability of attaining various neurobehavioral outcomes in adults with closed head injury. Maximum depth of lesion: None, no lesion; EXPAR, extraparenchymal; CTX, cortical; SUBCTX, subcortical white matter; CG/BST, Deep central gray matter/brain stem. Increasing depth of the lesion lowers the probability of a good outcome and raises the probability of severe disability. (Adapted from reference 156.)

sions, but was predicted by coma duration. Posttraumatic epilepsy predicted a worse eventual GOS score, even when the effects of injury severity as gauged by GCS score and coma duration were controlled.

Premorbid Intellectual Functioning

The interplay between premorbid capacity and the extent of neurobehavioral sequelae in head injury was captured by Sir Charles Symonds when he stated that "it is not only the kind of injury that matters, but the kind of head."[234] In keeping with Symonds' observations, it has been demonstrated that high levels of preinjury educational and occupational attainment are related to an improved prognosis for resumption of employment after closed head injury.[63,212] The level of premorbid intellectual functioning, which can be reliably predicted from demographic factors such as education and occupation,[256] affects the potential for neurobehavioral recovery and response to rehabilitation.

With regard to penetrating missile wounds, Weinstein and Teuber[249] reported that the degree of intellectual loss in soldiers was comparable across various levels of premorbid cognitive ability, which they estimated from premorbid test scores generated at the time of military induction. More recently, Grafman et al.[69] found that the level of premorbid cognitive functioning in Vietnam War veterans at military induction was a stronger predictor of performance after a penetrating missile wound than either brain tissue loss volume or locus of lesion. A stronger predictive relationship was apparent between premorbid intellect and postinjury performance on tests of complex cognition than was apparent between premorbid intellect and tests of narrower and more specific cognitive domains. The volume of brain tissue lost to missile injury was also more predictive of global cognition than of specific cognitive processes, whereas locus of lesion only predicted performance in specific cognitive domains.

Combinations of Predictive Variables

Multivariate models have been used to predict the outcome of severe head injury. Using a stepwise discriminant analysis on postresuscitation factors, Choi et al.[35] found that a combination of age, GCS motor score, and pupillary response comprised the best combination of predictive variables, with a correct classification rate of 78% for subsequent GOS category. Similar findings were reported by Braakman et al.,[17] who found that worst pupillary reactivity, age, and worst GCS motor score at 24 hours comprised the best combination of predictors. Although the use of clinical variables in combination can maximize the predictive accuracy of statistical models, the variables used in these combinations have different properties than they would if considered separately. Variables with high predictive value will be eliminated from the combination if they are highly intercorrelated with other predictors. Thus, these formulas do not indicate which individual factors are causal to the outcome; they only reflect the best combination of statistical predictors.

Neurobehavioral Outcome of Head Injury in Children

As in adults, there is a rostrocaudal gradient of severity of traumatic neuropathology in children, with lesions most frequently occurring in the orbitofrontal and dorsolateral frontal lobes and in the temporal poles (Fig. 11.5).[125,149,179] The quantitative MRI findings of Berryhill et al.[11] indicated reductions in orbitofrontal and dorsolateral frontal gray matter volumes even in the absence of focal brain lesions.

Like adults, children sustaining head injury are not a representive sample of the population.[64] Consistent with their higher rates of impulsivity, more boys than girls sustain head injuries, and there is a higher rate of premorbid learning disability, developmental delay, and poor academic achievement in children sustaining head injury than in those who avoid injury. In comparison with the question of recovery of mature brain systems and established cognitive abilities in adults, brain insult impacts cognitive development in children.

Cognitive Effects of Head Injury in Children

Memory

Recovery from head injury in children may involve an interval of posttraumatic amnesia with anterograde and retrograde components.[50] As with adults, memory is the cognitive domain most frequently

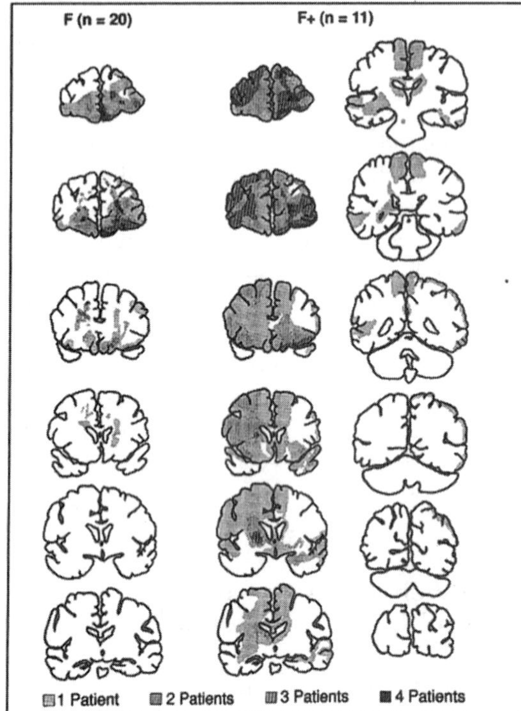

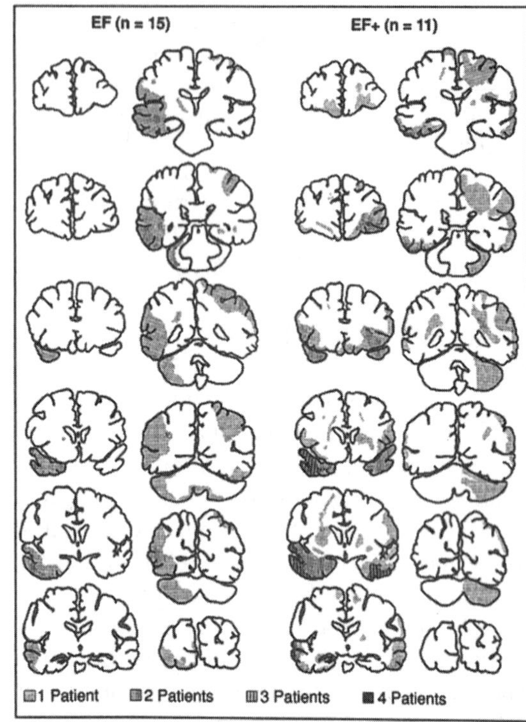

Figure 11.5. Distribution of magnetic resonance imaging lesions plotted on coronal templates in two experimental groups of children (n = 57) after closed head injury. A rostrocaudal gradient of lesion is seen in the children classified in the frontal (F) and predominantly frontal (EF) groups. A centripetal gradient of lesion is seen in the EF and predominantly EF (EF+) lesion groups. (From reference 125, with permission.)

and most severely affected by head injury.[126] Children's memory is typically at normal levels 1 year following mild to moderate head injury, although significant memory deficits may be seen in children 1 year following severe head injury.[142,165,190]

The addition of a *prospective* element to a memory task is especially difficult for children recovering from severe head trauma. That is, the task becomes much more difficult for these children when they must remember on their own to perform an intended element of the task, rather than having to simply follow the current demands of the examiner. McCauley and Levin[174] found that 71% of children recovered from orthopedic injuries remembered to perform a previous task instruction carried over to a current problem compared to only 7% of children recovered from severe head trauma.

Intelligence

Children recovering from moderate to severe head trauma typically have loss in IQ performance, as measured by the Wechsler Intelligence Scales for Children (the current revision is the WISC-IV). In the absence of a focal left hemisphere mass lesion, the VIQ is typically less severely affected than the PIQ,[30,54,92–95,165] and as with adults, the more severe loss of PIQ is likely secondary to the demands of novel problem solving on both mental capacity and motor speed.[51,109] Among children with severe head injury and coma duration of at least 1 week, 37% had Full Scale IQs in the mentally deficient range (<70 points) at 1 to 7 years postinjury.[20] Of these children, 77% were enrolled in special education classes. The severity of intellectual deficit was related to coma duration. Jaffe et al.[54,92–94] followed 72 children, ages 6 to 15 years, over a 3-year period following mild, moderate, or severe head injury. As show in Figure 11.6, there were significant effects of both head injury severity and recovery time, with the PIQ more severely affected than the VIQ. Consistent with the findings of other studies,[30,47] progressive recovery of intellect was apparent in the first 6 months to 1 year of recovery, with relatively modest gains in the 2 years thereafter.[94]

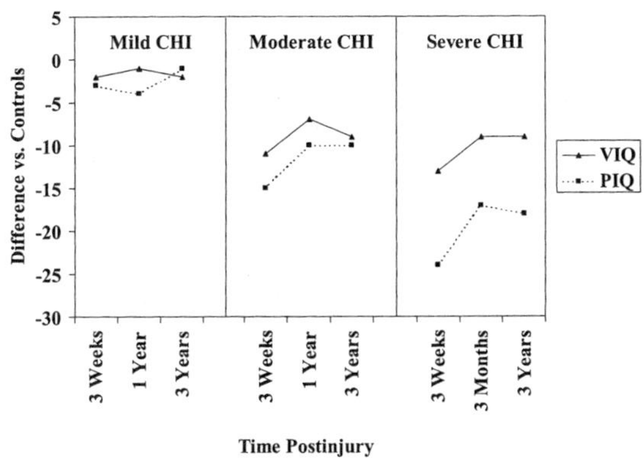

Figure 11.6. Relationship of intellect to severity of closed head injury (CHI) and recovery time following head injury in children. The data points represent mean standard score differences of patient cases versus uninjured controls. (Adapted from the series of Jaffe et al.[64,65] and from Fay et al.[35])

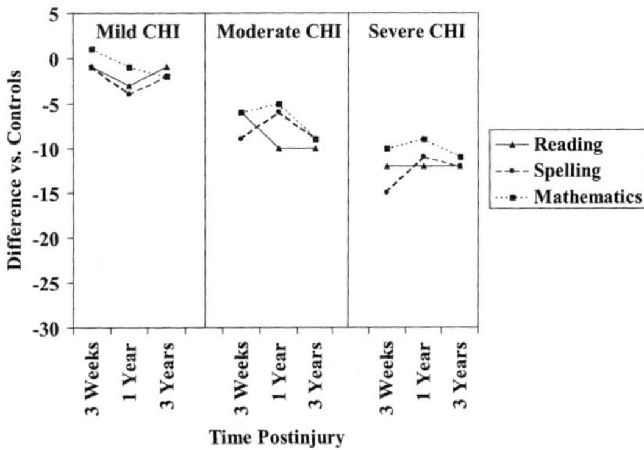

Figure 11.7. Relationship of Wide Range Achievement Test–Revised (WRAT-R) Reading, Spelling, and Arithmetic performances to severity of closed head injury (CHI) and recovery time. The data points represent mean standard score differences of patient cases versus uninjured controls. (Adapted from the series of Jaffe et al.[64,65] and from Fay et al.[35])

The WISC-IV is the current version of the most widely used test of intelligence for children ages 6 to 16 years.[248] Consistent with past studies, children recovered at least 6 months from both closed and open head injury typically demonstrated deficits in Processing Speed (-18 points) and Perceptual Reasoning (-12 points), whereas Verbal Conceptual (-9 points) and Working Memory (-7 points) indices remained relatively preserved.

Academic Performance

Levin et al.[130] found that single word reading and spelling skills tended to remain unchanged by severe head injury, whereas arithmetic performance was relatively impaired compared to both reading performance and premorbid achievement scores. These findings were thought to stem from the heavier demands of mathematics on sustained attention and concentration. The finding of relative impairment in arithmetic performance was replicated in the study of Ewing-Cobbs et al.[48] but not in the series of Jaffe and his colleagues[54,92–94] who found equivalent decrements in reading, spelling, and arithmetic achievement across a three year recovery interval (see Fig. 11.7).

Ewing-Cobbs et al.[48] investigated the placement and performance of children in school after head trauma. They found that only 23% of children and 18% of adolescents were performing without failure in a regular curriculum 2 years after severe head trauma compared to 88% of children and 92% of adolescents who were passing in a regular curriculum 2 years following mild head trauma. The high rates of failure, resource room placement, and special education placement in children recovered from severe head trauma occurred despite their generally average performance on achievement tests of reading and spelling and their low average performance on achievement tests of arithmetic. Similar findings were reported by Massagli et al.[166] who found that of children sustaining severe head trauma, 21% had preinjury placement in special education, but that this figure increased to a 79% rate of either special education placement or school dropout after injury.

Language

Levin and Chapman[123] reported that posttraumatic aphasia in children differs in its clinical characteristics from the pattern seen in adults after head injury. Mutism, lack of spontaneous speech, and poverty of expression are more characteristic of posttraumatic aphasia in children, whereas adults with posttraumatic aphasia tend to have fluent anomic speech. With regard to language performance on psychometric tests, Levin and Eisenberg[126] profiled children and adolescents following head injury and found the following rates of deficit: naming objects 13%, repetition 4%, and aural comprehension 11%.

A series of studies by Chapman and colleagues[24,31,32] investigated the discourse of children who had sustained a severe closed head trauma as young as age 1 year. Initial testing occurred at ages 6 to 8 years, with additional follow-up 3 years later. The general finding was that the discourse of children recovered from severe head trauma did not differ from that of controls or of children with mild to moderate head trauma in terms of linguistic structure, flow of information, or cohesiveness. Rather, significant deficits in information structure were consistently present in the discourse of children recovered from severe head trauma. Specifically, the recovered children related a lower quantity of overall information, and their selection, organization, and integration of information were also impaired compared to controls. Following head trauma, children communicated less of the *gist*, or essential meaning, of a sequence of events in their discourse. While children recovered from severe head trauma did not differ from controls in the sheer amount of language used in discourse, they tended toward the vague and concrete, whereas normal children gave much more concise, abstract, and generalized statements when attempting to convey information.[33] No effects were observed for age at injury, volume of lesion, or locus of lesion.[24] Significant correlations were found between measures of discourse and tasks of abstract problem solving (Wisconsin Card Sorting Test) and verbal associate fluency (Controlled Oral Word Association), suggesting that executive deficits may contribute to the abnormalities in discourse apparent in children recovered from severe head trauma.

Yorkston et al.[260] evaluated the written language of 76 children, ages 8 to 15 years, 1 month after the resolution of posttraumatic amnesia. Significant correlations with head injury severity were found for all written language variables, with efficiency (number of words and ideas per minute) and completeness (numbers of words and ideas, and maturity of ideas) the variables most affected. Written vocabulary was least severely affected.

Attention

Kaufmann et al.[106] tested attentional functioning in 36 children, ages 7 to 16 years, 6 months following closed head injury using both the WISC-R Digit Span and a continuous performance test that comprised 40 blocks of stimuli, with 21 stimuli in each block. Consistent with other reports,[9,30,257] Digit Span proved resistant to the effect of head injury severity. Thus, simple attentional capacity measured in discrete intervals is not a particularly sensitive task for children beyond the acute phase of recovery. In contrast, there was a strong effect of head injury severity on a continuous performance test, which demands sustained attention over a substantial time interval. Although the performance of patients with mild and moderate head injury was similar, and at a rate equivalent to normative expectations, the severe head injury group showed deficits in sustained attention across the duration of the continuous performance test.

Levin et al.[141] measured the ability of children recovered 5 years from severe head trauma to perform a task that demanded a selective response to a target that had occurred one, two, or three stimulus items previously (N-back procedure), which makes significant demands on sustained attentional capacity. Children who had sustained severe head trauma showed deficits in response to target items and produced an excessive number of false alarms, indicating both poor attentional functioning and response disinhibtion. Despite the putative importance of the frontal lobes in regulating attention, the performance of the one-third of the children with frontal lesions on MRI was no worse than that of the two-thirds of the children who had either no lesion or an extrafrontal lesion.

Children recovered from head trauma have particular difficulty when their attention is divided by having to perform two task conditions simultaneously[174]—for example, if they are asked to categorize a word while also notifying the examiner if a word appears in ink of a certain color. Under such conditions, children recovered from severe head trauma demonstrate marked slowing of reaction time compared to controls.

Wassenberg et al.[246] found that recovery time of children after head trauma predicted errors of omission (inattention) on a continuous performance (sustained-attention) task, and that commission errors (impulsiveness) were predicted by both injury severity and recovery time. Remarkably, omission errors were not predicted by injury severity, but were predicted by social background and preinjury adaptive functioning. This finding reinforces the idea that the behavioral manifestations of a neurological event will often be influenced by preexisting psychosocial factors on cognitive development.

Executive Functioning

Levin et al.[125] evaluated executive functioning in 76 children and adolescents (ages 6 to 16 years) with moderate to severe head injury and a mean recovery time of approximately 1.5 years. They found effects of injury severity on all executive tasks administered, including tests of concept formation/problem solving (Wisconsin Card Sorting Test; 20 Questions test), planning (Tower of London), verbal associative fluency (Controlled Oral Word Association; Design Fluency), response modulation (Go/No-Go), and abstraction (WISC-R Similarities). Levin et al.[155] studied executive functioning in 151 children with mild or severe closed head injury. Effects of injury severity were again apparent on all three tasks of concept formation/problem solving and planning. Level of executive functioning accounted for 21% of the variance in parental reports of adaptive behavior in the head-injured children. Even performance on relatively straightforward tasks such as the Porteus Mazes (performed with paper and pencil) is often impaired in children following severe head trauma.[153]

Ewing-Cobbs et al.[52] found persisting deficits in executive functioning even 5 to 8 years following severe head injury in children, particularly on a test of abstract problem solving (Wisconsin Card Sorting Test). Also suggestive of executive dysfunction was the tendency of children recovered from severe head injury to display response disinhibition by identifying target stimuli for which there was no previous exposure (i.e., an excessive false alarm rate on recognition memory). Nybo and Koskiniemi[194] found that the Wisconsin Card Sorting Test was the neurospsychological test that was most strongly associated with vocational outcome in adults 16 to 30 years after they sustained severe head trauma as children. With regard to the metacognitive, or self-appraisal, aspect of executive functioning, children recovered 3 years from severe head injury tend to significantly overestimate their own learning capacity compared to normal controls.[79]

Psychosocial Outcome of Head Injury in Children

Several studies have indicated that children who sustain head trauma have premorbid tendencies toward impulsive behavior, hyperactivity, and conduct problems.[12,39,64,161,223] Brown et al.[26] found that children sustaining mild head injury had a higher incidence of premorbid behavioral problems than did children with severe head injury or controls with orthopedic injuries. Likewise, Schachar et al.[228] found that parents described 42% of children sustaining closed head injury as suffering from preexisting behavioral problems such as short attention span and underachievement compared to a 25% rate of behavioral disorder for controls. Bloom et al.[13] found that 43% of children sustaining head trauma had preexisting undiagnosed psychiatric disorders, most commonly attention-deficit/hyperactivity disroder (ADHD).

Brown et al.[26] found that following 2 years of recovery, there was a 10% to 20% increase in the onset of psychiatric disorder in orthopedic controls or in children with mild head injury, whereas children with severe head injury had triple the rate of new psychiatric disorder compared to the other two groups. Rutter[223] found no specific set of symptoms or characteristic psychiatric syndrome caused by head injury in children, although there was a distinctive trend for these children to be described by others as socially disinhibited. Similar findings were reported by Fletcher et al.[55] They found that parental reports of children with severe head injury contained descriptions of reduced adaptive behavior, social withdrawal, and hyperactive, aggressive behavior, but they did not find consistent evidence of a severe behavioral disorder or of a specific and particular behavioral syndrome in these children. Cognitive performance and behavioral outcome variables were only weakly correlated.

Rutter[223] found that factors such as parental marital discord, parental psychiatric disorder, and socioeconomic disadvantage lead to an increased incidence of psychiatric disorder among children with head injury. Rivara et al.[214] also found that premorbid family and child functioning are significant predictors of a child's outcome 1 year following head injury. Although head injury severity affected the cognitive and academic outcome in a child, family variables predicted behavioral and social outcomes.[215]

Fletcher et al.[56] studied children with head injuries on a variety of behavioral dimensions. Parents of children with severe head injuries rated their children as having difficulties in cognition but not in self-control, social competence, or somatic symptoms. On the Vineland Adaptive Behavior

Scales for Children, an effect of injury severity was seen on the Communication and Socialization domains, but there was no effect on the Daily Living domain. Age at testing, GCS score, and MRI variables did not explain more than 21% of the variance in children's adaptive behavior following head injury. Brookshire et al.[25] found that neuropsychological tests of language, memory, executive functioning, processing speed, and motor speed were moderately predictive of adaptive behavior 3 years after severe head trauma as measured by the Vineland Scales, with correlations generally ranging from low (r = 0.27) to moderate (r = .54).

Max et al.[170] found novel (i.e., not present before the injury) psychiatric disorder in 15 of 42 (36%) children 2 years after head injury, but appreciation of the significance of this figure is limited by the lack of a control group. A variety of psychiatric disorders developed following head injury in these children including oppositional defiant disorder in 8 children, ADHD in 6, and organic personality disorder in 4, comorbid with ADHD. Severity of injury, family psychiatric history, premorbid psychiatric disorder, socioeconomic class, premorbid intelligence, and adaptive behavior all predicted the development of a novel psychiatric disorder at follow-up intervals of 3, 6, 12, and 24 months, but only the level of family functioning consistently predicted the psychiatric status in head-injured children across all follow-up intervals.

Gerring et al.[62] investigated the development of ADHD in children after closed head injury. Of 95 children ages 4 to 19 years, 20% had premorbid diagnoses of ADHD, a significantly higher incidence than the 4.5% in the general population. Of the 80 children in the study who did not have premorbid ADHD, 19% developed ADHD, an incidence rate that is again substantially higher than the population prevalence for the disorder. Compared with children whose ADHD was not diagnosed, children developing ADHD following closed head injury had significantly higher levels of family dysfunction, a finding similar to that of both Brown et al.[26] and Max et al.[170] Children who developed ADHD also had higher levels of posttraumatic affective lability and aggression, higher levels of posttraumatic psychiatric comorbidity, and higher levels of overall disability. Consistent findings were also reported by Schachar et al.,[228] who found that ADHD developed in approximately 20% of children who did not evidence behavioral disorder prior to injury. An even higher 36% rate of novel ADHD was observed when children who had some previous behavioral disturbance were included, and this rate significantly exceeds the 12% base rate of ADHD that was found in controls. Bloom et al.[13] found a 57% rate of novel psychiatric disorders in children following mild, moderate, and severe head trauma, with these disorders persisting at 1 year in 81% of the cases. Again, ADHD was most commonly seen, followed by depressive and then anxiety disorder. No relationship was apparent between the rate of novel disorder and injury severity.

Max et al.[169] found a relationship between trauma severity and the probability of developing subsequent ADHD. Following injury, 5% of orthopedic controls developed ADHD compared to 8% of children with mild head injury, 13% of children with moderate head injury, and 38% of children with severe head injury. Lowest postresuscitation GCS score and duration of impaired consciousness were related to the development of ADHD, but age and lesion area on CT were not significant. The ADHD resolved in almost one-third of the children within 18 months postinjury.

Inflicted Head Injury in Children

A number of investigators have focused on the neurobehavioral outcome in young children who are the victims of purposeful infliction of head injury by a caregiver. These victims of the *shaken baby syndrome* have typically been excluded from most outcome studies, as the repetitive rotational force induced by intentional shaking of a child differs from the single acceleration/deceleration or blunt impact forces imparted during accidental closed head injuries, and because these children are often the victims of chronic abuse that includes past unreported head injuries.

Duhaime et al.[44] located 14 children discharged from a hospital after violent shaking at age 2 years or younger, with a mean age at head injury of 6.4 months. Of these 14 children, 1 had died while vegetative, 6 survived as vegetative or severely disabled, 2 were moderately disabled, and 5 had a good recovery. Of the five children with a good recovery, three also had cognitive deficits or behavior problems. Haviland and Russell[82] studied 15 children who were victims of shaking at ages 1 to

30 months. At follow-up, which ranged from 3 months to 3 years, two children were dead, seven had major neurological handicaps, four had moderate neurological handicaps, one was mildly handicapped, and only one child had an apparently normal outcome.

Ewing-Cobbs et al.[49] investigated 20 children, ages 1 to 6 months, who were the victims of inflicted head injuries, and compared them to control children who were the victims of accidental closed head injuries. Cerebral atrophy consistent with a previous head injury was apparent only in the children presenting with acute inflicted head injuries, and several of the children in the inflicted head injury group also had subdural hygromas that may have evolved from previous subdural hematomas. Ex-vacuo ventricular abnormalities were apparent in 40% of the children with inflicted head injury, whereas the 15% of the children with accidental head injury had ventricular abnormalities consistent with mass effect or edema. The children with inflicted head injuries had a higher incidence of subdural hematoma and seizures, and retinal hemorrhages were found exclusively in these children. In contrast, children with accidental head injuries had higher incidences of extradural hematomas, parenchymal hematomas, and shear injury. With regard to neurobehavioral outcome, at an average of 1 month following resolution of posttraumatic amnesia, 45% of the children with inflicted injuries were mentally deficient compared to 5% of the children with accidental injuries. The GOS outcome in the children with inflicted head injuries was follows: 20% had a good recovery, 65% had moderate disability, and 15% had severe disability.

Similar findings were reported by Bonnier et al.,[16] who studied the effects of head trauma inflicted on 23 surviving babies ages 3 weeks to 13 months. They found that retinal hemorrhage, skull fracture, diffuse parenchymal lesions on MRI, and deceleration of cranial growth all predicted the global outcome, but it was not clear if any or all of these factors added incremental predictive value to the initial GCS score, which was also correlated with the outcome at least 2 years postinjury. Persistent vegetative state was seen in 13% of surviving children, severe disability in 48%, moderate disability in 35%, and good recovery in 4%. The majority of children were left with borderline or defective intellect, severe motor impairments such as hemiplegia or quadraplegia, and frequently visual impairment or blindness.

Predictors of the Neurobehavioral Outcome in Children

Age

The plasticity of the developing brain often permits dramatic recovery of function following a focal hemispheric insult in young children.[115,239,254] However, the effects of the diffuse insult produced by head injury result in greater cognitive impairment in the developing brain than in the mature brain.[129] Levin et al.[130] found that children are left with a global intellectual deficit (IQ <80) only if they were younger than 13 years at the time of severe head injury. Children under 10 years of age are at higher risk for significant cognitive impairment following head injury than adolescents,[20] and infants and toddlers are at greater risk than children of preschool and kindergarten age.[113] In the Finnish study of Koskiniemi et al.,[111] children who had sustained head injury at age 7 or less were followed into adulthood. None of those who were age 3 years or younger at the time of injury was subsequently able to work full time compared to 29% of those who were age 4 years or older at injury.

Among survivors of severe head injury, Levin et al.[116] found that patients from infancy to 4 years of age had the least probability of a good outcome 1 year following head injury, whereas the probability of a good outcome increased in a linear fashion between ages 5 to 10, 11 to 15, and adult cohorts. Heindl and Laub[86] studied 82 children and adolescents with head injury, ages infancy to 22 years, who had been unconscious for at least 1 month. At 12 months, 80% regained consciousness, although at 19 months only 16% had achieved independence in their daily activities, and no child had a complete recovery. Once in a persistent vegetative state, age of the was child not a significant prognostic factor in regaining consciousness.

Consistent with the idea that more devastating effects may be seen when head trauma is sustained at a younger age, performance on some neuropsychological tasks is affected by an interaction of age of injury with injury severity.[48] That is, worse performance is seen when injury is sustained at an earlier age. This is not seen on all tasks, and may only become apparent when the head trauma occurs during an age interval in which performance on a particular task is undergoing rapid development.

Acute Neurological Indices

Acute GCS scores are predictive of the cognitive outcome in children sustaining head injury.[126,130] In children with severe head injuries, Levin et al.[116] found that age, GCS score, and pupillary reactivity were all significant predictors of GOS score at 6 months, with an interaction present between GCS score and pupillary reactivity. The addition of percentage of time of increased intracranial pressure did not improve prediction beyond that provided by age, GCS score, and pupillary reactivity. Prasad et al.[205] studied children who sustained injury at less than 6 years of age and attained similar findings for the predictive relationship between lowest GCS score and 1-year GOS score (r = .54), pupillary reactivity (r = .31), and duration of imparied consciousness (r = .41).

Massagli et al.[166] investigated the relationship between acute neurological indices and outcome in children and adolescents at discharge and 5 to 7 years following severe head trauma in children and adolescents. They found that GOS score at discharge was strongly predicted by 24-hour GCS score (r = .75) and coma duration (r = .76). Significant prediction of the 5- to 7-year GOS category was also apparent, although the magnitude of the correlations had diminished for both 24-hour GCS score (r = .54) and coma duration (r = .54). In clinical terms, only 14% of children with a 24-hour GCS score of 3–8 attained good recovery on GOS at 5 to 7 years compared to a 50% rate of good recovery for children who achieved a 24-hour GCS score of 9–15. For children with up to one day of coma, there was a 56% rate of good recovery compared to a 17% rate of good recovery for children with more than 1 day of coma. The median coma duration for children ultimately attaining good recovery was 1 day, median coma duration for moderate disability was 6 days, and median coma duration for severe disability was 62 days.

Posttraumatic Amnesia

Duration of posttraumatic amnesia predicts the outcome in children.[50] A posttraumatic amnesia >1 week predicted poor verbal memory performances at 6 and 12 months. Good recovery was found in 67% of children with posttraumatic amnesia of <1 week, in 43% of children with posttraumatic amnesia of 1–2 weeks, and in 11% of children with posttraumatic amnesia >2 weeks. Similar results were reported by Rutter.[223] Definite psychiatric sequelae are only associated with posttraumatic amnesia of at least 7 days' duration.[224]

Neuroimaging

Levin et al.[116] found that in children with severe head trauma, the addition of CT variables did not improve prediction of the outcome at 6 months beyond information provided by age, GCS score, and pupillary reactivity. A diagnosis of diffuse swelling or a mass lesion on CT did lead to a higher probability of vegetative state in survivors. Different results were found by Ong et al.,[199] who found that the predictive value of the GCS was enhanced by hypoxia and the CT variables of subarachnoid hemorrhage, diffuse axonal injury, and brain swelling, whereas age and pupillary reactivity did not add predictive value. Prasad et al.[205] found that for children sustaining head trauma at less than 6 years of age, the number of lesions imaged on CT or MRI was not significantly correlated with GOS at 1 year but was moderately correlated with intellectual functioning (r = .45). The number of lesions was also highly correlated with the lowest GCS scores.

Levin et al.[149] performed MRI on 251 children ages 5 to 18 years. As the maximum depth of lesions present progressed from cortical to subcortical to brain stem level, there was a decreasing probability of achieving good recovery and an increasing probability of having severe disability at up to 3 years or recovery (Fig. 11.8). For children with moderate disability, maximum lesion depth was predominantly at the subcortical and cortical levels. Lower ratings on the Vineland Adaptive Behavior Scales for Children were also seen with increasing depth of lesion. As with adults, the presence of impaired pupils or deep lesions visible on MRI suggests that trauma severe enough to induce lesions in the brain stem will signal diffuse and massive shear strain throughout higher levels of the brain. The findings of Levin et al. were replicated by Woischneck et al.[258] They found that coma duration was longer in children with infratentorial lesions imaged on MRI compared to those with supratentorial lesions. Only the presence of brain stem lesions predicted GOS: of nonsurviving or vegetative children, 100% had an imaged brain stem lesion, and only 25% of children with a brain stem lesion attained good recovery. In contrast,

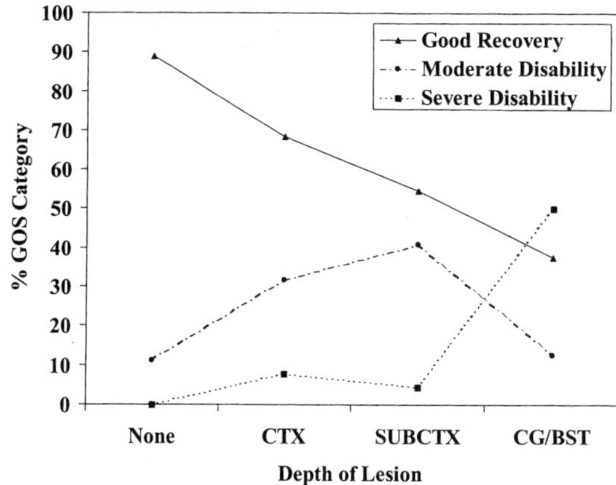

Figure 11.8. Relationship between depth of lesion and probability of obtaining various neurobehavioral outcomes in children with closed head injury. GOS, Glasgow Outcome Scale. Depth of lesion: None, no lesion; CTX, cortical; SUBCTX, subcortical; CG/BST, deep central gray/brain stem lesion. Increasing depth of the lesion lowers the probability of a good outcome and raises the probability of severe disability. (Adapted from reference 149.)

75% of children with cerebral lesions, but without brain stem lesions, attained good recovery.

Koelfen et al.[110] studied children ages 6 to 14 years who had achieved a GOS rating of good recovery after head injury. On follow-up 1 to 5 years after injury, children with negative MRI and negative neurological findings performed equivalently to controls on both cognitive and motor tasks. Deep white matter or multiple lesion findings on MRI were associated with worsened cognitive performances, whereas MRI findings of cortical or subcortical lesions were associated with motor but not cognitive deficits. Children with negative MRI findings but positive neurological findings (i.e., *soft signs*) had fine motor but not cognitive deficits.

Outcome as related to the area of corpus callosum imaged by midsagittal MRI slice has been studied because the massive white matter tracts in the corpus callosum present an opportunity to gauge diffuse axonal injury in a fairly discrete manner. Additional force may be imparted in the area of the splenium due to the proximity and architecture of the falx cerebri. Because myelinization continues into early adulthood, imaging of the corpus callosum may also reflect postinjury dysgenesis of the cerebral white matter. Levin et al.[118] found that the corpus callosum had grown in children 3 years following mild head injury. In contrast, the corpus callosum atrophied in children during the 3 years that followed severe head injury. Midsagittal corpus callosum area had a moderate correlation (r = 0.42) with level of adaptive behavior, as measured by the Vineland scale. A larger corpus callosum area was also associated with attainment of good recovery or moderate disability on the GOS.

With regard to the relationship between callosal MRI findings and specific neuropsychological performances, Verger et al.[243] found that midsagittal corpus callosum area correlated to a moderate degree with neuropsychological test performance. For example, corpus callosum area was significantly correlated with VIQ (r = .50), with PIQ (r = .68), and with Wisconsin Card Sorting Test categories achieved (r = .44). Lateral ventricular volume was only correlated with the Wisconsin Card Sorting Test (r = .53).

Levin et al.[124] found that prediction of verbal delayed recall was influenced by the presence of frontal, but not extrafrontal lesions. In view of the role of the hippocampus in memory functioning, Di Stefano et al.[43] studied the relationship between hippocampal volume and verbal memory performance in 183 children 1 to 3 years following mild, moderate, or severe head trauma. Despite expectations, hippocampal volume did not provide incremental prediction of the GCS score. Hippocampal volume did not differ for children with mild verus severe closed head injury, and improved prediction was found only for the relationship between left hippocampal volume and verbal recognition memory. Replicating the earlier study of Levin et al.,[124] left or right frontal lesion volume again predicted memory performance beyond the information provided by the GCS, but extrafrontal lesion volume did not provide additional predictive power.

Consistent with accepted functional localization, Levin et al.[154] found that the presence of a left frontal lesion predicted worse verbal associative fluency (Controlled Oral Word Association) performance in children 3 months and 3 years after injury. Furthermore, the presence of a left frontal lesion was associated with more impoverished verbal fluency in older children than in younger children, perhaps reflecting a more established functional commitment of the left frontal lobe in older than in younger children. The neuroplasticity of the younger brain may permit development of an alternative localization for word fluency in the context of a left frontal lesion sustained at an early age.

With regard to a nonverbal task such as the Porteus Maze, Levin et al.[153] found that in children recovered 3 years from severe head trauma, frontal lesion size in the orbital, rectal, and inferior frontal gyri provided incremental prediction of performance over the effects of GCS score and age. Other frontal lobe lesions and extrafrontal lesions did not provide incremental prediction.

Levin et al.[125] integrated MRI findings with GCS scores to determine if focal lesion size and localization contributed to level of executive functioning in children. Frontal MRI lesion size improved prediction of executive functioning on a variety of tasks, whereas extrafrontal lesion size did not improve prediction over GCS score alone for any task. Although statistically significant, the size of the correlations between executive functioning and MRI findings was modest, and there were several instances of inconsistency between the findings and generally accepted principles of cognitive localization.

More recently, Levin et al.[155] studied the association of lesion location and volume as determined by MRI with executive functioning in children with severe head injury. They found that left hemisphere and right prefrontal lesion volumes contributed to the prediction of executive functioning in children, with lesion volume adding predictive information beyond that provided by age and GCS score. Levin et al.[148] investigated the relationship between volume of frontal and nonfrontal lesions on MRI and performance on the Tower of London task. Lesion volume in nonfrontal regions did not provide incremental prediction of performance over the variables of age and injury severity. In contrast, orbitofrontal and frontal white matter lesion volumes provided incremental prediction of the number of rules broken by children on the Tower of London task, whereas dorsolateral frontal lesions increased prediction of whether children were able to solve the problem on the first trial of the task. These findings demonstrate that executive functioning in children is related to the structural integrity of frontal lobe regions following head injury, and that this relationship is robust even when more global indices of development and head injury severity are taken into account.

Mild Head Injury in Children

Most studies are in general agreement that uncomplicated mild head injury has no clinically significant long-term effects on children's cognitive, academic, or psychosocial functioning.[8,12,53,55,127,131,161,203,223,263] Ponsford et al.[203] found that the features and course of mild head injury in children tended to resemble those found in adults. The mild head injury group did not differ from controls on cognitive testing or in frequency of behavioral problems at 1 week, although the patient group did have more frequent complaints of headaches, dizziness, and fatigue. Although no group differences were observed at 3 months, 17% of children who had sustained mild head injury were *outliers* who had persisting cognitive and somatic complaints with behavioral problems. Inclusion in this group was not predicted by duration of posttraumatic amnesia, but was predicted by a history of a previous head injury and premorbid stressors such as family breakdown.

Another view was presented in a well-controlled study reported by McKinlay et al.[177] Similar to the studies above, they found no effect on academic outcome in 132 children sustaining mild head trauma from birth to age 10 years, when outcome was considered at age 10–13 years. They found no effect on attentional functioning or conduct, as rated by the mothers and teachers of those children who were not admitted to a hospital as result of their injuries or complications. They did find that children who had been admitted to a hospital because of the severity of their injuries tended to be rated as having more attentional difficulties by both mothers and teachers, and were rated by teachers as having worse conduct. The effect was more pronounced in children who had sustained mild head trauma from birth to 5 years compared to children injured from 6 to 10 years of age. The children with mild head trauma also differed significantly from controls on various measures of familial adversity. Once these variables were controlled for, only a small effect size was apparent for mild head trauma in the children who had been hospitalized.

Summary

Neurobehavioral sequelae of head injury typically reflect the diffuse cerebral insult, although cognitive and behavioral changes may also be caused by superimposed focal or mass lesions. The first 6 to 12 months of recovery produce the most rapid and substantial recovery of function, with smaller incremental gains following thereafter. Memory is the cognitive domain most severely affected by head injury, with reductions in executive functioning, problem solving and psychomotor speed also common. Social disinhibition, lack of judgment, irritability, and depression are the most prominent behavioral sequelae in conscious survivors of head injury. Mild head injury may have an acute effect on cognitive and behavioral functioning, but most adult and child patients attain a good recovery within 3 months, with little or no residual deficits apparent thereafter. Age, GCS score, pupillary reactivity, and duration of posttraumatic amnesia consistently provide the best predictions of global outcome.

REFERENCES

1. Adams JH, Graham D, Scott G, Parker LS, Doyle D: Brain damage in fatal non-missile head injury. J Clin Pathol 33:1132, 1980.
2. Adams JH, Scott G, Parker LS, Graham DI, Doyle D: The contusion index: A quantitative approach to cerebral contusion. Neuropathol Appl Neurobiol 6:319, 1980.
3. Alexander MP: Mild traumatic brain injury: Pathophysiology, natural history, and clinical management. Neurology 45:1253, 1995.
4. Alexander MP, Benson DF, Stuss DT: Frontal lobes and language. Brain Lang 37:656, 1989.
5. Alexandre A, Colombo F, Nertempi P, Benedetti A: Cognitive outcome and early indices of severity of head injury. J Neurosurg 59:751, 1983.
6. American Neurological Association Committee on Ethical Affairs: Persistent vegetative state. Ann Neurol 33:386, 1993.
7. Anderson CV, Bigler ED, Blatter DD: Frontal lobe lesions, diffuse damage, and neuropsychological functioning in traumatic brain-injured patients. J Clin Exp Neuropsychol 17:900, 1995.
8. Anderson V, Catroppa C, Morse S, et al: Outcome from mild head injury in young children: A prospective study. J Clin Exp Neuropsychol 23:705, 2001.
9. Anderson VA, Catroppa C, Rosenfeld J, et al. Recovery of memory function following traumatic brain injury in pre-school children. Brain Inj 14:679, 2000.
10. Benton AL: The prefrontal region: Its early history. In: Levin HS, Eisenberg HM, Benton AL (eds): Frontal Lobe Function and Dysfunction. New York, Oxford University Press, 1991, pp 3–32.
11. Berryhill P, Lilly MA, Levin HS, Hillman GR, Mendelsohn D, Brunder DG, Fletcher JM, Kufera J, Kent TA, Yeakley J, Bruce D, Eisenberg HM: Frontal lobe changes after severe diffuse closed head injury in children: A volumetric study of magnetic resonance imaging. Neurosurgery 37:392, 1995.
12. Bijur P, Kurzon M: Cognitive, behavioral, and motor sequelae of mild head injury in a national birth cohort. J Clin Exp Neuropsychol 15:21, 1993.
13. Bloom DR, Levin HS, Ewing-Cobbs L, et al. Lifetime and novel psychiatric disorders after pediatric traumatic brain injury. J Am Acad Child Adolesc Psychiatry 40: 572, 2001.
14. Blumer D, Benson DF: Personality changes with frontal and temporal lobe lesions. In: Benson DF, Blumer D (eds): Psychiatric Aspects of Neurologic Disease. New York, Grune & Stratton, 1975, pp 151–170.
15. Boake C, Millis SR, High WM Jr, et al. Using early neuropsychologic testing to predict long-term productivity outcome from traumatic brain injury. Arch Phys Med Rehabil 82:761, 2001.
16. Bonnier C, Nassogne MC, Saint-Martin C, et al. Neuroimaging of intraparenchymal lesions predicts outcome in shaken baby syndrome. Pediatrics 112:808, 2003.
17. Braakman R, Gelpke GJ, Habbema JDF, Maas, AIR, Minderhound M: Systematic selection of prognostic features in patients with severe head injury. Neurosurgery 6:362, 1980.
18. Braakman R, Jennett B, Minderhound JM: Prognosis of the post-traumatic vegetative state. Acta Neurochir 95:49, 1988.
19. Bricolo A, Turazzi S, Feriotti G: Prolonged traumatic unconsciousness: Therapeutic assets and liabilities. J Neurosurg 52:625, 1980.
20. Brink JD, Garrett AL, Hale WR, Woo-Sam J, Nickel VL: Recovery of motor and intellectual function in children sustaining severe head injuries. Dev Med Child Neurol 12:565, 1970.
21. Brooks DN: The head-injured family. J Clin Exp Neuropsychol 13:155, 1991.
22. Brooks DN, McKinlay W: Personality and behavioral change after severe blunt head injury—A relative's view. J Neurol Neurosurg Psychiatry 46:336, 1983.
23. Brooks DN, McKinlay W, Symington C, Beattie A, Campsie L: Return to work within the first seven years of severe head injury. Brain Inj 1:5, 1987.
24. Brookshire BL, Chapman SB, Song J, et al: Cognitive and linguistic correlates of children's discourse after closed head injury: A three-year follow-up. J Int Neuropsychol Soc 6:741, 2000.
25. Brookshire B, Levin HS, Song J, et al. Components of executive function in typically developing and head-injured children. Dev Neuropsychol 25:61, 2004.
26. Brown GW, Chadwick O, Shaffer D, Rutter M, Traub M: A prospective study of children with head injuries: III. Psychiatric sequelae. Psychol Med 11:63, 1981.
27. Brown SJ, Fann JR, Grant I: Postconcussional disorder: Time to acknowledge a common source of neuro-

behavioral morbidity. J Neuropsychiatry Clin Neurosci 6:15, 1994.

28. Capruso DX, Marasco DL, Hamsher KdeS: Chronic postconcussive syndrome: Relationship to simulation of malfunction and psychopathology. J Intl Neuropsychol Soc 3:75, 1997.
29. Cattelani R, Tanzi F, Lombardi F, et al: Competitive re-employment after severe traumatic brain injury: Clinical, cognitive and behavioural predictive variables. Brain Inj 16:51, 2002.
30. Chadwick O, Rutter M, Shaffer D, Shrout PE: A prospective study of children with head injuries: IV. Specific cognitive deficits. J Clin Neuropsychol 3:101, 1981.
31. Chapman SB, Levin HS, Wanek A, Weyrauch J, Kufera J: Discourse after closed head injury in young children. Brain Lang 61:420, 1998.
32. Chapman SB, McKinnon L, Levin HS, et al: Longitudinal outcome of verbal discourse in children with traumatic brain injury: Three-year follow-up. J Head Trauma Rehabil 16:441, 2001.
33. Chapman SB, Sparks G, Levin HS, et al: Discourse macrolevel processing after severe pediatric traumatic brain injury. Dev Neuropsychol 25:37, 2004.
34. Choi SC, Barnes TY, Bullock R, Germanson TA, Marmarou A, Young HF: Temporal profile of outcomes in severe head injury. J Neurosurg 81:169, 1994.
35. Choi SC, Narayan RK, Anderson RL, Ward JD: Enhanced specificity of prognosis in severe head injury. J Neurosurg 69:381, 1998.
36. Clifton GL, Miller ER, Choi SC, et al: Fluid thresholds and outcome from severe brain injury. Crit Care Med 30:739, 2002.
37. Cockburn J: Performance on the Tower of London test after severe head injury. J Intl Neuropsychol Soc 1:537, 1995.
38. Collins MW, Lovell MR, Iverson GL, et al. Cumulative effects of concussion in high school athletes. Neurosurgery 51:1175, 2002.
39. Craft AW, Shaw DA, Cartlidge NEF: Head injuries in children. BMJ 4:200, 1972.
40. Deb S, Lyons I, Koutzoukis C, et al: Rate of psychiatric illness 1 year after traumatic brain injury. Am J Psychiatry 156:374, 1999.
41. Dikmen S, Machamer J, Temkin N: Mild head injury: Facts and artifacts. J Clin Exp Neuropsychol 23:729, 2001.
42. Dikmen S, Machamer J, Temkin N, McLean A: Neuropsychological recovery in patients with moderate to severe head injury: 2 year follow-up. J Clin Exp Neuropsychol 12:507, 1990.
43. Di Stefano G, Bachevalier J, Levin HS, et al. Volume of focal brain lesions and hippocampal formation in relation to memory function after closed head injury in children. J Neurol Neurosurg Psychiatry 69:210, 2000.
44. Duhaime AC, Christian C, Moss E, Seidl T: Long-term outcome in infants with the shaking-impact syndrome. Pediatr Neurosurg 24:292, 1996.
45. Edwards JK, Larson EB, Hughes JP, Kukull WA: Are there clinical and epidemiological differences between familial and non-familial Alzheimer's disease? J Am Geriatr Soc 39:477, 1991.
46. Ellenberg JH, Levin HS, Saydjari C: Posttraumatic amnesia as a predictor of outcome after severe closed head injury. Prospective assessment. Arch Neurol 53:782, 1996.
47. Ewing-Cobbs L, Fletcher JM, Levin HS, et al: Longitudinal neuropsychological outcome in infants and preschoolers with traumatic brain injury. J Int Neuropsychol Soc 3:581, 1997.
48. Ewing-Cobbs L, Fletcher JM, Levin HS, et al: Academic achievement and academic placement following traumatic brain injury in children and adolescents: A two-year longitudinal study. J Clin Exp Neuropsychol 20:769, 1998.
49. Ewing-Cobbs L, Kramer L, Prasad M, Canales DN, Louis PT, Fletcher JM, Vollero H, Landry SH, Cheung K: Neuroimaging, physical, and developmental findings after inflicted and noninflicted traumatic brain injury in young children. Pediatrics 102:300, 1998.
50. Ewing-Cobbs L, Levin HS, Fletcher JM, Miner ME, Eisenberg HM: The Children's Orientation and Amnesia Test: Relationship to severity of acute head injury and to recovery of memory. Neurosurgery 27:683, 1990.
51. Ewing-Cobbs L, Miner ME, Fletcher JM, Levin HS: Intellectual, motor and language sequelae following closed head injury in infants and preschoolers. J Pediatr Psychol 14:531, 1989.
52. Ewing-Cobbs L, Prasad M, Fletcher JM, et al. Attention after pediatric traumatic brain injury: A multidimensional assessment. Child Neuropsych 4:35, 1998.
53. Fay GC, Jaffe KM, Polissar NL, Liao S, Martin KM, Shurtleff HA, Rivara JB, Winn HR: Mild pediatric traumatic brain injury: A cohort study. Arch Phys Med Rehabil 74:895, 1993.
54. Fay GC, Jaffe KM, Polissar NL, Liao S, Rivara JB, Martin KM: Outcome of pediatric traumatic brain injury at three years: A cohort study. Arch Phys Med Rehabil 75:733, 1994.
55. Fletcher JM, Ewing-Cobbs L, Miner ME, Levin HS, Eisenberg HM: Behavioral changes after closed head injury in children. J Consult Clin Psychol 58:93, 1990.
56. Fletcher JM, Levin HS, Lachar D, Kusnerik L, Harward H, Mendelsohn D, Lilly MA: Behavioral outcomes after pediatric closed head injury: Relationships with age, severity, and lesion size. J Child Neurol 11: 283, 1996.
57. Fratiglioni L, Ahlbom A, Viitanen M, Winblad B: Risk factors for late-onset Alzheimer's disease: A population-based, case-control study. Ann Neurol 33:258, 1993.
58. Friedman G, Froom P, Sazbon L, et al: Apolipoprotein E-epsilon4 genotype predicts a poor outcome in survivors of traumatic brain injury. Neurology 15:244, 1999.
59. Galski T, Tompkins C, Johnston MV: Competence in discourse as a measure of social integration and qual-

ity of life in persons with traumatic brain injury. Brain Inj 12:769, 1998.

60. Gentilini M, Nichelli P, Schoenhuber R, et al: Neuropsychological evaluation of mild head injury. J Neurol Neurosurg Psychiatry 48:137, 1985.
61. Gentry LR, Godersky JC, Thompson B: MR imaging of head trauma: Review of the distribution and radiopathologic features of traumatic lesions. Am J Roentgenol 150:663, 1988.
62. Gerring JP, Brady KD, Chen A, Vasa R, Grados M, Bandeen-Roche KJ, Bryan RN, Denckla MB: Premorbid prevalence of ADHD and development of secondary ADHD after closed head injury. J Am Acad Child Adolesc Psychiatry, 37:647, 1998.
63. Gilchrist E, Wilkinson M: Some factors determining prognosis in young people with severe head injuries. Arch Neurol 36:355, 1979.
64. Goldstein FC, Levin HS: Epidemiology of pediatric closed head injury: Incidence, clinical characteristics, and risk factors. J Learn Disabil 20:518, 1987.
65. Goldstein FC, Levin HS: Question-asking strategies after severe closed head injury. Brain Cogn 17:23, 1991.
66. Goldstein FC, Levin HS. Cognitive outcome after mild and moderate traumatic brain injury in older adults. J Clin Exp Neuropsychol 23:739, 2001.
67. Goldstein FC, Levin HS, Goldman WP, et al: Cognitive and behavioral sequelae of closed head injury in older adults according to their significant others. J Neuropsychiatry Clin Neurosci 11:38, 1999.
68. Goldstein FC, Levin HS, Goldman WP, et al: Cognitive and neurobehavioral functioning after mild versus moderate traumatic brain injury in older adults. J Int Neuropsychol Soc 7:373, 2001.
69. Grafman J, Salazar A, Weingartner H, Vance S, Amin D: The relationship of brain-tissue loss volume and lesion location to cognitive defict. J Neurosci 6:301, 1986.
70. Grafman J, Schwab K, Warden D, Pridgen A, Brown HR, Salazar AM: Frontal lobe injuries, violence, and aggression: A report of the Vietnam Head Injury Study. Neurology 46:1231, 1996.
71. Graham DI, Adams JH, Doyle D: Ischaemic brain damage in fatal non-missile head injuries. J Neurol Sci 39:213, 1978.
72. Greve KW, Sherwin E, Stanford MS, et al. Personality and neurocognitive correlates of impulsive aggression in long-term survivors of severe traumatic brain injury. Brain Inj 15:255, 2001.
73. Gronwall DMA: Advances in the assessment of attention and information processing after head injury. In: Levin HS, Grafman J, Eisenberg HM (eds): Neurobehavioral Recovery from Head Injury. New York, Oxford University Press, 1987, pp 355–371.
74. Gronwall DMA, Sampson H: The Psychological Effects of Concussion. Auckland, New Zealand, Auckland University Press, 1974.
75. Gronwall DMA, Wrightson P: Cumulative effects of concussion. Lancet 2:995, 1975.
76. Gronwall DMA, Wrightson P: Memory and information processing capacity after closed head injury. J Neurol Neurosurg Psychiatry 44:889, 1981.
77. Gurdjian ES, Gurdjian ES: Cerebral contusions: Reevaluation of the mechanism of their development. J Trauma 16:35, 1976.
78. Hall KM, Karzmark P, Stevens M, Englander J, O'Hare P, Wright J: Family stressors in traumatic brain injury: A two-year follow-up. Arch Phys Med Rehabil 75:876, 1994.
79. Hanten G, Dennis M, Zhang L, et al. Childhood head injury and metacognitive processes in language and memory. Dev Neuropsychol 25:85, 2004.
80. Harmsen M, Geurts AC, Fasotti L, et al: Positive behavioural disturbances in the rehabilitation phase after severe traumatic brain injury: An historic cohort study. Brain Inj 18:787, 2004.
81. Haselkorn JK, Mueller BA, Rivara FA: Characteristics of drivers and driving record after traumatic and non-traumatic brain injury. Arch Phys Med Rehabil 79:738, 1998.
82. Haviland J, Russell RI: Outcome after severe non-accidental head injury. Arch Dis Child 77:504, 1997.
83. Heaton RK: Wisconsin Card Sorting Test Manual. Odessa, FL, Psychological Assessment Resources, 1981.
84. Heiden JS, Small R, Caton W, Weiss MH, Kurze T: Severe head injury and outcome: A prospective study. In: Popp AJ, Bourke RS, Nelson LR, Kimelberg HK (eds): Neural Trauma. New York, Raven Press, 1979, pp 181–193.
85. Heilman KM, Safran A, Geschwind N: Closed head trauma and aphasia. J Neurol Neurosurg Psychiatry 34:265, 1971.
86. Heindl UT, Laub MC: Outcome of persistent vegetative state following hypoxic or traumatic brain injury in children and adolescents. Neuropediatrics 27:94, 1996.
87. Hibbard MR, Uysal S, Kepler K, et al: Axis I psychopathology in individuals with traumatic brain injury. J Head Trauma Rehabil 13:24, 1998.
88. Higashi K: Epidemiology of catastrophic brain injury: Findings from the Traumatic Coma Data Bank. In: Levin HS, Benton AL, Muizelaar JP, Eisenberg HM (eds): Catastrophic Brain Injury. New York, Oxford University Press, 1996, pp 15–34.
89. High WM Jr, Levin HS, Gary HE Jr: Recovery of orientation following closed-head injury. J Clin Exp Neuropsychol 12:703, 1990.
90. Holbourn AHS: Mechanics of head injuries. Lancet 2:438, 1943.
91. Hukkelhoven CW, Steyerberg EW, Rampen AJ et al. Patient age and outcome following severe traumatic brain injury: An analysis of 5600 patients. J Neurosurg 99:666, 2003.
92. Jaffe KM, Fay GC, Polissar NL, Martin KM, Shurtleff H, Rivara JB, Winn HR: Severity of pediatric traumatic brain injury and early neurobehavioral outcome: A cohort study. Arch Phys Med Rehabil 73:540, 1992.
93. Jaffe KM, Fay GC, Polissar NL, Martin KM, Shurtleff HA, Rivara JB, Winn HR: Severity of pediatric trau-

matic brain injury and neurobehavioral recovery at one year—a cohort study. Arch Phys Med Rehabil 74:587, 1993.

94. Jaffe KM, Polissar NL, Fay GC, Liao S: Recovery trends over three years following pediatric traumatic brain injury. Arch Phys Med Rehabil 76:17, 1995.
95. Jennett B: Clinical and pathological features of vegetative survival. In: Levin HS, Benton AL, Muizelaar JP, Eisenberg HM (eds): Catastrophic Brain Injury. New York, Oxford University Press, 1996, pp 3–14.
96. Jennett B, Bond M: Assessment of outcome after severe brain damage. Lancet 1:480, 1975.
97. Jennett B, Snoek J, Bond MR, Brooks N: Disability after severe head injury: Observations on the use of the Glasgow Outcome Scale. J Neurol Neurosurg Psychiatry 44:285, 1981.
98. Jennett B, Teasdale G: Management of Head Injuries. Philadelphia, FA Davis, 1981.
99. Jennett B, Teasdale G, Braakman R, Minderhound J, Heiden J, Kurze T: Prognosis in patients with severe head injury. Neurosurgery 4:283, 1979.
100. Jorge RE, Robinson RG, Arndt SV: Are there symptoms that are specific for depressed mood in patients with traumatic brain injury? J Nerv Ment Dis 181:91, 1993.
101. Jorge RE, Robinson RG, Arndt SV, Forrester AW, Geisler F, Starkstein SE: Comparison between acute- and delayed-onset depression following traumatic brain injury. J Neuropsychiatry Clin Neurosci 5:43, 1993.
102. Jorge RE, Robinson RG, Starkstein SE: Secondary mania following traumatic brain injury. Am J Psychiatry 150:916, 1993.
103. Jorge RE, Robinson RG, Starkstein SE, Arndt SV: Depression and anxiety following traumatic brain injury. J Neuropsychiatry Clin Neurosci 5:369, 1993.
104. Kampfl A, Franz G, Aichner F, Pfausler B, Haring HP, Felber S, Luz G, Schocke M, Schmutzhard E: The persistent vegetative state after closed head injury: Clinical and magnetic resonance imaging findings in 42 patients. J Neurosurg 88:809, 1998.
105. Kampfl A, Schmutzhard E, Franz G, Pfausler B, Haring HP, Ulmer H, Felber S, Golaszewski S, Aichner F: Prediction of recovery from post-traumatic vegetative state with cerebral magnetic-resonance imaging. Lancet 351: 1763, 1998.
106. Kaufmann PM, Fletcher JM, Levin HS, Miner ME, Ewing-Cobbs L: Attentional disturbance after pediatric closed head injury. J Child Neurol 8:348, 1993.
107. Kelly MP, Johnson CT, Knoller N, et al: Substance abuse, traumatic brain injury and neuropsychological outcome. Brain Inj 11:391, 1997.
108. Kilaru S, Garb J, Emhoff T, Fiallo V, Simon B, Swiencicki T, Lee KF: Long term functional status and mortality of elderly patients with severe closed head injuries. J Trauma 41:957, 1996.
109. Klonoff H, Low MD, Clark C: Head injuries in children: A prospective five year follow-up. J Neurol Neurosurg Psychiatry 40:1211, 1977.
110. Koelfen W, Freund M, Dinter D, Schmidt B, Koenig S, Schultze C: Long-term follow up of children with head injuries-classified as "good recovery" using the Glasgow Outcome Scale: Neurological, neuropsychological and magnetic resonance imaging results. Eur J Pediatr 156:230, 1997.
111. Koskiniemi M, Kyykka T, Nybo T, et al. Long-term outcome after severe brain injury in preschoolers is worse than expected. Arch Pediatr Adolesc Med 149:249, 1995.
112. Kotapka MJ, Graham DI, Adams JH, Gennarelli TA: Hippocampal pathology in fatal non-missile head injury. Acta Neuropathol 83:530, 1992.
113. Lange-Cosack H, Wider B, Schlesner HJ, Grumme T, Kubicki S: Prognosis of brain injuries in young children (one until five years of age). Neuropadiatrie 10:105, 1979.
114. Leininger BE, Gramling SE, Farrell AD, Kreutzer JS, Peck EA: Neuropsychological deficits in symptomatic minor head injury patients after concussion and mild concussion. J Neurol Neurosurg Psychiatry 53:293, 1990.
115. Lenneberg E: Biological Foundations of Language. New York, Wiley, 1967.
116. Levin HS, Aldrich EF, Saydjari C, Eisenberg HM, Foulkes MA, Bellefleur M, Luerssen TG, Jane JA, Marmarou A, Marshall LF, Young HF: Severe head injury in children: Experience of the Traumatic Coma Data Bank. Neurosurgery 31:435, 1992.
117. Levin HS, Amparo E, Eisenberg HM, Williams DH, High WM, McArdle CB, Weiner RL: Magnetic resonance imaging and computerized tomography in relation to the neurobehavioral sequelae of mild and moderate head injuries. J Neurosurg 66:706, 1987.
118. Levin HS, Benavidez DA, Verger-Maestre K, et al: Reduction of corpus callosum growth after severe traumatic brain injury in children. Neurology 8:647, 2000.
119. Levin HS, Benton AL, Grossman RG: Neurobehavioral Consequences of Closed Head Injury. New York, Oxford University Press, 1982.
120. Levin HS, Benton AL, Muizelaar JP, Eisenberg HM (eds): Catastrophic Brain Injury. New York, Oxford University Press, 1996.
121. Levin HS, Boake C, Song J, et al: Validity and sensitivity to change of the extended Glasgow Outcome Scale in mild to moderate traumatic brain injury. J Neurotrauma 18:575, 2001.
122. Levin HS, Brown SA, Song JX, et al. Depression and posttraumatic stress disorder at three months after mild to moderate traumatic brain injury. J Clin Exp Neuropsychol 23:754, 2001.
123. Levin HS, Chapman SB: Aphasia after traumatic brain injury. In: Sarno MT (ed): Acquired Aphasia, 3rd ed. New York, Academic Press, 1991, pp 481–589.
124. Levin HS, Culhane KA, Fletcher JM, Mendelsohn DB, Lilly MA, Harward H, Chapman SB, Bruce DA, Bertolino-Kusnerik L, Eisenberg HM: Dissociation between delayed alternation and memory after pediatric head injury: Relationship to MRI findings. J Child Neurol 9:81, 1994.

125. Levin HS, Culhane KA, Mendelsohn D, Lilly MA, Bruce D, Fletcher JM, Chapman SB, Harward H, Eisenberg HM: Cognition in relation to magnetic resonance imaging in head-injured children and adolescents. Arch Neurol 50:897, 1993.
126. Levin HS, Eisenberg HM: Neuropsychological impairment after closed head injury in children and adolescents. J Pediatr Psychol 4:389, 1979.
127. Levin HS, Eisenberg HM, Benton AL: Mild Head Injury. New York: Oxford University Press, 1989.
128. Levin HS, Eisenberg HM, Gary HE, Marmarou A, Foulkes MA, Jane JA Marshall LF, Portman SM: Intracranial hypertension in relation to memory functioning during the first year after severe head injury. Neurosurgery 28:196, 1991.
129. Levin HS, Eisenberg HM, Miner ME: Neuropsychologic findings in head injured children. In: Shapiro D (ed): Pediatric Head Trauma. New York, Futura, 1983, pp 223–240.
130. Levin HS, Eisenberg HM, Wigg NR, Kobayashi K: Memory and intellectual ability after head injury in children and adolescents. Neurosurgery 11:668, 1982.
131. Levin HS, Fletcher JM, Kusnerik L, et al: Semantic memory following pediatric head injury: Relationship to age, severity of injury, and MRI. Cortex 32:461, 1996.
132. Levin HS, Gary HE, Eisenberg HM, Ruff RM, Barth JT, Kreutzer J, High WM, Portman S, Foulkes MA, Jane JA, Marmarou A, Marshall LF: Neurobehavioral outcome 1 year after severe head injury: Experience of the Traumatic Coma Data Bank. J Neurosurg 73:699, 1990.
133. Levin HS, Goldstein FC: Closed head injury and Alzheimer's disease: Epidemiologic, neurobehavioral, and neuropathologic links. J Int Neuropsychol Soc 1: 183, 1995.
134. Levin HS, Goldstein FC, High WM Jr, Eisenberg HM: Disproportionately severe memory deficit in relation to normal intellectual functioning after closed head injury. J Neurol Neurosurg Psychiatry 51:1294, 1988.
135. Levin HS, Goldstein FC, Williams DH, Eisenberg HM: The contribution of frontal lobe lesions to the neurobehavioral outcome of closed head injury. In: Levin HS, Eisenberg HM, Benton AL (eds): Frontal Lobe Function and Dysfunction. New York, Oxford University Press, 1991, pp 318–338.
136. Levin HS, Grossman RG, Kelly PJ: Aphasic disorder in patients with closed head injury. J Neurol Neurosurg Psychiatry 39:1062, 1976.
137. Levin HS, Grossman RG, Kelly PJ: Impairment of facial recognition after closed head injuries of varying severity. Cortex 13:119, 1977.
138. Levin HS, Grossman RG, Rose JE, Teasdale G: Long-term neuropsychological outcome of closed head injury. J Neurosurg 50:412, 1979.
139. Levin HS, Grossman RG, Sarwar M, Meyers, CA: Linguistic recovery after closed head injury. Brain Lang 12:360, 1981.
140. Levin HS, Handel SF, Goldman AM, Eisenberg HM, Guinto FC: Magnetic resonance imaging after 'diffuse' nonmissile injury. Arch Neurol 42:963, 1985.
141. Levin HS, Hanten G, Chang CC, et al. Working memory after traumatic brain injury in children. Ann Neurol 52:82, 2002.
142. Levin HS, High WM Jr, Ewing-Cobbs L, Fletcher JM, Eisenberg HM, Miner ME, Goldstein FC: Memory functioning during the first year after closed head injury in children and adolescents. Neurosurgery 22: 1043, 1988.
143. Levin HS, High WM, Goethe KE, Sisson RA, Overall JE, Rhoades HM, Eisenberg HM, Kalisky Z, Gary HE: The Neurobehavioral Rating Scale: Assessment of the behavioural sequelae of head injury by the clinician. J Neurol Neurosurg Psychiatry 50:183, 1987.
144. Levin HS, High WM, Goldstein FC, Williams DH: Sustained attention and information processing speed in chronic survivors of severe closed head injury. Scand J Rehab Med Suppl 17:33, 1988.
145. Levin HS, High WM, Meyers CA, von Laufen A, Hayden ME, Eisenberg HM: Impairment of remote memory after closed head injury. J Neurol Neurosurg Psychiatry 48:556, 1985.
146. Levin HS, Madison CF, Bailey C, Meyers CA, Eisenberg HM, Guinto FC: Mutism after closed head injury. Arch Neurol 40:601, 1983.
147. Levin HS, Mattis S, Ruff RM, Eisenberg HM, Marshall LF, Tabaddor K, High WM, Frankowski RF: Neurobehavioral outcome following minor head injury: A three-center study. J Neurosurg 66:234, 1987.
148. Levin HS, Mendelsohn D, Lilly MA, Fletcher JM, Culhane KA, Chapman SB, Harward H, Kusnerik L, Bruce D, Eisenberg HM: Tower of London performance in relation to magnetic resonance imaging following closed head injury in children. Neuropsychology 8:171, 1994.
149. Levin HS, Mendelsohn D, Lilly MA, Yeakley J, Song J, Scheibel RS, Harward H, Fletcher JM, Kufera JA, Davidson KC, Bruce D: Magnetic resonance imaging in relation to functional outcome of pediatric closed head injury: A test of the Ommaya-Gennarelli model. Neurosurgery 40:432, 1997.
150. Levin HS, Meyers CA, Grossman RG, Sarwar M: Ventricular enlargement after closed head injury. Arch Neurol 38:623, 1981.
151. Levin HS, O'Donnell VM, Grossman RG: The Galveston Orientation and Amnesia Test: A practical scale to assess cognition after head injury. J Nerv Ment Dis 167:675, 1979.
152. Levin HS, Saydjari C, Eisenberg HM, Foulkes M, Marshall LF, Ruff RM, Jane JA, Marmarou A: Vegetative state after closed-head injury: A traumatic Coma Data Bank Report. Arch Neurol 48:580, 1991.
153. Levin HS, Song J, Ewing-Cobbs L, et al: Porteus Maze performance following traumatic brain injury in children. Neuropsychology 15:557, 2001.
154. Levin HS, Song J, Ewing-Cobbs L, et al: Word fluency

in relation to severity of closed head injury, associated frontal brain lesions, and age at injury in children. Neuropsychologia 39:122, 2001.

155. Levin HS, Song J, Scheibel RS, et al: Concept formation and problem-solving following closed head injury in children. J Int Neuropsychol Soc 3:598, 1997.
156. Levin HS, Williams DH, Crofford MJ, High WM, Eisenberg HM, Amparo EG, Guinto FC, Kalisky Z, Handel SF, Goldman AM: Relationship of depth of brain lesions to consciousness and outcome after closed head injury. J Neurosurg 69:861, 1988.
157. Levin HS, Williams DH, Eisenberg HM, High WM, Guinto FC: Serial MRI and neurobehavioral findings after mild to moderate closed head injury. J Neurol Neurosurg Psychiatry 55:255, 1992.
158. Lezak MD: Assessment of psychosocial dysfunctions resulting from head trauma. In: Lezak MD (ed): Assessment of the Behavioral Consequences of Head Trauma. New York, Alan R. Liss, 1989, pp 113–143.
159. Lezak MD, Howieson DB, Loring DW, Hannay HJ, Fischer JS: Neuropsychological Assessment, 4th ed. New York, Oxford University Press, 2004.
160. Lichtman SW, Seliger G, Tycko B, et al: Apolipoprotein E and functional recovery from brain injury following postacute rehabilitation. Neurology 28:1536, 2000.
161. Light R, Asarnow RF, Satz P, et al: UCLA studies of mild closed-ead injury in children and adolescents: III—Behavioral and academic outcomes. J Clin Exp Neuropsychol 5:20, 1993.
162. Macmillan MB: A wonderful journey through skull and brains: The travels of Mr. Gage's tamping iron. Brain Cogn 5:67, 1986.
163. MacMillan PJ, Hart RP, Martelli MF, et al: Pre-injury status and adaptation following traumatic brain injury. Brain Inj 16:41, 2002.
164. Mandleberg IA, Brooks DN: Cognitive recovery after severe head injury. I. Serial testing on the Wechsler Adult Intelligence Scale. J Neurol Neurosurg Psychiatry 38:1121, 1975.
165. Massagli TL, Jaffe KM, Fay GC, et al: Neurobehavioral sequelae of severe pediatric traumatic brain injury: A cohort study. Arch Phys Med Rehabil 77:223, 1996.
166. Massagli TL, Michaud LJ, Rivara FP: Association between injury indices and outcome after severe traumatic brain injury in children. Arch Phys Med Rehabil 77:125, 1996.
167. Matarazzo JD: Wechsler's Measurement and Appraisal of Adult Intelligence, 5th ed. New York, Oxford University Press, 1972.
168. Mataro M, Poca MA, Sahuquillo J, et al. Neuropsychological outcome in relation to the Traumatic Coma Data Bank classification of computed tomography imaging. J Neurotrauma 18:869, 2001.
169. Max JE, Lansing AE, Koele SL, et al: Attention deficit hyperactivity disorder in children and adolescents following traumatic brain injury. Dev Neuropsychol 25; 159, 2004.
170. Max JE, Robin DA, Lindgren SD, Smith WL Jr, Sato Y, Mattheis PJ, Stierwalt JA, Castillo CS: Traumatic brain injury in children and adolescents: Psychiatric disorders at two years. J Am Acad Child Adolesc Psychiatry 36:1278, 1997.
171. Mayeux R, Ottman R, Maestre G, Ngai C, Tang MX, Ginsberg H, Chun M, Tycko B, Shelanski M: Synergistic effects of traumatic head injury and apolipoprotein-epsilon 4 in patients with Alzheimer's disease. Neurology 45:555, 1995.
172. Mazaux JM, Masson F, Levin HS, Alaoui P, Maurette P, Barat M: Long-term neuropsychological outcome and loss of social autonomy after traumatic brain injury. Arch Phys Med Rehabil 78:1316, 1997.
173. Mazzini L, Cossa FM, Angelino E, et al: Posttraumatic epilepsy: Neuroradiologic and neuropsychological assessment of long-term outcome. Epilepsia. 44:569, 2003.
174. McCauley SR, Levin HS. Prospective memory in pediatric traumatic brain injury: A preliminary study. Dev Neuropsychol 25:5, 2004.
175. McCauley SR, Levin HS: Vanier M, et al: The Neurobehavioural Rating Scale–Revised: sensitivity and validity in closed head injury assessment. J Neurol Neurosurg Psychiatry 71:643, 2001.
176. McKinlay WW, Brooks DN, Bond MR: The short term outcome of severe blunt head injury as reported by relatives of the injured persons. J Neurol Neurosurg Psychiatry 44:527, 1981.
177. McKinlay A, Dalrymple-Alford JC, Horwood LJ, et al. Long term psychosocial outcomes after mild head injury in early childhood. J Neurol Neurosurg Psychiatry 73:281, 2002.
178. McLean A, Dikmen SS, Temkin NR: Psychosocial recovery after head injury. Arch Phys Med Rehabil 74: 1041, 1993.
179. Mendelsohn D, Levin HS, Bruce D, Lilly M, Harward H, Culhane KA, Eisenberg HM: Late MRI after head injury in children: Relationship to clinical features and outcome. Childs Nerv Syst 8:445, 1992.
180. Meyers CA, Levin HS: Temporal perception following closed head injury: Relationship of orientation and attention span. Neuropsychiatry, Neuropsychol, Behav Neurol 5:28, 1992.
181. Meyers CA, Levin HS, Eisenberg HM, et al: Early versus late lateral ventricular enlargement following closed head injury. J Neurol Neurosurg Psychiatry46:1092, 1983.
182. Millar K, Nicoll JA, Thornhill S, et al. Long term neuropsychological outcome after head injury: Relation to APOE genotype. J Neurol Neurosurg Psychiatry 74:1047, 2003.
183. Miller E: Simple and choice reaction time following severe head injury. Cortex 6:121, 1970.
184. Milner B: Hemisphere specialization: Scope and limits. In: Schmitt FO, Worden FG (eds): The Neurosciences: Third Study Program. Cambridge, MA, MIT Press, 1974, pp 75–89.
185. Mittenberg W, DiGiulio DV, Perrin S, Bass AE: Symptoms following mild head injury: Expectation as aetiology. J Neurol Neurosurg Psychol 55:200, 1992.

186. Mooney G, Speed J: The association between mild traumatic brain injury and psychiatric conditions. Brain Inj 15:865, 2001.
187. Mortimer JA, van Duijn CM, Chandra V, Fratiglioni L, Graves AB, Heyman A, Jorm AF, Kokmen E, Kondo K, Rocca WA, et al: Head trauma as a risk factor for Alzheimer's disease: A collaborative re-analysis of case-control studies. EURODEM Risk Factors Research Group. Int J Epidemiol 20 (Suppl 2):S28, 1991.
188. Mosenthal AC, Livingston DH, Lavery RF, et al: The effect of age on functional outcome in mild traumatic brain injury: 6-month report of a prospective multi-center trial. J Trauma 56:1042, 2004.
189. Nakase-Thompson R, Sherer M, Yablon SA, et al: Acute confusion following traumatic brain injury. Brain Inj 18:131, 2004.
190. Narayan RK, Greenberg RP, Miller JD, Enas GG, Choi SC, Kishore PRS, Selhorst JB, Lutz HA, Becker DP: Improved confidence of outcome prediction in severe head injury. J Neurosurg 54:751, 1981.
191. Newcombe F: Missile Wounds of the Brain: A Study of Psychological Deficits. New York, Oxford University Press, 1969.
192. Newcombe F, Rabbitt P, Briggs M: Minor head injury: Pathophysiological or iatrogenic sequelae? J Neurol Neurosurg Psychiatry 57:709, 1994.
193. Novoa OP, Ardila A: Linguistic abilities in patients with prefrontal damage. Brain Lang 30:206, 1987.
194. Nybo T, Koskiniemi M: Cognitive indicators of vocational outcome after severe traumatic brain injury (TBI) in childhood. Brain Inj 13:759, 1999.
195. Oddy M, Coughlan T, Tyerman A, Jenkins D: Social adjustment after closed head injury: A further follow-up seven years after injury. J Neurol Neurosurg Psychiatry 48:564, 1985.
196. Oddy M, Humphrey M, Uttley D: Subjective impairment and social recovery after closed head injury. J Neurol Neurosurg Psychiatry 41:611, 1978.
197. O'Meara ES, Kukull WA, Sheppard L, Bowen JD, McCormick WC, Teri L, Pfanschmidt M, Thompson JD, Schellenberg GD, Larson EB: Head injury and risk of Alzheimer's disease by apolipoprotein E genotype. Am J Epidemiol 1;373, 1997.
198. Ommaya AD, Gennarelli TA: Cerebral concussion and traumatic unconsciousness: Correlation of experimental and clinical observations on blunt head injuries. Brain 97:633, 1974.
199. Ong L, Selladurai BM, Dhillon MK, et al: The prognostic value of the Glasgow Coma Scale, hypoxia and computerised tomography in outcome prediction of pediatric head injury. Pediatr Neurosurg 24:285, 1996.
200. Pettigrew LEL, Lindsay-Wilson JT, Teasdale GM: Assessing disability after head injury: Improved use of the Glasgow Outcome Scale J Neurosurg 89:939, 1998.
201. Pierallini A, Pantano P, Fantozzi LM, et al: Correlation between MRI findings and long-term outcome in patients with severe brain trauma. Neuroradiology 42: 860, 2000.
202. Polin RS, Shaffrey ME, Phillips CD, et al: Multivariate analysis and prediction of outcome following penetrating head injury. Neurosurg Clin North Am 6:689, 1995.
203. Ponsford J, Willmott C, Rothwell A, et al: Cognitive and behavioral outcome following mild traumatic head injury in children. J Head Trauma Rehabil 14:360, 1999.
204. Ponsford J, Willmott C, Rothwell A, et al: Factors influencing outcome following mild traumatic brain injury in adults. J Int Neuropsychol Soc 6:568, 2000.
205. Prasad MR, Ewing-Cobbs L, Swank PR, et al: Predictors of outcome following traumatic brain injury in young children. Pediatr Neurosurg 36:64, 2002.
206. Prigatano GP: The relationship of frontal lobe damage to diminished awareness: Studies in rehabilitation. In: Levin HS, Eisenberg HM, Benton AL (eds): Frontal Lobe Function and Dysfunction. New York, Oxford University Press, 1993, pp 381–397.
207. Quigley MR, Vidovich D, Cantella D, Wilberger JE, Maroon JC, Diamond D: Defining the limits of survivorship after very severe head injury. J Trauma 42:7, 1997.
208. Rapoport MJ, Feinstein A: Age and functioning after mild traumatic brain injury: The acute picture. Brain Inj 15:857, 2001.
209. Rasmusson DX, Brandt J, Martin DB, Folstein MF: Head injury as a risk factor in Alzheimer's disease. Brain Inj 9:213, 1995.
210. Resnick DK, Marion DW, Carlier P: Outcome analysis of patients with severe head injuries and prolonged intracranial hypertension. J Trauma 42:1108, 1997.
211. Ribot T: Diseases of Memory: An Essay in the Positive Psychology. New York, Appleton, 1882.
212. Rimel RW, Giordani B, Barth JT, Boll TJ, Jane JA: Disability caused by minor head injury. Neurosurgery 9: 221, 1981.
213. Risser AH, Hamsher KdeS: Vigilance and distractibility on a continuous performance task by severely head-injured adults. J Clin Exp Neuropsychol 12:35, 1990.
214. Rivara JB, Jaffe KM, Fay GC, Polissar NL, Martin KM, Shurtleff HA, Liao S: Family functioning and injury severity as predictors of child functioning one year following traumatic brain injury. Arch Phys Med Rehabil 74:1047, 1993.
215. Rivara JB, Jaffe KM, Polissar NL, Fay GC, Martin KM, Shurtleff HA, Liao S: Family functioning and children's academic performance and behavior problems in the year following traumatic brain injury. Arch Phys Med Rehabil 75:369, 1994.
216. Rothweiler B, Temkin NR, Dikmen SS: Aging effect on psychosocial outcome in traumatic brain injury. Arch Phys Med Rehabil 79:881, 1998.
217. Russell WR: Cerebral involvement in head injury. Brain 55:549, 1932.
218. Russell WR: Amnesia following head injuries. Lancet 2:762, 1935.
219. Russell WR: The Traumatic Amnesias. New York, Oxford University Press, 1971.

220. Russell WR, Nathan PW: Traumatic amnesia. Brain 69:183, 1946.
221. Rutherford WM: Concussion symptoms: Relationship to acute neurological indices, individual differences, and circumstances of injury. In: Levin HS, Eisenberg HM, Benton AL (eds): Mild Head Injury. New York, Oxford University Press, 1989, pp. 217–228.
222. Rutherford WM, Merrett JD, McDonald JR: Symptoms at one year following concussion from minor head injuries. Injury 10:225, 1978.
223. Rutter M: Psychological sequelae of brain damage in children. Am J Psychiatry 138:1533, 1981.
224. Rutter M, Chadwick O, Shaffer D: Head injury, In: Rutter M (ed): Developmental Neuropsychiatry. New York, Guilford Press, 1983, pp 83–111.
225. Salazar AM, Grafman JH, Vance SC, Weingartner H, Dillon JD, Ludlow C: Consciousness and amnesia after penetrating head injury: Neurology and anatomy. Neurology 36:178, 1986.
226. Salib E, Hillier V: Head injury and the risk of Alzheimer's disease: A case control study. Int J Geriatr Psychiatry 12:363, 1997.
227. Sarno MT, Buonaguro A, Levita E: Characteristics of verbal impairment in closed head. Arch Phys Med Rehabil 67:400, 1986.
228. Schachar R, Levin HS, Max JE, et al: Attention deficit hyperactivity disorder symptoms and response inhibition after closed head injury in children: Do preinjury behavior and injury severity predict outcome? Dev Neuropsychol 25:179, 2004.
229. Schwab K, Grafman J, Salazar AM, Kraft J: Residual impairment and work status 15 years after penetrating head injury: Report from the Vietnam Head Injury Study. Neurology 43:95, 1993.
230. Spatt J, Zebenholzer K, Oder W: Psychosocial long-term outcome of severe head injury as perceived by patients, relatives, and professionals. Acta Neurol Scand 95:173, 1997.
231. Squire LR, Zola-Morgan S: The medial temporal lobe memory system. Science 253:1380, 1991.
232a. Steegmann AT: Dr. Harlow's famous case: The "impossible" accident of Phineas P. Gage. Surgery 52:952, 1962.
232b. Stuss DT, Binns MA, Carruth FG, et al: The acute period of recovery from traumatic brain injury: Post-traumatic amnesia or posttraumatic confusional state? J Neurosurg 90:635, 1999.
233. Sundstrom A, Marklund P, Nilsson LG, et al: APOE influences on neuropsychological function after mild head injury: Within-person comparisons. Neurology 8:1963, 2004.
234. Symonds C: Mental disorder following head injury. Proc R Soc Med 30:1081, 1937.
235. Teasdale TW, Engberg A: Duration of cognitive dysfunction after concussion, and cognitive dysfunction as a risk factor: A population study of young men. BMJ 315:569, 1997.
236. Teasdale G, Jennett B: Assessment of coma and impaired consciousness: A practical scale. Lancet 2:81, 1974.
237. Thomsen IV: Late psychosocial outcome in severe traumatic brain injury: Preliminary results of a third follow-up study after 20 years. Scand J Rehabil Med Suppl 26:142, 1992.
238. Tsuang MT, Boor M, Fleming JA: Psychiatric aspects of traffic aspects. J Psychiatry 142:538, 1985.
239. Uzzell BP, Dolinskas CA, Wiser RF, Langfitt TW: Influence of lesions detected by computed tomography on outcome and neuropsychological recovery after severe head injury. Neurosurgery 20:396, 1987.
240. van der Naalt J, van Zomeren AH, Sluiter WJ, et al: Acute behavioural disturbances related to imaging studies and outcome in mild-to-moderate head injury. Brain Inj 14:781, 2000.
241. van Zomeren AH, Deelman BG: Long-term recovery of visual reaction time after closed head injury. J Neurol Neurosurg Psychiatry 41:452, 1978.
242. Vanier M, Mazaux JM, Lambert J, et al: Assessment of neuropsychologic impairments after head injury: Interrater reliability and factorial and criterion validity of the Neurobehavioral Rating Scale–Revised. Arch Phys Med Rehabil 81:796, 2000.
243. Verger K, Junque C, Levin HS, et al: Correlation of atrophy measures on MRI with neuropsychological sequelae in children and adolescents with traumatic brain injury. Brain Inj 15:211, 2001.
244. Virkkunen M, Nuutila A, Huusko S: Brain injury and criminality: A retrospective study. Dis Nerv System 38:907, 1977.
245. Vollmer DG, Dacey RG, Jane JA: Craniocerebral trauma. In: Joynt RJ (ed): Clinical Neurology, vol 3, rev. ed. Philadelphia, JB Lippincott, 1994, pp 1–68.
246. Wassenberg R, Max JE, Lindgren SD, et al: Sustained attention in children and adolescents after traumatic brain injury: Relation to severity of injury, adaptive functioning, ADHD and social background. Brain Inj 18:751, 2004.
247. Wechsler, D: WAIS-III WMS-III: Technical Manual. San Antonio, TX, Psychological Corporation, 1997.
248. Wechsler D: WISC-IV: Technical Manual. San Antonio, TX, Psychological Corporation, 2003.
249. Weinstein S, Teuber H-L: The role of preinjury education and intelligence level in intellectual loss after brain injury. J Comp Physiol Psychol 50:535, 1957.
250. Whetsell LA, Patterson CM, Young DH, Schiller WR: Preinjury psychopathology in trauma patients. J Trauma 29:1158, 1989.
251. Whyte J, Cifu D, Dikmen S, et al: Prediction of functional outcomes after traumatic brain injury: A comparison of 2 measures of duration of unconsciousness. Arch Phys Med Rehabil 82:1355, 2001.
252. Whyte J, Polansky M, Cavallucci C, Fleming N, Lhulier J, Coslett HB: Inattentive behavior after traumatic brain injury. J Int Neuropsychol Soc 2:274–281, 1996.
253. Williams DH, Levin HS, Eisenberg HM: Mild head injury classification. Neurosurgery 27:422, 1990.

254. Wilson PJE: Cerebral hemispherectomy for infantile hemiplegia: A report of 50 cases. Brain 93:147, 1970.
255. Wilson JTL, Teasdale GM, Hadley DM, Wiedmann KD, Lang D: Posttraumatic amnesia: Still a valuable yardstick. J Neurol Neurosurg Psychiatry 56:198, 1993.
256. Wilson RS, Rosenbaum G, Brown G, Rourke D, Whitman D, Grisell J: An index of premorbid intelligence. J Consult Clin Psychol 46:1554, 1978.
257. Winogron HW, Knights RM, Bawden HN; Neuropsychological deficits following head injury in children. J Clin Neuropsychol 6:269, 1984.
258. Woischneck D, Klein S, Reissberg S, et al: Prognosis of brain stem lesion in children with head injury. Childs Nerv Syst 19:174, 2003.
259. Wong JL, Regennitter RP, Barrios F: Base rate and simulated symptoms of mild head injury among normals. Arch Clin Neuropsychol 9:411, 1994.
260. Yorkston KM, Jaffe KM, Polissar NL, Liao S, Fay GC: Written language production and neuropsychological function in children with traumatic brain injury. Arch Phys Med Rehabil 78:1096, 1997.
261. Zafonte RD, Mann NR, Millis SR, et al: Posttraumatic amnesia: Its relation to functional outcome. Arch Phys Med Rehabil 78:1103, 1997.
262. Zafonte RD, Wood DL, Harrison-Felix CL, et al: Penetrating head injury: A prospective study of outcomes. Neurol Res 23:219, 2001.
263. Zaucha K, Asarnow RF, Satz P, et al: The UCLA studies of mild closed-head injury in children and adolescents: II—Neuropsychological outcomes. J Clin Exp Neuropsychol 15:20, 1993.

Chapter 12

Neuropsychological Testing after Traumatic Brain Injury

GEORGE P. PRIGATANO
AND SUSAN R. BORGARO

Soon after the publication of the first edition of this book, the American Academy of Neurology[35] published its position on the utility of neuropsychological assessment. "Neuropsychological assessment is useful in the assessment of patients with traumatic brain injury (TBI) where it can aid in the detection of subtle deficits, provide information on outcome and prognosis, contribute to the construction of direct rehabilitation strategies, and facilitate rehabilitation that leads to more functional independence" (p. 594). As noted in the first edition of this book, neuropsychological testing can also aid in diagnosis, medical-legal testimony, and research.

The purpose of this chapter is to provide neurologists and neurosurgeons with a brief overview of what neuropsychological tests are, what factors seem to influence performance on neuropsychological tests after TBI, what common questions can be addressed by existing neuropsychological testing methods, and what aspects of higher cerebral functioning are commonly assessed after TBI. Recent research related to these questions is also addressed. The neuropsychological examination of children with TBI is not addressed in this chapter.[1,3]

Neuropsychological Tests: What Are They and What Do They Attempt to Do?

"At its most basic level, a neuropsychological test is a series of requests to perform a variety of tasks that may reveal something about the nature and level of higher cerebral functions and dysfunctions."[32]

Neuropsychological tests are essentially questions or tasks presented to a person with the intent of revealing something about the nature of higher integrative brain functions. Typically, the questions or tasks are administered in a standardized manner so that reliable and valid conclusions can be made regarding the patient's functioning.[17,32,43] The need for appropriate comparison groups has been emphasized by several authors, particularly in assessing patients with reported mild head injury.[11]

Neuropsychological tests have a long history and are not reviewed here (readers are referred to the previous edition of this book). Although neuropsychological tests attempt to sample a wide variety of higher integrated brain functions, 10 dimensions are crucial for a clinical neuropsychological examination[33] (Table 12.1).

Table 12.1. Ten Dimensions of a Clinical Neuropsychological Examination

1. Speech and language functions
2. Perceptual skills (auditory, visual, and tactual)
3. Attention and concentration skills
4. Learning capacity
5. Memory
6. Intellectual level and executive function
7. Speed of new learning
8. Speed and coordination of simple motor responses
9. Emotional and motivational characteristics
10. Self-awareness of level of functioning and judgments regarding psychosocial implications

Table 12.2. Factors That Influence Neuropsychological Test Results after Traumatic Brain Injury

Lesion location
Size (extent) of lesion
Severity of the initial brain injury
Pathological nature of the lesion
Developmental (biological and psychosocial) stage*
Chronicity of the lesion
Personal reactions to altered functioning
Materials (methods) used to elicit disturbances in higher cerebral functioning
Cooperation and motivation of the person to perform on the test
Sensitivity and sensibility of the examiner

*This variable includes such dimensions as age at injury, educational level, cognitive and affective status of the individual at the time of the injury, and level of psychosocial adaptation before the injury.

The tests used and the time spent to assess each of these dimensions are influenced by the patients' history, their present symptom picture, and their capacity to participate in various forms of testing, as well as concerns related to cost effectiveness and costs-benefits. At times, extensive neuropsychological testing is warranted. In other instances, it is not (see Prigatano et al.[33] for a discussion of this point). Parenthetically, psychologists have now developed methods for the meaningful assessment of the economic impact of psychological (including neuropsychological) assessments.[44]

Factors That Influence Neuropsychological Test Results after Traumatic Brain Injury

Citing Pavlov, Herbert Birch[6] listed four factors that influence the neurobehavioral outcome after brain injury: the lesion's location, the extent and distribution of the lesion (i.e., its size), the pathological nature of the lesion, and the person's developmental state. The last dimension includes the person's age, cognitive and affective status, and the degree to which handedness and language functions developed before brain injury.

Other factors also may influence neuropsychological test performance in children and adults with TBI (Table 12.2). These factors include the initial severity of the TBI, as measured by such indices as the Glasgow Coma Scale (GCS)[18,19] and the period of posttraumatic amnesia (PTA),[37,41,42] the chronicity of the brain lesion(s) (i.e., the elapsed time from the onset of brain injury to the time of testing,[12] the patient's personal reactions to his or her altered functioning (e.g., the level of anxiety, depression, and anger),[24,31] and the patient's cooperation and motivation to perform neuropsychological tasks.[27]

Other factors also can influence test scores. The types of tests administered and the level of difficulty can interact with the patient variables to influence test performance. The skill and clinical sensitivity of the examiner may influence not only what tests are given but also what patients experience when tested.[23,38] Such variables can indirectly affect a patient's motivation to perform to maximum capacity on the various tests presented.

Clinical neuropsychologists must consider all these factors when interpreting test findings.

Common Neuropsychological Questions after Traumatic Brain Injury

Chapter 11 highlights the many neurobehavioral changes that can be associated with TBI. This chapter focuses on a few of these changes to elucidate the various questions that neuropsychological testing can help answer.

Numerous questions are asked of clinical neuropsychologists involved in the evaluation of TBI patients. The questions vary, depending on the referral source and the clinical setting of the patient. When patients are in the hospital but not in a rehabilitation unit, nursing personnel often ask the neurosurgeon or neurologist for a neuropsychological consultation. These requests are typically prompted by some problematic behavior of the patient that is difficult for the nursing staff to understand and manage. The patient may be acting "strange," may be uncooperative, or may appear paranoid with no apparent reason. The nursing staff needs help in managing a behavioral problem.

At times, the family of a patient on an inpatient neurological unit requests a neuropsychological consultation. Family members may ask the physician questions he or she cannot answer directly, so a neuropsychological consultation is obtained. The following are common questions: How long will it take before the individual can return to his or her premorbid self? When can their son or daughter actually return to school? What kind of educational program will be most appropriate for them? Should a baseline assessment of their higher cerebral functions be obtained to monitor recovery and ability to return to school or work?

When physicians themselves, however, initiate the referral without indirect influence from nursing staff or the family, the questions frequently center on diagnostic issues or on easing the patient's transition from an inpatient neurological setting to another environment. At this time, physicians may request objective documentation of higher cerebral dysfunction.

Once the patient is in a neurorehabilitation setting, the questions asked by physicians and other health care professionals focus on how to use information about higher cerebral dysfunctions to guide the patient's rehabilitation activities and management in the home and the treatment environment. Physicians also may request information about higher cerebral dysfunction to help educate family members and others involved in the patient's long-term care.

Chronic or long-term neuropsychological disturbances in this patient population have been instrumental in the development of new approaches to rehabilitation. Prigatano and Fordyce,[29] for example, listed a series of neuropsychological problems and their psychosocial consequences that helped develop a milieu-oriented neuropsychological rehabilitation program.[30] Ben-Yishay and Prigatano[4] also identified several common neuropsychological deficits that needed to be addressed in the context of a holistic neuropsychological rehabilitation program.

Table 12.3 lists common questions that can and should be asked of the clinical neuropsychologist evaluating TBI patients. Case examples were presented in the first edition of this chapter.

Higher Cerebral Dysfunction Commonly Assessed after Traumatic Brain Injury

Over the past several years, various tests have been revised and restandardized and new tests have appeared. Neuroimaging and neuropsychological assessment of these patients have also entered the field. This section does not review the various tests that are available. The reader is referred to Lezak et al.[17] for a comprehensive list of such tests. This section emphasizes an approach to neuropsychological assessment and testing that may be helpful in the assessment of TBI patients.

Table 12.3. Common Questions Asked of Clinical Neuropsychologists When Evaluating Patients with Traumatic Brain Injury

- What is the nature and the severity of higher cerebral dysfunctions?
- Are there specific, perhaps unobvious, deficits that need to be kept in mind when managing this patient?
- Why is this patient acting in an unusual or difficult manner (e.g., why is he or she uncooperative, delusional, belligerent, or withdrawn?)
- Is the level of neuropsychological impairment compatible with the medical history? The following are corollaries to this question:
  - Are psychiatric factors major contributors to the symptom picture?
  - Is there an effort on the part of the patient to appear more impaired than she or he actually is for some type of secondary or financial gain?
- Given the neuropsychological test findings, how can they be used to help guide the following?
  - Rehabilitation activities
  - Return to work
  - Management in the home
  - Return to school
  - Decisions about whether driving should be attempted
- Can neuropsychological test findings help determine the potential benefits of certain forms of pharmacological or surgical intervention?
- Can neuropsychological test findings tell us something about the nature of cerebral organization and processes underlying the recovery of higher cerebral dysfunction?

Although neuropsychological testing provides objective information about patients' status, this information is best interpreted in light of the documented medical history. Secondarily, information obtained in a clinical interview is important in determining whether the pattern and level of neuropsychological test findings are compatible with patients' medical and social histories and present clinical condition. Luria[20] emphasized the importance of patients' attitudes toward their illness in formulating a diagnosis and a treatment plan. We reaffirmed this clinical observation. Patients with severe TBI often underestimate their symptoms and appear to show impaired self-awareness after brain injury.[26,39] In contrast, some patients with mild or concussive brain injuries tend to report cognitive impairments above and beyond what is measured by neuropsychological tests. This trend is especially true in patients who show persistent symptoms. Neuropsychological tests must be sensitive to the known and suspected disturbances commonly associated with any neurological condition. Thus, the tests are specifically chosen to help clinicians clarify whether patients are showing quantitative and qualitative features indicative of *brain dysfunction*, *psychiatric disturbance*, or a combination of the two.

All neuropsychological examinations should consider the 10 factors listed in Table 12.1. However, specific dimensions should be emphasized when evaluating individuals with TBI. First, one should attempt to record patients' admitting GCS score or whether loss or disruption of consciousness was documented.[13] Retrospective assessments of the period of PTA are notoriously unreliable. When prospective assessments are obtained, the information can be quite useful. In this regard, the Galveston Orientation Amnesia Test (GOAT) may be helpful.

During the early stages after a brain injury, brief assessment of higher cerebral functioning is not only useful but frequently warranted. Lengthy examinations are unwarranted. Borgaro and Prigatano[8] and Borgaro et al.[9] have shown that the BNI Screen for Higher Cerebral Functioning briefly assesses a combination of cognitive and affective disturbances after TBI. This screening test, for example, reliably demonstrated that TBI patients had significantly more memory impairment, less awareness, and greater affective disturbances than normal controls. As patients progress and can tolerate further testing, more extensive neuropsychological tests should be administered. Table 12.4 lists the neuropsychological functions that should be specifically assessed in TBI patients.

Neuropsychological Considerations When Assessing Patients with Mild Traumatic Brain Injury

In evaluating patients with a history of mild TBI, those whose symptoms rapidly improve must be separated from those whose symptoms persist months or years after injury. The neuropsychological examination of the former group is relatively routine and straightforward. Neuropsychologists typically assess orientation for time and place, memory, speed of information processing, verbal fluency, and overall problem-solving abilities. Patients often are asked to rate various symptoms. With appropriate management, these patients, particularly children, often make an excellent recovery.[2]

Patients with persistent symptoms often present considerable diagnostic challenges. Ruff and Richards[36] reviewed the issues involved in assessing this group of individuals and provided a model that they find useful in understanding why certain symptoms may persist. Examination of this patient group requires a careful assessment of medical history, premorbid adjustment, the potential role

Table 12.4. Specific Neuropsychological Functions That Should Be Assessed in Patients with Traumatic Brain Injury

- Orientation and duration of posttraumatic amnesia
- Primary and secondary language functions (e.g., fluency, auditory comprehension, naming, repetition, reading, writing, and spelling)
- Attention, concentration, and arousal level
- Visuospatial skills (e.g., the presence of hemi-inattention, and higher-order visuospatial deficits)
- Learning and memory (of verbal and nonverbal information)
- Speed of information processing, regardless of the modality in which information is presented
- Speed and accuracy of psychomotor skills
- Abstract reasoning and executive functions (i.e., verbal control of behavior, level of insight, and ability to monitor one's behavior)
- Affect expression, perception, and experience
- Awareness of impaired neuropsychological deficits

of psychiatric factors influencing the symptom picture, and the possible role of secondary gain.[5]

As in severe TBI, speed of information processing and memory impairments are at high risk after mild TBI. It is important to determine whether a patient with a history of mild TBI is showing a level of impairment in these areas that is compatible with his or her known or suspected medical history. There should be a rough *dose-response* relationship between the severity of brain injury and the level of neuropsychological test performance.[10] In other words, if a person lost consciousness only briefly or not at all, speed of information processing and memory should be within the lower ranges of normal, if not average, within 30 to 90 days of injury. If the patient's performance is two to three standard deviations below average on these dimensions during this time frame, factors other than reported mild TBI may be contributing to the symptom picture. This information has to be considered in the differential diagnosis and treatment plan.

Prigatano[25] recently described a professional athlete who suffered a concussion and made a good neuropsychological recovery. That report emphasized that not only do neuropsychological test findings improve with time, but patients' subjective complaints of cognitive, affective, and physical dysfunction also progressively improve. These two dimensions correlate, but physical recovery may actually take longer than cognitive recovery in some patients with concussions.

In patients with known or suspected concussive injuries and persistent neuropsychological impairments, retrospective assessment of the period of PTA is notoriously unreliable. Emergency room records and records from individuals who transport patients to the hospital provide the most objective information about the extent to which consciousness was disrupted and how long the disruption may have persisted.

Neuropsychological Considerations When Assessing Patients with Moderate to Severe Traumatic Brain Injury

Patients whose admitting GCS scores are between 9 and 11 or 3 and 8 are typically classified as having moderate and severe injuries, respectively.[13] Sherer and Novak[40] reviewed a number of studies dealing with the neuropsychological impairments associated with this heterogeneous group of patients. As would be expected, such patients may show a wide variety of neuropsychological impairments that often require extensive neuropsychological testing. They may exhibit disturbances of attention, decreased speed of information processing, memory impairments, compromised language function, disturbed visuospatial abilities, and a wide variety of disturbances described as *executive dysfunctions*. Typically, the latter include disturbances of working memory, self-awareness, and the ability to inhibit and to monitor one's behavior. The speed of simple finger tapping is clearly affected after moderate to severe TBI.[10,28]

Sherer and Novak[40] have suggested guidelines for assessing this patient group. They and others emphasize that the nature and duration of neuropsychological symptoms seen in moderate to severe TBI patients is complicated by the variety of neuropathological lesions observed in this patient group. Although many of these patients survive and resume some form of independent living, they frequently have persistent cognitive and behavioral difficulties that impede true social integration and psychosocial adjustment.[17] Studies have shown that the length of time that passes before the patient can be tested or meaningfully examined by neuropsychological methods is one of the strongest predictors of the long-term prognosis.[10,18] Boake et al.[7] emphasize this same point.

The Persistent Problem of Malingering

Many TBI patients are involved in litigation, raising the question of whether a given patient is exerting adequate effort when performing neuropsychological tests. There is no easy answer to this question. A number of methods have been developed to assess malingering, but all have limitations. Typically, how patients interact in the interview provides clues about whether they are motivated to perform. Patients' presentation of their premorbid status also provides useful information. For example, if patients describe themselves as "remembering everything" before the accident but are now devastated after a mild TBI, complaints are likely exaggerated or deficits are feigned. Tests such as the Digit Memory Test may help confirm the clinician's impressions obtained during the interview.[27] However, it typically takes years of experience examining various types of TBI patients in nonlitigious settings to determine whether their level and pattern of performance are compatible with their medical history. Binder[5] has reviewed the literature on mild TBI and discussed the problem of malingering in this patient group.

Advances in Neuropsychological Testing

Although new neuropsychological tests are appearing on a regular basis and old tests are being restandardized, true innovation in the assessment of these patients is difficult to find. Perhaps the most meaningful advance involves the role of neuroimaging techniques combined with neuropsychological testing.

Speed of information processing relates to severity of brain injury. Johnson et al.[14] demonstrated that the ventricle-to-brain ratio in TBI patients was related to the speed at which information was processed (using the Wechsler Adult Intelligence Scale–Revised [WAIS-R] Digit Symbol subtest). Interestingly, this finding was observed in males but not in females.

Kirkby et al.[15] studied physiological changes in a patient with frontal lobe damage after a TBI. Using positron emission tomography (PET), these authors showed that the pattern of activation observed when the patient performed the Wisconsin Card Sorting Test (WCST) differed from that of his uninjured monozygotic twin. "The impaired twin showed less activation in the inferior portion of the left inferior frontal gyrus while showing greater activation in the left hippocampus ($p < 0.04$)" (p. 689). The authors noted that this pattern differed from what is observed when normal individuals perform the WCST. They suggested that the differences in metabolic activity may "reflect the utilization of different neural systems when performing a frontal lobe task" (p. 689). This study and many like it suggest that one cannot rely purely on the level of neuropsychological test performance to know if recovery has occurred. Multiple measures of recovery must be considered. In the future, neuroimaging studies undoubtedly will be a part of the method of assessing whether recovery has been established.

McDowell et al.[22] have encouraged neuropsychologists to use theoretically driven tests to improve understanding of the nature of higher integrated brain dysfunction in TBI patients. They report that slowed reaction times in TBI patients are amplified when patients are required to perform two tasks at once. This finding is often observed in everyday life. McDowell et al. suggested that when an increased load is placed on *working memory*, the performance of TBI patients deteriorates even more. Using a different paradigm and functional magnetic resonance imaging (MRI) techniques, McAllister et al.[21] made a similar point. They noted different patterns of brain activation when patients with mild TBI performed a working memory task compared to normal controls. They observed different patterns of brain activation even when the actual level of performance on psychometric tests did not differ substantially between controls and patients with mild TBI.

Limits of Neuropsychological Testing

Clearly, neuropsychological tests are useful but have their limits. Patients with TBI experience important phenomena that neuropsychological tests do not measure adequately. For example, the problem of mental fatigue is common after TBI, and yet there is no test for it. Behavioral dyscontrol and emotional lability are also quite common after TBI, but there is no test for them.

Besides being unable to measure important phenomena after TBI, performance on psychometric tests is influenced by a wide variety of nonneurological factors (see Table 12.2). A common problem confronting many clinical neuropsychologists is the examination of individuals from another culture who speak languages other than English. Interpreting their test findings based on the typical normative databases associated with standardized neuropsychological tests is at best problematic and at worst misleading. Neuropsychologists have attempted to correct this problem, particularly when assessing individuals from Hispanic cultures who primarily speak Spanish.[16] Further work, however, is needed in this area.

Finally, neuropsychologists often lack a measure of the premorbid status of patients. Various formulas have been proposed for assessing premorbid IQ. However, these formulas often fail to capture the level and pattern of premorbid higher brain functional capacities in a given individual. Work with professional athletes has highlighted the importance of having a reasonable assessment of their premorbid status to determine whether neuropsychological functioning has returned to baseline. Clinical neuropsychologists must use considerable skill in judging whether patients' level and pattern of neuropsychological performance match premorbid estimates. For example, if an individual was a professional engineer in his mid-30s and suffered a moderate to severe TBI, one might find that his Performance IQ was still average or even above average. This finding, however, would not indicate that the patient's level of performance was normal for the individual. Furthermore, measures of speed of information processing (such as the Digit Symbol subtest of the WAIS-III) can be in the average range but still represent a drop from the premorbid status. Thus, interpreting the pattern and level of performance in light of the patient's medical history continues to be an important feature of a meaningful clinical neuropsychological examination, as Reitan[34] has long emphasized.

Concl\usions

Neuropsychological testing is an important component in the assessment of patients with known or suspected TBI. An understanding of the typical disturbances in higher integrated brain functions associated with these injuries will help develop better methods for assessing this patient group. This chapter provides background information that may be helpful to neurologists and neurosurgeons when evaluating neuropsychological test findings of TBI patients.

ACKNOWLEDGMENTS

The authors thank Shelley Kick, Ph.D., for her editorial assistance and Mary Henry for secretarial support while preparing this manuscript. Funding from the Newsome Chair in Clinical Neuropsychology to the first author provided time to prepare this manuscript.

REFERENCES

1. Appleton RE, Baldwin T: Management of Brain-Injured Children. New York, Oxford University Press, 1998.
2. Asarnow RF, Satz P, Light R, Zaucha K, Lewis R, McCleary C: The UCLA study of mild closed head injury in children and adolescents. In: Broman SH, Michel ME (eds): Traumatic Head Injury in Children. New York, Oxford University Press, 1995, pp 117–146.
3. Barron IS, Fennell EB, Voeller KKS: Pediatric Neuropsychology in the Medical Setting. New York, Oxford University Press, 1995.
4. Ben-Yishay Y, Prigatano GP: Cognitive remediation. In: Rosenthal M, Griffith ER, Bond MR, Miller JD (eds): Rehabilitation of the Adult and Child with Traumatic Brain Injury. Philadelphia, FA Davis, 1990, pp 393–409.
5. Binder LM: A review of mild head trauma. Part II: Clinical implications. J Clin Exp Neuropsycho 19(3):432–457, 1997.
6. Birch H: Brain Damage in Children: The Biological and Social Aspects. New York, Williams & Wilkins, 1964.
7. Boake C, Millis SR, High, WM, Delmonico RL, Kreutzer JS, Rosenthal M, Sherer M, Ivanhoe CB: Using early neuropsychologic testing to predict long-term productivity outcome from traumatic brain injury. Arch Phys Med Rehabil 82:761–768, 2001.
8. Borgaro SR, Prigatano GP: Early cognitive and affective sequelae of traumatic brain injury: A study using the BNI Screen for higher cerebral functions. J Head Trauma Rehabil 17(6):526–534, 2002.
9. Borgaro SR, Prigatano GP, Kwasnica C, Rexer JL: Cognitive and affective sequelae in complicated and uncomplicated mild traumatic brain injury. Brain Injury 17(3): 189–198, 2003.
10. Dikmen SS, Machamer JE, Winn HR, Temkin NR: Neuropsychological outcome at 1 year post head injury. Neuropsychology 9:80–90, 1995.
11. Dikmen SS, Temkin N, Armsden G: Neuropsychological recovery: Relationship to psychosocial functioning and postconcussional complaints. In: Levin HS, Eisenberg HM, Benton AL (eds): Mild Head Injury. New York, Oxford University Press, 1989, pp 229–241.
12. Fordyce DJ, Roueche JR, Prigatano GP: Enhanced emotional reactions in chronic head trauma patients. J Neurol Neurosurg Psychiatry 46:620–624, 1983.
13. Jennett B, Teasdale G: Management of Head Injuries. Philadelphia, FA Davis, 1981.
14. Johnson SC, Bigler ED, Burr RB, Blatter D: White matter atrophy, ventricular dilation, and intellectual functioning following traumatic brain injury. Neuropsychology 8(3):307–315, 1994.
15. Kirkby BS, Van Horn JD, Ostrem JL, Weinberger DR, Berman KF: Cognitive activation during PET: A case study of monozygotic twins discordant for closed head injury. Neuropsychologia 34(7):689–697, 1996.
16. LaRue A, Romero LJ, Ortiz IE, Hwa CL, Lidndem RD: Neuropsychological performance of Hispanic and non-Hispanic older adults: An epidemiologic survey. Clin Neuropsychol 13(4):474–486, 1999.
17. Lezak MD, Howieson, DB, Loring, DW: Neuropsychological Assessment, 4th ed. New York, Oxford University Press, 2004.
18. Levin HS, Gary HE, Eisenberg HM, Ruff RM, Barth JT, Kreutzer J, High WM, Portman S, Foulkes MA, Jane JA,

Marmarou A, Marshall L: Neurobehavioral outcome 1 year after severe head injury. J Neurosurg 73:699–709, 1990.

19. Levin HS, Mendelsohn D, Lilly MA, Fletcher JM, Culhane KA, Chapman SB, Harward H, Kusnerik L, Bruce D, Eisenberg HM: Tower of London performance in relation to magnetic resonance imaging following closed head injury in children. Neuropsychology 8(2):171–179, 1994.
20. Luria AR: Higher Cortical Functions in Man. New York, Basic Books, 1966.
21. McAllister TW, Sparling MB, Flashman LA, Guerin SJ, Mamourian AC, Saykin AJ: Differential working memory load effects after mild traumatic brain injury. NeuroImage 14:1004–1012, 2001.
22. McDowell S, Whyte J, D'Esposito M: Working memory impairments in traumatic brain injury: Evidence from a dual-task paradigm. Neuropsychologia 35:1341–1353, 1997.
23. Parsons OA, Stewart KD: Effects of supportive versus disinterested interviews on perceptual-motor performance in brain-damaged and neurotic patients. J Consult Psychol 30:260–266, 1966.
24. Prigatano GP: Principles of Neuropsychological Rehabilitation. New York, Oxford University Press, 1999.
25. Prigatano GP: Recovery after concussion: A case report of a professional athlete. Unpublished Manuscript.
26. Prigatano GP, Altman IM, O'Brien KP: Behavioral limitations that brain injured patients tend to underestimate. Clin Neuropsychol 4:163–176, 1990.
27. Prigatano GP, Amin K: Digit Memory Test: Unequivocal cerebral dysfunction and suspected malingering. J Clin Exp Neuropsychol 15(4):537–546, 1993.
28. Prigatano GP, Borgaro SR: Qualitative features of finger movement during the Halstead finger oscillation test following traumatic brain injury. J Int Neuropsychol Soc 9: 128–133, 2003.
29. Prigatano GP, Fordyce D: The neuropsychological rehabilitation program at Presbyterian Hospital, Oklahoma City. In: Prigatano GP et al (eds): Neuropsychological Rehabilitation After Brain Injury. Baltimore, Johns Hopkins University Press, 1986, pp 96–118.
30. Prigatano GP, Fordyce DJ, Zeiner HK, Roueche JR, Pepping M, Wood B: Neuropsychological Rehabilitation After Brain Injury. Baltimore, Johns Hopkins University Press, 1986.
31. Prigatano GP, Pepping M, Klonoff P: Cognitive, personality, and psychosocial factors in the neuropsychological assessment of brain-injured patients. In: Uzell BP, Gross Y (eds): Clinical Neuropsychology of Intervention. Boston, Martinus Nijhoff, 1986, pp 135–166.
32. Prigatano GP, Redner JR: The uses and abuses of neuropsychological testing in behavioral neurology. Neurol Clin 11(1):219–231, 1993.
33. Prigatano GP, Zigler LY, Rosenstein LD: The clinical neuropsychological examination: Scope, cost and health-care value: In: Prigatano GP, Pliskin NH (eds): Clinical Neuropsychology and Cost Outcome Research: A Beginning. New York, Psychology Press, 2003, pp 15–36.
34. Reitan RM: Theoretical and methodological bases of the Halstead-Reitan Neuropsychological Test Battery. In: Grant, II, Adams KM (eds): Neuropsychological Assessment of Neuropsychiatric Disorders. New York, Oxford University, 1986, pp 3–30.
35. Report of the Therapeutics and Technology Assessment Subcommittee of the American Academy of Neurology: Special Article. Assessment: Neuropsychological testing of adults. Considerations for neurologists. Neurology 47: 592–599, 1996.
36. Ruff RM, Richards PM: Neuropsychological assessment and management of patients with persistent postconcussional disorders: In: Prigatano GP, Pliskin NH (eds): Clinical Neuropsychology and Cost Outcome Research: A Beginning. New York, Psychology Press, 2003, pp 61–81.
37. Russell WR: The Traumatic Amnesias. New York, Oxford University Press, 1971.
38. Schafer R: Psychoanalytic Interpretation in Rorschach Testing. New York, Grune & Stratton, 1954.
39. Sherer M, Boake C, Levin E, Silver BV, Ringholz, G, High W: Characteristics of impaired awareness after traumatic brain injury. J Int Neuropsychol Soc 4:380–387, 1998.
40. Sherer M, Novak TA: Neuropsychological assessment after traumatic brain injury in adults: In: Prigatano GP, Pliskin NH (eds): Clinical Neuropsychology and Cost Outcome Research: A Beginning. New York, Psychology Press, 2003, pp 39–60.
41. Van Zomeren AH: Reaction Time and Attention After Closed Head Injury. Lisse, The Netherlands, Swets & Zeitlinger BV, 1981.
42. Van Zomeren AH, Van Den Burg W: Residual complaints of patients two years after severe head injury. J Neurol Neurosurg Psychiatry 48:21–28, 1985.
43. Weintraub S, Mesulam M-M: Mental state assessment of young and elderly adults in behavioral neurology. In: Mesulam M-M (ed): Principles of Behavioral Neurology. Philadelphia, FA Davis, 1985, pp 71–123.
44. Yates BT, Taub J: Assessing the cost, benefits, cost-effectiveness, and cost-benefit of psychological assessment: We should, we can, and here's how. Psychol Assess 15(4):478–495, 2003.

Chapter 13
Cognitive Rehabilitation

JAMES F. MALEC AND
KEITH D. CICERONE

As might be said about most areas of clinical care, professional interest in cognitive rehabilitation (CR) was motivated more by humanistic than by scientific concerns during its initial development. Increasing numbers of young people survived severe traumatic brain injuries (TBI) in the 1970s due to improved emergency and neurosurgical methods. Rehabilitation professionals responded by attempting to formulate procedures to assist these people in reentering the mainstream of life. These early rehabilitation efforts were strongly encouraged by family members of people with TBI and through the advocacy of the National Head Injury Association (later renamed the Brain Injury Association of America) and its affiliates.

During these early years, rehabilitation after TBI emphasized the rebuilding of cognitive processes rather than physical rehabilitation for several reasons. First, TBI most often resulted in primary damage to the brain's frontal and temporal areas, which, in turn, resulted in significant cognitive impairments. Because prominent trauma to the primary motor and sensory regions is less common in TBI, many people with TBI—even those with moderate to severe injuries—showed dramatic physical recovery. Impaired cognition, particularly impaired concentration and memory, were the most apparent and long-standing deficits after TBI. Second, many of the behavioral and emotional problems of people with TBI seemed to be based on cognitive impairments. Many rehabilitationists believed that improving the cognition of the person with TBI should result in improved behavioral and emotional self-management and associated gains in functional activities.[87] This viewpoint—that cognition provides an important avenue for emotional and behavioral self-management—is consonant with the basic assumptions of cognitive-behavioral psychotherapy, which was also emerging as a powerful clinical method in the 1970s. Furthermore, cognitive-behavioral methods to treat children with learning disabilities (another group with putative brain disorders) had shown initial success.[95] Finally, cognitive skills were becoming increasingly valued in American culture as employment opportunities shifted from blue collar to white collar. The importance of cognitive abilities was no less recognized by well-educated rehabilitation professionals. This cultural value probably also guided the early emphasis of TBI rehabilitation toward cognitive processes.

As TBI rehabilitation developed, however, these early assumptions were challenged by clinical experience. Emotional and behavioral dysfunctions were identified as barriers that are at least as problematic as cognitive impairments to psychosocial and vocational adaptation after TBI. Although a cognitive-behavioral approach remains a potent method for improving emotional and behavioral self-management,[135] other interpersonal, group-oriented psychotherapeutic approaches for improving mood and behavior also appeared beneficial in some cases. A multimodal psychotherapeutic approach has become the standard in comprehensive-holistic TBI rehabilitation methods developed by Ben-Yishay and Prigatano.[11]

Perhaps most significantly, it became apparent that functional gains relevant to effective daily living are not necessarily dependent on cognitive improvements. Good memory and reasoning abilities are only two elements in the formula for success in life. Other personal qualities, including sociability, agreeableness, and conscientiousness, as well as a supportive environment and some good luck, figure prominently in the equation for a rewarding life. For example, some survivors of TBI have become astute and powerful political advocates by virtue of their commitment and charisma despite having residual cognitive impairments. Other people with TBI have reentered the mainstream of society simply by realigning their expectations. Still others have successfully maintained relatively sophisticated employment positions based on well-established remote memory and with external adaptations to ensure that the working environment is relatively routine and predictable.

In addition to predictability and routinization, other beneficial environmental changes and aids include a system of memory prompts and other assistive devices to help compensate for cognitive deficits. Such interventions do not improve cognition itself but do reduce the disability associated with cognitive impairments, just as wheelchair use and ramping reduce the disability associated with paraplegia. As TBI rehabilitation developed over the past 30 years, outcome expectations became clearly focused on real-life results that significantly improve the capacity for independent living, socialization and family life, education and work.[28] While this focus took improved cognition per se from the center stage, CR remains a component of most postacute TBI rehabilitation programs. Ninety-five percent of rehabilitation facilities provide some form of CR.[94]

Even during the early stages of its development, humanistic and functional emphases of TBI rehabilitation were never divorced from scientific concerns. From the beginning of interest in CR, responsible professionals attempted to validate their clinical methods scientifically. In what provides as viable a list of ingredients for the scientific investigation of CR today as it did nearly 25 years ago, two seminal researchers in the field, Leonard Diller and Wayne Gordon,[33] outlined six elements of research and practice TBI rehabilitation:

1. neurologic information,
2. medical information,
3. psychometric and other neuropsychologic information to specify impairments,
4. functional competency information (i.e., measures of individual ability to act without assistance),
5. patterns of behaviors in natural settings (i.e., the relationships between acquired brain damage and activity choice or time usage; is it beyond the scope of intervention efforts to impact this domain?),
6. environment (i.e., effective ways of developing or using environmental supports)

During the 1980s, scientific interest in CR was encouraged by allegations of unethical practices against some TBI rehabilitation providers. Computer programs and other materials for CR were marketed and sold without any substantial clinical or scientific validation of their efficacy or usefulness, or, in some cases, without even a statement that their efficacy was not substantiated. Rehabilitation entrepreneurs discovered that CR exercises could be provided simultaneously to multiple clients by a single staff person, thereby minimizing expense and maximizing revenues. Too frequently, such enterprises did not evaluate the benefit to the patient (or lack thereof) of these lucrative practices.

The scientific community reacted to entrepreneurial abuses by emphasizing the unproven nature of CR.[14,81,164,170] Although clearly well intentioned and motivated to protect consumers from unscrupulous providers, the conservative response of some scientists to CR was at times overstated and probably slowed the development of potentially viable clinical techniques. More liberal clinical researchers also responded to alleged entrepreneurial abuses in TBI rehabilitation.[88] Neuropsychologists[93] and rehabilitationists[54] developed clinical guidelines for the practice of CR. These guidelines identified risks of these procedures (Table 13.1),

Table 13.1. Potential Risks of Cognitive Rehabilitation (CR)

1. False hopes may be raised, and denial of disability may be reinforced.
2. The development of an isolated or task-specific skill may serve as false evidence of general competency.
3. CR may divert attention from more important or problematic concerns.
4. CR may perpetuate social isolation.

Source: Adapted from Mathews et al.[93]

recommended clinical practices that evaluated outcomes in the individual case, recommended quality control and full disclosure in the development and marketing of CR materials, and emphasized the growing body of clinical and scientific work that support the effectiveness of CR in specific cases.

At the present time, this debate continues among CR researchers. More conservative CR researchers tend to set extremely high standards for methodology and evidence, in comparison to other researchers who understand science as an incremental process that characteristically moves from naturalistic observation through detailed study of specific cases and other limited experiments that provide the foundation for more sophisticated and well-controlled experimental designs leading to definitive demonstration of a phenomenon. For example, an independent panel led by Carney and Chestnut[18] that reviewed the CR literature between January 1988 and August 1998 noted the heterogeneity of subjects, interventions, and outcomes and the small sample sizes characteristic of CR studies. Because of these limitations, the panel concluded that there was only weak evidence for the efficacy of CR. Despite this very conservative conclusion, the panel also noted a group of studies, including randomized, controlled trials, that demonstrated significant improvements in attention, memory, and executive cognitive abilities under some conditions. A subsequent evidence-based review of the literature organized by Cicerone[23] through the Brain Injury Interdisciplinary Special Interest Group (BI-ISIG) of the American Congress for Rehabilitation Medicine included more recent studies and allowed for a more liberal interpretation of available data. For instance, while the Carney-Chestnut review excluded studies with small numbers of subjects, the Cicerone group endorsed results of small-group studies if these were replicated by other independent researchers in similar studies that in aggregate provided a substantial sample size.

Such evidence-based reviews have become popular in medicine during the past 10 years as an empirically based method to identify the best practices in specific clinical areas.[185] The evidence-based review method results in classification of studies into three levels of scientific rigor. Class I studies are well designed, prospective, randomized, controlled trials (RCTs). Class II studies include prospective, nonrandomized or uncontrolled cohort studies; retrospective case control studies; and clinical series with well-designed controls, such as multiple baseline studies of a series of subjects. Single-subject designs or uncontrolled case series investigations are considered Class III. The level of recommendation resulting from the review is linked to the class of supporting evidence. At least one Class I study with an adequate sample demonstrating treatment efficacy is required for a treatment standard. A *standard* indicates that the treatment should be applied to appropriate cases unless there are specific contraindications. Well-designed Class II studies with an adequate sample are required for a treatment guideline. A *guideline* indicates that the treatment should be considered in appropriate cases. More limited Class II or Class III evidence may support a treatment option. An *option* is a treatment that may be reasonably applied in appropriate cases, although there is not strong support for general efficacy.

In CR and TBI rehabilitation generally, skepticism and waning support by medical insurance providers have prodded scientific investigation and evidence-based reviews. Since the first publication of this chapter in the mid-1990s, the provision of CR and other TBI rehabilitation methods has become increasingly restricted by lack of adequate funding. In the year 2005, an absence of funding for rehabilitation services may have been the single largest obstacle to community reentry for people with significant disability following TBI. Despite the publication of the extensive BI-ISIG evidence-based review, which presented 29 well-designed RCTs supporting the efficacy of CR, many insurance providers continue to deny payment for such services based on claims of limited evidence of efficacy. Very recently, the BI-ISIG group completed an update[24] of their original evidence-based review of CR that identified 17 additional well-controlled Class I studies supporting the efficacy of CR procedures.

In the original version of this chapter, a series of clinical research questions in CR (see Table 13.2) served as an outline. These questions follow a traditional sequence for scientific inquiry in any clinical field, moving from demonstration of a phenomenon in any context, toward elaboration of necessary and sufficient conditions for the phenomenon, and culminating in the explication of underlying mechanisms that can predict or create the phenomenon.

For this second edition, these questions seem no less relevant. However, a stronger and more extensive body of scientific evidence of efficacy exists on which to base answers to these questions. This evidence has been summarized in the evidence-based reviews of the BI-ISIG.[23,24] We refer the reader to the original publications of these reviews for details of the review process and results. In this chapter, we will cite specific recommendations emanating from these reviews and describe exemplary studies supporting recommendations for best practices in CR. In keeping with the BI-ISIG reviews, we focus on evidence resulting from studies of people with TBI or stroke. Although results of these studies may generalize to groups of patients with other types of acquired brain dysfunction (ABD) (i.e., tumor, cerebral anoxia), specific application to such groups is largely absent from the literature. We consider only behavioral interventions and do not include pharmacological interventions to improve cognition. The study of pharmacologics to enhance cognition has burgeoned during the past 10 years and is considered beyond the scope of this chapter. For purposes of this chapter, we have adopted the BI-ISIG definition[23] of CR as

> a systematic, functionally oriented service of therapeutic activities that is based on assessment and understanding of the patient's brain-behavioral deficits. Specific interventions may have various approaches, including (1) reinforcing, strengthening, or reestablishing previously learned patterns of behavior; (2) establishing new patterns of cognitive activity through compensatory cognitive mechanisms for impaired neurologic systems; (3) establishing new patterns of activity through external compensatory mechanisms such as personal orthoses or environmental structuring and support; and (4) enabling persons to adapt to the cognitive disability, even though it may not be possible to directly modify or compensate for cognitive impairments, in order to improve their overall level of functioning and quality of life. (pp. 1596–1597)

Table 13.2. Clinical Research Questions in Cognitive Rehabilitation (CR)

1. Can any cognitive function be improved in any individual with cognitive impairments consequent to acquired brain dysfunction (ABD)?
2. Can specific cognitive functions (i.e., attention, memory, language, visuospatial skills, executive cognitive functions) be improved in any individual with impairments in these areas consequent to ABD? Are such procedures effective in most cases?
3. If improvements in cognitive functioning occur as a result of CR, are these improvements maintained in and generalized to nontraining conditions? Do maintenance and generalization vary among specific cognitive functions? Are improvement, maintenance, and generalization sufficient to support activities that are of functional value to the individual with ABD?
4. What environmental features affect the outcome (i.e., improvement, maintenance, generalization) of CR for specific cognitive functions?
5. What characteristics of people with acquired cognitive impairments (e.g., injury severity, type of cognitive impairment, emotional factors, personality, preinjury abilities) affect the outcome of CR?
6. What neurological, psychological, social, and environmental processes underlie positive outcomes in CR?

State-of-the-Art Answers to Clinical Research Questions in Cognitive Rehabilitation

Can Any Cognitive Function Be Improved in Any Individual with Impairments Consequent to Traumatic Brain Injury or Stroke?

A very large number of studies (29 Class I, 35 Class II, and 107 Class III studies in the initial BI-ISIG evidence-based review of CR and an additional 17 Class I, 8 Class II, and 62 Class III studies in the update) provide abundant evidence that, at least in some cases and under some circumstances, a variety of cognitive functions improve with CR.

Can Specific Cognitive Functions (i.e., Attention, Memory, Language, Visuospatial Skills, Executive Cognitive Functions) Be Improved in Any Individual with Impairments in These Areas Consequent to Traumatic Brain Injury or Stroke? Are Such Procedures Effective in Most Cases?

Sohlberg and Matter's 1989 volume[144] was a landmark text in many respects. It was the first comprehensive textbook for CR. More importantly, it integrated theory with practice and described a process-specific approach to CR. Before the late 1980s, CR was often discussed as a broadband intervention to address an equally broad range of cognitive impairments. In contrast, Sohlberg and Mateer applied specific elements of neuropsychological theory to the rehabilitation of equally specific cognitive processes. Now in its second edition,[146] the Sohlberg-Mateer text remains a comprehensive source for theory and practice in CR. The text published by Barbara Wilson and colleagues[180] at the Cambridge Cognition and Brain Sciences Unit provides an additional comprehensive source elaborating contemporary approaches to CR.

In an admittedly less comprehensive fashion, we will review the theoretical foundations of current practice in specific CR interventions in this section in addition to reviewing evidence-based best practices. Although the research evidence supporting CR applications is more extensive and sound than at the time of the first edition of the present chapter, much of the theory that provides the foundation for these practices remains classic and unchanged.

Attention

THEORY. Shum and colleagues[140,141] demonstrated that Sternberg's additive factor model of attention is applicable to patients with TBI. Sternberg's model identifies four sequential noninteractive phases of attention: (1) feature extraction: discriminating a target stimulus from background noise; (2) identification: recognizing the distinct meaning of the target stimulus in contrast to similar stimuli (i.e., matching the stimulus accurately to memory); (3) response selection: selection of the appropriate response to the stimulus; and (4) motor adjustment: appropriately delaying or otherwise inhibiting a response to the stimulus.

This model is compatible with other models of attention that have been applied to TBI[143,184] in that it discriminates between phases of perceptual processing (phases 1 and 2) and response determination (phases 3 and 4) in attention. Most importantly Shum's group has shown that a year or more after TBI, deficits in attention are typically confined to impairments in response organization (i.e., response selection and motor adjustment). Their research indicates that deficits in the perceptual processing phases of attention (specifically phase 2: identification) are present early after TBI but generally resolve with natural recovery. This is consistent with Ponsford and Kinsella's[115] failure to find distinct attentional impairments among TBI patients related to the stimulus demands of experimental tasks (i.e., focused or sustained attention), although subjects demonstrated impaired response speed.

These basic studies have implications for CR of attention in suggesting that the specific nature of attentional impairments varies among subjects and varies with the time since injury. Patients may show more complex attentional impairments involving both perceptual and response processes soon after injury. With natural recovery, attentional problems probably resolve in most cases, although response processes may remain impaired.

In this regard, chronic impairment of attention after TBI may be described more accurately as impairment of *intention*. Changes in attention as a result of treatment in the postacute period should be assessed in terms of response speed and accuracy rather than stimulus discrimination. Primary impairment of intention in the postacute period after TBI does not preclude the possibility that varying stimulus presentations is an important aspect of training to improve the speed and accuracy of response. However, it does suggest that attention training should also emphasize procedures that require progressively more complex response selection, delay, and execution.

EVIDENCE-BASED BEST PRACTICES

Practice Standards: *(1) Attention training is recommended during the postacute (posthospital) phase of rehabilitation after TBI and stroke. (2) Strategy training for attention deficits (including training with different stimulus modalities, levels of complexity, and response demands) is recommended during the postacute (posthospital) phase of rehabilitation after*

TBI and stroke. (3) *Insufficient evidence exists to distinguish the effects of specific attention training during acute recovery and rehabilitation from spontaneous recovery or from more general cognitive interventions.*

These recommendation are supported by four Class I[39,51,114,147] studies with a total of 93 subjects and three Class II studies[22,143,153] with a total of 57 subjects. Therapists providing treatment in these studies assisted the participants by monitoring performance, providing feedback, and teaching strategies. There was not sufficient evidence for the effectiveness of this type of intervention during the *acute* phase of recovery. In the acute period, recovery of attention occurs spontaneously to a degree that appears to obviate any potential treatment effect.

In one of the earliest demonstrations of effective treatment for attention deficits, Sohlberg and Mateer[143] conducted a Class II multiple-baseline study of four subjects that they described as *Attention Process Training*. Attention Process Training relies on discrete attention tasks organized according to a presumed hierarchy of five attention components (focused, sustained, alternating, selective, and divided attention) but also incorporates elements of task complexity and multiple-modality treatment that also characterizes Class I studies. A recent Class I study[147] compared Attention Process Training with an alternative condition of brain injury education and support. Using a crossover design, 14 subjects were randomly assigned to receive each treatment in different order. Most of the subjects had sustained a severe TBI, and the attention treatment was conducted with tasks selected on the basis of each participant's specific profile of attention deficits. Improvements on neuropsychological measures of attention and self-reported changes in attention and *working memory* were more common after Attention Process Training than after therapeutic support. Neuropsychological improvements were evident on the more complex aspects of attention but not on measures of vigilance or covert orienting, suggesting that the gains were not due to general cognitive stimulation.

Three postacute Class I studies contrasted attention training with an alternative treatment condition. Gray and colleagues[51] randomly assigned 31 subjects to either computerized attention retraining or an equivalent amount of recreational computing. Both TBI and stroke patients with mild or moderate/severe attentional deficits entered the study between approximately 2 months and 10 years postinjury/event. No effect on treatment of either diagnosis or severity was apparent, although the small number of subjects suggests that the study may have lacked power to identify a modest effect for these factors. Attention training tasks were selected that required sustained and divided attention and placed demands on working memory. Specific tasks included simple and complex reaction time and divided attention. Subjects were instructed in strategies involving self-talk and allocation of attention. Experimental subjects performed better than controls on psychometric measures of attention immediately after treatment and at 6-month follow-up. In another Class I study, Niemann and colleagues[105] randomly assigned 26 subjects with moderate/severe TBI to attention or memory retraining conditions. Subjects entered the study 12 to 72 months postinjury. Similar to the Gray study, the attention treatment condition involved computer-based training in focused and divided attention to auditory or visual stimuli, as well as strategy training and therapist feedback. Both groups improved on measures monitored during treatment, but the attention training group improved more than the memory training group on measures specific to attention. Fasotti and colleagues[39] compared an intervention intended to teach patients to compensate for slowed information processing and information overload (*time pressure management*) with more generic *concentration training*. The 22 subjects with severe or very severe TBI were, on average, 9 months postinjury, and all had evidence of slowed information processing. The subjects who received the experimental treatment were more likely to use self-management strategies to manage time pressure and demonstrated significantly greater improvements in attention and memory functioning compared with the participants who received generic concentration training. These benefits were apparent on more complex tasks that allowed for strategy use, but not on basic reaction time tasks in which such strategies could not be applied.

Two Class II studies have reported beneficial effects of similar attention training methods for a group of 45 subjects with TBI and stroke[153] or 8 subjects with mild TBI[22] compared to a nonrandomized control condition.

These and other studies of attention training suggest that the effects of treatment are most apparent on measures that closely resemble training tasks and that generalization to functional tasks may be weak. However, few studies carefully examined generalization to functional activities. There is some suggestion in this literature that training in strategies for attention and therapist feedback may enhance the potential for generalization.[105,114,178] Studies suggest greater benefit from training that involves manipulating complex stimulus arrays requiring selective or divided attention rather than from training with simpler tasks or tasks directed at increasing simple processing speed.[37,51,114,154,155] Applied research in this area appears to confirm theoretical expectations that the most effective treatment involves both perceptual and response components of attention/intention in discriminating and manipulating complex stimulus arrays.

Memory

THEORY. Various types of learning and memory disorders may be present after ABD. Impaired attention and impaired executive cognitive abilities, which are required to organize new, unstructured, or divergent information for memory storage, may interfere with learning apart from any primary impairment of specific memory systems. Within the domain of memory itself, multiple memory and learning systems exist. Patients with ABD typically show impairment of some and preservation of other memory functions (see Gliksy et al.[48] for review and discussion).

After ABD, patients very often demonstrate impairment in the acquisition and retention of discrete bits of information, such as recalling facts, recognizing faces, recalling a name in association with a recognized face, or recalling information represented in standardized memory tests. This type of memory, commonly called *declarative memory*, is an indexed system in which knowledge is stored as well as information about the store of knowledge itself. Thus, when one knows a fact, one also knows that one knows the fact.

Establishing new declarative memories is a complex process. Classically, two major stages in the encoding process have been identified. The initial stage, representing brief storage and processing of new information, was referred to as *short-term memory*. More contemporaneously, this initial memory processing stage is encompassed under the rubric of *working memory*. If information is to be remembered indefinitely, the information must be transferred from working memory to *long-term storage*. Once information is stored for long-term retention, retrieval processes become paramount in order to negotiate recall of information at times when the information is relevant or required.

Baddeley and Hitch's[4] theory of working memory provides an elaboration of the involvement of attentional and executive cognitive functions in the transfer of information to long-term storage. This theory is not reviewed in detail here. However, it is particularly relevant to memory rehabilitation for patients with frontal lobe injuries because it incorporates the interface between the regulation of attention and other executive cognitive functions, modulated by the frontal cerebrum, and memory processing. The theory of working memory is consistent with observations that impaired attention and executive cognitive functions interfere with memory processing and memory rehabilitation. Along these same lines, working memory theory would support a multimodal approach to memory rehabilitation that addresses attention, learning, and executive abilities. The interested reader is referred to other sources[4,9,45,131] for thorough reviews of working memory theory.

A number of brain areas contribute to declarative learning and memory processes. Adequate attention, modulated by the fronto-limbic-reticular axis, is necessary for both acquisition and retrieval of new information. Frontal lobe functions support working memory and the integration of new information for memory storage and later retrieval. The hippocampus, a structure in the mesial temporal lobes, is critical for the transfer of information to long-term storage. Classic Alzheimer's disease, which typically first attacks the hippocampus, provides an illustration of the devastating effect on forming new memories of hippocampal pathology. The saliency, and associated memorability, of new information is determined by the affective valence associated with the information by limbic arousal. The process of long-term storage very likely involves biochemical coding of the new information. Neuropsychometric evaluations attempt to distinguish impairment in initial learning and working memory from restricted capacity to transfer information to long-term storage, as evidenced by performance on delayed recall trials.

A second type of memory, *procedural memory*, is a skill-based, stimulus-response learning sytem in which behaviors contingent upon specific stimuli are acquired. Sequences of behaviors that are performed relatively automatically, such as driving, playing sports, and dressing, are examples of procedural learning. The acquisition of domain-specific knowledge, such as reciting the steps in fixing a packaged microwave dinner, may be a type of procedural learning. In such domain-specific learning, very specific information is acquired not through the associative processes normally involved in declarative memory, but through highly repetitive or specialized (e.g., vanishing cues) rehearsal processes. Procedural memory is not well indexed. Consequently, one's knowledge (declarative memory) of one's skill level may not always accurately represent one's actual skill (procedural memory). Over- and underestimates of skill levels are common in the non-ABD population. However, inaccurate estimation of personal abilities may be more dramatic after ABD because declarative memory coding of procedural skills is more impaired and because of complex, higher-order impairments that affect self-awareness.

Typically, procedural memory is less affected by ABD than declarative memory. Miller[98] found little difference in the rate or transfer of motor skill learning between patients with Alzheimer's disease and normal controls. Glisky et al.,[48] in a now classic demonstration, showed that severely amnestic patients were able to learn computer skills with specialized procedural training. Their patients' procedural learning appeared to be sequential and formatted in stimulus-response strings. If precise stimulus conditions were not present, access to learning faltered. In contrast, in normal learning, responses are accessible to multiple stimuli, including novel stimuli that only partially resemble the stimuli present during initial learning. Neuropsychometric methods to assess procedural memory are not well established. Typically, the capacity for procedural learning is judged through observation of skill acquisition and day-to- day carryover of new learning in rehabilitation therapies.

Our reading of the literature suggests to us that memory rehabilitation approaches may be classified along two dimensions (Fig. 13.1). The first dimension describes the degree to which the process that enhances memory is internal or external to the person. The second dimension is the degree to which the process is regulated by the person or by the environment, including other people. Figure 13.1 provides examples of memory rehabilitation interventions in each quadrant defined by these dimensions. Learning internalized memory

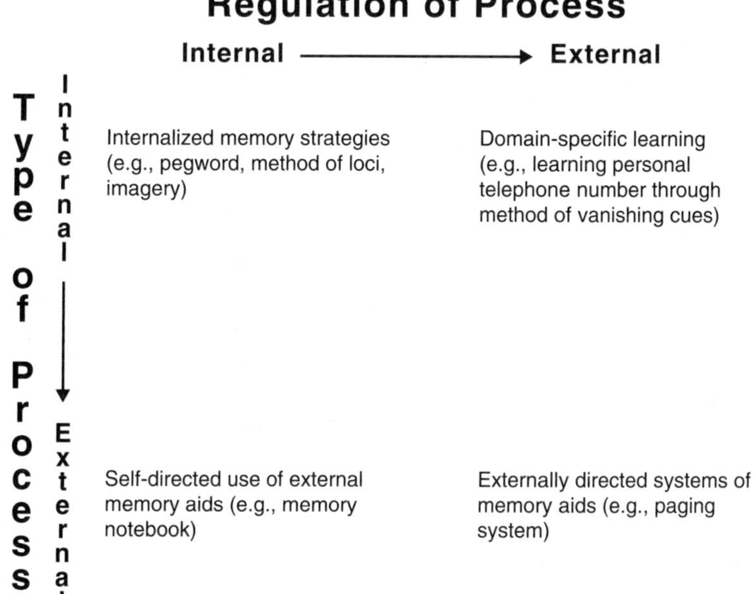

Figure 13.1. Dimensions of memory rehabilitation.

strategies that are self-regulated requires a degree of preservation of working and declarative memory and executive cognitive functions. Learning generalized, externally based procedures (such as use of an organized memory notebook) requires less declarative memory and executive cognitive abilities and relies more—but not exclusively—on procedural learning. Acquiring internalized, domain-specific knowledge (such as steps for preparing a specific type of microwave dinner) through externally directed overlearning or other specialized procedures, however, may rely entirely on procedural memory. External memory compensation methods that are entirely other-directed (such as a paging system or cue card) may require minimal declarative or procedural memory.

Within the approach of teaching learning strategies, neuropsychological theory suggests two types of techniques: (1) structuring and association techniques that support frontal lobe processing of new information and (2) techniques that enhance attention to and the saliency of information to be learned. The ability to remember these techniques, the extent of frontal lobe dysfunction required to implement these techniques in appropriate settings, and the extent of primary impairment of attention will determine the degree to which such techniques can be used successfully.

Acquiring procedural skills and, even more so, domain-specific knowledge does not necessarily require declarative memory (i.e., the ability to describe the procedures and their appropriate application). However, the generalization of new learning to new situations depends on both (1) executive functions that support abstraction and association of learned stimuli and (2) the capacity to retrieve procedural learning in response to multiple associated stimuli. People with ABD who depend primarily on procedural memory may not always be able to gain access to new learning in stimulus situations that deviate from the training situation. If declarative memory and executive cognitive abilities are not sufficiently preserved to support such generalization, environmental supports (such as prompts, cues, and other externally directed reminding systems) will be necessary.

Evidence-Based Best Practices

Practice Standard: *Compensatory memory strategy training is recommended for people with mild memory impairment due to TBI. This may include either internalized memory strategies (e.g., visual imagery) or the independent use of external memory compensations (e.g., memory notebooks).*

Learning Strategies. The first evidence-based review[23] combined research on learning strategies with teaching other compensatory mechanisms to support this practice standard, based on six Class I studies of 132 subjects with ABD. Four of the Class I studies supporting this standard specifically evaluated learning strategies. Berg and associates[13] compared learning strategy training in people with relatively mild cognitive impairment to a sham treatment control condition that involved playing memory games. The active treatment resulted in superior performance (compared to the control condition) on objective memory tests both immediately after treatment and at 4-month follow-up. Active treatment participants also reported improved everyday memory function. Kerner and Acker[69] showed similar results in people with mild memory impairment post-TBI on objective memory testing in a study comparing computer-based memory retraining with a sham control condition. However, gains from this limited 12-week intervention were not maintained 15 days later. Kaschel and colleagues[63] evaluated the use of visual imagery for subjects with mild memory impairment after ABD compared with the standard memory treatment used in seven different rehabilitation centers. For all of the patients, memory problems were considered to be of primary importance, although patients with severe memory impairment were excluded. The use of visual imagery led to significant improvements on verbal recall and ratings of memory functioning. Ryan and Ruff[129] evaluated the benefits of learning strategies, such as employing rehearsal and visual imagery, compared to a sham treatment (recreational computing). Differential benefit of memory retraining was observed only in those subjects who had mild memory impairment prior to treatment and not for the more severely impaired group. These studies offer strong support for the effectiveness of learning strategy training post-TBI but also indicate that this type of intervention is most effective with participants who are relatively independent in daily function, who recognize and are concerned about their memory problems, and who are motivated to continue the active and independent use of these strategies in daily life.

External Compensatory Strategies. Two Class I studies with 28 subjects evaluated the use of a memory notebook as a compensatory strategy for patients with mild memory impairments after TBI. Schmitter-Edgecombe and associates[136] found that a 9-week memory notebook training course resulted in fewer reports of everyday memory failures than a control condition. Unfortunately, this study involved only eight subjects. Three of the subjects who received memory therapy were still actively using the memory notebook to assist with their daily activities at 6-month follow-up. Ownsworth and McFarland[106] trained 20 patients with mild memory impairments to use a self-management strategy involving the use of a diary to compensate for their memory problems in their daily living situations. The use of the diary in conjunction with self-management techniques resulted in maintenance of strategy use during the treatment period and greater reduction in memory problems. These findings are consistent with a single-subject study[79] suggesting that self-instructional training may facilitate the use of memory compensations to a greater extent than task-specific training methods. These two studies of self-directed use of external compensatory strategies (e.g., notebook training) both suggest that this type of compensatory memory strategy training is effective primarily for patients with relatively mild memory impairment, and that patients' motivation and capacity for executive functioning contribute to the use and effectiveness of memory compensations.

Procedural and Domain-Specific Learning

Practice Guideline: *Use of external compensations with direct application to functional activities is recommended for people with severe memory impairment after TBI or stroke. These techniques appear effective when intended to facilitate acquisition of specific skills and knowledge rather than as an attempt to improve memory function per se.*

One RCT[181] extended the results of a previous uncontrolled study[182] that investigated the effectiveness of a portable pager to prompt memory in 173 subjects with mixed neurological diagnoses, all of whom had severe memory impairment. The pager was used to address specific aspects of subjects' daily responsibilities, such as taking medications on time or keeping appointments. Prompting with the pager produced significant improvement in the subjects' ability to carry out their everyday activities, particularly when the tasks occurred on a regular basis, compared with no treatment and baseline conditions. Diagnosis was not related to the effectiveness of the pager. The authors noted that the external paging system seemed particularly useful for those people with some insight and a need to carry out some tasks independently.

A number of additional uncontrolled studies have investigated the application of some form of external compensation for memory impairments, including the use of memory notebooks and various forms of technological assistance (e.g., mobile phones, portable voice organizers; see evidence-based reviews[23,24]). These studies suggest that extensive training may be required, and in many instances, the control of the compensation remains external. Despite these potential limitations, the use of these types of environmental interventions appears to hold promise as a means of enabling people with severe memory impairment to carry out a range of everyday activities.

Research with Older People. Although the focus of this review is on CR following TBI and stroke, it may be of interest that research investigating the use of similar approaches to address memory problems associated with normal aging or mild cognitive impairment in the elderly has resulted in similar findings. Organizational and other learning strategies[57,58,78,152] as well as multimodal training approaches[85a,151,162,163,187–190] may be of benefit to the elderly. However, methods to support generalization of these techniques to everyday life have not been documented,[2,101,137] and the efficacy of these interventions may decline with age.[91a] In an intriguing application of domain-specific learning, Leirer and colleagues[80] demonstrated that training in computer use to monitor medications had a positive effect on regular medication use in the elderly.

Visuospatial Abilities

Theory. The classic literature in this area[44,50,104,166,167] distinguishes three major types of visuospatial impairment: (1) primary visual field defects, (2) visual hemi-inattention or visual neglect, and (3) more complex visuoperceptual and visuomotor impairments. The empirical interventional research supports these distinctions. One group of researchers has provided evidence that specialized training may actually reduce primary visual field defects. However, their finding remains controversial because of the lack of replication in independent laboratories and because this finding is contrary to current wisdom regarding the permanence of visual field deficits due to neurological damage. A number of Class I studies have demonstrated the effectiveness of interventions that include scanning training for visual neglect. Because studies that include interventions directed at improving more complex visuospatial abilities typically include scanning training, it is difficult to determine whether this additional training adds to the positive effect of treatment of neglect on general visuospatial functioning. The relationship between visual neglect and visuospatial functioning and its implications for CR remains a salient theoretical as well as practical issue.

Evidence-based Best Practices: Visual Neglect

Practice Standard: *Visuospatial rehabilitation is recommended for people with visuoperceptual deficits associated with visual neglect after right hemisphere stroke.*

Practice Guideline: *Scanning training is recommended as an important, even critical, intervention element for people with severe visuoperceptual impairment that includes visual neglect after right hemisphere stroke.*

Eight Class I studies[3,49,62,102,171,172,177a,191] with a total of 327 subjects provide evidence to support the standard. Ten Class II studies[5,16,67,68,108,111,113,125,142,168] provide additional support. Interventions evaluated typically included visual scanning with additional exercises on more complex visuospatial constructional tasks. Visual scanning training may be the critical component of these interventions. However, the design of none of these studies provided for an explicit test of that hypothesis. Only one study[124] that provided visual scanning training on a small computer screen yielded a negative result. A more recent study,[168] however, demonstrated that, if the computer display is projected to a large enough area to challenge peripheral vision, a computer-based display can be effective. A critical element of a scanning intervention appears to be providing a large enough stimulus display to require scanning of the full visual field. Effective treatment is relatively intense and, and in most studies, involved 20 one-hour sessions over about four weeks.

Studies of visuospatial rehabilitation also document generalization of the effects of treatment[73,108,111,177a] resulting, for instance, in improved driving ability[74] and greater gains and shorter lengths of stay in acute rehabilitation facilities.[62] Maintenance of treatment gains for up to 1 year have been reported.[177a]

Evidence-Based Best Practices: Complex Visuospatial Skills

Practice Option: *Systematic training of visuospatial and organizational skills may be considered for people with visual perceptual deficits but without visual neglect after right hemisphere stroke as part of acute rehabilitation. Such interventions are not recommended for people with left hemisphere stroke or TBI who do not exhibit unilateral spatial inattention because no consistent evidence exists to support its specific effectiveness in these cases.*

Class I and Class II studies of visuospatial rehabilitation in the absence of visual neglect have yielded equivocal results.[19,84,103,156,173] Although these interventions appear to be effective in specific cases, the literature provides no guidance in selection of specific interventions. This type of intervention does not appear appropriate in cases of left hemisphere stroke or TBI in the absence of visual neglect. In such cases, impairment on visuospatial tasks is likely to be secondary to other cognitive impairments in attention, efficiency, and higher-order cognitive abilities. Among people with right hemisphere stroke, additional criteria have not been identified to select specific patients who may benefit from these treatments.

Evidence-Based Best Practices: Visual Field Deficits

Practice Option: *Computer-based interventions intended to produce extension of damaged visual fields may be considered for people with TBI or stroke.*

Several early investigations[34,67,68,193] reported reductions in visual field deficits with specialized rehabilitation procedures. These studies, however, stand in stark contrast to other evidence that such apparent improvement in visual fields is due to improved scanning and compensation for field deficits, and that the apparent reduction in visual field defects is insufficient to explain the associated reduction in functional visual impairments.[68,171]

A recent Class I study by Kasten and colleagues[65] evaluated a computer-based treatment of partial blindness due to optic nerve damage, or postchiasmal lesions due to TBI or stroke, compared with a sham treatment of visual fixation. The visual restitution training resulted in significant enlargement of the visual field in most of the subjects, although subjects with optic nerve damage showed much greater visual field enlargement than subjects with postchiasmal lesions. These changes were associated with subjective improvement in their functional vision, in contrast with the lack of change in either visual fields or subjective function after the sham treatment. These improvements appeared stable approximately 2 years later.[64] Given these findings, the use of computer-based interventions that have been designed to ameliorate visual field deficits due to pre- or postchiasmal damage may have beneficial effects. The combined use of interventions to enlarge visual fields and training in visual scanning to compensate for functional visual impairments has intuitive appeal but has not, to our knowledge, been directly investigated.

Language and Communication

THEORY. Cognitive-linguistic rehabilitation and aphasiology developed independently and prior to other forms of CR. These practices enjoy a rich theoretical and empirical basis, elaborated in other sources[1,31,123] but beyond the scope of this chapter. As in other areas of CR, language rehabilitation is most effective when based on a thorough assessment.[1] De Pedro-Cuesta and colleagues' meta-analytic review[31] suggested that once a language disorder has been described and appropriate rehabilitation methods determined by a speech pathologist, language therapy may be administered effectively by a nonprofessional under the direction of the speech pathologist.

Language rehabilitation for aphasia should be distinguished from other interventions designed to improve both verbal and nonverbal functional communication skills. These latter interventions typically target *pragmatic* communication abilities, such as organization and length of verbal communication, turn taking, listening, and facial and gestural expression.

EVIDENCE-BASED BEST PRACTICES: COGNITIVE-LINGUISTIC THERAPY

Practice Standard: *Cognitive-linguistic therapies are recommended during acute and postacute rehabilitation for people with language deficits secondary to left hemisphere stroke.*

Practice Guideline: *Cognitive interventions for specific language impairments, such as in reading comprehension and language formation, are recommended after left hemisphere stroke or TBI.*

Three Class I studies[52,66,175] comparing language therapy to no treatment, and three Class II studies[6,112,139] involving a total of 676 subjects, support the effectiveness of language remediation after left hemisphere stroke. These studies recorded gains for participants treated acutely, as well as for those treated long after a period of spontaneous recovery had occurred. Only one Class II study showed negative results.[120]

Two Class I studies[32,121] evaluated the effect of intensity of treatment for subjects with aphasia after stroke. These studies suggest that either increased frequency of treatment over an equal duration[32] or massed practice of language skills[121] increases the amount of functional improvement from treatment. Several uncontrolled studies have also indicated improved functional communication associated with increased intensity of treatment,[7,59,60] suggesting that treatment intensity should be considered in evaluating the effectiveness of rehabilitation for cognitive impairment after TBI or stroke.

Other Class I studies compared traditional language therapy to active treatment conditions. These active treatment control conditions were (1) group treatment to improve functional communication,[174] (2) nonspecific language stimulation by volunteers,[30] (3) group counseling provided by speech pathologists,[53] or (4) social and recreational activities.[186] Although subjects in these studies showed some benefit from the active treatment, these studies have typically failed to demonstrate a significant difference among treatment conditions. These latter studies suggest that nonspecific effects that include a focus on language and communication, stimulation, and therapist interest, support, and encouragement are an important component of language rehabilitation and may be as important as specific therapeutic techniques.

Two Class I studies, one conducted with people with stroke and one with people with TBI, support the effectiveness of interventions to remediate more specific language impairments. Katz and Wertz[66] demonstrated the effectiveness of a computerized reading remediation program in subjects with aphasia after left hemisphere stroke compared to both sham treatment and no-treatment conditions. Using a multimodal intervention, Thomas-Stonell et al.[161] demonstrated the efficacy of another computer-based intervention (TEACHware) that targets higher-level language skills as well as attention and memory. These Class I studies support a recommendation at the level of a guideline rather than a standard because of the diversity and relatively small number of subjects.

Evidence-Based Best Practices: Functional Communication Skills

Practice Standard: *Specific interventions for functional communication deficits, including pragmatic conversational skills, is recommended for people with TBI.*

A Class I study[55] supported by several case studies and case series[36,43,46,83,100,183] forms the basis for this practice standard recommending communication skill training that is more general in nature than specific language therapy. Most of this work has been conducted with patients with TBI, with an emphasis on the pragmatic and interpersonal aspects of communication (rather than specific changes in language functioning due to aphasia). The Class I study, conducted by Helffenstein and Wechsler,[55] emphasized the use of videotape feedback to develop effective interpersonal communication skills in the treatment condition. Participants in the treatment condition (compared to a sham control condition) reported better self-concepts, were rated by others as superior in interpersonal and communication skills, and demonstrated more effective interpersonal communication in nontherapeutic social situations. This form of intervention is also supported by a Class I study of patients after left hemisphere stroke. Elman and Berstein-Ellis[35] assigned 24 patients with chronic aphasia to receive either group communication treatment or deferred treatment; participants in the deferred treatment condition participated in various social activities to control for the effects of social contact. Subjects receiving group communication treatment were more likely to show clinically significant improvement in language and functional communication skills, suggesting that the active treatment rather than mere social contact was responsible for participants' improved communication skills. A number of studies previously mentioned[30,53,174,186] also indicate the potential benefits of nonspecific communication training and stimulation.

Executive Cognitive Abilities

THEORY. Executive cognitive abilities are "those integrative cognitive processes that determine goal-directed and purposeful behavior and are superordinate in the orderly execution of daily life functions."[23, p.1605] A broad range of abilities fall into this category, including goal development, behavioral initiation, organization and planning, self-monitoring, anticipation and recognition of consequences, decision making, and problem solving. These cognitive processes appear highly interrelated with emotional experiences that may either potentiate or interfere with cognitive components. Because they are second- and third-order processes (i.e., processes that involve a number of components), they are difficult to operationalize as observable behaviors. Consequently there is no clear consensus regarding the definition of a set of executive cognitive abilities, let alone specification of the interrelationships among such processes and noncognitive emotional components. With this limited theoretical basis on which to build interventions, treatment studies in this area have tended to focus on a relatively broad range of skills with hypotheses that such skill development will result in increased behavioral control and adaptability.

Evidence-based Best Practices

Practice Guideline: *Training in formal problem-solving strategies and their application to everyday situations and functional activities is recommended during postacute rehabilitation for people with stroke or TBI.*

Practice Option: *Interventions that promote internalization of self-regulation strategies through self-instruction and self-monitoring may be considered for people with deficits in executive functioning after TBI, including impairments in emotional self-regulation.*

Two Class I studies of 67 subjects investigated treatment of executive dysfunction through the training in formal problem-solving strategies. A quasi-

RCT conducted by von Cramen and Mathes-von Cramen[165] compared training in problem-solving strategies with a memory retraining intervention in a diverse sample of people with stroke, TBI, and other brain disorders. The problem-solving group performed better than the memory group on psychometric measures of problem solving and were rated as superior in awareness of deficits, goal-directed conceptualization, and appropriate behavioral inhibition. Levine and colleagues[82] evaluated the effect of training goal-directed behavior through a problem-solving model of intervention. Thirty subjects with TBI were randomly assigned to receive either *goal management training* or an equivalent amount of motor skills training. Goal management training was associated with improved performance on paper-and-pencil tasks that were designed to correspond to problem-solving activities in everyday situations. A Class II study[41] provides additional support for the effectiveness of practice in problem solving in functional situations. A Class III study[107] demonstrated improved strategy application and psychosocial functioning following treatment in problem solving. Taking a different approach to developing higher-order cognitive ablities, Constandinidou and colleagues[27b] conducted a nonrandomized trial in which participants received systematic training in categorization, that is, the ability to extract and use attributes of objects. Participants with TBI demonstrated improved categorization ability as well as improvement on functional measures, that is, the Mayo-Portland Adaptability Inventory[91b] and Community Integration Questionnaire.[177b]

The efficacy of self-instructional training in improving problem solving and planning was demonstrated in a Class II study[25] as well as in case and case series reports.[27a,61,79,85a,169] Other case reports have indicated that external cueing may be effective in supporting initiation.[38,148] Although sufficient evidence is available to support a practice guideline for these types of interventions, better-controlled and replicated research of more clearly specified interventions is required to advance practice in this area.

Multimodal Interventions

THEORY. Hermann and Parente[56] described three active (mental strategies, physical environment, social interaction) and five passive (physical state, chemical state, emotional state, attitudinal state, motivational state) modes that affect performances. These authors recommend that each of these modes be considered in developing a CR program. On a less abstract level, it seems reasonable to include multiple intervention modalities in CR programs for participants with impairments in multiple cognitive domains. Multimodal programs that include specific cognitive interventions that each enjoy empirical support (such as postacute programs combining training in attention, problem solving, and functional communication skills for appropriate participants) are expected to be effective. Research supporting the beneficial effects of each component of a multimodal program, however, leaves unanswered a remaining empirical question: Does the combination of such interventions have a synergistic effect?

EVIDENCE-BASED BEST PRACTICES. The small number of studies in this area (two Class II[8,20] and four Class III[42,77,96,127] studies) demonstrate the benefit of approaches that combine treatments in several cognitive areas in some cases. Combining CR techniques that have demonstrated efficacy is a viable treatment option. However, the limited research evaluating specific combinations of treatments does not allow for more specific recommendations.

Comprehensive-Holistic Rehabilitation

THEORY. Ben-Yishay and Prigatano[11] pioneered a comprehensive-holistic approach to rehabilitation after TBI. Because brain injury affects all aspects of the person (i.e., physical, cognitive, emotional) as well as the person's interpersonal systems (family, work, other social networks), the comprehensive-holistic approach advocates the evaluation and treatment of all these elements in an integrated treatment program. In its comprehensive focus, this model is similar to that advanced by Hermann and Parente. The comprehensive-holistic approach differs from other multimodal CR programs in that group treatment and development of a therapeutic milieu are essential parts of treatment. The group dynamic becomes a powerful tool in this form of treatment to assist participants in improving self-awareness of deficits; maintain motivation for participation in more specific CR treatments; develop communication, social, and interpersonal skills; and resolve interpersonal and emotional concerns. Prigatano[116] and Prigatano and colleagues[118] have described this model of rehabilitation in two books devoted to the topic. Defining features of the comprehensive-holistic approach, defined by a consensus group of experts, are listed in Table 13.3.

Evidence-based Best Practices

Practice Guideline: *Comprehensive-holistic neuropsychological rehabilitation is recommended to reduce cognitive and functional disability after TBI.*

Practice Option: *Integrated treatment, that is, both individualized cognitive and interpersonal therapies, may improve functioning within the context of a comprehensive-holistic neuropsychological rehabilitation program.*

Primarily Class II and Class III evidence supports the guideline and option in this treatment domain. The extended and complex nature of this type of treatment frustrates well-controlled trials and virtually precludes blinded clinical trials. Alternative research methodologies for assessing the effectiveness of extended rehabilitation interventions are under active discussion.[176] Experimental attempts to limit intervening variables often result in an experimental treatment that does not resemble the actual clinical application. For instance, in a controversial RCT, Salazar and associates[130] found that the results of a brief (8-week) comprehensive-holistic intervention were not superior to those of home-based rehabilitation. This study has been criticized on a number of counts.[47] A primary criticism is that the brevity of the treatment did not adequately reflect standard clinical practice. Standard practice typically involves participants in treatment for 5–6 months. Another important consideration in evaluating the Salazar et al. study is that post hoc analyses revealed that more severely disabled participants benefited more from the comprehensive-holistic intervention, whereas participants with mild impairments benefited equally from home-based and comprehensive-holistic rehabilitation. This finding supports clinical wisdom that an intensive comprehensive-holistic treatment program is not required in cases of mild disability after TBI but may be essential to assist people who are more severely and pervasively disabled after TBI to return to work and community participation. In a retrospective analysis of data on various levels of postacute TBI rehabilitation, Malec and Degiorgio[90] also showed that participants with relatively mild disabilities, particularly when treated within 1 year after injury, had a relatively high probability of return to work with limited medical and vocational rehabilitation. Those with more severe disabilities, particularly when entering treatment many years after injury, had a similarly high probability of returning to independent living and work only if they had participated in an intensive comprehensive-holistic rehabilitation program.

Table 13.3. Defining Features of Comprehensive-Holistic Traumatic Brain Injury Rehabilitation

I. Neuropsychological orientation focusing on:
   A. Cognitive and metacognitive impairments
   B. Neurobehavioral impairments
   C. Interpersonal and psychosocial issues
   D. Affective issues
II. Integrated treatment that includes:
   A. Formal staff meetings with core team in attendance four times per week
   B. A team leader or manager for each patient
   C. A program leader or manager with at least 3 years' experience in brain injury rehabilitation
   D. Integrated goal setting and monitoring
   E. Transdisciplinary staff roles
III. Group interventions to address:
   A. Awareness
   B. Acceptance
   C. Social pragmatics
IV. Dedicated resources including:
   A. An identified core team
   B. Dedicated space
   C. A patient: staff ratio no greater than 2:1
V. A neuropsychologist who is part of the treatment team, not just a consultant
VI. Formal and informal opportunities for involvement of significant others and systematic inclusion of significant others on a weekly basis
VII. Inclusion of a dedicated vocational or independent living trial
VIII. Multiple outcomes are assessed, including:
   A. Productive activity
   B. Independent living
   C. Psychosocial adjustment
   D. Emotional adjustment

Ruff and associates[126,128] conducted a brief quasi-RCT comparing two active components of the comprehensive-holistic approach. One group received treatment emphasizing cognitive skill development; the other group received treatment that emphasized coping and interpersonal skills. Both groups improved on cognitive measures and appeared less depressed following treatment. The cognitive group was marginally superior on cognitive measures. In a nonrandomized study, Rattok and colleagues[122] compared various combinations of interventions emphasizing attentional, other cognitive, or interpersonal skill training. As in the Ruff studies, all groups improved on measures of cognition and adaptation, with slight superiority on cognitive measures for those programs that emphasized cognitive skill development.

In their initial study of a comprehensive-holistic rehabilitation program, Prigatano and his group[117] reported improved cognitive and interpersonal functioning relative to historic controls. In a subsequent study,[119] Prigatano and associates reported that 87% of participants in their program graduated to gainful employment that was maintained for at least 2 years after injury. Malec[89] reported that more than 70% of comprehensive-holistic program participants maintained community-based employment for at least 1 year after program participation. In this study, a similarly high level of return to work was apparent even for cohorts entering the program after 1 to 10+ years of unsuccessful postinjury attempts at sustained employment. A number of factors have been identified in these studies that may affect treatment outcome, including severity of disability, time since injury, and therapeutic alliance.

If Improvements in Cognitive Functioning Occur as a Result of Cognitive Rehabilitation, Are These Improvements Maintained and Generalized to Nontraining Conditions?

If improvement in basic cognitive abilities through CR is to benefit treated patients, then these improvements must generalize to nontraining situations and support other cognitive functions and functional activities. For instance, improvement in attention would be expected to improve learning and memory, as well as everyday activities that require attention. Controversy remains as to whether this is a realistic expectation. Schachter and Glisky[133] recommended domain-specific training that emphasizes procedural learning. In this approach, clients are taught specific skills relevant to specific contexts without any expectation for this learning to generalize. A compromise position advocates domain-specific training of skills that have general application, such as use of a memory notebook, calculator, computer, or another cognitive-assistive device.

In each cognitive domain reviewed, a few studies have demonstrated the potential for generalization and maintenance of cognitive skill training. Strache[153] reported that attention training generalized to improved performance on memory and intelligence measures. Others[51,178] reported maintenance and generalization of attention strategy use in daily life. A number of studies[49,62,73,74,108,171,172,177a] provide evidence that visuospatial training generalizes to improved rehabilitation outcomes and functional activities. Gains in visuospatial training are maintained for at least 1 year.[177a] Language and communication training has been shown to generalize to everyday functional activities and increased feelings of self-worth.[55,161] In the memory domain, both strategy training[13] and notebook use[136] appear to be maintained by some subjects during a follow-up period and to have a long-term positive effect on everyday functioning. In the domain of executive cognitive abilities, studies of interventions emphasizing problem solving and self-instructional training[25,27a,41,61,79,85a,165,169] have also documented maintenance and generalization of these skills. Comprehensive-holistic programs have demonstrated improvements in social participation and community integration following treatment.[26,89,132,138] Studies of comprehensive-holistic CR have also reported generalized effects in psychosocial functioning, reduction in personal distress, increased independence in community living, and improved vocational achievement that are maintained for at least 1 year after completion of the program.[21,75,89,157,158]

These findings suggest that there is strong potential for generalization and maintenance of skills learned through various types of CR. What is lacking in the literature is elaboration of specific interventional elements that enhance generalization and maintenance (such as practice in real or simulated functional activities, a system of environmental cues and prompts, and self-instructional training). Evaluation of specific techniques to enhance generalization and maintenance of skills learned through CR is an important area for future research.

What Environmental Features Affect the Outcome (i.e., Improvement, Maintenance, Generalization) of Cognitive Rehabilitation for Specific Cognitive Functions?

More research is needed not only to identify specific elements of treatment that enhance maintenance and generalization, but also to identify environmental modifications that support and enhance the effectiveness of training and the positive impact of CR in real-world activities. Such research would extend the findings of previous studies demonstrating the value of external memory aids,[72] an external memory prompting system,[38] and environmental structuring to support executive cognitive problem solving and decision making.[38,148]

Prior studies have also suggested specific training elements that enhance the effectiveness of interventions. These merit further investigation. For instance, in attentional training, including tasks requiring selective or divided attention appears more effective than focusing on speed of processing.[37,51,114,154,155] Visual scanning training appears to require an apparatus that challenges peripheral vision.[49,62,124,171,172,177a,191] More generally, a positive therapeutic alliance and systematic feedback to the participant are elements that, in a number of studies,[30,51,53,105,114,174] appeared to be associated with greater treatment gains.

Computers

Kurlychek and Levin[76] identified several features of computer-assisted CR that may enhance learning for people with TBI: (1) the precision of presentation and feedback; (2) data gathering, analysis, and storage capacities to monitor progress; and (3) program modification to adapt to individual deficits, abilities, and attention spans. Although computers may facilitate CR in these ways, there is no evidence that computer assistance is necessary or sufficient for the effectiveness of CR. To the contrary, in the area of visuospatial CR, training that is restricted to a small computer screen appears less effective than noncomputerized treatment because of the imposed limitation on the visual field. Studies suggest that treatment delivered via computer interaction can serve as a valuable adjunct to treatment under the direction of a therapist.[40,110] However, there is no reason to believe—and no evidence—that the isolated use of computer-based exercises to treat cognitive impairments without therapist involvement is effective, and this is not recommended. Based on the comprehensive review of the literature, the CR Evidence-based Review Committee has stated:

> Computer-based interventions as an adjunct to clinician-guided treatment (that includes active therapist involvement to foster insight into cognitive strengths and weaknesses, to develop compensatory strategies, and to facilitate the transfer of skills into real-life situations) may be considered for people with TBI or stroke. Sole reliance on repeated exposure and practice on computer-based tasks without some involvement and intervention by a therapist is *not* recommended.

What Characteristics of People with Acquired Cognitive Impairments (e.g., Injury Severity, Type of Cognitive Impairment, Emotional Factors, Personality, Preinjury Abilities) Affect the Outcome of Cognitive Rehabilitation?

Specific participant characteristics that recommend specific CR interventions or affect the outcome of these interventions require further research elaboration. Studies that form the basis for such research include those suggesting that visuospatial retraining is most effective in participants with stroke who have severe visuoperceptual deficits with hemispatial negect.[171,172] Memory strategy retraining appears effective with highly motivated individuals with mild memory impairment;[129] whereas memory aid training and other domain-specific learning interventions may be more appropriate for people with moderate to severe memory deficits.[10,15,17,70–72,97,109,134,145,149,160,179,182,192] Severe and pervasive cognitive and behavioral impairments and impairment of self-awareness may limit the effectiveness of many CR treatments and require a more comprehensive-holistic approach.[12,92,119,159]

What Neurological, Psychological, Social, and Environmental Processes Underlie Positive Outcomes of Cognitive Rehabilitation?

In their early review, Kurlychek and Levin[76] provide a succinct summary of theories of brain recovery relevant to CR. Interested readers are referred to this and other primary sources.[86,99,150] Current theories are based on basic neurological science and animal models, with little consideration of psychosocial and environmental factors. Research is probably years away from specifying the complex biopsychosocial processes (as outlined 15 years ago by Diller and Gordon[33]) that subserve improvement as a result of various CR interventions. Nonetheless, pioneering efforts, such as Laatsch and colleagues'[77] demonstration of changes in functional neuroimaging associated with effective CR, form the basis for these more fundamental lines of research.

Conclusions

The field of rehabilitation, including the rehabilitation of cognitive disorders for people with ABD, has entered an era of evidence-based medicine where it is expected that controlled clinical studies serve as the basis for clinical practice. This review suggests that there is now substantial evidence to support the application of CR after TBI and stroke. While there is evidence to support the use of specific interventions for specific cognitive impairments, it is also apparent that so-called nonspecific factors, such as psychological support and the nature of the therapeutic alliance, contribute to the effectiveness of CR.

Ideally, the goal of evidence-based practice is to inform clinical decision making regarding which interventions are most appropriate for what problems for which patients in what settings under what conditions and toward what outcomes. There is still limited information on the latter aspects of this equation. It is likely that different types of intervention, or different complex rehabilitation pathways, will prove appropriate for patients with varying characteristics, such as severity of impairment and time postinjury.[90]

Despite the increased evidence for the effectiveness of CR, these findings have not necessarily been translated into clinical practice or policy. A recent survey of 1802 people with TBI indicated that 80% believed that their need to improve their cognition had not been met at 1 year postinjury.[29] While there is a general clinical consensus that the goal of cognitive and other rehabilitation is to improve people's level of autonomy, social participation, and productivity, most studies of CR have emphasized treatment outcomes at the impairment level. There is even less information about whether CR improves patients' subjective well-being and quality of life. Documentation of relevant outcomes from CR represents a continuing challenge to the professional clinical and research community. At the same time, there remains a compelling need to increase access to services, and to provide adequate funding for both clinical services and research in this area. Our review of 258 research studies involving several thousand patients indicates that CR for people with TBI or stroke offers unquestionable benefits compared with conventional rehabilitation, and is most certainly beneficial when compared with the alternative of receiving no rehabilitation at all.

REFERENCES

1. Albert ML, Helm-Estabrooks N: Diagnosis and treatment of aphasia. Part II. JAMA 259:1205–1210, 1988.
2. Anschutz L, Camp CL, Markley RP, Kramer JJ: Remembering mnenomics: A three-year follow-up on the effects of mnemonics training in elderly adults. Exp Aging Res 13:141–143, 1987.
3. Antonucci G, Guariglia C, Judica A, Magnotti L, Paolucci S, Pizzamiglio L, et al: Effectiveness of neglect rehabilitation in a randomized group study. J Clin Exp Neuropsychol 17:383–389, 1995.
4. Baddeley AD, Hitch GJ: Developments in the concept of working memory. Neuropsychology 8:485–493, 1994.
5. Bailey MJ, Riddoch MJ, Crome P: Treatment of visual neglect in elderly patients with stroke: A single-subject series using either a scanning and cueing strategy or a left-limb activation strategy. Phys Ther 82:782–797, 2002.
6. Basso A, Capitani E, Vignolo LA: Influence of rehabilitation of language skills in aphasic patients: A controlled study. Arch Neurol 36:190–196, 1979.
7. Basso A, Caporali A: Aphasia therapy or the importance of being earnest. Aphasiology 15:307–332, 2001.
8. Batchelor J, Shores EA, Marosszeky J, Sandanam J, Lovarini M: Cognitive rehabilitation of severely head-injured patients using computer assisted and non-computerized treatment techniques. J Head Trauma Rehabil 3:78–83, 1988.
9. Becker JT: Introduction to the special section: Working memory and neuropsychology—interdependence of clinical and experimental research. Neuropsychology 8:483–484, 1994.
10. Benedict RH: The effectiveness of cognitive remediation strategies for victims of traumatic brain injury: A review of the literature. Clin Psychol Rev 9:605–626, 1989.
11. Ben-Yishay Y, Prigatano GP: Cognitive remediation. In: Rosenthal, M, Griffith ER, Bond MR, Miller JD (eds): Rehabilitation of the Adult and Child with Traumatic Brain Injury. Philadelphia, FA Davis, 1990, pp 393–400.

12. Ben-Yishay Y, Silver SM, Piasetsky E, Rattock J: Relationship between employability and vocational outcome after intensive holistic cognitive rehabilitation. J Head Trauma Rehabil 2:35–48, 1987.
13. Berg I, Konning-Haanstra M, Deelman B: Long term effects of memory rehabilitation: A controlled study. Neuropsychol Rehabil 1:97–111, 1991.
14. Berrol S: Issues of cognitive rehabilitation. Arch Neurol 47:219–220, 1990.
15. Burke JM, Danick JA, Bemis B, Durgin CJ: A process approach to memory book training for neurological patients. Brain Inj 8:71–81, 1994.
16. Butter CM, Kirsch N: Combined and separate effects of eye patching and visual stimulation on unilateral neglect following stroke. Arch Phys Med Rehabil 73:1113–1119, 1992.
17. Cancelliere AEB, Moncuda C, Reid DT: Memory training to support educational reintegration. Arch Phys Med Rehabil 72:148–151, 1991.
18. Carney N, Chestnut RM, Maynard H, Mann NC, Hefland M: Effect of cognitive rehabilitation on outcomes for persons with traumatic brain injury: A systematic review. J Head Trauma Rehabil 14:277–307, 1999.
19. Carter LT, Howard BE, O'Neill WA: Effectiveness of the cognitive skill remediation in acute stroke patients. Am J Occup Ther 37:320–326, 1983.
20. Chen SHA, Glueckauf RL, Bracy OL: The effectiveness of computer-assisted cognitive rehabilitation for persons with traumatic brain injury. Brain Inj 2:197–209, 1997.
21. Christensen AL, Pinner EM, Moller-Pederson P, Teasdale TW, Trexler LE: Psychosocial outcome following individualized neuropsychological rehabilitation of brain damage. Acta Neurol Scand 85:32–38, 1992.
22. Cicerone KD: Remediation of "working attention" in mild traumatic brain injury. Brain Inj 16:185–195, 2002.
23. Cicerone KD, Dahlberg C, Kalmar K, Langenbahn DM, Malec JF, Bergquist TF, Felicetti T, Giacino JT, Harley JP, Harrington DE, Herzog J, Kneipp S, Laatsch L, Morse PA: Evidence-based cognitive rehabilitation: Recommendations for clinical prctice. Arch Phys Med Rehabil 81:1596–1615, 2000.
24. Cicerone KD, Dahlberg C, Malec JF, Langenbahn DM, Felicetti T, Kneipp S, Ellmo W, Kalmar K, Giacino JT, Harley JP, Laatsch L, Morse PA, Catanese J: Evidence-based cognitive rehabilitation: Updated review of the literature 1998–2002. Arch Phys Med Rehabil 86:1681–1692, 2005.
25. Cicerone KD, Giacino JT: Remediation of executive function deficits after traumatic brain injury. Neurorehabilitation 2:12–22, 1992.
26. Cicerone KD, Mott T, Azulay JA, Friel J: Community integration and satisfaction with functioning after intensive cognitive rehabilitation for traumatic brain injury. Arch Phys Med Rehabil 85:1644–1650, 2004.
27a. Cicerone KD, Wood JC: Planning disorder after closed head injury: A case study. Arch Phys Med Rehabil 68: 111–115, 1987.
27b. Constantinidou F, Thomas RD, Scharp VL, Laske KM, Hammerly MD, Guitonde, S: Effects of categorization training in patients with TBI during postacute rehabilitation: Preliminary findings. J. Head Trauma Rehabil 20:143–157, 2005.
28. Cope DN, O'Lear J: A clinical and economic perspective on head injury rehabilitation. J Head Trauma Rehabil 8:1–14, 1993.
29. Corrigan JD, Whiteneck G, Mellick MA: Perceived needs following traumatic brain injury. J Head Trauma Rehabil 19:205–216, 2004.
30. David R, Enderby P, Bainbton D: Treatment of acquired aphasia: Speech therapists and volunteers compared. J Neurol Neurosurg Psychiatry 45:957–961, 1982.
31. de Pedro-Cuesta J, Widen-Holmquist L, Bach-y-Rita P: Evaluation of stroke rehabilitation by randomized controlled studies: A review. Acta Neurol Scand 86:433–439, 1992.
32. Denes G, Perazzola C, Piani A, Piccione F: Intensive versus regular speech therapy in global aphasia: A controlled study. Aphasiology 10:385–394, 1996.
33. Diller L, Gordon WA: Interventions for cognitive deficits in brain injured adults. J Consult Clin Psychol 49:822–834, 1981.
34. Diller L, Weinberg J: Hemi-inattention in rehabilitation: The evaluation of a rational remediation program. Adv Neurol 18:63–82, 1977.
35. Elman RJ, Bernstein-Ellis E: The efficacy of group communication treatment in adults with chronic aphasia. J Speech Lang Hear Res 42:411–419, 1999.
36. Erlich J, Sipes A: Group treatment of communication skills for head trauma patients. Cogn Rehabil 3:32–37, 1985.
37. Ethier M, Braun CMJ, Baribeau JMC: Computer-dispensed cognitive perceptual training of closed head injury patients after spontaneous recovery. Study 1: Speeded tasks. Can J Rehabil 2:223–233, 1989.
38. Evans JJ, Emslie H, Wilson BA: External cueing systems in the rehabilitation of executive impairments of action. J Int Neuropsychol Soc 4:399–408, 1998.
39. Fasotti L, Kovacs F, Eling P, Brouwer WH: Time pressure management as a compensatory strategy training after closed head injury. Neuropsychol Rehabil 10:47–65, 2000.
40. Fink RB, Brecher A, Schwartz MF, Robey RR: A computer-implemented protocol for treatment of naming disorders: Evaluation of clinician-guided and partially self-guided instruction. Aphasiology 16:1061–1086, 2002.
41. Fox RM, Martella RC, Marchand-Martella NE: The acquisition, maintenance and generalization of problem-solving skills by closed head injured adults. Behav Ther 20:61–76, 1989.
42. Franzen MD, Harris CV: Neuropsychological rehabilitation: Application of a modified baseline design. Brain Inj 7:525–534, 1993.
43. Gajar A, Schloss PJ, Schloss CN, Thompson CK: Effects of feedback and self-monitoring on head trauma

youths' conversational skills. J Appl Behav Anal 17:353–358, 1984.
44. Gansler DA, McCaffrey RJ: Remediation of chronic attention deficits in traumatic brain injured patients. Arch Clin Neuropsychol 6:335–353, 1991.
45. Gathercole SE: Neuropsychology and working memory: A review. Neuropsychology 8:494–505, 1994.
46. Giles GM, Fussey I, Burgess P: The behavioral treatment of verbal interaction skills following severe head injury: A single case study. Brain Inj 2:75–77, 1988.
47. Glenn MB, Yablon SA, Whyte J, Zafonte R: Letter to the editor. J Head Trauma Rehabil 16:vii–viii, 2001.
48. Glisky EL, Schacter DL, Tulving E: Computer learning by memory-impaired patients: Acquisition and retention of complex knowledge. Neuropsychologia 24: 313–328, 1986.
49. Gordon WA, Hibbard M, Egelko S, et al: Perceptual remediation in patients with right brain damage: A comprehensive program. Arch Phys Med Rehabil 66:353–359, 1985.
50. Gouvier D, Webster JS, Blanton PD: Cognitive retraining with brain damaged patients. In: Wedding, D, Horton AM, Webster J (eds): The Neuropsychology Handbook: Behavioral and Clinical Perspectives. New York, Springer, 1986, pp 278–324.
51. Gray JM, Robertson I, Pentland B, Anderson S: Microcomputer-based attentional retraining after brain damage: A randomized group controlled trial. Neuropsychol Rehabil 2:97–115, 1992.
52. Hagen C: Communication abilities in hemiplegia: Effect of speech therapy. Arch Phys Med Rehabil 54:454–463, 1973.
53. Hartman J, Landau WM: Comparison of formal language therapy with supportive counseling for aphasia due to acute vascular accident. Arch Neurol 44:646–649, 1987.
54. Head Injury Special Interest Group of the American Congress of Rehabilitation Medicine: Guidelines for cognitive rehabilitation. Neurorehabilitation 2:62–67, 1992.
55. Helffenstein D, Wechsler R: The use of interpersonal process recall (IPR) in the remediation of interpersonal and communication skill deficits in the newly brain injured. Clin Neuropsychol 4:139–143, 1982.
56. Hermann D, Parente R: The multimodel approach to cognitive rehabilitation. Neurorehabilitation 4:133–142, 1994.
57. Hill RD, Allen C, Gregory K: Self generated mnemonics for enhancing free recall performance in older learners. Exp Aging Res 16:141–145, 1990.
58. Hill RD, Allen C, McWhorter P: Stories as a mnemonic aid for older learners. Psychol Aging 6:484–486, 1991.
59. Hillis AE: Treatment of naming disorders: New issues regarding old therapies. J Int Neuropsychol Soc 4:648–660, 1998.
60. Hinckley JJ, Craig HK: Influence of rate of treatment on the naming abilities of adults with chronic aphasia. Aphasiology 12:989–1006, 1998.
61. Hux K, Reid R, Lugert M: Self-instruction training following neurological injury. Appl Cogn Psychol 8:259–271, 1994.
62. Kalra L, Perez I, Gupta S, Wittink M: The influence of visual neglect on stroke rehabilitation. Stroke 28:1386–1391, 1997.
63. Kaschel R, Della Salla S, Cantagallo A, Fahlbock A, Laaksonen R, Kazen M: Imagery mnemonics for the rehabilitation of memory: A randomized group controlled trial. Neuropsychol Rehabil 12:127–153, 2002.
64. Kasten E, Mueller-Oehring E, Sabel BA: Stability of visual field enlargements following computer-based restitution training—results of a follow-up. J Clin Exp Neuropsychol 23:297–305, 2001.
65. Kasten E, Wuerst S, Behrens-Famann W, Sabel BA: Computer-based training for the treatment of partial blindness. Nature Med 4:1084–1087, 1998.
66. Katz RC, Wertz RT: The efficacy of computer-provided reading treatment for chronic aphasic adults. J Speech Lang Hear Res 40:493–507, 1997.
67. Kerkhoff G, Munbinger U, Eberle-Strauss G, Stogerer E: Rehabilitation of hemianopsic alexia in patients with postgeniculate visual field disorder. Neuropsychol Rehabil 2:21–42, 1992.
68. Kerkhoff G, Munbinger U, Eberle-Strauss G, Stogerer E: Rehabilitation of homonymous scotoma in patients with post-geniculate damage of the visual system. Saccadic compensation training. Restor Neurol Neurosci 4:245–254, 1992.
69. Kerner JJ, Acker M: Computer delivery of memory retraining with head injured patients. Cogn Rehabil Nov/Dec:26–31, 1985.
70. Kime S, Lamb D, Wilson G: Use of a comprehensive programme of external cueing to enhance procedural memory in a patient with dense amnesia. Brain Inj 10: 17–25, 1996.
71. Kirsch NL, Levine SP, Fallon-Krueger M, Jaros LA: The microcomputer as an "orthotic" device for patients with cognitive deficits. J Head Trauma Rehabil 2:77–86, 1987.
72. Kirsch NL, Levine SP, Lajiness-O'Neil R, Schnyder M: Computer-assisted interactive task guidance: Facilitating the performance of a simulated vocational task. J Head Trauma Rehabil 7:13–25, 1992.
73. Klavora P, Gaskovski P, Martin K, Forsyuch TD, Heslegrave RJ, Young M: The effects of Dynavision rehabilitation on behind the wheel driving ability and selected psychomotor abilities after stroke. Am J Occup Ther 29:534–542, 1995.
74. Klavora P, Warren M: Rehabilitation of visuomotor skills in post-stroke patients using the Dynavision apparatus. Percept Motor Skills 86:23–30, 1994.
75. Klonoff PS, Lamb DG, Henderson SW: Milieu-based neurorehabilitation in patients with traumatic brain injury: Outcome at up to 11 years post-discharge. Arch Phys Med Rehabil 81:1535–1537, 2000.
76. Kurlychek RT, Levin W: Computers in the cognitive rehabilitation of brain injured persons. Crit Rev Med Inform 1:241–257, 1987.

77. Laatsch L, Jobe T, Sychra J, Lin Q, Blend M: Impact of cognitive rehabilitation therapy on neuropsychological impairments as measured by brain perfusion SPECT: A longitudinal study. Brain Inj 11:837–850, 1997.
78. Lachman ME, Weaver SL, Bandura M, et al: Improving memory and control beliefs through cognitive restructuring and self generated strategies. J Gerontol 47:293–299, 1992.
79. Lawson MJ, Rice DN: Effects of training in use of executive strategies on a verbal memory problem resulting from closed head injury. J Clin Exp Neuropsychol 11:842–854, 1989.
80. Leirer VO, Morrow DG, Pariante GM, Sheikh JI: Elders' nonadherence, its assessment, and computer assisted instruction for medication recall training. J Am Geriatr Soc 36:877–884, 1988.
81. Levin HS: Cognitive rehabilitation. Unproved but promising. Arch Neurol 47:223–224, 1990.
82. Levine B, Robertson IH, Clare L, Carter G, Hong J, Wilson BA, Duncan J, Stuss DT: Rehabilitation of executive functioning: An experimental-clinical validation of goal management training. J Int Neuropsychol Soc 6:299–312, 2000.
83. Lewis FD, Nelson J, Nelson C, Reusink P: Effects of three feedback contingencies on the socially inappropriate talk of a brain injured adult. Behav Ther 19:203–211, 1988.
84. Lincoln NB, Whiting SE, Cockburn J, Bhavnani G: An evaluation of perceptual retraining. Int Rehabil Med 7:99–101, 1985.
85a. Lira FT, Carne W, Masri AM: Treatment of anger and impulsivity in a brain damaged patient: A case study applying stress inoculation. Clin Neuropsychol 5:159–160, 1983.
85b. Loewenstein, DA, Acevedo A, Czaja SJ, Duara R: Cognitive rehabilitation of mildly impaired Alzheimer's disease patients on cholinesterase inhibitors. J Geriatric Psychiat 12:395–402, 2004.
86. Luria AR: Restoration of Function After Brain Injury. New York, MacMillan, 1963.
87. Malec J: Training the brain-injured client in behavioral self-management skills. In: Edelstein, BA, Couture ET (eds): Behavioral Assessment and Rehabilitation of the Traumatically Brain-Damaged. New York, Plenum, 1984, pp 121–150.
88. Malec J: Ethics in brain injury rehabilitation: Existential choices among Western cultural beliefs. Brain Inj 7:383–400, 1993.
89. Malec JF: Impact of comprehensive day treatment on societal participation for persons with acquired brain injury. Arch Phys Med Rehabil 82:885–895, 2001.
90. Malec JF, Degiorgio L: Characteristics of successful and unsuccessful completers of 3 postacute brain injury rehabilitation pathways. Arch Phys Med Rehabil 83:1759–1764, 2002.
91a. Malec JF, Ivnik RJ, Smith GE: Neuropsychology and normal aging: Clinicians' perspective. In: Parks RW, Zec RF, Wilson RS (eds): Neuropsychology of Alzheimer's Disease and Other Dementias. New York, Oxford University Press, 1993, pp 81–111.
91b. Malec JF, Kragness M, Evans RW, Finlay KL, Kent A, Lezak MD: Further psychometric evaluation and revision of the Mayo-Portland Adaptability Inventory in a national sample. J Head Trauma Rehabil 8:479–492, 2003.
92. Malec JF, Smigielski JS, DePompolo RW, Thompson JM: Outcome evaluation and prediction in a comprehensive-integrated post-acute outpatient brain injury rehabilitation programme. Brain Inj 7:15–29, 1993.
93. Matthews CG, Harley JP, Malec JF: Guidelines for computer-assisted cognitive neuropsychological rehabilitation and cognitive rehabilitation. Clin Neuropsychol 5:3–19, 1991.
94. Mazmanian PE, Kreutzer JS, Devany CW, Martin KO: A survey of accredited and other rehabilitation facilities: Education, training and cognitive rehabilitation in brain injury programmes. Brain Inj 7:319–331, 1993.
95. Meichenbaum D: Cognitive Behavior Modification. New York, Plenum, 1977.
96. Middleton DK, Lambert MJ, Weggar LB: Neuropsychological rehabilitation: Microcomputer-assisted treatment of brain injured adults. Percept Motor Skills 72: 527–530, 1991.
97. Milders M, Deelman B, Berg I: Rehabilitation of memory for people's names. Memory 6:21–36, 1998.
98. Miller E: The training characteristics of severely head-injured patients: A preliminary study. J Neurol Neurosurg Psychiatry 43:525–528, 1980.
99. Miller E: Recovery and Management of Neuropsychological Impairments. New York, Wiley, 1984.
100. Milton SB: Management of subtle communication deficits. J Head Trauma Rehabil 3:1–11, 1988.
101. Neely AS, Backman L: Long-term maintenance of gains from memory training in older adults: Two 3½ year follow-up studies. J Gerontol 48:233–237, 1993.
102. Neimeier JP: The Lighthouse Strategy: Use of visual imagery technique to treat visual inattention in stroke patients. Brain Inj 12:399–406, 1998.
103. Neistadt ME: Occupational therapy treatments for constructional deficits. Am J Occup Ther 46: 141–148, 1992.
104. Neistadt ME: Perceptual retraining for adults with diffuse brain injury. Am J Occup Ther 48:225–233, 1994.
105. Niemann H, Ruff RM, Baser CA: Computer-assisted attention retraining in head-injured individuals: A controlled efficacy study of an outpatient program. J Consult Clin Psychol 58:811–817, 1990.
106. Ownsworth TL, McFarland KA: Memory remediation in long-term acquired brain injury: Two approaches in diary training. Brain Inj 13:605–626, 1999.
107. Ownsworth TL, McFarland KA, Young RMCD: Self-awareness and psychosocial functioning following acquired brain injury: An evaluation of a group support programme. Neuropsychol Rehabil 10:465–484, 2000.
108. Pantano O, DiPeiero V, Fieschi C, Judica A, Guariglia C, Pizzamiglio L: Pattern of CBF in the rehabilitation of visuospatial neglect. Int J Neurosci 66:153–161, 1992.

109. Parente R: Effect of monetary incentives on performance after traumatic brain injury. Neurorehabilitation 4:198–203, 1994.
110. Pederson PM, Vinter K, Olsen TS: Improvement of oral naming by unsupervised computerized rehabilitation. Aphasiology 15:151–170, 2001.
111. Pizzamiglio L, Antonucci G, Judica A, Montenero P, Razzano C, Zoccolotti P: Cognitive rehabilitation of the hemineglect disorder in chronic patients with unilateral right brain damage. J Clin Exp Neuropsychol 14: 901–923, 1992.
112. Poeck K, Huber W, Willmes K: Outcome of intensive language treatment in aphasia. J Speech Hear Disord 54:471–479, 1989.
113. Pommeranke K, Markowitsch JH: Rehabilitation training of homonymous visual field defects in patients with postgeniculate damage of the visual system. Restor Neurol Neurosci 1:47–63, 1989.
114. Ponsford JL, Kinsella G: Evaluation of a remedial programme for attentional deficits following closed-head injury. J Clin Exp Neuropsychol 10:693–703, 1988.
115. Ponsford JL, Kinsella G: Attentional deficits following closed head injury. J Clin Exp Neuropsychol 14:822–838, 1992.
116. Prigatano GP: Principles of Neuropsychological Rehabilitation. New York, Oxford University Press, 1999.
117. Prigatano GP, Fordyce DJ, Zeiner HK, Roueche JR, Pepping M, Wood BC: Neuropsychological rehabilitation after closed head injury in young adults. J Neurol Neurosurg Psychiatry 47:505–513, 1984.
118. Prigatano GP, Fordyce DJ, Zeiner HK, Roueche JR, Pepping M, Wood RC: Neuropsychological Rehabilitation after Brain Injury. Baltimore, Johns Hopkins University Press, 1986.
119. Prigatano GP, Klonoff PS, O'Brien KP, Altman IM, Amin K, Chiapello D, et al: Productivity after neuropsychologically oriented milieu rehabilitation. J Head Trauma Rehabil 9:91–102, 1994.
120. Prins RS, Schoonan R, Vermeulen J: Efficacy of two different types of speech therapy for aphasic stroke patients. Appl Psychol 10:85–123, 1989.
121. Pulvermuller F, Neininger B, Elbert T, Mohr B, Rockstroh B, Koebbel P, Taub E: Constraint induced therapy of chronic aphasia after stroke. Stroke 32:1621–1626, 2001.
122. Rattok J, Ben-Yishay Y, Ezrachi O, et al: Outcome of different treatment mixes in a multidimensional neuropsychological rehabilitation program. Neuropsychology 6:395–415, 1992.
123. Rimmele CT, Hester RK: Cognitive rehabilitation after traumatic brain injury. Arch Clin Neuropsychol 2:353–384, 1987.
124. Robertson IH, Gray JM, Pentland B, Waite LJ: Microcomputer-based rehabilitation for unilateral left visual neglect: A randomized controlled trial. Arch Phys Med Rehabil 71:663–668, 1990.
125. Robertson IH, Tegner R, Tham K, Lo A, Nimmo-Smith I: Sustained attention training for unilateral neglect: Theoretical and rehabilitation implications. J Clin Exp Neuropsychol 17:416–430, 1995.
126. Ruff RM, Baser CA, Johston JW, et al: Neuropsychological rehabilitation: An experimental study with head injured patients. J Head Trauma Rehabil 4:20–36, 1989.
127. Ruff RM, Mahaffey R, Engel JB: Efficacy study of THINKable in the attention and memory retraining of traumatically head-injured patients. Brain Inj 8:3–14, 1994.
128. Ruff RM, Neimann H: Cognitive rehabilitation versus day treatment in head-injured adults: Is there an impact on emotional and psychosocial adjustment? Brain Inj 4:339–347, 1990.
129. Ryan TV, Ruff RM: The efficacy of structured memory retraining in a group comparison of head trauma patients. Arch Clin Neuropsychol 3:165–179, 1988.
130. Salazar AM, Warden DL, Schwab K, Spector J, et al: Cognitive rehabilitation for traumatic brain injury: A randomized trial. JAMA 283:3075–3081, 2000.
131. Salthouse T: The aging of working memory. Neuropsychology 8:535–543, 1994.
132. Sander AM, Roebuck TM, Struchen MA, Sherer M, High WM: Long-term maintenance of gains obtained in postacute rehabilitation by persons with traumatic brain injury. J Head Trauma Rehabil 16:356–373, 2001.
133. Schachter DL, Glisky EL: Memory remediation: Restoration, alleviation, and the acquisition of domain-specific knowledge. In: Uzzell, B, Gross Y (eds): Clinical Neuropsychology of Intervention. Boston, Martinus Nijhoff, 1986, pp 257–282.
134. Schacter DL, Rich SA, Stampp MS: Remediation of memory disorders: Experimental evaluation of the spaced retrieval technique. J Clin Exp Neuropsychol 7:79–96, 1985.
135. Schefft BK, Malec JF, Lehr BK, Kanfer DH: The role of self-regulation therapy with the brain-injured patient. In: Maruish, M, Moses JA (eds): Theoretical Foundations of Clinical Neuropsychology for Clinical Practitioners. New York, Erlbaum, 1995, pp 237–282.
136. Schmitter-Edgecomb M, Fahy J, Whelan J, Long C: Memory remediation after severe closed head injury. Notebook training versus supportive therapy. J Consult Clin Psychol 63:484–489, 1995.
137. Scogin F, Bienias JL: A three-year follow-up of older adult participants in a memory skills training program. Psychol Aging 3:334–337, 1988.
138. Seale GS, Caroselli JS, High WM, Becker CL, Neese LE, Scheibel R: Use of the Community Integration Questionnaire (CIQ) to characterize changes in functioning for individuals with traumatic brain injury who participated in a post-acute rehabilitation programme. Brain Inj 16:955–967, 2002.
139. Shewan CM, Kertesz A: Effects of speech language treatment on recovery from aphasia. Brain Lang 23: 272–299, 1985.
140. Shum DHK, McFarland KA, Bain JD: Effects of closed head injury on attentional processes: Generality of Stern-

berg's additive factor model. J Clin Exp Neuropsychol 16:547–555, 1994.

141. Shum DHK, McFarland KA, Bain JD, Humphreys MS: Effects of closed head injury on attentional processes: An information processing stage analysis. J Clin Exp Neuropsychol 12:247–264, 1990.
142. Soderback I, Bengtsson I, Ginsburg E, Elkholm J: Video feedback in occupational therapy: Its effect in patients with neglect syndrome. Arch Phys Med Rehabil 73:1140–1146, 1992.
143. Sohlberg MM, Mateer CA: Effectiveness of an attention training program. J Clin Exp Neuropsychol 98:117–130, 1987.
144. Sohlberg MM, Mateer CA: Introduction to Cognitive Rehabilitation: Theory and Practice. New York, Guilford Press, 1989.
145. Sohlberg MM, Mateer CA: Training use of compensatory memory books: A three-stage behavioral approach. J Clin Exp Neuropsychol 11:871–891, 1989.
146. Sohlberg MM, Mateeer CA: Cognitive Rehabilitation: An Integrative Neurpsychological Approach. New York, Guilford Press, 2001.
147. Sohlberg MM, McLaughlin KA, Pavese A, Heidrich A, Posner MI: Evaluation of attention process training and brain injury education in persons with acquired brain injury. J Clin Exp Neuropsychol 22:656–676, 2000.
148. Sohlberg MM, Sprunk H, Metzelaar K: Efficacy of an external cueing system in an individual with severe frontal lobe damage. Cogn Rehabil 6:36–41, 1988.
149. Squires EJ, Hunkin NM, Parking AJ: Memory notebook training in a case of severe amnesia: Generalizing from paired associate learning to real life. Neuropsychol Rehabil 6:55–65, 1996.
150. Stein DG, Rosen JJ, Butters N: Plasticity and Recovery of Function in the Central Nervous System. New York, Academic Press, 1974.
151. Stigsdotter A, Backman L: Multifactorial memory training with older adults: How to foster maintenance of improved performance. Gerontology 35:260–267, 1989.
152. Storandt M: Memory skills training for older adults. Nebraska Symp Motiv 39:39–62, 1991.
153. Strache W: Effectiveness of two modes of training to overcome deficits of concentration. Int J Rehabil Res 10:141S–145S, 1987.
154. Sturm W, Wilmes K: Efficacy of a reaction training on various attentional and cognitive functions in stroke patients. Neuropsychol Rehabil 1:259–280, 1991.
155. Sturm W, Wilmes K, Orgass B: Do specific attention deficits need specific training? Neuropsychol Rehabil 7:81–103, 1997.
156. Taylor M, Schaeffer JN, Blumenthal FS, Grissel JL: Perceptual training in patients with left hemiplegia. Arch Phys Med Rehabil 52:163–169, 1971.
157. Teasdale TW, Caetano C: Psychopathological symptomatology in brain injured patients before and after a rehabilitation program. Appl Neurophysiol 2:116–123, 1995.
158. Teasdale TW, Christensen A, Pinner EM: Psychosocial rehabilitation of cranial trauma and stroke patients. Brain Inj 7:535–542, 1993.
159. Teasdale TW, Hansen HV, Gade A, Christensen A-L: Neuropsychological test scores before and after brain injury rehabilitation in relation to return to employment. Neuropsychol Rehabil 7:23–42, 1997.
160. Thoene AIT, Glisky EL: Learning of name-face associations in memory impaired patients: A comparison of different training procedures. J Int Neuropsychol Soc 1:29–38, 1995.
161. Thomas-Stonell N, Johnson P, Schuller R, Jutai J: Evaluation of a computer based program for cognitive-communication skills. J Head Trauma Rehabil 9:25–37, 1994.
162. Treat NJ, Poon LW, Fozard JL, Popkin SJ: Toward applying cognitive skill training to memory problems. Exp Aging Res 4:305–319, 1978.
163. Verhaegen P, Marcoen A, Goossens L: Improving memory performance in the aged through mnemonic training: A meta-analytic study. Psychol Aging 7:242–251, 1992.
164. Volpe BT, McDowell FH: The efficacy of cognitive rehabilitation in patients with traumatic brain injury. Arch Neurol 47:220–222, 1990.
165. von Cramen DY, Mathes-von Cramen MN: Problem solving deficits in brain injured patients. A therapeutic approach. Neuropsychol Rehabil 1:45–64, 1991.
166. Warren M: A hierarchical model for evaluation and treatment of visual perceptual dysfunction in adult acquired brain injury, Part 1. Am J Occup Ther 47:42–54, 1993.
167. Warren M: A hierarchical model for evaluation and treatment of visual perceptual dysfunction in adult acquired brain injury, Part 2. Am J Occup Ther 47:55–66, 1993.
168. Webster JS, McFarland PT, Rapport LJ, Morril B, et al: Computer-assisted training for improving wheelchair mobility in unilateral neglect patients. Arch Phys Med Rehabil 82:769–775, 2001.
169. Webster JS, Scott RR: The effects of self-instructional training of attentional deficits following head injury. Clin Neuropsychol 5:69–74, 1983.
170. Webster JS, Scott RR: Behavioral assessment and treatment of the brain injured patient. Progr Behav Modif 22:48–87, 1988.
171. Weinberg J, Diller L, Gordon WA, et al: Visual scanning training effect on reading related tasks in acquired right brain damage. Arch Phys Med Rehabil 58:479–496, 1977.
172. Weinberg J, Diller L, Gordon WA: Training sensory awareness and spatial organization in people with right brain dmage. Arch Phys Med Rehabil 60:491–496, 1979.
173. Weinberg J, Piasetsky E, Diller L, Gordon WA: Treating perceptual organization deficits in non-neglecting RBD stroke patients. J Clin Neuropsychol 4:59–75, 1982.
174. Wertz RT, Collins MJ, Weiss DG, Kurtzke JF, Friden

T, Brookshire RH, et al: Veterans Administration cooperative study on aphasia: Comparison of individual and group treatment. J Speech Hear Res 24:580–594, 1981.

175. Wertz RT, Weiss DG, Aten JTL, Brookshire RH, Garcia-Bunuel L, Holland AL, et al: Comparison of clinic, home, and deferred language treatment for aphasia: A Veterans Administration cooperative study. Arch Neurol 43:653–658, 1986.

176. Whyte J: Traumatic brain injury rehabilitation: Are there alternatives to randomized clinical trials? Arch Phys Med Rehabil 83:1320–1322, 2002.

177a. Wiart L, Bon Saint Come ADS, Petit H, Joseph PA, Mazaus JM, et al: Unilateral neglect syndrome rehabilitation by trunk rotation and scanning training. Arch Phys Med Rehabil 78:424–429, 1997.

177b. Willer B, Rosenthal M, Kreutzer JS, Gordon WA, Rempel R: Assessment of community intehgration following rehabilitation for traumatic brain injury. J Head Trauma Rehabil 8:75–87, 1993.

178. Wilson B, Robertson IH: A home based intervention for attentional slips during reading following head injury: A single case study. Neuropsychol Rehabil 2:193–205, 1992.

179. Wilson BA: Success and failure in memory training following a cerebral vascular accident. Cortex 18:581–594, 1982.

180. Wilson BA: Neuropsychological Rehabilitation: Theory and Practice. The Netherlands, Lisse, Swets & Zeitlinger, 2003.

181. Wilson BA, Emslie HC, Quirk K, Evans JJ: Reducing everyday memory and planning problems by means of a paging system: A randomized controlled crossover study. J Neurol Neurosurg Psychiatry 70:477–482, 2001.

182. Wilson BA, Evans JJ, Emslie H, Malinek V: Evaluation of NeuroPage: A new memory aid. J Neurol Neurosurg Psychiatry 63:113–115, 1997.

183. Wiseman-Hakes C, Stewart ML, Wasserman R, Schuller R: Peer group training of pragmatic skills in adolescents with acquired brain injury. J Head Trauma Rehabil 13:23–38, 1998.

184. Wood RL: Attention disorders in brain injury rehabilitation. J Learn Disabil 21:327–332, 1988.

185. Woolf SH: Practice guidelines, a new reality in medicine: II: Methods of developing guidelines. Arch Intern Med 152:956–962, 1992.

186. Worrel L, Yui E: Effectiveness of functional communication therapy by volunteers for people with aphasia follwing stroke. Aphasiology 14:911–924, 2000.

187. Yesavage JA: Nonpharmacologic treatments for memory losses with normal aging. Am J Psychiatry 142:600–605, 1985.

188. Yesavage JA, Rose TL: Concentration and mnemonic training in elderly subjects with memory complaints: A study of combined therapy and order effects. Psychiatr Res 9:157–167, 1983.

189. Yesavage JA, Sheikh JI, Friedman L, Tanke ED: Learning mnemonics: Roles of aging and subtle cognitive impairments. Psychol Aging 5:133–137, 1990.

190. Yesavage JA, Sheikh JI, Tanke ED, Hill R: Response to memory training and individual differences in verbal intelligence and state anxiety. Am J Psychiatry 145: 636–639, 1988.

191. Young GC, Collins C, Hren M: Effect of pairing scanning training with block design training in the remediation of perceptual problems in left hemiplegics. J Clin Exp Neuropsychol 5:201–212, 1983.

192. Zencius A, Wesolowski MD, Burke WH: A comparison of four memory strategies with traumatically brain injured clients. Brain Inj 4:33–38, 1990.

193. Zihl J, von Cramen D: Visual field recovery from scotoma in patients with postgeniculate damage. Brain 108:439–469, 1985.

Part II

Spinal Trauma

Chapter 14
Spinal Cord Injury

DAVID S. BASKIN

The management of the spinal cord–injured patient poses special challenges that begin at the instant that the patient is seen in the field and continue throughout the patient's life. This chapter discusses the principles of management of acute spinal cord injury (SCI), considering the initial evaluation at the scene of the accident, treatment in the emergency department, mechanisms of injury, assessment techniques, and presenting clinical syndromes. Initial diagnostic studies and their merits are also considered.

Traction and reduction and other interventions are then reviewed. Problems unique to the spinal cord–injured patient that may manifest later in the illness are considered, including such late sequelae as posttraumatic syringomyelia and myelomalacia with progressive neurological deficit. A discussion of the status of research in spinal cord injury concludes the chapter, with consideration of therapies that have already come to clinical trials, as well as those that hold promise for treatment in the near future.

Epidemiology

The incidence of acute SCI is relatively uncommon, affecting about 1 in 40 patients who present to a major trauma center.[12] Estimates of the annual incidence in developed countries vary from 11.5 to 53.4 per million population.[28,53] This by no means minimizes the impact of acute SCI on the individual patient and his or her family, as the case fatality rate is approximately 48%, with 79% of the fatalities occurring at the scene of the accident or on arrival at the hospital.[27] Among survivors of hospital admissions, mortality rates range from 4% to 17%, with very high morbidity.[28a] The financial burden to society is great, as one must consider not only the expenses for acute and chronic treatment, but also indirect costs from lost income and impaired productivity. Total direct cost for caring for all SCI patients exceeds $7 billion annually in the United States.[28b]

In developed nations, traffic accidents are the most common cause of SCI, whereas in many less developed countries, the most common cause is trauma from falls.[56] Violence as a causative factor varies quite a bit, depending on the location; in urban locations, gunshot wounds are one of the most frequent causes of SCI.[53]

The cervical spinal cord receives 55% of all injuries, with approximately 15% of injuries occurring in each of the other three regions of the spine.[54] Since 1969, there has been a change in the relative incidence of complete and incomplete SCI.[56] In the past, approximately two-thirds of SCIs were complete, whereas more recent reports indicate that approximately 45% are complete. This decrease in complete injuries may be due both to the increasing use of prophylactic measures, such as seat belts and airbags, and to better on-the-scene resuscitative efforts that limit secondary damage.[54] Alcohol continues to play an important role in SCI; 25% of all injuries have alcohol consumption as a factor influencing the mode of injury.[56]

In almost all large published series of spinal cord–injured patients, 80% to 85% of patients with SCI are male and 15% to 20% are female.[56] Young patients account for the majority of victims, with the usual mean ages ranging from the late 20s to the early 30s in series of patients from most countries.

Mechanisms of Injury

Various types of injury can produce damage to the spinal cord. What constitutes appropriate management will differ, depending on the mechanism of injury. Osseous disruption is the most common mechanism of injury and includes fracture dislocation, flexion distraction–associated fractures, burst fractures, and wedge compression fractures. In such cases, osseous disruption produces malalignment and subsequent bony compressive force and pressure that are distributed to the spinal cord and adjacent nerve roots. In some cases, the malalignment is temporary, and radiographs subsequently do not show ongoing compression. More commonly, however, obvious compression and mechanical deformation persist.

Ligamentous injury and disruption can also result in spinal cord injury. In some cases, the bony anatomy before injury may already be abnormal, so that ligamentous integrity is a primary determinant of spinal stability. In other circumstances, the degree of ligamentous disruption may be so severe that either transient or permanent osseous malalignment may occur, producing damage to the cord. A potential pitfall exists in the pediatric patient, in whom ligamentous disruption may lead to significant instability, yet the alignment on a static radiograph may be perfectly acceptable. This syndrome of spinal cord injury without radiological abnormality has been given the eponym SCIWORA.[36] The condition underscores the value of careful assessment of radiographs and the judicious use of flexion and extension views before assuming spinal stability.

Another common clinical entity is an injury due to preexisting spondylosis. As spondylitic disease progresses, there is compromise of the spinal canal and/or neural foramina, which often is asymptomatic. When force is transmitted to the spinal column, these spondylitic abnormalities compress and deform either the spinal cord or the nerve roots, producing subsequent neurological injury.

Disc herniation with associated spinal cord or nerve root compromise has traditionally been regarded as an uncommon problem in acute SCI, but this notion bears reexamination. Magnetic resonance imaging (MRI) scanning has demonstrated that traumatic disc herniation is a surprisingly common occurrence, often in conjunction with fracture or ligamentous injury. Flanders et al.[19] report that up to 54% of traumatic SCIs have associated disc herniations, and that demonstration of the herniation may affect the type of surgical approach chosen to achieve adequate decompression and stabilization.

Classification of Spinal Cord Injury

Optimal management of the spinal cord–injured patient requires a thorough assessment of the type of injury sustained. This, in turn, depends on accurate and detailed neurological examination and classification of the neurological injury that has been produced, followed by detailed radiological assessment of the spinal canal.

Neurological assessment and classification should be sufficiently thorough and reliable to allow for accurate comparisons of serial observations by either the same or differing examiners. A variety of standardized grading scales have been proposed over the years. The American Spinal Injury Association (ASIA) in conjunction with the International Medical Society of Paraplegia (IMSOP) has published the *International Standards for Neurological and Functional Classification of Spinal Cord Injury* (Fig. 14.1). This classification is a good assessment tool and should be used by all who evaluate spinal cord injury, just as the Glasgow Coma Scale is used to assess and track the progress of patients with acute head injuries.[1]

The ASIA/IMSOP classification provides precise definitions of the neurological, sensory, and skeletal levels, as well as zones of partial preservation of function. It also encourages the examiner to

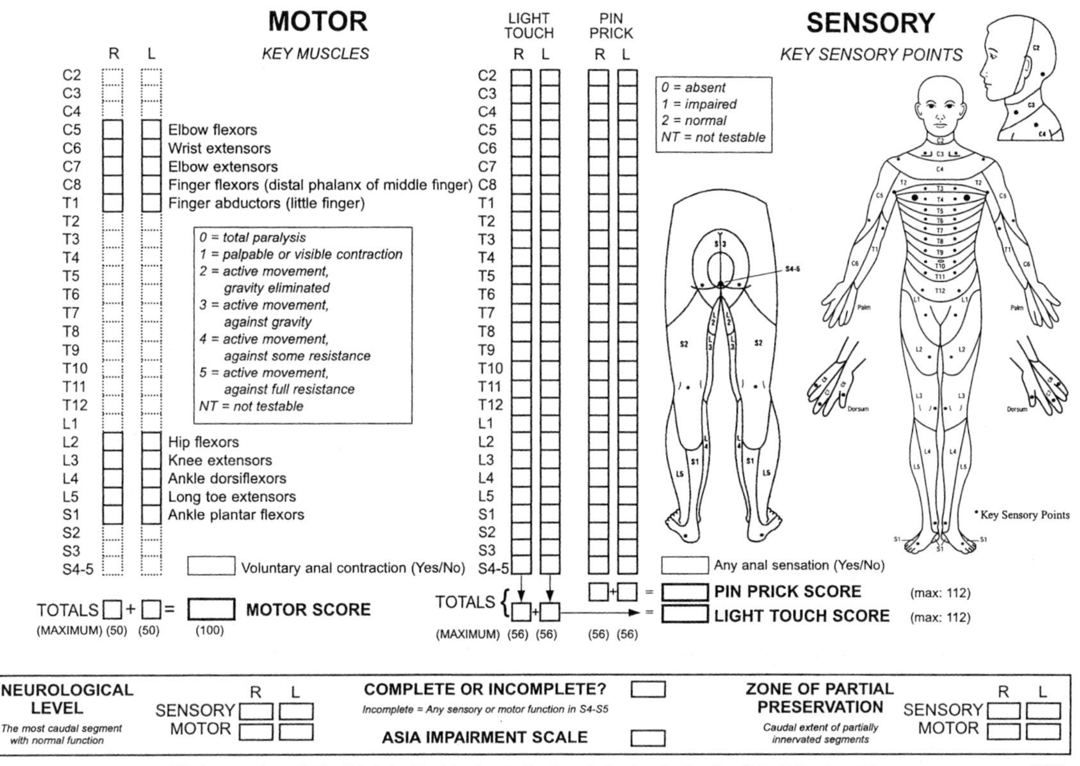

Figure 14.1. Standard Neurological Classification of Spinal Cord Injury. (From ASIA).

perform the kind of detailed neurological examination that is paramount to proper assessment and management. For this reason, many centers have adopted this form.

The ASIA/IMSOP has also developed an impairment scale for the spinal cord–injured patient (Table 14.1). This scale defines function more precisely than previous scales and is a useful tool when deciding on the ultimate level of long-term caregiver intervention that will be required for the individual patient.

Once thorough clinical and radiological assessment has occurred, it is possible to classify acute SCI into a variety of recognizable syndromes. Although the prognosis for recovery is much better for patients with incomplete injuries than for those with complete injuries, even complete cord injuries have some potential for recovery. Most large series of acute SCI patients include a small percentage of initially completely cord-injured patients (approximately 1% to 2%) who experience significant recovery of distal cord function.[24] It is felt that this phenomenon is not simply due to the confounding effects of drugs, altered levels of consciousness, or the presence of spinal shock, but rather represents a real potential for recovery.

Spinal Cord Injury Syndromes

Several incomplete injury syndromes have been delineated, and recognition of these syndromes is helpful to the clinician for several reasons. First, recognition provides some information on the likely mechanism of injury, which may determine the treatment and its timing. Furthermore, the various incomplete injury syndromes have different prognoses for recovery.

Cervicomedullary Syndrome

Many injuries to the upper aspect of the cervical cord also damage lower and middle brain stem structures, either because of direct trauma or because of vascular injury to the vertebral arteries. The main features of these syndromes include

Table 14.1. ASIA Impairment Scale

A = Complete: No motor or sensory function is preserved in the sacral segments S4-5.
B = Incomplete: Sensory but not motor function is preserved below the neurological level and includes the sacral segments S4-5.
C = Incomplete: Motor function is preserved below the neurological level, and more than half of key muscles below the neurological level have a muscle grade of less than 3.
D = Incomplete: Motor function is preserved below the neurological level, and at least half of key muscles below the neurological level have a muscle grade of 3 or more.
E = Normal: motor and sensory function are normal.

Clinical Syndromes

Central cord
Brown-Sequard
Anterior cord
Conus medullaris
Cauda equina

respiratory dysfunction, hypotension, varying degrees of tetraparesis and hyperesthesia from C1-4, and sensory loss in the face consistent with the onion skin or Dejerine pattern.[43,45]

Mechanisms of injury include traction injury from atlantoaxial dislocation, interior-posterior compression from a burst fracture or odontoid fracture, and dysfunction from a ruptured disc. More of these patients have survived such injuries in recent years because of more rapid access to rescue squads, and improved emergency medical care in the field, which allows for prompt resuscitation.

Evaluation of facial sensation can be very useful in such patients, as the pattern can help determine the rostral extent of the injury.[43,45] The pattern of topographic representation of the descending spinal tract of the trigeminal nerve is such that a perioral distribution of sensory loss indicates a lesion in the lower medulla and high cervical cord, whereas a more peripheral facial distribution of sensory loss indicates a lesion at C3 or C4. Cervicomedullary syndromes can mimic a central cord injury because of greater weakness in the arms than in the legs, but the absence of respiratory problems, normal cranial nerve function, and normal facial sensation are helpful distinguishing features.

Central Cord Syndrome

Schneider et al.[44] first described the acute central cervical cord injury syndrome, characterized by a greater loss of motor power in the lower extremities and associated with varying degrees of sensory loss. They hypothesized that acute compression was an etiological factor in many cases, such as cord compression between bony bars or spurs anteriorly and infolded ligamentum flavum posteriorly (Fig. 14.2). Schneider et al. emphasized the need to delay surgical intervention in most cases because most patients tend to improve spontaneously. Indeed, for many years, the teaching has been to delay intervention until the patient had reached a plateau in improvement. Recent experience has called this concept into question, although there is still no consensus on this matter.[50]

Anterior Cord Syndrome

The anterior cord syndrome was also originally described in the setting of acute cervical trauma

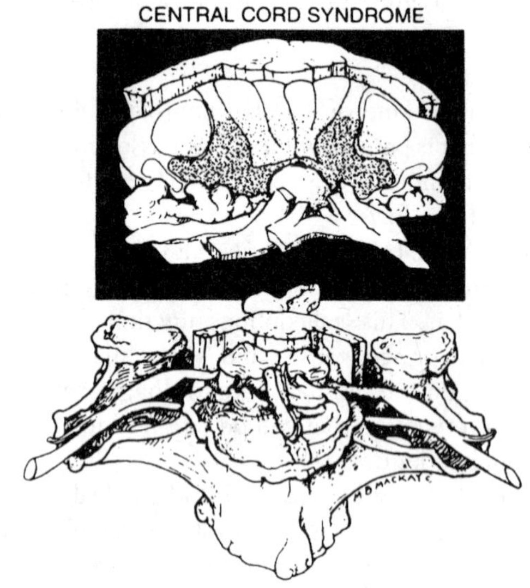

Figure 14.2. The central cord syndrome. The drawing depicts a case of preexisting cervical spondylosis with anterior and posterior osteophytes. Superimposed on this is an acute injury, with a central disc herniation that is compressing the spinal cord. The spinal cord is compressed anteriorly and posteriorly. The damaged areas include the medial segments of the corticospinal tracts, thought to control arm function. (From reference 55, with permission.)

by Schneider et al.,[42] who presented two cases of immediate complete paralysis with hyperesthesias at the level of the lesion and an associated sparing of touch and some vibration sense. Both patients had a ruptured disc and made a substantial recovery after operative removal. The syndrome in general is due to relatively focal and central anterior cord compression without associated posterior compression (Fig. 14.3). Patients present with varying degrees of motor loss and relatively normal sensory function. The extent of motor loss depends in part on the degree of compression, for some motor function can be preserved in smaller lesions because of sparing of the lateral corticospinal tracts. Schneider et al. felt that patients presenting with this syndrome were usually in need of early operative intervention. Most would agree with this concept today.

Brown-Sequard Syndrome

In 1849, Brown-Sequard first described a constellation of symptoms as a consequence of a knife injury causing hemisection of the spinal cord.[10] Subsequent reports have well documented the relationship of this syndrome to both penetrating[37] and blunt trauma.[35] It has been estimated that 2% to 4% of all traumatic spinal cord injuries have the features of the Brown-Sequard syndrome.[40] The syndrome is caused by a lesion of the lateral half of the spinal cord (Fig. 14.4), and is characterized by ipsilateral motor and proprioceptive loss and contralateral pain and body temperature loss. The syndrome can be associated with a variety of mechanisms of injury. In the series of Braakman and Penning,[6] the most common injury was associated with severe hyperextension, although patients with flexion injuries, locked facets, and compression fractures also had this problem. The syndrome has also been described in association with cervical disc herniation.[41]

Although the syndrome may be apparent at the time of the initial examination, it is also possible to see it evolve over time. Hybrid or mixed-type injuries may occur, with features of the Brown-Sequard syndrome coupled with other neurological deficits. The syndrome most often occurs in association with cervical injuries but can be seen throughout the course of the spinal cord.

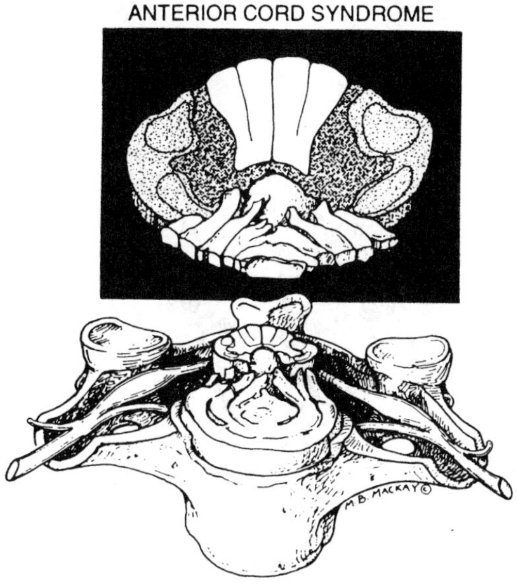

ANTERIOR CORD SYNDROME

Figure 14.3. The anterior cord syndrome. A large disc herniation is depicted that is compressing the anterior aspect of the cord and producing damage to the anterior and lateral white matter tracts and to the gray matter. The posterior columns, however, remain intact, in contrast to the previous example of central cord injury. (From reference 55, with permission.)

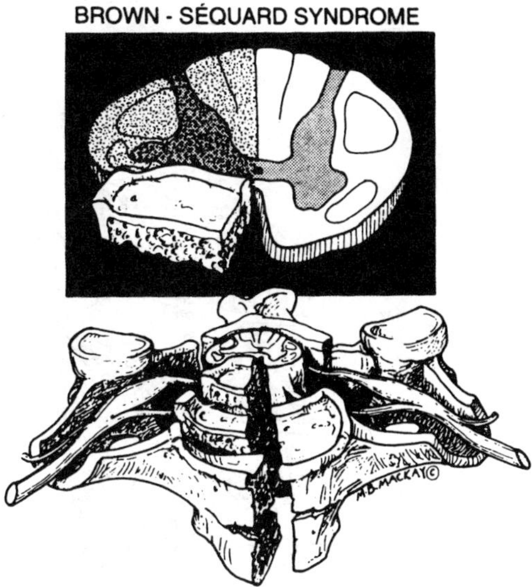

Figure 14.4. The Brown-Séquard syndrome. In this example, a burst fracture of the vertebral body is shown, with posterior displacement of both disc and bone fragments. The mechanics of the injury are such that unilateral damage to one-half of the spinal cord has been produced. (From reference 55, with permission.)

Conus Medullaris Syndrome

This syndrome is based on the anatomical fact that most of the lumbar cord segments are opposite the T12 vertebral body, and almost all of the sacral cord segments are opposite the LI vertebral body.[55] Because injuries at the thoracolumbar junction are relatively common, this syndrome is seen frequently (Fig. 14.5). Patients with this injury present with a combination of lower motor neuron deficits with a flaccid paralysis of the legs and anal sphincter. In the chronic phase, there is a combination of some degree of muscle atrophy and spasticity and reflex hyperactivity, occasionally with extensor plantar responses. Sensory deficits are variable, and in some cases the only evidence of retained function is the retention of perianal sensation, an example of sacral sparing.

Cauda Equina Syndrome

As the spinal cord usually terminates at the L1-2 disc space, injuries below this area involve the roots of the cauda equina. In general, the motor fibers tend to be more sensitive to injury, and the roots are more resistant to trauma than is the spinal cord. There is a consensus that cauda equina injuries have a much better prognosis for recovery than other incomplete injury syndromes. This is most likely due to the fact that the nerve roots are more resilient to injury, and because many of the biochemical processes occur in the spinal cord and produce secondary damage occur to a much less extent in the nerve roots.

Evaluation at the Accident Scene

Even though prehospital trauma care has markedly improved, 29% of patients with a spinal cord injury still die before reaching the hospital.[31] Furthermore, in every part of the initial evaluation and treatment, special consideration must be given using routine resuscitative measures; otherwise, further deterioration in function is likely to occur. It is important to remember that any trauma victim who is difficult to assess must be assumed to have a spinal cord injury and be treated appropriately until definitive diagnostic studies can be performed and can demonstrate otherwise.[14] It is prudent to assume that a spinal cord injury is present in such situations in order to avoid inadvertent worsening of the deficit by inappropriate mobilization of the patient. Such patients include every patient with a head injury, every unconscious patient, every patient with multiple trauma, every motor vehicle accident

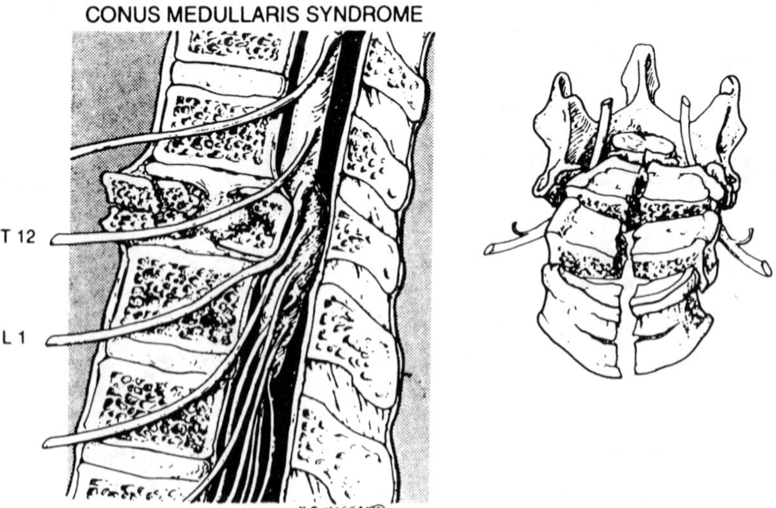

Figure 14.5. The conus medullaris syndrome. In this example, a burst fracture of the body of T12 is shown. There is posterior displacement of bone fragments from the vertebral body into the spinal canal. These fragments compress the conus medullaris. Recall that almost all the lumbar cord segments are opposite the T12 vertebral body. Therefore, a severe compression here could produce dysfunction in any or all the lumbar segments, as well as the sacral segments. (From reference 55, with permission.)

victim, every victim of a fall at home, and every severely injured worker. The presence of a high index of suspicion for spinal cord injury in any trauma victim improves the treatment outcome. Retrospective analysis demonstrates that an increased awareness of the need for stabilization before mobilization at the scene is associated with a decline in complete spinal cord lesions of almost 11%.[23]

If a spinal injury is suspected, immediate neck immobilization is vital. The usual technique is to pass a firm backboard beneath the victim. After the thoracic spine is immobilized, the cervical spine should be similarly restrained before it is moved. Sandbags are placed alongside the head and neck and secured by 3-inch tape passed from one edge of the backboard across the forehead to the other edge of the backboard. This allows free motion of the jaw and lower face for airway control while still providing stability that is (surprisingly) equal to that of rigid external orthoses.[11] Soft cervical collars are not valuable, as they do not provide sufficient immobilization.[25,63] A variety of other considerations apply, including airway, breathing, and resuscitative efforts, and are described in the next section.

Evaluation and Treatment in the Emergency Department

Much like the patient in the field, any patient who arrives at the hospital with a history of trauma or who is unconscious and cannot give an adequate history must be assumed to have a spinal injury until proven otherwise. Irreversible spinal cord injury with tragic consequences can occur from even trivial motion of such a patient whose neck has been inadequately stabilized. Therefore, if there is any chance of a spinal injury, the usual emergency protocol of an ABC (airway, breathing, circulation) survey should be appropriately modified to consider the spinal cord–injured patient.

As always, evaluation of the airway is the first step of treatment. If the airway is adequate on initial assessment, the patient should be stabilized and left secured "as he lies." Oxygen should be administered via face mask or nasal cannula. If the airway is compromised, the first maneuver should be a chin lift rather than a jaw thrust or neck extension. This reduces the chance of inadvertent mobilization of an unstable cervical spine injury, which could result in quadriplegia. If simply lifting the chin is not adequate to establish the airway, intubation should be considered.

Although one might be inclined to perform a tracheotomy or a cricothyroidotomy, this procedure should be avoided whenever possible. This is because if surgery is required for stabilization of the spine, an anterior operation may be required. With a cricothyroidotomy or tracheotomy in place, the chances for infection increase dramatically.

Consequently, intubation is the preferable technique. Nasotracheal intubation is much easier than oral intubation in this setting.[47] This procedure does not require hyperextension of the neck and therefore diminishes the likelihood of aspiration. However, the patient must have spontaneous respirations for this procedure to be successful. If not, laryngoscopically guided oral intubation should be performed gently, with the head and neck immobilized by an assistant. Intubation can almost always be accomplished without neck extension.[14] Tracheotomy or cricothyroidotomy should then be performed in those few cases in which intubation is not possible.

Once the airway is cleared and breathing is established, attention should be given to the circulatory status. Hypotension is a significant complication associated with spinal cord injury, and if the neurogenic basis for it is not recognized, inappropriate therapy may be administered. Hypotension associated with the spinal cord injury in multiple trauma can be either hypovolemic, cardiogenic, or both.[32] Hypovolemic hypotension can be a sequela of simple hemorrhage; in many cases, the acute spinal injury produces a loss of peripheral sympathetic drive with a marked decrease in peripheral vascular resistance. This, in turn, produces significant venous pooling in the arms and legs and a decreased cardiac preload.[14]

Initial therapy for hypovolemic shock should include volume expansion and placement of thigh-high compressive stockings or simple wrapping of the legs with Ace bandages to reduce peripheral venous pooling. Intravenous access should be obtained, and administration of isotonic fluid should be initiated. Placing the patient in a Trendelenburg position will increase central venous return and spinal cord perfusion pressure. Cardiogenic shock, which is caused by the loss of sympathetic antagonism of tonic vagal influence, usually presents with bradycardia despite hypotension. Increasing cardiac filling pressures may not counteract this effect.

If volume expansion does not adequately improve the situation, intravenous atropine, 0.5 to 1.0 mg, or glycopyrrolate, 0.1 mg IV, should be administered.[14] If the presumed spinal shock does not respond to the above measures, one should be concerned about either inadequate intravascular volume expansion or intrathoracic or abdominal bleeding that has not been recognized. If the blood pressure remains low, a pressor such as dopamine or Neo-Synephrine can be very useful. If no internal bleeding is present, pressors are the mainstay of therapy for spinal shock, as volume expansion alone will not increase the blood pressure because of the loss of peripheral vascular resistance secondary to the loss of sympathetic outflow. Early placement of a central venous line or a Swan-Ganz catheter to monitor cardiac filling pressures is helpful in guiding therapy. A Foley catheter should be placed to monitor urine output and to prevent bladder distention.

A rapid head-to-toe survey should be performed in order to establish the presence or absence of other injuries. If the patient is awake and alert, a detailed and careful neurological examination is of paramount importance, both to establish the deficit that is present and to serve as a useful baseline to assess the success or failure of subsequent interventions. This point cannot be emphasized enough. For example, if a patient is subsequently transported and suddenly reports that his or her function has deteriorated, this is a very serious concern both medically and, much later on, medicolegally. If it indeed turns out that the patient has deteriorated, consideration must immediately be given to inadequately treated instability, progressive subluxation in the spine, or another new injury. On the other hand, it is entirely possible that the patient is now becoming much more aware of the deficit and that no deterioration has occurred. For diagnostic, therapeutic, and subsequent medicolegal reasons, there is no substitute for an early, careful, and thorough neurological examination.[3]

Occasionally, a patient will position the head in an unusual and nonneutral position. If the patient is awake and alert and resists reduction of the neck into a neutral position, such reduction should be avoided at all costs. Remarkable as it may seem, an awake and alert patient will always position the neck in a manner that minimizes further damage. Until the nature of the spinal injury and the associated vertebral body disruption is clear, the head should be left in this position.[14]

Pharmacological Intervention

Even before the initiation of diagnostic x-rays, as soon as a spinal cord injury is even remotely suspected, pharmacotherapy is indicated. After over 30 years of exhaustive research involving tens of millions of dollars, a landmark study has demonstrated that the use of high-dose methylprednisolone is efficacious in the treatment of spinal cord injury. The National Acute Spinal Cord Injury Study II (NASCIS II)[7] compared the effects of high-dose methylprednisolone, naloxone, and placebo in spinal cord–injured patients. The study documented that the use of high-dose methylprednisolone can reduce the severity and improve the functional outcome in human spinal cord injury.[7] While the study has been criticized for a variety of reasons, most would agree that the use of methylprednisolone is indicated within the first 8 hours.

The study included 387 spinal cord–injured patients, with injuries most commonly due to motor vehicle accidents, falls, or water-related injuries. Even patients with "complete" spinal injuries improved after the initiation of therapy. Although at times this improvement only includes recovery of several adjacent spinal segments, it can be of great significance for a patient who starts out with a spinal level at C5 or C6 and improves to a C7 or TI level. Patients who were treated 8 hours after injury did not improve and actually did worse than patients treated with placebo.[8] Therefore, administration within 8 hours from the time of injury is crucial. Patients should receive a 30 mg/kg bolus of methylprednisolone IV as soon as a spinal injury is suspected. For patients in the field in whom weight estimation is difficult, a 2-g bolus is recommended. Once the loading dose is given, continuous infusion of 5.4 mg/kg/hr should be started 1 hour later and continued for 23 hours. The results of treatment after 24 hours are not clear. Each clinician should decide how to best handle treatment. As there are deleterious effects of high-dose methylprednisolone over an extended period of time, the author slowly tapers the continuous infusion dosage over 72 hours. Further research is ongoing to determine how this therapy can be improved. The consensus is that the primary mechanism of action of methylprednisolone in the spinal cord–injured patient involves the inhibition of lipid peroxidation.

Radiological Evaluation

Once the patient has been resuscitated, the airway, breathing, and circulation controlled, and an initial dose of methylprednisolone administered, timely radiological evaluation is essential to establish definitive therapy. Particularly in the patient with an incomplete spinal cord injury, it is of paramount importance to diagnose rapidly all conditions in which spinal cord compression is present. It is generally thought that early reduction of the spinal canal to its normal configuration can improve the outcome significantly and even, at times, allow the patient to return to a normal or near-normal state. It cannot be overemphasized that although one wants to take the time required for the initial stabilization and assessment, the evaluation should proceed rapidly to clearly image the spine.

Plain Radiographs

The first step is to obtain a lateral radiograph of the cervical spine. This should be done with the patient still on the stretcher, and all handling of the patient should be delayed until the results of the examination are known. Great care must be taken to ensure that the lower part of the cervical spine is adequately seen on these films. Superimposition of the shoulders must be overcome, which can usually be achieved by downward traction on the arms. If this is unsuccessful, careful elevation of the arm into the swimmer's position will allow for imaging down to the first thoracic vertebra in almost every case. Tragic consequences due to inadequate visualization of the lower cervical spine are unfortunately common. In almost every circumstance, the initial imaging of the lower cervical area was difficult, and for whatever reason, it was decided that such visualization was not critical.

After it has been ascertained that all seven cervical vertebrae have been visualized on the x-ray, the outlines of the bony canal are studied, and additional films of the thoracic and lumbar spine in the anterior-posterior (AP) and lateral projections are made. An open-mouth odontoid view is also part of the initial evaluation, for fracture of the odontoid process is usually best seen in this projection. For a suspected cervical spine injury, if AP, lateral, and odontoid views are normal, oblique views are obtained. If these show no fracture, a computed tomography (CT) scan is the next study of choice if an injury is still suspected.

At this point, clinical judgment is paramount. Clearly, many patients who are awake and alert, and who can accurately report the presence or absence of pain and discomfort at the site of injury and undergo a detailed neurological examination, may not require further imaging studies. From a practical point of view, many unconscious patients may not receive further study. It is important to note, however, that plain spine radiographs alone do not rule out the presence of either a bony fracture or a spinal cord injury, so clinical judgment and discretion are needed at this point in the evaluation algorithitm

Computed Tomography Scanning

Computed tomography has become the mainstay for imaging of spinal injuries. The major advantage of the CT scan is that bone is imaged rapidly and in exquisite detail. The technique is especially helpful in depicting the size and shape of the bony spinal canal and of the pedicles, lamina, and spinous processes. The configuration of the canal and the extent of bony encroachment usually become immediately obvious. Nonetheless, fractures parallel to the scan plane can be missed, and the spinal canal contents cannot be assessed completely without intrathecal contrast agents. However, opacification of the subarachnoid space by intrathecal contrast injection allows excellent visualization of the spinal cord and nonosseous masses within the canal. Intrathecal contrast enhancement may be performed to augment the CT scan, or the CT scan can follow a conventional radiographic myelogram. In the case of acute spinal cord injury, routine CT scanning without dye is often sufficient to establish a diagnosis, and the injection of dye (usually via a lateral C1-2 puncture) with the patient maintained in a stabilized position can be reserved for those cases in which the further delineation of anatomy is required.[4]

Sagittal, coronal, and oblique reconstruction of the spine is usually performed for demonstrations of fractures in the plane of the section and for evaluation of alignment. The usual protocol for routine examination of the cervical spine consists of a 3-mm slice thickness and 2-mm longitudinal spacing of slices, allowing for a 1-mm overlap. This provides a high-quality image and allows for subsequent reformatting. Similar imaging can be performed in the thoracic and lumbar spine, in the areas where a fracture is either diagnosed or suspected on the basis of the clinical information or plain film imaging. It is usually possible to obtain a detailed picture of the nature of the bony disruption, which is critical for further treatment.

Magnetic Resonance Imaging Scanning

For soft tissue contrast resolution, the MRI scan is superior to the CT scan or conventional noninvasive x-ray techniques. Since the spinal cord is well visualized without the use of intrathecal contrast agents, intra-axial spinal cord lesions are best studied by MRI scanning. Myelopathy due to an extra-axial lesion compressing the cord is also well evaluated by MRI, particularly when the process is poorly localized by clinical findings. Magnetic resonance imaging scanning is particularly useful in the craniocervical junction, where commonly encountered streak artifacts due to x-ray beam hardening seen with CT scanning are eliminated. The clear visualization of the medulla and cervical spinal cord provided by the sagittal and coronal images is extremely helpful. The direct sagittal image plane usually best displays many of the important anatomical relationships in this area. Furthermore, when the CT scan is normal, MRI may demonstrate a significant cord contusion, a hematomyelia, and even a central disc herniation not well visualized by CT. Disadvantages of the MRI study include the long examination time, as well as the fact that if the patient is to be immobilized with skeletal traction, nonmetallic hardware is required. The enclosed space often required in most machines also makes it more difficult to manage the patient in the acute setting, as well as presenting problems with some patients because of claustrophobia. Nonetheless, if the plain x-rays and the CT scan do not demonstrate clearly the nature of the spinal lesion, MRI scanning can be invaluable.

Immobilization

Once plain radiographic images are obtained, immobilization is essential before patient transfer to CT scanning, MRI scanning, or CT myelography. Immobilization is particularly essential when the cervical spine is involved.

In cervical spine fractures, the gold standard of initial mobilization involves the placement of Gardner-Wells tongs.[3] The tongs are placed with the pins just above the pinnae of the ears on an imaginary plane connecting the mastoid processes and the external auditory canals. Once the tongs have been applied under local anesthesia, traction is initiated in a neutral plane. The initial amount of weight to be applied varies considerably with the level of injury and the amount of suspected disruption of the cervical ligaments. If there is significant ligamentous damage, a minimal amount of weight should be used to avoid distraction and potentially significant neurological deterioration. If there is any uncertainty whatsoever, it is best to start with 5 to 6 lb for upper cervical levels and 10 lb for lower levels and then await the initial radiographic evaluation.

After traction is applied, additional diagnostic studies are usually required before making therapeutic decisions regarding reduction of the fracture using either open or closed techniques. In such cases, the patient can be transferred to the CT scanning area in traction, and traction can be maintained throughout the study. If myelography is required, a lateral C1-2 puncture can be performed, with the patient's neck immobilized. In MRI scanning the problem is more difficult, although systems using nonmetallic traction devices now exist.

For thoracic and lumbar fractures, immobilization is more difficult. Although a variety of orthoses do exist, simple bed rest with log rolling of the patient is generally used initially. Halo tibial or halo pelvic traction and/or immobilization is occasionally used in special cases.

Reduction of Spinal Fractures

Several cervical injuries can be initially treated via closed reduction using Gardner-Wells tongs and the addition of weights. The initial goal of therapy is simply to restore the alignment of the spinal canal to normal. Such injuries as fracture subluxation without locked facets, unilaterally locked facets, or even occasionally bilaterally locked facets can initially be treated with an attempt at closed reduction. The advantage of such treatment is that a general anesthetic and surgical intervention are avoided during a time of potential medical instability.

Specific treatment protocols depend upon the nature of the injury. For example, hyperextension injuries, where the anterior longitudinal ligament is disrupted, require application of traction posterior to the neutral plane to maintain normal anatomical alignment. Management of unilaterally or bilaterally locked facets may also require posterior or flexion movement of the traction vector. If the fracture and the malalignment are reduced successfully, application of a rigid external orthosis, such as a halo vest, usually immediately follows the reduction procedure.

The use of muscle relaxants is common and useful during such procedures, although one must guard against clouding of the sensorium and therefore reduction of the ability to perform an adequate neurological examination. Other concerns include respiratory compromise, particularly in high cervical injuries, as well as a sudden reduction in muscle tone that allows overdistraction to occur.

Surgical Intervention: Patient Selection and Timing

As the management of the spinal cord–injured patient has evolved over the years, the thrust of change has been toward earlier intervention. The development of better and more sophisticated emergency medical systems, with more rapid transport of patients to the hospital, has given us a better understanding of the advanced trauma life support techniques needed to resuscitate patients in the field and in the emergency department. Advanced radiological imaging techniques provide both rapid and exquisitely sensitive images of the spine. Pharmacotherapy that is effective if instituted early is now available, and we have made tremendous advances in the technical aspects of surgery, including the development of complex and efficient instrumentation to better fixate and stabilize even the most complex spinal fractures. Unfortunately, despite the firm belief among many spinal surgeons (including the author) that early intervention is of benefit, available data do not support this contention. The results of recent animal studies investigating the timing of intervention in SCI suggest that early relief of compression clearly enhances neurological recovery.[16,24,39] The problem is that no prospective, randomized study incorporating the most recent advances in treatment has evaluated the efficacy of early versus late surgery in human SCI.[50]

Surgeons who advocate early surgery still encounter resistance of two types—from those who think that early surgery is unnecessary and from those who think that early surgery is contraindicated because of the increase in risk. Those who advocate early surgery believe that it decreases both the length of hospitalization and the risks associated with prolonged bed rest. Most important, however, is the firm belief that in incomplete injuries, restoration of the spinal canal and its contents to normal alignment and the resulting cessation of compression of the spinal cord and other neural elements are more likely to be beneficial when accomplished as soon as possible after the injury. Furthermore, early surgery permits earlier mobilization and institution of physical therapy, which decrease the incidence of medical complications associated with prolonged immobility.

There is little debate that until recently, the preponderance of literature supported delayed operative intervention to treat patients with SCI. In fact, even those who advocated early surgery consistently failed to present convincing data to support their opinion. However, with advances in neuroanesthesia and critical care, the risk of perioperative complications has been reduced greatly. In fact, there now is a higher risk of systemic complications, such as pneumonia, deep venous thrombosis, pulmonary embolism, and formation of decubitus ulcers, in patients for whom surgery is delayed.

Furthermore, the results of the NASCIS II study, in which pharmacological intervention before 8 hours after injury produced improvement in function and intervention after 8 hours did not, strongly suggest that early intervention using modern techniques is a superior approach. Clinical judgment in the individual patient should still ultimately dictate surgical timing, but the author, among others,[3] believes that early intervention is likely to be most beneficial, when it is feasible.

Posttraumatic Syringomyelia and Related Entities

Syringomyelia has challenged neurologists and neurosurgeons for as long as the entity has been recognized. Although the management of the patient with symptomatic syringomyelia with an associated Arnold-Chiari malformation is relatively standardized, patients with posttraumatic syringomyelia are more problematic.

The reported incidence of posttraumatic syringomyelia ranges from 0.3% to 3.0%,[58] although MRI scanning can detect this abnormality in up to 22% of patients with SCI.[51] The interval between spinal trauma and the appearance of neurological symptoms varies from 2 months to 36 years. The entity occurs with equal frequency in patients with complete and incomplete lesions, and there is no relation to the intensity of the initial trauma.[58] The syrinxes occur more often in patients with thoracic and lumbar injuries than in those with cervical lesions and may be associated with arachnoid cysts.[2]

The etiology of the posttraumatic syrinx is not well understood. Many believe that it arises as the result of initial hematomyelia, with subsequent resorption and formation of a cyst cavity. Other proposed mechanisms include vascular lesions remote from the initial site of injury; coalescence of ischemic microinfarcts with the formation of ischemic cores of tissue; the action of cellular enzymes, particularly of lysosomes; and the possible role of arachnoiditis and adhesions in producing a chronic ischemic state.[59] All of these processes can produce loss of spinal cord substance, with subsequent formation of a cystic cavity within the parenchyma of the spinal cord.

Van den Bergh[59] writes that four kinds of trauma should be considered in order to understand this entity: repeated microtrauma, arachnoiditis, severe single trauma, and minor single trauma. Repeated microtrauma can occur in some physically demanding occupations and may contribute to chronic spinal cord damage and syrinx formation. Arachnoiditis, either traumatic or inflammatory, can cause syringomyelia, both by local cord tethering and by obstruction of the foramina of the fourth ventricle. Severe single trauma is thought to lead to syrinx formation via contusion, hemorrhage, or partial section of the cord. Minor single trauma is an uncommon cause, but can occasionally contribute to the formation of a syrinx when there is initial intramedullary bleeding.

Part of the confusion regarding treatment arises from the controversy surrounding the pathophysiology of the condition. A major unanswered question is whether the progressive neurological deficits seen are caused by increased pressure within the syringomyelic cavity or by late deterioration due to other causes. In support of the pressure hypothesis is the fact that anecdotal surgical reports have described increased pressure inside the syrinx cavity at the time of surgical exploration and drainage, as well as subsequent improvement after drainage and decompression. However, the results of surgical treatment of posttraumatic syrinxes in general have been disappointing, and often the intrasyrinx pressure at the time of surgery is not elevated. In every patient with a syrinx, the question arises of whether increased pressure within the syrinx itself plays any role in the additional loss of neurological function that can be associated with the syrinx. Although there are no unequivocal guidelines in this regard, the patients with elevated pressure for whom surgery has the greatest benefit are either those with very large syrinxes or those in whom serial MRI scans have documented progressive significant enlargement.

It is the author's experience that although surgical intervention can occasionally be helpful, unless the syrinx is large, the results of surgical treatment are usually disappointing. Furthermore, exploration itself carries a risk of creating additional deficits, although these can be minimized by avoiding a midline myelotomy and making the cord incision at the dorsal root entry zone. Simple drainage is usually inadequate, even in cases where the pressure is clearly elevated. It would appear that the outcome of surgery is improved by insertion of a shunt tube into the syrinx cavity. Shunting to the subarachnoid space,[57] the peritoneum,[61] and the pleural space has been described; there is no consensus on which procedure is best. In the author's experience, syringo-pleural shunts seem to have the best outcome, most likely because the flow of fluid from the syrinx to the cavity in question is very slow and driven by very low pressure. Consequently, there is a tendency for the shunt tubing to become occluded, and it is felt that the negative pressure in the pleural space helps prevent such occlusion. Further study including a prospective, randomized trial is needed before definitive conclusions can be drawn about the success of surgery in the treatment of this condition.

A separate but related entity of posttraumatic myelomalacia has been described.[18] Often this diagnosis is simply based on the MRI appearance of the spinal cord in a patient with a previous traumatic injury to the cord. In such cases, cord atrophy, microcyst formation, and a heterogeneous signal within the cord substance are seen. At times, the distinction between syringomyelia and this entity can be difficult, as it may be difficult to distinguish between a single larger cyst and numerous microcysts that appear to be more or less confluent. A challenging patient is one with the MRI finding of posttraumatic myelomalacia, as described above, and the development of a progressive neurological deficit months to years after the injury, after a long period of time has elapsed with completely stable neurological deficits. Some feel that such late deterioration is due to a tethering of the spinal cord in local scar and advocate surgical intervention for neurolysis and placement of a dural patch graft.[18] Others feel that surgical intervention is futile and may often lead to a worsening of the preoperative deficit. No consensus exists, although most surgeons (including the author) consider surgical intervention to be a last resort in these patients.

Research and the Future

As research in the field of spinal cord injury has advanced and become more sophisticated, it has become increasingly apparent how complex the problem is and how many different factors must be considered. Strategies for early intervention have focused on neuroprotection, as well as interventions that consider vascularization and closure of the blood spinal cord barrier. At later times after injury, efforts have focused on stimulation of remyelination and axonal activity, axon regeneration at the site of injury, plasticity and reconnection strategies both at the site of injury and in areas distant from it, and replacement of lost neurons and/or glia. There is increasing appreciation for the temporal dimensions of injury, and for the fact that for any proposed intervention, there is a period of time during which it is most likely to be effective.

Windows for intervention are being more clearly defined, each with its own therapeutic strategies. Compression, hemorrhage, and vascular damage occur within seconds to minutes of the onset of injury, for which decompression and stabilization, as well as blood pressure control, are helpful. Within hours to days, edema, inflammation, necrosis, and apoptosis play important roles. At this point, different interventions are more likely to be successful. Steroids to control edema, cooling, steroids and immunosuppresion to control inflammation, and specific antiapoptotic drugs such as minocycline are under study.

Later on, the focus of intervention changes. At the stage of cavitation and glial scar formation, drugs that affect the extracellular matrix as and chondroitinase and decorin hold promise, as does artificial scaffolding with extracellular matrix proteins.

The role that glial scarring plays in inhibiting recovery should not be underestimated. The observation that axon growth fails within the glial scar has been known since the early twentieth century. Silver and Miller[48] have demonstrated that glial scar contains inhibitory proteoglycans. Bradbury et. al.[9] have shown that enzymatic degradation of acute scar proteoglycans promotes axon regeneration. Davies et al.[15] found that suppression of inflammation, astrogliosis, and multiple inhibitors promotes axon growth across acute spinal cord injuries. A number of scar-associated inhibitors of axon growth have been identified, which are rapidly expressed within 24 hours of injury, peaking about 8 days later.

At much later stages, research has focused on stimulating neural regeneration.[49] Strategies influencing axonal sprouting and guidance, remyelination, and increasing conductance are under intense studies. At this point, interventions with stem cells are considered.

There are a number of factors that prevent axon regeneration in human spinal cord. These include a lack of trophic factor support, intrinsic limitation of adult neuronal cells, and a number of myelin-associated inhibitors, such as Nogo-A and myelin-associated glycoprotein.[30] Strategies to promote axon regeneration include blockade of signaling from myelin-associated inhibitors, suppression of synthesis of enzymatic degradation of scan proteoglycans, bridging sites of injury with a variety of transplant constructs including biopolymers and biodegradable implants,[34] infusion of neurotropins at either the site of injury or in neuronal cell bodies, or increasing neuronal cAMP levels.

Considering the above factors, the effect of any one intervention is likely to be small, and if it is to be effective, the timing of treatment must be carefully considered. The motor and sensory outcomes to be measured should be chosen to be sensitive to the therapy applied. For example, if the therapy is expected to cause sprouting of the cervical spinal cord in the injured segment, the motor neurons of that segment must be tested.

Any successful trial in humans must carefully consider the heterogeneity of the mechanisms of injury and repair and the large number of factors that influence the outcome. Factors known to influence the outcome include the age of the patient, preexisting medical conditions, associated injuries and infection, hypoxia, hypotension, genetic polymorphisms, the spinal cord level of injury, variation in cord anatomy and blood supply, and the variety of medical and surgical treatments prior to and after the experimental therapy is administered.

Several large-scale clinical trials in human spinal cord injury have been completed. The NASCIS study with methylprednisolone has demonstrated an improved outcome with treatment.[7,8] Treatment with GM 1 ganglioside, while initially encouraging,[21,22] proved to be ineffective, as did blockade of *N*-methyl-D-glutamate (NMDA) glutamate receptors. Studies now underway include a study of surgical treatment of acute spinal cord injury, a study of Procord, an autologous activated macrophage therapy,[5,38,46] Cethrin, a recombinant protein that inactivates Rho,[29] and fampridine (4-AP), a potassium channel blocker.[60] Erythropoietin, a hematopoietic growth factor that stimulates proliferation and differentiation of erythroid precursor cells, is also known to stimulate neurotrophic activity in the central nervous system and is under intense study for use in spinal cord injury.[13] Other studies include transplantation of human fetal olfactory ensheathing glia to the site of injury,[26] transplantation of human autologous olfactory mucosa to the injury site, and use of autologous blood or neural-derived stem cells at the site of injury.[20]

The exponentially increasing level of sophistication and the appreciation for the complexities of spinal cord structure and function bode well for the future of research in this area. It is the author's belief that a significant intervention that alters the lives of spinal cord–injured patients will be available in the first half of this century.

ACKNOWLEDGMENTS

This work was supported in part by the Methodist Hospital Neurological Institute, the Henry J.N. Taub Fund for Neurosurgical Research, the George R. Robinson Foundation, and the Neurological Research Foundation.

REFERENCES

1. American Spinal Injury Association, International Medical Society of Paraplegia: International Standards for Neurological and Functional Classification of Spinal Cord Injury–Revised 1992. Chicago, ASIA/IMSOP, 1992.
2. Andrews BT, Weinstein PR, Rosenblum ML, Barbaro NM: Intradural arachnoid cysts of the spinal canal associated with intramedullary cyst. J Neurosurg 68:544–549, 1988.
3. Baskin DS: Treatment of spinal cord injury. In: Grotta J (ed): Management of the Acutely Ill Neurological Patient. New York, Churchill Livingstone, 1993, pp 75–91.
4. Baskin DS, Azordigan P: Non-neurological complications of spinal cord injury. In: Piepmeier JM (ed): The Outcome Following Traumatic Spinal Cord Injury. Mt. Kisco, NY, Futura, 1992, pp 119–138.
5. Bomstein Y, Marder JB, Vitner K, Smirnov I, Lisaey G, Butovsky O, Fulga V, Yoles E: Features of skin-coincubated macrophages that promote recovery from spinal cord injury. J Neuroimmunol 142(1–2):10–16, 2003.
6. Braakman R, Penning L: Injuries of the cervical spine. In: Vinken PJ, Bruyn GW (eds): Handbook of Clinical Neurology, vol 25. New York, Elsevier, 1996, pp 227–380.
7. Bracken MB, Shephard MJ, Collins WF, et al: A randomized, controlled trial of methylprednisolone or naloxone in the treatment of acute spinal cord injury. N Engl J Med 322:1405, 1990.
8. Bracken MB, Shephard MJ, Collins WF, et al: Methylprednisolone or naloxone treatment after acute spinal cord injury: 1-year follow-up data. J Neurosurg 76:23, 1992.
9. Bradbury EJ, Moon LD, Popat RJ, King VR, Bennett GS, Patel PN, Fawcett JW, McMahon SB: Chondroitinase ABC promotes functional recovery after spinal cord injury. Nature 416(6881):589–590, 2002.
10. Brown-Sequard CE: De la transmission des impressions sensitives par la moelle epiniere. CR Soc Biol 1:192–194, 1849.
11. Buller HR, Ockelford PA, Hull RD: Strategies of diagnosis and screening of deep venous thrombosis and pulmonary embolism. Neth J Surg 35:121–128, 1983.
12. Burney RE, Maio RF, Maynard F, et al: Incidence, characteristics, and outcome of spinal cord injury at trauma centers in North America. Arch Surg 128:596–599, 1992.

13. Celik M, Gokmen N, Erbayraktar S, Akhisaroglu M, Konakc S, Ulukus C, Genc S, Genc, Sagiroglu E, Cerami A, Brines M: Erythropoietin prevents motor neuron apoptosis and neurologic disability in experimental spinal cord ischemic injury. PNAS 99:2258–2263, 2002.
14. Chestnut RM, Marshall LF: Early assessment, transport, and management of patients with post-traumatic spinal instability. In: Cooper PR (ed): Management of Posttraumatic Spinal Instability. Parkridge, IL, American Association of Neurological Surgeons, 1990.
15. Davies JE, Tang X, Denning JW, Archibald SJ, Davies SJ: Decorin suppresses neurocan, brevican, phosphacan and NG2 expression and promotes axon growth across adult rat spinal cord injuries. Eur J Neurosci 19(5):1226–1242, 2004.
16. Dolan EJ, Tator CH, Endrenyi L: The value of decompression for acute experimental spinal cord compression injury. J Neurosurg 53:749–755, 1980.
17. Dykstra DD, Sidi AA: Treatment of detrusor-sphincter dyssynergia with botulinum a toxin: A double-blind study. Arch Phys Med Rehabil 71:24–26, 1990.
18. Falcone S, Quencer RM, Green BA, Patchen SJ, Post MJD: Progressive posttraumatic myelomalacic myelopathy: Imaging and clinical features. Am J Neuroradiol 15:747–754, 1994.
19. Flanders AE, Schaefer DM, Doan HT, et al: Acute cervical spine trauma: Correlation of MR imaging findings with degree of neurologic deficit. Radiology 177:25–33, 1990.
20. Galvin K, Jones D: Adult human neural stem cells for cell-replacement therapies in the central nervous system. Med J Aust 177:316–318, 2002.
21. Geisler FH, Dorsey FC, Colenaan WP: Recovery of motor function after spinal cord injury: A randomized placebo-controlled trial with GM-1 ganglioside. N Engl J Med 324:1829–1838, 1991.
22. Geisler FH, Dorsey FC, Coleman WP: GM-1 ganglioside in human spinal cord injury. J Neurotrauma 9(suppl): S165–S172, 1992.
23. Gunby P: New focus on spinal cord injury. JAMA 245: 1201, 1981.
24. Hansebout RR: A comprehensive review of methods of improving cord recovery after acute spinal cord injury. In: Tator CH (ed): Early Management of Acute Spinal Cord Injury. New York, Raven Press, 1982, pp 181–196.
25. Johnson RM, Hart DL, Simmons EF, et al: Cervical orthoses: A study comparing their effectiveness in restricting cervical motion in normal subjects. J Bone Joint Surg Am 59A:332, 1977.
26. Keyvan-Fouladi, N, Raisman G, Li Y: Development/plasticity/repair—functional repair of the corticospinal tract by delayed transplantation of olfactory ensheathing cells in adult rats. Neurosci 23(28):9428–9434, 2003.
27. Kraus JF: Injury to the head and spinal cord: The epidemiological relevance of the medical literature published from 1960 to 1978. J Neurosurg 53(suppl):S3–S10, 1980.
28a. Kraus JF, Franti CE, Riggins RS, et al: Incidence of traumatic spinal cord lesions. J Chronic Dis 28:471–492, 1975.
28b. McDonald JW, Sadowsky C: Spinal-cord injury. Lancet 359:417–425, 2002.
29. McKerracher L, Winton MJ: Targeting rho to stimulate repair after spinal cord injury. Top Spinal Cord Inj Rehabil 8(4):69–75, 2003.
30. Merkler D, Oertle T, Buss A, Pinschewer D, Schnell L, Bareyre F, Kerschensteiner M, Buddeberg B, Schwab M: Rapid induction of autoantibodies against Nogo-A and MOG in the absence of an encephalitogenic T cell response: Implication for immunotherapeutic approaches in neurological diseases. FASEB J express article 10.1096, published online October 16, 2003.
31. Mesard L, Carmody A, Mannarino E, et al: Survival after spinal cord trauma: A life table analysis. Arch Neurol 35:78, 1978.
32. Meyer GA, Berman IR, Doty DB, et al: Hemodynamic responses to acute quadriplegia with or without chest trauma. J Neurosurg 34:168, 1971.
33. Mielants H, Vanhove E, Neels J, et al: Clinical surgery of and pathogenic approach to paraarticular ossificans in long-term coma. Acta Orthop Scand 46:190–197, 1975.
34. Novikova LN, Novikov LN, Kellerth JO, Biopolymers and biodegradable smart implants for tissue regeneration after spinal cord injury. Curr Opin Neurol 16(6): 711–715, 2003.
35. Oiler DW, Boone S: Blunt cervical spine Brown-Sequard injury. Am Surg 57:361–365, 1991.
36. Pang D, Wilberger JE: Spinal cord injury without radiographic abnormalities in children. J Neurosurg 57:114–129, 1982.
37. Peacock WJ, Shrosbree RN, Key AG: A review of 450 stab wounds of the spinal cord. S Afr Med J 51:961–964, 1977.
38. Rapalino O, Lazarov-Spiegler O, Agranov E, Velan GJ, Yoles E, Fraidakis M, Solomon A, Gepstein R, Katz A, Belkin M, Hadani M, Schwartz M. Implantation of stimulated homologous macrophages results in partial recovery of paraplegic rats. Nature Med 4(7):814–821, 1998.
39. Rivlin AS, Tator CH: Effect of duration of spinal cord compression in a new acute injury model in the rat. Surg Neurol 10:39–43, 1978.
40. Roth EJ, Park T, Pang T, Yarkony GM, Lee MY: Traumatic cervical Brown-Sequard and Brown-Sequard plus syndromes: The spectrum of presentations and outcomes. Paraplegia 29:582–589, 1991.
41. Rumana CS, Baskin DS: Brown-Sequard syndrome produced by cervical disc herniation: Case report and literature review. Surg Neurol 45:359–361, 1996.
42. Schneider RC: A syndrome in acute cervical injuries for which early operation is indicated. J Neurosurg 8:360–367, 1951.
43. Schneider RC: Concomitant craniocerebral and spinal trauma with special reference to the cervicomedullary region. Clin Neurosurg 17:266–309, 1970.

44. Schneider RC, Cherry G, Pantek H: The syndrome of acute central cervical spinal cord injury. J Neurosurg 11:546–577, 1954.
45. Schneider RC, Crosby EC, Russo EH, et al: Traumatic spinal cord syndromes and their management. Clin Neurosurg 20:424–492, 1973.
46. Schwartz M: Helping the body to cure itself: Immune modulation by therapeutic vaccination for spinal cord injury. J Spinal Cord Med 26(suppl.):S6–S10, 2003.
47. Sellick BA: Cricoid pressure to control regurgitation of stomach contents during induction of anesthesia. Lancet 2:40–46, 1961.
48. Silver J, Miller JH. Regeneration beyond the glial scar. Nat Rev Neurosci 5(2):146–156, 2004.
49. Skaper SD, Leon A: Monosialogangliosides, neuroprotection, and neuronal repair processes. J Neurotrauma 9(suppl):S507–S516, 1992.
50. Sonntag VKH, Francis PM: Patient Selection and Timing of Surgery in Contemporary Management of Spinal Cord Injury. Park Ridge, IL, AANS Publication Committee, 1995, pp 97–107.
51. Squier MV, Lehr RP: Post-traumatic syringomyelia. J Neurol Neurosurg Psychiatry 57:1095–1098, 1994.
52. Stripling TE: The cost of economic consequences of traumatic spinal cord injury. Paraplegia News 8:50–54, 1990.
53. Sutherland MW: The prevention of violent spinal cord injuries. Spinal Cord Inj Nurs 10:91–95, 1993.
54. Tator CH: Epidemiology and general characteristics of the spinal cord injury patient. In: Benzel EC, Tator CH (eds): Contemporary Management of Spinal Cord Injury. Park Ridge, IL, AANS Publication Committee, 1995, pp 9–13.
55. Tator CH: Clinical manifestations of acute spinal cord injury. In: Benzel EC, Tator CH (eds): Contemporary Management of Spinal Cord Injury. Park Ridge, IL, AANS Publication Committee, 1995, pp 15–26.
56. Tator CH, Duncan EG, Edmonds VE, et al: Changes in epidemiology of acute spinal cord injury from 1947 to 1981. Surg Neurol 40:207–215, 1993.
57. Tator CH, Meguro K, Rowed DW: Favorable results with syringosubarachnoid shunts for treatment of syringomyelia. J Neurosurg 56:517–523, 1982.
58. Umbach I, Heilporn MD: Review article: Post-spinal cord injury syringomyelia. Paraplegia 29:219–221, 1991.
59. Van den Bergh R: Pathogenesis and treatment of delayed post-traumatic syringomyelia. Acta Neurochir 110:82–86, 1991.
60. Van der Bruggen MA, Huisman HB, Beckerman H, Bertelsmann FW, Polman CH, Lankhorst GJ: Randomized trial of 4-aminopyridine in patients with chronic incomplete spinal cord injury. J Neurol 248:665–671, 2001.
61. Vassilouthis J, Papandreou A, Anagnostaras S: Thecoperitoneal shunt for post-traumatic syringomyelia. J Neurol Neurosurg Psychiatry 57:755–756, 1994.
62. Vroemen M, Aigner L, Winkler J, Weidner N: Adult neural progenitor cell grafts survive after acute spinal cord injury and integrate along axonal pathways. Eur J Neurosci 18:743, 2003.
63. White AA, Panjabi MM: Clinical Biomechanics of the Spine. Philadelphia, JB Lippincott, 1978, p 345.

Chapter 15
Complications of Spinal Cord Injury

OKSANA VOLSHTEYN
AND JOHN W. McDONALD

The epidemiology of spinal cord injury (SCI) has been studied extensively over the past three decades. The most accurate epidemiological data are derived from the database of the National Spinal Cord Injury Statistical Center (NSCISC), established in 1973. To date, 25 federally funded Model Spinal Cord Injury Care Systems have contributed information to this SCI database, which contains nearly 23,000 cases of traumatic SCI.[81]

The estimated annual incidence of traumatic SCI injury in the United States is ~40 cases per million population, with ~11,000 new cases each year. The estimated prevalence is ~270,000 persons. Over the past decade, new trends in the etiology of SCI have emerged: a decrease in motor vehicle accidents (40.9%) and increases in violence (21.6%) and falls (22.4%). Nearly 60% of injuries occur in persons under age 30. The male:female ratio is 4:1.[81] Table 15.1 shows the distribution of neurological level and severity of injury.

Table 15.1. Neurological Level and Severity of Injury

Severity of Injury	Tetraplegia	Paraplegia
Complete	18.6	26.6
Incomplete	30.8	19.7

The estimated lifetime cost of treating an individual with traumatic SCI ranges from $500,000 to $2 million, depending on the severity of the neurological injury, associated medical complications, and age at the time of injury.[75] The life expectancy of individuals with SCI has been steadily increasing over the past decade because of advances in medical knowledge, improved quality of care, and new advanced rehabilitative therapies.

Spinal cord injury causes complex multisystem impairments. This chapter will focus on the most common medical complications and their management with traditional and advanced therapeutic approaches to rehabilitation. To achieve optimal outcomes, SCI patients should be managed in a specialized SCI rehabilitation center that offers a multidisciplinary rehabilitation team with the necessary expertise in SCI care, the required resources, and the technologically advanced equipment that can facilitate neurological recovery and optimize functional restoration.

Pulmonary Complications

Pulmonary complications in SCI are highly dependent on the neurological level of injury. Thus, cervical and upper thoracic lesions profoundly impact pulmonary function, whereas midthoracic and lumbar injuries have little or no effect.

Atelectasis, pneumonia, aspiration, mucus plugging, and failed ventilation are the most common causes of morbidity after SCI. Pneumonia remains the leading primary cause of death in this population.[23]

Patients with high tetraplegia at C1-C3 require mechanical ventilation because of bilateral paralysis of the diaphragm. In the absence of chest trauma, these patients do better if they are ventilated with high tidal volumes at low respiratory rates.[65] Tetraplegia at C4-C5 is usually associated with partial diaphragmatic and abdominal wall dysfunction leading to paradoxical breathing. Individuals with a high level of tetraplegia have a restrictive pattern of pulmonary dysfunction, with reduced chest wall and lung compliance and a decrease in all lung volumes except residual volume.[1] Parasympathetic activity is increased, causing bronchial constriction and overproduction of mucus, which leads to atelectasis. The presence of ileus, or of G-tube or gastroesophageal reflux, are risk factors for recurrent aspiration.[47]

Rehabilitation strategies for managing pulmonary complications in SCI patients include frequent suctioning, postural drainage, chest percussion and vibration, intermittent positive-pressure breathing, (IPPB), assisted coughing (*quad coughing*),[10] mechanical insufflation/exsufflation, incentive spirometry, and therapy with a beta agonist(s).

Patients with complete C3 and C4 neurological levels can be successfully weaned from mechanical ventilation by intermittent mandatory ventilation, pressure support ventilation, and progressive ventilator-free breathing.[3] For those who require lifelong respiratory support, the alternative to invasive translaryngeal intubation and tracheostomy is to use respiratory muscle aids to maintain alveolar ventilation and manage airway secretions. The main functions of respiratory muscle aids include applying mechanical forces directly to the body (rocking bed ventilators and intermittent abdominal pressure ventilators [IAPV]) and changing airway pressure intermittently (noninvasive IPPB). Oral IPPB through a mouthpiece is effective for total ventilation and usually does not interfere with eating, speaking, or operating a wheelchair unless a mouth stick is used for some activities. Nasal IPPB can be delivered through continuous positive airway pressure (CPAP) masks or bilevel positive airway pressure (BIPAP) machines.

Glossopharyngeal breathing (GPB) assists both inspiratory and expiratory effort. It is performed by pushing boluses of air through the outward movement of the glottis. Glossopharyngeal breathing is useful if the mechanical ventilator fails because it allows patients to sustain alveolar ventilation for some time. Expiratory muscle aids include manually assisted coughing, which is evoked by pushing in the upper abdominal area with the hand during expiration.[10] Mechanical insufflation-exsufflation is an effective method for producing adequate peak cough flows to help remove mucus plugs.

For patients with SCI above C3 and intact phrenic nerves, an implantable system for functional electrical stimulation (FES) of the phrenic nerve(s) can produce diaphragmatic contractions.[16,24,33,34] Phrenic nerve integrity is best evaluated by nerve conduction studies that assess both the conduction velocity and amplitude of the compound muscle action potential, a function of the diaphragmatic muscle mass.[49] The latter can be assessed by fluoroscopy during supramaximal stimulation of the phrenic nerve. As well as meeting physiological selection criteria, the patient needs to be psychologically stable and highly motivated, and must understand the potential risks and complications associated with implantation.[33,34] Benefits of this system include improved speech, transfers, and mobility; fewer respiratory tract infections; and an improved comfort level and a psychosocial sense of well-being.

The most common complications of phrenic nerve FES are mechanical failure of the implanted components, phrenic nerve injury during implantation, and scar formation. Most patients continue to require tracheostomy to clear excessive secretions. A backup mechanical ventilator is required in the event of system failure.[24,33] Phrenic nerve FES is an innovative way to manage respiratory impairment in tetraplegic patients and has significant advantages over traditional mechanical ventilation. However, the risks of the surgical procedure, post-implantation complications, and high cost remain limiting factors.

Cardiovascular Complications

Epidemiological studies in individuals with SCI demonstrated accelerated and premature coronary heart disease.[5,6,33,87] Cardiovascular disease is reported to be the most frequent cause of death among persons with SCI older than 30 years after injury (46%) and among those older than 60 years (35%).

Direct cardiovascular complications after SCI result from interruption of communication between the brain stem centers and the receptors and effectors in the heart and the vascular system.[60] There is also derangement of the autonomic nervous system leading to loss of coordination between sympathetic response and conditions demanding changes in heart rate and vascular tone.[2] Sympathetic innervation to the heart originates from T1-T5 and reaches the heart through the sympathetic chain branches. Splanchnic vasculature is innervated from the T5-T7 spinal cord segments. Parasympathetic innervation is provided through the vagus nerve, which originates in the medulla and innervates ventricles, sinoatrial and atrioventricular nodes and is intact in SCI patients. Activation of the sympathetic system increases the heart rate, causes vasoconstriction below the level of injury, and elevates arterial blood pressure.[52] Spinal cord injury at or above T6 (above the major splanchnic outflow) causes autonomic imbalance secondary to intact parasympathetic innervation and an impaired sympathetic response; these abnormalities lead to an exaggerated or hyperreflexic sympathetic reaction. Because of paralysis and the absence of muscular contractions in the lower extremities, venous return and cardiac output are diminished.[2]

Reduced central inhibition of spinal sympathetic outflow also impairs humoral mechanisms, resulting in elevated aldosterone levels and increased activity of angiotensin II and plasma rennin.[76] The higher the SCI lesion, the more severe the cardiovascular problems are. In the acute phase after SCI, patients suffer neurogenic shock, which presents as hypotension, bradycardia, and hypothermia and results from a reduction in the preload to the heart following loss of sympathetic tone and dilation of the venous vessels.[52] In patients with multiple traumas, hypovolemic shock is frequently an associated complication. The best approach is judicious fluid resuscitation and awareness of the risk of neurogenic pulmonary edema. For adequate tissue perfusion, it is important to maintain systolic blood pressure at around 90 mm Hg.[66]

Bradycardia results from the unopposed effect of the vagus nerve and disruption of cardiosympathetic influences. It is usually most pronounced within the first 3 weeks after SCI and generally resolves as spinal shock abates. It is important to avoid procedures that can stimulate an abnormal vagal response, such as suctioning, insertion of a nasogastric tube, and rapid changes in position, especially in high tetraplegic patients.[52] Usually, bradycardia in SCI patients does not require specific treatment, though atropine or permanent demand pacemakers may be required if it becomes severe and persistent.[29]

Orthostatic hypotension is common after SCI. It is usually most severe in the acute phase, though it can persist into more chronic phases. In chronic SCI, adaptation occurs through renal mechanisms and increased rennin secretion in response to position change; however, baseline pressure in patients with tetraplegia remains low—usually around 90/60 mm Hg. The baseline heart rate is also low (50–60/minute), exacerbating the problem.[66] Patients frequently complain of dizziness, blurred vision, palpitations, sweating above the level of the lesion, generalized weakness, and frequent fainting during positional changes, especially while in the shower or having a bowel movement on the toilet or commode. The best approach is prevention, which includes the use of compression garments, such as abdominal binders, elastic stockings, and Ace bandages wrapped around the lower extremities, as well as gradual mobilization of the patient during transfer activities. If an orthostatic episode occurs while a patient is in the wheelchair, tilting the wheelchair back usually stops symptom progression. Some patients will require pharmacological management with adrenergic alpha-agonist drugs such as ephedrine and proamatine (Midodrine), which increase vascular tone and elevate blood pressure by contracting the arterial and venous vascular beds. Fludrocortisone (Florinef) is a mineralocorticoid that promotes sodium and water retention, which expands the intravascular volume.[52] The rehabilitation team and caregivers should receive appropriate education so that such preventive measures can be implemented during day-to-day activities of SCI patients who experience orthostasis.

Thermoregulation is impaired in SCI patients because compromise of autonomic pathways to the hypothalamus causes either hyperthermia or hypothermia.[55] Mechanisms to increase the core body temperature include shivering and vasoconstriction, while sweating and vasodilation increase heat loss and reduce the core temperature. However, these mechanisms are impaired in SCI patients, who therefore assume the temperature of the environment, becoming poikilothermic. Tetraplegic patients should avoid extreme temperatures whenever possible and should be in a climate-controlled environment.

One of the most significant and potentially life-threatening cardiovascular complications of SCI is autonomic dysreflexia (AD), which results in a massive and uninhibited reflex sympathetic discharge in individuals with injuries above the T6 level. The incidence of AD varies from 48% to 85%.[20] It is triggered by various noxious stimuli below the level of neurological injury. It usually occurs when spinal shock resolves and the spinal-mediated sympathetic vasomotor reflexes return. There is unopposed sympathetic outflow since the sensory nerves transmitting impulses to the spinal cord are intact, while sympathetic inhibitory impulses originating above the T6 level are blocked as a result of SCI. This imbalance leads to significant vasoconstriction below the injury level, elevating the blood pressure. Associated tachycardia is usually down-regulated by a vagal response, often producing bradycardia.[20] The causes of AD are numerous, but the most common triggers are listed in Table 15.2.

Table 15.2. Most Common Causes of Autonomic Dysreflexia

Urological	Bladder overdistention, catheter plugging, urethral distention, urological manipulations, urinary tract infection, bladder or renal calculi, epididymitis
Gastrointestinal	Fecal impaction, bowel distention, ileus, gastroesophageal reflux, gallstones, gastric ulcers, hemorrhoids, or any acute abdominal pathology
Dermatological	Ingrown toenails, pressure ulcers, burns, restrictive clothing
Musculoskeletal	Fractures, heterotopic ossification, acute tendinitis, stretching of spastic muscles
Cardiopulmonary	Deep vein thrombosis, pulmonary embolism, pneumonia, angina
Gynecological	Uterine contractions, pelvic exam, sexual intercourse

Clinical symptoms of dysreflexia are pounding headache, a rise in blood pressure (20–40 mm Hg above the normal baseline), bradycardia, profuse sweating, piloerection and flushed skin above the injury level, blurred vision, nasal congestion, and feelings of anxiety and apprehension. Blood pressure elevation is the most significant complication of AD because it can lead to intracranial hemorrhage, seizures, myocardial infarction, and, potentially, death.[20]

Autonomic dysreflexia should be treated as a medical emergency; therefore, treatment should be initiated immediately. All vital signs should be continuously monitored. A patient who is supine needs to be immediately helped to sit up, and all constrictive clothing must be removed or loosened. Potential sites of noxious stimuli should be identified, beginning with the urinary system, since that is the most common cause of AD. If the patient is on a catheterization program, the bladder needs to be catheterized after instillation of 2% lidocaine in the urethra to avoid additional stimuli caused by advancement of the catheter. If the patient has an indwelling catheter, it needs to be checked for kinking or blockage. If the catheter is not draining, it is best to remove it and catheterize the bladder. Otherwise, irrigation should be performed gently and with small amounts of fluid at body temperature to avoid further overdistending the bladder and aggravating the symptoms of AD. If the urinary system is intact, the second most common cause of AD is fecal impaction. The rectal wall should be lubricated with lidocaine gel for up to 5 minutes before performing a gentle rectal exam. If stool is present, it needs to be gently removed. If symptoms of AD persist and blood pressure remains elevated, pharmacological management should be considered. It is advisable to use antihypertensive medications with rapid onset of action and short duration while further causes of AD are being identified. Topical and sublingual nitrates are appropriate initial drugs of choice. One inch of 2% nitroglycerin paste is applied to the chest above the level of injury. Topically applied nitroglycerin has the advantage of being easily removed if blood pressure falls precipitously. Another drug of choice is nifedipine 10 mg, administered to bite and swallow. If needed, the dose can be repeated every 15 minutes until blood pressure is controlled. Other agents can also be used, including phenoxybenzamine, diazoxide, mecamylamine, and hydralazine.[20]

Patients with episodes of severe dysreflexia that respond poorly to the above measures need to be admitted to the hospital for further management and workup. Usually, an intravenous drip of sodium nitroprusside applied under close monitoring in the intensive care unit is effective.

As with many other complications after SCI, prevention is the best management. Educating patients, family members, and emergency room physicians is critical for identifying early symptoms and proper management. For patients with recurrent episodes of dysreflexia associated with the bowel routine or sexual intercourse, prophylaxis with medication is warranted.

Cardiovascular Response to Exercise

Patients with SCI have an impaired cardiovascular response to exercise.[26] Even though their heart rate and oxygen uptake increase, they do not reach the same parameters as people without SCI. Moreover, the response to exercise is even more impaired in patients with tetraplegia than in those with paraplegia. After SCI, especially in patients with high complete tetraplegia, there is reduced central nervous system vasoconstrictor efferent output, which decreases venous return and reduces end-diastolic ventricular volume. At the same time, heart rate and myocardial contractility increase only marginally. Obviously, these deficits reduce cardiac performance and contribute to exercise intolerance in the population with SCI.[26] Patients with SCI who engage in athletic activities practice *boosting* to improve their performance—intentionally increasing blood pressure and inducing hyperreflexia.[15]

Thromboembolism after Spinal Cord Injury

Deep venous thrombosis (DVT) and pulmonary embolism (PE) are common complications after SCI, and they continue to be major causes of morbidity in this population. The incidence of DVT ranges from 23% to 100%, being greatest within the first 2 weeks after SCI. In the acute rehabilitation setting, DVT occurs in nearly 10% of patients and PE in 2.6%.[17]

Greater awareness of thromboembolism after SCI, more advanced diagnostic techniques, and early treatment have significantly reduced morbidity and mortality in the SCI population. Options for diagnosing DVT include Doppler ultrasound, which is noninvasive and has high sensitivity for proximal DVT. Although it compares favorably with venography and is commonly used to diagnose DVT, its accuracy is highly dependent on the expertise of the technician. The I-125 fibrinogen scan has greater sensitivity for calf vein DVT, though it is used infrequently in the clinical setting.[19] Venography remains the gold standard, but it is invasive and carries side effects (phlebitis, an allergic reaction).

A number of risk factors contribute to the development of DVT in SCI patients. They include obesity, trauma to the pelvis and lower extremities, congestive heart failure, a history of malignancy, and previous thromboembolism.[71]

Diagnosis of PE is frequently delayed in patients with SCI because of a nonspecific presentation.[19] Frequently, initial symptoms are similar to those of pneumonia or atelectasis. However, clinical suspicion should be very high in the population with SCI, since PE is associated with very high mortality if diagnosis is delayed. A ventilation-perfusion (VQ) lung scan is the diagnostic test of choice. The diagnosis is based on a mismatch between blood flow and airway ventilation. The accuracy of VQ scanning exceeds 90% when high-probability scans accompany high clinical suspicion.[82] Pulmonary angiography is considered the gold standard for diagnosing PE, but it is invasive and is usually recommended only when there is a high clinical suspicion in patients with complex injuries.[19] Recently, spiral computed tomography (CT) has been used to diagnose PE, especially when angiography is unavailable or contraindicated.

Given that thromboembolism is a significant issue in SCI patients, early implementation of preventive measures is critical. Prophylaxis should be started within 72 hours after injury and should include high-grade compression stockings, pneumatic compression sleeves, early patient mobilization such as passive range-of-motion exercises, out-of-bed mobility exercises, electrical stimulation for lower extremity ankle dorsiflexion and plantar flexion, and pharmacological prophylaxis with either low molecular weight heparin or unfractionated heparin.[70] Placement of vena cava filters is indicated for PE prevention in high-risk patients.

However, this procedure is usually reserved for patients with contraindications to anticoagulation prophylaxis, those with a history of PE, or high-risk trauma patients with extensive chest and lower extremity injuries. The most significant complications of filters include thrombosis, perforation, and filter migration.[44]

The Consortium for Spinal Cord Medicine has established guidelines for preventing thromboembolism after SCI. These guidelines consider the desired intensity of prophylaxis based on SCI severity (complete vs. incomplete) and the presence of other risk factors. In general, pneumatic compression sleeves should be used for 2 weeks after injury. For motor incomplete injuries, anticoagulation should continue for 8 weeks for American Spinal Injury Association (ASIA) Class C patients and during hospitalization for ASIA Class D patients. For patients with more complete injuries, anticoagulation should continue for at least 8 weeks. For those with complete injuries with high risks, especially tetraplegia, anticoagulation should continue for 12 weeks.[19]

Thromboembolism prophylaxis should also be initiated if patients with chronic SCI are readmitted to the hospital with an acute medical condition that necessitates prolonged bed rest or if they undergo surgical procedures.

Metabolic and Endocrine Changes after Spinal Cord Injury

Spinal cord injury impacts the endocrine system and leads to a number of metabolic changes.

Changes in *carbohydrate metabolism* are consistent with glucose intolerance secondary to reduction of glucose uptake by peripheral tissues. It has been reported that patients with complete tetraplegia have significantly lower carbohydrate tolerance than those with incomplete tetraplegia or paraplegia.[6] Impaired glucose tolerance is usually associated with insulin resistance.[4] It is unknown whether this leads to diabetes in patients with SCI. Since insulin works predominantly at the muscle level, paralysis of the muscles, especially skeletal muscle denervation, and prolonged inactivity causing loss of lean body mass and obesity are likely primary causes for insulin resistance.[87] Individuals with SCI who are genetically predisposed to diabetes and are glucose intolerant should be closely monitored for the development of diabetes.[4,6] Management is similar to that in the population without SCI. Diet, medications, and an appropriate level of physical activity should be part of the treatment strategy.

Lipid metabolism is also impaired after SCI, leading to accelerated cardiovascular disease. From 24% to 40% of patients with SCI have a low level of high-density lipoprotein (HDL) compared with 10% of the general population.[4] Patients with motor complete injuries have lower levels of serum HDL than those with incomplete injuries, and HDL level is related inversely to triglyceride level.[87] Decreased HDL in patients with SCI is also associated with increased body mass index.

The goal of treating hyperlipidemia is to reduce the morbidity and mortality associated with coronary heart disease. A complete lipid profile should be obtained annually, and risk factors for coronary artery disease should be identified, especially a family history of premature heart disease, hypertension, cigarette smoking, and diabetes. A low-fat, low-cholesterol diet should be implemented and continued indefinitely. Guidelines for using pharmacological agents to lower serum low-density lipoprotein (LDL) and triglycerides are similar as those for the population without SCI. Acid binding resins are probably not a good choice for patients with SCI because they increase constipation and abdominal flatulence and interfere with the absorption of nutrients and medications. An exercise program should be part of any comprehensive management of patients with SCI. Improved cardiopulmonary fitness has been shown to increase serum HDL levels in this population and should be part of any long-term physical fitness program.[4,6] Abstinence from alcohol is beneficial, as is smoking cessation.

Several *endocrine changes* also occur after spinal cord injury.[35] Acute SCI may be associated with a reduction in serum triiodothyronine (T3), resulting in *low T3 syndrome*.[67] It has been reported that both T3 and thyroxine (T4) levels remain depressed 6 months after traumatic tetraplegia. Levels of thyroid stimulating hormone (TSH), however, are usually within the normal range, indicating a euthyroid state. The current consensus is that low T3 syndrome does not require replacement treatment, though the patient might present with symptoms suggesting hypothyroidism.[14] This syndrome can also be seen in patients with active medical conditions such as urinary tract infection, pulmonary infection, and pressure ulcers.

Spinal cord injury also affects *anabolic hormones*, particularly testosterone and growth hormone.[84] In some patients, an absolute androgen deficiency state is observed. The etiology of testosterone deficiency after SCI is not clear, though prolonged sitting and an elevated temperature of the scrotal sac and testes certainly can produce a local effect on testosterone production. In the population with SCI, the testosterone level usually does not decrease with age; however, it decreases significantly with the duration of injury. No associated elevation of gonadotropin is found.[84]

Growth hormone is also reported to be decreased in individuals with SCI, and levels are lower in nonambulatory patients than in those who ambulate. It is possible that a decreased growth hormone level negatively affects patients' functional abilities.[84] Replacement of growth hormone reduces fat mass, increases lean body tissue, lowers LDL, and elevates HDL, thus reducing the cardiovascular risk.[84]

There is a direct relationship between serum growth hormone and serum total testosterone, with mutual potentiation. Replacement therapy for testosterone usually improves body composition, particularly by reducing fat mass and increasing lean body mass.[84,87] In young individuals, however, testosterone replacement has been associated with an adverse lipid profile, though in older individuals it decreased LDL without significantly changing serum levels of HDL.[6]

Another anabolic steroid, oxandrolone, has been shown to increase the diaphragm mass, which improves pulmonary function in subjects with tetraplegia. It also accelerates healing of refractory pressure ulcers.[6] However, caution should always be exercised when using anabolic steroids, which generally are associated with hepatotoxicity and adversely affect lipid profiles. Nevertheless, a brief therapeutic trial for a patient population with a specific SCI injury could be beneficial.

Awareness of metabolic abnormalities after SCI is extremely important in improving the quality of care. Timely implementation of proper therapies, including a lifelong exercise program, reduces morbidity and improves survival and the quality of life.

Pressure Ulcers

Patients with SCI are at significant risk for pressure ulcers, which are defined as localized areas of tissue necrosis that develop when soft tissue is compressed between a bony prominence and an external surface for a prolonged period. The incidence and prevalence of pressure ulcers depend upon patient-care settings. It has been reported that pressure ulcers develop in up to 40% of SCI patients during initial acute care and rehabilitation and in up to 30% in each 5 years thereafter.[46,53] The prevalence is high in complete injury compared with incomplete injury and in tetraplegia compared with paraplegia. The cost of treating pressure ulcers is estimated at more than $70,000 for complex full-thickness pressure ulcers and up to $30,000 for less serious ulcers.[9]

The etiology of pressure ulcers is multidimensional. Tissue ischemia and skin breakdown result from direct pressure on bony prominences that exceeds capillary pressure. Shearing, friction, maceration, elevated tissue temperature, and moisture compromise tissue further. Other contributory factors include poor nutrition, anemia, contractures, spasticity, urinary and fecal incontinence, decreased mobility, and smoking.[9,68,89] During acute rehabilitation, pressure ulcers are most commonly found over the sacrum, followed by the heels and ischium. In the chronic phase, they are more common over the sacrum, followed by the ischium, heels, and trochanter.

To develop a proper treatment plan, it is important to accurately assess a pressure ulcer. Its dimensions should be measured, including areas of undermining, tunneling, and tracks. Surrounding tissue should be evaluated to establish the extent of induration, capillary refill, and warmth. The extent of tissue necrosis, the color, and the odor of the exudate should be described. At times, x-rays or CT, magnetic resonance imaging (MRI) or bone scans are needed to define the depth and severity of the wound, especially if osteomyelitis is suspected. Table 15.3 shows the classification of pressure ulcers recommended by the National Pressure Ulcer Advisory Panel.

Treatment should include management of general health issues, local wound treatment, and use of overlay surfaces to reduce pressure and shearing forces. For general medical management, it

Table 15.3. Classification of Pressure Ulcers

Pressure Ulcer Stage	Description
Stage I	Nonblanching erythema of anatomically intact skin
Stage II	Partial-thickness skin loss involving epidermis and dermis
Stage III	Full-thickness skin loss including subcutaneous tissue, but not through underlying fascia
Stage IV	Full-thickness skin loss with destruction of the fascia, muscle, bone, or joint

Table 15.4. Dressings for Pressure Ulcers

Dressing Type	Indication for use
Transparent polymeric membrane dressings	Nondraining, clean, granulating wounds; allow oxygen exchange, prevent bacterial entry, promote epithelial migration, and reduce shear and friction
Hydrocolloids	Provide occlusive barrier, form gels with wound exudate, create moist wound environment, aid autolytic debridement, and appropriate for wounds with minimal to moderate exudate
Polymeric foam dressings	Provide high absorbency and indicated for moderatly to heavily exudating wounds; do not adhere to the wound and can be used with other topical agents
Hydrogels dressings	Provide primary wound covering, require secondary dressing, maintain moist wound; indicated for dry wounds or those with minimal drainage
Alginate dressings	Highly hydrophilic, converts to gel, used for moderately to heavily exudating wounds.

is important to provide aggressive nutritional support, especially adequate protein intake (1.25–1.5 g/kg), to treat anemia, and to provide vitamin and mineral supplements, especially vitamin A, vitamin C and zinc, which promote collagen synthesis and stimulate the growth of epithelial tissue, thus facilitating wound healing.[62] Local management of pressure ulcers is based on the principle of maintaining a wound that is clean, moist, and appropriately debrided. Sharp debridement is the most effective method and is indicated when the wound contains necrotic tissue. Enzymatic and autolytic processes can also be used for debridement; however, they are much slower and selective and are contraindicated when the wound is infected. Acetic acid, hydrogen peroxide, iodine, and bleach solutions are no longer considered appropriate for wound care, except for briefly reducing the bacterial load, since they impair fibroblast formation and wound healing. The wet-to-dry method for mechanical debridement of necrotic tissue is still widely used, given its simplicity and low cost.

The choice of wound dressing should be based on wound stage and the amount of exudate. Various commercially available wound dressings are listed in Table 15.4. Several adjunctive treatments for pressure ulcers are available: electrical stimulation, vacuum-assisted closure (wound VAC), and hydrotherapy.

Chronic Stage III and IV pressure wounds may require surgical intervention. The following procedures are available: split-thickness skin grafts, fasciacutaneous flaps, myocutaneous flaps, and skin grafts.[68] The success of such surgery is highly dependent on postoperative care, proper nutrition, and management of comorbid conditions.[77] Specialty beds and proper positioning are critical, and a *sitting protocol* should be initiated when sitting is resumed.

When wound infection is suspected, the granulation tissue within the wound should be biopsied to confirm infection and determine which systemic antibiotics would be appropriate. Topical silver sulfadiazine can be applied to the wound to help reduce the bacterial load. Osteomyelitis can be confirmed only by bone biopsy.

Prevention of skin ulcers is the best treatment. Therefore, daily skin inspection is essential. All patients at high risk for skin breakdown should use appropriate wheelchair cushions, bed overlays, and specialty beds.[11] Pressure should be relieved every 15 minutes while patients are sitting in a wheelchair. While in bed, a patient's position needs to be changed every 2–3 hours. Excessive moisture and exposure of the skin to urine or stool should be addressed immediately. Special precautions should be taken when a patient is traveling or is in an unfamiliar environment. Sun exposure should be limited, and dry skin should be avoided. Educating patients about preventing pressure ulcers is essential for long-term success.

Musculoskeletal Impairment

Spinal cord injury leads to widespread morphological changes in skeletal muscle below the injury level. Thus, metabolic and contractile changes in muscle fibers lead to muscle fiber atrophy, focal degeneration, and impairment of capillary flow. Within a few months after SCI, muscle fiber atrophy is predominantly Type I. Six to 8 months after the injury, however, it shifts to Type II due to fiber remodeling and plasticity.[37,80] Understanding these changes allows proper selection of the most appropriate rehabilitative program for patients with SCI.

Changes in Bone Metabolism

Spinal cord injury leads to significant bone loss, with subsequent osteoporosis, though the exact etiology is unclear. Immobilization as a result of paralysis and rapid bone turnover secondary to increased bone resorption significantly elevate serum calcium (hypercalcemia) and increase urinary calcium (hypercalciuria). This phenomenon, immobilization hypercalcemia, can present as an acute medical emergency, especially in male adolescents and young adults who usually have a large active bone mass.[51] When serum calcium rises above a certain level—usually about 12 mg/dl—these patients present with acute onset of abdominal pain, nausea and vomiting, behavioral changes, and progressive lethargy.

Management of clinically symptomatic hypercalcemia includes adequate hydration and thiazide diuretics such as furosemide to increase urinary excretion of calcium. Medications that reduce bone resorption by suppressing osteoclastic activity are also indicated (calcitonin, mitomycin, biphosphonates). Intravenous use of pamidronate 60–90 mg administered over 4 hours usually resolves hypercalcemia.[58] Untreated hypercalcemia can cause nephrocalcinosis, urolithiasis, and renal failure.

Osteoporosis

The specific mechanism of osteoporosis after SCI is unclear. Most likely, it is multifactorial and includes immobilization and a significant increase in osteoclastic activity with only a slight increase in osteoblastic activity.[63] Increased bone resorption increases the serum ionized calcium level, suppressing parathyroid hormone and likely causing secondary vitamin D deficiency, which also may be an important contributor to osteoporosis after SCI.[6,85] Whether a specific neurogenic effect causes bone hyperresorption and osteoporosis after SCI remains unclear. Other factors, such as loss of active muscle traction on bone and reduced absorption of calcium from the gastrointestinal tract, further enhance bone loss.

The extent of bone loss correlates with the severity of SCI: greater with complete than incomplete SCI and greater with longer time since injury than with shorter time. Approximately 30% of bone loss occurs within the first 4 months after SCI, but bone density continues to decline significantly over the following 2 to 3 years. More rapid loss occurs in the distal femur and proximal tibia, followed by the femoral neck and midshaft.[27] No significant loss from vertebral bone has been reported, probably because the spine continues to bear weight as patients sit in a wheelchair.

Progressive bone loss continues slowly during the 10 years after injury, reaching more than 50% of total bone content in the distal bones of the lower extremities, especially in the proximal and distal tibia and calcaneus.[6,63,74] The most significant complication of osteoporosis is long bone fractures. It is important to quantify the severity of osteoporosis and follow it over time. The most commonly used diagnostic test is bone density dual energy x-ray absorptiometry (DEXA).

Treatment of osteoporosis after SCI has not been successful, though there are a number of promising therapies: early mobilization; weight-bearing exercises such as standing in a standing frame; ambulation with lower extremity orthoses; and treadmill walking using either partial weight-supported systems or robotic devices. The latter allows autoambulation through passive mobilization of the lower extremities with a reciprocating alternating pattern resembling stepping. Functional electrical stimulation (FES) has been shown to significantly retard bone loss,[7,8] and it can be used in association with cycling or ambulation (Table 15.5). These treatments are effective if they are introduced early in the rehabilitation program and continue for months after the injury with a consistent intensity of training.[28,30,36,40]

No pharmacological treatment can restore lost bone mass in patients with SCI. However, drugs

Table 15.5. Functional Electrical Stimulation Application for Mobility in Patients with Spinal Cord Injury

Stationary leg-cycle ergometer—ERGYS, StimMaster
Surface electrical stimulation for standing and stepping—Parastep system
Functional nerve stimulation—FNS-Hybrid orthoses
Implantable systems for standing, transfers, and stepping

that reduce osteoclast activity and inhibit bone resorption are promising. The parathyroid hormone teriparatide, which promotes new bone formation, is another option. Calcium and vitamin D supplementation should also be part of treatment.

Preventing and treating osteoporosis in patients with SCI most likely will require multiple approaches: early implementation of pharmacological therapy and rehabilitative programs that include aggressive FES and weight-bearing activities.

Heterotopic Ossification

Heterotopic ossification (HO) is the formation of mature bone in soft tissue surrounding joints. In SCI patients, it occurs below the neurological level of injury. The incidence of HO is 16% to 53%, and 30% of cases are considered clinically significant.

The pathophysiology of HO is not well understood. It is believed to be initiated by unknown triggers that prompt pluripotential mesenchymal stem cells to change into osteoprogenitor cell lines that further differentiate into osteoblasts within adipose and muscle tissue. Risk factors include local trauma that causes soft tissue inflammation, hypoxia, and necrosis; spasticity; pressure ulcers; complete SCI; and age over 30. In most cases, HO begins between 4 and 12 weeks after injury. The most common location is the hip region followed by the knee, shoulder, and elbow. Clinically, HO presents as decreased range of motion, swelling, tenderness, erythema, and pain in the involved area. Differential diagnoses should include DVT, cellulitis, abscess, fracture, and hematoma.

A triple-phase bone scan is essential for early diagnosis. It becomes positive 2 to 4 weeks after injury. The first two phases are the most sensitive indicators of HO. The scan usually returns to normal when HO matures at 12 to 18 months after injury.

Serum alkaline phosphatase (AP), a marker for osteoblastic activity, rises early, peaks ~10 weeks after injury, and returns to normal when HO matures. However, the AP level is not specific for HO and does not always correlate with HO activity. Plain x-rays are not sensitive in the early stages, since they require the presence of calcification. They usually become positive 6 to 8 weeks after injury.

Ultrasound may be used as an early diagnostic tool and is usually positive before x-rays. Other diagnostic studies, such as CT scans, can be useful for evaluating the volume of the bone mass at later stages if surgery is planned.

Once HO is diagnosed, early pharmacological intervention should be initiated. Nonsteroidal anti-inflammatory drugs (NSAIDs) are helpful during the initial osteoid stage, especially when significant soft tissue erythema, swelling, and tenderness are present. Biphosphonates, especially etidronate disodium (Didronel), are effective in the mineralization stage, preventing the conversion of amorphous calcium phosphate to hydroxyapatite crystals. Didronel has anti-inflammatory effects as well because it reduces cytokine production. The recommended starting oral dose is 20 mg/kg/day for 2 weeks, followed by 10 mg/kg/day for up to 6 months or longer to prevent a rebound of HO. The most common side effects of Didronel are nausea, vomiting, and diarrhea, which usually are reduced if the medication is given in divided doses. An intravenous loading dose of 300 mg etidronate disodium/day for the first 3 days, followed by oral therapy as stated above, is more effective for reducing early symptoms and inhibiting mineralization. Radiation therapy, of 10 to 20 Gy dose, has been shown to arrest the progression of HO with no significant side effects.

Surgical intervention is appropriate only in the minority of patients (3% to 5%) whose HO is so severe that it results in joint ankylosis. Indications for surgical intervention include neurovascular compromise by massive HO and significant functional limitation in mobility and self-care. Goals are to improve the patient's positioning, sitting, grooming, hygiene, and dressing. Unfortunately, HO recurs frequently after surgical resection, so it is important to implement appropriate treatment with NSAIDs, radiation, and etidronate disodium for 3 to 6 months postoperatively.

A rehabilitation program must be an integral part of the management of HO. Physical therapy should include gentle range-of-motion and stretching exercises, and dynamic and static bracing should be used to maintain a functional range of motion.

Neurogenic Bladder

Management of neurogenic bladder is one of the most important issues to be addressed during both the acute and chronic phases of SCI.[41] This lifelong issue is correlated strongly with the perceived quality of life.[39]

Over the past several decades, there has been a significant reduction in mortality associated with renal complications in SCI patients. Introduction of intermittent catheterization, use of diagnostic urodynamic studies, and more aggressive management of urinary tract infections are credited.[86] However, morbidity due to neurogenic bladder remains high and contributes to more than 30% of readmissions to acute care hospitals.[45]

Management of neurogenic bladder immediately after SCI is best achieved with an indwelling urethral catheter. During this phase, patients are still in spinal shock and are frequently medically and hemodynamically unstable. Once their medical condition stabilizes, they no longer require a significant volume of IV fluids to maintain adequate hydration and electrolyte balance, and their total urinary output is less than 2000 cc over 24 hours, intermittent catheterization should be initiated. However, prolonged use of an indwelling catheter carries the risk of urinary tract infections and early antibiotic resistance.[83]

Spinal cord injury above the sacral micturition center usually results in an upper motor neuron (UMN) hyperreflexic bladder pattern characterized by small capacity, reduced compliance, uninhibited detrusor contractions, and elevated detrusor and intravesical pressure. Detrusor sphincter dyssynergia (DSD) is often observed. It causes a functional obstruction to urinary flow, which results in poor detrusor emptying and high detrusor pressure. Sustained high detrusor pressure causes deterioration of the upper urinary tract, with hydronephrosis and subsequent renal failure. Detrusor sphincter dyssinergia is more marked in complete injury than in incomplete injury and in male than in female SCI patients.

Sacral SCI results in lower motor neuron (LMN) areflexic detrusor of large capacity and overflow incontinence. Because the external urethral sphincter is also flaccid and the bladder neck is usually open, patients are highly susceptible to stress incontinence.

Patients with incomplete SCI have various patterns of voiding dysfunction. While considering a particular method for managing neurogenic bladder, it is important to remember that the dynamics of the urinary system change over time after injury. It may take up to 12 months to establish a stable pattern of voiding.

Intermittent catheterization (IC) has become the standard of care for managing neurogenic bladder. It is usually performed every 4–6 hours to achieve a bladder volume of 300–500 cc with each catheterization. Fluid intake should be reduced after dinner to prevent bladder overdistention during the night. During hospitalization, sterile technique is preferred for IC; however, clean self-intermittent technique does not produce significantly more infections if the patient is in a private room. In the home, the clean catheterization technique has essentially become the standard of care.

When an IC program is initiated, it is critical that the patient and family members receive appropriate education regarding bladder physiology, catheterization technique, catheter management, and potential complications. The patient's compliance is a significant factor in successful bladder management.

Many patients are able to achieve adequate bladder emptying by reflex voiding. However, this method carries a high risk of complications, such as vesicoureteral reflux and hydronephrosis, due to sustained elevation of detrusor pressure and substantial postvoid residuals. Urodynamic studies are important to assess reflex voiding and provide critical guidance in management.

Specific cutaneous reflex triggers can facilitate the voiding reflex: light tapping of the lower abdomen, scratching the inner thigh, or pulling the pubic hair. These triggers should be used every time voiding occurs. This method synchronizes, strengthens, and habituates the detrusor reflex, allowing the patient to empty the bladder more completely. Continence is maintained by collecting urine in external catheters.

For LMN bladder, Valsalva and Crede maneuvers facilitate bladder emptying by increasing intra-abdominal pressure.

Patients who are unable to perform self-catheterization frequently choose urethral or suprapubic indwelling catheters for long-term management. Complications include a high incidence of urinary tract infections, bladder calculi, incontinence around the catheter, bladder spasms, urethral erosions, fistulas, and a high incidence of squamous cell carcinoma of the bladder.[45] Other options include surgical or laser sphincterotomy in male patients, especially if DSD is present.[41] After sphincterotomy, 70% to 90% of patients have improved bladder emptying. Stent placement at the level of the proximal urethra has also been used to reduce sphincter resistance to urinary outflow.[73]

Botulinum toxin injected into the detrusor muscle or sphincter has been found effective for managing high-pressure hyperreflexic bladder and DSD.[25] Urinary diversion, augmentation cystoplasty, detrusor myomectomy, and continent and incontinent urostomies are more complex alternative surgical procedures[38] that are usually reserved for patients who have persistent and progressive hydronephrosis or recurrent pyelonephritis with sepsis and in whom all other therapies have failed. The approach to LMN bladder may include periurethral injection of collagen or Teflon, surgical implantation of an artificial sphincter, and fascia bladder neck sling procedures.

Bladder neuroprostheses are available for more advanced management of UMN neurogenic bladder. These prostheses use FES of the detrusor to initiate micturition on demand.[42] Commercially available systems were first introduced in Europe (Finetech-Brindley stimulator). In the United States, the Food and Drug Administration approved the VoCare System in 1998. This implantable FES system is indicated for patients with complete SCI above the sacral segments, and it requires intact peripheral innervation to the bladder. Implantation requires additional procedures, including laminectomy L3-S2 and dorsal selective rhizotomy S2-S5 to inhibit sensory input from the bladder and eliminate the afferent pathway of voiding reflex. Benefits and disadvantages of the VoCare system are listed in Table 15.6. This system is more appropriate for female patients with complete paraplegia who are able to use a wheelchair for mobility and for activities of daily living.

The type of pharmacology used to manage neurogenic bladder depends on the pattern of urinary dysfunction. For patients who have detrusor hyperreflexia, anticholinergic drugs that block parasympathetic postganglionic receptors are indicated. The most commonly used drugs are oxybutynin, tolterodine, hyoscyamine, imipramine, and propantheline.

Table 15.6. VoCare System Benefits and Disadvantages

Benefits	Disadvantages
Voiding on demand	Need for major surgery
Increased bladder capacity	Loss of reflex erection and ejaculation
Elimination of incontinence	Loss of sensation in sacral dermatomes
Improved bladder emptying	Decreased bowel motility
Decreased urinary tract infections	
Elimination of detrusor shincter dyssinergia	
Decreased episodes of autonomic dysreflexia	
Prevention of upper urinary tract complications	
Improved quality of life	

When using anticholinergic drugs, it is preferable to use extended-release preparations, which have fewer side effects and comparable efficacy. The most significant side effects include dry mouth, blurred vision, constipation, dizziness, headache, and somnolence.

For patients with significant DSD, alpha-adrenergic antagonists that reduce internal sphincter tone are indicated. They include terazosin, tamsulosin, prazosin, and phenoxybenzamine. Antispasticity drugs such as baclofen, diazepam, and dantrolene might be of value to those with severe spasticity of perineal muscles.

For a hyporeflexic bladder, pharmacological management is limited. Bethanechol chloride, a cholinergic agonist, has only a limited effect on detrusor contractility in SCI. Sphincter resistance can be increased with alpha-adrenergic agonists such as ephedrine, pseudoephedrine, and phenylpropanolamine. These drugs are not very effective, however, and their side effects include high blood pressure, tremor, cardiac arrhythmias and palpitations, anxiety, and insomnia.

Before designing a specific rehabilitation program for managing neurogenic bladder, it is important to obtain a premorbid urological history, perform a thorough physical examination, establish the type of neurological bladder dysfunction, and evaluate the patient's functional abilities, especially with regard to hand function and dexterity. In addition, the patient's cognitive status and psychosocial issues such as lifestyle and support system should be considered. Other important factors include cultural issues and patient motivation. Patient and family participation in rehabilitation is crucial because the program's long-term success will depend on the patient's compliance with recommendations.

Urinary tract infection is the most frequent medical complication of neurogenic bladder, reported in 80.4% of individuals with SCI.[83] Due to the high frequency of resistant organisms, urinalysis with Gram stain, urinary culture, and sensitivity should be obtained whenever possible before initiating antibiotic therapy. Uncomplicated urinary tract infection can be successfully treated with oral antibiotics, and treatment can often be initiated empirically with such drugs as quinolones, trimethoprim-sulfamethoxazole, and nitrofurantoin. Subsequent treatment should be modified according to the sensitivity results from the culture. The usual duration of treatment is 7–14 days. In cases of asymptomatic bacteriuria, pyuria may be used as an indication for treatment even though it is usually a poor indicator of tissue invasion in SCI patients. The current consensus stipulates that asymptomatic bacteriuria does not require routine antibiotic treatment in otherwise healthy persons with SCI. Use of prophylactic antibiotics in SCI patients has not been shown to prevent recurrent urinary tract infection. Use of urine acidifiers is controversial but may be warranted in some cases.[83]

Urinary stones are another common and serious complication in SCI patients due to immobilization and recurrent urinary tract infections. Twenty-five percent of SCI patients develop stones within 10 years of injury,[18] and bladder stones are more common than kidney stones. The most common type of stone is struvite (magnesium-ammonium-phosphate). The presence of urea-splitting bacteria (*Proteus*, *Serratia*, *Klebsiella*, *Pseudomonas*, and *Staphylococcus*) increases the risk of urinary stones. Bladder stones usually require cystoscopic removal.

Renal stones are followed conservatively in many instances and are frequently asymptomatic. However, stones that obstruct the renal pelvis should be treated aggressively. Shock wave lithotripsy is usually the treatment of choice.

Routing urinary tract surveillance is essential in all SCI patients and has contributed significantly to the reduction in mortality and morbidity in this population.[45,83] Initial baseline studies should be obtained within 3 months of injury and include renal ultrasound, renal scan, urodynamic testing, serum creatinine, and 24-hour urinary creatinine clearance. For the first 3–5 years after injury, annual evaluations are appropriate. After that time, testing frequency should be determined by the patient's symptoms and complications. Intravenous pyelograms are no longer routinely performed and should be reserved for cases that require a more specific workup for renal calculi, obstruction, or suspicion of tumor or other lesions. Cystoscopy is recommended for patients with recurrent episodes of hematuria, frequent urinary tract infections, and bladder stones, as well as for those with indwelling catheters for more than 10 years or a history of smoking, which increases the risk of bladder cancer.[45]

Managing neurogenic bladder is a challenging and dynamic process. It is important to reassess bladder management programs regularly to ensure their effectiveness and timely prevention of complications.

Neurogenic Bowel

Neurogenic bowel dysfunction is another impairment that results from SCI. More than one-third of SCI patients rank neurogenic bowel dysfunction as one of their major quality of life limiting problems. For many SCI patients, colonic dysfunction is a source of continued inconvenience and frustration. An inadequately managed bowel has a far-reaching psychosocial impact.

Rehabilitation goals include achievement of predictable bowel evacuation without bowel accidents and prevention of gastrointestinal complications. Bowel programs should be individualized and usually combine diet, oral medications, procedures to facilitate defecation, and an adequate level of physical activity. Depending on the level and completeness of SCI, various patterns of bowel dysfunction are seen. In suprasacral lesions, bowel dysfunction is hyperreflexic. The intrinsic motility of the bowel remains intact and is maintained by the reflex. The external anal sphincter and colonic wall show increased tone, which leads to overactive segmental peristalsis, underactive propulsive peristalsis (colonic transit time is prolonged), and a hyperactive holding reflex. These impairments produce fecal distention of the colon, fecal retention, and constipation.

For lesions at or below the conus medullaris, parasympathetic innervation to the colon and somatic innervation to the external anal sphincter are affected. The spinal cord–mediated colonic reflex for peristalsis is absent. Segmental colonic peristalsis is under the influence of the myenteric plexus alone. The external anal sphincter is flaccid, presenting a high risk for incontinence.

Bowel assessment in SCI patients should include documentation of premorbid bowel function, evaluation for any other bowel pathology unrelated to SCI, dietary history, the patient's functional abilities, lifestyle, and job-related or other activities outside the home. Having the patient take charge of developing a bowel routine will promote long-term success of the program.

For most patients, bowel evacuation every other day is adequate. The bowel routine should be scheduled shortly after a meal to capitalize on the natural gastrocolic reflex.

The patient's diet should include adequate fiber (20–30 g/day) and adequate fluids (2000–3000 ml/day). Proper positioning during the bowel routine takes advantage of gravity and places the abdominal muscles at maximum mechanical advantage to facilitate the passage of stool. Oral medications are frequently necessary to modify bowel habits and include stool softeners (Colace, Surfak, Dialose); bulk-forming agents (Metamucil, Perdiem, Konzyl, FiberCon, Citrucel); colonic irritants or stimulant laxatives (Senokot, Bisacodyl, Lactulose, Milk of Magnesia); and prokinetic agents (Reglan, Propulsid, Cicapride).

Rectal agents are usually necessary for triggering reflex peristalsis and initiation of defecation. They chemically stimulate the mucus membrane in the upper rectum and provide mechanical stimulation. Many patients also require digital stimulation to facilitate stool evacuation and reduce the time required for the bowel routine. For those who have established bowel routine, digital stimulation may be sufficient to complete bowel evacuation. Digital stimulation and stretching of the external anal sphincter reduces sphincter spasticity and resistance to rectal outflow. Rectal preparations usually include suppositories, mini-enemas, and enemas.

For patients with LMN injury, bowel care usually consists of manual removal of stool with some digital stimulation to enhance local segmental peristalsis. Many patients use the Valsalva maneuver and massage the abdominal wall in a clockwise manner to advance the stool. Since the external anal sphincter is flaccid, patients choose to perform the bowel routine daily to prevent incontinence.

The most frequent complication associated with neurogenic bowel in the acute stage of SCI is paralytic ileus, which usually resolves spontaneously within several days. In chronic SCI, partial bowel obstruction with fecal impaction is common. It presents as an alternation of diarrhea and constipation resulting from the ball-valve effect of an intermittently obstructing fecal mass. Impaction requires complete evacuation of the bowel with oral osmotic or saline stimulants and enemas, with pulsed irrigation to enhance stool evacuation.

Long-term use of stimulant laxatives containing anthraquinones, such as Senna, produces neuropathic damage to the myenteric plexus. Osmotic laxatives are preferred because there is no organ damage and patients do not develop tolerance with long-term use.

For patients with SCI who have repeated fecal impaction and excessively long bowel care time, surgical intervention may be warranted. Ileostomy or colostomy is usually the procedure of choice.

Pain after Spinal Cord Injury

Pain after SCI presents a significant diagnostic and management challenge. Its prevalence varies significantly and is reported to be 34% to 94%, with one-third of patients experiencing severe pain.[12]

The prevalence of pain is higher in paraplegics than in tetraplegics. It is reported to be more severe in incomplete than complete injuries and in SCI from a gunshot wound than in SCI from other types of trauma.[13] The presence of pain at 6 weeks is the most significant predictor of pain 1 year after injury. Pain significantly impacts function and quality of life in SCI patients, being frequently associated with depression, increased stress, poor morale, and self-perceived poor health.[61]

There is no consensus on SCI pain classification, definition, and terminology. From a clinical standpoint, it makes sense to categorize pain in relation to the neurological level of injury, with further subtypes of nociceptive and neuropathic pain at each level. This approach allows for more systematic assessment and management of SCI pain.[12,78]

Nociceptive or musculoskeletal pain usually results from damage to nonneural tissue in partially or fully enervated areas. It usually originates from damage to the muscle, joint, or bone due to trauma, inflammation, mechanical instability, or overuse. This pain is usually dull and aching, worsens with activity, and improves with rest and immobilization.

Neuropathic pain can originate from either peripheral or central neurogenic structures. It is described as tingling, sharp, burning, shooting, stabbing, piercing, crushing, and electric pain.

Above the injury level, pain frequently is associated with compressive neuropathies, such as compression of the median nerve in the carpal tunnel or of the ulnar nerve in Guyon's canal or cubital tunnel. Radicular pain is not uncommon in SCI and has an etiology and a clinical presentation similar to those in the non-SCI population. It is more often unilateral and more common in comminuted spinal fractures. Cauda equina injuries produce the most devastating pain, which is usually symmetric and affects sacral dermatomes.[12]

At the injury level, neuropathic pain can be radicular, arising from damaged nerve roots, or can arise from spinal cord segments. In the latter case, it is defined as central pain of the transitional or border zone and is usually bilateral, involving single or multiple adjacent dermatomes.[78]

Below the injury level, neuropathic pain is described as central pain, though other terminology has been used, such as *deafferentation central pain*, *spinal cord pain*, or *phantom pain*. The mechanism of central pain is not well understood, but the proposed *central pattern-generating mechanism* is supported by the increase in spontaneous abnormal neuronal activity in *pain-generating regions*, such as thalamic somatosensory nuclei and sensory neurons at segmental levels in the spinal cord. Other possible mechanisms include loss of spinal and cortical inhibition and loss of balance between different sensory and motor channels.[12]

Central pain is the most common type of SCI pain. It is typically diffuse and nondermatomal. Exacerbating factors include depression, stress, anxiety, adverse psychosocial situations, reduced activity, bladder and bowel complications, pressure sores, spasticity, overexertion and fatigue, changes in the weather, and smoking. Managing central neuropathic pain is challenging because this pain is usually persistent and refractory to common treatments.[13] Accurate diagnosis is essential to achieving a favorable outcome. However, the subjective nature of pain hampers studies of a treatment's effectiveness. Therefore, the treatment approach is often empirical and seldom eliminates the pain completely. The key to success is a systematic and multidisciplinary approach, thorough assessment of all of the factors that might potentially influence pain, and perseverance, active involvement, and commitment on the part of the patient.[43] A general approach includes a trial of various pharmacological agents, modification of social factors, psychological intervention, and general measures related to health and physical activity.[70]

Pharmacological intervention should be reserved for patients with moderate to severe pain that interferes with function and impairs the quality of life.[13] Medications offer some relief for some patients, but considerable time and effort are needed to optimize the pharmacological regimen. Medications should be prescribed by only one physician and should be administered regularly. Long-term efficacy is limited to a rather small percentage of patients. Pharmacological options for managing SCI pain include nonopioid analgesics, tricyclic antidepressants with adrenergic reuptake inhibition, and selective serotonin reuptake inhibitors. A number of studies have found anticonvulsants to be the most effective class of drugs for various types of neuropathic pain, including central pain. Among these are gabapentin, carbamazepine, and topiramate. Other options include opioids and benzodiazepines, the GABA agonist baclofen, and the adrenergic agonists clonidine and tizanidine.[13] Intrathecal administration of morphine, baclofen, and clonidine should be considered for severe intractable pain.[48,56] Nonsteroidal anti-inflammatory drugs and muscle relaxants usually are not effective for central pain.

Transcutaneous electrical nerve stimulation is another possible treatment, though its success in SCI patients is mixed. Functional electrical stimulation has been reported to decrease pain by reducing spasticity, increasing activity levels, and improving overall physical conditioning.[31] Epidural dorsal column high-frequency electrical stimulation demonstrated few long-term successful outcomes.[54] Neurosurgical destructive procedures, such as cordotomy and tractotomy, demonstrated no predictable long-term benefits for SCI central pain.[72] The dorsal root entry zone microcoagulation procedure

(DREZ) proposed by Nashold and Bullitt[59] was shown to have some effectiveness in reducing radicular and central pain at the neurological level of injury, but results have been disappointing for central pain below the injury level.

Other surgical procedures such as stabilization, fusion, and decompression for managing spinal instability, herniated nucleus pulposus, associated spinal stenosis, and cord tethering are usually successful in addressing pain in SCI patients. Aggressive pain management in SCI patients should always be considered, especially if there is a change in the character, intensity, or quality of the pain or if the patient describes new pain.

Pain of musculoskeletal origin is quite prevalent in both tetraplegia and paraplegia. The upper extremities become weight-bearing limbs in SCI patients for such repetitive functions as transfers, wheelchair propulsion, and weight shifts for pressure relief, which places joints and soft tissue at significant risk for overuse and injury. The shoulder is by far the most common site of pain in the upper extremities in both acute and chronic SCI.[22] In acute tetraplegia, the incidence of shoulder pain is reported to be as high as 75% for unilateral pain and 61% for bilateral pain.[21] The most frequent cause is repeated trauma of the shoulder by improper handling, poor positioning, or the presence of cervical orthoses. The shoulder joint becomes vulnerable when the scapula and glenohumeral joint lose stability due to muscle paralysis, spasticity, and early development of contractures. Factors that predispose SCI patients to an early onset of shoulder pain include injury above the C6 level, associated trauma to the shoulder girdle complex, lack of early range of motion, preexisting degenerative pathology, and age over 50. Shoulder pain is usually related to rotator cuff pathology, bicipital tendinitis, shoulder subluxation, acromioclavicular joint pathology, and myofascial pain.[22]

In chronic SCI, the prevalence of shoulder pain ranges from 30% to 73%. It is more common in tetraplegia than in paraplegia, in women than in men, and in complete than in incomplete injury. The most common cause of shoulder pain in tetraplegia is rotator cuff injury; in paraplegia, it is bicipital tendinitis. Other shoulder pathologies include adhesive capsulitis, osteonecrosis of the humeral head, subacromial bursitis, and instability.[21,22]

Musculoskeletal pain in the forearm usually relates to medial or lateral epicondylitis. Both overuse conditions result from repetitive flexion/extension of the wrist during wheelchair use and transfers. For lateral epicondylitis, the extensor carpi radialis brevis is the most common offending muscle, while in medial epicondylitis it is usually the flexor carpi ulnaris.[70]

Neck pain is a common problem in patients with tetraplegia as well. It usually originates at the site of the spinal fracture or results from spinal instability, soft tissue injury, and myofascial pain.

Pain in the lower extremities in SCI patients occurs most frequently in incomplete injuries and results from pelvic girdle muscular instability. Pathology is often localized to the sacroiliac and hip joints. This type of pain is frequently seen with SCI above the L3 level, with an incidence of more than 50%.[50] The most significant contributing factors are poor wheelchair posture, inadequate bracing in ambulatory patients, spasticity, and frequent urinary tract infections.

Management of musculoskeletal pain requires accurate diagnosis and localization of the site and origin and should include a thorough examination, imaging studies, and electrodiagnosis. Treatment of musculoskeletal conditions in patients with SCI is the same as in the noninjured population. However, it is critical to implement preventive measures early during rehabilitation. For patients with tetraplegia, proper positioning, early mobilization exercises, supportive splinting and bracing, proper transfer skills, and a proper arrangement for sitting in a wheelchair are needed.

In patients with paraplegia, a vigorous exercise program for strengthening the upper extremities, postural education, and selection of an appropriate wheelchair are important.

If shoulder pain persists or recurs in paraplegic patients who use a manual wheelchair, strong consideration should be given to powered wheelchairs and assisted transfers, especially in aging SCI patients.

Pharmacological management with NSAIDs, steroid injections and therapeutic modalities should be started early. Analgesics, both nonopioid and opioid, can be included in treatment. Electrical stimulation should be implemented to strengthen muscles that are too weak to oppose gravity and to reduce spasticity in antagonistic muscles.

Pain in SCI remains a challenging problem. In many instances, diagnosis and management are quite complex. Clearly, more clinical and basic research is needed to further define mechanisms of pain and develop clear outcome guidelines for interventions.

Spasticity

Spasticity is one of the most common clinical problems encountered by individuals with SCI. Spasticity is a component of UMN syndrome and is characterized by a velocity-dependent increase in tonic stretch reflexes (muscle tone) with exaggerated tendon jerks resulting from hyperexcitability of the stretch reflex.

The pathophysiology of spasticity remains unclear. Spasticity is believed to result from loss of suprasegmental inhibition, increased motor neuron excitability, changes in the intrinsic electrical properties of neurons, denervation hypersensitivity, and collateral sprouting. Both alpha motor neuron pathways and the gamma efferent system may contribute.[88] Spasticity does not develop immediately after SCI but appears after the spinal shock phase resolves. As it develops, associated cutaneomuscular and flexion withdrawal reflexes emerge, causing muscle spasms. Flexor and extensor muscles often demonstrate spasticity and spasms.

Clinical evaluation of spasticity must include quantitative assessments of a patient's muscle tone, functional abilities (transfers, ambulation, activities of daily living), and risk for musculoskeletal complications. The frequently used Ashworth Scale quantifies spasticity severity.[79,88]

Spasticity is exacerbated by associated medical conditions, such as urinary tract infection, pressure sores, intra-abdominal pathology, or virtually any noxious stimulus below the injury level. It frequently interferes with hygiene, sexual function, and sleeping pattern, leads to joint and muscle contractures, promotes skin breakdown, and contributes to muscle fibrosis and atrophy.[69]

Spasticity does not require treatment in all cases. The decision should be based on whether it causes significant discomfort, interferes with a patient's functioning, or is associated with medical complications.

Initial management includes avoidance of noxious stimuli, proper positioning in the bed and wheelchair, and daily range-of-motion and stretching exercises. Physical modalities such as superficial heat or cold, biofeedback, electrical stimulation, splinting, serial casting, and orthoses are also important.[69,79] Weight-bearing activities such as standing in a standing frame facilitate stretching of the lower extremities.

When conservative measures fail to control spasticity, pharmacological intervention is instituted. Generalized spasticity with severe spasms should be treated with systemic medications. Regional spasticity is best managed by chemical nerve blocks with neurochemical agents and neurotoxins.[32,88]

Several classes of antispasticity medications are currently available. Baclofen, the most commonly used first-line agent, is a structural analog of gamma-aminobutyric acid (GABA), the primary inhibitory neurotransmitter in the spinal cord. Baclofen binds to GABA-B receptors at presynaptic terminals, inhibiting calcium influx and suppressing the release of excitatory neurotransmitters. It also increases potassium conductance, which is responsible for the postsynaptic inhibitory effect. Both monosynaptic and polysynaptic reflexes are inhibited by baclofen. Although the recommended maximum dose is 80 mg, patients with SCI usually require much higher doses (up to 160 mg/day). Oral baclofen is well tolerated, though common side effects include fatigue, weakness, dizziness, gastrointestinal irritation, and mental changes. Baclofen should not be stopped abruptly because that can cause seizures, fever, and palpitations.

Diazepam (benzodiazepine) binds to GABA-A receptors, enhancing postsynaptic inhibition. It has the potential for dependency and abuse and frequently causes sedation, impairs cognitive function, precipitates depression, and increases muscle weakness.

Antispasticity drugs with adrenergic properties include the alpha-adrenergic agonists tizanidine and clonidine, which inhibit excitatory interneurons at both spinal and supraspinal levels. The most significant side effects of tizanidine are dry mouth and lethargy. Because tizanidine is metabolized by the liver, it should be given with caution to patients with impaired liver function.

Clonidine has limited utility because of its hypotensive effect. The transdermal form of clonidine appears to be better tolerated, though its effectiveness is limited. Both tizanidine and clonidine demonstrate better effectiveness with fewer side effects when used in combination with baclofen or diazepam.[57]

Among peripherally acting agents, dantrolene sodium is frequently considered. It directly affects muscle by inhibiting calcium reuptake into the sarcoplasmic reticulum. The most significant side effects are muscle weakness and hepatotoxicity, but the drug may also cause nausea, vomiting, and diarrhea. Hepatotoxicity is dose-dependent and reversible. Liver function enzymes should be monitored periodically as long as a patient takes this medication.

Other medications such as gabapentin (Neurontin), vigabatrin (Sabril), cyproheptadine (Periactin), glycine, and cannabinoids (Marinol) reportedly are useful for spasticity, but there are insufficient clinical or scientific data to demonstrate their effectiveness.

For patients with SCI who continue to have severe spasticity, demonstrate a poor response to oral medications, or experience severe side effects, intrathecal baclofen infusion therapy should be considered.[64] It delivers baclofen directly into the spinal fluid, achieving a higher concentration than is possible with oral baclofen. Intrathecal baclofen is delivered through a surgically implanted pump infusion system. Before the pump is implanted, all patients are screened to assess baclofen's effectiveness. After implantation, the intrathecal dose is slowly titrated until a therapeutic effect is achieved. Depending on the pattern of spasticity, the pump can be programmed to deliver a continuous dose of baclofen or periodic boluses or to achieve complex delivery rates throughout the day or night. Side effects of intrathecal baclofen are dose-dependent. Overdose causes drowsiness, weakness, nausea, respiratory depression, bradycardia, progressive hypotonia, and loss of consciousness progressing to coma.[79]

Physostigmine, the anticholinesterase inhibitor, usually reverses respiratory depression when given intravenously 1–2 mg over 5–10 minutes. When patients withdraw from intrathecal baclofen abruptly, as when they fail to refill the pump in a timely manner or when mechanical problems develop in the pump or catheter (a kink, blockage, disconnection, dislodgement), they develop progressive spasticity, acute agitation, extreme fever, tachycardia, and severe itching. Intrathecal baclofen withdrawal and overdose are medical emergencies, and patients should have access to immediate medical attention. Some patients decrease their response to intrathecal baclofen with time. In this case, a drug *holiday* might be necessary to restore effectiveness.

When patients with SCI develop severe localized spasticity, a nerve block with alcohol, phenol, or local anesthetics or an intramuscular injection of botulinum toxin A should be considered.[32,88] A nerve block can be performed on any anatomically accessible nerve. The duration of chemical neurolysis is variable but on average lasts between 3 and 9 months. The musculocutaneous nerve is blocked to treat severe elbow spasticity; the median and ulnar nerves are blocked to treat severe wrist spasticity. Obturator nerve block is effective for hip adductor spasticity; a tibial nerve block is effective for equinovarus deformity of the foot. Most nerve blocks are performed on sensorimotor nerves, which can result in unwanted dysesthesias. Thus, it is critical to localize the relevant nerve precisely.[32]

Spinal blocks using intrathecal phenol or alcohol may be beneficial in cases of severe, intractable, generalized spasticity, though these procedures usually lead to urinary and fecal incontinence, and need to be considered carefully and only after a full explanation to patients and their families.

Botulinum toxin can also be used in SCI patients to reduce focal muscle tone in specific muscle groups.[88] Its effect is dose-dependent and usually wears off within 3 months. The toxin has essentially no systemic side effects, and its local effectiveness is attributed to muscle weakness.

The success of treating regional spasticity in patients with SCI depends on proper patient selection, proper dosage, and the physician's skill and experience.

Surgical treatment of spasticity is usually destructive. Neurectomy, rhizotomy, and myelotomy should be avoided, especially in view of the significant progress that is being made in the field of spinal cord regeneration.

Orthopedic surgical procedures such as tendon release, tendon transfers, and tenotomies may be useful in association with other therapeutic interventions.

Conclusion

Rehabilitation of patients with complications of spinal cord injury is a challenging task. The rehabilitation team and all other health care providers must have an extensive knowledge of the physiological impairments and psychosocial consequences of this devastating injury.

It is important to maintain continuity of care for patients with SCI, both to ensure timely management of their medical issues and to focus on preventive and health maintenance issues, especially since the SCI population is surviving longer and now has to cope with the problems of aging. Physicians should strive to provide patients with access to innovative advanced rehabilitative therapies and new adaptive technologies with the ultimate goal of enhancing neurological recovery and functional outcomes, improving the quality of life, and promoting meaningful social reintegration.

REFERENCES

1. Anke A: Lung volumes in tetraplegic patients according to cervical spinal cord injury level. Scand J Rehabil Med 25:73–77, 1993.
2. Arrowood M, Mohanty P, Thames M: Cardiovascular problems in the spinal cord injured patient. Phys Med Rehabil: State Art Rev 1:443–456, 1987.
3. Bach JR: Update and perspective on noninvasive respiratory muscle aids: Parts 1 and 2 the inspiratory and expiratory muscle aids. Chest 105:1230–1240, 1538–1544, 1994.
4. Bauman WA: Carbohydrate and lipid metabolism after spinal cord injury. Top Spinal Cord Inj Rehabil 2:1–22, 1997.
5. Bauman WA, Adkins RH, Spungen AM, et al: The effect of residual neurological deficit on serum lipoproteins in individuals with chronic spinal cord injury. Spinal Cord 36:13–17, 1998.
6. Bauman WA, Spungen AM: Metabolic changes in persons after spinal cord injury. Phys Med Rehabil Clin North Am 11:109–140, 2000.
7. BeDell KK, Scremin AM, et al: Effects of functional electrical stimulation-induced lower extremity cycling on bone density of spinal cord-injured patients. Am J Phys Med Rehabil 75:29–34, 1996.
8. Belanger M, Stein RB, Wheeler GD, Gordon T, Leduc B: Electrical stimulation: Can it increase muscle strength and reverse osteopenia in spinal cord injured individuals? Arch Phys Med Rehabil 81:1090–1098, 2000.
9. Bergstrom N, Bennett MA, Carlson CE, et al: Clinical Practice Guideline No. 15: Treatment of Pressure Ulcers. AHCPR Pub. 95-0652. Rockville, MD, U.S. Department of Health and Human Services, Agency for Health Care Policy and Research, 1994.
10. Braun SR, Giovannoni R, O'Connor M: Improving the cough in patients with spinal cord injury. Am J Phys Med 63:1–10, 1984.
11. Breslow RA: Nutrition and air-fluidized beds: A literature review. Adv Wound Care 7:57–62, 1994.
12. Bryce T, Ragnarsson K: Pain after spinal cord injury. In: Kraft G, Hammond M (eds): Topics in Spinal Cord Injury Medicine (pp 77–99). Physical Medicine and Rehabilitation Clinics of North America. Philadelphia, WB Saunders, 2000, pp 157–168.
13. Bryce TN, Ragnarsson KT: Pain management in persons with spinal cord disorders. In: Lin V (ed.): Spinal Cord Medicine. New York, Demos, 2001, pp
14. Bugaresti JM, Tator CH, Silverberg JD, et al: Changes in thyroid hormones, thyroid stimulating hormone and cortisol in acute spinal cord injury. Paraplegia 30:401–409, 1992.
15. Burnham R, Wheeler G, et al: Intentional induction of autonomic dysreflexia among quadriplegic athletes for performance enhancement: Efficacy, safety and mechanism of action. Clin J Sport Med 4:1–10, 1994.
16. Carter RE, Dono WH, Halstead L, Wilkerson MA: Comparative study of electrophrenic nerve stimulation and mechanical ventilatory support in traumatic spinal cord injury. Paraplegia 25:86, 1987.
17. Chen D, Apple DA, Hudson LM, Bode R: Medical complications during acute rehabilitation following spinal cord injury—current experience of the model systems. Arch Phys Med Rehabil 80:1397–1401, 1999.
18. Chen Y, DeVivo MJ, Stover SL, Lloyd LK: Recurrent kidney stone: A 25-year follow-up study in persons with spinal cord injury. Urology 60:228–232, 2002.
19. Consortium for Spinal Cord Medicine: Prevention of Thromboembolism in Spinal Cord Injury, 2nd ed. Washington, DC, Paralyzed Veterans of America, 1999.
20. Consortium for Spinal Cord Medicine: Acute Management of Autonomic Dysreflexia: Individuals with Spinal Cord Injury Presenting to Healthcare Facilities. Washington, DC, Paralyzed Veterans of America, 2001.
21. Curtis KA, Drysdale GA, et al: Shoulder pain in wheelchair users with tetraplegia and paraplegia. Arch Phys Med Rehabil 80:453–457, 1995.
22. Dalyan M, Cardenas DD, Gerard B: Upper extremity pain after spinal cord injury. Spinal Cord 37(3):191–195, 1999.
23. DeVivo MJ, Black KJ, Stover SL: Causes of death during the first 12 years after spinal cord injury. Arch Phys Med Rehabil 74:248–254, 1993.
24. Dobelle WH: 200 cases with a new breathing pacemaker dispel myths about diaphragm pacing. Trans Am Soc Arif Intern Organs 40:244, 1994.
25. Dykstra DD, Sidi AA: Treatment of detrusor-sphincter dysynergia with botulinum A toxin: A double-blind study. Arch Phys Med Rehabil 71(1):24–26, 1990.
26. Figoni S: Exercise responses and tetraplegia. Med Sci Sports Exerc 25:433–441, 1993.
27. Frey-Rindova P, de Bruin ED, et al: Bone mineral density in upper and lower extremities during 12 months after

spinal cord injury measured by peripheral quantitative computed tomography. Spinal Cord 38:26–32, 2000.
28. Gallien P, Brissot R, Eyssette M, et al: Restoration of gait by functional electrical stimulation for spinal cord injured patients. Paraplegia 33:660–664, 1995.
29. Gilgoff IS, Ward SL, Hohn AR: Cardiac pacemaker in high spinal cord injury. Arch Phys Med Rehabil 72:601–603, 1991.
30. Glaser RM: Physiology of functional electrical stimulation-induced exercise: Basic science stimulation-induced exercise: Basic science perspective. J Neurol Rehabil 5:49–61, 1991.
31. Glaser RM: Functional neuromuscular stimulation: Exercise conditioning of spinal cord injured patients. Int J Sports Med 15:142–148, 1994.
32. Glen MB: Nerve blocks for treatment of spasticity. Phys Med Rehabil State Art Rev 8(3):481–505, 1994.
33. Glenn WWL, Brouillette RT, Dents B: Fundamental considerations in pacing of the diaphragm for chronic ventilatory insufficiency: A multi-center study. PACE 11:2121, 1988.
34. Glenn WWL, Phelps ML, Elefteriades JA, Dents B, Hogan JF: Twenty years' experience in phrenic nerve stimulation to pace the diaphragm. PACE 9:781, 1986.
35. Gomberg-Maitland M, Frishman WH: Thyroid hormone and cardiovascular disease. Am Heart J 135:187–196, 1998.
36. Graupe D, Kohn K: Functional Electrical Stimulation for Ambulation by Paraplegics. Malabar, FL, Krieger, 1994.
37. Grimby G, Broberg C, Krotkiewsky M: Muscle fibre composition in patients with traumatic spinal cord lesion. Scand J Rehab Med 8:37–42, 1976.
38. Gudziak MR, Tiguert R, et al: Management of neurogenic bladder dysfunction with incontinent ileovesicotomy. Urology 54(6):1008–1011, 1999.
39. Hicken BL, Putzke JD, Richards JS: Bladder management and quality of life after spinal cord injury. Am J Phys Med Rehabil 80(12):916–922, 2001.
40. Jaeger R, Yarkony G, Smith R: Standing the spinal cord injured patient by electrical stimulation: Refinement of a protocol for clinical use. IEEE Trans Biomed Eng 36: 720–728, 1989.
41. Jamil F: Towards a catheter free status in neurogenic bladder dysfunction: A review of bladder management options in spinal cord injury (SCI). Spinal Cord 39(7):355–361, 2001.
42. Jezernik S, Craggs M, Grill WM, Creasey G, Rijkhoff NJ: Electrical stimulation for the treatment of bladder dysfunction: Current status and future possibilities. Neural Res 24(5):413–430, 2002.
43. Kennedy P, Frankel H, Gardner B, Nuseibeh I: Factors associated with acute and chronic pain following traumatic spinal cord injuries. Spinal Cord 35:814–817, 1997.
44. Khansarinia S, Dennis JW, Veldenz HC, et al: Prophylactic Greenfield filter placement in selected high-risk trauma patients. J Vasc Surg 22:231–236, 1995.
45. Kirshblum SC, Groah SL, McKinley WO, Gittler MS, Steins SA: Spinal cord injury medicine. 1. Etiology, classification and acute medical management. Arch Phys Med Rehabil 83(suppl 1):S50–S57, 2002.
46. Kraft CF: Skin care. Top Spinal Cord Inj Rehabil 2(1):1–20, 1996.
47. Lemons VR, Wagner FC Jr: Respiratory complications after cervical spinal cord injury. Spine 19:2315–2320, 1994.
48. Loubser PG, Akman NM: Effects of intrathecal Baclofen on chronic spinal cord injury pain. J Pain Symptom Manage 4:241–247, 1996.
49. MacLean IC, Mattioni TA: Phrenic nerve conduction studies: A new technique and its application in quadriplegic patients. Arch Phys Med Rehabil 62:70–73, 1981.
50. Maldjian C, Mesgrzadeh M, Tehranzadeh J: Diagnostic and therapeutic features of facet and sacroiliac joint injection. Radiol Clin North Am 36(3):497–508, 1998.
51. Maynard FM: Immobilization hypercalcemia following spinal cord injury. Arch Phys Med Rehabil 67:41–44, 1986.
52. McKinley WO, Gittler MS, Kirshblum SC: Spinal cord injury medicine. 2. Medical complications after spinal cord injury: Identification and management. Arch Phys Med Rehabil 83:S58–S64, 2003.
53. Meehan M: Multisite pressure ulcer prevalence survey. Decubitus 3:14–17, 1990.
54. Meglio M, Cioni B, Prezioso A, Talamonti G: Spinal cord stimulation in deafferentation pain. Pacing Clin Electrophysiol 12:709–712, 1989.
55. Menard MR, Hahn G: Acute and chronic hypothermia in a man with spinal cord injury: Environmental and pharmacologic causes. Arch Phys Med Rehabil 72:421–424, 1991.
56. Middelton B, Kuipers-Upmeijer H, Bouma J, et al: Intrathecal clonidine and baclofen in the management of spasticity and neuropathic pain following spinal cord injury: A Case study. Arch Phys Med Rehabil 77(8):824–826, 1996.
57. Nance PW: A comparison of clonidine, cyprohepatadine and baclofen in spastic spinal cord injured patients. J Am Paraplegia Soc 17:151–157, 1994.
58. Nance PW, Schryvers O, et al: Intravenous pamidronate attenuates bone density loss after acute spinal cord injury. Arch Phys Med Rehabil 80:243–251, 1999.
59. Nashold BS, Bullitt E: Dorsal root entry zone lesions to control central pain in paraplegics. J Neurosurg 55:414–419, 1981.
60. Naso F: Cardiovascular problems in patients with spinal cord injury. Phys Med Rehabil Clin North Am 3(4):741–749, 1992.
61. Nepomuceno C, Fine P, Richards J, et al: Pain in patients with spinal cord injury. Arch Phys Med Rehabil 60:605–609, 1979.
62. Nutritional support after spinal cord injury. Neurosurgery 50(3 suppl):S81–S84, 2002.
63. Peck WA, Burckhardt P, et al: Consensus development conference: Diagnosis, prophylaxis and treatment of osteoporosis. Am J Med 94:646–650, 1993.
64. Penn RD, Kroin JS: Continuous intrathecal baclofen for severe spasticity. Lancet 2(8447):125–127, 1985.

65. Peterson P: Pulmonary physiology and medical management. In: Whiteneck G (ed.): The Management of High Quadriplegia. New York, Demos, 1989, pp 35–50.
66. Piepmeier JM, Lehmann KB, Lane JG: Cardiovascular instability following acute cervical spinal cord trauma. Cent Nerv Syst Trauma 2:153–160, 1985.
67. Prakash V, Lin M, Song C, Perkash I: Thyroid hypofunction in spinal cord injury patients. Paraplegia 1856–1863, 1980.
68. Priebe MM: Pressure ulcers. In: O'Young B, Young M (eds): Physical Medicine and Rehabilitation Secrets. Philadelphia, Hanley & Belfus, 1997, pp 493–497.
69. Priebe MM, Sherwood AM, et al: Assessment of spasticity in spinal cord injury with a multidimensional problem. Arch Phys Med Rehabil 77:713–716, 1996.
70. Ragnarsson K: Management of pain in persons with spinal cord injury. J Spinal Cord Med 20:186–199, 1997.
71. Ragnarsson K, Hall KM, Wilmot CB, et al: Management of pulmonary, cardiovascular, and metabolic conditions after spinal cord injury. In: Stover S, DeLisa JA, Whiteneck GG (eds): Spinal Cord Injury: Clinical Outcomes from the Model Systems. Gaithersburg, PA, Aspen, 1995, pp 79–99.
72. Rawlings C, Rossitch E, Nashold BS: The history of neurosurgical procedures for the relief of pain. Surg Neurol 38:454–463, 1992.
73. Ricottone AR, Pranikoff K, Steinmetz JR, Constantino G: Long-term follow-up of sphincterotomy in the treatment of autonomic dysreflexia. Neurouradiol Urodyn 14(1):43–46, 1995.
74. Rochester L, Barron MJ: Influence of electrical stimulation of the tibialis anterior muscle in paraplegic patients. Morphological and histochemical properties. Paraplegia 33:514–522, 1995.
75. Sadowsky CL, Margherita A: The cost of spinal cord injury care. Spine 13:593–606, 1999.
76. Schmitt J, Alder R: Endocrine-metabolic consequences of spinal cord injury. Phys Med Rehabil State Art Rev 1:425, 1987.
77. Shin K, Priebe MM, Rossi D: Follow-up of surgically managed pressure ulcers in persons with SCI. Predictive factors for recurrence. J Am Paraplegia Soc 17:129, 1994.
78. Siddall P, Taylor D, Cousins M: Classification of pain following spinal cord injury. Spinal Cord 35:69–75, 1997.
79. Stein AB, Pomerantz F, Schechtman J: Evaluation and management of spasticity in spinal cord injury. Top Spinal Cord Inj Rehabil 2(4):70–83, 1997.
80. Stilwill EW, Sahgal V: Histochemical and morphologic changes in skeletal muscle following cervical cord injury: A study of upper and lower motor neuron lesions. Arch Phys Med Rehabil 58:201–206, 1977.
81. The National SCI Statistical Center: Facts and Figures at a Glance. Birmingham, University of Alabama Press, 2003.
82. The PIOPED Investigators: Value of the ventilation/perfusion scan in acute pulmonary embolism. Results of the prospective investigation of pulmonary embolism diagnosis (PIOPED). JAMA 263:2753–2759, 1990.
83. The prevention and management of urinary tract infections among people with spinal cord injuries. National Institute on Disability and Rehabilitation Research consensus statement. January 27–29, 1992. J Am Paraplegia Soc 15(3):194–204, 1992.
84. Tsitouras PD, Zhong YG, Spungen AM, et al: Serum testosterone and growth hormone/insulin-like growth factor in adults with spinal cord injury. Horm Metab Res 27: 287–292, 1995.
85. Vaziri ND, Pandian MR, et al: Vitamin D, parathyroid hormone, and calcitonin profiles in persons with long-standing spinal cord injury. Arch Phys Med Rehabil 75: 766–769, 1994.
86. Wein AJ, Raezer DM, Benson GS: Management of neurogenic bladder dysfunction in the adult. Urology 8:432, 1976.
87. Whiteneck G: Learning from empirical investigations. In: Menter R, Whiteneck G (eds): Perspectives on Aging with Spinal Cord Injury. New York, Demos, 1992, pp 23–37.
88. Worldwide Education and Awareness for Movement Disorders (WE MOVE): Spasticity: Diagnosis and Treatment. New York, Mount Sinai Medical Center, 1995.
89. Young JS, Burns PE: Pressure sores and the spinal cord injured. SCI Digest 3:9–25, 1981.

Chapter 16

Low-Back Pain and Sciatica: Evaluation and Treatment

JAMES F. HOWARD, JR.

Unquestionably, the patient with low-back pain often is a diagnostic challenge for the physician irrespective of whether the physician is a neurologist, neurosurgeon, orthopedist, physiatrist, internist, or generalist.

This is due, in part, to the fact that the patient's complaint is a symptom, not a clinical sign or diagnosis, and the anatomical substrates for causing the problem are myriad (Fig. 16.1). The etiologies are diverse, if not legion, and there is poor correlation with symptoms, laboratory study findings, and pathological findings. This accounts for the fact that in 85% of patients with acute low-back pain and in 50% of patients with chronic low-back pain, no diagnosis is ever established.[64,156,209] Further the problem may be complicated by other factors, resulting in an exaggeration of symptoms by nonphysiological processes (psychological, remunerative, occupational, etc.). However, despite this, one can establish a logical approach to the diagnosis and management of

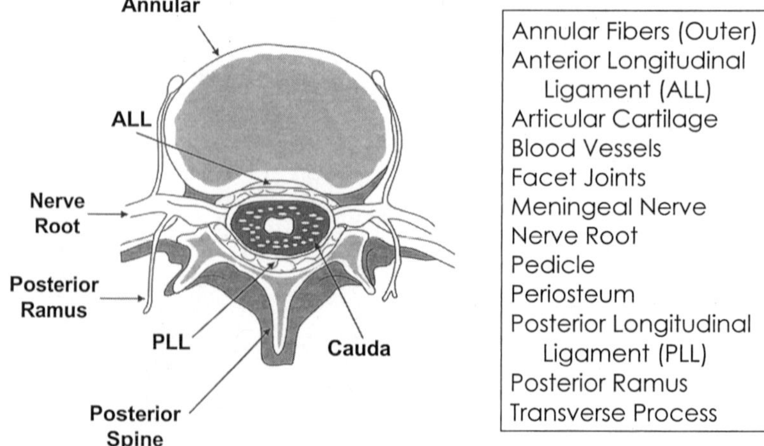

Figure 16.1. Pain-sensitive structures in the lumbar spine.

low-back pain. For this review, low-back pain is defined as pain located between the lower thoracic spine and the gluteal folds. Sciatica is defined as low-back pain that radiates below the gluteal folds in the distribution of a specific nerve root(s).

Demographics of Low-Back Pain

Low-back pain and sciatica are socioeconomic problems of epidemic proportions and the foremost cause of disability in young patients, as evidenced by the activities of the advertising sector.[168] They are the primary reasons that young adults limit physical activity.[33,130] They are second only to the common cold for work time lost, the third most common cause for surgical procedures, and the fifth most common cause for hospitalizations.[98,192,223] Lifetime prevalence rates range from 49% to 80% of adults.[74,137,180] The monthly prevalence for those between 10 and 85 years of age is 40%. Only 25% of these individuals will seek medical care, and while 90% will ultimately recover within 6 weeks, the number of those so afflicted without recovery constitutes a severe economic burden on society.[160] About 85% of the U.S. population will be affected at some time during their lives (about 75 million Americans), and 7 million new patients will develop low-back pain each year.[130] As expected, the costs are staggering for everyone. Some simple demographics include the following:

- 2–3 million people unable to work at any point in time
- 149 million work days lost each year[89]
- Approximately $15 billion per year spent on diagnosis and treatment[75]
- Estimated cost of work time lost: $28 to 56 billion annually[132,151]

Of the 85% of patients who develop low-back pain, an estimated 14% will have episodes that persist longer than 2 weeks and only 1.5% will have sciatica.[63] Recurrent low-back pain is common. Estimates suggest that 20% to 44% of patients will have a recurrence within 1 year and 80% will have a recurrence within 10 years of their initial episode.[164] Of more concern is that 5% of the population will develop chronic, disabling low-back pain.[51]

Several risk factors have been identified that influence the prevalence of low-back pain and are elaborated on by Loeser and Volinn.[131] These include age, with an increasing incidence up to about age 60.[22] Men and women have a similar risk to about age 60; afterward, women are more likely to have low-back pain, perhaps due to their risk of osteoporosis.[78] Occupations that require severe physical labor or long-distance driving also increase the risk of future back pain.[100] The size and shape of the lumbar spinal canal are probable risk factors. Interestingly, smoking appears to increase the risk of low-back pain, perhaps through the vasoconstrictive effects of nicotine.[100,172]

Anatomy and Biomechanics of the Lumbosacral Spine

The lumbar spine is composed of five vertebrae, between which are the intervertebral discs. Each vertebral spine consists of a body, lamina, and neural arch. The neural arch has a pedicle and a transverse process on either side, and a spinous process projects posteriorly. The spinal cord passes between these elements and ends at the L1 level in the majority of patients. The vertebral bodies are bordered by two supporting ligaments: (1) the anterior longitudinal ligament, a strap-like band originating at the atlas and ending at the sacrum, is firmly attached to the anterior surface of the vertebral bodies; (2) the posterior longitudinal ligament, which lies within the vertebral canal along the posterior surface of the vertebral bodies. The sacrum is composed of five fused vertebrae. The intervertebral discs comprise 25% of the length of the lumbar spine. They function as a universal joint and are composed of gelatinous fibrocartilage, the nucleus pulposus that is surrounded by concentric layers of fibrous tissue, the annulus fibrosus. The intervertebral discs are interposed between the cartilaginous end plates of the vertebral body.

Nerve roots exit from the spinal canal through intervertebral foramina. Each foramen is bordered by:

1. Pedicles (superiorly and inferiorly)
2. Intervertebral disc and a vertebral body (anteriorly)
3. A lamina and a facet joint (posteriorly)

The stability of the spine depends upon two supporting structures: muscles that provide most of the support via voluntary and reflex contractions of the abdominal, gluteus maximus, hamstring, and sacrospinal musculature, and the ligaments that offer some support but are passive in nature.

Patient History

Because it is often difficult to obtain good physical or laboratory confirmation of low-back pain disorders, the importance of an accurate clinical history cannot be stressed enough. The general aspects of history taking are straightforward, with attention to the circumstances surrounding the onset of the pain, its location, its intensity, the quality of the pain, factors that precipitate (aggravate) or relieve the pain, the effect of medications, previous episodes, and prior surgery. In addition, the patient should be questioned carefully about fever, weight loss, headache, other medical problems, and habits regarding medication, drug, and alcohol use and work activities.

Understanding Pain Complaints

Pain syndromes can be distinguished by individual characteristics and classified in a number of ways. There are four main types of low-back pain; *local*, *referred*, *radicular*, and *other*.

Local Pain
Local pain results from irritation of local sensory nerve endings at the site of involvement. Examples include the following:

1. *Skin and subcutaneous tissue* produce pain covering a territory that correlates with the degree of tissue injury (e.g. laceration, burns, infection). This should not pose diagnostic difficulties to anyone. One exception is the pain of herpes zoster, which is in the distribution of a dermatome and is characterized as burning.
2. *Muscular spasm* produces a dull aching, sometimes cramping, and discomfort in the low back due to a reflex contraction of muscle surrounding an area of injury. This produces spasm and tightness of the muscles that is appreciated best by visual inspection and palpation. Muscular trigger points may be present.
3. *Vertebral spine disease* is pain free unless there is involvement of the periosteum. Tumor involvement of the vertebral body alone will *not* produce pain per se. The pain produces a deep, dull, aching discomfort that is maximal at the site of involvement.

The symptoms of local pain are exacerbated by movement and improved with rest (lying down), and are often associated with paraspinal muscle spasm and tenderness to palpation. Pain due to tendon disruption is more severe than pain due to muscle injury itself. Low-back pain that does not improve with rest should raise the possibility of tumor or infection.

Referred Pain
Referred pain is of two types; that projected from the spine to viscera in the dermatomes of the lumbar and sacral regions, and that projected from the abdominal and pelvic viscera to the spine. Examples include:

1. *Spinal pain*. Pain from disease of the upper lumbar spine refers to the anterior thigh, groin, or flank. The mechanism of this pain is due to irritation of the cuneal nerves that derive from the L1-L3 nerve roots. Pain from disease of the lower lumbar spine refers to the posterior thigh, or buttocks. The mechanism of this pain is due to irritation of the nerves derived from the L5-S1 nerve roots. Both produce a dull, deep, aching discomfort. The symptoms are exacerbated by manipulation of the spine.
2. *Visceral pain*. This occurs in association with symptoms of systemic illness, particularly with gastrointestinal (GI) or genitourinary (GU) disease (e.g., hematochezia, hematuria). Gastrointestinal disorders produce a severe, colicky discomfort that is sometimes recurrent (e.g., peptic ulcer disease). These disorders may produce variable degrees of discomfort ranging from a deep, aching quality to a severe pain. Often the pain is related to the degree of visceral activity, with little exacerbation or relief with postural change. Of note, one must not confuse this pain with that of an expanding abdominal aortic aneurysm.

Radicular Pain
Radicular pain has many of the characteristics of referred pain but differs in its intensity, its radia-

tion to distal structures, and the processes that aggravate it. The mechanism of pain is due to stretching, irritation, or compression of the proximal portion of the nerve or nerve root usually proximal to or within the intervertebral foramina. This pain is described as a shooting, lancinating, burning, sharp discomfort that radiates from the back to a distal site in the lower extremity. The radiation is in the distribution of the involved nerve root. It is often associated with a dull, aching discomfort due to referred pain. This type of pain is referred to as *sciatica*. It is exacerbated by any movement that increases tension on the nerve root (e.g., twisting, bending, stooping, coughing). It improves with recumbency. It is often associated with focal neurological findings (see below).

Other Types of Pain

Neurogenic pain results from disorders of the peripheral nerve and/or the sympathetic nervous system. This type of pain produces a severe, excruciating discomfort similar to that seen with complex regional pain syndromes (reflex sympathetic dystrophy or causalgia). It is described as burning, tingling, unpleasant, crawling, and so on. Autonomic disturbances may be evident, including swelling, sweating, pallor, or rubor.

Psychogenic pain produces a poorly defined, vague, discomfort not respecting the anatomy of a nerve root or peripheral nerve. It is often superficial but may be deep, dull, or sharp, radicular or nonradicular, severe or mild. The duration of pain does not follow true patterns, lasting for moments or for years. It is resistant to most therapies and never disappears.

Key Elements of the History

The physician must establish a chronological history of the patient's low-back pain. Often specific details or earlier episodes and evaluations are lost as the patient concentrates on the immediate problem. Selected aspects of the review of systems and family history will give important clues as well.

1. *Role of Age.* Some clues to the etiology are gained when one takes into account the patient's age. Acute disc herniation, ankylosing spondylitis, Reiter's syndrome, and benign bone tumors have a peak incidence between the third and fourth decades, whereas malignant disease, spinal stenosis, osteoporosis, and degenerative joint disease have a peak incidence beyond the sixth decade.
2. *Role of Gender.* Low-back pain predominates in men due to the occupational hazards of robust labor. Numerous illnesses also predominate in men, including spondyloarthropathies, infection, and tumor, whereas metabolic disorders predominate in women, such as osteoporosis, parathyroid disorders, and polymyalgia rheumatica.
3. *Role of Family History.* Familial disorders include ankylosing spondylosis, Reiter's syndrome, psoriatic spondylosis, and spondylosis associated with inflammatory bowel disease.
4. *Role of Occupation.* Obtaining an occupational history is critical for establishing the risk of low-back pain. The greatest risk is in heavy-duty laborers, truck drivers, and nursing personnel.
5. *Present Illness.* Details of the history are directed toward the characteristic features of the low-back pain as outlined below, as well as the chronologic history of the problem. Such details are forgotten if the problem has existed for a few years or if multiple evaluations are involved. It is necessary to scrutinize outside information carefully for clues.
6. *Onset of Illness.* Acute mechanical injuries, including disc disease, are abrupt in onset and are often associated with a specific movement or task. Nonmechanical etiologies are usually slower in onset, with a gradual worsening of pain. One exception to this is pathological fractures or osteopenic fractures of the vertebral spine.
7. *Duration and Frequency of Pain.* Medical illness will cause pain that persists rather than being episodic, whereas mechanical causes of low-back pain are intermittent, with each episode lasting for a few days to several weeks. If there is chronic disc degeneration, the patient may experience low-grade discomfort that is periodically exacerbated during an acute attack. The frequency of each attack is related to the exposure of the patient to the mechanical stresses that worsen the symptoms. Psychogenic pain never ceases; it is constant

and unrelenting. The progression of symptoms even after a long interval of stability should warrant consideration of a repeat evaluation to rule out a new cause or worsening of an old one.

8. *Location of Pain.* The majority of medical and mechanical causes of low-back pain localize to the lumbosacral spine. Referred pain often will occur to the paraspinal region. Bilateral pain is common in patients with sacroiliac disease. Radicular pain or pain restricted to a lower extremity is suggestive of nerve root irritation, especially if the pain goes below the knee. Disruption of the annulus relieves the low-back pain component because pressure is relieved and the patient has restricted leg pain due to root involvement. Spinal stenosis can cause radicular pain but it is not present typically at rest, whereas nerve root disease from disc herniation is. Radicular pain is worse with walking. Psychogenic pain is not well localized, and the patient will report nonanatomical localization (i.e., not root or nerve).
9. *Quality and Intensity of Pain.* It is best to let the patient describe the characteristics of pain in his or her own words. The McGill Pain Questionnaire is helpful If the patient cannot describe the pain. Visual analog scales, denoting maximum, least, and average pain intensity, are helpful in determining the severity of pain over time.
10. *Aggravating Factors.* Mechanical causes of low-back pain improve with the patient supine. Those patients who feel better with absolutely no movement are more likely to have a localized process, including infection, compression fracture, or pathological fracture. Radicular root pain will worsen with upright activity, particularly with sitting and with forward flexion. Spinal stenosis will have worsened pain with standing and truncal extension. Increased intraspinal pressure (e.g., with coughing, sneezing, stooling, and other Valsalva maneuvers) will worsen root pain. The pain will be of a radicular type, thus differentiating it from muscle strain that remains localized with an abrupt Valsalva maneuver. Psychogenic pain is often difficult to relate to particular aggravating factors or is enhanced greatly by minimal physical exertion.

Clinical Examination

The examination of the patient with low-back pain is performed to answer questions about the spine, peripheral nerves, nerve roots, cauda equina, and spinal cord. One should not exclude the general examination lest one miss significant systemic illness (e.g., a pulsatile abdominal aneurysm, infection, or joint disease) that may be causing the patient's symptoms. The examination begins with *observation* of the patient—his or her mannerisms as they relate to the pain, the way the patient moves, and so on. Gait, turns, and balance should be observed. The patient who has difficulty squatting or arising from a chair is more likely to have rheumatological disease or neuromuscular disease rather than radiculopathy.

Examination of the vertebral spine should be performed with the patient standing and disrobed. The spine should be examined from behind and from a lateral position to determine alterations in alignment (scoliosis) and posture (lordosis). The gluteal folds and popliteal crease should be at similar heights. The patient with paravertebral muscle spasm may tilt in one direction while attempting to protect the site of injury. The patient will often lose the lumbar lordosis as well. The spine is palpated and percussed to identify any area of focal tenderness, and observations are made for congenital anomalies (e.g., excessive dimpling, diastematomyelia, or tuft of hair, cafe-au-lait spots). Spinal motion should be assessed from a standing position. Full range of motion (forward flexion, 40° to 60°; extension, 20° to 35°; lateral bending, 15° to 20°; rotation, 5° to 15°) should occur without discomfort. Normal forward flexion should result in at least a 5-cm expansion between a mark placed between the sacral dimples and a point 10 cm anteriorly (Schober Test). Musculoskeletal disease (i.e., spondylosis) will have limited flexion, and the expansion will be less than 4 cm.

Straight leg raising (SLR) should be done with the patient supine and, if there is concern about psychogenic disease, in the sitting position as well. In this latter maneuver, the leg is brought to 90° under the pretense that the clinician is examining the sole of the foot. Patients with true back pain will extend at the hips as they try to keep the angle greater than 90°. Sciatic notch tenderness implies that the nerve root is irritated but does not give any clues as to the cause of the irritation. Patrick's test assesses the hip and the sacroiliac (SI) joint. The test is performed by placing the lateral malleolus of one leg on the patella of the other leg while applying downward pressure to the knee. Acute pain with rapid downward pressure suggests disease of the SI joint, whereas pain produced with slow downward movement suggests hip disease.

The neurological examination should be detailed in an attempt to determine the presence or absence of abnormality and the segmental level of involvement. Elements of this exam should include the following:

1. *Muscle testing* is performed comparing the findings on one side to those on the other and to the examiner's expected norms. Inspect muscle bulk carefully, looking for atrophy. Palpate the muscle for spasm and trigger points. Observe for spontaneous movements (fasciculations) as well. Pay particular attention to the small muscles of the foot, especially the extensors of the great toe (extensor hallucis longus), which is a L5 marker. Give-away weakness suggests nonorganic disease. Remembered that the patient may not use full effort in the presence of pain.
2. *Sensory examination* should include all of the primary modalities (pain, light touch, temperature, position sense, and vibratory sensation). Patients may experience an abnormality in one sensation and not another. Pay careful attention to the distribution of abnormality; does it respect a peripheral nerve, a nerve root, or a spinal level? Accurate testing cannot be done if the patient is fatigued, in severe pain, or hostile.
3. *Muscle stretch reflexes* are carefully assessed to determine any asymmetry. The following chart is helpful in determining common reflex–nerve root correlations:

Nerve Root	Reflex
L4	Knee
L5	*None*
S1	Ankle

Note that L5 does not have an easily elicitable reflex. One must rely on other markers (extension of the great toe) for clues. The demonstration of hyperreflexia and pathological reflexes (the presence of a Babinski response) suggests the presence of central nervous system involvement.

Elements of the examination that are painful should be done last in order to maintain patient cooperation throughout the majority of the exam. The uncomfortable patient is less likely to cooperate. One must carefully determine the presence or absence of a sensory level, the integrity of sphincter function, and the presence of accentuated muscle stretch reflexes if there is concern about an intraspinal lesion.

The clinical examination should provide the examiner with a list of potential diagnostic etiologies. Abnormalities of spinal motion in the absence of discrete neurological findings suggest that the patient has primary disease of the spine or joints. Abnormalities of the neurological examination should be defined in terms of the level of the neuraxis involved: the spinal cord, conus medullaris, cauda equina, nerve root, or peripheral nerve. Peripheral neuropathies typically exhibit symmetrical loss of sensation (stocking-glove distribution), distal muscle weakness and atrophy, and diminished reflexes. Lesions of the peripheral nerve roots will manifest with discrete motor abnormalities in the distribution of the involved nerve root, sensory disturbances in the dermatomal distribution of the involved nerve root, and an asymmetrical or absent muscle stretch reflex appropriate to the involved nerve root. Lesions of the cauda equina and conus medullaris will produce asymmetrical findings of muscle weakness, saddle anesthesia, and bowel and bladder disturbances.

Diagnostic Studies

The goal of diagnostic studies is to further confirm the clinical hypothesis. Studies should be requested to answer specific questions and should proceed in a logical fashion rather than using the shotgun approach. *It should be remembered that 20% to 30% of normal, asymptomatic individuals have evidence of disc herniation on radiographic studies.*[25,219] Weinstein and colleagues note that imaging studies have improved the diagnostician's ability to view disc anatomy, but these studies have not improved the ability to predict which patients with low-back pain will benefit from intervention.[218] Intra- and interobserver disagreement compounds the difficulties in determining a diagnosis with many of these studies.[29,162] Therefore, careful correlation of the patient's complaints, and neurological and musculoskeletal findings, with the results of diagnostic studies is necessary before treatment is initiated.[59] However, in the vast majority of cases, no definable cause is identified.[162] Regrettably, many diagnostic tests have no scientific validity demonstrating their utility to pinpoint the cause of the pain source.[161]

1. *Routine Blood Work*. Most often, routine blood work is not helpful unless there is a suspicion of systemic illness.
2. *Plain Radiographs*. Patients should be screened with radiographs of the spine to assess spinal stability and anatomical correlates, with the following caveats: Unless there is concern about systemic illness or congenital spinal disorder, plain radiographs will not add significant information about a specific etiology. The Quebec Task Force on Spinal Disorders states that plain radiographs are necessary only in patients with lateralizing findings, below the age of 20 or over the age of 50, in the presence of fever, trauma, or evidence of neoplasia.[186] Spine radiographs will give information on the presence or absence of spondylosis, disc space narrowing, vertebral body compression, and metabolic or neoplastic disorders. There is a tendency to *overread* changes that occur due to the normal aging process, particularly disc space narrowing. Attention should focus on the following features:
   a. *Intervertebral Disc Space*. This should be divergent anteriorly on a lateral film. Each disc space should increase in width from L1 through L5.
   b. *Bone Density*. Lytic lesions of bone suggest tumor or an infectious process. Discrete blastic lesions of bone will suggest a neoplastic process.
   c. *Foraminal Size*. Nerve root foramina should be free from osteophyte formation; their appearance is ovoid to round.
3. *Computed Tomography (CT) Scanning*. There are several advantages to CT scanning:
   a. It is an excellent tool to determine bony architecture.
   b. Transverse images establish the relationship of the spinal cord to the spinal canal and are therefore helpful in diagnosing spinal stenosis.
   c. It is more sensitive than plain radiographs in establishing subtle bony destruction due to tumor or infection.

   There are, however, several potential pitfalls:
   a. Computed tomography scanning produces lower resolution of the anatomical structures when compared to magnetic resonance imaging.
   b. The ability to identify a herniated disc without concurrent myelography is poor.
4. *Magnetic Resonance Imaging (MRI)*. The correlation between symptoms of low-back pain and MRI remains to be established, although it is becoming the initial study of choice at some centers. It is the study of choice in evaluating intramedullary lesions of the spinal cord. There are several advantages to its use:
   a. It can establish an excellent relationship of the spinal cord to the spinal canal.
   b. It is more accurate than CT in characterizing extramedullary tumors and focal infection (abscess).
   c. It is more sensitive than CT in establishing subtle bony destruction due to tumor or infection.

   There are, however, several potential pitfalls:
   a. Localization of external landmarks to spinal images is difficult.
   b. The extent of the lesion may be overestimated.
   c. It is not as reliable technically as myelography.
   d. Its usefulness in evaluating vascular disorders of the spine and spinal cord is not very good.
   e. It is not as useful as CT in establishing bony detail.
6. *Myelography*. Myelography should be used to confirm the clinical diagnosis. It is useful in determining the presence of lesions at other spinal levels and inflammatory complications of surgery, and in identifying disc

fragments. It is less sensitive in defining disorders of L5-S1 due to the tapering of the dural sac. Reports abound that 20% to 25% of asymptomatic patients have an abnormal myelogram; therefore, an abnormal study in the absence of clinical symptoms is not meaningful. It should also be borne in mind that myelography is an invasive procedure with the attendant risks of infection, bleeding, and so on. Tricyclic antidepressant medication should be discontinued prior to myelography because of the risk of seizures. The study should include the following views:

a. Frontal—to evaluate cauda equina and nerve root exit zones.
b. Lateral—to evaluate the relationship of the subarachnoid space to the posterior wall of the spinal canal.
c. Oblique—to evaluate nerve roots and the associated nerve root sheaths.

7. *Electrophysiology*. Electrodiagnostic studies (neurography [NCV], late responses, electromyography [EMG]) are used to evaluate the presence of abnormalities of the peripheral nerve, nerve root, cauda equina, and spinal cord. Unlike radiographic techniques, these studies give information on the severity of the physiological dysfunction. They should be performed *prior to* myelography to minimize the chance of dye-induced abnormalities. There is about a 70% to 80% agreement with clinical and radiological studies.[115] Most often, standard NCV studies are normal, with one exception: the H-reflex. Its absence or asymmetry suggests an S1 root lesion. Electromyographic findings in nerve root disease include the presence of denervation potentials (fibrillations, positive sharp waves) acutely and reduced motor unit recruitment, a reduced interference pattern, and polyphasic motor unit potentials chronically. Abnormality of the paraspinal musculature is clear evidence of a lesion at or proximal to the dorsal root.[67] There is a delay between the onset of injury and the presence of abnormal EMG findings, often taking as long as 2 weeks to become apparent. Somatosensory evoked potential (SSEP) studies remain controversial concerning their utility in the evaluation of nerve root disease.
8. *Lumbar Discography*. Discography involves radiography of the spine following injection of radiopaque material into the disc. The goal is to reproduce the patient's symptoms, as well as to assess the characteristics of the disc anatomy. It is most useful in the evaluation of the L5-S1 level, though its use is not widespread.
9. *Radionucleotide Bone Scanning*. Bone scanning involves the use of a radiopharmaceutical in small doses to assess the metabolic activity of bone. It is most useful in the evaluation of infiltrating tumor, infectious processes, and blood flow. Inflammatory arthropathies may be imaged due to increased blood flow to the area. Its advantages include the facts that it is a rapid, easy screen of metabolic bone function, and it is better than plain radiographs in establishing infiltrating or inflammatory disease. Its disadvantages include the fact that it has less specificity than other radiographic procedures in establishing a pathological process.
10. *Thermography*. Infrared thermography is the measurement of the relative emission of infrared energy (skin temperature). Its use in the diagnosis of low-back pain syndromes has been very controversial and the subject of numerous reviews and white papers[7,77,171] Proponents of its use in low-back pain and lumbar radiculopathy argue that it is noninvasive, painless, and cheaper than electrodiagnosis, myelography, and other imaging studies.[97,110,200] Other investigators disagree, citing the lack of specificity, sensitivity, and clinical usefulness.[7,77,97,108,133,134,184] There are no data to support the role of thermography in the diagnosis and management of low-back pain syndromes.

Diagnostic Etiologies

Congenital Disorders of the Spine

Most congenital disorders of the spine (asymmetrical facets, abnormalities of the transverse processes, sacralization L5, etc.) do not produce low-back pain syndromes. They may however, predispose the individual to future disc disease.

Spondylolisthesis

Spondylolisthesis is the anterior displacement of one vertebral body over another. There are several forms of spondylolisthesis. The majority result from degenerative change; other forms occur as a congenital disorder, tumor invasion with secondary instability, or traumatic injury. Because of the similarity of symptoms, they are discussed as one.

HISTORY. Patients present with complaints of low-back pain: dull and boring in quality, with radiation into the thighs and stiffness of movement. The pain improves with extension of the spine and worsens with anterior flexion. More than half of the patients associate the onset of symptoms with minor trauma. Discomfort is nearly constant and is of variable severity.

EXAMINATION. Patients exhibit some tenderness with palpation or percussion over the affected area. They may have some associated paraspinal muscle spasm. There is an accentuation of the lumbar lordosis, and occasionally one can palpate the bony displacement. Many patients exhibit hamstring tightness, the pathogenesis of which is not clear. Neurological examination is normal unless there has been nerve root compression by fibrocartilage formation at the site of the lesion.

LABORATORY TESTS. Standard blood tests are normal. Plain radiographs demonstrate the abnormal displacement (subluxation) of the vertebral body. Most commonly, L5 is displaced forward of the sacrum in congenital disease and L4 on L5 in degenerative disease.

Mechanical Disorders of the Lumbosacral Spine

Mechanical disorders of the lumbosacral spine are the most frequent cause of low-back pain and range from simple muscle strains to vertebral fractures with secondary spinal cord injury. By definition, this group of disorders results from the overuse of a normal anatomical structure or is secondary to injury or deformity of an anatomical structure. These disorders should not pose a problem for the clinician. Mechanical disorders of the spine are usually aggravated by particular activities and relieved by rest. Such movements may be helpful in differentiating the cause of pain; for example, flexion worsens disc disease but improves facet disease.

Muscle Strain

Muscle strain results from injuries to muscle and ligamentous structures associated with lifting heavy objects, from falls, and from other unexpected movements. These are usually self-limited injuries.

HISTORY. The patient will usually complain of abrupt, severe low-back pain confined to the low-back region either in the midline or in the paravertebral regions. The patient should be able to report a temporal association with an above precipitating activity.

EXAMINATION. The patient will exhibit significant point tenderness to palpation over the affected area. There is accentuation of the discomfort with postural change and improvement with relaxation. Marked paraspinal muscle spasm is present, and trigger points may be evident.

LABORATORY TESTS. All laboratory studies will be normal.

Herniated Nucleus Pulposus

Herniated nucleus pulposus protrudes into the spinal canal due to thinning of the annulus fibrosus or rupture through the annulus with extrusion of the nuclear material into the spinal canal. Most often these lesions occur between L5-S1 > L4-L5 >> L3-L4, and a single disc herniation may involve more than one spinal root. Sensory complaints are frequent. Objective motor and sensory findings may be few, and while reflex abnormalities are common, their absence does not preclude disc disease. It is in this group of patients with convincing histories and unconvincing exams that ancillary studies, particularly of physiological function, are helpful. Most patients, particularly younger ones, will report minor trauma, and the onset of symptoms coincides with the activity or closely follows it.

HISTORY. The patient will complain of intermittent radicular pain into the buttocks and leg. The pain is worsened by flexion or rotation of the spine, straining, and so on. The precise symptoms depend upon the segmental level of involvement.

L3-L4 disc with L4 nerve root involvement will produce pain in the low back radiating into the posterior-lateral thigh and the anterior portion of the leg. The patient may complain of weakness in extending the knee, with some instability of gait and disturbed sensation in the anteromedial portion of the thigh.

L4-L5 disc with L5 nerve root involvement will produce pain over the sacroiliac joint in the hip with radiation into the lateral thigh and leg. The patient may complain of difficulty walking on the heels and lifting the toes. He or she may report disturbed sensation along the lateral border of the leg and in the web space of the great toe.

L5-S1 disc with S1 nerve root involvement will produce pain over the sacroiliac joint in the hip with radiation down the posterior lateral thigh, down the leg, and into the heel. The patient may complain of weakness in walking on the toes. He or she may report disturbed sensation along the back of the calf and the lateral border of the foot.

Central disc herniation will produce pain, often bilateral, in the low back, thighs, legs, and perineum. The patient may report variable degrees of weakness and sensory disturbances that can also be bilateral. Depending upon the level of involvement, the patient may also report sphincter disturbances.

EXAMINATION. The examination of the patient with a herniated disc will reflect the segmental level of involvement, but objective motor and sensory findings are often minimal.

L3-L4 disc with L4 nerve root involvement may demonstrate weakness of the quadriceps muscle. This may be associated with atrophy of the thigh. The patient may report diminished sensation in the distribution noted in the above section. The knee jerk may be reduced or absent.

L4-L5 disc with L5 nerve root involvement may demonstrate weakness of foot dorsiflexion and extension of the great toe. The patient may report diminished sensation in the distribution noted in the above section. There is no reflex abnormality.

L5-S1 disc with S1 nerve root involvement may demonstrate weakness of gastrocnemius muscles. Often weakness will not be detectable on manual muscle testing, and the examiner will have to rely on functional assessments such as walking on the toes. The patient may report diminished sensation in the distribution noted in the above section. The ankle jerk may be reduced or absent.

Central disc herniation will produce a variable pattern of muscle weakness and sensory disturbance. Depending upon the level of involvement, the patient may also demonstrate reduced anal sphincter tone. The ankle jerk may be reduced or absent.

Examination of the spine will demonstrate decreased range of motion with anterior flexion due to pain, and the patient may exhibit a tilt to the side of the lesion. Movement of the spine will often accentuate the patient's discomfort, as will Valsalva maneuvers.

Straight leg raising will reproduce radicular pain, the distribution of which will determine the nerve root involved. Tension is applied to the tethered nerve at 30°, with little additional tension beyond 70°. Back pain alone is not considered a positive test finding. A modification of this test involves lifting the leg to the point of pain, lowering the leg slightly, and then performing dorsiflexion of the foot. This will re-create the pain. If radicular pain is produced on the nonlifted side, the implication is that of a medial disc herniation; the pain is produced by the downward movement of the nerve root around the disc. Another modification of the test is the *crossed SLR*. Lifting the unaffected limb will reproduce the patient's symptoms. This variation is highly specific but less sensitive than the standard SLR test.[92,111]

LABORATORY TESTS. Plain radiographs are of little value but may show degenerative change at various levels. Computed tomography imaging may demonstrate a disc bulge or soft tissue fragment within the spinal canal. At times, there seems to be a poor correlation between radiographic images and clinical symptomatology. Myelography is a excellent way to visualize the level of involvement and is better than CT imaging. Magnetic resonance imaging will detect a herniated disc easily, though the degree of abnormality may be exaggerated. Electrodiagnostic studies are extensions of the neurological examination, and are performed to map the distribution of involvement and to determine the physiological severity of the problem. Electromyographic abnormalities are found in about 90% of patients. The diagnosis of a radiculopathy is supported by the demonstration of an abnormality in several muscles innervated by the same nerve root but of different peripheral nerves. Abnormalities found in the associated paraspinal muscles will localize the problem to the nerve root.

Lumbar (Spinal) Stenosis
Lumbar (spinal) stenosis is broadly defined as any condition resulting in any type of spinal canal narrowing by soft tissue or bony structures. Patients are usually in their sixth decade. There are four common etiologies:

1. Idiopathic spinal stenosis
2. Degenerative spinal stenosis
3. Degenerative spondylolisthesis (see above)
4. Postoperative spinal stenosis

HISTORY. The patient will usually complain of intermittent, dull, aching discomfort (claudication) in the legs that is quite distinct from the radicular pain of nerve root disease. The muscle cramping typical of vascular claudication is not present. Low-back pain, of variable severity, is present in the majority of patients. This tends to be more common in the early stages of the illness, when there is joint laxity, and decreases with osteophyte formation. The claudication is worsened by walking or standing and is quickly relieved by sitting or leaning forward. Some patients will report numbness of the affected leg. True radicular pain is very uncommon but is found in the lateral recess syndrome (see below).

EXAMINATION. The neurological examination will be normal in more than 50% to 65% of patients with lumbar stenosis. About 25% to 40% will demonstrate an asymmetrical ankle jerk or knee jerk. About 33% will demonstrate some weakness in the most affected limb. Maneuvers to worsen the pain of root disease (SLR, etc.) are normal. Backward bending results in marked worsening in about 50% of patients.

LABORATORY TESTS. Plain radiographs are of little value in this patient population but may show degenerative change at L4. Computed tomography imaging with transverse views of the spine is most helpful. Measurements of the anterior-posterior and transverse diameters will establish the diagnosis. Myelography or MRI will also establish the extent of canal narrowing. Electromyographic abnormalities are found in patients who have associated radiculopathies.

Lateral Recess Syndrome
Lateral recess syndrome results from osteophyte formation on the superior articular facet that encroaches on the nerve root canal, with subsequent compression of the nerve root itself. It is similar to other radiculopathies, with some important differences.

HISTORY. The patient will usually complain of pain typical of nerve root disease that is precipitated by standing and walking and improves with sitting. This is the opposite of what patients report with radiculopathies from herniated discs. Coughing, sneezing, and stooling (Valsalva maneuvers) do not aggravate the pain in this syndrome, in contrast to a herniated disc.

EXAMINATION. See above.

LABORATORY TESTS. See above.

Vertebral Body Compression Fracture
Vertebral body compression fracture in general occurs in patients who are elderly and often have an underlying predisposing disorder, such as osteopenia, chronic corticosteroid use, bony malignancy, or parathyroid disorders.

HISTORY. The patient will usually complain of abrupt, severe low-back pain that is confined to the low-back region either in the midline or in the paravertebral regions. The patient will often report a temporal association with a specific movement or activity. The vast majority of patients do not have a history of trauma.

EXAMINATION. The patient will exhibit significant point tenderness to palpation over the affected area. There is accentuation of the discomfort with postural change. The patient reports pain even with relaxation in the acute phase. Marked paraspinal muscle spasm is also present.

LABORATORY TESTS. Findings will depend upon the underlying etiology. Spine radiographs will demonstrate the compression fracture. Osteopenia or blastic or lytic lesions of bone may be evident. Abnormalities of serum and urine proteins, an elevated erythrocyte sedimentation rate (ESR), and so will be present, depending upon the etiology.

Rheumatological Disorders with Low-Back Pain

Low-back pain is a common symptom of a variety of rheumatological disorders of the spine due to involvement of the vertebral bodies, ligaments, muscles, tendons, and joints. The most common disorders in this group are the seronegative spondyloarthropathies. Characteristically, the pain is present upon awakening and improves throughout the day.

Ankylosing Spondylitis

Ankylosing spondylitis is a chronic inflammatory process characterized by progressive arthritic change of the sacroiliac joints and the vertebral spine. It affects about 2% of Caucasians in a 10:1 male:female ratio. The pathogenesis remains unknown.[31]

HISTORY. Typically, the patient is a middle-aged white male complaining of intermittent, dull, aching low-back pain associated with stiffness that slowly worsens over several months. The pain is most severe in the morning and usually improves throughout the day. Remember that these inflammatory symptoms (morning stiffness, improvement with exercise, and nocturnal pain), while sensitive, are not specific for ankylosing spondylitis. Rarely, the pain will be severe enough to mimic an acute radiculopathy with radiation into the lower extremities. A few patients may report arthritic symptoms elsewhere. Calin et al.[38] have defined five questions to screen for this illness, and positive responses to four of them are defined as positive in 95% of cases.

EXAMINATION. The examination of spine mobility demonstrates limitation in forward flexion or lateral bending. There is tenderness to palpation of the paraspinal muscles in the region of involvement. The neurological examination is normal.

LABORATORY TESTS. Most laboratory test findings are nonspecific (minimal elevation of the ESR, mild anemia). Notably, the rheumatoid factor is absent. Patients will exhibit HLA-B27 antigens, but this finding is not diagnostic. Plain radiographs of the spine are most helpful in demonstrating the symmetrical changes of ankylosing spondylitis, but often these changes are not present in the early stages of the illness. Radiographic changes are noted first in the sacroiliac joints, with later involvement of the lumbar spine. The diagnostic criteria for staging are beyond the scope of this discussion. Electrodiagnostic studies have no role in the diagnosis.

Reiter's Syndrome

Reiter's syndrome occurs typically in a young male with associated symptoms of urethritis, conjunctivitis, and arthritis.

HISTORY. The patient will usually complain of back pain, and nearly 95% of patients will experience pain at some time during their illness. Pain is usually aching in quality; occasionally it will radiate into the thighs, but this radicular symptom is clearly distinct from the radicular pain of a true radiculopathy.

EXAMINATION. The examination will demonstrate restriction of spine movement with forward flexion. There will be involvement of other joints, usually of the legs in men and the arms in women. Tenderness to percussion of the sacroiliac joints is common. Plantar fasciitis is also a common complaint. The examination will also demonstrate mild conjunctivitis and mucocutaneous lesions of the oropharynx. Rarely, there will be evidence of constitutional and neurological disease (neuropathy, cranial nerve palsies).

LABORATORY TESTS. While these patients may have a variety of abnormalities, most are nonspecific (elevated sedimentation rate, anemia and thrombocytosis). Presence of HLA-B27 will differentiate the patient form rheumatoid arthritis. Radiographs will demonstrate asymmetrical joint destruction, that is most severe in hands and feet. Usually there is sparing of hips and shoulders. Variable amounts of bony erosion are seen. Electrodiagnostic studies have no role in the diagnosis of Reiter's Syndrome but may be abnormal when there are associated neurological complications.

Diffuse Idiopathic Skeletal Hyperostosis

Diffuse idiopathic skeletal hyperostosis (DISH) occurs in about 25% of autopsy series. It predominates in Caucasian men (2:1 ratio) and typically occurs over the age of 50.[31]

HISTORY. The patient will usually complain of a mild, dull, aching discomfort in the back associated with stiffness. The stiffness may precede the onset of pain by several years. There may be a previous history of a minor accident or occupational spine trauma.

EXAMINATION. The examination of the spine demonstrates mild limitation of lumbar spine mobility. Few patients will have tenderness to percussion; when present, the tenderness localizes to the sacroiliac joints. Occasionally there is extraspinal involvement of the shoulders, knees, and elbows.

LABORATORY TESTS. Most laboratory parameters are normal. Radiographs of the spine will demonstrate a characteristic calcification/ossification of the anterolateral border of the vertebral bodies, preservation of disc space height, and absence of other bony abnormalities. Electrodiagnostic studies have no role in this disorder.

Osteochondritis

Osteochondritis of the vertebral spine results from an irregular ossification and endochondral growth of the vertebral body at the junction of the disc. It is estimated that nearly 10% of the population suffers from this disorder. The male:female patient ratio is 1:2. The pathogenesis is unknown.

HISTORY. The patient often complains of back pain associated with increasing kyphosis. With lumbar spine involvement there is local pain, with radiation into the hips but not below the gluteal folds. The pain is dull, aching, occasionally sharp, and severe.

EXAMINATION. The examination of the spine will demonstrate limitation of forward flexion, extension, and lateral rotation. The patient will have paraspinal muscle spasm and tenderness to palpation. Typically, the patient will demonstrate kyphosis, primarily in the thoracic region, but in 25% this may involve lumbar spine. The neurological examination is normal.

LABORATORY TESTS. Blood test findings are normal. Plain radiographs of the spine demonstrate the characteristic anterior wedging of the vertebral bodies by more than 5°, Schmorl's nodes, and kyphosis.

Fibromyalgia

Fibromyalgia (fibrositis) is a soft tissue disorder characterized by relapsing and remitting pain and stiffness with no associated abnormality of anatomical structures.[39,227] It tends to occur more frequently in the type A personality and is more frequent in women than men. The pathogenesis is unknown.

HISTORY. Patients complain of severe, diffuse pain and aches associated with severe stiffness of joints. Stiffness tends to be more severe in the morning, though some report it in the evening or as occurring in an unrelenting fashion. Many patients have associated fatigue and a number of other nonspecific constitutional complaints including disturbed sleep. Inactivity and overactivity, cold weather, and increased humidity are reported to exacerbate the symptoms.

EXAMINATION. The examination demonstrates discrete areas of tenderness, commonly at the upper border of the trapezius muscle, the medial aspect of the knees, the elbows, the posterior iliac crest, and the lumbar spine. Some patients will have fibrocystic nodules: discrete, firm, mobile, tender nodules that are of indeterminate significance.

LABORATORY TESTS. No laboratory test findings are abnormal, including, routine tests, radiographs and electrophysiological tests.

Infectious Diseases with Low-Back Pain

Infections of the lumbar spine are uncommon causes of low-back pain and are easily treatable if recognized. The clinical symptoms relate to the type of organism involved. Fungal and tubercular infections have an indolent course. Bacterial infections are abrupt in onset and worsen, with a rapid course. The etiology is quite varied, and an extensive discussion is beyond the scope of this chapter. The majority of bacterial infections are hematogenously spread. Their source is often a urinary tract infection, an indwelling catheter, a focal site of cellulitis, or an injection site (i.e., an illicit drug user).[211]

Osteomyelitis

Osteomyelitis of the vertebral spine is caused by a number of pathogens, usually from hematogenous spread. Rarely, there is direct spread from an adjacent focus.

HISTORY. The patient presents with a history of progressive low-back pain lasting for several days to a few weeks. Initially the pain is intermittent, becomes constant, and is worsened by movement. Often there is a history of a recent infection or an invasive procedure. Occasionally, there may be signs of meningeal or nerve root irritation, and the pain is similar to that of an acute radiculopathy.

EXAMINATION. These patients are systemically ill, with fever (often low-grade), and complain of tenderness to percussion or palpation over the affected area. Examination of the spine demonstrates diminished spinal mobility to flexion, extension, and lateral rotation. Neurological findings may be common due to nerve root irritation or compression of the caudal sac or spinal cord. The specifics will reflect the segmental level of involvement.

LABORATORY TESTS. Standard blood tests findings are usually normal or are nonspecific. The ESR is often elevated, particularly during the acute phase of the illness and more so with bacterial infections. Blood cultures are positive in 50% of patients. However, in patients with normal blood cultures, it may be necessary to obtain tissue by needle or surgical biopsy of bone. Skin test antigens will be positive in appropriate infections. Radiographic studies will demonstrate early bone loss, decreased disc height, and, later, soft tissue swelling of adjacent structures. Radiographic findings will lag behind the clinical picture by 4 to 8 weeks. Magnetic resonance imaging and CT are more sensitive in detecting inflammatory lesions of bone or adjacent tissue. Bone scanning may be very useful early in the course of the illness or in those patients suspected of having more indolent infections such as tuberculosis or fungal infections.

Disc Infection

Disc infection (infections of the intervertebral disc space) is uncommon but does produce severe low-back pain when present. Infection occurs as the result of hematogenous spread of an organism or by contamination of the site at the time of disc surgery.

HISTORY. The character of the pain is often acute, severe, and restricted to the low back. Infrequently, it may be mild and have a more insidious onset. Minimal movement exacerbates the pain, and it is relieved by strict rest.

EXAMINATION. Examination of the spine demonstrates paraspinal muscle spasm and a guarding of all movement. There is tenderness to palpation/percussion over the involved interspace. The neurological examination is normal unless there has been compression of adjacent nerve roots by the inflammatory reaction.

LABORATORY TESTS. Other than an elevation of the ESR, blood test findings are normal or nonspecific. Culture of disc space contents is rewarding, but blood cultures are rarely positive. Plain radiographs demonstrate an early reduction in the height of the disc space that later increases, with a loss of vertebral bone. There is reactive bone formation at adjacent vertebral bodies. Magnetic resonance imaging is more sensitive for demonstrating an inflammatory reaction as is radionucleotide bone scanning.

Epidural Abscess

Epidural abscess results from the hematogenous spread of infection from a remote site to the epidural space or by direct extension from a primary site in proximity to the vertebral spine.[12] Hematogenous spread from a known source of infection occurs in about 50% of case and from nonidentifiable sources in nearly 40% of cases.[53] Direct extension may occur as the result of osteomyelitis, perinephric abscess, indwelling catheters, or surgical wounds.[53,206] While rare, this disorder can be a diagnostic nightmare because it may mimic other common disorders.[6]

HISTORY. Characteristically patients report the acute, subacute, or chronic development of fever, headache, and malaise in association with low-back pain, radicular pain, and percussion tenderness over the affected area. In actuality, the clinical presentation is quite varied, and this accounts for the delay in diagnosis that commonly occurs. It should be remembered that in chronic epidural abscesses, fever and evidence of systemic illness may not be present; uncommonly, pain and spinal tenderness may be absent as well.[206]

EXAMINATION. The findings on examination will be varied and reflect the level of involvement of the neuraxis. Tenderness to percussion of the vertebral spine is nearly pathognomonic in the setting of fever and back pain given the caveats above.

LABORATORY TESTS. Routine blood tests will often show elevation of the white blood cell count and marked elevation of the ESR (although there are cases in which this has been normal).[53] Bacteriological studies will reflect the underlying organism, *Staphylococcus aureus* being the most common isolate. Cerebrospinal fluid examination should be performed cautiously using a cisternal approach if the abscess is in the path of a lumbar approach. Plain radiographs are commonly unrevealing but may show evidence of an inflammatory process

Herpes Zoster

Herpes zoster (shingles) results from the reactivation of the varicella virus and is characterized by an erythematous, vesicular rash accompanied by pain in the distribution of the affected nerve root

HISTORY. Patients report the onset of local pain, often burning in quality and associated with dysesthesias following a vague illness. These symptoms respect the territory of a sensory dermatome. Touch, light pressure, and movement of clothes across the region will aggravate the pain or heighten the dysesthesias. As the characteristic rash appears, the pain will abate until the rash begins to crust over. The pain then becomes a deep, boring, constant ache. The symptoms localize to the lumbar and sacral regions in 15% to 18% of patients. The pain will resolve with the resolution of the cutaneous rash in the majority of patients. However, in some, particularly the elderly, the pain may persist indefinitely (postherpetic neuralgia). Recently, gabapentin has gained approval for the treatment of postherpetic pain with significant benefit.[19]

EXAMINATION. There may be no findings on examination despite intense pain prior to the development of the skin rash. Some patients will describe hyperesthesia on sensory testing in the distribution of the affected sensory nerve root. The rash is erythematous, plaque-like, and associated with scattered vesicles. These are found at the distal portion of the dermatome initially and subsequently develop more proximally along the same sensory nerve root.

LABORATORY TESTS. Routine blood tests are normal, other than the occasional elevation in the ESR. Plain radiographs are normal. Imaging studies are normal in the uncomplicated case. They may demonstrate changes of spinal cord gray–white matter in situations where there are neurological sequelae. Electrophysiological studies are usually normal.

Neoplasms Associated with Low-Back Pain

Tumors of the spine are an uncommon cause of low-back pain (less than 1%), though there are a few situations in which they must be considered.[63] Many of the rare benign tumors will not be discussed here except in the most general terms. Pain that increases in the supine position is characteristic of tumors of the spine, though not of all tumors in this region. Neurological abnormalities, when present, reflect the encroachment by tumor on neural elements. This may take the form of root disease or compressive lesions of the spinal cord. As a rule, benign tumors involve the posterior elements of the spine (transverse process, spinous process) whereas malignant tumors tend to involve the vertebral body. In all situations, radiographic studies are the best way to define the anatomical abnormality for the cause of pain, and it is necessary to obtain tissue to establish a definitive diagnosis.

Metastatic Disease

Metastatic disease to the vertebral spine results from direct extension of tumor or hematogenous spread. These tumors are more common than primary tumors of the spine, and their incidence increases with age.

HISTORY. The typical patient will be one with a prior history of malignancy, over the age of 50, who has back pain without previous trauma. The pain is insidious in onset, increasing over time, and has a deep, aching quality. While localized initially, it may develop a radicular pattern. Lumbar pain is worsened with movement as well as with Valsalva maneuvers. Patients will report that their pain is not relieved with rest, but this is a nonspecific finding.[60]

EXAMINATION. The examination will demonstrate pain to palpation/percussion over the affected vertebral body (bodies). Many patients will have some limitation of movement. Neurological examination is critical to establish, if present, the segmental level of involvement and to differentiate between root compression and a more ominous problem such as the cauda equina syndrome, the conus medullaris syndrome, or spinal cord compression. Attention must be paid to sphincter function, which, if abnormal, would suggest a cauda equina, conus medullaris, or spinal cord lesion.

LABORATORY TESTS. Standard blood tests may be normal or nonspecific in many instances. Specific tumors may produce abnormalities in blood chemistries, such as increased alkaline phosphatase with metastatic prostatic carcinoma.

Multiple Myeloma

HISTORY. Pain is the most common presenting complaint in patients with multiple myeloma. The majority will have low-back pain, though pain can occur in any of the bones. Its quality is often aching, intermittent, and mild in severity. It is worse with upright posture and improves with recumbency. A small percentage of patients will have radicular pain that will be diagnosed as lumbar disc disease. Twenty percent of patients will report minor trauma that results in a pathological fracture of the vertebral spine producing severe local pain.

EXAMINATION. The examination of the spine may be normal in the earliest stages of the illness. With progression there will be limitation of spinal movement, particularly if there are pathological fractures. There will be discrete tenderness to palpation over areas of fracture. The neurological examination will be abnormal and will emonstrate the features of root disease or spinal cord compression, depending upon the segmental level of involvement. These findings may result from compression of the vertebral body or compression by a plasmacytoma.

LABORATORY TESTS. Nonspecific changes are seen in blood chemistries, elevation of the ESR, thrombocytopenia, and so on. Characteristic abnormalities of serum and urine immunoglobulins are found. Bone marrow examination will demonstrate increased numbers of plasma cells, typical of this disorder. Plain radiographs will demonstrate changes due to osteopenia, usually diffusely. Lytic lesions with the absence of sclerosis are found. Destruction is preferentially seen in the vertebral bodies, sparing the transverse and spinous processes and pedicles. Computed tomography scanning may demonstrate these changes earlier than those seen with standard radiographs. Electrophysiological testing will demonstrate changes of root compression if such involvement is present.

Intraspinal Tumors

Intraspinal tumors account for 10% of all central nervous system tumors. They may be extradural (outside of the meninges), intradural but extramedullary (within the meninges but outside of the spinal cord proper), or intramedullary (within the substance of the spinal cord). The quality of the pain and its location are summarized in Table 16.1.

HISTORY. The history of patients with an intraspinal tumor is varied. Many patients will report that their pain is accentuated when lying down, and reduced with sitting—a feature that distinguishes it from pain due to mechanical disorders of the spine. Pain will be the primary complaint in patients with extradural tumors. Typically, the pain is local, severe, progressing with time, and worse at night with the patient recumbent. The patient will report radicular discomfort in an appropriate dermatome if there is nerve root compression, and this pain worsens with activity. Neurological abnormalities occur early in the course of the disease and the patient will report a number of symptoms, including weakness, disturbances of sensation, and bladder and bowel dysfunction.

Table 16.1. Location and Quality of Tumor-Associated Spinal Pain

Location of Tumor	Quality of Pain	Frequency of Pain	Location of Pain
Extradural	Deep ache	Very common	Lumbar spine
Intradural-Extramedullary	Referred	Common	Low back and leg
Intramedullary	Radicular	Rare	Low back and leg

Source: Modified from Borenstein and Wiesel.[31]

Intradural-extramedullary tumors will produce radicular pain due to the proximity of the tumor to nerve roots. The specific symptoms will depend upon the root involved (see the previous discussion on herniated disc). Typically, progression is slow though constant.

Intramedullary tumors of the spinal cord rarely produce pain. When present, the pain is radicular in character, insidious in progression, and frequently associated with complaints characteristic of spinal cord dysfunction.

EXAMINATION. Examination of the spine will demonstrate local pain to palpation/percussion of the spine in the region of the abnormality and associated paraspinal muscle spasm. Neurological examination will demonstrate abnormalities referable to the segmental level of involvement. Extradural tumors will produce motor, sensory, and reflex abnormalities in the distribution of one or a few nerve roots. Intradural-extramedullary tumors will produce varied neurological findings, while intramedullary lesions will produce changes due to muscle weakness with spasticity, the sensory level, and hyperreflexia.

LABORATORY TESTS. Standard blood chemistries are normal, other than an increased ESR with extradural tumors. Radiographic studies will give the physician information regarding the location of the tumor, its configuration, and its relationship to the spinal cord and nerve roots. Plain radiographs will be helpful in assessing bone destruction, as might occur with a neurofibroma widening the neural foramina or metastatic disease with destruction of the vertebral body or posterior elements. Myelography with or without CT scanning will be helpful in establishing the relationship of the tumor to the spinal canal as well as the rostral-caudal extension. Similarly, MRI will give excellent information regarding intramedullary abnormalities (this is the study of choice), as well as the size and scope of other tissue abnormalities. Electromyographic studies will be abnormal when there is involvement of the nerve root, cauda equina, or anterior horn cell. Somatosensory evoked potentials will be helpful in identifying abnormalities of central pathways within the spinal cord.

Visceral Disease with Referred Low-Back Pain

Occasionally, back pain may be the first symptom of visceral pain from pelvic and abdominal structures. Typically, disease of the pelvis will refer pain to the sacral region. Lower abdominal disease will refer pain to the lumbar region, particularly L2-L4.

HISTORY. The patient's complaints of pain tend to reflect the characteristics of the underlying problem. For example, endometrial disease of the pelvis will follow a menstrual pattern. Pancreatic disease will refer to the back; involvement of the head of the pancreas is perceived in the right paravertebral region; disease in the tail of the pancreas refers to the left of the spine. Retroperitoneal disease (e.g., hemorrhage) will refer pain to the lumbar region and thighs. Gynecological disease often has referred pain to the sacral region, most often due to involvement of the uterosacral ligaments. Examples include prolapse of the uterus, malposition of the uterus, and endometriosis.

EXAMINATION. There are usually no focal findings on examination of the spine or on neurological exam. The abdominal exam or pelvic and rectal exams will give clues as to the diagnosis.

LABORATORY TESTS. The laboratory findings will reflect the underlying cause of the problem. Laboratory studies of the spine, nerve, root, and so on are normal.

Other Causes of Low-Back Pain

Postural Low-Back Pain Syndromes

This group of syndromes occurs in either very slender or moderately to severely obese individuals.

HISTORY. The patient's pain is typically vague, diffuse, and primarily localized to the low thoracic or midlumbar regions of the back. It is relieved by rest and aggravated by assuming a given posture for a period of time.

EXAMINATION. Examination of the back demonstrates poor posture. The spine and neurological examinations are normal.

LABORATORY TESTS. There are no abnormal laboratory test findings.

Psychiatric Back Pain Syndromes

Low-back pain may be an initial and major symptom of depressive illness. In addition, it is seen in patients with anxiety, hysteria, or malingering. The physician must be cautious about jumping to conclusions, as even the embellished symptom or sign may reflect significant underlying organic disease.

HISTORY. Typically, the pain is vague and diffuse, and may seem out of proportion to the problem at hand, an attitude termed *la belle indifférence*. Often the description of pain will vary from examination to examination. The pain is relieved by rest and aggravated by assuming a given posture for a period of time.

EXAMINATION. The spine and neurological examinations may be normal. In certain situations, the reported findings on examination do not fit an anatomical pattern; for example, the patient reports severe proximal leg weakness but is able to climb up to the exam table, or sensory examinations do not respect the territory of a peripheral nerve or nerve root. Some patients will fail to demonstrate the motor abnormality if both sides are tested simultaneously (Hoover's sign) and will fail sensory testing if visual-spatial clues are not present. The reader is directed to an excellent paper by Waddell et al.[210]

LABORATORY TESTS. There are no abnormal laboratory test findings.

Treatment of Low-Back Pain Syndromes

The treatment of low-back pain has been likened to an ongoing fashion show, with seductive fads taking the place of reason and enlightenment.[58] To a large degree, our dependence upon these therapeutic fads is due to inadequate knowledge about the problem. Many speculate that this is due to the diagnostic ambiguity of the problem, the poor correlation between symptoms and pathology, and the paucity of scientifically rigorous randomized clinical trials.[156,220] As has been pointed out, these fads involve significant cost to the health care system, and some are associated with significant morbidity.[58] The therapeutic objectives in the treatment of low-back pain disorders are as follows:

To promote rest
To reduce spasm
To reduce inflammation
To alter neurological structures
To increase functional capacity
To reduce pain
To increase strength
To increase spinal range of motion
To increase endurance
To alter mechanical structures
To increase work capacity
To modify the work environment
To modify the social environment
To treat psychological aspects

Source. Modified from Sptizer et al.[186]

It must be remembered that 85% of patients with low-back pain will not have a definitive diagnosis, and the majority of patients with acute low-back pain will get better with minimal symptomatic intervention on the part of the physician.[74,220]

Acupuncture

Acupuncture, the insertion of small-gauge needles into specific points of the skin, has only relatively recently been used in the West for treatment of low-back pain syndromes. Its use is rooted in Chinese medicine dating back many centuries.[96] The mode of action is unknown, but it is theorized that the twirling motion of the acupuncture needle blocks nociceptive afferent impulses (gate control theory of pain) or that there are alternative inhibitory pathways in the dorsal horn that are stimulated by afferent activity generated by the motion of the needle. Others propose that acupuncture may stimulate the production of endorphins, serotonin, and acetylcholine within the central nervous system, enhancing analgesia.[16,139,188,214] Its role is growing in specific centers, but its application is not widespread to date. Small series have demonstrated some lessening of pain.[82,146] However, there have been no studies demonstrating its superiority to more conventional modes of therapy. Studies comparing acupuncture with no treatment have yielded conflicting results.[46,88,194] Similarly, no conclusive efficacy has been demonstrated for acupuncture compared to conventional treatment.[81,126] A recent Cochrane Review states that acupuncture is no more effective than placebo for the treatment of chronic low-back pain.[202]

Nonnarcotic Analgesics

Nonnarcotic analgesics, that is acetaminophen, are the most commonly prescribed treatment for the majority of low-back pain syndromes. There are numerous formulations but all are capable of relieving pain to some degree. Many of these compounds will not alleviate the associated inflammation that may occur in some of the pain syndromes. Aspirin will do so, however. Their use is adjunctive and symptomatic. At no time should the physician prescribe narcotic analgesics without a clear understanding of their potential for addiction and abuse.

Anesthetic Block

Local anesthetics with or without the concomitant use of steroids have been used to block nociceptive responses locally in muscles, ligaments, facet joints, and regionally as a caudal epidural block.[154,224] Some authors have reported that trigger point injections or infiltrations into areas of intense muscle spasm have been beneficial, providing some pain relief for several hours.[26,196] Others have argued that the response is no better than that provided by placebo alone.[40,52,183] To date, trigger point injections remain controversial, without definitive support in the literature.

Antidepressants (Tricyclics)

The mechanism of action of antidepressant medications in patients with chronic low-back pain syndromes is not understood. Their effects may be related to treatment of the commonly associated depression (particularly if it is part of a chronic pain syndrome). They may provide pain relief independent of their antidepressant effect and, in some instances, may improve sleep due to their sedating properties in patients with nighttime pain. In the few studies that have been done, it appears that their use may be of benefit, though they have not been compared to other modalities of conservative therapy.[5,71,114,179,213]

Anti-Inflammatory Agents

The mechanism of action of the anti-inflammatory agents is not fully known. As a class, their major role is to relieve pain. All have the ability to relieve pain, and the choice of agent remains empirical.[205] Several low-quality studies have compared nonsteroidal anti-inflammatory agents (NSAIDs) with other drugs. No difference was found between NSAIDs, narcotic analgesics, and muscle relaxants.[17,35,189,207] There is suggestive evidence that the combination of an NSAID with a muscle relaxant is better than an NSAID alone.[21,30] In summary, there is conflicting evidence that NSAIDs are more effective than other minor analgesics in the treatment of acute low-back pain or bed rest.[205] There is some evidence that they are no more effective than other types of analgesics, spinal manipulation, and physical therapy.[205]

Anti-inflammatory compounds have been shown to be useful in acute pain syndromes, but their role, if any, in the continuing management of chronic low-back pain has yet to be determined.[20,57,105,179] Their success is dependent upon time-contingent dosing patterns in order to achieve a constant blood level. Pain-contingent protocols will not be successful. The potential side effects of gastric irritation, renal and hepatic toxicity, and altered coagulation must be kept in mind. Gastric irritation is common, though some drugs are tolerated better than others. It should be remembered that the simultaneous use of aspirin and an NSAID results in a competitive inhibition of each other and an overall reduction in the efficacy of each.[37]

Many physicians will empirically treat the patient with acute radicular low-back pain with a 7-day tapering course of steroids. It is felt that this will reduce inflammation around the entrapped nerve root. To date, there has been no controlled study demonstrating the validity of this presumption.

Controversy also exists as towhether injection with analgesics and/or corticosteroids is an effective treatment for patients with chronic low-back pain. These therapies have targeted facets, the epidural space and into the paravertebral regions of the spine. Evidence of their short-term and long-term effects is lacking. Conflicting results have been reported by Watts and Silagy[215] and Koes et al.[120] concerning the efficacy of epidural injections, and no conclusions can be drawn. Similarly, there is no reported significant difference between the results of local injections and placebo.[47,81] In summary, a Cochrane Review states that there is no evidence to make a recommendation regarding the use of facet joint, epidural, or local injection therapy for low-back pain. Injection therapies should not be abandoned because these studies suggest a possible benefit and because of the paucity of side effects.[165]

Bed Rest

Nearly all patients are prescribed bed rest at some time in the course of their illness. Controversy remains as to the efficacy of bed rest in the treatment of low-back pain. The mechanism of action is unclear, although some authors postulate that diffuse skin pressure will inhibit C-fiber conduction by promoting A-fiber stimulation. Others state that recumbency will reduce intradiscal pressure. The majority of reported studies do not differentiate between simple low-back pain and sciatica. Some authors firmly believe that bed rest on a firm surface is an effective and integral part of the conservative treatment program for an acute radiculopathy.[80,217] What remains controversial is the duration of bed rest necessary for optimal results. Deyo et al.[61] and Szpalski and Hayez[190] found no outcome difference in patients treated with 2 days' compared with 7 days' rest for acute low-back pain. Others believe that there is no difference between bed rest and the advice to remain active.[135,208] In summary, high-quality studies have not conclusively demonstrated that bed rest is effective in reducing pain or shortening the disability time.[91] While there are no contraindications to its use, bed rest may increase the risk of deep venous thrombosis and deconditioning in patients who are bedridden for prolonged periods.[48] Another concern in patients treated with prolonged bed rest is that there may be reinforcement of pain behaviors.

Biofeedback

Biofeedback encompasses a number of training techniques whose goal is to reduce pain and muscle spasm through relaxation. This is achieved by displaying the patient's muscular activity on a visual or auditory scale. While there are numerous studies enumerating the benefits of these techniques in headache syndromes, the studies addressing their role in low-back pain are poorly designed and flawed because of the lack of long-term follow-up.[57] To date, there has been no substantial proof that biofeedback alters the long-term course of low-back pain.[167] Many patients achieve a sense of some control over the problem. However, most experts do not discount its possible role in the treatment of the chronic pain patient.[144]

Chemonucleolysis

Chemonucleolysis involves the injection of a proteolytic enzyme (chymopapain) into a herniated disc to enzymatically digest the nucleus pulposus and thereby reduce pressure on the ligamentous structures surrounding the disc protrusion. Its precise mechanism of action is not known, but it is postulated that chymopapain reduces the water content of the nucleus pulposus, thereby reducing intradiscal pressure.[191] The efficacy of chemonucleolysis in reducing pain has been demonstrated.[87,112] However, there are few blinded, randomized clinical trials comparing its efficacy with that of other modalities of pain relief in patients with low-back pain syndromes. Gogan and Fraser have demonstrated its benefit over a 10-year period compared to placebo injections, with nearly 80% of patients reporting benefit compared to 40% receiving saline injections.[87] Muralikuttan et al., in a study flawed with nearly 40% of the patient population excluded, reported no benefit of chemonucleolysis over lumbar surgery for periods of 3 months or less and similar responses when the populations were compared at 1 year.[155] A recent Cochrane Review using a meta-analysis clearly showed that chymopapain was superior to placebo, and fewer patients required lumbar discectomy after chymopapain injection.[83]

The use of chemonucleolysis may be complicated by severe allergic and anaphylactic reactions and subarachnoid hemorrhage.[1,2]

The literature does not demonstrate the relative efficacy of different doses of chymopapain, chymopapain compared with collagenase, and collagenase compared with placebo.[83]

Cold/Heat Massage, Diathermy

The application of heat and cold by a variety of methods has been advocated by many authors. However, to date, there has been no controlled study demonstrating the efficacy of these techniques in the treatment of low-back pain syndromes. The physiological basis for their effect is unknown. Some feel that it is related to relaxation of muscle (heating) or to increasing muscle spindle activity (cooling).[125,147] Others suggest that there may be stimulation of endorphins.[163] It is know that cold application as an irritant will increase pain thresholds. In one comparative study with transcutaneous nerve stimulation, both modalities were equally effective.[143]

Corsets and Braces

Lumbar corsets and braces are widely used to prevent or relieve low-back pain.[65,201] While there are numerous reasons for their purported effectiveness, the methodology reported in several recent studies is poor, and each study design was severely flawed.[203] Authors argue that such devices produce postural correction and abdominal support and restrict lumbosacral motion, thereby reducing intradiscal pressure.[148,158,221] There is no evidence to suggest the use of lumbar support in the workplace to prevent low-back pain[203] and no indication for its use in acute low-back pain.[70] Its use in the treatment of chronic low-back pain remains controversial.[121] Corsets were found to be less effective than autotraction, and their effectiveness compared to a placebo has yet to be demonstrated.[123] A recent Cochrane Review reports that the use of corsets, braces, and other lumbar supports is not effective in preventing low-back pain.[203]

Exercise Therapy

Exercise therapy is designed to strengthen paravertebral and abdominal muscles and produce a corset-like effect (see above). Numerous exercise programs have been advocated and include isometric flexion, hyperextension, and general strengthening programs. In general, the majority of the studies suffer from design flaws.[57] Several studies have not shown any benefit over other conventional forms of therapy.[54,128] Many authors, however, advocate isometric flexion programs as safer than other forms of exercise, such as isotonic exercise, which will increase intradiscal pressure.[116,157] A recent Cochrane Review states that no specific exercises are effective for the treatment of acute low-back pain. The data show that exercise therapy is no more effective than any other treatment or inactivity; also, specifically, flexion and extension exercises have no role in the treatment of acute pain.[204] The data on chronic low-back pain are less dogmatic. Evidence suggests that exercise therapy is more effective than the conservative therapy prescribed by most general practitioners and conventional physical therapy.[204] Controversy remains as to whether specific types of exercise are more beneficial than others. Perhaps the more important benefit of exercise therapy is not its alleged ability to reduce pain, but rather its use as a tool for behavior modification—teaching the patient proper body mechanics, ergonomics, and so on.

Intradiscal Electrothermal Treatment

Intradiscal electrothermal treatment is an invasive procedure in which the posterior annulus of the painful disc is heated to 90°C for 15 to 17 minutes. The heat contracts and thickens the collagen fibers of the annulus, thus promoting closure of tears and cracks while cauterizing nerve endings, making them less sensitive to painful stimuli. Although this technique was originally thought to produce excellent results, its efficacy is now questioned.[72,170,178]

Lumbar Disc Surgery

Discectomy, involving complete or partial removal of the intervertebral disc, has a limited role in the treatment of low-back pain and of sciatica specifically. There is no literature to support the role of this form of surgery in patients with simple low-back pain. Surgery should be restricted to patients with pain who in addition have pain radiating into a limb(s), in those who have focal neurological findings that have not responded to conservative forms of therapy, or in those in whom there is a progression of neurological abnormalities. Even in this last population, the key to surgical success is in the choice of the patient. Those patients who have the appropriate syndromatic complaints, associated clinical findings, and correlated imaging findings have a nearly 90% success rate if their surgery is performed early.[106] Motor complaints are more likely to be improved than sensory complaints.[136] Some studies have shown that a delay in surgery for as much as 3 months, particularly if there are focal neurological findings, reduces the likelihood of a good outcome.[193] Other have found that while the short-term success rate of lumbar disc surgery (about 90%) is good, the long-term rate is no better than that of conservative therapy at 5 years.[76,217] Weber also demonstrated that in patients with uncertain clinical indications, postponing surgery to further assess the clinical course may delay recovery from low-back pain but does not produce long-term harm.[217]

A recent Cochrane Review has found that the type of surgery (microscopic discectomy vs. conventional discectomy) does not appear to be a factor in the ultimate result.[83] While the use of the microscope often lengthens the operative procedure, the complication rates, the length of inpatient hospital stay, and the development of scar formation do not appear to be different.[101] Poorer outcomes are associated with the automated percutaneous technique compared to conventional discectomy or chymopapain injection.[42] There are no studies that conclusively demonstrate the superiority of laser discectomy. Insufficient evidence prevents comparison between video-assisted microdiscectomy and standard discectomy, although it is suggested that the former procedure may have less perioperative complications and disability.[103]

One study suggests that a good response to a preoperative nerve block is associated with a much higher success rate in patients with a lateral stenosis syndrome.[159] Several studies have demonstrated that surgical failure in these patients can be predicted. Patients with significant psychological disarray (hypochondriasis, hysteria, somatization), pending litigation, and nonanatomical findings on examination are more likely to have a poor result after surgery.[166,185,210,222] Spinal fusion has no role in the treatment of lumbar disc herniation.[76]

The role of surgery for treatment of lumbar spondylosis is less clear, and controversy persists. There are no controlled trials assessing the efficacy of surgical spinal root decompression in lumbar stenosis or spondylosis.[45,198] No difference in outcomes has been reported in the comparison of laminectomy with laminotomy, posterolateral fusion, or fusion with laminectomy.[34,41,102,173] A Cochrane Review states that there is no conclusive evidence to support surgery as more beneficial than natural history, placebo, or conservative management.[84]

There is considerable discussion regarding the merits internal fixation. Recent data suggest that the use of a variety of fixation procedures for one- or two-level fusions for chronic low back pain offers no advantage in pain reduction or ultimate clinical outcome even though they have a higher fusion rate.[56,140] The complication rates of such procedures are higher that in those without internal fixation or the use of a prosthesis.[23,28,73,153,161]

Similarly, there is a growing body of evidence suggesting the role of nucleus pulposus replacement, vertebroplasty, kyphoplasty, and total disc replacement procedures.[44,49,117,127,129,141] Each of these studies is seriously flawed, and each has significant complications. The precise role of these procedures in the armamentarium of surgeons remains to be seen. Rigorous evidence-based studies are needed.

Multidisciplinary Biopsychosocial Rehabilitation

Research has addressed the role of education in the rehabilitation for patients with chronic, disabling low-back pain because of its epidemic proportions and major socioeconomic burden to society. There are over 100 nonrandomized studies on this subject. Only a few methodologically poor studies exist.[90] *Low-back schools* use intensive functional restoration protocols consisting of didactic training, behavioral modification, and exercise programs. The goal is to improve performance of daily activities and job performance. A recent Cochrane Review identifies strong evidence that multidisciplinary approaches (in excess of 100 hours) that use functional restoration are of benefit compared to nonmultidisciplinary inpatient and outpatient programs. This approach will improve function but does not reduce pain significantly.[90] Evidence is contradictory when one compares accumulated sick time from work at 5 years.[4,152] It is unclear whether the economic costs of these programs can be rationalized by the small degree of benefit derived.

Massage

Massage is a common therapy for acute back pain, particularly pain arising from musculoskeletal strain injuries. Its use is based on theories that soft tissue massage produces symptomatic relief of pain. This pain relief is thought to be mediated by mental and physical (muscle) relaxation and by increasing the pain threshold by activating endorphin release.[68] Its popularity is growing among those seeking alternative medicine strategies and has been a standard of care in Eastern cultures. There is only one study in subacute low-back pain comparing comprehensive massage therapy, soft-tissue manipulation, remedial exercise with posture education, or a placebo involving sham laser therapy. Reductions were seen in the amount of residual pain but not in the quality of pain.[174] Some authors report that no significant difference was seen when message was compared to spinal manipulation.[86,107] These studies are seriously flawed, however. Others have demonstrated that massage does not compare favorably to chiropractic manipulation when measures of pain quality, pain intensity, and range of motion are considered.[109] Similarly negative results have been shown when message was compared to electrical stimulation, bracing, exercise, acupuncture, and education.[79]

Muscle Relaxants

Muscle relaxants have been in use for years as adjunctive therapy in nonspecific low-back pain, and primary care physicians have prescribed them to 35% of patients seeking intervention.[43] Muscle relaxants can be divided into two main categories: antispasmodic and antispasticity. Antispasmodics are subclassified into benzodiazepines and nonbenzodiazepines. A recent Cochrane Review reports that there is strong evidence to support the use of nonbenzodiazepines for acute low-back pain.[197] The evidence for the use benzodiazepines for acute low-back pain and nonbenzodiazepines for chronic low-back pain is less convincing. Whether there is significant muscle spasm in low-back pain remains controversial. Some authors believe that muscle relaxants, in appropriate oral doses, result in more sedation than any degree of muscle relaxation.[57] Baclofen has gained some favor, though studies have yet to demonstrate this. Methocarbamol and carisoprodol have been reported to be of some benefit, but these studies have been severely criticized for design flaws.[14,50,57] Benzodiazepines should be avoided in these patients because of the significant abuse potential with moderate to long-term use. Caution must be used when prescribing muscle relaxants given their significant side effects (drowsiness and dizziness). The physician must carefully weigh the pros and cons, taking into account the needs and preferences of the individual patient to determine whether a specific patient is a suitable candidate for these agents.

Prolotherapy

Prolotherapy (sclerotherapy) is an injection into surrounding ligaments of the spine and is purported to reduce pain by strengthening stretched or torn ligaments.[118] It is believed that ligamentous injections promote the infiltration of granulocytes, macrophages, and fibroblasts. These, in turn, release growth factors, resulting in the deposition of collagen. Different classes of proliferants are used, including irritants, chemotactics, and osmotic agents.[13] Irritants—pumice flour, phenol, guaiacol, and tannic acid—act by direct or indirect cell injury that activates macrophages and secretes growth factors. Chemotactics—sodium morrhuate—function by attracting inflammatory cells as well. Osmotics—solutions of glucose, glycerin, and zinc—create an osmotic state that releases proinflammatory substances. Adverse reactions include a transient increase in pain and severe headaches. Only a few studies have addressed the efficacy of prolotherapy as a treatment for chronic low-back pain. Conflicting evidence exists. Two studies comparing prolotherapy to placebo found no evidence of superiority, although one study demonstrated reduced pain but no change in disability.[55,119,226] Many of the reported studies are not interpretable due to the use of cointerventions.[225] A recent Cochrane Review failed to find substantive evidence that prolotherapy alone is efficacious in the treatment of chronic low-back pain but may have some role in a multimodality program.[225]

Spinal Manipulation

Spinal manipulation, involving abrupt movement of the spine beyond its physiological range, has received much publicity of late as an often-maligned form of treatment for low-back pain disorders. Previously, in the domain of the chiropractor, it gained some favor in the United States and Great Britain among osteopaths and orthopedists, though its use remains highly controversial. This is due, in part, to the lack of methodological standardization of studies. The physiological basis for the use of spinal manipulation is unknown. Two basic theories exist, one of mechanical and one of neurological origin. Authors supporting a mechanical basis suggest that there is a tightening of the posterior longitudinal ligaments, rupturing of adhesions, and inhibition of nociceptive fibers.[69,113] Proponents of the neurological theory suggest that manipulation reduces nerve root compression, alters function, and impairs afferent and efferent electrophysiological function, resulting in venular, capillary, and arteriolar constriction with the extravasation of proteins.[94] No studies exist to suggest that manipulation alters spinal alignment resulting in relief of nerve root compression. Manipulation is thought to modify or activate spinal reflexes and induce tendon, muscle, and ligamentous afferents.[104] Spinal manipulation has been extensively reviewed in the literature. Some authors suggest that there may be short-term benefit with pain reduction, but there have been no conclusive studies demonstrating its efficacy over the long term.[36,57,93] Most studies are methodologically flawed. A recent Cochrane Review states that spinal manipulation has clinically significant benefit compared to placebo or sham manipulation but is not of proven benefit when compared to other therapies for low-back pain (e.g. analgesics, physical therapy, exercises).[10]

Contraindications for spinal manipulation include bony, joint, or ligamentous abnormalities, bleeding diathesis, and conditions in which the diagnosis is unknown.[11] Side effects, while uncommon, have been reported.[187] In one study, nearly 34% of patients experienced benign transient discomfort (radiating discomfort, fatigue, headache).[181] More serious reversible complications are rare but include herniated disc, dizziness, loss of consciousness, and a worsening neurological deficit.[66] Catastrophic complications are ever rarer but remain a concern. Stroke, cauda equina syndrome, and anterior spinal artery syndrome have been reported with lumbar spinal manipution.[9,95,182]

Transcutaneous Electrical Nerve Stimulation

Transcutaneous electrical nerve stimulation (TENS) is a noninvasive therapeutic modality used for pain relief. Electronic stimulation of peripheral nerves is done via skin surface pad electrodes.[15] Its purported mechanism of action is based on the gating theory of Melzack and Wall and on the demonstration that prolonged nerve stimulation alters C-fiber responses to noxious stimuli.[145,212] Early, uncontrolled studies suggest that TENS may relieve pain in nearly 60% of patients with acute low-back pain and in 30% of patients with chronic pain syndromes. This has not been borne out by more recent randomized control studies and a Cochrane Review.[150] There is marked variation in patient response relative to stimulation duration, current intensity, and stimulus frequency. However, a meta-analysis of reported studies failed to demonstrate any difference between high- and low-frequency stimulation parameters.[150] A single randomized study did demonstrate a placebo effect in patients whose stimulator was not functioning.[195] Review of the literature finds this report in accordance with other systematic reviews of the use of TENS in chronic low-back pain but in contrast to the recommendations of the Quebec Task Force (QTF).[176] Of note, the QTF did not address TENS in isolation from other electroanesthesia modalities.[150]

Traction

The goal of traction is to distract adjacent vertebral bodies from each other in order to reduce intradiscal pressure. A reduction in intradiscal pressure is thought to allow retraction of the herniated disc, reducing pressure against adjacent ligaments and nerve roots, thereby relieving pain. There are a number of techniques to accomplish this: auto-traction, gravity traction, and manual traction. Its use as a treatment modality for low-back pain is nearly universal, but the data on its efficacy remain to be proven. Authors have suggested that 25% to 60% of the body weight must be applied before one sees distraction of the vertebral bodies and changes in the lumbar disc configuration, respectively.[74,175] Auto-traction has been shown to produce some short-lived benefit, although others have suggested that traction merely reinforces the need for bed rest.[85,123,169] Many other studies report little or no benefit of traction over other conventional forms of therapy.[113,138,216] The majority of studies are flawed because of design failure, and studies cannot be compared to each other because of variations in the type of traction used, the amount of weight used for distraction, the duration of treatment, and other parameters. At this time, there is no evidence that traction therapy is of benefit in the treatment of low-back pain.[32,99]

Common Low-Back Pain Scenarios

Acute Low-Back Pain

Nonspecific low-back pain is the most common low-back syndrome the health care professional will encounter. Typically, the patient is under the age of 45 and associates the onset of pain with a specific episode or activity. However, some patient will be unaware of any precipitating event. The initial symptoms of pain are acute in onset; sharp, severe, or stabbing in quality; nonradiating (although migration or perception of pain in the gluteal region may be noted); and worsened with activity but relieved with rest.

On examination patients are uncomfortable, unwilling to make rapid changes in body position, and guarded in gait and may exhibit a tilt to the side of the pain. They will have flattening of the normal spinal lordosis, marked paravertebral muscle spasm, and tenderness to all but the most minimal palpation of the paravertebral region. There will be no lateralizing findings on neurological examination.

In the vast majority of these patients no diagnostic evaluation is necessary, as the pain is derived from musculoskeletal injury.

Treatment is symptomatic, as shown in Table 16.2. Aspirin or NSAIDs, heat, and a minimum of bed rest will often suffice until the acute injury has resolved.

Acute Radicular Low-Back Pain

The etiology of acute radicular low-back pain (sciatica) is varied, though the most common cause in the middle-aged population is a herniated intervertebral disc with compression of an adjacent nerve root. Other etiologies include degenerative disease of the lumbar spine with compression of the cauda equina or nerve roots, tumors of the lower spinal canal, herpes zoster, traumatic injuries to the sciatic nerve, or intrapelvic disease with involvement of the lumbosacral plexus. Historically, the patient will report abrupt onset of symptoms, with or without recognized precipitating events. The initial pain is severe; often the patient cannot straighten the back, and by the next day will have difficulty getting out of bed and performing daily activities. Often, over a period of several days, the intense pain will wane, leaving the patient with a gnawing discomfort more proximally in the buttock region. Neurological symptoms and signs will usually evolve over a few days to a week.

Examination will be variable, depending upon the level of involvement of the spinal axis. It should be focused to demonstrate evidence of nerve root irritation and the level of nerve root involvement and to exclude intraspinal pathology, that is, of the cord or cauda equina.

The diagnostic studies will depend upon the clinical constellation of symptoms and signs. Plain radiographs of the spine are the initial choice when there is a history of trauma. Computed tomography scanning is probably the initial imaging study of choice if one is concerned about nerve root impingement from disc disease. Its sensitivity is increased if one also uses contrast media. Magnetic resonance imaging is the imaging procedure of choice if one's concern is an intraspinal lesion or a lesion involving the lumbosacral plexus. These imaging studies need not be done immediately during the conservative phase of treatment unless one is concerned about trauma, systemic illness, or malignancy. Electrodiagnostic studies will be useful in determining the level and extent of abnormality in those patients who have evidence of multilevel disease or plexus involvement. Abnormalities may not be seen for 10 to 14 days following the injury. In addition, these studies are helpful in determining the degree of acute abnormality and chronic injury in patients who have had multiple

Table 16.2. Scientific Efficacy of Common Treatments of Nonspecific Low-Back Pain

Modality	<7 Days	1–6 Weeks	7 Weeks–3 Months	> 3 Months
Bed rest <2 days	Conclusive	Conclusive	Low	Low
Bed rest >7 days	None	None	None	Negative
Medication: NSAID	Conclusive	Conclusive	Conclusive	Low
Heat/cold massage	Low	None	None	None
Exercise		Low	Conclusive	Low
Facet injection		Negative	Negative	Negative
Traction	None	None	None	None
Surgery		None	None	None

Source: Modified from Nachemson.[159]

episodes of radicular pain. *Remember: if the diagnostic findings do not fit with the clinical picture, then rethink the problem.*

Initial treatment should be conservative. Less than 10% of patients with acute radicular back pain will require surgery. More than 50% of patients will recover within 6 weeks with conservative treatment.[8,177] Nonsteroidal anti-inflammatory agents and perhaps a muscle relaxant should be employed for up to 6 weeks so long as there is no progression of neurological findings or evidence of cauda equina involvement. Strict bed rest for 2 days may be employed in those individuals who are more comfortable being inactive. In the 5% of patients with significant focal neurological findings, surgery can be considered if there is a failure to respond to conservative measures. Weber has found no adverse effects in waiting for up to 12 weeks before operating.[217] Emergency surgery is required in the 1% to 3% of patients who have a massive disc herniation syndrome, intraspinal tumor, epidural abscess, or hemorrhage.[74] It should be emphasized that many authors feel that the use of surgery in radicular pain syndromes is for short-term benefit. There appears to be no difference in outcome when compared to conservative treatment at intervals greater than 5 years.[76,199,217]

Low-Back Pain Associated with Claudication-Like Symptoms

Spinal stenosis will produce a clinical pain syndrome characterized by pain precipitated or aggravated by walking or prolonged standing and improved with rest. This pain often exacerbated by extension of the spine, and most often not associated with focal neurological findings on examination. Many patients will have had vague backache for years, often due to arthritic changes in the spine. Most patients will report discomfort upon arising that will improve with initial activity. They will also report that their legs "do not feel right," or are "rubbery" or "cold." Typically, their pain will not be present when sitting or when standing in a forward flexed posture.

Examination of the patient often is very nonspecific. In many patients, there will be a reduction in spinal range of motion, though not to the degree found in patients with lumbar root disease and often commensurate with their age. Discomfort to palpation is absent, and there are no lateralizing neurological findings. If the patient is exercised (walking, prolonged standing) and becomes symptomatic, one may find signs referable to a nerve root(s) that will disappear with rest.

Treatment consists composed of intermittent bed rest, NSAIDs, and, in some patients, epidural injections of corticosteroids (Table 16.3). In the rare patient who does not benefit from these therapies, surgical decompression should be considered.

Low-Back Pain with Bladder/Bowel Dysfunction

Patients who present with low-back pain and sphincter disturbances have evidence of an intraspinal disorder such as the cauda equina syndrome. The symptoms and signs include low-back pain with bilateral radicular pain, disturbed perineal sensation, and an inability to void. Pain is often

Table 16.3. Scientific Efficacy of Common Treatments of Radicular Low-Back Pain

Modality	Disc Herniation <4 Weeks	Disc Herniation 5–12 Weeks	Disc Herniation > 3 Months	Lateral Stenosis	Spinal Stenosis
Bed rest <2 days	High		None	Low	None
Bed rest >7 days	None	None	None	Negative	Negative
Corset/Brace	None	None			High
Exercise	None	Low	Conclusive	Low	High
Traction	Low	Negative	Negative	None	None
Medication: NSAID	Conclusive	Conclusive	Low	Low	Low
Steroid injection	Low	Low	Low	Low	Negative
Chemonucleolysis	Low	Conclusive	Low	Negative	Negative
Surgery	None	Low	Low	Low	Conclusive

Source: Modified from Nachemson.[159]

relieved in a sitting position or by bending forward from the waist. The presentation may be either acute or chronic. Patients in the former group are typically younger than those with the chronic form of the illness. One must be ever wary of patients with acute low-back pain who develop urinary retention and not ascribe the symptom to the use of narcotic medications and bed rest. The etiology of the cauda equina syndrome varies in the acute and chronic forms. Acutely, central disc herniation (accounting for 1% to 2% of disc herniation), epidural abscess, and hemorrhage are most likely. In more chronic forms, intraspinal tumors, ankylosing spondylitis, and chronic abscess (tuberculous, fungal) should be considered.

The examination of the patient with a cauda equina syndrome will reveal many of the elements of an acute radiculopathy, as described above, though the findings suggest multilevel involvement. One must search carefully for disturbances of sensation on the buttocks and recognize that forme frustes of the syndrome are the rule, that is, posterior thigh hypesthesia, minimally reduced sphincter tone and variable weakness, and so on. Nearly all patients will have evidence of urinary retention, a dilated bladder, and lower abdominal discomfort. In addition, there may be evidence of systemic illness in more chronic forms.

Laboratory investigations will depend upon whether the illness is acute or chronic. In the acute cauda equina syndrome, urgent MRI or, if not available, myelography is the procedure of choice. Additional imaging studies may be necessary, depending upon the etiology of the problem. In the chronic form, these studies are not as urgently needed and MRI is the procedure of choice.

Treatment of the cauda equina syndrome should be regarded as a medical emergency. This holds true more for the acute form of the illness than for the chronic form. Decompression laminectomy is the treatment of choice. If decompression surgery is performed very early (within 24 hours) relative to the onset of symptoms, the results are often beneficial; delay in excess of 48 hours usually results in severe residual deficits, that is, bladder dysfunction.[3]

Chronic Low-Back Pain

The patient with chronic low-back pain will be the most problematic for the physician. It is this group of patients that accounts for the vast expenditure of time, money, and health care resources and has the greatest socioeconomic impact on society. Chronic low-back pain, a symptom, is defined by Bonica and Chapman as pain lasting for more than 3 months or pain that chronically recurs over months and years that has not responded to treatment modalities.[27] The differential diagnosis encompasses all that has been discussed in previous sections, but in many cases a single definitive diagnosis will not and cannot be made. In this subpopulation of patients, pain is no longer a direct result of nociceptive stimulation alone, or at all, but rather results primarily from the interplay of emotions and behavior. Several chronic pain models have been developed, but their discussion is beyond the scope of this chapter.

The findings on examination of the patient with chronic low-back pain will vary and reflect the diversity of the complaints. Patients may or may not have lateralizing neurological or musculoskeletal findings on examination. It is important to carefully review the patient's history and to perform detailed musculoskeletal, neurological, and general examinations. It is also important to determine whether or not the patient's pain is associated with demonstrable findings; if it is, the physician will have to decide whether previous diagnostic studies are adequate or whether additional studies are needed. In most instances, it is not necessary to repeat previous studies. Neuropsychological testing will often be helpful in this group of patients. The Minnesota Multiphasic Personality Inventory (MMPI) is the most common test battery used, although the McGill Pain Questionnaire and the Garron Low-Back Pain Questionnaire are more specific and more easily administered to this population.[124,142]

The primary goal in treating patients who have a chronic low-back pain syndrome in the absence of lateralizing findings is to initiate behavior modification in an attempt to reduce medication consumption and decrease the dependency on health care resources. Retrospective studies suggest that less than one-half of patients disabled for 6 months due to chronic pain will be rehabilitated. Those disabled for 18 months have less than a 25% chance of significant rehabilitation, and those disabled for 2 years have virtually no chance at all.[18,24,149] To accomplish rehabilitation requires a multifaceted approach. It is important to *educate* the patient that the pain is not the result of an underlying disease process but rather is the mnadmixture of an illness behavior that is reinforced by a psychosocial reaction to the previous pain syndrome and modified by a number of extraneous factors. Many of these patients have been treated with narcotics, hypnotics, and minor tranquilizers. When possible, these medications should be tapered and discontinued. Admission to a hospital and detoxification may be necessary. Pharmacological treatment should consist of minor analgesics (aspirin, NSAIDs) and perhaps tricyclic antidepressants.[5,213] It should be stressed to patients that maximum benefit will occur if their medications are taken in a timely manner to maintain a therapeutic blood level rather than in a pulsed manner when they feel pain. Bed rest should be avoided or minimized, as it will promote deconditioning, a sedentary lifestyle, and increased pain. Graded exercise programs under the direction of a physical therapist should be initiated and tailored to the individual. Patients should be taught proper body mechanics and ergonomics with the goal of increasing muscle strength and endurance. Work-hardening exercises to increase task-specific activities should be incorporated into the overall program. Psychological support is critical to the success of the program. Patients should be encouraged to pace their activity, recognizing that overactivity is as much of a problem as too little activity. Individuals in whom specific tasks are likely to exacerbate their pain should be counseled and programs developed to minimize the fear-avoidance response.[122]

Other patients with chronic pain syndromes will have lateralizing neurological or musculoskeletal findings. In these patients, treatment should be directed to the underlying cause. Despite such efforts, pain may persist. Treatment with NSAIDs, tricyclic antidepressants, and physical therapy should be undertaken. Trigger point injections may be helpful in myofascial pain syndromes.[196] It is important for patients to realize that the pain syndrome may not be "cured" but that the goal is to maximize their functional state through alterations in work/lifestyle and medication. Surgical intervention has a very small role in these patients and should be limited to those who have progressive neurological abnormalities, bladder or bowel dysfunction, persistent neurogenic claudication, and myelographic blocks of the spinal canal.[74] Spinal fusion is useless in the patient with chronic low-back pain without a proven cause. "The emphasis of research efforts should shift from examining how to fuse or replace [the spine] to examining who really should have an operation.[62]

Summary

Nondescript low-back pain is an epidemic symptom that, for the most part, is self-limited and of minimal importance. More severe symptoms of low-back pain are accompanied by sciatica and have definable and recognized risk factors. Disabling low-back pain is primarily a psychosocial phenomenon whose socioeconomic impact is growing exponentially and is of greatest concern.[75] The approach to the patient with low-back pain need not be the usual frustrating experience. Elicitation of a careful history should provide the clinician with those clues necessary to develop a differential diagnosis. The history must include a chronology of the pain, associated risk factors and those features that modify the problem, and associated symptoms that might affect the outcome or management of the low-back syndrome. The findings (or lack of) on examination should further strengthen the clinician's suspicions and allow the ordering (if necessary) of appropriate diagnostic tests to confirm the clinical impression. Laboratory studies should *never* replace a good history and a thorough examination.

In the majority of patients (80% to 90%) with acute low-back pain, symptoms will resolve within 4 weeks.[81] They should be treated symptomatically with reduced activity, gentle exercise, and a 2- to 4-week course of NSAIDs and a muscle relaxant. When conservative measures fail to help the patient and radicular symptoms are present after a 4- to 6-week trial, and/or if neurological signs are present, electrodiagnostic, imaging, and other studies (as deemed appropriate) should be considered. In patients whose pain has persisted in excess of 3 months and in whom there may or may not be lateralizing findings, one must take into account the psychosocial aspects of the illness and address them. In this population, a multidisciplinary approach is invaluable.

Low-back pain places a major socioeconomic burden on society. The pleomorphic causes and the lack of consensus regarding management hinder the physician's ability to develop diagnostic and treatment pathways and best practices. A thorough review and further study of the cost effectiveness of current treatment strategies is necessary if the physician is to be able to affect this societal burden.

REFERENCES

1. Agre K: Serious adverse neurological events associated with administration of Cymodiaction. In: Brown JE, Nordby EJ, Smith L (eds): Chemonucleolysis. Thorofare, NJ, Slack, 1985, pp
2. Agre K, Wilson RR, Brim M, McDermott DJ: Chymodiactin postmarketing surveillance. Demographic and adverse experience data in 29,075 patients. Spine 9:479–485, 1984.
3. Aho AJ, Auranen A, Pesonen K: Analysis of cauda equina symptoms in patients with lumbar disc prolapse. Acta Chir Scand 135:413–420, 1969.
4. Alaranta H, Rytokoski U, Rissanen A, Talo S, Ronnemaa T, Puukka P, et al: Intensive physical and psychosocial training program for patients with chronic low back pain. A controlled clinical trial. Spine 19(12):1339–1349, 1994.
5. Alcoff J, Jones E, Rust P, Newman R: Controlled trial of imipramine for chronic low back pain. J Fam Pract 14:841–846, 1982.
6. Altocchi PH. Acute spinal epidural abscess vs. acute transverse myelopathy. Arch Neurol 9:17–25, 1963.
7. American Academy of Neurology: Assessment: Thermography in neurologic practice. Neurology 40:523–525, 1990.
8. Andersson GJB, Svensson H-O, Odén A: The intensity of work recovery in low back pain. Spine 8:880–884, 1983.
9. Assendelft WJ, Bouter LM, Knipschild PG: Complications of spinal manipulation: a comprehensive review of the literature. J Fam Pract 42(5):475–480, 1996.
10. Assendelft WJ, Morton SC, Yu IE, Suttorp MJ, Shekelle PG: Spinal manipulative therapy for low back pain (Cochrane Review). The Cochrane Library, Issue 3. Chichester, UK, Wiley, 2004.
11. Atchinson JW: Manual medicine: An evidence-based medicine review. The Best Darn Spine Program . . . Period! Rochester, MN, American Association of Electrodiagnostic Medicine, 2004, pp 7–16.
12. Baker AS, Ojemann RJ, Swartz NM, Richardson EP: Spinal epidural abscess. N Engl J Med 293:463–468, 1975.
13. Banks AR: A rational for prolotherapy. J Orthop Med 13(3):54–59, 1991.
14. Baratta RR: A double-blind comparative study of carisoprodol, proxyphene, and placebo in the management of low back sydrome. Curr Ther Res 20:233–240, 1976.
15. Barr JO: Transcutaneous electrical nerve stimulation for pain management. In: Nelson RM, Hayes KW, Currier DP (eds): Clinical Electrotherapy. Stamford, CT, Appleton & Lange, 1999, pp 291–354.
16. Basbaum AI, Fields HL: Endogenous pain control mechanisms. Review and hypothesis. Ann Neurol 4:451–462, 1978.
17. Basmajian JV: Acute back pain and spasm. A controlled multicenter trial of combined analgesic and antispasm agents. Spine 14(4):438–439, 1989.
18. Beals RK, Hickman NW: Industrial injuries of the back and extremities: Comprehensive evaluation—an aid in prognosis and management: A study of one hundred and eighty patients. J Bone Joint Surg Am 54-A:1593–1561, 1972.
19. Berger A, Dukes E, McCarberg B, Liss M, Oster G: Change in opioid use after the initiation of gabapentin therapy in patients with postherpetic neuralgia. Clin Ther 25(11):2809–2821, 2003.
20. Berry H, Bloom B, Hamilton EBD, Swinson DR: Naproxen sodium, diflunisal, and placebo in the treatment of chronic back pain. Ann Rheum Dis 41:129–132, 1982.
21. Berry H, Hutchinson DR: Tizanidine and ibuprofen in acute low-back pain: Results of a double-blind multicentre study in general practice. J Int Med Res 16:83–91, 1988.
22. Biering-Sorensen F: Low back trouble in a general population of 30-, 40-, 50- and 60-year old men and women: Study design, representativeness and basic results. Dan Med Bull 29:289–299, 1982.
23. Bjarke CF, Stender HE, Laursen M, Thomsen K, Bunger CE: Long-term functional outcome of pedicle screw instrumentation as a support for posterolateral spinal fusion: Randomized clinical study with a 5-year follow-up. Spine 27(12):1269–1277, 2002.
24. Blumer D, Heilbronn M: Chronic pain as a variant of depressive disease: The pain-prone disorder. J Nerv Ment Dis 170:381–406, 1982.
25. Boden SD, Davis DO, Dina TS, Patronas NJ, Wiesel SW: Abnormal magnetic-resonance scans of the lumbar spine in asymptomatic subjects. A prospective investigation. J Bone Joint Surg [Am] 72:403–408, 1990.
26. Bonica JJ: Other painful disorders of the low back. In: Bonica JJ (ed): The Management of Pain. Philadelphia, Lea & Febiger, 1990, pp 1484–1514.
27. Bonica JJ, Chapman CR: Biology, pathophysiology, and therapy of chronic pain. In: Berger PA, Keith H, Brodie M (eds): American Handbook of Psychiatry. New York, Basic Books, 1986, pp 711–761.
28. Bono CM, Lee CK: Critical analysis of trends in fusion for degenerative disc disease over the past 20 years: Influence of technique on fusion rate and clinical outcome. Spine 29(4):455–463, 2004.
29. Boos N, Rieder R, Schade V, Spratt KF, Semmer N, Aebi M: 1995 Volvo Award winner in clinical studies: The diagnostic accuracy of magnetic resonance imaging, work perception, and psychosocial factors in identifying symptomatic disc herniations. Spine 20:2613–2625, 1995.
30. Borenstein DG, Lacks S, Wiesel SW: Cyclobenzaprine and naproxen versus naproxen alone in the treatment of acute low back pain and muscle spasm. Clin Ther 12:125–131, 1990.

31. Borenstein DG, Wiesel SW: Low Back Pain. Medical Diagnosis and Comprehensive Management. Philadelphia, WB Saunders, 1989.
32. Borman P, Keskin D, Bodur H: The efficacy of lumbar traction in the management of patients with low back pain. Rheumatol Int 23(2):82–86, 2003.
33. Bratton RL: Assessment and management of acute low back pain. Am Fam Physician 60:2299–2308, 1999.
34. Bridwell KH, Sedgewick TA, O'Brien MF, Lenke LG, Baldus C: The role of fusion and instrumentation in the treatment of degenerative spondylolisthesis with spinal stenosis. J Spinal Disord 6(6):461–472, 1993.
35. Brown FL Jr, Bodison S, Dixon J, Davis W, Nowoslawski J: Comparison of diflunisal and acetaminophen with codeine in the treatment of initial or recurrent acute low back strain. Clin Ther 9 (suppl C):52–58, 1986.
36. Brunarski DJ: Clinical trials of spinal manipulation: A critical appraisal and review of the literature. J Manip Physiol Ther 7:243–249, 1984.
37. Butler SH: Pharmacologic treatment of low back pain. Neurosurg Clin North Am 2:891–897, 1991.
38. Calin A, Porta J, Fries JF, Schurman DJ: Clinical history as a screening test for ankylosing spondylitis. JAMA 237:2613–2614, 1977.
39. Campbell SM, Bennett RM: Fibrositis. Dis Mon 32:653–722, 1986.
40. Carette S, Marcoux S, Truchon R, Grondin C, Gagnon J, Allard Y, et al: A controlled trial of corticosteroid injections into facet joints for chronic low back pain. N Engl J Medicine 325:1002–1007, 1991.
41. Carragee EJ: Single-level posterolateral arthrodesis, with or without posterior decompression, for the treatment of isthmic spondylolisthesis in adults. A prospective, randomized study. J Bone Joint Surg Am 79(8):1175–1180, 1997.
42. Chatterjee S, Foy PM, Findlay GF: Report of a controlled clinical trial comparing automated percutaneous lumbar discectomy and microdiscectomy in the treatment of contained lumbar disc herniation. Spine 20(6): 734–738, 1995.
43. Cherkin DC, Wheeler KJ, Barlow W, Deyo RA: Medication use for low back pain in primary care. Spine 23(5): 607–614, 1998.
44. Cherng A, Takagi S, Chow LC: Effects of hydroxypropyl methylcellulose and other gelling agents on the handling properties of calcium phosphate cement. J Biomed Mater Res 35(3):273–277, 1997.
45. Ciol MA, Deyo RA, Howell E, Kreif S: An assessment of surgery for spinal stenosis: Time trends, geographic variations, complications, and reoperations. J Am Geriatr Soc 44(3):285–290, 1996.
46. Coan R, Wong G, Ku SL, Chan YC, Ozer FT, Coan PL: The acupuncture treatment of low back pain: A randomized controlled study. Am J Chinese Med 8:181–189, 1980.
47. Collee G, Dijkmans BA, Vandenbroucke JP, Cats A: Iliac crest pain syndrome in low back pain. A double blind, randomized study of local injection therapy. J Rheumatol 18:1060–1063, 1991.
48. Convertino VA, Bloomfield SA, Greenleaf JE: An overview of the issues: Physiological effects of bed rest and restricted physical activity. Med Sci Sports Exerc 29(2): 187–190, 1997.
49. Cotten A, Dewatre F, Cortet B, Assaker R, Leblond D, Duquesnoy B, et al: Percutaneous vertebroplasty for osteolytic metastases and myeloma: Effects of the percentage of lesion filling and the leakage of methyl methacrylate at clinical follow-up. Radiology 200(2):525–530, 1996.
50. Cowan IC, Mapes RE: Carisoprodol in the management of musculoskeletal disorders: A controlled trial. Ann Phys Med 7:140–143, 1963.
51. Croft P, Papageorgious A, McNally R: Health Care Needs Assessment. Series 2. Oxford, Radcliffe Medical Press, 1997, pp 129–181.
52. Cuckler JM, Bernini PA, Weisel SW, Booth RE, Rothman RH, Pickens GT: The use of epidural steroids in the treatment of lumbar radicular pain. J Bone Joint Surg 67A:63–66, 1985.
53. Danner RL, Hartman BJ: Update of spinal epidural abscess: 35 cases and review of the literature. Rev Infect Dis 9:265–274, 1987.
54. Davies JE, Gibson T, Tester L: The value of exercises in the treatment of low back pain. Rheumatol Rehabil 18:243–247, 1979.
55. Dechow E, Davies RK, Carr AJ, Thompson PW: A randomized, double-blind, placebo-controlled trial of sclerosing injections in patients with chronic low back pain. Rheumatology (Oxford) 38(12):1255–1259, 1999.
56. Delamarter RB, Fribourg DM, Kanim LE, Bae H: ProDisc artificial total lumbar disc replacement: Introduction and early results from the United States clinical trial. Spine 28(20):S167–S175, 2003.
57. Deyo RA: Conservative therapy for low back pain. Distinguishing useful from useless therapy. JAMA 250:1057–1062, 1983.
58. Deyo RA: Fads in the treatment of low back pain [editorial]. N Engl J Med 325:1039–1040, 1991.
59. Deyo RA, Bigos SJ, Maravilla KR: Diagnostic imaging procedures for the lumbar spine. Ann Intern Med 111: 865–867, 1989.
60. Deyo RA, Diehl AK: Cancer as a cause of back pain: Frequency, clinical presentation, and diagnostic strategies. J Gen Intern Med 3:230–238, 1988.
61. Deyo RA et al: How many days' bed rest for acute low back pain? N Engl J Med 325:1039–1040, 1991.
62. Deyo RA, Nachemson A, Mirza SK: Spinal-fusion surgery—the case for restraint. N Engl J Med 350(7): 722–726, 2004.
63. Deyo RA, Rainville J, Kent DL: What can the history and physical examination tell us about low back pain? JAMA 268:760–765, 1992.
64. Dillane JB, Fry J, Kalton G: Acute back syndrome: A study from general practice. BMJ 2:82–84, 1966.
65. Dillingham TR: Lumbar supports for prevention of low back pain in the workplace. JAMA 279(22):1826–1828, 1998.

66. Dvorak J, Dvorak V, Schneider W, Tritschler T: [Manual therapy in lumbovertebral syndromes]. Orthopäde 28(11): 939–945, 1999.
67. Eisen AA: Radiculopathies and plexopathies. In: Brown WF, Bolton CF (eds): Clinical Electromyography. Boston, Butterworths, 1987, pp 51–73.
68. Ernst E: Massage therapy for low back pain: A systematic review. J Pain Symptom Manage 17(1):65–69, 1999.
69. Evans DW: Mechanisms and effects of spinal high-velocity, low-amplitude thrust manipulation: Previous theories. J Manip Physiol Ther 25(4):251–262, 2002.
70. Faas A, Chavannes AW, Koes BW, Van den Hoogen HMM, Mens JMA, Smeele LJM, et al: Guidelines for low back pain of the College of General Practitioners [NHG-Standaard Lage-Rugpijn]. Huisarts Wet 39:18–31, 1996.
71. Fishbain D: Evidence-based data on pain relief with antidepressants. Ann Med 32(5):305–316, 2000.
72. Freeman BJ, Walters RM, Moore RJ, Fraser RD: Does intradiscal electrothermal therapy denervate and repair experimentally induced posterolateral annular tears in an animal model? Spine 28(23):2602–2608, 2003.
73. Fritzell P, Hagg O, Nordwall A: Complications in lumbar fusion surgery for chronic low back pain: Comparison of three surgical techniques used in a prospective randomized study. A report from the Swedish Lumbar Spine Study Group. Eur Spine J 12(2):178–189, 2003.
74. Frymoyer JW: Back pain and sciatica. N Engl J Med 318:291–300, 1988.
75. Frymoyer JW, Cats-Baril WL: An overview of the incidences and costs of low back pain. Orthop Clin North Am 22:263–271, 1991.
76. Frymoyer JW, Hanley E, Howe J, Kuhlmann D, Matteri R: Disc excision and spine fusion in the management of lumbar disc disease: A minimum ten-year followup. Spine 3:1–6, 1978.
77. Frymoyer JW, Haugh LD: Thermography: A call for scientific studies to establish its diagnostic efficacy. Orthopedics 9:699–700, 1986.
78. Frymoyer JW, Pope MH, Clements JH, Wilder DG, MacPherson B, Ashikaga T: Risk factors in low back pain. J Bone Joint Surg [Am] 65-A:213–218, 1983.
79. Furlan AD, Brosseau L, Imamura M, Irwin E: Massage for low-back pain (Cochrane Review). The Cochrane Library, Issue 3. Chichester, UK, Wiley, 2004.
80. Garfin SR, Pye SA: Bed design and its effect on chronic low back pain—a limited controlled trial. Pain 10:87–91, 1981.
81. Garvey TA, Marks MR, Wiesel SW: A prospective, randomized, double-blind evaluation of trigger-point injection therapy for low-back pain. Spine 14(9):962–964, 1989.
82. Ghia JN, Mao W, Toomey TC, Gregg JM: Acupuncture and chronic pain mechanisms. Pain 2:285–299, 1976.
83. Gibson JNA, Grant IC, Waddell G: Surgery for lumbar disc prolapse (Cochrane Review). The Cochrane Library, Issue 3. Chichester, UK, Wiley, 2004.
84. Gibson JNA, Waddell G, Grant IC: Surgery for degenerative lumbar spondylosis (Cochrane Review). The Cochrane Library, Issue 3. Chichester, UK, Wiley, 2004.
85. Gillström P, Ehrnberg A: Long-term results of autotraction in the treatment of lumbago and sciatica: An attempt to correlate clinical results with objective parameters. Acta Orthop Trauma Surg 104:294–298, 1985.
86. Godfrey CM, Morgan PP, Schatzker J: A randomized trial of manipulation for low back pain in a medical setting. Spine 9:301–304, 1984.
87. Gogan WJ, Fraser RD: Chymopapain. A 10-year, double-blind study. Spine 17:388–394, 1992.
88. Gunn CC, Milbrandt WE, Little AS, Mason KE: Dry needling of muscle motor points for chronic low-back pain: A randomized clinical trial with long-term follow-up. Spine 5(3):279–291, 1980.
89. Guo HR, Tanaka S, Halperin WE, Cameron LL: Back pain prevalence in U.S. industry and estimates of lost workdays. Am J Public Health 89(7):1029–1035, 1999.
90. Guzmán J, Esmail R, Karjalainen K, Malmivaara A, Irvin E, Bombardier C: Multidisciplinary bio-psycho-social rehabilitation for chronic low back pain (Cochrane Review). The Cochrane Library, Issue 3. Chichester, UK, Wiley, 2004.
91. Hagan KB, Hilde G, Jamtvedt G, Winnem M: Bed rest for acute low-back pain and sciatica (Cochrane Review). The Cochrane Library, Issue 3. Chichester, UK, Wiley, 2004.
92. Hakellus A, Hindmarsh J: The comparative reliability of preoperative diagnostic methods in lumbar disc surgery. Acta Orthop Scand 43:234–238, 1972.
93. Haldeman S: Spinal manipulative therapy: A status report. Clin Orthop 179:62–70, 1983.
94. Haldeman S: Neurological effects of the adjustment. J Manip Physiol Ther 23(2):112–114, 2000.
95. Haldeman S, Rubinstein SM: Cauda equina syndrome in patients undergoing manipulation of the lumbar spine. Spine 17(12):1469–1473, 1992.
96. Han JS: The neurochemical basis of pain relief by acupuncture. A collection of papers 1973–1987. Beijing Medical University, 1987 (unpublished).
97. Harper CMJ, Low PA, Fealey RD, Chelimsky TC, Proper CJ, Gillen DA: Utility of thermography in the diagnosis of lumbosacral radiculopathy. Neurology 41:1010–1014, 1991.
98. Hart LG, Deyo RA, Cherkin DC: Physician office visits for low back pain: Frequency, clinical evaluation, and treatment patterns from a U.S. national survey. Spine 20:11–19, 1995.
99. Harte AA, Baxter GD, Gracey JH: The efficacy of traction for back pain: A systematic review of randomized controlled trials. Arch Phys Med Rehabil 84(10):1542–1553, 2003.
100. Heliovaara M: Risk factors for low back pain and sciatica. Ann Med 21:257–264, 1989.
101. Henriksen L, Schmidt K, Eskesen V, Jantzen E: A controlled study of microsurgical versus standard lumbar discectomy. Br J Neurosurg 10(3):289–293, 1996.
102. Herkowitz HN, Kurz LT: Degenerative lumbar

spondylolisthesis with spinal stenosis. A prospective study comparing decompression with decompression and intertransverse process arthrodesis. J Bone Joint Surg Am 73(6): 802–808, 1991.

103. Hermantin FU, Peters T, Quartararo L, Kambin P: A prospective, randomized study comparing the results of open discectomy with those of video-assisted arthroscopic microdiscectomy. J Bone Joint Surg Am 81(7): 958–965, 1999.
104. Herzog W, Scheele D, Conway PJ: Electromyographic responses of back and limb muscles associated with spinal manipulative therapy. Spine 24(2):146–152, 1999.
105. Hickey RFJ: Chronic low back pain: A comparison of diflunisal with paracetamol. NZ Med J 95:312–314, 1982.
106. Hirsch C, Nachemson A: The reliability of lumbar disc surgery. Clin Orthop 29:189–194, 1963.
107. Hoehler FK, Tobin JS, Buerger AA: Spinal manipulation for low back pain. JAMA 245:1835–1838, 1981.
108. Hoffman RM, Kent DL, Deyo RA: Diagnostic accuracy and clinical utility of thermography for lumbar radiculopathy. A meta-analysis. Spine 16:623–628, 1991.
109. Hsieh CY, Phillips RB, Adams AH, Pope MH: Functional outcomes of low back pain: Comparison of four treatment groups in a randomized controlled trial. J Manip Physiol Ther 15:4–9, 1992.
110. Hubbard JE, Hoyt C: Pain evaluation by electronic infrared thermography: Correlation with symptoms, EMG, myelogram and CT scan. Thermology 1:26–35, 1985.
111. Hudgins RW: The crossed straight leg raising test: A diagnostic sign of herniated disc. J Occup Med 21:407–408, 1979.
112. Javid MJ: A 1- to 4-year follow-up review of treatment of sciatica using chemonucleolysis or laminectomy. J Neurosurg 76:184–190, 1992.
113. Jayson MIV, Sims-Williams H, Young S, Baddeley H, Collins E: Mobilization and manipulation for low back pain. Spine 6:409–416, 1981.
114. Jenkins DG, Ebbutt AF, Evans CD: Tofranil in the treatment of low back pain. J Int Med Res 4(suppl 2):28–40, 1976.
115. Johnson EW, Melvin JL: Value of electromyography in lumbar radiculopathy. Arch Phys Med Rehabil 52:239–243, 1971.
116. Kendall PH, Jenkins JM: Exercise for backache: A double-blind controlled trial. Physiotherapy 54:154–157, 1968.
117. Klara PM, Ray CD: Artificial nucleus replacement: Clinical experience. Spine 27(12):1374–1377, 2002.
118. Klein RG, Dorman TA, Johnson CE: Proliferant injections for low back pain: Histologic changes of injected ligaments and objective measurements of spinal mobility before and after treatment. J Neurol Orthop Med Surg 10(2):123–126, 1989.
119. Klein RG, Eek BC, DeLong WB, Mooney V: A randomized double-blind trial of dextrose-glycerine-phenol injections for chronic low back pain. J Spinal Disord 6(1): 23–33, 1993.
120. Koes BW, Scholten RJ, Mens JM, Bouter LM: Efficacy of epidural steroid injections for low-back pain and sciatica: A systematic review of randomized clinical trials. Pain 63(3):279–288, 1995.
121. Koes BW, Van den Hoogen HMM: Efficacy of bed rest and orthoses of low-back pain. Eur J Phys Med Rehabil 4(3):86–93, 1994.
122. Kriegler JS, Ashenberg ZS: Management of chronic low back pain. A comprehensive approach. Semin Neurol 7:303–312, 1987.
123. Larsson U, Chöler U, Lidström A, Lind G, Nachemson A, Nilsson B, et al: Auto-traction for treatment of lumbago-sciatica: A multicentre controlled investigation. Acta Orthop Scand 51:791–798, 1980.
124. Leavitt F, Garron DC: Validity of a back pain classification scale among patients with low back pain not associated with demonstrable organic disease. J Psychosom Res 23:301–306, 1979.
125. Lehmann JF, De Lateur BJ: Cryotherapy. In: Lehmann JF (ed): Therapeutic Heat and Cold. Baltimore, Williams & Wilkins, 1990, pp 590–632.
126. Lehmann TR, Russell DW, Spratt KF, Colby H, Liu YK, Fairchild ML, et al: Efficacy of electroacupuncture and TENS in the rehabilitation of chronic low back pain patients. Pain 26:277–290, 1986.
127. Lemaire JP, Skalli W, Lavaste F, Templier A, Mendes F, Diop A, et al: Intervertebral disc prosthesis. Results and prospects for the year 2000. Clin Orthop Relat Res 337:64–76, 1997.
128. Lidstrom A, Zachrisson M: Physical therapy on low back pain and sciatica: An attempt at evaluation. Scand J Rehabil Med 2:37–42, 1970.
129. Lieberman IH, Dudeney S, Reinhardt MK, Bell G: Initial outcome and efficacy of "kyphoplasty" in the treatment of painful osteoporotic vertebral compression fractures. Spine 26(14):1631–1638, 2001.
130. Lively MW: Sports medicine approach to low back pain. South Med J 95:642–646, 2004.
131. Loeser JD: Volinn E: Epidemiology of low back pain. Neurosurg Clin North Am 2:713–718, 1991.
132. Maetzel A, Li L: The economic burden of low back pain: A review of studies published between 1996 and 2001. Best Pract Res Clin Rheumatol 16:23–30, 2002.
133. Mahoney L, McCulloch J, Csima A: Thermography in back pain: 1. Thermography as a diagnostic aid in sciatica. Thermology 1:43, 1985.
134. Mahoney L, Patt N, McCulloch J, Csima A: Thermography in back pain: 2. Relation of thermography to back pain. Thermology 1:51, 1985.
135. Malmivaara A, Hakkinen U, Aro T, Heinrichs ML, Koskenniemi L, Kuosma E, et al: The treatment of acute low back pain—bed rest, exercises, or ordinary activity? N Engl J Med 332(6):351–355, 1995.
136. Malter AD, Weinstein J: Cost-effectiveness of lumbar discectomy. Spine 21(24 suppl):69S–74S, 1996.
137. Maniadakis N, Gray A: The economic burden of back pain in the UK. Pain 84:95–103, 2000.
138. Mathews JA, Hickling J: Lumbar traction: A double blind controlled study for sciatica. Rheumatol Rehabil 14:222, 1975.

139. Mayer DJ, Price DD: Central nervous system mechanisms of analgesia. Pain 2:379–404, 1976.
140. McAfee PC, Fedder IL, Saiedy S, Shucosky EM, Cunningham BW: Experimental design of total disk replacement—experience with a prospective randomized study of the SB Charite. Spine 28(20):S153–S162, 2003.
141. McAfee PC, Fedder IL, Saiedy S, Shucosky EM, Cunningham BW: SB Charite disc replacement: Report of 60 prospective randomized cases in a U.S. center. J Spinal Disord Tech 16(4):424–433, 2003.
142. Melzack R: The McGill questionnaire. Major properties and scoring methods. Pain 1:277–299, 1975.
143. Melzack R, Jeans ME, Stratford JG, Monks RC: Ice massage and transcutaneous stimulation: Comparison of treatment for low back pain. Pain 9:209–217, 1980.
144. Melzack R, Perry C: Self-regulation of pain: The use of alpha feedback and hypnotic training for the control of chronic pain. Exp Neruol 46:452–463, 1975.
145. Melzack R, Wall PD: Pain mechanisms: A new theory. Science 150:971–979, 1965.
146. Mendelson G, Selwood RG, Krantz H, Loh TS, Kidson MA, Scott DS: Acupuncture treatment of chronic low back pain: A double-blind placebo-controlled trial. Am J Med 74:49–55, 1983.
147. Miglietta O: Action of cold on spasticity. Am J Phys Med 52:198–205, 1973.
148. Million R, Haavik HN, Jayson MIV, Baker RD: Evaluation of low back pain and assessment of lumbar corsets with and without back supports. Ann Rheum Dis 40: 449–454, 1981.
149. Million R, Hall W, Nilsen KH, Baker RD, Jayson MIV: Assessment of the progress of the back-pain patient. Spine 7:204–212, 1982.
150. Milne S, Welch V, Brosseau L, Saginur M, Shea B, Tugwell PWG: Transcutaneous electrical nerve stimulation (TENS) for chronic low back pain (Cochrane Review). Cochrane Library, Issue 3. Chichester, UK, Wiley, 2004.
151. Mitchell LV, Lawler FH, Bowen D, Mote W, Asundi P, Purswell J: Effectiveness and cost-effectiveness of employer-issued back belts in areas of high risk for back injury. J Occup Med 36(1):90–94, 1994.
152. Mitchell RI, Carmen GM: The functional restoration approach to the treatment of chronic pain in patients with soft tissue and back injuries. Spine 19(6):633–642, 1994.
153. Moller H, Hedlund R: Instrumented and noninstrumented posterolateral fusion in adult spondylolisthesis—a prospective randomized study: Part 2. Spine 25(13):1716–1721, 2000.
154. Mooney V, Robertson J: The facet syndrome. Clin Orthop 115:149–156, 1976.
155. Muralkiuttan KP, Hamilton A, Kernohan WG, Mollan RAB, Adair IV: A prospective randomized trial of chemonucleolysis and conventional disc surgery in single level lumbar disc herniation. Spine 17:381–387, 1992.
156. Nachemson AL: The lumbar spine: An orthopedic challenge. Spine 1:59–71, 1976.
157. Nachemson AL: Disc pressure measurements. Spine 6:93–97, 1981.
158. Nachemson AL: Lumbar spine instability: A critical update and symposium summary. Spine 10:290–291, 1985.
159. Nachemson AL: Newest knowledge of low back pain. Solutions in sight. Clin Orthop Related Res 279:8–20, 1992.
160. Nachemson AL: Epidemiology and the economics of LBP. In: Herkowitz HN, Dvorak J, Bell G, Nordin M, Grob D (eds): The Lumbar Spine. Philadelphia, Lippincott, Williams & Wilkins, 2004, pp 3–10.
161. Nachemson AL: Surgery for chronic low back pain in the era of evidence-based medicine. In: The Best Darn Spine Program . . . Period! Rochester, MN, American Association of Electrodiagnostic Medicine, 2004, pp 1–5.
162. Nachemson AL, Jonsson E: Neck and Back Pain: The Scientific Evidence of Causes, Diagnosis, and Treatment. Philadelphia, Lippincott Williams & Wilkins, 2000.
163. Nagi SZ, Riley LE, Newby LG: A social epidemiology of back pain in a general population. J Chronic Dis 26: 769–779, 1973.
164. National Institutes of Health: Research on low back pain and common spinal disorders, vol 26, PA97-058. Bethesda, MD, National Institutes of Health, 1997.
165. Nelemans PJ, de Bie RA, de Vet HCW, Sturmans F: Injection therapy for subacute and chronic benign low-back pain (Cochrane Review). Cochrane Library, Issue 3. Chichester, UK, Wiley, 2004.
166. Norton WL: Chemonucleolysis versus surgical discectomy: Comparison of costs and results in workers' compensation claimants. Spine 11:440–443, 1986.
167. Nouwen A, Solinger JW: The effectiveness of EMG biofeedback training in low back pain. Biofeedback Self-Regul 4:103–111, 1979.
168. Orava S: Medical treatment of acute low back pain. Diflunisal compared with indomethacin in acute lumbago. Int J Clin Pharmacol Res 6:45–51, 1986.
169. Pal B, Mangion P, Hossain MA, Diffey BL: A controlled trial of continuous lumbar traction in the treatment of back pain and sciatica. Br J Rheumatol 25:181–183, 1986.
170. Pauza KJ, Howell S, Dreyfuss P, Peloza JH, Dawson K, Bogduk N: A randomized, placebo-controlled trial of intradiscal electrothermal therapy for the treatment of discogenic low back pain. Spine J 4(1):27–35, 2004.
171. Pawl RP: Thermography in the diagnosis of low back pain. Neurosurg Clin North Am 2:839–850, 1991.
172. Pope MH: Risk indicators in low back pain. Ann Med 21:387–392, 1989.
173. Postacchini F, Cinotti G, Perugia D, Gumina S: The surgical treatment of central lumbar stenosis. Multiple laminotomy compared with total laminectomy. J Bone Joint Surg Br 75(3):386–392, 1993.
174. Preyde M: Effectiveness of massage therapy for subacute low-back pain: A randomized controlled trial. CMAJ 162(13):1815–1820, 2000.
175. Quinet RJ, Hadler NM: Diagnosis and treatment of backache. Semin Arthritis Rheum 8:261–287, 1979.
176. Reeve J, Menon D, Corabian P: Transcutaneous electrical nerve stimulation (TENS): A technology assessment. Int J Technol Assess Health Care 12(2):299–324, 1996.

177. Rutkow IM: Orthopaedic operations in the United States, 1979 through 1983. J Bone Joint Surg Am 68-A:716–719, 1986.
178. Saal JA, Saal JS: Intradiscal electrothermal treatment for chronic discogenic low back pain: Prospective outcome study with a minimum 2-year follow-up. Spine 27(9):966–973, 2002.
179. Schnitzer TJ, Ferraro A, Hunsche E, Kong SX: A comprehensive review of clinical trials on the efficacy and safety of drugs for the treatment of low back pain. J Pain Symptom Manage 28(1):72–95, 2004.
180. Scovron ML, Szalski M, Nordin M, Melot C, Cucier D: Socioeconomic factors and back pain. Spine 19:129–137, 1994.
181. Senstad O, Leboeuf-Yde C, Borchgrevink CF: Side-effects of chiropractic spinal manipulation: Types, frequency, discomfort and course. Scand J Prim Health Care 14(1):50–53, 1996.
182. Shekelle PG, Adams AH, Chassin MR, Hurwitz EL, Brook RH: Spinal manipulation for low-back pain. Ann Intern Med 117(7):590–598, 1992.
183. Snoek W, Weber H: Double-blind evaluation of extradural methyl prednisolone for herniated lumbar discs. Acta Orthop Scand 48:635–641, 1977.
184. So YT, Aminoff MJ, Olney RK: The role of thermography in the evaluation of lumbosacral radiculopathy. Neurology 39:1154–1158, 1989.
185. Spengler DM, Freeman C, Westbrook R, Miller JW: Low-back pain following multiple lumbar spine procedures: Failure of initial selections? Spine 5:356–360, 1980.
186. Spitzer WO, LeBlanc FE, Dupuis M, et al: Scientific approach to the assessment and management of activity-related spinal disorders: A monograph for clinicians: Report of the Quebec Task Force on Spinal Disorders. Spine 12(suppl):S1–S59, 1987.
187. Stevinson C, Ernst E: Risks associated with spinal manipulation. Am J Med 112:566–571, 2002.
188. Stux G, Hammerschlag R: Clinical Acupuncture: Scientific Basis. New York, Springer, 2001.
189. Sweetman BJ, Baig A, Parsons DL: Mefenamic acid, chlormezanone-paracetamol, ethoheptazine-aspirin-meprobamate: A comparative study in acute low back pain. Br J Clin Pract 41(2):619–624, 1987.
190. Szpalski M, Hayez JP: How many days of bed rest for acute low back pain? Objective assessment of trunk function. Eur Spine J 1:29–31, 1992.
191. Takahashi K, Inoue S, Takada S, Nishiyama H, Mimura M, Wada Y: Experimental study on chemonucleolysis with special reference to the change of intradiscal pressure. Spine 11:617–620, 1986.
192. Taylor VM, Deyo RA, Cherkin DC, Kreuter W: Low back pain hospitalization: Recent United States trends and regional variations. Spine 19:1207–1213, 1994.
193. Thomas M, Grant N, Marshall J, Stevens J: Surgical treatment of low backache and sciatica. Lancet ii:1437–1439, 1983.
194. Thomas M, Lundberg T: Importance of modes of acupuncture in the treatment of chronic nociceptive low back pain. Acta Anaesthesiol Scand 38:63–69, 1994.
195. Thorsteinsson G, Stonnington HH, Stillwell GK, Elueback LR: The placebo effect of transcutaneous electrical stimulation. Pain 5:31–41, 1978.
196. Travell JG, Simons DG: Myofascial Pain and Dysfunction: The Trigger Point Manual. The Lower Extremities. Baltimore, William & Wilkins, 1992.
197. Tulder MW van, Touray T, Furlan AD, Solway S, Bouter LM: Muscle relaxants for non-specific low-back pain (Cochrane Review). The Cochrane Library, Issue 3. Chichester, UK, Wiley, 2004.
198. Turner JA, Ersek M, Herron L, Deyo R: Surgery for lumbar spinal stenosis. Attempted meta-analysis of the literature. Spine 17:1–8, 1992.
199. Turner JA, Ersek M, Herron L, Hasselkorn J, Kent D, Ciol MA, et al: Patient outcomes after lumbar spinal fusions. JAMA 268:907–911, 1992.
200. Uematsu S, Jankel WR, Edwin DH, Kim W, Kozikowski J, Rosenbaum A, et al: Quantification of thermal asymmetry. Part 2: Application in low-back pain and sciatica. J Neurosurg 69:556–561, 1988.
201. van Poppel MN, Koes BW, van der PT, Smid T, Bouter LM: Lumbar supports and education for the prevention of low back pain in industry: A randomized controlled trial. JAMA 279(22):1789–1794, 1998.
202. van Tulder MW, Cherkin DC, Berman B, Lao L, Koes BW: The effectiveness of acupuncture in the management of acute and chronic low back pain. A systematic review within the framework of the Cochrane Collaboration Back Review Group. Spine 24(11):1113–1123, 1999.
203. van Tulder MW, Jellema P, van Poppel MNM, Nachemson AL, Bouter LM: Lumbar supports for prevention and treatment of low-back pain (Cochrane Review). The Cochrane Library, Issue 3. Chichester, UK, Wiley, 2004.
204. van Tulder MW, Malmivaara A, Esmail R, Koes BW: Exercise therapy for low-back pain (Cochrane Review). The Cochrane Library, Issue 3. Chichester, UK, Wiley, 2004.
205. van Tulder MW, Scholten RJPM, Koes BW, Deyo RA: Non-steroidal anti-inflammatory drugs for low-back pain (Cochrane Review). The Cochrane Library, Issue 3. Chichester, UK, Wiley, 2004.
206. Verner EF, Musher DM: Spinal epidural abscess. Med Clin North Am 69:375–384, 1985.
207. Videman T, Heikkila J, Partanen T: Double-blind parallel study of meptazinol versus diflunisal in the treatment of lumbago. Curr Med Res Opin 9(4):246–252, 1984.
208. Vroomen PC, de Krom MC, Wilmink JT, Kester AD, Knottnerus JA: Lack of effectiveness of bed rest for sciatica. N Engl J Med 340(6):418–423, 1999.
209. Waddell G: An approach to backache. Br J Hosp Med 28:187–219, 1982.
210. Waddell G, McCulloch JA, Kummel E, Wenner RM: Nonorganic physical signs in low-back pain. Spine 5:117–125, 1980.
211. Waldvogel FA, Vasey H: Osteomyelitis: The past decade. N Engl J Med 33:360–370, 1980.

212. Wall PD, Sweet WH: Temporary abolition of pain in man. Science 155:108–109, 1967.
213. Ward NG: Tricyclic antidepressants for chronic low back pain: Mechanisms of action and predictors of response. Spine 11:661–665, 1986.
214. Watkins LR, Mayer DJ: Organization of endogenous opiate and nonopiate pain control systems. Science 216:1185–1192, 1982.
215. Watts RW, Silagy CA: A meta-analysis on the efficacy of epidural corticosteroids in the treatment of sciatica. Anaesth Intens Care 23(5):564–569, 1995.
216. Weber H: Traction therapy in sciatica due to disc prolapse. J Oslo City Hosp 23:167–176, 1973.
217. Weber H: Lumbar disc herniation: A controlled, prospective study with ten years of observation. Spine 8:131–140, 1983.
218. Weinstein JN, Boden SD, An H: Emerging technology in spine: Should we rethink the past or move forward in spite of the past? Spine 28:S1, 2003.
219. Weisel SE, Tsourmas N, Feffer H, Citrin CM, Patronas N: A study of computer-assisted tomography, I: The incidence of positive CAT scans in an asymptomatic group of patients. Spine 9:549–551, 1984.
220. White AA, Gordon SL: Synopsis: Workshop on idiopathic low back pain. Spine 7:141–149, 1982.
221. Willner S: Effect of a rigid brace on back pain. Acta Orthop Scand 56:40–42, 1985.
222. Wiltse LL, Rocchio PD: Preoperative psychological tests as a predictor of success of chemonucleolysis in the treatment of the low-back syndrome. J Bone Joint Surg Am 57-A:478–483, 1975.
223. Wolsko PM, Eisenberg DM, Davis RB, Kessler R, Phillips RS: Patterns and perceptions of care for treatment of back and neck pain: Results of a national survey. Spine 28:292–297, 2003.
224. Yates DW: A comparison of the types of epidural injections commonly used in the treatment of low back pain and sciatica. Rheumatol Rehabil 17:181–186, 1978.
225. Yelland MJ, Del Mar C, Pirozzo S, Schoene ML, Vercoe P: Prolotherapy injections for chronic low-back pain (Cochrane Review). The Cochrane Library, Issue 3. Chichester, UK, Wiley, 2004.
226. Yelland MJ, Glasziou PP, Bogduk N, Schluter PJ, McKernon M: Prolotherapy injections, saline injections, and exercises for chronic low-back pain: A randomized trial. Spine 29(1):9–16, 2004.
227. Yunus M, Masi AT, Calabro JJ, Miller KA, Feigenbaum SL: Primary fibromyalgia (fibrositis): Clinical study of 50 patients with matched normal controls. Semin Arthritis Rheum 11:151, 1981.

Chapter 17
Zygapophysial Joint Trauma

NIKOLAI BOGDUK

The zygapophysial joints are paired synovial joints formed between the neural arches of consecutive vertebrae. Five pairs are represented in the lumbar spine and six pairs in the cervical spine.

Each joint is formed by the articulation of an inferior articular process with the superior articular process of the next vertebra (Figs. 17.1 and 17.2). Each process is lined by articular cartilage, and the joint is enclosed in a fibrous capsule lined with synovial membrane. Ventrally, the capsule is formed by the ligamentum flavum. The joints contain intra-articular inclusions, the most prominent of which are fibroadipose meniscoids located at the superior and inferior poles of each joint.[19]

Like all synovial joints, the zygapophysial joints are subject to arthropathies, such as osteoarthrosis, rheumatoid arthritis, and ankylosing spondylitis. They are also susceptible to injury from trauma. The evidence on traumatic injury, however, differs for the lumbar spine and cervical spine.

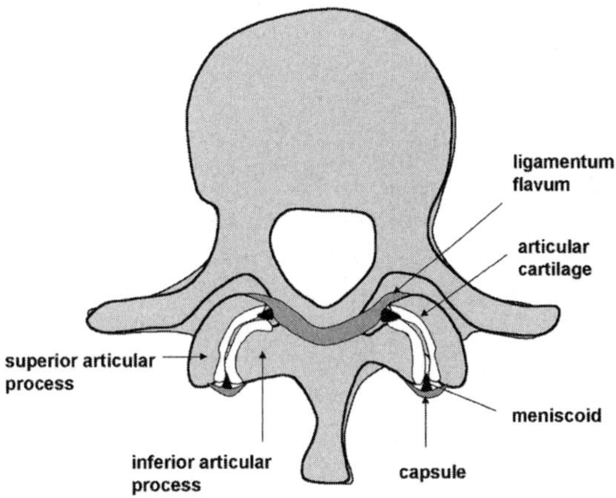

Figure 17.1. Axial view of a lumbar motion segment illustrating the appearance and structure of the lumbar zygapophysial joints.

Lumbar Spine

Injuries to the zygapophysial joints of the lumbar spine have been produced in laboratory experiments. Either of two mechanisms can operate.

Extension coupled with forced posterior rotation can injure the capsule of a lumbar zygapophysial joint.[28] Extension is limited by impaction of the tip of an inferior articular process on the underlying lamina (Figure 17.3). If posterior rotation is then added, the point of impaction acts as a pivot point around which the vertebra rotates. Posterior rotation causes the inferior articular process on the opposite side to move backwards and medially. This results in distraction of the joint on that side. The injuries that can occur are tears of the joint capsule or avulsions of the capsule insertion.

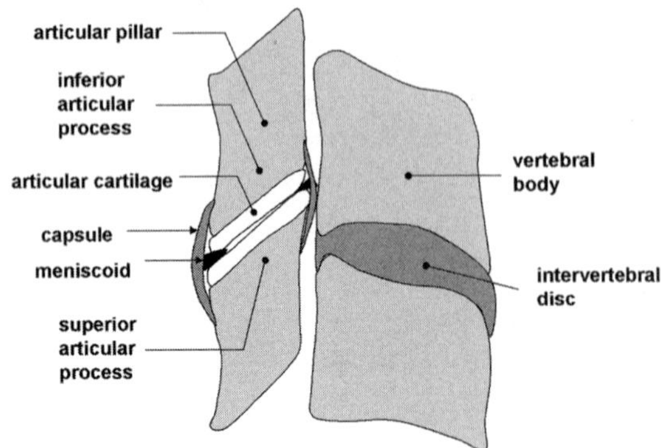

Figure 17.2. Lateral view of a cervical motion segment illustrating the appearance and structure of a cervical zygapophysial joint.

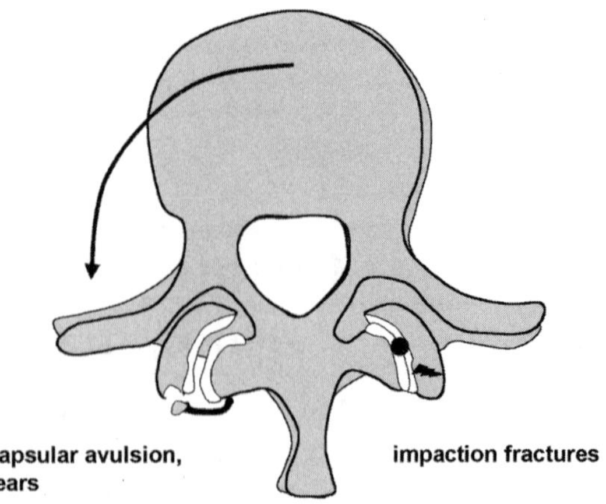

Figure 17.4. Axial view of a lumbar motion segment illustrating the types of injuries that can befall the lumbar zygapophysial joints during forced axial rotation. During axial rotation the segments pivots around an impaction point (block dot) in the contralateral zygapophysial joint, and the opposite joint is distracted backwards and medially.

Forced axial rotation can injure the joints on either side of the moving segment[11] (Fig. 17.4). Axial rotation initially occurs around an axis located in the posterior third of the vertebral body but is rapidly limited by impaction of the contralateral zygapophysial joint. If the rotatory force continues to be applied, further rotation occurs about the impaction point. This results in posterior distraction of the joint on the opposite side. In the impaction joint, impaction fractures or transarticular fractures can occur. In the distraction joint, tears or avulsions of the joint capsule can occur.

Postmortem studies have demonstrated injuries reflective of those produced in laboratory experiments.[24,25] The samples were harvested from subjects who had died in motor vehicle accidents or whose death otherwise involved serious trauma. Control samples were obtained from subjects whose death did not involve trauma. Evident in the trauma subjects were such injuries as subchondral fractures, fractures of articular processes, and avulsions of the articular cartilage. The presence of intra-articular hemorrhage indicated that the lesions were not postmortem artifacts. These lesions were not present in the control samples.

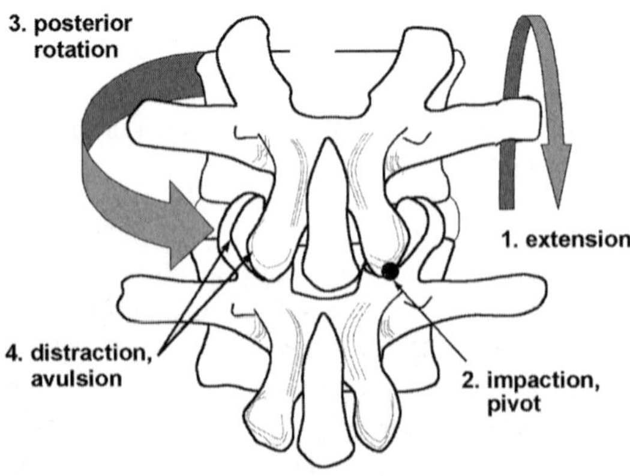

Figure 17.3. Posterior view of a lumbar motion segment illustrating the sequence of movements underlying extension-rotation injury of a lumbar zygapophysial joint.

In contrast to the laboratory and postmortem studies, traumatic lesions of the lumbar zygapophysial joints have rarely been reported in the clinical literature, for perhaps understandable reasons. Lesions of the capsule or of intra-articular meniscoids cannot be detected by any currently available technology. Small fractures are not demonstrated by plain radiography. Indeed, none of the lesions seen in postmortem studies were evident even in postmortem radiographs.[24,25] In routine conventional computed tomography (CT) scans, small fractures can escape notice because of sampling limitations. Fractures may be smaller than the slice thickness used, and conventional scans may sample a given joint at only one to three levels. Fractures located elsewhere, therefore, may escape detection. For CT or magnetic resonance imaging (MRI) to detect, or to exclude, small fractures in the lumbar zygapophysial joints, the joints would need to be subjected to serial scans of narrow width. An alternative is to use stereoradiography. At least one study[21] has reported small fractures demonstrable by this technique, which indicates that fractures of the lumbar zygapophysial joints do occur.

Symptomatic traumatic lesions of the lumbar zygapophysial joints are probably uncommon. In patients with a history of low-back pain and some sort of injury, zygapophysial joint pain appears to be uncommon. Among such patients, studies have shown that the prevalence of zygapophysial joint pain, defined as complete relief of pain following diagnostic blocks, is 10%[7] or less.[9,13] Thus, even if patients with low-back pain were thoroughly screened for small fractures, the likelihood of finding a symptomatic lesion would be very low.

Cervical Spine

The classical forms of injury to the zygapophysial joints are fractures and dislocations sustained in compression injuries of the cervical spine combined with flexion. The compression phase accounts for fractures of the articular pillars or the vertebral bodies, and the flexion accounts for the dislocation.[10,27] These injuries are well understood, and readily recognized on medical imaging.

More elusive have been the injuries associated with whiplash. However, relatively recent studies, using a variety of approaches, have identified both the types of injuries that can occur and their mechanism.[8]

Injuries to the cervical zygapophysial joints were initially implicated by clinical studies, in which the source of neck pain after whiplash was traced to the zygapophysial joints. These studies used controlled diagnostic blocks of the medial branches of the cervical dorsal rami, which innervate these joints.[4]

The first study investigated 100 patients with chronic neck pain and headache after whiplash.[17] Using comparative local anesthetic blocks[2,16] of the third occipital nerve, which innervates the C2-3 joint, the study found that in some 27% of patients, the C2-3 zygapophysial joint was the source of pain. Among those patients in whom headache was the dominant symptom, the prevalence of C2-3 zygapophysial joint pain was 53%.

A companion study of 50 patients, also using comparative local anesthetic blocks, established that in 54% of patients the source of neck pain could be traced to one or more of the cervical zygapophysial joints.[3] The segments most commonly affected were C5-6 and C2-3. A later study, of 68 patients, using placebo-controlled blocks, established two figures.[18] Excluding patients with headache, the prevalence of zygapophysial joint pain at segments below C2-3 was 49%. If patients with headache stemming from C2-3 pain were included, the prevalence of zygapophysial joint pain rose to 60%. Among drivers involved in high-speed collisions, the prevalence was at least 75%.[12]

These clinical studies drew attention to the cervical zygapophysial joints as the single most common source of pain in patients with chronic neck pain after whiplash. However, they were not accompanied by any imaging studies. They relied on controlled diagnostic blocks to pinpoint the source of pain but did not explore its cause.

The first data on lesions of the cervical zygapophysial joints came from opportunistic postmortem studies. In these studies, the investigators harvested the cervical spines of individuals who had died in motor vehicle accidents. The cause of death was head injury or suboccipital spinal cord injury, but the lower cervical spines were studied to provide insight into the injuries that can occur at typical cervical levels.[14,22,23,26]

The studies, conducted independently in Sweden[14] and Australia,[22,24] both revealed the same features. Apart from injuries to the intervertebral discs, transverse processes, and uncovertebral regions, the cervical spines exhibited several types of injury to the zygapophysial joints. These encompassed intra-articular hemorrhage, contusions and bruising of the meniscoids, small fractures of the articular cartilage and subchondral bone, and larger fractures of the articular processes or articular pillars (Fig. 17.5). Conspicuously and significantly, virtually none of these lesions could be seen on plain radiographs of the cervical spine even on retrospective review. These postmortem studies were not conducted explicitly on victims of whiplash accidents. The subjects had been involved in lethal, and therefore major, motor vehicle accidents. However, the studies do provide prima facie evidence of what might occur in sublethal accidents.[6,26]

A third line of evidence has come from studies of normal volunteers. In these studies, volunteers were subjected to equivalents of minor rear-end collisions while undergoing cineradiography.[15] The

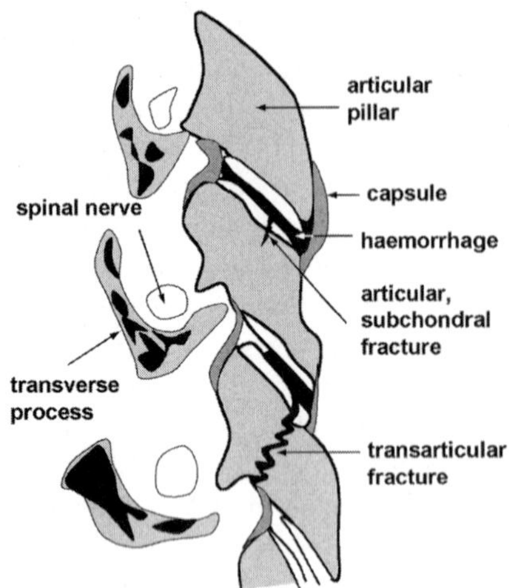

Figure 17.5. Lateral section through the cervical spine illustrating the types of lesions encountered in the cervical zygapophysial joints during motor vehicle accidents.

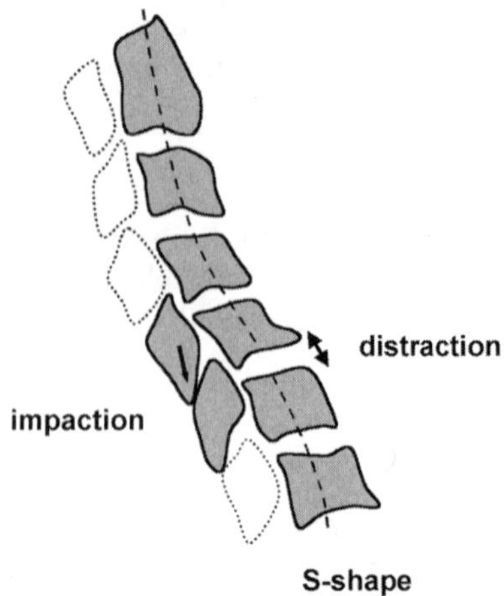

Figure 17.6. Sigmoid deformation of the cervical spine that occurs about 110 milliseconds after impact during a whiplash injury and the posterior impaction and anterior distraction that occur at C5-6 as that segment undergoes abnormal extension.

radiographs reveal the potential mechanism of injury during whiplash.

During the first 150 milliseconds after impact, the cervical spine undergoes compression from below.[8] Ostensibly because of straightening of the thoracic kyphosis, the base of the neck rises, exerting a compression load on the cervical spine, whose displacement is temporarily prevented by the inertia of the head. As a result, the cervical spine undergoes a sigmoid deformation in which the upper cervical spine is relatively flexed while the lower spine is extended[8] (Fig. 17.6).

Normally, extension involves a posterior sagittal rotation of the vertebral body accompanied by a posterior translation. This combination of movements results in the vertebra moving in an arcuate fashion around an axis located below the disc of the segment.[1] Because of the large radius of the arc, the facets of the zygapophysial joints glide across one another; that is, the inferior articular process moves tangential to the surface of the superior articular process (Fig. 17.7*A*). During normal movement, the posterior neck muscles are responsible for drawing the vertebrae backwards, and thus they are responsible for the tangential movement of the zygapophysial joints.

During the sigmoid deformation that occurs in whiplash, the lower cervical segments undergo extension in an abnormal manner.[15] Muscles are not responsible for the extension. Therefore, posterior translation does not occur. Instead, extension is caused by eccentric compression of the segment by the weight of the head. As a result, extension occurs around an abnormally high axis of rotation, located in the vertebral body (Fig. 17.7*B*). In essence, the vertebral body spins around this high axis without translating backwards. This motion results in a short radius of movement.

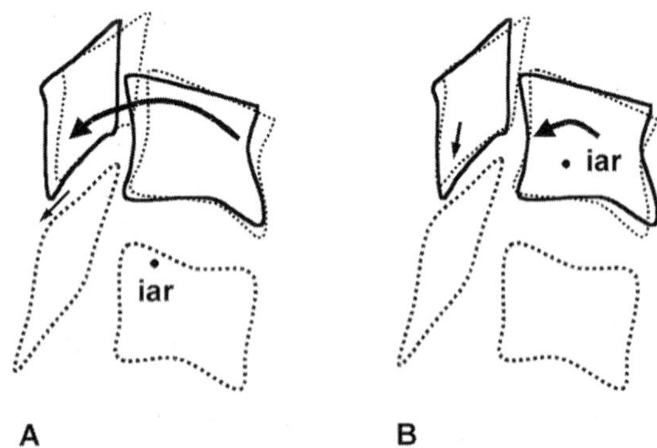

Figure 17.7. (*A*) Normal extension of a cervical motion segment. The vertebra moves in an arcuate pattern, with a large radius about an instantaneous axis of rotation (iar) located below the intervertebral disc. The inferior articular process glides tangentially across its oposing superior articular process (arrow). (*B*) Extension during whiplash. The vertebra moves in a tight arcuate fashion around an axis located within the vertebral body. As a result, the inferior edge of the inferior articular process chisels into the superior articular process (arrow).

Because of the short radius, the articular processes do not glide. Instead, the posterior edge of the inferior articular process chisels into the surface of the underlying superior articular process (Fig. 17.7*B*). Meanwhile, the anterior ends of the vertebral bodies are separated beyond their normal limits, exerting an abnormal strain on the anterior longitudinal ligament and anterior anulus fibrosus.

The chiseling motion of the inferior articular process predicts several possible types of injury. The inferior articular process could compress and injure a posterior meniscoid. If it is forceful enough, the chiseling impact could fracture the cartilage and subchondral bone of the superior articular process. With even greater force, the chisel could fracture the articular pillar. These are the lesions evident in the postmortem studies.

When several lines of evidence, using totally independent techniques, lead to the same conclusion, they provide convergent validity.[5] Under these conditions, acceptance of a concept does not depend on a single line of evidence, which alone might be contentious. Rather, the validity is increased because multiple different lines of evidence are independent of one another's respective limitations.

Zygapophysial joint injury has convergent validity. Clinical studies have shown that the joints are commonly painful in patients who report a whiplash injury. Postmortem studies show that lesions can occur in these joints. Biomechanics experiments show how these joint can be injured.

This evidence does not mean that all patients who suffer a whiplash accident incur a joint injury. Indeed, the natural history of whiplash is such that most patients probably suffer few or no injuries.[5,7,8] Zygapophysial joint pain is common only in the 10% of patients who develop chronic pain. Accordingly, zygapophysial joint injury is most likely to have occurred in that subset of patients.

The last step in refining the paradigm of cervical zygapophysial joint injury has not been taken. It consists of demonstrating lesions with high-resolution imaging. This has not been possible to date for a variety of reasons.

Investigators who conducted the clinical studies with diagnostic blocks did not have access to imaging facilities suitable for high-resolution studies. Nor would the studies have been valid had they been undertaken. Prior to any study looking for small lesions on the zygapophysial joints, it would have been necessary to establish a normative database stratified by age. Only by those means could the inference be refuted that the observed abnormalities were no more than normal changes due to aging.

In the past, only CT was available for high-resolution studies. Conventional MRI lacked the resolution for detailed studies of small lesions in small structures like the cervical zygapophysial joints. With the advent of three tesla magnets with spectroscopic facilities, the technology has become available by which the cervical zygapophysial joints can be studied in detail. Moreover, the need for normative data can be circumvented if diagnostic blocks are applied to determine, in given patients, which of their joints hurt and which do not.

At the time of writing, a Swiss group has applied for a grant to study patients with whiplash at inception through chronic phases, using high-resolution spectroscopic MRI coupled with controlled diagnostic blocks of the zygapophysial joints in those patients whose pain persists.

REFERENCES

1. Amevo B, Worth D, Bogduk N: Instantaneous axes of rotation of the typical cervical motion segments: a study in normal volunteers. Clin Biomech 6:111–117, 1991.
2. Barnsley L, Lord S, Bogduk N: Comparative local anaesthetic blocks in the diagnosis of cervical zygapophysial joints pain. Pain 55:99–106, 1993.
3. Barnsley L, Lord SM, Wallis BJ, Bogduk N: The prevalence of chronic cervical zygapophysial joint pain after whiplash. Spine 20:20–26, 1995.
4. Bogduk N: The clinical anatomy of the cervical dorsal rami. Spine 7:319–330, 1982.
5. Bogduk N: Acute and chronic whiplash. SpineLine 11(5): 8–11, 2001.
6. Bogduk N: Point of view. Spine 27:1940–1941, 2002.
7. Bogduk N: Neck pain and whiplash. In: Jensen TS, Wilson PR, Rice ASC (eds): Clinical Pain Management: Chronic Pain. London, Arnold, 2003, pp 504–519.
8. Bogduk N, Yoganandan N: Biomechanics of the cervical spine Part 3: Minor injuries. Clin Biomech 16:267–275, 2001.
9. Carette S, Marcoux S, Truchon R, Grondin, Gagnon J, Allard Y, Latulippe M: A controlled trial of corticosteroid injections into facet joints for chronic low back pain. N Engl J Med 325:1002–1007, 1991.
10. Cusick JF, Yoganandan N: Biomechanics of the cervical spine 4: Major injuries. Clin Biomech 17:1–20, 2002;
11. Farfan HF, Cossette JW, Robertson GH, Wells RV, Kraus H: The effects of torsion on the lumbar intervertebral

joints: The role of torsion in the production of disc degeneration. J Bone Joint Surg 52A:468–497, 1970.
12. Gibson T, Bogduk N, Macpherson J, McIntosh A: Crash characteristics of whiplash associated chronic neck pain. J Musculoskeletal Pain 8:87–95, 2000.
13. Jackson RP, Jacobs RR, Montesano PX: Facet joint injection in low back pain. A prospective study. Spine 13:966–971, 1988.
14. Jónsson H, Bring G, Rauschning W, et al: Hidden cervical spine injuries in traffic accident victims with skull fractures. J Spinal Disord 4:251–263, 1991.
15. Kaneoka K, Ono K, Inami S, Hayashi K: Motion analysis of cervical vertebrae during whiplash loading. Spine 24: 763–770, 1999.
16. Lord SM, Barnsley L, Bogduk N: The utility of comparative local anaesthetic blocks versus placebo-controlled blocks for the diagnosis of cervical zygapophysial joint pain. Clin J Pain 11:208–213, 1995.
17. Lord SM, Barnsley L, Wallis B, Bogduk N: Third occipital headache: A prevalence study. J Neurol Neurosurg Psychiatry 57:1187–1190, 1994.
18. Lord SM, Barnsley L, Wallis BJ, Bogduk N: Chronic cervical zygapophysial joint pain after whiplash: A placebo-controlled prevalence study. Spine 21:1737–1745, 1996.
19. Mercer S, Bogduk N: Intra-articular inclusions of the cervical synovial joints. Br J Rheumatol 32:705–710, 1993.
20. Schwarzer AC, Aprill CN, Derby R, Fortin J, Kine G, Bogduk N: Clinical features of patients with pain stemming from the lumbar zygapophysial joints. Is the lumbar facet syndrome a clinical entity? Spine 19:1132–1137, 1994.
21. Sims-Williams H, Jayson MIV, Baddeley H: Small spinal fractures in back pain patients. Ann Rheum Dis 37:262–265, 1978.
22. Taylor JR, Taylor MM: Cervical spinal injuries: An autopsy study of 109 blunt injuries. J Musculoskeletal Pain 4:61–79, 1996.
23. Taylor JR, Twomey LT: Acute injuries to cervical joints: An autopsy study of neck sprain. Spine 9:1115–1122, 1993.
24. Taylor JR, Twomey LT, Corker M: Bone and soft tissue injuries in post-mortem lumbar spines. Paraplegia 28:119–129, 1990.
25. Twomey LT, Taylor JR, Taylor MM: Unsuspected damage to lumbar zygapophyseal (facet) joints after motor-vehicle accidents. Med J Aust 151:210–217, 1989.
26. Uhrenholt L, Grunnet-Nilsson N, Hartvigsen J: Cervical spine lesions after road traffic accidents. A systematic review. Spine 27:1934–1941, 2002.
27. Winkelstein BA, Myers BS: Determinants of catastrophic neck injury. In: Yoganandan N, Pintar FA, Larson SJ, Sances A (eds): Frontiers in Head and Neck Trauma. Amsterdam, IOS Press, 1998, pp 266–295.
28. Yang KH, King AI: Mechanism of facet load transmission as a hypothesis for low-back pain. Spine 9:557–565, 1984.

Part III

Plexus and Peripheral Nerve Injuries

Chapter 18
Plexus Injuries

ASA J. WILBOURN

The peripheral nervous system (PNS) plexuses are intricate networks of nerve fibers located between the spinal cord or primary roots (proximally) and the proximal peripheral nerves (distally). The three major neural plexuses—brachial, lumbar, and sacral—are traversed by almost all the nerve fibers that supply the upper and lower extremities, the shoulder and hip girdles, and the pelvic floor.[13,85]

The anatomy of each plexus is unique. Nonetheless, all of them respond to injury with the same types of pathophysiological reactions, and lesions of them are identified and localized, to a greater or lesser extent, by the same diagnostic procedures. These two features, common to all the PNS plexuses, will now be discussed.

Pathology/Pathophysiology of Plexopathies

The axons that comprise the elements of the various neural plexuses, similar to those that constitute the peripheral nerves, can be injured by a great variety of processes. However, fundamentally they are very limited, both pathologically and pathophysiologically, in the manner in which they can respond to such injuries. When subjected to a focal insult of sufficient severity, nerve fibers of all sizes, both the small unmyelinated and the large myelinated, are killed at the lesion site, causing the segments of the axons distal to that point to undergo Wallerian, or axonal, degeneration. With injuries of lesser severity—those not sufficient to cause axon degeneration—the myelinated fibers have an additional method of response: they can undergo focal demyelination limited to the lesion site.[97]

Pathophysiologically, axon degeneration is manifested as conduction failure along the affected nerve fibers from the lesion site distally, with the exception that during the first 7 to 10 days after injury, an ever-diminishing number of the axons can still transmit impulses. In contrast to axon loss, the effects of demyelination remain focal, restricted to the relatively small portion of the large nerve fibers where the myelin has been compromised. Conduction along the nerve segments distal (and proximal) to that point is not altered in any manner.[97]

Axon Degeneration

Axon degeneration is the pathological substrate for most plexopathies. In any given plexus element, any percentage of axons, ranging from 1% to 100%, can be injured enough to degenerate. If only a few are affected, clinical changes may not be apparent. Whenever axon loss is substantial, however, clinical deficits are obvious: weakness and subsequent wasting whenever motor fibers are involved and sensory loss involving all modalities (including pain and temperature sensations) whenever sensory fibers are affected.[10,97]

Focal Demyelination

Focal demyelination along a segment of either motor or sensory fibers can produce two different types of pathophysiological abnormalities that functionally are quite dissimilar: conduction slowing and conduction block. With conduction slowing, all the nerve impulses ultimately reach their destination, even though their speed through the site of injury is reduced. Clinically, conduction slowing per se causes no symptoms: neither weakness nor wasting results when conduction is slowed along the motor nerve fibers, and no detectible sensory deficits are associated with uniform slowing along sensory axons. Conduction slowing, however, manifests itself on the formal neurological examination if it is present to different degrees along the various large, myelinated fibers (differential or desynchronized slowing) and synchronized volleys of impulses are required, as in vibratory testing and deep tendon reflex assessment. Synchronized demyelinating conduction slowing, in which the rate of conduction is reduced along all the affected axons to the same extent, generally is devoid of clinical symptomatology. Demyelinating conduction slowing is not included in any of the clinical classifications of peripheral nerve disorders, even though it helps localize lesions in the electrodiagnostic (EDX) laboratory whenever it is present.[8,10,97]

Demyelinating conduction block, although it shares the same underlying pathology with demyelinating conduction slowing, is a very different process pathophysiologically. Because transmission is stopped, rather than merely slowed, at the lesion site, nerve impulses do not reach their destinations. As a result, demyelinating conduction block in its clinical manifestations is very similar to axon degeneration: it can affect any percentage (1% to 100%) of the nerve fibers of any particular plexus element. Whenever it involves a sufficient number of motor axons, it produces clinical weakness that is identical to that manifested when the same number of motor axons undergo degeneration; in the same vein, when it affects a sufficient number of sensory fibers, it causes sensory deficits. There are at least two significant distinctions, however, between abrupt-onset demyelinating conduction block and axon loss: the former: (1) produces sensory deficits that are limited to those mediated over large myelinated fibers, consisting essentially of those responsible for position, vibration, and light touch senses—specifically, it does not cause pain or temperature abnormalities; (2) causes symptoms that typically are of relatively brief duration (because nerve impulse transmission throughout the lesion site resumes, and therefore motor and sensory functions are restored, as soon as the myelin damage is repaired; this can happen within several days after injury and seldom requires more than a few weeks).[10,97]

Demyelinating conduction block is the type of pathophysiology responsible for the relatively short-lived weakness manifested by many traumatic plexopathies, principally brachial plexopathies, such as those caused by mild closed traction injuries, gunshot wounds, and malpositioning on the operating table.[100] In these instances, the demyelinating conduction block lesion is clinically labeled *neurapraxia*,[75] or a *first degree injury*.[85] It is pertinent to note that not all demyelinating conduction blocks that affect the plexuses have this benign nature. With both radiation-induced lesions and multifocal conduction block syndrome, focal demyelinating conduction blocks may persist for years and then gradually convert to axon degeneration rather than resolving.[97]

Demyelinating conduction block occasionally is the sole type of pathophysiology present with a particular plexopathy. Much more frequently, however, it coexists with axon degeneration. Nonetheless, in some patients it is the predominant process operative, and thus is responsible for most of the clinical symptoms present. Demyelinating conduction block is far more commonly found with brachial plexopathies than with lumbar and sacral plexopathies because of the differing nature of the processes that produce them.[98,100]

This section has focused on the negative manifestations of plexus lesions, that is, the deficits that they produce. Positive phenomena, however, are also very common with plexopathies. Most of these relate to sensory fiber involvement. The only noteworthy positive motor manifestations encountered are the fasciculation potentials and especially the myokymic discharges that often are seen with radiation-induced lesions; these, however, are not relevant to this discussion. Positive sensory phenomena, such as pain and paresthesias, not only occur much more frequently than motor phenomena with plexopathies but at times are the cardinal symptoms; for example, from the patient's perspective, the severe pain associated with brachial plexus avulsion injuries often is the most intolerable aspect of these lesions. The mechanism whereby damaged sensory axons at the lesion site become ectopic generators, producing pain or paresthesias (small- and large-fiber manifestations, respectively), is independent of any functional deficit present.[76,97]

Recovery Potential

When produced by trauma, demyelinating conduction block plexus lesions always recover completely and generally fairly rapidly. Most authorities state that recovery should be beginning, if not completed, between 3 weeks and 6–8 weeks postinjury.[75,85]

The degree of ultimate recovery with axon degenerating lesions, in contrast, is extremely variable, even with injuries of the same initial severity. Obviously, other factors are operative.

A major factor is the degree of damage sustained at the lesion site by the nonconducting, supporting structures of the nerve: the endoneurium, perineurium, and epineurium. Progressively severe involvement of them causes the regenerating axons to experience increasing difficulty advancing through the damaged segment. With the mildest grade of axon degenerating lesion, Seddon's *axonotmesis* and Sunderland's *second-degree injury*, the axons are killed at the lesion site and their distal segments degenerate, but all the supporting structures of the nerve are intact. As a result, the regenerating axons encounter no obstacles as they advance distally. Intermediate grades of injury include Seddon's lesser degrees of *neurotmesis* injuries and Sunderland's *third-degree* and *fourth-degree injuries*, in which the endoneurium alone, or both the endoneurium and epineurium, are disrupted. With fourth-degree neurotmesis lesions the perineurium is still intact, so that on visual inspection the nerve remains in continuity, but its internal architecture has been so deranged that it cannot be bridged by an appreciable number of regenerating axons; consequently, spontaneous recovery essentially does not occur. With the highest grade of injury, Seddon's worst neurotmesis lesion and Sunderland's *fifth-degree injury*, both the axons and all of their supporting structures are disrupted at the lesion site, thereby eliminating any likely possibility of substantial spontaneous regeneration.[75,85] Whenever complete physical separation of a plexus element occurs, it is referred to as an *interruption* or a *rupture*. Whenever a primary root is torn from the spinal cord, it is labeled an *avulsion injury*; the latter is a special type of plexus lesion, nearly unique to the brachial plexus. Root avulsion lesions are not only fifth-degree neurotmesis injuries, but also the most severe traction lesions the plexus can sustain. They produce essentially irreversible loss of function and often severe pain as well. Brachial plexus root avulsions, unfortunately, are distressingly common. Ironically, some measures taken by the authorities to make highway travel safer—such as mandatory helmet laws for motorcyclists—have increased the incidence and severity of brachial plexus root avulsions (i.e., resulted in more roots avulsed per accident), as cyclists who formerly would have been killed on impact now survive with permanent deficits.[100] Usually these lesions are accompanied by injuries to other structures, particularly fractures, but they can occur in isolation. In contrast, so-called avulsion injuries of the lumbar and sacral plexuses are quite rare and almost always coexist with severe trauma to other pelvic structures (see below). In almost every series, most avulsion injuries are caused by violent high-velocity trauma, especially roadway accidents. Other causes of damage common to both brachial and lumbosacral plexus are industrial injuries and falls, often from a height.[100] Because most root avulsions affect brachial plexus fibers, these will be further discussed under closed supraclavicular traction lesions.

A second major factor in the degree of recovery from axon loss injuries is the nature of the injury. Some lesions, such as focal pressure, affect a relatively small axon segment. Others, however, damage a substantially greater length of nerve fiber, making satisfactory regeneration through the site of damage much more difficult, even with lesser degrees of injury. In this regard, traction lesions typically are much more injurious than compressive ones because they affect the axon over a far more extensive segment.[98,100]

The third and fourth major factors, which are interrelated, are the distance the regenerating fibers must grow to restore the lost function and the completeness of the lesion. After they have traversed the lesion site, axons regenerate distally quite slowly, advancing approximately 1 inch per month. Unfortunately, most muscle fibers can survive for only about 20–24 months in the denervated state before they, in turn, degenerate. As a result, whenever the site of injury and the motor point of the completely denervated muscle are separated by more than 20–24 inches, muscle reinnervation via progressive proximodistal regeneration typically is very unsatisfactory, having been severely compromised by an adverse *time-distance factor*. Another reinnervating process, however, is available: collateral sprouting. Via this mechanism, denervated structures are reinnervated by axon branches arising from nearby unaffected nerve fibers in the muscles or skin. To be effective, however, this process requires that a substantial number of axons supplying the muscle or skin region survive the initial injury so that they can serve as donor fibers. Consequently, collateral sprouting is of value only when axon loss has been incomplete. The fact that the plexuses are so proximal is the main reason why, following very severe axon loss lesions, the intrinsic hand muscles with lower trunk and medial cord brachial plexopathies, and the muscles below the knee with sacral plexopathies, reinnervate so poorly: the excessive regeneration distance prevents effective proximodistal regeneration, while the severity of the lesion precludes collateral sprouting.[1,98,100]

Laboratory Diagnostic Procedures

The plexuses are located quite proximally, and their anatomy is complex. Lesions of various plexus elements are readily mislocalized to both more proximal and more distal sites, that is, to the primary roots from which they originate or to one or more peripheral nerves that originate from them. Employing just the clinical examination alone, even skilled clinicians can encounter difficulties in separating injuries of one of these proximal PNS structures from those of another. Hence, ancillary diagnostic procedures usually are performed whenever the question of a plexopathy arises. The two most helpful of these are EDX examinations and various imaging studies. The general features of each of these will now be discussed.[95,100,101]

Electrodiagnostic Studies

Electrodiagnostic (EDX) studies have two uses in assessing patients with suspected plexopathies. First, they can exclude other PNS lesions with which a plexopathy can be confused. Second, if a plexus lesion is present, they often can provide reliable information regarding its location, pathophysiology, extent, and severity. Of the various components of the EDX examination, the two basic ones, the nerve conduction studies (NCSs) and needle electromyography (EMG), are of the most benefit. With both the motor and sensory NCSs, the amplitudes of the responses, rather than their latencies and conduction velocities, are the useful component. The sensory NCS responses can aid in distinguishing extraforaminal axon loss lesions from those of the primary roots; they are unaffected by the latter, since the nerve fiber injuries are proximal to the dorsal root ganglia (DRG), whereas they are low in amplitude or unelicitable with even moderate axon loss postganglionic disorders. The motor NCS amplitudes can determine whether a recorded muscle is weak because of demyelinating conduction block or axon degeneration; if the latter, then they provide information regarding its severity. Seven days or more after injury, a normal or near-normal motor NCS amplitude recorded from a weak muscle indicates that the muscle has not been substantially denervated. Consequently, if a lower motor neuron abnormality is present it must be, by default, a demyelinating conduction block lesion located proximal to the most proximal stimulation point. Conversely, if the motor NCS response is low in amplitude or unelicitable at that time, then axon loss is present; the approximate amount that has occurred can be determined by comparing that amplitude with the one obtained by performing the same NCS on the contralateral, asymptomatic side. The needle EMG, by revealing minimal axon loss and by permitting assessment of motor nerves that cannot be evaluated by motor NCSs, may demonstrate the full extent of PNS involvement and therefore help in localization. Also, depending on the timing of the examination, it can show either residual innervation or early reinnervation.[95,98,100]

Although several other EDX procedures can be performed on patients with suspected plexopathies, including tests of F-waves, H-responses, and somatosensory evoked potentials, generally all are of quite limited value compared to the two basic components. Most of them seek evidence primarily of focal slowing, which is rarely the type of pathophysiology responsible for plexus lesions.

Moreover, even when they are abnormal, they frequently cannot separate lesions of the proximal peripheral nerves, plexus, and roots from one another, and usually this is precisely why such studies are being performed.[102]

Because of the sheer number of axons that traverse the plexuses to reach the limbs, the EDX studies typically must be extensive if lesions of these structures are to be localized, or even diagnosed, accurately. Multiple motor and sensory NCSs are the rule, often with the identical studies performed on the contralateral limb for control purposes. The needle EMG must be detailed as well, generally with muscles sampled at all levels of the peripheral neuraxis, ranging from the distal limb to the neck or back.[98,100]

In spite of the extensiveness of the EDX examination, under some circumstances the results may be suboptimal or even valueless. There are at least three reasons.

First, the EDX examination has its greatest utility when most of the motor and sensory axons traversing the plexus can be assessed with NCSs and when muscles innervated by the motor axons are accessible for needle EMG. The various plexuses differ enormously in this regard. The brachial plexus is by far the most amenable to evaluation. A great number of motor and sensory NCSs can be performed, including many nonstandard ones, and a multitude of muscles are available for needle EMG sampling. The superior portion of the sacral plexus is the next best. The major limitation in assessing it is that, in many elderly persons, the lower limb sensory NCSs are unelicitable bilaterally, presumably due to age rather than pathology. Without reliable sensory NCSs, differentiating a sacral plexopathy from ipsilateral L5 and S1 radiculopathies that are not manifesting paraspinal fibrillation potentials is impossible. Assessing the lumbar plexus falls into an intermediate, but suboptimal, position. There are no reliable sensory NCSs and only one motor NCS (femoral motor NCS) available for assessment; in addition, relatively few muscles can be sampled on needle EMG, and almost all of them are located proximally in the limb and, therefore, reinnervate fairly soon after injury with incomplete axon loss lesions. Assessing the cervical plexus is quite suboptimal. Very few of the axons comprising it can be evaluated with NCSs (sensory: greater auricular NCS; motor: phrenic NCS) and, excluding the diaphragm, which is technically difficult to sample, no muscles can be studied on needle EMG. Assessing the inferior portion of the sacral plexus, which innervates the pelvic floor, is extremely suboptimal. It cannot be evaluated at all, except for needle EMG of the anal sphincter, unless quite specialized procedures are performed, and few EDX physicians are skilled at doing them.[95,98,101]

Second, after injury, there is a distinct time window for optimal EDX assessment of traumatic plexus lesions, which ranges from approximately 3 weeks to 12–16 weeks. Studies performed sooner than this are likely to be falsely negative or misleading, whereas studies performed after this period may be falsely negative, or they may erroneously localize the lesion to a more distal location than where it actually is.[100]

Third, a large number of confounding factors can render the EDX examination suboptimal, either because critical studies cannot be performed or because the results are difficult to interpret. These factors include casts, bandages and open wounds overlying stimulation and recording points necessary for NCSs and overlying muscles that need to be sampled during the needle EMG, coexisting PNS lesions such as coincidental carpal tunnel syndrome (CTS), traumatic peripheral nerve injuries, and generalized polyneuropathies; and the inability of patients to cooperate for various reasons, including pain, associated fractures or dislocations, and reduced mentation secondary to drugs or coexisting central nervous system (CNS) injury.

Imaging Studies

Several different imaging techniques are available for plexus assessment, depending upon the particular plexus involved, the mechanism of injury, and the size and location of the lesion. These include, but are not limited to, plain X-rays, venography, arteriography, myelography, computed tomography (CT), CT myelography, magnetic resonance imaging (MRI), and MRI myelography.

Plain X-rays can reveal humeral head dislocations, as well as fractures of various bony structures near the plexuses, such as the clavicle, scapula, proximal humerus, cervical transverse processes, first thoracic rib, cervical and lumbosacral vertebrae, and pelvic ring; in addition, foreign objects such as metal fragments, bullets, and errant hardware can be visualized, as can radiation changes of bone and disruptions of the sacroiliac and pubic joints.[2,18,100]

Myelography essentially evaluates the structures within and near the thecal sac: the spinal cord, the surrounding dura, and the nerve roots. Thus, its value is principally in differentiating preganglionic avulsion injuries from postganglionic lesions in the presence of rather severe trauma secondary to traction. For this reason, it is more often used with brachial plexopathies than with lumbosacral plexopathies. Although for many years it was considered by many to be the best indirect method for demonstrating root avulsions, an appreciable number of both falsely positive and falsely negative studies were reported with it, at least in regard to brachial plexopathies.[2,4,44,74] In addition, this technique is potentially hazardous to use in the presence of a coexisting head injury.[4] More recently, myelography has been combined with CT (see below).

Computed tomography has many limitations in evaluating the neural plexuses, especially for traumatic lesions.[2,25,26] Although CT alone has limited value in assessing the extraforaminal portions of the brachial plexus, when it is combined with myelography (CT myelography) it is considered by many to be the most sensitive imaging procedure for assessing the intraspinal canal components. In contrast to the restricted use of CT with brachial plexopathies, for several years it was the procedure of choice in lumbosacral plexus assessment, although principally for detecting mass lesions. Nonetheless, MRI has for the most part supplanted CT for evaluating this plexus as well.[4,18,25,28,44,81]

Magnetic resonance imaging currently is considered, overall, the optimal neuroimaging technique for brachial plexus and lumbosacral plexus evaluations. It lacks many of the limitations of CT in that it offers superior soft tissue contrast resolution and multiplanar capability. It can reveal posttraumatic hemorrhage and swelling, such as traumatic meningoceles as well as abnormalities caused by root avulsions. In this regard, it is more sensitive than myelography for detecting C5, C6 root avulsions. Not all traumatic plexopathies, however, even those associated with substantial clinical deficits, produce MRI changes.[4,28,31,44,56,66,81] Magnetic resonance myelography is a special noninvasive imaging technique for assessing the primary roots of the brachial plexus. It creates a myelogram-like image without the use of contrast material. For this reason, it can be employed in the acute phase of brachial plexus lesions. In some centers it is now the neuroimaging procedure of choice for assessing patients with proximal brachial plexopathies.[2,55,100]

In certain instances, primarily when combined lesions of the plexus and blood vessels are suspected, both arteriograms and venograms can be helpful. Similarly, whenever a possible C5 root avulsion exists, fluoroscopy of the diaphragm may reveal ipsilateral weakness due to involvement of the C5 phrenic contribution. With some lumbosacral plexus lesions, urethrograms and cystograms may be of assistance.[100]

Brachial Plexus

Anatomy

The brachial plexus has the form of a triangle, with its vertically aligned base resting on either the vertebral column or the spinal cord (see "Roots" below) and its apex located laterally and inferiorly in the axilla. The brachial plexus universally is reported to have five components: roots, trunks, divisions, cords, and terminal nerves (Fig. 18.1). There is not universal agreement, however, regarding certain aspects of both its first and fifth components, that is, the roots and the terminal nerves. Regarding the roots, anatomists consider the brachial plexus to be a strictly extraforaminal structure, and envision its "roots" actually to be the anterior primary rami (APRs).[10] In contrast, most surgeons who deal extensively with plexus lesions consider the roots, at least in regard to traction injuries, to include not only the APRs, located extraforaminally, but also the mixed spinal nerves, located intraforaminally, as well as the anterior and posterior primary roots, located within the intraspinal canal. Thus, to them, avulsions of the roots of the brachial plexus are just as much "plexus lesions" as are disorders of the trunks and cords.[1,4,44,45,74,85] Concerning the terminal nerves, neither anatomists nor clinicians ever discuss their precise extent: that is, exactly where do the terminal nerves end and the peripheral nerve trunks, with which they are continuous, begin? Noteworthy is that this is an arbitrary dividing line not marked by any anatomical alteration. Apparently, only one investigator, Narakas, has addressed this question, and the answer he provided is somewhat imprecise. In his view, injuries of the peripheral nerve trunks in the axilla, "at their

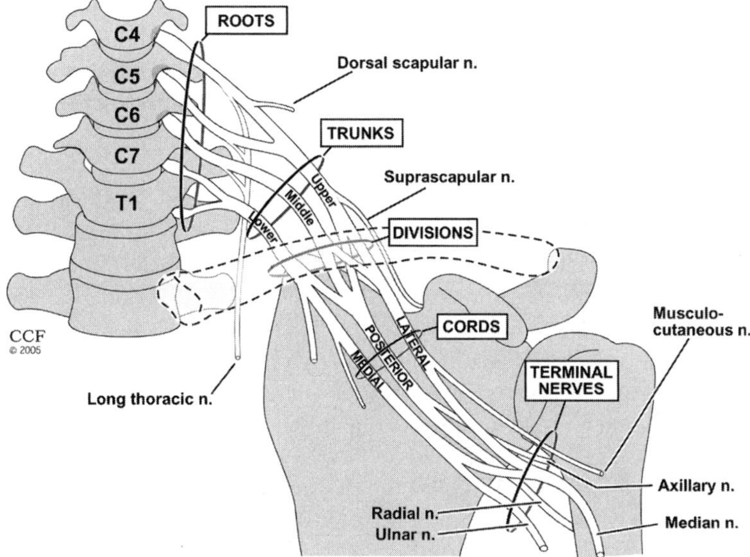

Figure 18.1. The brachial plexus; left side, anterior view. (Copyright Cleveland Clinic Foundation, used with permission)

origins and a few centimeters below," are brachial plexus lesions.[56] A practical, convenient distinction is to label the structures within the axilla as *terminal nerves* and those beyond the axilla as the proximal portions of the nerve trunks.[100]

The average adult length of the brachial plexus, measuring from the C5 vertebral foramen to the origin of the median nerve, is 15.3 cm, or slightly over 6 inches. If the intraspinal and intraforaminal root segments and the terminal nerves are included, then its total length is probably well over 9–10 inches. This relatively short space contains one of the largest PNS structures and the most complex of them. Two-thirds of the cross-sectional area of the brachial plexus is connective tissue. The other one-third is composed of at least 102,000–166,000 axons, grouped into fascicles that vary significantly in diameter and that are only approximately 5 mm in length due to constant fusion and division. The nerve fascicles also vary in number between one person and another and among the various elements of a single plexus, being fewer at the root level and more numerous distally.[77,100]

The gross anatomy of the brachial plexus will now be reviewed.

Roots

The roots consist of either (1) the C5 through T1 APRs (limited view) or (2) the C5 through T1 anterior and posterior primary roots (arising from the spinal cord), the mixed spinal nerves they form, and the APRs derived from them (expanded view). The latter definition will be used in this discussion.

Occasionally, the C4 root also contributes to the brachial plexus. When this occurs, the T1 contribution often is small and the root origins are thus shifted cephalad, producing a *prefixed* plexus. In contrast, in other instances there is a T2 root contribution while the C5 contribution is diminished, and a *postfixed* plexus results. The amount of actual clinical impact these plexus anomalies have is debated, but it probably is minimal.[100]

Of the various root subdivisions, the primary roots are most vulnerable to traction forces because of their structure: they lack both epineural and perineural sheaths, and internally they are arranged in parallel bundles, rather than in a lattice network, as are the more distal plexus portions.[85] The C5 and C6 primary roots are more readily injured by traction forces than are the C8 and T1 roots because they are already under tension at rest. However, they, and the C7 root to a lesser extent, are more protected from severe traction injuries than their C8 and T1 counterparts because the APRs derived from them are securely anchored immediately on leaving the intervertebral foramina, in the gutters of the transverse processes, by prevertebral fascia, by their epineural sheaths, and by fibrous slips of the transverse processes. Because the APRs of the C8 and T1 roots, and the C7 APR to a variable extent, are not similarly bound, traction forces placed upon them are transmitted directly to the primary roots, which may be avulsed from the spinal cord.[85]

The APRs are located deep in the lateral neck, between the anterior and middle scalene muscles. Several branches, consisting principally of motor fibers, arise from the APRs, including (1) the nerves to the scalene muscles and the longus colli; (2) the long thoracic nerve; (3) a branch of the phrenic nerve; and (4) the dorsal scapular nerve. The long thoracic and dorsal scapular nerves aid in the longitudinal localization of lesions involving the more superior portions of the brachial plexus. Whenever the muscles they innervate, the serratus anterior and rhomboids, respectively, are denervated, the lesion can be localized to some very proximal point, probably within the intraspinal canal. Although no somatic nerve branches arise from the T1 APR, some autonomic fibers do: the preganglionic sympathetic fibers destined for the head and neck. They are components of the C8 and T1 mixed spinal nerves, and as soon as the latter exit the intervertebral foramen, they pass from them to the inferior cervical ganglion by the white ramus communicans. If the C8 and T1 roots are injured proximally, where they contain these autonomic fibers, Horner syndrome—ipsilateral miosis, ptosis, head vasodilation, and head anhydrosis—results. Conversely, if the same roots are injured more laterally, the majority of the postganglionic sympathetic fibers destined for the arm, and particularly the hand, are compromised, but those supplying the head are not affected.[32,100]

Trunks

The second component of the brachial plexus consists of three trunks, which are named for their relationship to one another: upper, middle, and lower. The C5 and C6 APRs fuse to form the upper trunk, the C8 and T1 APRs join to form the lower trunk, and the C7 APR continues as the middle trunk. The trunks are located in the lowest anterior part of the posterior cervical triangle.

Only two nerves arise from the plexus at the trunk level, and both originate from the very proximal upper trunk: (1) the subclavius nerve and (2) the suprascapular nerve. Similar to the long thoracic and dorsal scapular nerves, the status of the suprascapular nerve and the muscles it innervates, the supraspinatus and infraspinatus, has important clinical implications for determining the proximal extent of an upper trunk lesion.[13,100]

Divisions

Each trunk ends by dividing into one anterior and one posterior division. Thus, there are six divisions in all, three anterior and three posterior. No branches arise from the divisions. However, this, the midportion of the plexus, has both anatomical and clinical significance. Anatomically, a profound change in the internal architecture of the brachial plexus occurs at this level because, with few exceptions, the motor fibers destined to supply the flexor muscles pass into the anterior divisions, whereas those that will supply extensor muscles enter the posterior divisions. As a result, plexus injuries proximal to the divisions present clinically as lesions of one or more roots, whereas those distal to the divisions present as lesions of multiple peripheral nerves or portions of peripheral nerves. Also, clinically, the divisions mark the boundary between the supraclavicular plexus and the infraclavicular plexus, so named because, when the arm is at the side, the clavicle overlies the divisions. For this reason, lesions of the roots and trunks are referred to as *supraclavicular plexopathies*, whereas lesions of the cords and terminal nerves are labeled *infraclavicular plexopathies* (Fig. 18.2). Lesions of the divisions themselves are referred to as *subclavicular plexopathies* or *retroclavicular plexopathies*, but these are discussed infrequently because they seldom occur in isolation.[98,100]

Subdividing brachial plexus lesions into supraclavicular plexopathies and infraclavicular plexopathies has significant clinical implications, because lesions affecting these two plexus regions tend to differ in incidence, severity, and prognosis. Both the anatomy of the brachial plexus and the nature of the disorders that affect these two subdivisions are responsible for this dichotomy.

The supraclavicular plexus is also subdivided, in regard to lesion location, on both a longitudinal and a vertical basis. Longitudinally, lesions are classified as *preganglionic* (*intradural*) or *postganglionic* (*extradural*, *extraforaminal*), depending upon whether they are located within the intraspinal canal or external to it. These terms literally apply only to the site of the damage along the sensory axons in relationship to their posterior root ganglia, but by convention they are used to localize lesions

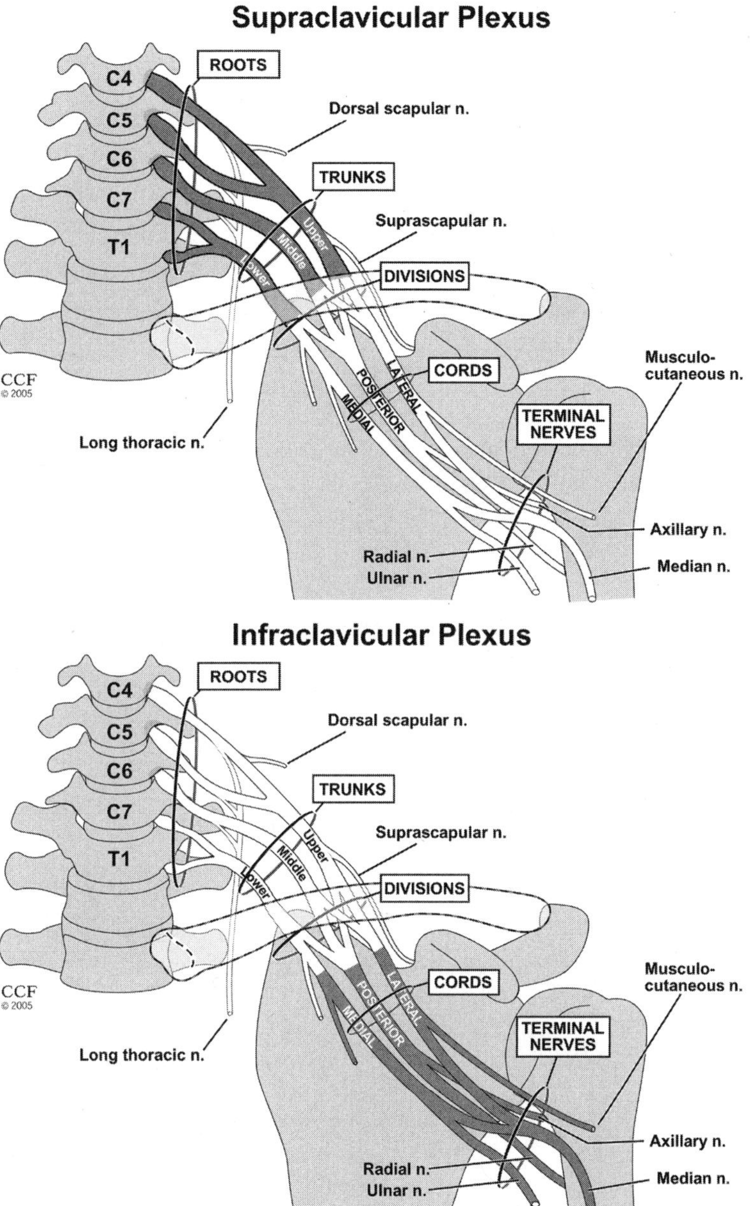

Figure 18.2. The supraclavicular and infraclavicular plexuses. The supraclavicular plexus consists of the roots and trunks, whereas the infraclavicular plexus is composed of the cords and terminal nerves. (Copyright Cleveland Clinic Foundation, used with permission)

of both the motor and sensory fibers. Vertically, the supraclavicular plexus is subdivided into three groups: *upper plexus*, *middle plexus*, and *lower plexus*. Each includes a trunk and the root fibers from which it derives. Thus, the upper plexus includes the C5, C6 primary roots, mixed spinal nerves, and APRs, as well as the upper trunk, whereas the lower plexus consists of the C8, T1 primary roots, mixed spinal nerves, APRs, and the lower trunk (Fig. 18.3). These designations are particularly helpful during the initial evaluations of many supraclavicular traction lesions, when often it is difficult to determine exactly which supraclavicular component has been injured.[98,100]

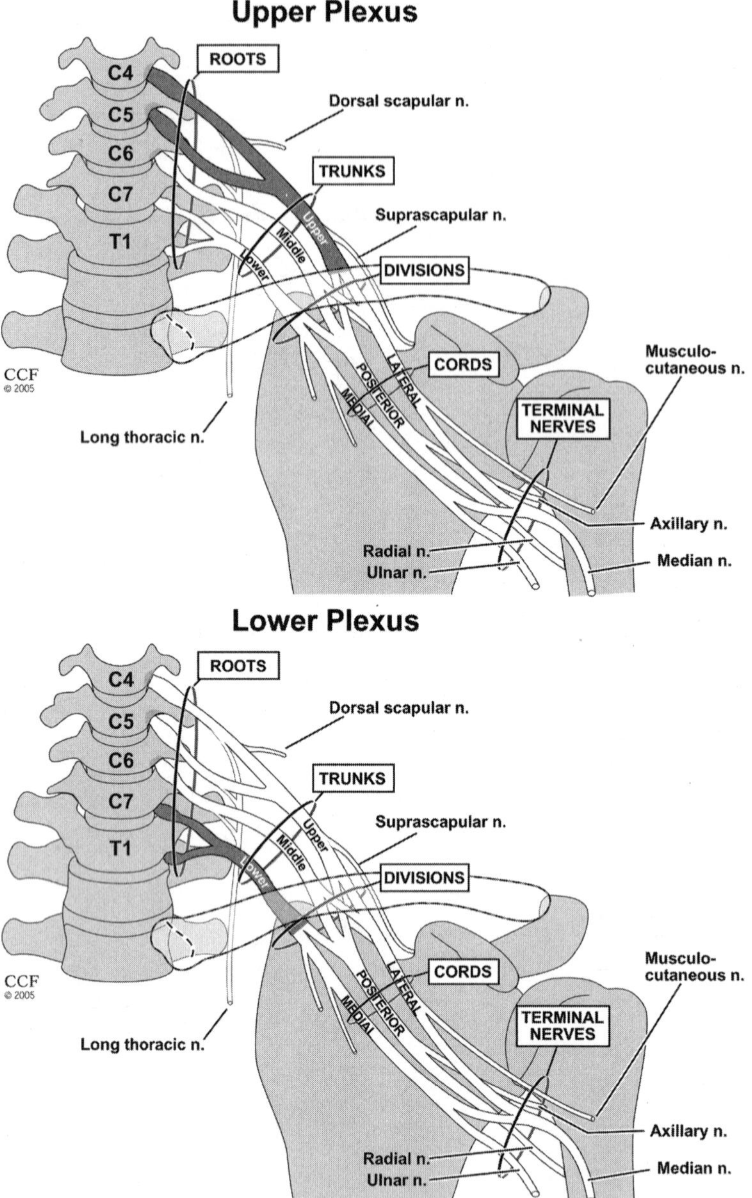

Figure 18.3. The upper and lower plexuses. Each of these consists of a trunk and the roots from which it is formed. Note that the lower plexus is the inferior component of the supraclavicular plexus, not the infra-clavicular plexus. (Copyright Cleveland Clinic Foundation, used with permission)

Cords

There are three cords—lateral, posterior, and medial—named for their positions relative to the second portion of the axillary artery, with which they are contiguous. The cords are situated in the proximal axilla. They are the longest components of the brachial plexus, and most of the peripheral nerves that arise from the brachial plexus do so at the cord level; virtually all of the upper extremity (as opposed to the shoulder girdle) muscles are innervated by motor axons that traverse one or more of the cords. The lateral and medial pectoral nerves, which supply the pectoralis muscles, arise from the proximal portion of the lateral and medial cords, respectively.[100]

Terminal Nerves

There is no consensus among anatomists regarding how many of the various peripheral nerves that originate from the cords merit the designation *terminal nerves*. All agree that the three major nerves of the arm—the median, radial, and ulnar—do so. In addition, some anatomists also include the axillary nerve, the musculocutaneous nerve, or both. Hence, depending upon the source, there are three to five terminal nerves. Along with the cords, these are located in the axilla and are components of the infraclavicular plexus.[100]

Brachial Plexus Injuries

The brachial plexus is one of the most vulnerable portions of the PNS. Because of this vulnerability, the majority of brachial plexopathies are traumatic in origin, and the incidence of brachial plexopathies is much higher than that of lumbosacral plexopathies. The proximity of the brachial plexus to the very mobile structures of the neck and shoulder make it particularly susceptible to traction. Moreover, its close association throughout much of its length with major blood vessels—which, like it, are responsible for supplying the upper extremity—places it at risk of being injured secondarily, by hematoma or pseudoaneurysm formation, following primary vascular trauma.[100]

All traumatic brachial plexopathies can be considered under one of two categories: closed and open. Closed lesions are by far the more common of the two, with traction being the principal etiology. These affect the supraclavicular more than the infraclavicular plexus, almost solely if there is no associated fracture or dislocation. Open lesions most often affect the infraclavicular plexus. With them, accompanying injuries to vital structures adjacent to the brachial plexus, especially the major limb vessels and the lung, frequently occur and are of more immediate concern.[4,44,72,98,100]

Brachial plexus injuries will now be discussed under two broad categories: supraclavicular and infraclavicular. These categories admittedly are somewhat artificial, not only because sometimes both the supraclavicular and infraclavicular plexus are injured simultaneously (e.g., some traction lesions; neoplasms; radiation), but also because the same type of lesion may involve the supraclavicular plexus on some occasions and the infraclavicular plexus on others (e.g., gunshot wounds, compression by hematomas). Regarding the latter, the discussion of a particular lesion will appear under the plexus subdivision that it most often affects. Thus, gunshot wounds, which can involve any portion of the brachial plexus, are reviewed under infraclavicular plexus lesions, because the majority of them injure the cords and peripheral nerves.[43]

Supraclavicular Plexus Lesions

High-Velocity Closed Injuries. These are the most common types of traumatic brachial plexopathies. The majority occur in men, and most are due to traction. The principal causes are roadway accidents, industrial mishaps, and falls. Any portion of the supraclavicular plexus can be involved, but the C5, C6 roots/upper trunk, that is, the upper plexus, fibers are the ones most frequently traumatized. Not only are they under slight tension at rest, but of the various supraclavicular fibers, they are injured initially and most severely by trauma in which there is abrupt widening of the angle between the neck and the shoulder, the most common mechanism for traction injury.[14,72,100] The plexus fibers that traverse the C8 and T1 roots and lower trunk, that is, the lower plexus fibers, also can be injured in isolation, although this happens far less often. In contrast, the C7 root/middle trunk fibers, or middle plexus fibers, are rarely injured alone; far more commonly, they are damaged in association with injuries of either the upper plexus, the lower plexus, or both. Traction can cause all grades of injury, ranging from demyelinating conduction block when mild to root avulsions and trunk ruptures when severe.[98,100]

Regarding demyelinating conduction block, few articles concerned with supraclavicular traction lesions specifically mention that it can be responsible for variable amounts of the initial clinical deficits; rather, this is acknowledged indirectly, with the recommendation that no decisions be reached regarding the severity of the lesion until repeat clinical examinations can be performed a month or two after onset, that is, until demyelinating conduction block has had time to resolve, if it is present. As would be expected, lesions having this underlying pathophysiology have an excellent prognosis.[98,100] Regarding traction-induced axon loss supraclavicular brachial plexopathies, in which the nerve fibers are still in continuity (i.e., second- to fourth-degree neurotmesis lesions), their prognosis is extremely variable, depending on several factors. These include (1) the specific brachial plexus elements damaged (upper trunk injuries recover much better than do lower trunk injuries, because the time distance factor is so much more favorable for them); (2) the amount of injury sustained by each plexus element (partial lesions, compared to total ones, are far more likely to show substantial recovery); and (3) the extensiveness of the lesion. (Kline and coworkers reported that, 3–4 months after injury, some spontaneous recovery was seen with 30% of lesions affecting the upper plexus alone, 12% involving both the upper and middle plexuses, and just 4% when pan trunk injuries were present[42,88,100]).

Whenever severe deficits persist in the distribution of one or more supraclavicular plexus elements, surgical exploration is indicated. The optimal time for these operations is 2–4 months after injury. Many surgeons refuse to operate (at least on adults) when the lesions are of more than 6 months' duration, because poor results are almost inevitable.

The surgical procedures performed are variable, ranging from neurolysis to resection of the damaged elements, with the placement of nerve grafts.[4,42,44,88]

Regarding root avulsions and extraforaminal ruptures, while any of the supraclavicular structures can sustain these injuries, the upper plexus has a predilection for extraforaminal ruptures, whereas the middle and lower plexuses more often sustain root avulsions. The reason for this, as previously noted, is that the C5 and C6 APRs are firmly anchored in the gutters of their transverse processes after they exit the intervertebral foramina, whereas the C7, C8, and T1 APRs are not.[69,100] Although some authorities report that the C8 and T1 roots most often sustain avulsion injuries,[14,85] in at least two articles concerned with motorcycle accidents, the C7 root most commonly was avulsed.[68,86]

As noted, a considerable majority of brachial plexus avulsion injuries result from roadway accidents, especially motorcycle accidents, and most occur in young men who can ill afford to be functionally one-armed.[3,68,86] Other causes include industrial accidents, birthing (i.e., obstetric paralysis), falls, objects falling onto the shoulder, and various sporting accidents, such as those that can occur with skiing.[100] The roots of the brachial plexus can be avulsed any time impact velocity exceeds 22 miles per hour. Impact velocities several times this amount often are achieved during head-on collisions involving two moving vehicles or even one moving vehicle and a stationary, unyielding object.[56] Simultaneous injuries of other portions of the body—head, thorax, abdomen, spine—are common; associated limb fractures are particularly frequent.[4,44,56,100]

Brachial plexus root avulsions can be difficult to distinguish from severe axon loss trunk lesions initially (see Fig. 18.1). However, a number of features do tend to set them apart from one another (Table 18.1). Moreover, they have a dismal prognosis because they do not recover spontaneously and they cannot be surgically repaired. Although they produce sensory loss and, if the T1 root is affected, a Horner syndrome, their most disabling effects are loss of motor function and pain. Both of these become more prominent as the number of avulsed roots increases.[7] On EDX examination,

Table 18.1. Findings Suggestive of Preganglionic (Root Avulsion Injuries)

Historical
Violent, high-velocity trauma
Flail, anesthetic upper limb
Early severe burning pain in hand
Physical Examination
Paralysis of serratus anterior, rhomboids, and spinati
Horner syndrome
Sensory loss supraclavicularly (cervical plexus distribution)
No Tinel's sign supraclavicularly
Coexisting spinal cord injury
Electrodiagnostic Examination
Unelicitable CMAPs with normal SNAPs
F-waves unelicitable
Paraspinal fibrillation potentials
Negative SEP (N9 to contralateral cortex)
Neuroimaging Studies
Fracture of transverse processes
Traumatic meningoceles
Root pouch obliterations
Roots absent in intraspinal canal

CMAP, compound muscle action potential; SEP, somatosensory evoked potentials; SNAP, sensory nerve action potential.

the sensory NCS responses are spared (unless ganglionic or extraforaminal lesions coexist along the same fibers), because the peripheral sensory fibers are still in continuity with their cell bodies in the DRG. Also, on needle EMG, fibrillation potentials may be detected in the cervical and high thoracic paraspinal muscles as well as in limb muscles. On neuroimaging studies, various associated injuries to bone, if present, may be seen on routine x-rays, while myelography, CT myelography, MRI, and MR myelography of the cervical roots usually reveal the lesions.[4,44,100]

Both the motor deficits and the sensory symptoms resulting from these plexopathies typically are difficult to manage. When only some of the motor roots are avulsed, various orthopedic procedures, such as shoulder arthrodesis and tendon transfers, may restore some motor function. However, when all or most of the roots are avulsed, producing a flail, anesthetic, and often painful limb, few options remain. In an attempt to partially restore at least one proximal limb function, usually elbow flexion, *neurotization* procedures may be performed. With this technique, intact nerve fibers, usually components of extraplexal nerves, are sectioned, and their proximal stumps are attached to plexus elements that have been separated from the spinal cord by avulsion.[100] Intercostal nerves, the phrenic nerve, the spinal accessory nerve, and even the contralateral C7 root have served as donor nerves.[57] Severe pain is also a frequent symptom of root avulsion. Root avulsion pain is distinct from all other types of persistent severe pain, including causalgia. Its characteristic presentation is a constant, intense burning or crushing background pain, upon which paroxysmal shock-like pains of very brief duration but extremely severe intensity are superimposed at infrequent and unpredictable intervals. The likelihood of avulsion pain being present increases with the number of roots avulsed, and when it is present for more than 3 years after injury, it usually persists indefinitely. This pain has proved resistant to almost all medical regimens and most surgical therapies, with the exception of coagulation of the dorsal root entry zones of the avulsed roots (DREZ procedure; Nashold's procedure).[7,87,100,104]

Regardless of their severity, most traumatic supraclavicular brachial plexopathies (excluding those sustained by infants at delivery, i.e., obstetric paralysis) occur in adults. On occasion, however, children also sustain such lesions. One report concerned 25 children, average age 6.2 years, all with closed traction injuries. Most were due to roadway accidents; usually the child had been a pedestrian struck by a vehicle. More than half of the children had pan-trunk lesions, while most of the remainder had upper plexus or upper and middle plexus involvement. Almost two-thirds of them had root avulsions.[19]

Although the majority of traumatic supraclavicular plexopathies are due to high-velocity trauma, a distinct minority have other specific causes. Some of these will now be reviewed.

Obstetric Paralysis (Congenital Brachial Plexus Palsy). These supraclavicular plexopathies are typically classified as iatrogenic, although this designation at times is debatable, not only because recent evidence suggests that in some cases they begin in utero, and that maternal propulsive forces may be at fault, but also because they can occur when medical personnel are not in attendance.[39,71] Obstetric paralysis affects male and female infants about equally and is usually unilateral. It tends to involve the right upper limb more than the left. Predisposing factors include breech births; large (increased birth weight) babies; multiparous, diabetic, heavy mothers; shoulder dystocia (i.e., difficulty in delivering the shoulder, after delivering the head, because of impaction of the anterior shoulder on the mother's pubic symphysis), and prolonged, difficult labor, often requiring forceps deliveries. In the majority of cases, the upper plexus fibers are affected, either alone or with middle plexus involvement. Diffuse supraclavicular pan-plexus lesions are less common, while isolated involvement of the lower plexus is rare. The underlying pathophysiology ranges from demyelinating conduction block to root avulsion, with intermediate grades of axon loss being most common. Demyelinating conduction block most commonly occurs with upper plexus lesions, whereas root avulsions usually are associated with lower plexus or pan-plexus lesions.[29,30,100]

How often obstetric paralysis recovers satisfactorily is debated. Nonetheless, because upper plexus fibers are most often involved, and because demyelinating conduction block is the frequent predominant underlying pathophysiology, initial conservative treatment is almost universally recommended. The minority (approximately 25%) of infants with these lesions who show no recovery after

3 months, particularly when one or more plexus elements are totally affected due to either lesions in continuity, ruptures, or avulsions, should undergo surgical exploration, with repair of the injured elements if necessary (or possible). Such surgery appreciably helps about 50% of patients. Operative treatment of obstetric paralysis, after experiencing a brief period of popularity around the turn of the twentieth century, fell into disfavor. Only relatively recently has it been rediscovered, primarily because of the pioneering work of Gilbert.[29,30,33,78]

Classic Postoperative Paralysis. This was the first reported type of postoperative brachial plexopathy. The term *postoperative* is a misnomer: the lesion develops during the operation and is recognized after it. Classic postoperative paralysis was described by Budinger in 1894 and was initially thought to result from some *toxic* property of the general anesthetic used. Soon it was appreciated, however, that it is due to malpositioning of the patient during the operation. The primary injury, traction or compression, is debated, although traction appears to be more likely. Patients under general anesthesia are particularly susceptible to malpositioning injuries, not only because their muscle tone has been reduced by the anesthesia (or abolished if muscle relaxants were added), but also because they have been rendered insensible to limb placements that would not be tolerated, due to pain, if they were conscious. Almost every patient position has been linked to this type of brachial plexopathy, although the majority of patients have been supine and often one or more of the following has occurred: (1) one or both arms have been abducted 90°or more; (2) the head has been rotated and laterally flexed to the opposite side; (3) the arm has been restrained on a board in abduction, extension, and external rotation; or (4) a steep Trendelenburg position has been used.

Classic postoperative paralysis presents in a rather stereotyped fashion. An operation is performed under general anesthesia on a body structure, most often one that is at a distance from the brachial plexus, such as the gallbladder, colon, uterus, or bladder, but sometimes on the ipsilateral shoulder. When the patient regains consciousness, one or occasionally both upper extremities are weak. The particular plexus element involved varies, but the two most common presentations by far are either upper plexus alone or initial total plexus involvement, with rapid resolution of the middle and lower plexus symptoms, leaving upper plexus symptoms. Paresthesias, primarily in an upper plexus distribution, sometimes are present, but pain is distinctly rare.[15,41,46,47,100] The lesions appear to be located along the distal upper trunk fibers because, in the relatively few EDX reports on such patients, conduction blocks characteristically have been demonstrated on supraclavicular (midtrunk) stimulation while recording from the biceps and deltoid.[54,89] Recovery usually begins promptly, often within a few days of onset, and is frequently complete after just a few weeks. Nonetheless, a few reports have described some persistence of symptoms for almost a year.[15,89,100]

Unfortunately, most surgeons appear to be aware of only this type of postoperative brachial plexopathy. As a result, when they have produced other types they often reassure their patients, without justification, that the symptoms will resolve rapidly and completely; all too often, they do neither, and malpractice suits follow.

Post-Median Sternotomy Brachial Plexopathy. This type of brachial plexopathy has some features in common with classic postoperative paralysis, in that it is an indirect supraclavicular plexus lesion sustained during surgery, and traction is the most likely mechanism of injury. However, it is caused by one particular surgical procedure, median sternotomy, and it characteristically involves the lower plexus fibers rather than the upper ones.

Coronary artery bypass surgery has become a very popular operation since it was first introduced in 1968. Access to the heart usually is gained by the median sternotomy approach, whereby the sternum is split lengthwise and both halves are then retracted laterally. A small minority of patients develop brachial plexopathies, nearly all unilateral, during the procedure.[100] The incidence is 10-fold higher when internal mammary artery grafts are used.[93] The etiology of these plexopathies has not been firmly established, but based on the clinical and EDX findings, it is probable that they are caused by the sternal retraction. The immediate cause probably is the very proximal portion of the first thoracic rib moving superiorly, following either a fracture or subluxation of that bony structure to impact on the C8 APR[49] (Fig. 18.4). The severity

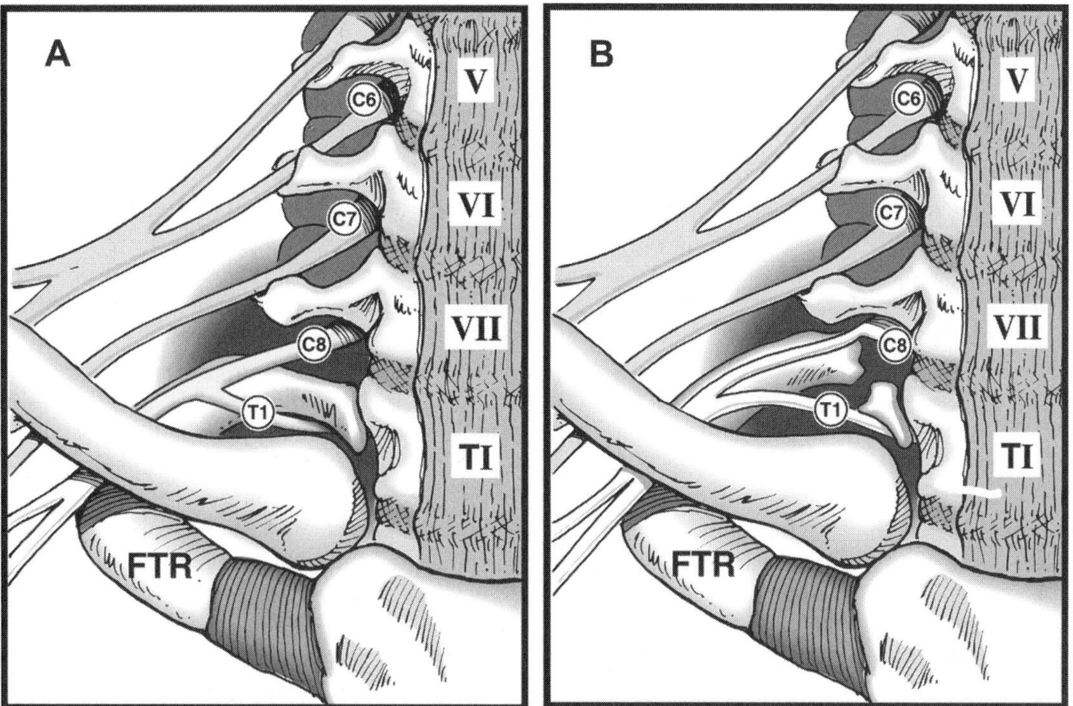

Figure 18.4. The presumed etiology of postmedian sternotomy brachial plexopathy. Illustrated is the lower cervical region (anterior views). A = Normal, B = C8 anterior primary ramus injured inferiorly by the proximal portion of the first thoracic rib. FTR, first thoracic rib. (Copyright Cleveland Clinic Foundation, used with permission)

of the lesion varies significantly from one patient to another. Some patients experience only transient paresthesias in a lower trunk distribution. Others, however, have substantial symptoms, consisting of hand weakness and paresthesias along the medial hand. Pain sometimes is present in the same distribution, occasionally prominent. Typically, the ulnar nerve fibers traversing the lower plexus are involved more than the median nerve fibers, because the ulnar fibers derive principally from the C8 APR, rather than from the T1 APR, as the median fibers do. The radial nerve fibers that derive from the C8 APR are also affected. Nonetheless, these lesions are often mistaken, on both cursory clinical and EDX examinations, for postoperative ulnar neuropathy at the elbow. Unnecessary and unhelpful ulnar nerve operations sometimes are performed on these patients for this reason. The pathophysiology usually consists of a mixture of demyelinating conduction block (neurapraxia) and axon loss, often with the former predominating. The lesion is quite proximal, however, because a conduction block cannot be demonstrated in the EDX laboratory on supraclavicular (midtrunk level) stimulation. Consequently, it must be affecting the proximal lower trunk or the C8 APR.[98,100] Noteworthy is that these lesions are high supraclavicular in location and not infraclavicular (i.e., involving the medial cord), as reported in one article.[35] As noted, for several reasons we believe that the lesion actually involves predominantly, if not solely, the C8 APR and thus is, in a sense, a *pre-lower trunk* disorder.

In contrast to the EDX examination, neuroimaging studies typically are normal with this entity (abnormalities of the very proximal portion of the first thoracic rib are difficult to visualize).

The appropriate management of these lesions, with very few exceptions, is conservative (i.e., nonoperative) treatment. A few surgeons have performed transaxillary first rib resections on these patients to treat them, reasoning that their symptoms are attributable to a type of thoracic outlet syndrome.[52] This therapeutic approach seems particularly ill-advised for at least three reasons: (1) the lesion is due to traction, not compression;

(2) demyelinating conduction block often is the predominant pathophysiology; and (3) the lesion characteristically is partial rather than complete. Consequently, not only is the stress of this additional surgical procedure itself likely to delay the patient's recovery from heart surgery, but the only brachial plexus alteration possible with the operation is an undesired one: an additional lower trunk surgical injury superimposed (see "Post-Disputed Thoracic Outlet Syndrome Surgery Plexopathy," below).[16,79,93,100]

Burner Syndrome (Stinger Syndrome). This is a well-defined clinical syndrome experienced by athletes who engage in contact sports, particularly football players and wrestlers. All authorities agree that the burner syndrome is a manifestation of an upper plexus traction injury. However, there is some disagreement regarding the exact site of the lesion, with the upper trunk favored by the majority and the C6 root by a distinct minority.[98,100]

The clinical presentation is characteristic. After the athlete has his shoulder abruptly, forcibly depressed, with or without his neck being forced to the contralateral side (such as can occur when one football player tackles another), he suddenly experiences a burning dysesthesia throughout his entire ipsilateral upper extremity. When it is severe, the arm hangs limply at the side. The episode is transient, typically lasting for a few minutes or less; several can occur during a single sporting event. Usually, the athletes are asymptomatic between attacks, and neurological examinations during these periods are unrevealing. However, a minority of athletes, most often those with recurrent severe episodes, develop persistent weakness, often just subjective, in an upper trunk distribution. Electrodiagnostic studies of these patients usually show modest active denervation in the deltoid, biceps, brachioradialis, pronator teres, and occasionally the spinati muscles. Neuroimaging studies are unrevealing. A number of preventative measures have been recommended, including neck and shoulder strengthening exercises and the use of neck pads and rolls, as well as high shoulder pads. The relatively few athletes whose recurrent burners cause demonstrable objective weakness typically have their participation in contact sports restricted.[34,65,100]

Pack Palsy (Rucksack Paralysis). Occasionally persons using backpacks or their equivalent (e.g., child or book carriers) develop upper extremity PNS disorders, presumably from pressure caused by the shoulder straps of the pack. Parents of young children, students, scouts, campers, hikers, and especially military personnel are at risk. Several factors favor the development of pack palsies, including heavy weights being carried, long periods of use, considerable distances being traversed, especially over irregular terrain (which requires much upper limb movement at the shoulder to achieve stability), and nonuse of pack frames or waist belts. The latter shift much of the weight of the pack to the hips, thereby reducing the pressure of the shoulder straps. The presence of bony anomalities about the shoulder, especially remote clavicular fractures with resulting deformities, also plays a role.

Clinically, pack palsies most often present as unilateral lesions (although some have been not only bilateral, but also symmetrical), involving either the dominant or non-dominant upper limb and shoulder region. They manifest as weakness, sometimes with atrophy, paresthesias and sensory loss, but seldom pain. The specific symptoms and signs present depend on the particular PNS structure(s) affected. Most often this is predominantly the upper trunk of the brachial plexus, but more extensive plexus lesions have occurred, as well as mononeuropathies, including spinal accessory, long thoracic and dorsal scapular neuropathies. The underlying pathophysiology with the majority of pack palsies is demyelinating conduction block (neurapraxia). However, in many other instances, conduction failure caused by axon loss is the predominant or sole pathophysiology. Thus, the recovery time can be quite variable; moreover, some patients with axon loss lesions have permanent disabilities. Neuroimaging studies are typically unhelpful with pack palsies (unless a bony lesion is present). In contrast, EDX examinations can establish their underlying pathophysiology, and identify the exact PNS structures affected. No specific treatment is available, except refraining from pack use; this is particularly important if the person has already experienced one or more transient episodes of symptoms.

Pack palsy has a tenuous relationship to two other entities: traumatic TOS and neuralgic amyotrophy. With traumatic TOS, most often related to a fractured clavicle, the PNS symptoms typically develop spontaneously, either immediately after the injury or some time later, frequently after a large clavicular callus has developed; characteristically these are in the distribution of one or more cords of the brachial plexus. Patients with neuralgic amyotrophy, in contrast to those with pack palsy, generally have severe pain, usually over the lateral shoulder, as their initial symptom; most often this appears abruptly, awakening them from sleep. The PNS structures characteristically involved are one or more peripheral nerves supplying proximal muscles, similar to those often affected with pack palsy; however, frequently this includes some nerves, such as the axillary and anterior interosseous, which are not compromised by pack palsy.[98,100]

TRAUMATIC THORACIC OUTLET SYNDROME. The term *traumatic* (or *posttraumatic*) *thoracic outlet syndrome* (TOS) is used in two separate contexts. First, the relatively rare patient who develops a brachial plexopathy, either immediate or delayed, secondary to a primary injury of the clavicle—most often a midshaft fracture—is described as having a traumatic TOS (discussed under infraclavicular lesions below). The term (or a similar one, such as *trauma-related TOS*) also is used to denote a highly controversial syndrome that some physicians believe commonly is triggered by relatively minor accidents, particularly roadway accidents and repetitive work. Characteristically, the clavicle, as well as all other bony structures about the shoulder, remain intact with this type of traumatic TOS, which customarily is identified by a more generic term, such as *disputed neurogenic TOS* or *nonspecific neurogenic TOS*.[20,92,100] To prevent confusion, the discussion of disputed neurogenic TOS must be preceded by a brief review of the general topic of TOS.

Under the title TOS are included a number of distinct entities, all of which are attributed to compromise of blood vessels, the brachial plexus, or both at some point between the base of the neck and the axilla. The term *thoracic outlet syndrome* was popularized in 1956 as an umbrella designation for a number of syndromes then in vogue (Table 18.2). Typically, these were based on, and named for, various structures that reputedly compressed one or more of the neurovascular elements in the thoracic outlet (brachial plexus; subclavian/axillary artery; subclavian axillary vein). Many of the original subdivisions have little current clinical relevance because they have been modified or abandoned with the passing of time. Consequently, another classification more recently has been adopted, based on the presumed structure affected[16,103] (Table 18.3). This seems appropriate since seldom is more than one structure (plexus, artery, vein) involved in any particular patient. The arterial, venous, and true neurogenic types of TOS are universally acknowledged, well-defined disorders. All are rare, and none is caused by trauma per se, although the venous type often follows excessive arm use. The arterial and true neurogenic types are due to a congenital anomaly: a large cervical rib and a rudimentary cervical rib (or an elongated C7 transverse process) with a taut band extending from its tip to the first thoracic rib, respectively. The disputed type of neurogenic TOS (disputed N-TOS) essentially lacks the objective findings (clinical, radiographic, and EDX) of true N-TOS; this is why it is such a controversial entity. Nonetheless, many physicians believe that it is a common disorder, caused by compression of various elements of the brachial plexus in the thoracic outlet. A variety of pathophysiological mechanisms have been proposed by its proponents to explain this compression. They can be grouped under three

Table 18.2. Thoracic Outlet Syndrome: Original Classification

Cervical rib syndrome
First thoracic rib syndrome
Scalenus anticus syndrome
Subcoracoid-pectoralis minor syndrome
Costoclavicular syndrome

Table 18.3. Thoracic Outlet Syndrome: Current Classification

Vascular
Arterial
Venous
Neurologic
True (classic)
Disputed (symptomatic, nonspecific)
Neurovascular
Traumatic

headings: (1) posttraumatic, (2) congenital anomalies, and (3) postural factors.[16,92,100] Many proponents believe that two or even all three of these frequently coexist. When disputed N-TOS first evolved from the discredited scalenus anticus syndrome in the 1960s, it was attributed to trauma in only a minority of instances. With each passing decade, however, a progressively increasing percentage of cases were considered posttraumatic. Currently, a sizable majority are included in this category by many proponents. The initiating trauma generally is of two main types: (1) a single event, such as a whiplash injury sustained in an automobile accident or fall or (2) repetitive work, such as is performed by assembly line workers, keyboard operators, and some musicians.[20,48,100] In one published series, single-event trauma, particularly related to automobile accidents, was responsible for 80% of all posttraumatic N-TOS.[20] Among the congenital anomalies considered responsible for disputed N-TOS, a number of fibromuscular bands in the thoracic outlet region have been implicated.[67,92] "There are no standard diagnostic criteria" for disputed N-TOS. Instead, diagnosis usually is based on what the physician considers to be "suggestive symptomatology," one or more confirming procedures, and the exclusion of other disorders.[92] A multitude of symptom complexes have been ascribed to disputed N-TOS by its various proponents; most have included pain in one or more forequarter regions, particularly in a lower trunk distribution. Many different procedures are used to confirm the diagnosis, depending upon the personal preference of each proponent. A variety of laboratory tests, including several different neuroimaging and EDX studies, have been employed for this purpose. However, probably the most popular are certain physical examination procedures, particularly those that seek symptom reproduction with plexus palpation or exercise tests (such as the elevated arm stress test of Roos), and those that detect radial pulse alterations with various shoulder girdle manipulations.[92,100,103] All proponents agree that once a diagnosis is made, conservative treatment should be tried initially. Nonetheless, many patients undergo surgery (far too many, in the opinion of the skeptics). A number of surgical procedures are performed to treat disputed N-TOS. Transaxillary first rib resection was almost the sole operation used for almost 20 years. Currently, however, anterior and middle scalenectomies often are done; frequently, they are combined with transaxillary first rib resection. The reported results of surgery, similar to all other aspects of disputed N-TOS, are quite controversial. Some surgeons, typically evaluating their own work after short periods of observation, have reported very high success rates. Others surgeons, however, have found that surgery did not help even the majority of operated patients, particularly when long-term follow-up was done.[50] A retrospective survey of workmen's compensation cases focusing on workers operated on in one state, covering a 6-year period, reported "dismal" results when the judgment was based on the very reliable criterion of whether the patient had or had not been able to return to work.[23] One of the many reasons so many physicians have serious reservations about disputed N-TOS, particularly its surgical treatment, is that the most common major complication of these operations is an intraoperative brachial plexus injury (discussed below). In contrast to the situation with disputed N-TOS, no physician contends that these latter lesions do not exist.

Post-Disputed Thoracic Outlet Syndrome Surgery Brachial Plexopathy. Some patients who undergo surgery for disputed N-TOS sustain intraoperative brachial plexopathies. Most of these lesions have been associated with transaxillary first rib resection, which is also the most common type of surgery performed. The typical patient awakens from anesthesia with ipsilateral paresis, paresthesias, and often pain involving either the entire upper extremity (pan-trunk involvement) or principally the hand (lower trunk distribution). Within a week or so, the upper trunk and middle trunk symptoms in those patients with initial pan-trunk involvement regress (suggesting that their underlying pathophysiology was demyelinating conduction block), leaving essentially an axon loss, lower trunk lesion. Also, during the first week or two after operation, pain characteristically develops in a lower trunk distribution in those patients in whom it was initially absent. Electrodiagnostic studies confirm the presence of a rather severe axon loss, lower trunk brachial plexopathy. Neuroimaging studies usually are normal. This open type of brachial plexus lesion most often is due to traction-contusion injury of the lower trunk or lower trunk to medial cord fibers; less often, it results from transection of these elements. Permanent residuals are common. Some patients, particularly those with severe, persistent pain, benefit from surgical repair or neurolysis.[44,98,100]

Little detailed information is available regarding the brachial plexopathies that are sustained during scalenectomies. In our limited experience with such injuries, they more often involve the upper plexus, or upper and middle plexus, rather than the lower plexus, in contrast to the characteristic lower plexus presentations that result from transaxillary first rib resections. Nonetheless, they are axon loss in type and are usually severe.

MISCELLANEOUS SUPRACLAVICULAR PLEXUS DISORDERS. In addition to the above, several other etiologies for primarily supraclavicular traumatic plexopathies have been mentioned in one or a few reports. Most have been closed lesions and have involved the upper plexus. These include lesions caused by (1) prolonged firing of shotguns and rifles (with the butt of the weapon recoiling against the clavicle); (2) the weight of a coffin suddenly shifting onto the shoulder of a pallbearer; (3) prolonged pressure sustained during alcohol or drug-induced coma; (4) traumatic asphyxia produced by crowd-crush disasters; (5) cadets assuming military brace positions for excessive time periods; (6) the wearing of body armor by soldiers; and (7) vest restraints on patients and seat belts on automobile passengers. Finally, a few patients have developed brachial plexopathies due to electrical injuries.[100] One report concerned an adolescent who, following an accidental electrical shock (100 volts AC) to the fifth finger of one hand, developed progressive weakness and anesthesia of his ipsilateral upper extremity over a period of a few hours, which was attributed to a total brachial plexopathy. The majority of the symptoms regressed by 1 week and almost all by 3 months,[84] suggesting that conduction block was the underlying pathophysiology.

Open injuries of the supraclavicular plexus have been caused by gunshots, knives, chainsaws, dog bites, and glass, among other etiologies. (These are discussed below.) An iatrogenic etiology for open injuries are biopsies performed on masses at the base of the neck, which subsequently are shown to be benign primary tumors, often involving the upper trunk elements.[100]

Infraclavicular Plexus Lesions

Brachial Plexopathies Caused By Orthopedic Injuries and Treatments

Brachial plexus lesions, usually of the closed traction variety, can occur with or follow various musculoskeletal injuries about the shoulder region. Typically, the infraclavicular plexus elements are affected. The most common of these are the traction injuries sustained with scapular and proximal humeral fractures and with humeral head dislocations. Most are due to falls, vehicular accidents, or direct blunt trauma to the shoulder. The reported incidence of brachial plexus involvement complicating these injuries varies. Several reports suggest that traumatic brachial plexopathies occur with approximately one-third or more of both humeral neck fractures and humeral head dislocations. Age plays an important role: older patients are two to three times more likely to sustain plexus injuries than are younger patients. The axillary terminal nerve is the plexus element most often injured, with posterior cord lesions and diffuse infraclavicular plexopathies being less common. Nonetheless, almost any terminal nerve, cord element, or combination of both can be damaged. Both neuroimaging and EDX studies are helpful in making the diagnosis.[5,6,59,94] With axillary nerve involvement, two very distinct types of pathophysiology are noted: in about 80% of patients, demyelinating conduction block (neurapraxia) is the principal pathophysiology, and recovery is not only fairly rapid but invariably complete. In contrast, in the remaining 20%, axon loss is present. At times this is caused by a lesion in continuity; recovery may occur spontaneously, albeit slowly, and may often be incomplete. At other times, however, the axillary nerve has been ruptured and no recovery occurs unless the nerve is surgically repaired. The infraclavicular plexus elements can also be injured secondarily by shoulder fractures and dislocations, resulting from an expanding hematoma produced by a tear in the axillary artery or one of its branches. Secondary brachial plexus lesions can also occur with humeral head dislocations when attempts are made to reduce the latter. Usually the infraclavicular plexus elements are traumatized during these procedures. However, before motorized vehicles became the standard means of transportation, and the main cause of root avulsions, one of the etiologies for such severe supraclavicular plexus injuries was forced reduction of humeral head dislocations —for example, having several persons simultaneously pull on the upper extremity while the trunk was restrained. Infraclavicular plexopathies can also be caused by the use of crutches, either through direct pressure or by their producing axillary hematomas in anticoagulated patients.[100]

Brachial plexus injuries have occurred, almost solely in adults, as a result of clavicular fractures. These nerve injuries can be produced at the time of the fracture, either directly (due to traction or compression) or indirectly (as the result of hematoma or pseudoaneurysm formation with secondary compression.) Their appearance may also be delayed. Typically, they are due to the patient's midshaft clavicular fracture being treated with inadequate external fixation, most often a figure-of-eight bandage. Because of nonunion and excess callus formation, aneurysm development, or motion of fragments at the fracture site, the costoclavicular space is narrowed and the plexus is damaged. All of these lesions have been designated *traumatic TOS*.[11,16,17,100]

Several different diagnostic and therapeutic orthopedic procedures are performed about the shoulder girdle region, and the brachial plexus can sustain open injury during many of them. Characteristically, the infraclavicular plexus elements are involved. The suprascapular and axillary nerves have been injured during shoulder joint replacement, and various terminal nerves have been traumatized during shoulder arthroscopy. In one study, more than 8% of patients who had surgery for anterior shoulder dislocations had some type of neurological deficit postoperatively. Even though the suprascapular nerve arises from the supraclavicular plexus, it often is injured by disorders that generally affect only infraclavicular elements—such as shoulder dislocations—because it is anchored at the supraclavicular notch and thereby is vulnerable to traction forces.[14] Some of the operations performed to treat chronic, recurrent anterior shoulder dislocations, especially the Putti-Platt and Bristrow procedures, have resulted in extensive damage to various infraclavicular plexus elements, particularly the musculocutaneous terminal nerve. Moreover, a few patients experienced delayed brachial plexopathies, which first appeared years after they had Bristrow procedures, when the bone screw holding the coracoid process to the glenoid rim came loose, penetrated the axillary artery, and produced a pseudoaneurysm. Finally, brachial plexus injuries can occur when the interval between the clavicle and first rib is reduced due to surgical causes, such as removal of the midportion of the clavicle with subsequent regeneration and the correction of Sprengel's deformity.[100]

Gunshot Wounds

The majority of gunshot wounds principally affect infraclavicular plexus elements. In Kline's series of 141 patients (85% male), the infraclavicular or retroclavicular plexus was involved 77% of the time, and the supraclavicular plexus was injured in 23%.[43] The amount of damage the brachial plexus sustains from a gunshot wound depends on a number of factors, including the velocity of the projectile, whether it is cased or uncased, its particular track through the plexus, and whether it injures the plexus primarily or secondarily after ricocheting off bone or other structures. High-velocity projectiles produce more extensive damage by causing the formation of transient, large cavities, via pressure waves, in the tissues they traverse. Gunshot wounds can produce any grade of damage to plexus elements, ranging from neurapraxia to fifth-degree neurotmesis injuries.[100] Intuitively, it would seem that the latter, that is, nerve ruptures, would predominate. In fact, however, gunshot wounds characteristically do not interrupt plexus fibers. In Kline's series of 90 patients who underwent surgical exploration, only 14 of the 221 total elements assessed (6%) were interrupted, and those were limited to 6 of the 90 patients (6.6%) explored. Although most injured elements were still in continuity, the majority of them had sustained fourth-degree neurotmesis lesions; consequently, more than half required surgical repair.[43] Although gunshot wounds usually cause immediate onset of symptoms, occasionally the latter are delayed for up to several hours. In these instances, almost always the plexus has been compromised secondarily because of initial blood vessel damage, with subsequent hematoma or pseudoaneurysm formation.[100]

Laceration Injuries

These plexus lesions can be divided into *sharp* and *blunt* injuries. Sharp lacerating injuries are principally due to knives and glass. They are more common than blunt lacerating injuries, which have various causes, including dog bites, moving mechanical objects, and chainsaws. Lacerations of the subclavian or axillary blood vessels frequently coexist with plexus lesions in this category. In these situations, limb salvage is of paramount importance, with vascular repair taking priority over plexus repair even when the plexus elements have sustained sharp lacerating injuries and could conceivably be repaired primarily. Although the plexus elements may escape initial injury with penetrating lesions of the infra- or supraclavicular regions, they can be damaged secondarily by the formation of hematomas or pseudoaneurysms if the adjacent blood vessels were injured. In contrast to gunshot wound injuries, in which only 6% of the injured plexus element are interrupted, with laceration injuries 66% of the injured plexus elements sustain fifth-degree neurotmesis lesions. Nonetheless, a sizable minority (34%) do not, although it would appear that all should.[4,44,45,100]

Injection Injuries

A specific type of open injury the brachial plexus sustains results from injections, or attempted injections, of various substances near it (e.g., regional anesthetics) or into the blood vessels contiguous with it (e.g., contrast material). Most often the infraclavicular elements are damaged.

The medial brachial fascial compartment, which extends along the medial side of the upper limb from the axilla to the elbow, contains the neurovascular bundle. A *medial brachial fascial compartment syndrome* results when the axillary artery is damaged and a hematoma develops, which compromises one or more terminal nerves; almost always this includes the medial terminal nerve and often is limited to it. Typically, this syndrome is caused by a penetrating injury. The two major noniatrogenic causes are gunshot wounds and stab wounds (discussed above), whereas the two principal iatrogenic causes are axillary arteriograms and axillary regional blocks. With the latter group, leakage of blood at the arterial puncture site may be so slow that symptoms are markedly delayed in onset. Thus, the time that can elapse between the injection of contrast material or an anesthetic agent and the first appearance of symptoms is extremely variable, ranging from almost immediately to nearly 3 weeks. The initial symptom characteristically is pain, usually in a median nerve distribution in the hand, which becomes progressively severe. As with all compartment syndromes, prompt recognition and surgical decompression are mandatory if permanent residuals are to be prevented. Those patients who are treated conservatively, or who are operated on weeks to months after onset, generally experience no appreciable improvement and, consequently, are left with substantial permanent residuals, particularly involving the hand.[90,91]

Axon loss brachial plexopathies, usually manifesting severe pain, have also resulted when alcohol inadvertently has been substituted for the local anesthetic agent during attempted axillary regional blocks and when cisplatin has been injected in the axillary artery to treat cancer of the humerus.[100]

There are a few descriptions of brachial plexopathies resulting from percutaneous cannulation of the subclavian and internal jugular veins. Both the supra- and infraclavicular plexus elements have been injured during these procedures, probably due either to instrumentation or to bleeding with hematoma formation.[100]

Miscellaneous Non-orthopedic Surgical Procedures

The brachial plexus, most often its infraclavicular elements, occasionally is injured during various surgical procedures, including radical mastectomies; upper thoracic sympathectomies (to treat palmar hyperhidrosis); creation of transaxillary bypasses to treat limb ischemia; formation of axillary arteriovenous fistulas for renal dialysis; and during biopsies, both of unknown masses that prove to be normal plexus elements and of brachial plexus tumors (which are usually benign).[100]

Lumbosacral Plexus

The lumbar plexus and the sacral plexus are separate structures linked by the lumbosacral trunk. They essentially originate from different roots, have different anatomical relationships, and innervate different, although sometimes adjacent, structures. Moreover, concomitant lesions of both are relatively uncommon.[80] Nonetheless, they most often are viewed as a single PNS structure, the *lumbosacral plexus*, or *pelvic plexus*,[44] and disorders of them, even when only one is involved, usually are discussed as *lumbosacral plexopathies*. For these reasons, in this chapter this format will be followed.

Anatomy

The lumbar plexus is the more superior component of the lumbosacral plexus (Fig. 18.5). It is formed from the APRs of L1, L2, L3, and a portion of L4. (The remaining portion of L4 joins with the L5 root to form the lumbosacral trunk, which passes inferiorly and joins the sacral plexus.) Sometimes the T12 APR also contributes to the lumbar plexus. Compared to that of the brachial plexus, the configuration of the lumbar plexus is much simpler, consisting only of APRs, branches (upper and lower), divisions (anterior and posterior), and terminal nerves. The innervation of the psoas and the quadratus lumborum muscles arises from the L1 through L4 APRs. The L1, L2, and L4 APRs then divide into upper and lower branches. The upper branch of L1, joined by the T1 contribution when it is present, terminates as the iliohypogastric and ilioinguinal nerves. The lower branch of the L1 APR and the upper branch of the L2 APR join to form the genitofemoral nerve. The lower branch of the L4 APR joins with the L5 APR to form the lumbosacral trunk. The lower branch of L2, the entire L3 APR, and the upper branch of L4 each divide into anterior and posterior divisions. The three anterior divisions then fuse to form the obturator nerve, whereas the L2 and L3 posterior divisions first give off branches that unite to create the lateral femoral cutaneous nerve and then join with the L4 posterior division to form the femoral nerve. The L1 and L2 APRs give off white rami communicants to the chain of sympathetic ganglia, while the L1 through L5 APRs receive gray rami communicants from the sympathetic chain. The lumbar plexus is formed and contained within the substance of the psoas major muscle.[12,13]

The sacral plexus is the more inferior component of the lumbosacral plexus (Fig. 18.6). It is formed from the L5, S1, S2, and S3 APRs, as well as the lower branch of the L4 APR and a portion of the S4 APR. Similar to the lumbar plexus, its composition is rather simple, consisting of APRs, divisions (anterior and posterior), and terminal nerves. No branches arise at the APR level. Each APR divides into an anterior and a posterior division. The S1, S2, and S3 anterior divisions and the S1 and S2 posterior divisions contribute fibers to form the posterior femoral cutaneous nerve. Fibers from the S2, S3, and S4 anterior divisions fuse to form the pudendal nerve. Fibers from the L4, L5, and S1 posterior divisions join to form the superior gluteal nerve, while other fibers from the L5, S1, and S2 posterior divisions combine to form the inferior gluteal nerve. A small branch also arises from the posterior division of S1 or S2 (or both) to innervate the piriformis muscle. The remaining fibers (L4, L5, S1, and S2) composing the anterior divisions then merge to form the tibial nerve, whereas those of the posterior divisions (L4, L5, S1, and S2) converge to make up the common peroneal nerve. The APRs of S2–S4 supply parasympathetic fibers

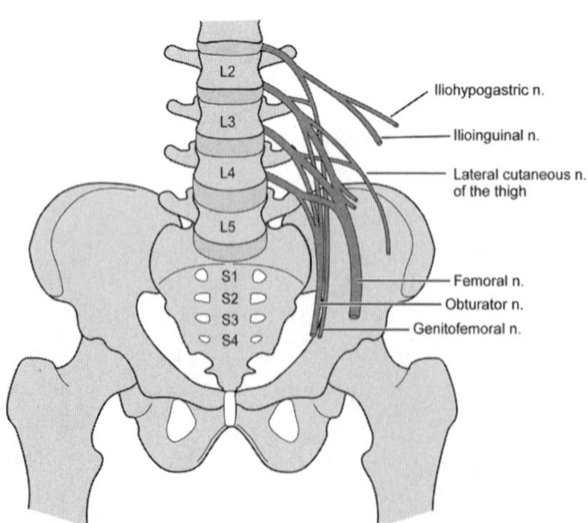

Figure 18.5. The lumbar plexus: left side, anterior view. (Copyright Cleveland Clinic Foundation, used with permission)

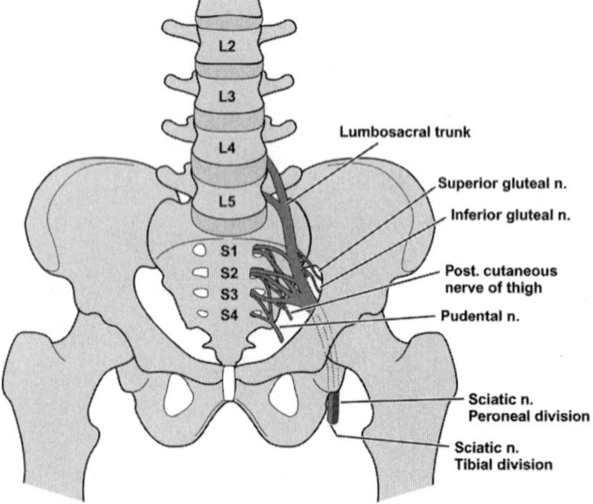

Figure 18.6. The sacral plexus: left side, anterior view. (Copyright Cleveland Clinic Foundation, used with permission)

to the urinary, bladder, and anal sphincters, while all of the APRs contributing to the sacral plexus receive postganglionic sympathetic fibers. The sacral plexus rests against the posterior and lateral walls of the true pelvis, between the piriformis muscle laterally and the internal iliac blood vessels medially.[12,13] Noteworthy is that only the superior portion of the sacral plexus (i.e., that derived from the L4, L5, and S1 roots) can be adequately assessed by laboratory diagnostic procedures such as EDX and neuroimaging studies. It is quite difficult to detect abnormalities involving the inferior portion of the sacral plexus (S2, S3, and S4 derived), which supplies principally the pelvic floor. Excluding needle electrode examination of the anal sphincter, none of the standard procedures performed in the typical EDX laboratory evaluates this part of the sacral plexus; moreover, neuroimaging studies often reveal no abnormalities when the clinical symptoms suggest that the inferior portion of the sacral plexus has been damaged.[101]

Lumbosacral Plexus Injuries

In contrast to the brachial plexus, the lumbosacral plexus is much less vulnerable to trauma, in large part because much of it is encased within the pelvic bony ring (either the false or true pelvis). Thus, it is much more protected from external trauma than the brachial plexus.[9] In addition, unlike the brachial plexus, most of it (including all of the sacral plexus) is rarely injured by external trauma, either direct or indirect, without concomitant fracture or dislocation of various bony or ligamentous structures. For these reasons, the majority of lumbosacral plexopathies are nontraumatic in origin. Thus, in one report of 86 cases of lumbosacral plexopathies, less than 6% were due to trauma, whereas over 50% were caused by neoplasms.[53] Because traumatic lumbosacral plexopathies occur infrequently, the relative incidence of lumbosacral plexopathies compared to brachial plexopathies is quite low.

Lumbosacral Plexopathies Due to Violent Trauma

Lesions of this nature compose only a fraction of all lumbosacral plexopathies. Nonetheless, they will be reviewed in some detail here because they are discussed only very briefly, if at all, in most sources concerned with plexopathies. Because they usually coexist with pelvic fractures and dislocations, some features of the bony pelvis and some of the injuries that befall it merit discussion.

The two principal functions of the bony pelvis are weight bearing and protection of the structures it contains. It is viewed as a *pelvic girdle* or *pelvic ring*, consisting of three bones linked together by ligaments. The two paired lateral components are the innominate bones (each composed of an ilium, an ischium, and a pubis); they articulate anteriorly with each other at the pubic symphysis. The third bone of the group, the sacrum, forms the posterior aspect of the pelvic ring; it articulates with both innominate bones (Fig. 18.7). The anterior third of the pelvic ring does not bear weight; therefore, fractures of it are usually stable. Moreover, isolated fractures in this region rarely result in PNS injuries. In contrast, the posterolateral two-thirds of the pelvic ring serves as an arch connecting the trunk with the lower limbs, through which the weight load is transmitted. Both the weight-bearing and protective properties of the pelvic ring can be severely compromised by fractures or dislocations involving its posterolateral aspect. Bony injuries in this area often are unstable, and structures near or adjacent to the posterior pelvic girdle, such as the genitourinary tract, blood vessels, lumbosacral nerves, and rectum, can sustain damage.[36,51]

Pelvic fractures constitute approximately 5% of all fractures requiring hospitalization. Three etiologies are responsible for over 80% of them: (1) high-velocity traffic accidents, often with the victims

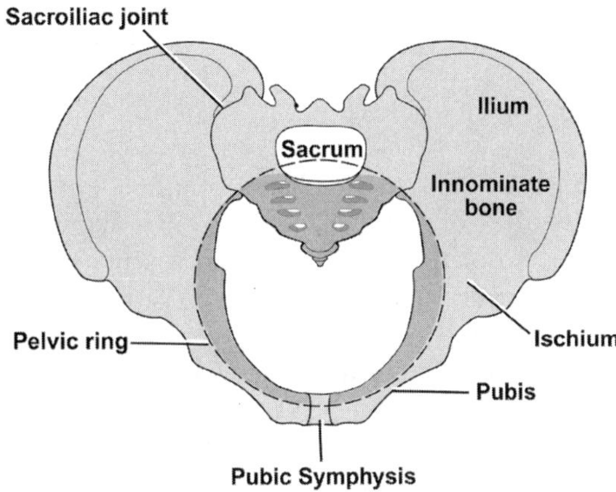

Figure 18.7. The pelvic bony structures, cross-sectional view (from above), illustrating the pelvic ring. (Copyright Cleveland Clinic Foundation, used with permission)

being pedestrians struck by moving vehicles; (2) industrial accidents, typically with the victims being crushed between heavy objects (e.g., logs, vehicles); and (3) falls from a height. Pelvic fractures are one of the markers of injury severity with high-speed traffic accidents: they are present in 2% to 4.5% of nonfatal accidents, in 22% of fatal accidents in general, and in 45% of fatal accidents involving pedestrians. Almost two-thirds of them are complicated by other fractures or by soft tissue injuries.[37,60–62] The most common and the most devastating complications of pelvic fractures are hemorrhage with subsequent shock, and genitourinary injuries.[37]

The incidence of PNS injuries with pelvic fractures overall is relatively low: less than 7.5% in several large series. However, this incidence increases substantially with certain types of pelvic fractures and dislocations, such as transverse sacral fractures and double-vertical fractures. Moreover, these neurological injuries are frequently overlooked, even though they are an important cause of delayed and often unsatisfactory recovery. Some investigators have commented on the difficulty of determining the level of the PNS lesion: lumbosacral roots, lumbosacral plexus, or proximal peripheral nerves. However, several studies, particularly the detailed autopsy series reported by Huittinen, suggest that the lumbosacral plexus frequently is injured.[36,38,60]

Several classifications of pelvic fractures and dislocations have been proposed. Only some of the types of injury they describe are relevant to this discussion because many are not associated with PNS disorders. Two that are pertinent, however, are (1) sacral fractures and (2) double-vertical pelvic fractures; certain sacral fractures are frequently a component of the latter.

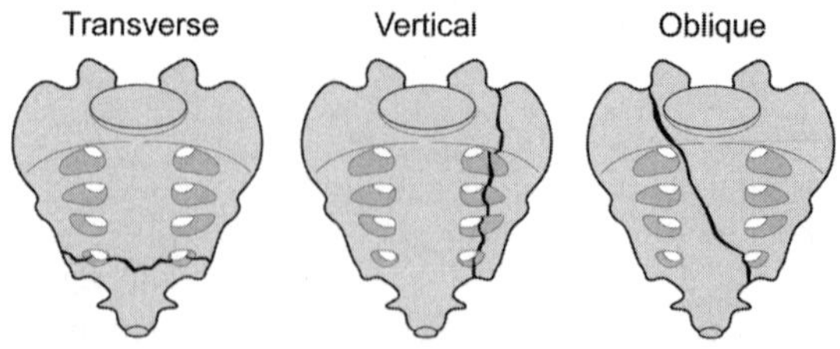

Figure 18.8. The three major types of sacral fracture. Oblique fractures often are considered a type of vertical fracture. (Copyright Cleveland Clinic Foundation, used with permission)

SACRAL FRACTURES. These compose approximately 17% of all pelvic fractures. Only about 9% occur in isolation; in the other 91% other pelvic ring bones also are fractured. Of the various bones composing the pelvic ring, fractures of the sacrum are most likely to be associated with neurological symptoms; in one series, 34% of patients with these injuries had neurological deficits.[27,69,73]

Sacral fractures can be classified as transverse (horizontal) or vertical (Fig. 18.8). Transverse sacral fractures are uncommon. They can be caused by both direct and indirect trauma and may occur in isolation. Marked displacement of the fractured fragment may occur. Overall, the major cause of sacral fractures is motor vehicle accidents.[27,73] Nonetheless, a substantial number of high transverse sacral fractures are due to falls from a height; in one series, most were the result of failed suicide jumps.[69] Major neurological injuries are uncommon with transverse fractures at or below the S4 foramina. In contrast, they often are substantial with fractures above that level; damage to the pudendal nerve and autonomic nerves causes principally bowel and genitourinary abnormalities, including bladder dysfunction and impotence. As would be anticipated, transverse sacral fractures are particularly likely to cause intraspinal and intraforaminal injury to nerve roots.[27,69,73] Most so-called lumbosacral root avulsions are associated with transverse sacral fractures. However, the term *avulsion* actually is incorrect, because the lumbosacral roots are ruptured within the cauda equina rather than torn from the lumbar enlargement of the spinal cord. (Ruptures, rather than avulsions, occur in these instances because the traction being applied to the lumbosacral roots is almost parallel to the long axis of the spinal cord, rather than at a more horizontal angle, as it is when brachial plexus roots are avulsed.[36,73]) Treatment of transverse sacral fractures often consists of operative decompression, with reduction and fixation; this is required for pain control, to aid in recovery of the damaged roots, and to prevent further injury to them.[27,69,73] The majority of sacral fractures are vertical fractures, with oblique sacral fractures being included in this category. Most sacral fractures of this type are associated with injuries of other portions of the pelvic ring. Vertical sacral fractures that are strictly unilateral, either lateral to the foramina or passing through them, tend to produce ipsilateral abnormalities of the L5 root, the

S1 root, or both. Oblique vertical fractures that involve the central canal, similar to transverse sacral fractures, tend to affect the middle and lower sacral roots (i.e., S2, S3, S4) bilaterally, producing bowel and genitourinary dysfunction.[27,69]

Double Vertical Pelvic Fractures. With this type of presentation, there are combined separation injuries of both the anterior and posterior pelvic rings. As a result, the middle segment, containing the hip joint, is often displaced.[35,36,58] The anterior ring injury is usually a pubic fracture (unilateral or bilateral) or a rupture of the pubic synthesis. The posterior ring injury most often is a vertical sacral fracture, but it can be a vertical fracture through the adjacent ilium or a rupture of the sacroiliac joint. Sacroiliac joint ruptures are more common in young adults and are especially likely to be associated with injuries of the sacral plexus, which rests on the joint. In one large series (407 consecutive patients) with pelvic fractures, over 27% were double vertical pelvic fractures; they were the second most common fracture type, trailing only pubic ramus fractures. Most (60% to 77%) double-vertical pelvic fractures are sustained in traffic accidents. They have a relatively high (12%) mortality associated with them, usually due to hemorrhagic shock or renal failure. There is also a high incidence of PNS lesions with them, ranging from 18% to 46%. Neurological complications are seen most often when the posterior ring injuries are vertical sacral fractures and least often with vertical ilium fractures. With sacral fractures, as previously noted, the neurological deficits usually result from injury of the middle and lower sacral roots. In contrast, sacroiliac joint ruptures often produce sacral plexopathies. In over two-thirds of patients with these injuries, the sacral plexus fibers affected derive from multiple roots.[37,64] In a detailed postmortem study, which included pelvic x-rays and autopsies of 42 victims of fatal accidents (traffic, industrial, or domestic) who had sustained pelvic fractures, Huittinen determined that 38 had unstable double vertical fractures of the pelvis. Of these, the majority had two fractures involving the posterior pelvic ring, with the most common combination by far being bilateral fractures that were near the sacroiliac joint region. Twenty of the 42 bodies (48%) had PNS lesions. Combined injuries of more than one neural structure were more common than isolated injuries; there was a total of 40 injuries among the 20 bodies (Fig. 18.9). The single most common PNS lesion found was a traction injury of the lumbosacral trunk, seen in 12 of the 20 bodies (60%). This was always associated with fractures involving the ipsilateral sacroiliac joint and frequently was accompanied by traction lesions of the ipsilateral superior gluteal nerve. There were 15 instances of actual rupture of nerve fibers, involving cauda equina roots in 6, the obturator and superior gluteal nerves in 3, and the fifth lumbar root in 2. Only four compressive lesions were seen, of which all resulted from comminuted fractures of the sacral foramina, and involved the APRs of S1 through S4.[36]

Intrapartum Maternal Lumbosacral Plexopathy
This rare maternal intrapartum PNS disorder was first recognized more than 150 years ago and has been identified by a number of terms in the interim, including *maternal paralysis*, *maternal birth palsy*, *traumatic neuritis of the puerperium*, *maternal lumbosacral plexopathy*, and, based on its most obvious and persistent feature, *postpartum footdrop*.[40,96] Clinically, it is characterized by pain, paresthesias, and later weakness, typically restricted to one lower extremity. Pain, sometimes cramping in nature, is the initial symptom, although it is not present in some instances. It usually begins during

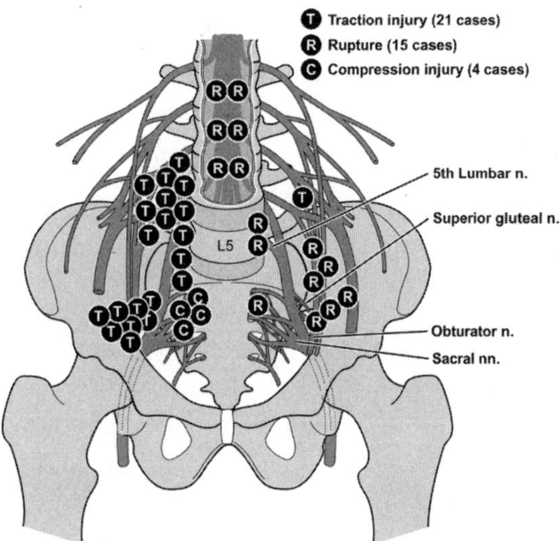

Figure 18.9. Distribution of associated PNS injuries found by Huittinen in his autopsy series of trauma victims with pelvic fractures. Note that traction lesions were the most common, and they almost exclusively affected the lumbosacral trunk and the superior gluteal nerve. (From reference 36, used with permission.)

early labor and radiates down the lower limb in an L5 (*sciatic nerve*) distribution. Initially, it may be intermittent, occurring only with contractions, but it tends to become more severe and more persistent as labor progresses. Following delivery, the patient usually notices paresthesias, sensory loss, and lower limb weakness in an L5 distribution, mainly distal to the knee. The most prominent motor disability is footdrop, which frequently is initially noted when the patient first attempts to walk in the early postpartum period. In contrast, pain generally is not present after delivery. The right lower limb is preferentially affected.[40]

The predisposing factors for this disorder include small (short stature) patients; large babies; prolonged or arrested labor; and malpresentations. Often, these complicating factors have resulted in forceps deliveries or cesarean sections.

Intrapartum maternal lumbosacral plexopathy very likely is due to direct pressure on the lumbosacral trunk (sometimes accompanied by similar pressure on the superior gluteal nerve and occasionally the obturator nerve) during the second stage of labor by the descending fetal head; the latter compresses the PNS structure(s) against the rim of the pelvis. The symptoms characteristically are on the same side as the brow of the infant was during the descent (usually the right, as noted above)[21,40] (Fig. 18.10).

Without exception, involvement of the lumbosacral trunk fibers that distally will contribute to the peroneal nerve dominates the clinical presen-

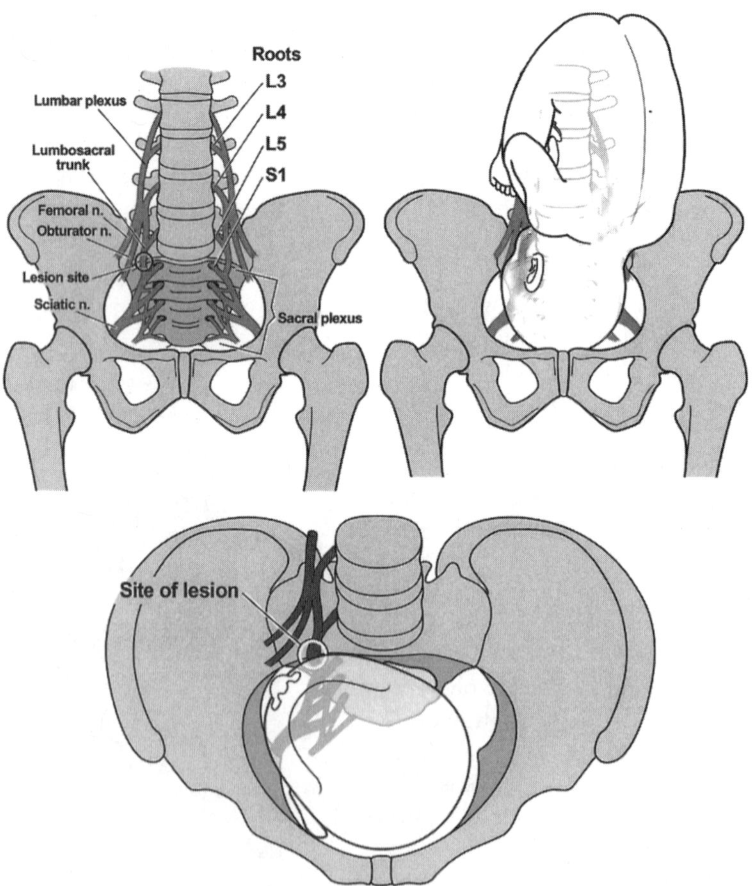

Figure 18.10. Diagrams of the lumbosacral plexus and surrounding bony pelvic structures, anterior view (upper left), showing the site of the compressive nerve injury (circle) in intrapartum maternal lumbosacral plexopathy. This is caused by the lumbosacral trunk being compressed between the underlying pelvic brim and the fetal head, illustrated with anterior (upper right) and superior (lower center) views. (Copyright Cleveland Clinic Foundation, used with permission)

tation. Thus, the only weakness sometimes noted is that of foot dorsiflexion and eversion; for this reason these patients often are thought to have a peroneal neuropathy. However, a detailed neurological examination typically reveals abnormalities of other L5-innervated muscles.[21,40]

The underlying pathophysiology generally consists of variable amounts of demyelinating conduction block and axon loss. In most patients, the former predominates and the postpartum motor symptoms regress fairly rapidly. In a few patients, however, the weakness persists for several months and, occasionally, never resolves completely, indicating that total or near-total axon loss has occurred.

It should be noted that even though one of the synonyms for this disorder is *postpartum footdrop*, a more common cause for foot dorsiflexion weakness in the postpartum period is a peroneal neuropathy at the fibular head caused by the mother's legs being in stirrups during the parturition.[21,40,81,96]

Postoperative Lumbosacral Plexopathy

Infrequently, various components of the lumbosacral plexus are injured during abdominal and pelvic operations. Probably the most common of these are lumbar plexus injuries sustained during renal surgery, which most likely are due to instrumentation. A single report described three patients, all of whom were in a modified lithotomy position for at least 2 hours, as having sustained "lumbosacral plexus stretch injuries"; in one patient the lumbar plexus was affected, in the second the sacral plexus, and in the third both plexuses. The clinical and EDX details provided, however, are equally consistent with multiple lower extremity peripheral nerve injuries.[18,22,95]

Surgical repair of aortic aneurysms can cause ischemic injury of the lumbosacral plexus (and the spinal cord). In the majority of reports on the subject, the exact site of injury has been debatable. This is because at times it can be extremely difficult to distinguish one proximal PNS lesion from another on clinical, EDX, and neuroimaging examinations. The problem is the considerable degree of overlap of nerve fiber involvement among L2–L4 radiculopathies, lumbar plexopathies, and femoral neuropathies on the one hand and L5–S1 radiculopathies, sacral plexopathies (superior aspect), and high sciatic neuropathies on the other. Moreover, very often the nature of the injury is such that all three of the neural structures at risk are about equally likely to sustain damage.[99]

There have been descriptions of lumbosacral plexopathies occurring during hip operations. One concerned 22 patients who reportedly developed such plexopathies, primarily during total hip replacements; 7 had lumbar plexus lesions, 4 had sacral plexus lesions, and 11 had both plexuses involved.[82] Unfortunately, it is not clear from the information provided exactly how the authors localized these lesions to the lumbar and sacral plexuses, as opposed to various nerves derived from those neural structures. Thus, after total hip replacement, abnormalities present in obturator and femoral nerve distributions are just as likely to be due to coexisting injuries of those peripheral nerves as to a lumbar plexopathy. Similarly, postoperative abnormalities found in the distributions of the high sciatic nerve and the gluteal nerves seem just as likely to be the result of a proximal sciatic neuropathy combined with local surgical injury to the gluteal nerves as to a sacral plexopathy. In fact, when the mechanics of the operation are considered, the sciatic and gluteal nerves appear to be at far greater risk than the sacral plexus.

Injection Injuries

A few reports have described patients developing lumbosacral plexopathies, presumably on an ischemic basis, following the injection of drugs, often pain medication, into the buttocks. Typically, local pain developed immediately, but the complete clinical presentation of limb pain, weakness, and paresthesias usually evolved over minutes to hours. The small number of available reports on the topic have described involvement of the lumbar plexus alone, and simultaneous involvement of both the lumbar and sacral plexuses. Presumably, these plexus lesions result from the injurious injections inadvertently being given into the inferior gluteal artery and causing toxic vasospasm and thrombosis, which spread in a retrograde fashion to involve the blood supply of the plexus fibers. Consistent with this theory is the fact that many of these patients develop characteristic skin lesions over the buttocks, called *embolia cutis medicamentosa*, which consist of swelling and a bluish discoloration and which frequently progress to gangrene.[83]

Some patients have developed a lumbosacral plexopathy following intra-arterial injection of antimetabolites (cisplatin, fluorouracil) through the internal iliac arteries to treat pelvic cancer. Clinical details have been provided on two such patients. Both experienced the immediate onset of paresthesias in the ipsilateral lower limb, but neither complained of pain and, apparently, neither developed motor deficits. Presumably, these symptoms were either ischemic in nature, caused by thrombosis of the arterial supply to the involved portion of the plexus, or the result of lumbosacral plexus demyelination due to the chemotherapeutic agents. Considering their mild nature, the latter seems the most likely possibility. Although very few lesions of this type have been reported, one group of authors has stated that intra-arterial injection of chemotherapy is one of the four major causes of lumbosacral plexopathies seen at their cancer center, suggesting that this PNS complication is underreported.[63]

Rather severe PNS lesions involving the lower limb, causing principally pain but sometimes weakness as well, have been described as following paracervical block anesthesia. This type of regional anesthesia is used prior both to deliveries, and to dilatation and curettage of the uterus. The cause is unclear, although it is most likely hematoma formation in the region of the sacral plexus. Such an etiology is consistent with the fact that (1) the symptoms, at least in most patients, often are delayed in onset (up to 10 days) and then evolve over several hours and (2) in some patients, a tender mass is palpable over the sacroiliac joint on pelvic examination. In the majority of the reported patients, the most constant symptom has been severe buttock pain. Typically, the symptoms regress after 1 or 2 months, leaving no residuals, so axon loss cannot be the predominant underlying pathophysiology.[24,70]

Retroperitoneal Hemorrhage

Bleeding into the retroperitoneal space is a well-known cause of isolated femoral neuropathies and lumbar plexopathies. When the bleed is within the iliacus muscle, or in the intramuscular groove between the iliacus and psoas muscles, the femoral nerve is affected. Conversely, when the bleed is within the psoas muscle itself, the lumbar plexus is involved. The majority of these lesions are complications of anticoagulation, hemophilia, or some acquired bleeding disorder, but on rare occasions they can develop in otherwise normal patients who sustain blunt trauma to the lower abdomen. Severe pain typically is the initial symptom with lumbar plexus involvement. It begins in the lower abdomen or groin and radiates into the buttock, thigh, and medial leg (saphenous distribution). The pain is accentuated by hip flexion and attenuated by hip extension and external rotation. Weakness and paresthesias then appear in the distributions of both the femoral and obturator nerves, usually followed by atrophy. This is one of the very few types of established compartment syndromes that probably is best treated conservatively. Because these lesions almost always are the result of axon loss, recovery typically is slow and sometimes incomplete.[18,53,81]

REFERENCES

1. Alnot JY: Traumatic paralysis of the brachial plexus: Preoperative problems and therapeutic indications. In: Terzis JK (ed): Micro-reconstruction of Nerve Injuries. Philadelphia, WB Saunders, 1987, pp 325–346.
2. Amrami KK, Port JD: Imaging the brachial plexus. Hand Clin 21:25–37, 2005.
3. Birch R: Traction lesions of the brachial plexus. Br J Hosp Med 32:140–143, 1984.
4. Birch R, Bonney G, Wynn-Parry CB: Surgical Disorders of Peripheral Nerves. London, Churchill-Livingston, 1998.
5. Blom S, Dahlback LO: Nerve injuries in dislocations of the shoulder joint and fractures of the neck of the humerus. Acta Chir Scand 136:461–466, 1970.
6. Boardman ND, Cofield RH: Neurological complications of shoulder surgery. Clin Orthop, 368:44–53, 1999.
7. Bruxelle J, Travers V, Thiebaut JB: Occurrence and treatment of pain after brachial plexus injury. Clin Orthop Related Res 237:87–95, 1988.
8. Burke D: Value and limitations of nerve conduction studies. In: Delwaide PJ, Gorio A (eds): Clinical Neurophysiology in Peripheral Neuropathies. Amsterdam, Elsevier, 1985, pp 91–102.
9. Buruma OJS, Maat GJR: Lumbosacral plexus lesions. In: Vikin PJ, Bruyn GW, Klawans HL, Matthews WB (eds): Handbook of Clinical Neurology: Neuropathies, vol 51. Amsterdam, Elsevier, 1987, pp 157–170.
10. Chavin JM, Brown WF: Negative signs and symptoms in neurogenic and muscle disease. In: Brown WF, Bolton CF, Aminoff MJ (eds): Neuromuscular Function and Disease: Basic, Clinical and Electrodiagnostic Aspects, vol 1. Philadelphia, WB Saunders, 2002, pp 369–385.
11. Chen D-J, Chuang DCC, Wei F-C: Unusual thoracic outlet syndrome secondary to fractured clavicle. J Trauma 52:393–399, 2002.
12. Chusid JG: Correlative Neuroanatomy and Functional Neurology, 16th ed. Los Altos, Lange Medical, 1976.
13. Clemente CD: Gray's Anatomy, 30th ed (American). Philadelphia, Lea & Febiger, 1985.
14. Coene LNJEM: Mechanisms of brachial plexus lesions. Clin Neurol Neurosurg 95(suppl):S24–S29, 1993.

15. Cooper DE: Nerve injury associated with patient positioning in the operating room. In: Gelberman RH (ed): Operative Nerve Repair and Reconstruction, vol 2. Philadelphia, JB Lippincott, 1991, pp 1231–1242.
16. Dawson D, Hallett M, Wilbourn AJ: Thoracic outlet syndromes. In: Dawson D, Hallett M, Wilbourn AJ (eds): Entrapment Neuropathies, 3rd ed. Philadelphia, Lippincott-Raven, 1998, pp 227–250.
17. Della Santa D, Narakas A, Bonnard C: Late lesions of the brachial plexus after fracture of the clavicle. Ann Hand Surg 10:531–540, 1991.
18. Donaghy M: Lumbosacral plexus lesions. In: Dyck PJ, Thomas PK (eds): Peripheral Neuropathy, vol 2. 3rd ed, Philadelphia, WB Saunders 1990, pp 951–959.
19. Dumontier C, Gilbert A: Traumatic brachial plexopathy in children. Ann Hand Surg 9:351–357, 1990.
20. Ellison DW, Wood VE: Trauma-related thoracic outlet syndrome. J Hand Surg 19B:424–426, 1994.
21. Feasby JE, Burton SR, Hahn AF: Obstetrical lumbosacral plexus injury. Muscle Nerve 15:937–940, 1992.
22. Flanagan WF, Webster GD, Brown MW, Massey EW: Lumbosacral plexus stretch injury following the use of the modified lithotomy position. J Urol 134:567–568, 1985.
23. Franklin GM, Gulton-Kehoe D, Smith-Waller T: Outcome of surgery for thoracic outlet syndrome in Washington Workers' Compensation, 1986–1991. Neurology 44(suppl 2):A380, 1994.
24. Gaylord TG, Pearson JW: Neuropathy following paracervical block in obstetric patients. Obstet Gynecol 60: 521–524, 1982.
25. Gebarski KS, Gebarski SS, Glazer GM, et al: The lumbosacral plexus: Anatomic-radiologic-pathologic correlation using CT. Radiographics 6:401–425, 1986.
26. Gebarski KS, Glazer GM, Gebarski SS: Brachial plexus: Anatomic, radiologic and pathologic correlation using computer tomography. J Comput Assist Tomogr 6:1058–1063, 1982.
27. Gibbons KJ, Soloniuk DS, Razack N: Neurological injury and patterns of sacral fractures. J Neurosurg 72: 889–893, 1990.
28. Gieradà DS, Erickson SJ: MR imaging of the sacral plexus: Abnormal findings. Am J Roentgenol 160:1067–1071, 1993.
29. Gilbert A, Brockman R, Carlioz H: Surgical treatment of brachial plexus birth palsy. Clin Orthop Related Res 264:39–47, 1991.
30. Gilbert A, Whitaker I: Obstetrical brachial plexus lesions. J Hand Surg 16B:489–491, 1991.
31. Glass RF: The brachial plexus. In: Edelman RR, Hesselink JR (eds): Clinical Magnetic Response Imaging. Philadelphia, WB Saunders, 1990, pp 653–666.
32. Haymaker W, Woodhall B: Peripheral Nerve Injuries, 2nd ed. Philadelphia, WB Saunders, 1953.
33. Hentz VR, Meyer RD: Brachial plexus microsurgery in children. Microsurgery 12:175–185, 1991.
34. Hirshman EB: Brachial plexus injury. Clin Sports Med 9:311–329, 1990.
35. Hudson DA, Boome R, Sanpera I: Brachial plexus injury after median sternotomy. J Hand Surg 18A:282–284, 1993.
36. Huittinen V-M: Lumbosacral nerve injury in fracture of the pelvis. Acta Chir Scand 138(suppl 429):1–43, 1972.
37. Huittinen V-M, Slatis P: Fractures of the pelvis. Acta Chir Scand 138:563–569, 1972.
38. Huittinen V-M, Slatis P: Nerve injury in double vertical pelvic fractures. Acta Chir Scand 138:571–575, 1972.
39. Jennett RJ, Tarby TJ, Kreinick CJ: Brachial plexus palsy: An old problem reinvestigated. Am J Obstet Gynecol 166:1673–1677, 1992.
40. Katirji B, Wilbourn AJ, Scarberry SL, Preston DC: Intrapartum maternal lumbosacral plexopathy. Muscle Nerve 26:340–347, 2002.
41. Kiloh LG: Brachial plexus lesions after cholecystectomy. Lancet 1:103–105, 1950.
42. Kim DH, Cho Y-L, Tiel RL, Kline DG: Outcomes of surgery in 1019 brachial plexus lesions treated at Louisiana State University Health Sciences Center. J Neurosurg 98:1005–1016, 2003.
43. Kline DG: Civilian gunshot wounds to the brachial plexus. J Neurosurg 70:166–174, 1989.
44. Kline DG, Hudson AR: Nerve Injuries. Philadelphia, WB Saunders, 1995.
45. Kline DG, Judice DJ: Operative management of selected brachial plexus lesions. J Neurosurg 58:631–640, 1983.
46. Kroll DA, Caplan RA, Posner K, Ward RJ, Cheney FW: Nerve injury associated with anesthesia. Anesthesiology 73:202–207, 1990.
47. Kwaan JH, Rapoport I: Postoperative brachial plexus palsy: A study of the mechanism. Arch Surg 101:612–615, 1970.
48. Lederman R: Neuromuscular and musculoskeletal problems in instrumental musicians. Muscle Nerve 27:549–561, 2003.
49. Levin K, Wilbourn AJ, Maggiano HJ: Cervical rib and median sternotomy-related plexopathies: A reassessment. Neurology 50:1407–1012, 1998.
50. Lindgren KA, Oksala I: Long-term outcome of surgery for thoracic outlet syndrome. Am J Surg 169:358–360, 1995.
51. Marshall RW, DeSilva RDD: Computerized axial tomography in traction injuries of the brachial plexus. J Bone Joint Surg 68B:734–738, 1986.
52. Morin JE, Long R, Elleker MG, et al: Upper extremity neuropathy following medial sternotomy. Ann Thorac Surg 34:181–184, 1982.
53. Mumenthaler M, Schliack H: Peripheral Nerve Lesions. New York, Thieme Medical, 1991.
54. Murray B, Wilbourn AJ: The clinical and electrodiagnostic features of "classic" postoperative brachial plexopathy. Neurology 54(suppl 3):A325–A326, 2001.
55. Nakamura T, Yabe Y, Horiuchi Y, Takayama S: Magnetic resonance myelography in brachial plexus injury. J Bone Joint Surg 79B:764–769, 1997.
56. Narakas AO: Traumatic brachial plexus lesions. In: Dyck PJ, Thomas PK, Lambert EH, et al (eds): Peripheral

Neuropathy, vol 2, 2nd ed. Philadelphia, WB Saunders, 1984, pp 1394–1409.

57. Narakas AO: Thoughts on neurotization of nerve transfers. In: Terzis JK (ed): Micro-reconstruction of Nerve Injuries. Philadelphia, WB Saunders, 1987, pp 447–454.
58. Ochi M, Ikuta Y, Watunabe M, Kimori K, Itoh K: The diagnostic value of MRI in traumatic brachial plexus injury. J Hand Surg 19B:55–59, 1994.
59. Pasila M, Jaroma H, Kiviluoto O, Sundholm A: Early complications of primary shoulder dislocations. Acta Orthop Scand 49:260–263, 1978.
60. Patterson FP, Morton KS: Neurological complications of fractures and dislocations of the pelvis. J Trauma 12: 1013–1023, 1973.
61. Peltier LF: Complications associated with fractures of the pelvis. J Bone Joint Surg 47A:1060–1069, 1965.
62. Perry JF, McClellan RJ: Autopsy findings in 127 patients following fatal traffic accidents. Surg Gynecol Obstet 119:586–590, 1964.
63. Pettigrew LC, Glass JP, Maor M, Zornoza J: Diagnosis and treatment of lumbosacral plexopathies in patients with cancer. Arch Neurol 41:1282, 1984.
64. Raf L: Double vertical fractures of the pelvis. Acta Chir Scand 131:298–305, 1966.
65. Robertson WC, Eichman PL, Clancy WG: Upper trunk brachial plexopathy in football players. JAMA 241:1480–1482, 1979.
66. Roger B, Travers V, Laval-Jeantet M: Imaging of post-traumatic brachial plexus injury. Clin Orthop Related Res 237:57–61, 1988.
67. Roos DB: The place for scalenectomy and first rib resection in thoracic outlet syndrome. Surgery 92:1077–1085, 1982.
68. Rosson JW: Disability following closed traction lesions of the brachial plexus sustained in motorcycle accidents. J Hand Surg 12B:353–355, 1987.
69. Roy-Camille R, Saillant G, Gagna G, Mazel C: Transverse fractures of the sacrum: Suicidal jumper's fracture. Spine 10:838–845, 1985.
70. Sanchetee PC, Madan VS, Dhamija RM, Venkataraman S: Lumbosacral plexopathy following regional paracervical block anesthesia. J Assoc Physicians India 38:302–303, 1990.
71. Sandmire HF, DeMott RK: Erb's palsy: Concepts of causation. Obstet Gynecol 95:941–942, 2000.
72. Schaafma SJ: Plexus injuries. In: Vinkin PJ, Bruyn GW (eds): Handbook of Clinical Neurology: Diseases of Nerves, Part 1, vol 7. Amsterdam, North-Holland, 1970, pp 402–429.
73. Schmidek HH, Smith DA, Kristiansen TK: Sacral fractures. Neurosurgery 15:735–746, 1984.
74. Sedel L: The management of supraclavicular lesions: Clinical examination, surgical procedures, results. In: Terzis JK (ed): Micro-reconstruction of Nerve Injuries. Philadelphia, WB Saunders, 1987, pp 385–392.
75. Seddon HJ: Three types of nerve injury. Brain 66:237–281, 1943.
76. Sivak M, Ochoa J, Fernandez JM: Positive manifestations of nerve fiber dysfunction: Clinical, electrophysiologic and pathologic correlates. In: Brown WF, Bolton CF (eds): Clinical Electromyography, 2nd ed. Boston, Butterworth-Heinemann, 1993, pp 117–148.
77. Slingluff CL, Terzis JK, Edgerton MT: The quantitative microanatomy of the brachial plexus in man: Reconstructive relevance. In: Terzis JK (ed): Micro-reconstruction of Nerve Injuries. Philadelphia, WB Saunders, 1987, pp 285–324.
78. Sloff ACJ: Obstetric brachial plexus lesions and their neurosurgical management. Clin Neurol Neurosurg 95(suppl):S73–S77, 1993.
79. Stangl R, Alterdorf-Hofmann A, von der Emde J: Brachial plexus lesions following median sternotomy in cardiac surgery. Thorac Cardiovasc Surg 39:360–364, 1991.
80. Stevens JC: Lumbosacral plexus lesions. In: Dyck PJ, Thomas PK, Lambert EH, et al (eds): Peripheral Neuropathy, 2nd ed, vol 20 Philadelphia, WB Saunders, 1984, pp 1425–1434.
81. Stewart JD: Focal Peripheral Neuropathies, 3rd ed. Philadelphia, Lippincott Williams & Wilkins, 2000.
82. Stohr M: Traumatic and postoperative lesions of the lumbosacral plexus. Arch Neurol 35:757–760, 1978.
83. Stohr M, Dichgans J, Dorstelmann D: Ischaemic neuropathy of the lumbosacral plexus following intragluteal injection. J Neurol Neurosurg Psychiatry 43:489–494, 1980.
84. Suematsu N, Matsuura J, Atsuta Y: Brachial plexus injury caused by electric current through the ulnar nerve. Arch Orthop Trauma Surg 108:400–402, 1989.
85. Sunderland S: Nerve and Nerve Injuries, 2nd ed. London, Churchill-Livingstone, 1978.
86. Terzis JK, Liberson WT, Maragh HA: Motorcycle brachial plexopathy. In: Terzis JK (ed): Micro-reconstruction of Nerve Injuries. Philadelphia, WB Saunders, 1987, pp 361–384.
87. Thomas DGT: Brachial plexus injury: Deafferentation pain and dorsal root entry zone (DREZ) coagulation. Clin Neurol Neurosurg 95(suppl):S48–S49, 1993.
88. Thomeer RTWM: Recovery of brachial plexus injuries. Clin Neurol Neurosurg 93:3–11, 1991.
89. Trojaborg W: Electrophysiological findings in pressure palsy of the brachial plexus. J Neurol Neurosurg Psychiatry 40:1116–1164, 1977.
90. Tsao BE, Wilbourn AJ: The medial brachial fascial compartment syndrome following axillary arteriography. Neurology; 61:1037–1041, 2003.
91. Tsao BE, Wilbourn AJ: Infraclavicular brachial plexus injury following axillary regional block. Muscle Nerve 30:44–48, 2004.
92. Urschel JD, Hameed SM, Grewal RP: Neurogenic thoracic outlet syndromes. Postgrad Med J 70:785–789, 1994.
93. Vahl CF, Carl I, Müller-Vahl C, Struck E: Brachial plexus injury after cardiac surgery. J Thorac Cardiovasc Surg 102:724–729, 1991.
94. Visser CPJ, Coene LNJEM, Brand R, Tavy DLJ: The incidence of nerve injury in anterior dislocation of the

shoulder and its influence on functional recovery. J Bone Joint Surg 81B:679–685, 1999.
95. Weber M: Lumbosacral plexopathies. In: Brown WF, Bolton CF, Aminoff MJ (eds): Neuromuscular Function and Disease: Basic, Clinical and Electrodiagnostic Aspects, vol 1. Philadelphia, WB Saunders, 2002, pp 852–864.
96. Whittaker WG: Injuries to the sacral plexus in obstetrics. Can Med Assoc J 79:622–627, 1958.
97. Wilbourn AJ: Nerve conduction studies: Types, components, abnormalities, and value in localization. Neurol Clin 20:305–333, 2002.
98. Wilbourn AJ: Brachial plexopathies. In: Brown WF, Bolton CF, Aminoff MJ (eds): Neuromuscular Function and Disease: Basic, Clinical and Electrodiagnostic Aspects, vol 1. Phildelphia, WB Saunders, 2002, pp 852–864.
99. Wilbourn AJ: Peripheral neuropathies associated with vascular diseases and the vasculitides. In: Brown WF, Bolton CF, Aminoff MJ (eds): Neuromuscular Function and Disease: Basic, Clinical and Electrodiagnostic Aspects, vol 2. Philadelphia, WB Saunders, 2002, pp 1229–1249.
100. Wilbourn AJ: Brachial plexus lesions. In: Dyck PJ, Thomas PK (eds): Peripheral Neuropathy, 4th ed, vol 2. Philadelphia, (Saunders) Elsevier, 2005, pp 1339–1373.
101. Wilbourn AJ: Lumbosacral plexopathies. In: Kamura J (ed): Clinical Neurophysiology of Peripheral Nerves (vol 7 of the Handbook of Clinical Neurophysiology). Amsterdam, Elsevier, in press.
102. Wilbourn AJ, Aminoff MJ: The electrodiagnostic examination with radiculopathies. *Muscle Nerve* 21:1612–1631, 1998.
103. Wilbourn AJ, Porter JM: Thoracic outlet syndromes. In: Weiner MA (ed): Spine: State of the Art Review. Philadelphia, Hanley and Belfus, 1988, pp 597–626.
104. Wynn Parry CB: Pain in avulsion lesions of the brachial plexus. Pain 9:41–53, 1980.

Chapter 19

Occupational and Use-Related Mononeuropathies

TIMOTHY M. MILLER
AND MICHAEL J. AMINOFF

General Considerations

Occupational and use-related mononeuropathies cause significant morbidity. Although the full impact of these syndromes is difficult to assess, the major consequences of carpal tunnel syndrome (CTS) alone provide some insight. The prevalence of CTS in the general population is 2% to 3%. In comparison to other work-related injuries and illnesses, median days away from work are highest for CTS. The average worker undergoing carpal tunnel surgery requires 27 days off work, and the estimated cost of carpal tunnel surgery in the United States is $2 billion.[32]

The reason that some individuals are injured by certain activities is unknown. When the mononeuropathy and the inciting activity are linked, the pathophysiological route to nerve injury often seems obvious. Yet that cannot be the full explanation, because other workers in a similar situation may be doing the exact same thing without experiencing ill effects. The protective mechanisms of peripheral nerves must be truly remarkable given the number of circumstances in which the nerve is percussed, stretched, angulated, or compressed without loss of function. This is especially true given the superficial course of many peripheral nerves. Do certain individuals have less protective covering or, perhaps, nerves that recover less well? There are clear situations, such as inebriation, in which the loss of the typical arousal and movement that would protect the nerve apparently leads to nerve injury. Similarly, ignoring warning signs of nerve injury, such as paresthesias, may lead to more severe nerve damage. Certain diseases predispose to nerve injury. For example, diabetics have a higher risk of CTS than nondiabetics.[30,80] Multiple compressive neuropathies raises the possibility of disorders such as hereditary liability to pressure palsies, in which a deletion in PMP-22 leads to unusual sensitivity of the nerves to pressure.[20]

Most of the mononeuropathies discussed here are characterized by chronic low-level trauma that eventually causes damage to the nerve and significant dysfunction. Compression of the nerve is the most common proposed mechanism of injury in mononeuropathies associated with activity. Compression may occur from pressure on the nerve by forces outside the body or by entrapment of the nerve in a tight compartment. Compression of the ulnar nerve at the elbow and compression of the median nerve within the carpal tunnel are two prototypic examples. These mechanisms of injury are not mutually exclusive. Overuse of the limbs causing compression within a muscular compartment is another proposed but less common mechanism of nerve injury often associated with excessive use of the arms or shoulder muscles. One example of this is the radial neuropathy associated with overwork of the triceps muscle.[73]

Once identified, the inciting activity should be discontinued. However, the pattern of nerve injury must first be recognized and correlated with the causal activity. Since continued activity is likely to provoke continued nerve injury and may result in permanent nerve damage, it is important to establish the correct diagnosis as soon as possible. The goal of this chapter is to aid clinicians in assessing patients with occupational or use-related mononeuropathies by providing an understanding of common patterns of activity-related nerve injury and of certain occupational hazards. We will not focus on plexus lesions, polyneuropathies, spinal root disorders, back pain, acute nerve injuries, or treatment for the various disorders described.

Recognition of an occupational or use-related mononeuropathy is not always easy. In rare instances the patient identifies the offending activity. More often, the patient presents with complaints of uncertain cause referable to a single nerve. Inquiry about occupational activities may provide the first clue. The next step is to identify specific activities that may predispose to nerve injury. These are usually related to work, exercise, hobbies, or habits. The "gold standard" is probably to accompany patients to the workplace or observe them exercising or performing their regular activities to identify any activities that commonly cause nerve injury. This is usually impractical. However, much information may be gained by asking patients to demonstrate the nature of their activities during the day, especially among manual laborers. Hobbies and athletic activities are also important lines of questioning and should lead to a similar demonstration of requisite activity. Note should also be taken of the clothes, instruments, or straps that the patient wears; the site of any pressure applied to the limb is also important. In some circumstances, knowledge of the habits of a given occupation is important. In fact, the "activity" causing nerve injury may be the least active part of the job. For example, a truck driver simulating driving may use exaggerated motions to demonstrate turning of the steering wheel or changing of gears. However, the most likely cause of left-sided ulnar neuropathy in this context is leaning the elbow against the side of the door when doing the least amount of physical activity.

The function of the clinical examination is mainly to confirm the existence of the mononeuropathy and to exclude other neuropathies. In some cases, evidence of unrecognized pressure points may be obtained, as by the presence of calluses. In the case of nerve injury, the electromyogram (EMG) and nerve conduction studies (NCSs) are an extension of the physical examination that allows more precise localization of the site of nerve injury and helps to quantify objectively the degree of axon loss or conduction slowing (see Chapter 20). The electrophysiological examination also clarifies the nature of reported symptoms (such as pain or paresthesias) that may be associated with significant nerve injury. The EMG/NCS may not be particularly useful in the first few days following traumatic injury (except to confirm the continuity of the nerve) since the signs of damage to the nerve (and associated electrical changes in the muscle) are most apparent 10 days to several weeks after injury. In most cases of occupational and use-related mononeuropathies, the injury is chronic and the timing of the examination is therefore not an issue. Although most patients with severe mononeuropathies will show changes on NCSs and on EMG, a "normal" result does not necessarily imply that the nerve in question is unharmed for several reasons. First, a mild degree of axon loss or slowing may be abnormal for a given individual, yet may not reach the threshold of abnormality for a particular laboratory. Skilled electromyographers routinely perform interside comparisons for this reason, especially in nerves with greater variability, such as when studying radial sensory fibers. Second, a nerve may be irritated and cause either pain or discomfort without providing clear electrophysiological evidence of damage to the nerve, since neither small-diameter nerve fibers nor nerve irritation are assessed well by NCS. One common example of this is full recovery of a nerve by NCS criteria after traumatic injury despite persistent pain in the affected area.

Finally, a word of caution is required concerning these evaluations. The apparent association between mononeuropathies and certain activities can be so compelling as to erroneously sway the evaluation in that direction. Those who have picked strawberries in a field in a crouching position will have an immediate understanding of and affinity for the peroneal neuropathy experienced by professional strawberry pickers. Despite this, lumbar disc disease and other musculoskeletal disorders remain much more common problems affecting the leg than this rare cause of peroneal neuropathy.

Specific Neuropathies

In the next several sections, mononeuropathies associated with specific activities or occupations are discussed. Many of these are listed in Tables 19.1 and 19.2. No effort has been made to provide a complete list of all possible associations between nerve damage and various activities. Instead, a more general account is provided to familiarize the reader with the types of activities that lead to nerve injury. In some instances, technological or other advances may have eliminated or reduced the incidence of certain disorders, although this is difficult to determine from a review of the literature. For example, improvements in biking gloves and seats in the past two decades may have decreased the multiple compression neuropathies associated with this sport, but this is unclear. The medical literature caters to novel findings, and therefore a lack of reported cases does not necessarily imply a decreased incidence. For most occupational and use-related mononeuropathies, the published literature relates to reports of single cases or small series rather than to large series. Thus, the association implied by the case reports that comprise the bulk of this literature may, in fact, be random associations.

Table 19.1. Occupational and Use Mononeuropathies of the Upper Extremities

Nerve	Location of Injury	Presumed Mechanism	Examples of Activity/Occupation
Long thoracic	Shoulder	Sudden forceful movement	Sports, carrying loaded backpack
Suprascapular	Suprascapular notch/foramen	Excessive use of shoulder	Baseball pitchers, volleyball players, weight lifters, wrestlers, cameramen
Axillary	Shoulder	Repeated minor trauma	Football and ice hockey
Lateral cutaneous nerve of the forearm	Forearm	Unusually long, strenuous activity	Any associated with prolonged activity
Median	Upper arm	Compression in pronator teres muscle	Women using milking machines
Carpal tunnel syndrome	Wrist	Overuse of hands	Many (see text)
Recurrent motor branch	Hand	Pressure from certain tools or excessive hand pressure	Shiatsu massage
Ulnar	Elbow	Flexion and compression	Leaning/resting elbow on hard surface, talking on phone, sleeping with arms flexed, jobs with repetitive elbow flexion
	Wrist and hand	Compression at base of hand	Using certain tools, bicycle riding, pizza cutting, prolonged video game playing, using computer mouse, wheelchair racing
Dorsal cutaneous branch of the ulnar nerve		Repetitive pronation	Use of code-sensing machine
Radial	Upper arm	Compression/overuse	Rifle firing, excessive triceps exercise
Posterior interosseous neuropathies	Forearm	Excessive pronation/supination	Repetitive twisting motion with hand
Superficial radial nerve	Wrist	Compression	Watches, bracelets, gloves, handcuffs
Digital nerves	Fingers	Compression	Bowler's thumb, musicians, certain tools, wrist splints

Table 19.2. Occupational and Use Mononeuropathies of the Lower Extremities

Nerve	Location of Injury	Presumed Mechanism	Examples of Activity/Occupation
Sciatic	Gluteal region	Compression	Sitting on hard surface, bicycling
Pudendal	Perineum	Compression	Bicycling
Common peroneal	Fibular head	Compression	Leg crossing, squatting for long periods of time (farm workers, carpet layers)
Deep peroneal	Ankle	Compression	Tight-fitting shoes
Superficial peroneal	Within peroneal compartment	Compression/inflammation	Excessive exercise
Tibial	Tarsal tunnel	Compression/minor trauma	Poorly fitting shoes, jogging, other athletes
Sural	Calf	Compression	Resting leg against hard surface, ski boots
Femoral	Upper thigh	Hyperextension/stretch	Gymnasts/dancers during hyperextension of hip
Saphenous	Medial knee	Compression	Surfing (gripping board between legs), kneeling to work
Lateral cutaneous nerve of the thigh	Inguinal Ligament	Compression	Wearing heavy belt (carpenter) or tight-fitting clothes
Ilioinguinal neuropathies	Inguinal region	Compression	Ice hockey
Iliohypogastric	Inguinal region	Compression	Belts, tight-fitting pants

Nerves of the Arm and Shoulder

Median Nerve

Carpal tunnel syndrome is the prototypical occupational and use-related mononeuropathy. In an autopsy study in 1913, Marie and Foix first focused attention on the carpal tunnel as a site of compression of the median nerve.[70] Numerous studies have expanded on this observation, showing kinking, stretching, or compression of the nerve within the carpal tunnel, as well as increased pressure within the tunnel with repetitive hand motions.[3,4,88,90,97,100] It is not possible to cite all the relevant studies on this topic because there are so many. Many occupations associated with repetitive hand movements have been linked to CTS: for example, housekeeper (commercial and domestic), data processor, packager, food and beverage workers (both processing and service workers), dental technician, secretary, and factory worker.[88,90,97,100]

Is CTS truly work-related? Authors who have reviewed the literature agree that many of the available studies on occupation and CTS are flawed. Not surprisingly, there is some disagreement regarding the conclusions. The 1997 summary statement from the National Institutes for Occupational Safety and Health concluded: "There is evidence of a positive association between highly repetitive work alone or in combination with other factors and CTS based on the currently available epidemiological data. . . . There is strong evidence of a positive association between exposure to a combination of risk factors (e.g., force and repetition, force and posture) and CTS."[10] Other authors agree.[93,95] A contrasting conclusion is: "except in the case of work that involves very cold temperatures, possibly in conjunction with load and repetition, work is less likely than demographic and disease-related variables to cause CTS."[32] Other authors agree.[102]

It is clear that other factors besides the work itself influence the likelihood of developing CTS. Such factors include working in a cold environment, age, obesity, weight gain, diabetes, and psychosocial factors.[7,62,78,80,85,92,99] Other conditions associated with CTS are pregnancy, thyroid disease, acromegaly, amyloidosis, rheumatoid arthritis, and long-term renal dialysis. These should be considered in all patients with or without presumed work-related symptoms. Indeed, more than one cause may be present. Among athletes, elite wheelchair athletes are particularly susceptible to CTS.[14] Cycling has also been associated with this condition.

Although the most well-known site of compression of the median nerve is the carpal tunnel, more proximal lesions associated with overuse have also been described. For example, the median nerve may be compressed as it passes through the heads of the pronator teres.[75] The distinction between compression of the nerve in this forearm compartment and nonspecific aching and pain in this area has sometimes been blurred. In the most clear cases, symptoms, signs, and electrodiagnostic findings show evidence of a median neuropathy that localizes to the forearm. If this were the case in the setting of excessive use of the forearm, it would be highly suggestive of what some authors have termed the *true neurogenic* pronator syndrome.[93] Nonspecific aching/pain in the arm may or may not be linked to median nerve damage.

In some cases, the distal branches of the median nerve may be selectively damaged. The anterior interosseous nerve (a branch of the median nerve) has been associated with excessive forearm exercise.[47] Use of certain tools and shiatsu massage can compress the recurrent motor branch of the median nerve.[46,103]

Ulnar Nerve

The ulnar nerve is particularly vulnerable at the elbow, where the nerve takes a superficial course through the condylar groove with little external padding, and through a tunnel (cubital tunnel) that narrows with elbow flexion. These vulnerabilities, combined with the convenience of resting the arm on the elbow, leads to repeated minor trauma and ulnar neuropathy in some individuals. This may relate to, for example, leaning the elbow on hard chair-arms, frequent or prolonged use of the telephone, and resting the arm on automobile door or window frame. Prolonged flexion with mild pressure, such as occurs in some individuals who sleep with the arms tightly flexed, may be enough to cause a neuropathy.[18] Repetitive flexion at the elbow in the workplace is sometimes associated with ulnar neuropathy.[17,65] The left arm of musicians, which is frequently held in a flexed position for long periods of time, may be at particular risk for ulnar neuropathy at the elbow.[63]

The ulnar nerve may also be damaged at the wrist and in the hand, both by recreational and occupational activities. Destot described the phenomenon in bicycle riders at the end of the nineteenth century,[26] and Hunt recognized that tools pressing into the base of the hand may damage the palmar branches of the nerve.[51] With time, different tools have been added to the list of those responsible for ulnar neuropathies, such as the computer mouse, video game controllers, and pizza cutters.[25,36,55] Bicycle riding[43,50,69] and wheelchair racing are also important causes. Distinguishing between ulnar neuropathies at the wrist and at the elbow based on patterns of weakness can be challenging since the forearm flexors are often spared even with lesions at the elbow. The most striking finding in ulnar nerve damage at the wrist is often sparing of sensory loss on the back of the hand since the dorsal ulnar cutaneous nerve branches proximal to the wrist.

The dorsal cutaneous branch of the ulnar nerve may be damaged exclusively. A combination of flexor position of the wrist and repetitive pronation of the arm likely contributed to *pricer palsy*, a dorsal ulnar cutaneous nerve palsy in workers using a code-reading machine.[107] In karate training, the distinction between a use-related neuropathy and trauma may be somewhat blurred; one patient developed a dorsal ulnar cutaneous neuropathy presumably from repeated blows to the side of the hand.[22]

Radial Nerve

Although injuries of the radial nerve near the humerus are relatively common (Saturday night palsy, or fracture of the humerus), they do not figure prominently in occupational and use-related mononeuropathies. However, some occupations place workers at risk. The radial nerve may be compressed between the humerus and a rifle sling[76] or when firing in the kneeling position with the medial arm pressing against the knee.[87] On rare occasions, strenuous abrupt use of the triceps has been associated with radial neuropathy.[68,73,83,89,96] Prolonged muscle activity from using a walker[8] has also been described.

Excessive pronation/supination has been associated with damage to the posterior interosseous nerve (PIN), a branch of the radial nerve.[23,33,44] This is not surprising given that the PIN courses through the supinator muscle. The opening in the proximal border of the superficial head of the muscle is distinctive enough to have earned its own eponym: the *arcade of Frohse*. Almost any type of band around the wrist, if tight enough, can cause damage to the superficial radial nerve, an exclusively sensory nerve. Well-known examples include handcuffs, bracelets, and watch straps. Pain and uncomfortable paresthesias are often more troublesome than the numbness or minor functional consequences of reduced sensation on the back of the hand.[19]

Other Mononeuropathies of the Arm and Shoulder

The long thoracic nerve innervates the serratus anterior, which stabilizes the scapula, an anchor point for several muscles that move the upper arm and shoulder. Thus, *long thoracic neuropathy* causes weakness and difficulty in moving the shoulder and arm. Winging of the scapula may be apparent to both patient and examiner and is exaggerated by raising the arm. Excessive use of the shoulder may damage the long thoracic nerve, as occurs in a variety of athletic activities.[9,38,53,56,79,82] Compression of the long thoracic nerve from a knapsack in soldiers was described at the beginning of World War ll.[52] Carrying a knapsack may injure the brachial plexus as well.[39,54]

The *suprascapular nerve*, a C5-6 branch off the upper trunk of the brachial plexus, innervates the supraspinatus and infraspinatus muscles. Complaints associated with suprascapular neuropathy may include pain in the shoulder, asymptomatic wasting of one or both spinati muscles, and weakness of shoulder abduction. Various athletic activities associated with prolonged, intense use of the arms have been associated with damage to this nerve. Thus, suprascapular neuropathy has been described in baseball pitchers,[67,84] volleyball players,[5,34,35,48,74,101,105] and weight lifters.[1,11,13,109] The neuropathy produces a curious pattern in these athletes: the infraspinatus is predominantly, if not exclusively, involved. While this might imply a lesion within the spinoglenoid notch through which the branch to the infraspinatus passes, suprascapular notch lesions may also produce exclusive infraspinatus weakness.[12,59,98]

Occupations requiring carrying heavy objects on the shoulder may be associated with suprascapular nerve impingement. Suprascapular neuropathies in meat packers, a livestock farmer loading sheep onto his shoulder,[6] and newsreel cameramen[57] have been described. Although volleyball and camera toting are remarkable causes of suprascapular neuropathy, other musculoskeletal injuries of the shoulder and acute brachial neuritis remain more common diagnoses.

Most *axillary nerve* injuries are secondary to shoulder dislocations or fracture of the proximal humerus. However, axillary nerve injury has also been described in ice hockey and football players without evidence of more than routine trauma to the shoulder involved in the sport.[81] Sleeping with the arms above the head in the prone position has been associated with axillary neuropathy.[2] Axillary neuropathy results in wasting of the deltoid muscle and weakness of shoulder abduction. The limitation in shoulder abduction may not be complete in some patients who maintain some function by using the supraspinatus as a shoulder abductor. Brachial plexopathies, including a lesion of the posterior cord or acute brachial neuritis, are important differential considerations.

Digital nerves run superficially, with little padding, in an area susceptible to constant minor trauma, that is, the hands. In this setting, it is remarkable that digital neuropathies are not more common. However, many different activities and professions in which significant pressure is placed on the digits have been associated with damage to digital nerves. The most common one is bowler's thumb.[29,49] A partial list of other digital neuropathies includes frisbee finger, jeweler's thumb, cheerleader's hand, harpist's hand, guitar finger, pen pusher's paresthesia, batter's thumb, tennis player's finger, violinist's finger, surgeon's finger, dental hygienist's finger, dentist's thumb, and wire twister's digit.[28]

Nerves of the Legs

As might be expected, the arms bear the brunt of occupational and use-related mononeuropathies compared with the legs. Nevertheless, the nerves in the lower extremities are sometimes involved.

Sciatic Nerve

There is considerable individual variation in the amount of padding that protects the sciatic nerve in the buttock region. Despite this cushioning, sciatic neuropathies may occur from sitting on hard benches, sitting in the yoga lotus position, or carrying a thick wallet in the back pocket.[24,27,41,94,104,108]

Peroneal Nerve

Squatting probably compresses the peroneal between the biceps femoris tendon, the lateral head of the gastrocnemius, and the head of the fibula. Workers who squat for long periods of time, such as strawberry pickers or carpet layers, may develop a peroneal neuropathy.[60,86] It is not clear if those who develop neuropathies have ignored premonitory paresthesias in the superficial peroneal distribution. The common habit of crossing the legs has been associated with common peroneal neuropathy. Tight-fitting boots may damage the distal sensory branch of the superficial peroneal nerve.[37,66] Damage to the terminal branch of the deep peroneal nerve to the extensor digitorum brevis is common and usually of limited functional significance. The presumed cause in many cases is tight-fitting shoes.[58]

Tibial Nerve

When the tibial division of the sciatic nerve is affected by an occupational or use-related mononeuropathy, it is most often damaged distally—for example, in the tarsal tunnel or near the metatarsal head. Though not common, tarsal tunnel syndrome has been described in athletes, especially joggers.[71] Compression of the interdigital nerve of the foot between adjacent metatarsals (Morton's neuroma) or damage to the medial plantar proper digital nerve near the first metatarsalphalangeal joint (Joplin's neuroma) results in pain and paresthesias in the affected area. Since these conditions may be associated with wearing poor-fitting shoes, and given that standing for long periods of time is required in many occupations, these syndromes may be considered occupational mononeuropathies.

Other Mononeuropathies of the Legs

Pressing the calf against any hard surface has potential to damage the *sural nerve*. The discomfort and tight fit of some ski boots is well known. In a few cases, this lead to sural nerve injury.[42,64] In the ankle, compression against tight-fitting boots or frequent, prolonged squatting may result in a similar injury.

An ever-evolving seat cushioning industry has been trying to avoid the discomfort of sitting on a bicycle seat for long periods of time. For most, temporary discomfort is the only problem. For a few, compression of the *pudendal nerve* leads to numbness of the genitals (on one side or both) and erectile impotence. [21,40,45,91,106]

Though uncommon, hyperextension stretch injuries of the *femoral nerve* have been described in gymnasts and dancers.[72]

Pressure on the medial edge of the knees may lead to damage of the *saphenous nerve*, the distal sensory branch of the femoral nerve. Prolonged kneeling at work or gripping a surf board between the knees are examples.[31]

The *lateral femoral cutaneous nerve* is prone to injury as it crosses the inguinal ligament. Wearing a heavy belt, as do many carpenters, electricians, and police personnel, or wearing tight-fitting clothing may cause compression of the nerve.[77]

Chronic groin pain in some athletes has been linked to *obturator nerve* entrapment within a thickened fascia of the short leg adductors. In these reports, the presenting complaint was exercise-induced medial thigh pain. The EMG showed denervation of adductor muscles.[15,16]

In a small group of professional ice hockey players whose lower abdominal pain was refractory to the conventional diagnostic approach, the pain was linked to entrapment of the *ilioinguinal nerve* in a torn external oblique aponeurosis and muscles. Surgical repair of the external oblique and ablation of the ilioinguinal nerve returned the players to the ice.[61]

Concluding Comments

Occupational and use-related mononeuropathies may occur in those with certain hobbies, sports, and jobs, and may impair the ability to work productively and comfortably. Recognition of these disorders will help patients prevent further injury and return to their normal activities more quickly.

REFERENCES

1. Agre JC, Ash N, Cameron MC, House J: Suprascapular neuropathy after intensive progressive resistive exercise: Case report. Arch Phys Med Rehabil 68:236–238, 1987.
2. Aita JF: An unusual compressive neuropathy. Arch Neurol 41:341, 1984.
3. Anonymous: From the Centers for Disease Control. Occupational disease surveillance: Carpal tunnel syndrome. JAMA 262:886, 889, 1989.
4. Anonymous: Occupational disease surveillance: Carpal tunnel syndrome. MMWR 38:485–489, 1989.
5. Antoniadis G, Richter HP, Rath S, Braun V, Moese G:

Suprascapular nerve entrapment: Experience with 28 cases. J Neurosurg 85:1020–1025, 1996.
6. Arboleya L, Garcia A: Suprascapular nerve entrapment of occupational etiology: Clinical and electrophysiological characteristics. Clin Exp Rheumatol 11:665–668, 1993.
7. Atcheson SG, Ward JR, Lowe W: Concurrent medical disease in work-related carpal tunnel syndrome. Arch Intern Med 158:1506–1512, 1998.
8. Ball NA, Stempien LM, Pasupuleti DV, and Wertsch JJ: Radial nerve palsy: A complication of walker usage. Arch Phys Med Rehabil 70:236–238, 1989.
9. Bateman JE: Nerve injuries about the shoulder in sports. J Bone Joint Surg Am 49:785–792, 1967.
10. Bernard B: Musculoskeletal Disorders and Workplace Factors: A Critical Review of the Epidemiological Evidence for Work-Related Musculoskeletal Disorders of the Neck, Upper Extremities, and Low Back. Washington, DC, National Institutes for Occupational Safety and Health Pub. 97-141, 1997.
11. Berry H, Kong K, Hudson AR, Moulton RJ: Isolated suprascapular nerve palsy: A review of nine cases. Can J Neurol Sci 22:301–304, 1995.
12. Biedert RM: Atrophy of the infraspinatus muscle caused by a suprascapular ganglion. Clin J Sport Med 6:262–263; discussion 264, 1996.
13. Bird SJ, Brown MJ: Acute focal neuropathy in male weight lifters. Muscle Nerve 19:897–899, 1996.
14. Boninger ML, Robertson RN, Wolff M, Cooper RA: Upper limb nerve entrapments in elite wheelchair racers. Am J Phys Med Rehabil 75:170–176, 1996.
15. Bradshaw C, McCrory P: Obturator nerve entrapment. Clin J Sport Med 7:217–219, 1997.
16. Bradshaw C, McCrory P, Bell S, Brukner P: Obturator nerve entrapment. A cause of groin pain in athletes. Am J Sports Med 25:402–408, 1997.
17. Bradshaw DY, Shefner JM: Ulnar neuropathy at the elbow. Neurol Clin 17:447–461, 1999.
18. Campbell WW: Ulnar neuropathy at the elbow. Muscle Nerve 23:450–452, 2000.
19. Carlson N, Logigian EL: Radial neuropathy. Neurol Clin 17:499–523, 1999.
20. Chance PF, Alderson MK, Leppig KA, Lensch MW, Matsunami N, et al: DNA deletion associated with hereditary neuropathy with liability to pressure palsies. Cell 72:143–151, 1993.
21. Cherington M: Hazards of bicycling: from handlebars to lightning. Semin Neurol 20:247–253, 2000.
22. Chiu DT: "Karate kid" finger. Plast Reconstr Surg 91: 362–364, 1993.
23. Cravens G, Kline DG: Posterior interosseous nerve palsies. Neurosurgery 27:397–402, 1990.
24. Crisci C, Baker MK, Wood MB, Litchy WJ, Dyck PJ: Trochanteric sciatic neuropathy. Neurology 39:1539–1541, 1989.
25. Davie C, Katifi H, Ridley A, Swash M: "Mouse"-trap or personal computer palsy. Lancet 338:832, 1991.
26. Destot M: Paralysie cubitale par l'usage de la bicyclette. Gaz Hop 69:1176–1177, 1896.
27. Deverell WF, Ferguson JH: An unusual case of sciatic nerve paralysis. JAMA 205:699–700, 1968.
28. Dobyns JH: Digital nerve compression. Hand Clin 8: 359–367, 1992.
29. Dobyns JH, O'Brien ET, Linscheid RL, Farrow GM: Bowler's thumb: Diagnosis and treatment. A review of seventeen cases. J Bone Joint Surg Am 54:751–755, 1972.
30. Dyck PJ: Peripheral Neuropathy, 3rd ed. Philadelphia, Saunders, 1993.
31. Fabian RH, Norcross KA, Hancock MB: Surfer's neuropathy. N Engl J Med 316:555, 1987.
32. Falkiner S, Myers S: When exactly can carpal tunnel syndrome be considered work-related? ANZ J Surg 72:204–209, 2002.
33. Fardin P, Negrin P, Sparta S, Zuliani C, Cacciavillani M, Colledan L: Posterior interosseous nerve neuropathy. Clinical and electromyographical aspects. Electromyogr Clin Neurophysiol 32:229–234, 1992.
34. Ferretti A, Cerullo G, Russo G: Suprascapular neuropathy in volleyball players. J Bone Joint Surg Am 69: 260–263, 1987.
35. Ferretti A, De Carli A, Fontana M: Injury of the suprascapular nerve at the spinoglenoid notch. The natural history of infraspinatus atrophy in volleyball players. Am J Sports Med 26:759–763, 1998.
36. Friedland RP, St John JN: Video-game palsy: Distal ulnar neuropathy in a video-game enthusiast. N Engl J Med 311:58–59, 1984.
37. Gatens PF, Saeed MA: Combat boot palsy: Case reports. Mil Med 147:664–666, 1982.
38. Goodman CE, Kenrick MM, Blum MV: Long thoracic nerve palsy: A follow-up study. Arch Phys Med Rehabil 56:352–358, 1975.
39. Goodson JD: Brachial plexus injury from light tight backpack straps. N Engl J Med 305:524–525, 1981.
40. Goodson JD: Pudendal neuritis from biking. N Engl J Med 304:365, 1981.
41. Gould N: Letter: Back-pocket sciatica. N Engl J Med 290:633, 1974.
42. Gross JA, Hamilton WJ, Swift TR: Isolated mechanical lesions of the sural nerve. Muscle Nerve 3:248–249, 1980.
43. Hankey GJ, Gubbay SS: Compressive mononeuropathy of the deep palmar branch of the ulnar nerve in cyclists. J Neurol Neurosurg Psychiatry 51:1588–1590, 1988.
44. Hashizume H, Nishida K, Nanba Y, Shigeyama Y, Inoue H, Morito Y: Nontraumatic paralysis of the posterior interosseous nerve. J Bone Joint Surg [Br] 78:771–776, 1996.
45. Hershfield NB: Pedaller's penis. Can Med Assoc J 128: 366–367, 1983.
46. Herskovitz S, Strauch B, Gordon MJ: Shiatsu massage–induced injury of the median recurrent motor branch. Muscle Nerve 15:1215, 1992.
47. Hill NA, Howard FM, Huffer BR: The incomplete anterior interosseous nerve syndrome. J Hand Surg [Am] 10:4–16, 1985.
48. Holzgraefe M, Kukowski B, Eggert S: Prevalence of latent and manifest suprascapular neuropathy in high-

performance volleyball players. Br J Sports Med 28:177–179, 1994.
49. Howell AE, Leach RE: Bowler's thumb. Perineural fibrosis of the digital nerve. J Bone Joint Surg [Am] 52: 379–381, 1970.
50. Hoyt CS: Letter: Ulnar neuropathy in bicycle riders. Arch Neurol 33:372, 1976.
51. Hunt J: The thenar and hypothenar types of neural atrophy of the hand. Am J Med Sci 141:224–241, 1911.
52. Ilfeld F, Holder H: Winged scapula: Case occurring in soldier from knapsack. JAMA 120:448–449, 1942.
53. Johnson JT, Kendall HO: Isolated paralysis of the serratus anterior muscle. J Bone Joint Surg [Am] 37-A:567–574, 1955.
54. Johnson RJ: Anatomy of backpack-strap injury. N Engl J Med 305:1594, 1981.
55. Jones HR Jr: Pizza cutter's palsy. N Engl J Med 319:450, 1988.
56. Kaplan PE: Electrodiagnostic confirmation of long thoracic nerve palsy. J Neurol Neurosurg Psychiatry 43:50–52, 1980.
57. Karatas GK, Gogus F: Suprascapular nerve entrapment in newsreel cameramen. Am J Phys Med Rehabil 82:192–196, 2003.
58. Katirji B: Peroneal nerve. In: Brown WF, Bolton CF, Aminoff MJ (eds): Neuromuscular Function and Disease: Basic, Clinical, and Electrodiagnostic Aspects, vol. I. Philadelphia, Saunders, 2002, pp 981–995.
59. Kiss G, Komar J: Suprascapular nerve compression at the spinoglenoid notch. Muscle Nerve 13:556–557, 1990.
60. Koller RL, Blank NK: Strawberry pickers' palsy. Arch Neurol 37:320, 1980.
61. Lacroix VJ, Kinnear DG, Mulder DS, Brown RA: Lower abdominal pain syndrome in national hockey league players: A report of 11 cases. Clin J Sport Med 8:5–9, 1998.
62. Leclerc A, Franchi P, Cristofari MF, Delemotte B, Mereau P, Teyssier-Cotte C, Touranchet A: Carpal tunnel syndrome and work organisation in repetitive work: A cross sectional study in France. Study Group on Repetitive Work. Occup Environ Med 55:180–187, 1998.
63. Lederman RJ: Neuromuscular and musculoskeletal problems in instrumental musicians. Muscle Nerve 27:549–561, 2003.
64. Levy AS, Smith RH: Neurologic injuries in skiers and snowboarders. Semin Neurol 20:233–245, 2000.
65. Lewis MB: Telesales neuropathy. Postgrad Med J 76:793–794, 2000.
66. Lindenbaum BL: Ski boot compression syndrome. Clin Orthop 140:109–110, 1979.
67. Liveson JA, Bronson MJ, Pollack MA: Suprascapular nerve lesions at the spinoglenoid notch: Report of three cases and review of the literature. J Neurol Neurosurg Psychiatry 54:241–243, 1991.
68. Lotem M, Fried A, Levy M, Solzi P, Najenson T, Nathan H: Radial palsy following muscular effort. A nerve compression syndrome possibly related to a fibrous arch of the lateral head of the triceps. J Bone Joint Surg [Br] 53:500–506, 1971.
69. Maimaris C, Zadeh HG: Ulnar nerve compression in the cyclist's hand: Two case reports and review of the literature. Br J Sports Med 24:245–246, 1990.
70. Marie P, Foix C: Atrophie isolee de l'eminence thenar d'origine neuritique:role du ligament annulaire anterieur dans la localization de la lesion. Rev Neurol (Paris) 26: 647–649, 1913.
71. McCrory P, Bell S, Bradshaw C: Nerve entrapments of the lower leg, ankle and foot in sport. Sports Med 32:371–391, 2002.
72. Miller EH, Benedict FE: Stretch of the femoral nerve in a dancer. A case report. J Bone Joint Surg [Am] 67:315–317, 1985.
73. Mitsunaga MM, Nakano K: High radial nerve palsy following strenuous muscular activity. A case report. Clin Orthop 234:39–42, 1988.
74. Montagna P, Colonna S: Suprascapular neuropathy restricted to the infraspinatus muscle in volleyball players. Acta Neurol Scand 87:248–250, 1993.
75. Morris HH, Peters BH: Pronator syndrome: Clinical and electrophysiological features in seven cases. J Neurol Neurosurg Psychiatry 39:461–464, 1976.
76. Muntz H, Conrad R, Murchison R: Rifle-sling palsy. Armed Forces Med J 8:1189–1194, 1957.
77. Nahabedian MY, Dellon AL: Meralgia paresthetica: Etiology, diagnosis, and outcome of surgical decompression. Ann Plast Surg 35:590–594, 1995.
78. Nordstrom DL, Vierkant RA, DeStefano F, Layde PM: Risk factors for carpal tunnel syndrome in a general population. Occup Environ Med 54:734–740, 1997.
79. Packer GJ, McLatchie GR, Bowden W: Scapula winging in a sports injury clinic. Br J Sports Med 27:90–91, 1993.
80. Perkins BA, Olaleye D, Bril V: Carpal tunnel syndrome in patients with diabetic polyneuropathy. Diabetes Care 25:565–569, 2002.
81. Perlmutter GS, Leffert RD, Zarins B: Direct injury to the axillary nerve in athletes playing contact sports. Am J Sports Med 25:65–68, 1997.
82. Petrera JE, Trojaborg W: Conduction studies along the accessory nerve and follow-up of patients with trapezius palsy. J Neurol Neurosurg Psychiatry 47:630–636, 1984.
83. Prochaska V, Crosby LA, Murphy RP: High radial nerve palsy in a tennis player. Orthop Rev 22:90–92, 1993.
84. Ringel SP, Treihaft M, Carry M, Fisher R, Jacobs P: Suprascapular neuropathy in pitchers. Am J Sports Med 18:80–86, 1990.
85. Roquelaure Y, Mechali S, Dano C, Fanello S, Benetti F, et al: Occupational and personal risk factors for carpal tunnel syndrome in industrial workers. Scand J Work Environ Health 23:364–369, 1997.
86. Seppalainen AM, Aho K, Uusitupa M: Strawberry pickers' foot drop. Br Med J 2:767, 1977.
87. Shyu WC, Lin JC, Chang MK, Tsao WL: Compressive radial nerve palsy induced by military shooting training: Clinical and electrophysiological study. J Neurol Neurosurg Psychiatry 56:890–893, 1993.
88. Siegel DB, Kuzma G, Eakins D: Anatomic investigation

of the role of the lumbrical muscles in carpal tunnel syndrome. J Hand Surg [Am] 20:860–863, 1995.
89. Sinson G, Zager EL, Kline DG: Windmill pitcher's radial neuropathy. Neurosurgery 34:1087–1089; discussion 1089–1090, 1994.
90. Smith EM, Sonstegard DA, Anderson WH Jr: Carpal tunnel syndrome: Contribution of flexor tendons. Arch Phys Med Rehabil 58:379–385, 1977.
91. Solomon S, Cappa KG: Impotence and bicycling. A seldom-reported connection. Postgrad Med 81:99–100, 102, 1987.
92. Stallings SP, Kasdan ML, Soergel TM, Corwin HM: A case-control study of obesity as a risk factor for carpal tunnel syndrome in a population of 600 patients presenting for independent medical examination. J Hand Surg [Am] 22:211–215, 1997.
93. Stewart JD: Focal Peripheral Neuropathies, 3rd ed. Philadelphia, Lippincott Williams & Wilkins, 2000.
94. Stewart JD, Angus E, Gendron D: Sciatic neuropathies. Br Med J (Clin Res Ed) 287:1108–1109, 1983.
95. Stock SR: Workplace ergonomic factors and the development of musculoskeletal disorders of the neck and upper limbs: A meta-analysis. Am J Ind Med 19:87–107, 1991.
96. Streib E: Upper arm radial nerve palsy after muscular effort: Report of three cases. Neurology 42:1632–1634, 1992.
97. Szabo RM, Chidgey LK: Stress carpal tunnel pressures in patients with carpal tunnel syndrome and normal patients. J Hand Surg [Am] 14:624–627, 1989.
98. Takagishi K, Maeda K, Ikeda T, Itoman M, Yamamoto M: Ganglion causing paralysis of the suprascapular nerve. Diagnosis by MRI and ultrasonography. Acta Orthop Scand 62:391–393, 1991.
99. Tanaka S, Wild DK, Seligman PJ, Halperin WE, Behrens VJ, Putz-Anderson V: Prevalence and work-relatedness of self-reported carpal tunnel syndrome among U.S. workers: Analysis of the Occupational Health Supplement data of 1988 National Health Interview Survey. Am J Ind Med 27:451–470, 1995.
100. Tanzer RC: The carpal-tunnel syndrome; a clinical and anatomical study. J Bone Joint Surg [Am] 41–A:626–634, 1959.
101. Tengan CH, Oliveira AS, Kiymoto BH, Morita MP, De Medeiros JL, Gabbai AA: Isolated and painless infraspinatus atrophy in top-level volleyball players. Report of two cases and review of the literature. Arq Neuropsiquiatr 51:125–129, 1993.
102. Vender MI, Kasdan ML, Truppa KL: Upper extremity disorders: A literature review to determine work-relatedness. J Hand Surg [Am] 20:534–541, 1995.
103. Vinken PJ, Bruyn GW: Diseases of nerves. In: Vinken PJ, Bruyn GW (eds): Handbook of Clinical Neurology. Amsterdam, New York, North-Holland, American Elsevier 1970.
104. Vogel CM, Albin R, Alberts JW: Lotus footdrop: Sciatic neuropathy in the thigh. Neurology 41:605–606, 1991.
105. Wang DH, Koehler SM: Isolated infraspinatus atrophy in a collegiate volleyball player. Clin J Sport Med 6:255–258, 1996.
106. Weiss BD: Nontraumatic injuries in amateur long distance bicyclists. Am J Sports Med 13:187–192, 1985.
107. Wertsch JJ: Pricer palsy. N Engl J Med 312:1645, 1985.
108. Yuen EC, So YT, Olney RK: The electrophysiologic features of sciatic neuropathy in 100 patients. Muscle Nerve 18:414–420, 1995.
109. Zeiss J, Woldenberg LS, Saddemi SR, Ebraheim NA: MRI of suprascapular neuropathy in a weight lifter. J Comput Assist Tomogr 17:303–308, 1993

Chapter 20

Electrodiagnostic Studies in the Evaluation of Peripheral Nerve Injuries

BASHAR KATIRJI

Injuries to peripheral nerves are most prevalent in young adults between the age of 18 and 35 years and result in substantial disability. These lesions are much more common during wartime, but they also often accompany civilian trauma that results from motor vehicle accidents, motorcycle accidents, industrial accidents, and gunshot or knife wounds.[12,13,15] Traumatic nerve injuries may be direct (such as with stab wounds) or indirect (such as with radial neuropathy following humeral fracture). Also, a significant percentage of peripheral nerve injuries encountered in clinical practice are iatrogenic, occurring in the setting of surgical or radiological procedures, needle injuries, and, occasionally, following medical therapy, such as with the use of anticoagulation.[1,8,14,24]

The incidence of peripheral nerve, plexus, or root injury among patients admitted to Level 1 trauma centers during peacetime is about 5%.[12,13] Peripheral nerve injury is often accompanied by other bodily injuries including fractures, dislocations, and other soft tissue damage. Also, head injury is commonly associated with peripheral nerve trauma, and in the setting of severe head or spine injury, peripheral nerve lesions are often overlooked.[18] Unfortunately, the long-term prognosis for the majority of peripheral nerve injuries remains poor. However, recent advances in diagnostic techniques (including intraoperative studies) and surgical techniques (including nerve grafting) have improved the outcome in some patients, particularly when evaluated and treated in tertiary hospitals with specialized peripheral nerve centers.[5,9,10,17,19,22]

Anatomically, the peripheral nerve is composed of unmyelinated and myelinated axons surrounded by Schwann cells and a supporting tissue.[19] The unmyelinated axon is surrounded only by the plasma membrane of Schwann cells. The myelinated axon is wrapped around several times by Schwann cells that insulate the axon by multiple layers of their sphingomyelin-rich cell membrane. Nerve fibers are surrounded by three supportive layers that are highly elastic and serve as shields to protect the myelin and axon from external pressure and tension. These layers include the endoneurium, perineurium, and epineurium. The myelinated axon is completely surrounded by myelin and Schwann cells except at certain gaps, called the *nodes of Ranvier*, where sodium channels are highly concentrated. In adults, the length of myelinated segments, called the *internodal segments*, is approximately 1 mm, while the nodes of Ranvier measure approximately 1 μm. Saltatory conduction occurs in myelinated axons through the nodes of Ranvier due their high sodium channel concentration and the low capacitance and large resistance of the internodal myelin.

Classification of Nerve Injuries

Compression, traction, laceration, and thermal or chemical injury may damage one or more components of the peripheral nerves, while the pathophysiological responses to these peripheral nerve injuries have a limited repertoire, that is, axon loss, demyelination, or a combination of both. In practice, most traumatic peripheral nerve lesions result in some degree of axonal damage with variable destruction to the supporting structures, while pure demyelination plays a relatively minor role in the pathophysiology of these lesions.

Peripheral nerve injuries are classified on the basis of the functional status of the nerve and histological findings. Seddon proposed a classification of peripheral nerve injury that remains popular, particularly among surgeons, because of its correlation to the outcome.[15] Later, Sunderland revised the classification into five degrees that have better prognostic implications (Table 20.1).[19]

a. *Neurapraxia (first-degree nerve injury)*. This usually results from brief or mild compression of the nerve that distorts the myelin, resulting in segmental demyelination but leaving the axons intact. The nerve conducts normally distal to the lesion but not across the lesion, resulting in conduction block, which is the electrophysiological correlate of neurapraxia (see below). With this type of injury, there is little or no change in the muscles, and recovery is usually complete following remyelination, which occurs within 1–3 months if the cause (such as a hematoma) is removed.
b. *Axonotmesis*. This type of injury is characterized by axonal damage that results in wallerian degeneration; distal to the of injury, the axons and their investing myelin sheath degenerate (wallerian degeneration) and the end organs (muscle fibers and sensory receptors) become denervated. However, with this type of injury, there is variable disruption of the supporting structures (endoneurium, perineurium, and epineurium) that, in turn, predicts variable degrees of improvement. Sunderland proposed that these lesions should be divided into three further subtypes,[19] since peripheral nerve injury may at times affect one or several components of the surrounding nerve stroma:
   1. *Second-degree nerve injury*, in which axon loss is associated with intact endoneurial tubes, as well as intact perineurium and epineurium. These lesions have a fairly good prognosis that depends mostly on the distance between the site of nerve injury and the muscles.
   2. *Third-degree nerve injury*, in which the axons, Schwann cell tubes, and endoneurium are damaged while leaving the perineurium and epineurium intact. These lesions have a fair prognosis and may require surgical intervention, mostly because of axonal misdirection and formation of neuromas.
   3. *Fourth-degree nerve injury*, in which the perineurium is also disrupted but the epineurium is intact. These lesions have a poor prognosis, and often require surgical repair.
c. *Neurotmesis (fifth-degree nerve injury)*. This is the most severe type of nerve injury, manifesting as complete disruption of the nerve with all the supporting structures. The nerve is transected, with loss of continuity between its proximal and distal stumps.

Scope, Indications for, and Limitations of the Electrodiagnostic Study in Nerve Injury

The electrodiagnostic (EDX) examination comprises a group of tests that are usually complementary to each other and often necessary for a final diagnosis. These include the nerve conduction studies (NCS), which include sensory, motor, and mixed NCS, and the needle electromyographic (EMG) examination.[6,7] Other special studies, which are occasionally useful in the evaluation of peripheral nerve injury, include F-waves and H-reflexes.[6,7]

Sensory NCS evaluates sensory axons by stimulating a peripheral nerve while recording the compound sensory nerve action potential (SNAP) from

Table 20.1. Classification of Peripheral Nerve Injury

Seddon classification	Neurapraxia	Axonotmesis			Neurotmesis
Sunderland classification	First degree	Second degree	Third degree	Fourth degree	Fifth degree
Electrodiagnostic findings	Conduction block		Axonal loss		
Pathological findings	Segmental demyelination with intact axons and supporting structures	Loss of axons and myelin with intact supporting structures	Loss of axons and myelin with disrupted endoneurium only	Loss of axons and myelin with disrupted endoneurium and perineurium	Loss of axons and myelin with disruption of all supporting structures (transection)
Prognosis	Excellent; recovery is usually complete in 2–3 months	Slow but good recovery; dependent on sprouting and reinnervation	Protracted improvement that may fail due to misdirected axonal sprouts	Unlikely improvement without surgical repair	Improvement impossible without surgical repair

the same nerve at a different site. This can be done antidromically (recording SNAP directed toward the sensory receptors) or orthodromically (recording SNAP directed away from these receptors). The SNAP amplitude, measured in microvolts, is a semiquantitative measure of the number of sensory axons that conduct between the stimulation and recording sites, while latencies and conduction velocity reflect the speed of the fastest (largest) sensory conducting axons.

Motor NCS is performed by stimulating a peripheral nerve while recording the compound muscle action potential (CMAP) from a muscle innervated by that nerve. This technique produces a useful magnification effect, since activation of a single motor axon results in action potentials in up to several hundred individual muscle fibers, depending upon the innervation ratio of the recorded muscle. Hence, surface-recorded CMAP amplitude and area are relatively large and are measured in millivolts. They are semiquantitative measurements of the number of axons conducting between the stimulating and recording points, while distal latencies and conduction velocities assess the speed of the largest (fastest) motor axons.

Mixed NCS is performed by stimulating and recording from a mixed nerve trunk with sensory and motor axons. Often, these tests are done by stimulating a nerve trunk distally and recording more proximally, since the reverse testing is often contaminated by large CMAP that obscures the relatively low-amplitude mixed nerve action potentials (MNAPs). In situations where the nerve is deep and considerable tissue is interposed between the nerve and the electrode (such as at the elbow or knee), the MNAP may be very low in amplitude or unelicitable. Hence, these studies are now restricted to evaluating mixed nerves in distal nerve segments, such as in the hand or foot (e.g., for carpal tunnel or tarsal tunnel syndrome).

Needle EMG is performed by inserting a concentric or monopolar needle electrode into individual muscles of interest and evaluating their spontaneous and insertional activities, as well as voluntary motor unit action potential (MUAP) recruitment and activation and MUAP morphology. In normal conditions, muscle exhibit silence at rest with no spontaneous activities. With voluntary contraction, MUAPs normally fire in a semirhythmic pattern. As force is increased, the firing rate as well as the number of MUAPs recruited increase. As this process continues, the ratio of firing frequency to the number of MUAPs firing is usually maintained at approximately 5:1. For example, when a third unit get recruited, the firing rate of the first unit should not exceed about 15 Hz (15:3 = 5:1). Motor unit action potential morphology (duration, amplitude, and phases) varies, depending on the muscle tested and the age of the patient. The duration of MUAP depends primarily on the number of muscle fibers within a motor unit and is typically between 5 and 15 msec. Motor unit action potentials have more variable amplitudes, depending on how close the recording electrode is to activated muscle fibers, but they are usually greater than 100 μV and less than 2 mV. Normally, MUAPs have up to four phases, though up to 10% of MUAPs in distal muscles and up to 25% of MUAPs in proximal muscles (such as the iliacus or deltoid) may have increased polyphasia.

The EDX examination is the most important test in the evaluation of patients with peripheral nerve injury. The *indications* for an EDX examination depend on the clinical situation. Sometimes, the study is requested to verify that a focal peripheral nerve lesion has occurred, such in a patient whose clinical examination may preclude confirming or excluding a focal peripheral neuropathy due to multiple bodily injuries, tendon rupture, head trauma, or severe pain. For example, a patient with a ruptured flexor pollicis longus tendon may not be able to flex the thumb (mimicking an anterior interosseous neuropathy) but will have, on needle EMG, normal insertional and spontaneous activities, as well as normal MUAP recruitment and morphology. Apart from diagnosis, the other major roles of the EDX examination in patients with peripheral nerve injury are to accurately localize the site of injury, determine the pathophysiology, semiquantitate the extent and severity of the injury, estimate the prognosis, and assess the progress of reinnervation.

Despite their useful role in peripheral nerve trauma, EDX studies have several *limitations* that should be considered before a test is requested or interpreted. Three limitations apply to EDX studies in general. First, these studies only assess the extrafusal (alpha) motor axons and the large myelinated sensory axons (that conduct position, vibration, and light touch). They cannot evaluate thinly myelinated or unmyelinated axons (that transmit pain and temperature sensation). Second, some muscles are inaccessible to needle EMG (e.g., the psoas muscle), and certain nerves are not amenable to NCS (e.g., genitofemoral and ilioinguinal nerves). Third, several other factors may prevent accurate localization of nerve lesions, such as the presence of an underlying peripheral polyneuropathy (such as in diabetics) or inability to record SNAPs (such with severe limb edema and in older patients in the lower limbs). In addition to these general shortcomings , there are additional EDX limitations that are pertinent to patients with peripheral nerve injuries. First and most important, the EDX studies have a limited range of findings, since they only evaluate the integrity of the myelin sheath and axon. They cannot assess the extent of the damage to the supporting structure of the peripheral nerve, since injury to these structure has no discernible effect on physiology. Hence, EDX examinations can only distinguish a neurapraxic injury (first-degree nerve injury), where only the myelin is damaged while the axons remain intact, from all other degrees of injury that are associated with axonal damage and wallerian degeneration (second through fifth degrees of nerve injury). A second disadvantage of the EDX studies is specific to patients with peripheral nerve injury associated with other bodily trauma. In those patients, nerves and muscles may become inaccessible to the NCSs or needle EMG due to compounding factors such as large scars, casts, or metal hardware.

Evolution of Wallerian Degeneration

Following focal axon loss, the distal axons undergo a degenerative process known as *wallerian degeneration*. This occurs because all the necessary building blocks needed for maintaining the axon are made in the cell body (peikaryon) and cannot reach the distal stump. The rate at which wallerian degeneration proceeds varies, depending on the nerve injured, the axon diameter, and the length of the distal stump (the larger and longer the distal stump, the more time is needed for wallerian degeneration to be completed).[11] Within hours of most nerve injuries, myelin begins to retract from the axons at the nodes of Ranvier. This is followed by swelling of the distal nerve segment, leakage of axoplasm, and, subsequently, the disappearance of neurofibrils. Within days, the axon and myelin fragment, and digestion of nerve components starts. By the end of the first week, the axon and myelin become fully digested and Schwann cells start to bridge the gap between the two nerve segments. In chronic nerve lesions, the endoneurial tubes in the distal stump shrink, the nerve fascicles distal to the lesion atrophy, and, in complete nerve transection, the severed ends retract away from each other.[11]

In addition to the severe changes that occur distal to the lesion, proximal nerve fibers degenerate for a variable distance, depending on the severity of the lesion, usually up to several centimeters from the site of injury (retrograde degeneration).[19] Also, the Nissl bodies (rough endoplasmic reticulum) within the perikaryon disintegrate into fine particles, and by the third week, the nucleus becomes displaced eccentrically and the nucleolus is also eccentrically placed within the nucleus. These cell body changes are more dramatic with proximal than distal nerve injuries.

On NCS, wallerian degeneration manifests by a progressive decline in the distal CMAP and SNAP amplitudes and areas.[2,4,23] Soon after the insult, the CMAP and SNAP obtained by stimulation distal to the lesion are normal, while their proximal counterparts are lower in amplitude (in partial lesions) or absent (in complete lesions). The distal CMAP remains normal for 1–2 days postinjury and then falls precipitously, reaching its nadir by 5–6 days. In contrast to the motor NCS, the distal SNAP remains normal for 5–6 days and then decreases rapidly, reaching its nadir in 10–11 days (Fig. 20.1). This discrepancy between the distal CMAP and SNAP is best explained by the early failure of neuromuscular transmission, which affects recording the CMAP while having no bearing on the SNAP.

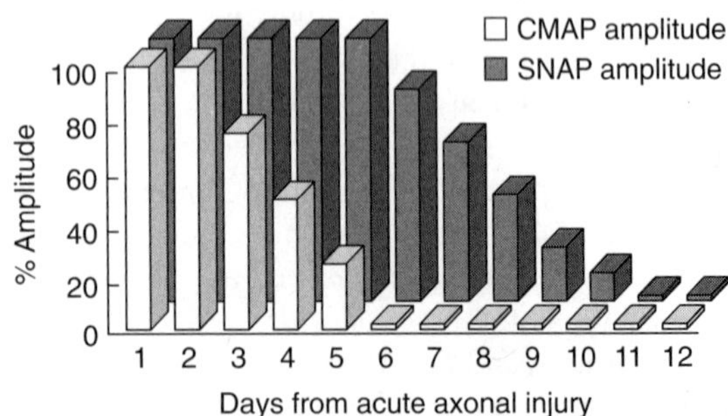

Figure 20.1. The effect of wallerian degeneration on the distal compound muscle action potential (CMAP) and sensory nerve action potential (SNAP) amplitudes overtime.

Needle EMG of muscles innervated by the damaged nerve reveals several changes that have a more protracted time course compared to the NCS changes (Table 20.2). The earliest finding is a loss of voluntary activity (in a complete lesion) or a decrease in the number of MUAPs that recruit rapidly at rates reaching 25–40 Hz (in a partial lesion). The rapid firing rate of the residual MUAPs is highly specific for a lesion that involves the lower motor neuron (i.e., a peripheral nervous system lesion), resulting in axon loss, demyelinating conduction block, or both. The rapid rate of MUAP firing also helps to distinguish the dropout of MUAPs from that which accompanies poor patient effort or a central disorder of motor unit control. In these situations, there is poor activation of MUAPs, which fire at slow or moderate rates (usually less that 10 Hz) despite apparent full patient effort.

Soon after partial peripheral nerve injury, the residual MUAPs have normal morphology (amplitude, duration, and phases). However, following the completion of wallerian degeneration, the trophic influence of the nerve on muscle disappears and denervation changes appear. At about the second week, there is increased insertional activity and fibrillation potentials begin to appear in denervated muscles. Fibrillation potentials are spontaneous action potentials generated by denervated muscle fibers. They always reflect evidence of axonal injury, though they are also seen in certain necrotizing myopathies that are associated with segmental muscle degeneration and denervation. In acute axonal lesions, fibrillation potentials appear first in proximally situated muscles and proceed distally. For example, following an ulnar nerve injury at the elbow, fibrillation potentials may appear as early as 10–15 days in the flexor digitorum profundus but require about 3 weeks before they are detected in the hand muscles. Similarly, with C5 root avulsion, fibrillation potentials may be seen in the midcervical paraspinal muscles as early as 1 week postinjury but will not appear in muscles innervated by the C5 myotome (such as the biceps, brachioradialis, deltoid, and spinati) until 2–3 weeks postinjury. In general, fibrillation potentials become widespread in all denervated muscles by 3 weeks and are most abundant at about 4–6 weeks after axonal nerve injury (see Table 20.2). They ultimately decrease in number due to either reinnervation of muscle fibers or fatty degeneration of chronically denervated muscle fibers.

Electrodiagnostic Findings in Peripheral Nerve Injuries

The EDX studies are the cornerstone in the diagnosis and management of nerve injuries. Soon after injury, these studies provide valuable information on the location, severity, and pathophysiology of the lesion. Intraoperatively, EDX studies guide the surgeon and help assess the status of the regenerating axons within the injured nerve segment. During the recovery stage of peripheral nerve injury, EDX studies are also essential in the evaluation of remyelination, regeneration, and reinnervation that may occur spontaneously or following surgical intervention.

Initial Diagnostic Studies

The diagnosis of peripheral nerve injury often requires a detailed history and a neurological examination, with the EDX studies and surgical findings playing very important roles in diagnosis and management. Although the site of the nerve injury may occasionally be remote from the location of the external injury, the history and physical examination are extremely important in predicting the location, type, and severity of the nerve lesion. For example, a history of stab wound injury to the sciatic nerve in the buttock is often associated with axonal interruptions and grade 3 to 5 nerve injuries, while intraoperative peroneal nerve compression at the fibular neck is either a grade 1 (neurapraxic) or 2 (axonotmetic) nerve injury.

Localization of Nerve Lesions Using Nerve Conduction Studies

In general, there are three electrophysiological manifestations of peripheral nerve injury that can be assessed by NCSs. These include conduction block, focal slowing of conduction, and axon loss (conduction failure).[25] The first two are due to disruption of myelin, and are benign and often resolve spontaneously. The third is due to axonal damage, is more severe, and may be irreversible. Combined patterns may also occur.

Conduction block is caused by blockage of transmission of action potentials across the injured nerve segment. Normally, the action potential travels in a saltatory fashion, passing the nodes of Ranvier without failure. Conduction block is usually the result of loss of one or more myelin segments (seg-

Table 20.2. Evolution of the Electrodiagnostic Changes in Moderate to Severe Axon Loss Focal Nerve Injury

Time of EDX Study in Relation to Time of Injury	Sensory NCS	Motor NCS	Insertional Activity	Spontaneous Activity	MUAP Recruitment	MUAP Morphology
Immediately to days 1–2	Normal distal SNAP	Normal distal CMAP with proximal conduction block (partial or complete)	Normal	Normal	Decreased (partial lesion) or no voluntary activity (complete lesion)	Normal
Between day 2 and day 5	Normal distal SNAP	Low-amplitude distal CMAP with conduction block or absent CMAPs at all stimulation sites	Normal	Normal	Decreased (partial lesion) or no voluntary activity (complete lesion)	Normal
Between day 6 and day 11	Low-amplitude distal SNAP	Low-amplitude (partial lesion) or absent (complete lesion) CMAPs at all stimulation sites	Normal or slightly increased	Normal	Decreased (partial lesion) or no voluntary activity (complete lesion)	Normal
Between day 12 and day 30	Absent distal SNAP	Low-amplitude (partial lesion) or absent (complete lesion) CMAPs at all stimulation sites	Increased	Scattered fibrillation potentials appearing in proximal muscles	Decreased (partial lesion) or no voluntary activity (complete lesion)	Normal
Between 1 and 3 months	Absent distal SNAP	Low-amplitude (partial lesion) or absent (complete lesion) CMAPs at all stimulation sites	Increased	Abundant fibrillation potentials in all denervated muscles	Decreased (partial lesion) or no voluntary activity (complete lesion)	Polyphasic with satellites and unstable
Months to years (with reinnervation)	Low-amplitude to absent distal SNAP	Low-amplitude CMAPs at all stimulation sites	Normal or decreased (with atrophy)	Absent or rare fibrillation potentials	Decreased	Long-duration, high amplitudes, but stable

CMAP, compound muscle action potential; EDX, electrodiagnostic; MUAP, motor unit action potential; NCS, nerve conduction study; SNAP, sensory nerve action potential.

mental or internodal demyelination) and is the electrophysiological counterpart of neurapraxia (first-degree nerve injury). During NCSs, conduction block manifests as a significant drop in CMAP amplitude and area with stimulation proximal to the injury site, when compared with the CMAP distal to it, without evidence of significant temporal dispersion (i.e., prolongation of CMAP duration). Conduction block may be complete (involving all the myelinated axons) or partial (involving some myelinated fibers while leaving others normal) (Table 20.3). A nerve lesion manifesting with conduction block is best localized when it can be bracketed by two stimulation points, one distal to the site of injury (resulting in a normal CMAP) and one proximal (resulting in a partial or complete drop in CMAP) (Fig. 20.2).

Focal slowing of conduction reflects nerve fibers that have undergone widening of the nodes of Ranvier (paranodal demyelination). When isolated, focal slowing is not associated with weakness or sensory loss. However, in a mixed lesion where some fibers have undergone paranodal demyelination and others axon loss, focal slowing is a convenient method for accurate localization of the exact site of the peripheral nerve injury. When the large myelinated fibers are slowed to essentially the same degree, *focal slowing (synchronized slowing)* of conduction across the involved nerve segment is evident on NCSs, while other segments of the same nerve as well as neighboring nerves remain normal. This is shown by either a prolongation of distal latencies (in distal lesions) or slowing in conduction velocities (in proximal lesions). In contrast,

Table 20.3. Electrodiagnostic Criteria for Conduction Block

Definite°
1. ≥50% drop in CMAP amplitude with ≤15% prolongation of CMAP duration, or
2. ≥50% drop in CMAP area, or
3. ≥20% drop in area or amplitude over a short nerve segment (10 cm or less)

Possible°
1. 20%–50% drop in CMAP amplitude with ≤15% prolongation of CMAP duration, or
2. 20%–50% drop in CMAP area

CMAP = compound muscle action potential.

°Caution should be used in evaluating the tibial nerve, where stimulation at the knee may yield ≥ 50% drop in amplitude, especially in obese patients.

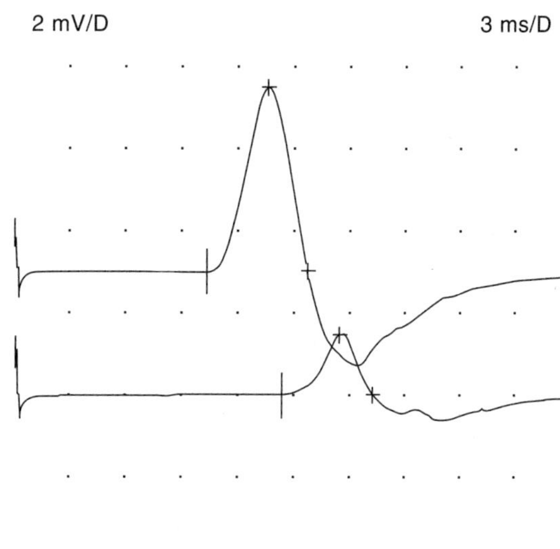

Figure 20.2. Partial conduction block of the ulnar nerve across the elbow in a patient who awoke after abdominal surgery with weakness of the hand. The top response followed stimulation below the elbow, and the bottom response followed stimulation above the elbow. Note the significant (>50%) drop across the elbow of compound muscle action potential amplitudes (from 4.5 to 1.5 mV) and areas (from 11.4 to 2.9 mVms), findings that confirmed an ulnar neuropathy across the elbow. Since the study was performed 2 days after symptom onset, the findings could be due to segmental demyelination (neurapraxia or first-degree nerve injury), axon loss, or both. A repeat nerve conduction studies after 10–11 days from injury would answer this question.

CMAP amplitude and duration are not affected and do not change when the nerve is stimulated proximal to the lesion. When the speed of impulse transmission is reduced at the lesion site along a variable number of medium-sized or small nerve fibers (average- or slower-conducting axons), *differential slowing (desynchronized slowing)* of conduction across the nerve segment is evident. In this situation, CMAP is dispersed on stimulation proximal to the lesion and has prolonged duration, with a normal (nondispersed) response on distal stimulation. If this finding is isolated, the speed of conduction along the injury site (distal latency or conduction velocity) is normal, since at least some of the fastest-conducting axons are spared. However, since the large fibers are often involved as well, differential slowing is usually accompanied by focal slowing of distal latency or conduction velocity.

In cases where there has been *axonal damage following the completion of wallerian degeneration*, the NCSs characteristically result in unelicitable or uniformly low CMAP amplitude, which is not dispersed, at all stimulation points. This pattern unfortunately cannot localize the site of injury to a specific segment of the nerve, and other measures need to be considered such the history, clinical examination, and needle EMG.

Nerve conduction studies, done on patients with *axonal damage before the completion of wallerian degeneration*, require special attention since they can be a source of error in localizing, characterizing, or prognosticating about nerve lesions. However, these studies are useful, since they often help localize lesions better than if NCSs are done after the completion of wallerian degeneration. Early after axonal damage, the distal stump remains excitable for a variable period, with some differences between the motor and sensory responses. The distal CMAP remains normal for 1 to 2 days after injury, giving rise to a pattern of conduction block on NCS that mimics the one seen with segmental demyelination (see Fig. 20.2). This pattern, sometimes referred to as *axonal noncontinuity, early axon loss, and axon discontinuity* conduction block, is important to recognize since it carries a poor prognosis, in contrast to the conduction block caused by segmental demyelination, which usually recovers rapidly and completely. As wallerian degeneration progresses following axon injury, the distal CMAP then falls precipitously, reaching its nadir by 5–6 days postinjury, and the conduction block pattern is replaced by unelicitable CMAPs in complete lesions or uniformly low-amplitude CMAPs in partial lesions that are independent of the stimulation sites. In contrast to the findings on motor studies, the distal sensory nerve remains excitable for a longer period. The distal SNAP remains normal for 5–6 days and then decreases rapidly, reaching its nadir in 10–11 days (see fig. 20.1).

Mixed lesions exhibit a variety of pathophysiology including axon loss and segmental demyelination. In acute nerve lesions, this often manifests as axon loss and conduction block, while focal slowing tends to be a feature of more chronic lesions (e.g., entrapment neuropathies). By analyzing distal and proximal CMAPs as well as distal SNAPs, the EDX study can estimate semiquantitavely the number of axons that have undergone wallerian degeneration and those that have segmental demyelination.

Another important role of NCS, particularly sensory NCS, is to distinguish between preganglionic (intraspinal canal) lesions (e.g., avulsion injuries) and postganglionic (extraspinal canal) lesions (e.g., brachial plexus injuries). Since SNAPs assess sensory axons, or their cell bodies in the dorsal root ganglia (DRGs), sensory axonal loss located proximal to the DRG does not affect SNAP amplitude, because the peripheral sensory axons originating from the unipolar DRG neurons remain intact. Since the DRGs are usually located outside of the spinal canal and within the intervertebral foramina, traumatic root avulsions have no effect on SNAP amplitudes. These lesions, however, often result in motor axon degeneration, as reflected by abnormal needle EMG and, when severe, by low-amplitude CMAP. In contrast to these intraspinal canal lesions, axon loss brachial plexopathies affect CMAP as well as SNAP amplitudes when mixed nerves undergo wallerian degeneration. This is discussed in detail in chapter 18.

Localization of Nerve Lesions Using Needle Electromyography

The earliest finding on needle EMG following a nerve injury is a complete loss of voluntary activity (in a complete lesion) or a decrease in MUAP recruitment (in a partial lesion) in weak muscles. This is the result of failure of nerve action potentials to reach the target muscle that follows nerve lesions associated with axon loss or segmental demyelination. Hence, a decrease in MUAP recruitment per se cannot distinguish between axon loss and demyelinating lesions. Also, the degree of impaired MUAP recruitment correlates with the extent of clinical weakness and is proportional to the number of lost or demyelinated axons.

Axon loss lesions studied by NCSs prior to wallerian degeneration, as well as demyelinating (neurapraxic) lesions, are often precisely localized to a short segment of the nerve due to the presence of conduction block across that segment. Hence, localization of lesions by needle EMG is most important in axon loss lesions that are first studied following the completion of wallerian degeneration of motor axons (more than 5–6 days postinjury). These lesions are associated with nonlocalizable NCSs that are characterized by low-amplitude or unelicitable CMAPs from all nerve simulation sites.

The concept of localization by needle EMG is similar to that of clinical localization using manual muscle strength testing that is part of the neurological examination. It is assumed that muscles innervated by branches arising from the nerve distal to the lesion are weak, while those innervated by branches proximal to the lesion are normal. Clinical localization of the site of the lesion is usually accurate in sharp, well-defined penetrating injuries such as laceration of the median or ulnar nerves. However, this may not be possible in patients with extensive trauma that may involve several nerves or elements of a plexus. In these cases, EDX studies play a major role in localization.

Localization by needle EMG alone follows the same rules as the manual muscle examination but relies on electrophysiological changes detected during the study, namely, fibrillation potentials, reduced MUAP recruitment, and MUAP changes characteristic of reinnervation. Unfortunately, several type of axon loss lesions may pose problems when attempting to localize the site of the injury solely by needle EMG.[25]

1. *Nerve lesions along segments with no motor branches*. The anatomy of the injured nerve plays an important role in the precise localization of nerve lesions. Many nerves travel substantial distances without giving out any motor branches. Examples include the median and ulnar nerves, which have very long segments in the arm from which no motor branches arise. Hence, long segment localization along one of these nerves may be of relatively little assistance to the clinician simply because the focal lesion may be at any point along the nerve segment. In contrast to the median and ulnar nerves, the radial nerve is more useful for localization by needle EMG, since it gives off multiple motor branches at fairly regular and short intervals.
2. *Fascicular nerve lesions.* Occasionally, peripheral nerve lesions spare one or two nerve fascicles, resulting in muscles that escape denervation despite being located distal to the lesion site. This usually results in an erroneous localization that is more distal to the actual site of the lesion. The explanation for this phenomenon is not always satisfactory, but one theory suggests that the spared fascicle occupies a protected location on the nerve at the lesion site or that the intact fascicle exits the nerve at or near the lesion site. Examples of this fascicular involvement include sparing of ulnar muscles in the forearm (flexor carpi ulnaris and ulnar part of the flexor digitorum profundus) following development of an axon loss ulnar nerve lesion at the elbow, and sparing the superficial peroneal innervated muscles (peroneus longus and brevis) following development of an axon loss common peroneal nerve lesion at the knee or fibular neck.
3. *Chronic nerve lesions.* The process of reinnervation include proximodistal regeneration of nerve fibers, from the site of the injury, collateral sprouting, or both (see below). Often with partial axon loss lesions that are mild or modest, proximodistal regeneration and reinnervation can be extremely efficient in proximally located muscles, resulting in remodeling of the motor units. Hence, a needle EMG done several years after the development of such lesions may only detect the neurogenic changes in the more distal muscles and result in mislocalizing the lesion more distally.

Timing of Initial Electrodiagnostic Studies

The ideal timing of the initial EDX study in a patient with peripheral nerve injury depends on the clinical situation. The physician should be aware of the limitations of EDX studies and know that abnormalities that develop progressively during the first 2–3 weeks postinjury on NCS and needle EMG are critical to the accurate interpretation of the location and severity of the lesion.

In patients with closed nerve trauma or severe limb trauma at several sites, where the exact site of injury is not clear, early NCSs are very useful in attempting to identify the presence of conduction block across the site of the lesion. These studies should be done before 3–5 days postinjury since the distal CMAP reaches its nadir after that time (see Fig. 20.1).[2,23] Detecting conduction block is extremely useful in precise localization of the site of the lesion, though at this early time, the block cannot reveal whether the lesion is due to axon loss, demyelination, or both. A repeat study after the completion of motor and sensory wallerian degeneration (after 10–11 days postinjury) will make the pathophysiological diagnosis, as well as estimate the degree of injury and the prognosis. When NCSs are repeated, three scenarios may occur. If the conduction block does not change, the lesion is purely demyelinating (neurapraxia), whereas if the distal CMAP drops to equal the proximal CMAP, the lesion is axon loss (axonotmesis or neurotmesis). When the CMAP amplitude drops distally but there is a further drop proximally (i.e., the distal CMAP is low but significantly higher than the proximal CMAP), a mixed demyelinating and axon loss lesion is identified.

In axon loss lesions, waiting to obtain NCSs until after the completion of wallerian degeneration (after 10–11 days postinjury) will result in diffusely low-amplitude or absent CMAPs and SNAPs (regardless of the stimulation site), which does not allow for precise localization of the injury site. This is accepted in many circumstances where the site of the lesion is clear and the lesion is likely axon loss (e.g., in a stab wound). Not infrequently, the patient presents to the peripheral nerve specialist after the time expected for completion of wallerian degeneration (after 10–11 days postinjury). In this situation, localization will depend on needle EMG. Hence, the optimal timing of the EDX study would be 3–5 weeks after injury, when fibrillation potentials are fully developed in all denervated muscles and reinnervation has not yet started.

Determining the Severity of Nerve Injury by Electrodiagnostic Studies

An important role of EDX studies is to estimate the degree of nerve injury, since this has a direct effect on prognosis and long-term disability. In demyelinating conduction block lesions, one can approximate the number of blocked motor axons by comparing the distal and proximal CMAPs. For example, in a patient with a common peroneal nerve lesion across the fibular neck, a 6 mV response from tibialis anterior obtained from distal stimulation below the fibular neck and a 3 mV response from proximal stimulation above the fibular neck implies that about 50% of the axons are blocked (demyelinated), while the remaining 50% conduct normally.

In axon loss lesions, the CMAP amplitude, obtained during NCS, is the best estimate of the presence and degree of motor axon loss. In contrast, fibrillation potentials, observed on needle EMG, are the most sensitive indicator of motor axon loss, since loss of a single axon results in up to 200 denervating muscle fibers (depending on the innervation ratio of the innervated muscle). The SNAP amplitude, however, reflects the degree of sensory axon loss, though it has a less important implication for disability. The changes seen on EDX studies with increasing severity of axon loss follow a certain pattern that is predictable and applies to most nerve lesions. With mild lesions, there are usually only fibrillation potentials in affected muscles, with normal or slightly reduced MUAP recruitment and normal CMAP and SNAP. With moderate axon loss lesions, fibrillation potentials and decreased recruitment are coupled with a low-amplitude or absent SNAP, while the CMAP usually remains normal or is borderline in amplitude. Following severe lesions, the SNAP is absent and the CMAP is either very low in amplitude or absent. This picture is accompanied by profuse fibrillation potentials and marked reduction in MUAP recruitment. The sensitivity of the various EDX parameters of axon loss is inversely related to the time when these abnormalities become apparent after an acute lesion develops. For example, fibrillation potentials that are most sensitive to axon loss loss do not become fully developed until 3–5 weeks postinjury, and CMAP amplitude becomes abnormal only after significant axon loss (i.e., insensitive) 2–5 days postinjury. Hence, it is important to perform needle EMG about 3–5 weeks postinjury on all patients with suspected acute peripheral nerve trauma to look for fibrillation potentials and assess for the presence of axon loss.[25]

In axon loss lesions, estimating the extent of motor axon loss after the completion of wallerian degeneration (more than 10–11 days) requires comparison of the distal CMAP to its contralateral counterpart. Optimally, motor and sensory NCSs should be done bilaterally and compared, though there is up to 30% side-to-side variability in normal controls. In a complete neurotmetic lesion, distal and proximal CMAPs are absent. In a partial axonotmetic lesions, the low distal CMAP amplitude reflects the number of axons lost. For example, in a patient with median nerve laceration in the forearm, a 2 mV response from abductor pollicis brevis obtained from distal stimulation at the wrist in the presence of a 10 mV response from the contralateral side implies that about 80% of the axons were injured and have undergone wallerian degeneration.

In mixed lesions, a guestimate of the percentage of axons that were demyelinated versus those that underwent wallerian degeneration is possible but more tricky. A combination of calculations that assess the degree of conduction block and axon loss is required and should be done only after wallerian degeneration is completed. For example, in a patient with radial injury at the spiral groove, if a 6 mV response was obtained from the extensor digitorum longus following distal stimulation at the elbow and a 3 mV response was obtained from proximal stimulation above the spiral groove, coupled with a 10 mV response from distal stimulation on the contralateral side, one can estimate that 40% of the axons are lost, 30% of the axons are blocked (demyelinated), and 30% remain intact and are conducting through the lesion.

Intraoperative Studies

The indication for surgical repair of a peripheral nerve lesion depend on the type and severity of the nerve lesion.[9,17,22] In situations associated with a sharp nerve transection (such as with glass, knife, or razor blade injuries), immediate (primary) repair is often indicated, and should be done at the same time as the soft tissue repair. This primary repair may be delayed several weeks if infection complicates the wound or when the nerve transection is blunt and the anatomy is distorted (such as with propeller blade or power saw injuries or compound fractures). In these situations, the amount of tissue to be trimmed from each stump is more evident several weeks postinjury. When peripheral nerve lesions remain in continuity, the decision to operate is delayed for several months and is usually based on whether functional recovery and reinnervation have occurred. If the nerve fails to regenerate or exhibits poor regeneration, surgery is often indicated.

Operative exploration of the site of injury allows visual inspection of the injured nerve. This is useful in determining the extent of injury to the nerve, particularly to its supporting nerve structure, but is notoriously inadequate in determining the severity of nerve injuries that are in continuity. More importantly, visual inspection cannot establish whether some axons have regenerated and bridged across the injured segment. Injured nerves may look good by inspection but show no evidence of regeneration due to endoneurial damage and fibrosis. In contrast, a nerve may look very bad at the time of exploration, with fibrosis and enlargement, yet have satisfactorily regenerating axons. The former nerve may need resection or neurolysis, while the latter is better left alone or at least not resected.

Intraoperative recordings are becoming increasingly important in the surgical management of patients with severe nerve injuries. Surgery provides a unique opportunity for direct recording of *compound nerve action potentials* (*CNAPs*) across the injured segment of the nerve.[5,9,10,17] These studies are most helpful in nerve lesions associated with severe or total axon injury, since the clinical and EDX studies cannot accurately classify the degree of nerve injury. Recordings of intraoperative CNAPs are most useful in nerve lesions that remain in continuity (second- through fourth-degree nerve injuries). In contrast, intraoperative CNAP studies are not useful in neurapraxia (first-degree injury), since remyelination is expected and surgical intervention is rarely indicated, or in complete nerve transection (neurotmesis or fifth-degree injury), since these studies will have no role in the choice of surgical intervention (reanastomosis or grafting).

Intraoperative recordings are performed using two electrode pairs that hook on the exposed nerve and are used for stimulating the nerve proximal to the lesion while recording distal to it.[9,10,17] The purpose of this study is to try to record a CNAP across the lesion and establish if some axons have crossed the injured segment, and, if so, how many. If there is no distal CNAP, the recording electrode should be moved proximally until a CNAP is recorded. This indicates the distal end of conduction axons. This is most important in lesions that seem to extend a considerable distance, such as with extensive fibrosis due to hemorrhage, infection, or ischemia, since this technique helps to identify the proximal end of the nerve lesion.

Follow-up Studies During Recovery

Recovery following peripheral nerve injury is due to remyelination, reinnervation, or both. The latter may follow collateral sprouting (in partial axon loss lesions only), proximodistal axon regeneration, or both. Once the diagnosis of the nerve injury is secure, the optimal timing of the repeat EDX studies depends mostly on the pathophysiology of the lesion, the nerve injured, and the location of the nerve injury. Recovery is quick with demyelinative conduction block lesions, while improvement is protracted in axon loss lesions and biphasic in mixed lesions. Axon loss lesions that affect proximal nerve structures, such as the lower brachial plexus or the sciatic nerve, have to be restudied earlier than others. In these situations, the target muscles to be reinnervated (hand or leg muscles) are far from the site of injury. Early surgical intervention is often necessary, since muscles that do not reinnervate after 18–24 months will undergo atrophy and fibrosis, and their fibers will not be more viable.[16]

Remyelination

In patients with a neurapraxic (first-degree) nerve injury that is due to segmental demyelination and manifests as conduction block, the process of remyelination is usually rapid and may take up to 2–3 months for completion, provided that the cause (such as compression by hematoma or a bony structure) has been removed. For example, a patient who develops foot drop due to a purely demyelinating peroneal nerve injury at the fibular neck will often recover completely in 2–3 months. Hence, on follow-up NCSs done at that time, remyelination is confirmed by resolution of the conduction block and restoration of the proximal CMAP. During and for a short period after reversal of the conduction block, NCSs not uncommonly reveal focal slowing of the injured nerve segment that was not present on the initial EDX study. This is best explained by the presence of newly formed thin myelin that was laid out by the Schwann cells. As the myelin thickens with time, focal slowing also disappears.

Reinnervation by Collateral Sprouting

Collateral sprouting is a process in which the surviving (intact) axons send axon terminals (sprouts) to the denervated muscles in an attempt to reinnervate these muscle fibers and restore muscle power. This is a quick and effective method of reinnervation that applies only to partial axon loss lesions where some axons escape injury and wallerian degeneration. Collateral sprouting is clinically effective in restoring function when only a modest number of axons have been injured. In practice, it is most effective when less than 80% of the axons were damaged. In very severe lesions, collateral sprouting may lead to little or no change of motor function.

Collateral sprouting in partial axon loss lesions starts as early as 1–2 days after injury. However, the early signs of reinnervation first become evident on needle EMG by 1 month after the injury and are usually definite by 2–3 months postinjury.[13] Immediately following nerve injury, there is a decrease in MUAP recruitment in affected muscles that is proportional to the number of lost axons. In the first few weeks after injury, MUAPs of surviving axons with a normal morphology remain. As collateral sprouting proceeds, muscle fibers become progressively incorporated in the territory of the motor unit. Early on, the collateral axons (sprouts) are immature; they have thin or incomplete myelin. Hence, action potentials along collateral sprouts conduct slowly. This is often reflected on needle EMG by MUAPs with *satellite potentials* (linked or parasite potentials). The satellite potential is a late spike of the MUAP that is distinct and time-locked with the main potential. The satellite potential trails the main MUAP because the newly formed nerve terminal may be long, or small and thinly myelinated, or both, resulting in slower conduction. When a satellite potential is suspected on needle EMG, it is useful to use a trigger line to demonstrate that this potential is time-locked to the main potential (Fig. 20.3).

Reinnervation MUAPs, including satellite potentials, may be unstable. Collateral sprouts may show evidence of intermittent conduction blocking or neuromuscular junction blocking due insecure transmission at the end plate. This results in individual muscle fibers being either blocked or coming to action potentials at varying intervals, leading to a MUAP that changes in configuration from impulse to impulse (amplitude or number of phases or both). Often, the sprout matures over time, the conduction velocity increases, and the satellite potential then fires more closely to the main potential, and ultimately fuses with it to become an additional phase or serration within the main MUAP complex. In general, MUAPs become more stable, more polyphasic, and longer in duration as collateral sprouting continues. In very chronic lesions, MUAPs are typically stable, with long duration, high amplitude, and little polyphasia, reflecting the maturity of all the nerve sprouts. Also, as reinnervation proceeds, there is a decline in the number of fibrillation potentials, since reinnervated muscle fibers will cease to generate these potentials (see Table 20.2).

On NCSs, the CMAP amplitude slowly increases in size over time as reinnervation of the recorded muscle continues. The SNAP often parallels the CMAP. In mild to moderate nerve lesions, effective reinnervation may bring the CMAP within

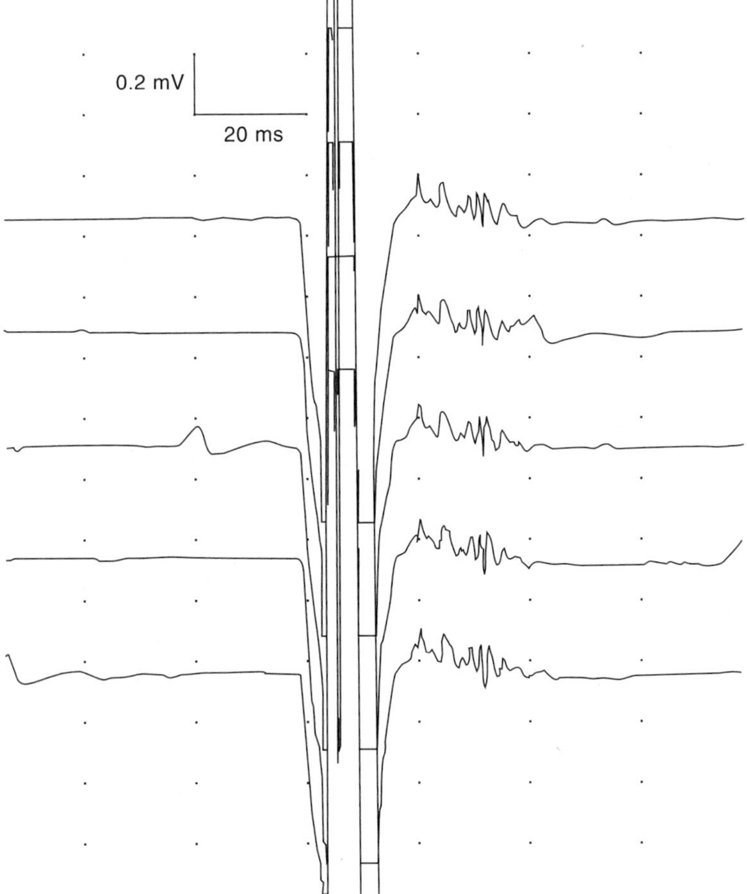

Figure 20.3. Reinnervated muscle unit action potential (MUAP) with long duration and several linked potentials (satellites) that follow the main potential recorded from the extensor digitorum communis in a patient with a severe partial axon loss radial lesion in the arm following a humeral fracture 6 months earlier. The tracings are shown in a raster format using a trigger line. Note that the main MUAP and all of its satellites are stable; that is, they do not vary between impulses.

normal values and result in NCSs that do not show evidence of a remote nerve injury. In these situations, however, needle EMG will continue to confirm the existence of the old injury by exhibiting large MUAPs that fires rapidly.

Reinnervation by Axon Regeneration

In complete axon loss peripheral nerve lesions, improvement is completely dependent on axon regeneration, which may occur spontaneously or following surgical repair. Unfortunately, in most cases of nerve injury, regeneration is slow and incomplete. The axons first have to traverse the injured segment; this can be achieved in 8–15 days when the endoneurial tubes are intact (second-degree nerve lesion).[19] In more severe axon loss lesions, the regenerating axons may not find intact endoneurial tubes and sometimes form a neuroma with tangled axons at the site of injury. In such lesions as well as in neurotmetic lesions, surgical repair is often needed.

In humans, once the axons cross successfully the injured nerve segment, they continue to regenerate at a slow rate, averaging 1 to 2 mm per/day (about 1 inch per/month).[15,16,19] Based on this rate, the timing of repeat EDX studies in complete lesions depends on the site of injury in relation to the most proximal muscle that is expected to be reinnervated first. For example, following a median nerve injury in the middle of the arm, the first muscle expected to show reinnervation is the pronator teres muscle with its branch arising from the nerve in the antecubital fossa. If the distance between this lesion and the muscle is 5 inches, then the repeat study should be done about 6 months after the injury.

On needle EMG, the early signs of regeneration can be confirmed by the appearance of small, complex, unstable MUAPs, sometimes referred to as *nascent MUAPs*, that precede the onset of visible voluntary contraction. These units appear first in muscles nearest the site of the injury and progress distally. Hence, they are useful in assessing the progress of this proximodistal regeneration. Nascent MUAPs are very low in amplitude and extremely polyphasic, with a normal or increased duration. These small nascent MUAPs mimic the MUAPs seen with myopathies. Nascent MUAPs are often unstable due to conduction or neuromuscular junction blocking and are associated with decreased MUAP recruitment (Fig. 20.4). As reinnervation proceeds, nascent MUAPs that are unstable become transformed into stable, long-duration, polyphasic MUAPs, reflecting increased numbers of muscle fibers per motor unit, full myelination of the regenerating axons, and the maturity of the neuromuscular junctions. Similar to what is seen in reinnervation by collateral sprouting, there is also a decline in the number of fibrillation potentials and the progressive improvement of the SNAP and CMAP on NCS. However, in these severe or complete nerve lesions, the CMAP and SNAP usually never return to baseline values. In addition, there is often permanent slowing and dispersion of the CMAPs due to the extreme variability in the diameter and myelination of the regenerated axons, which results in significant differential slowing of conduction velocities (Fig. 20.5).

Aberrant Regeneration

Aberrant regeneration occurs when regenerating axons are misdirected into new end organs. It is most common in axon loss nerve injuries that distort the endoneurial tubes (third-degree injury or more) and in proximal peripheral nerve or root injuries. Misdirected fibers may not find endoneurial tubes and generate a neuroma at the site of the lesion. Regenerating motor axons in a mixed sensorimotor nerve may elongate into sensory nerves or vice versa. Motor axons may also be misdirected into the wrong muscles and result in cocontraction of muscles that can interfere with the intended function or cause abnormal movements. Aberrant regeneration may also account for some of the poor functional recovery such as poor dexterity.

The most common neurological sequelae of aberrant reinnervation occurs after facial nerve injury, including after idiopathic Bell's palsy. Aberrant regeneration between motor axons results in facial synkinesis, mainly contraction of the lower facial muscles on the affected side whenever there is an eye blink or vice versa. Other much less common, yet more widely publicized, abnormal regeneration patterns are *crocodile tears*, manifested as lacrimation of the ipsilateral eye during chewing, and the Marin-Amat syndrome, or *jaw winking*, manifested as closure of the ipsilateral eyelid when the jaw opens.

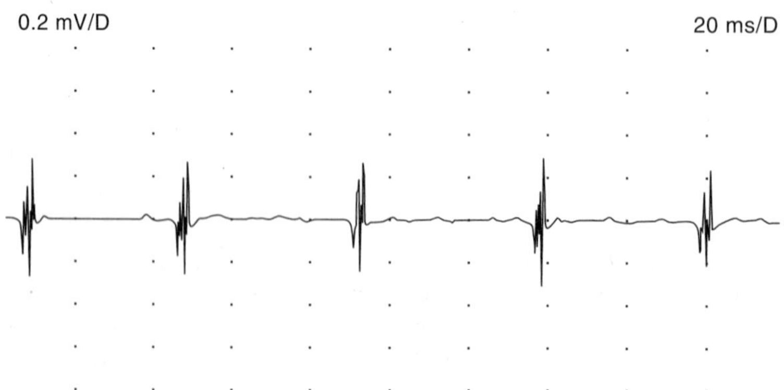

Figure 20.4. Nascent unit (polyphasic with a low-amplitude muscle unit action potential) that fires very rapidly (firing rate = 25 Hz) and is unstable, with moment-to-moment variation in configuration. This was recorded from the flexor carpi ulnaris in a patient with complete transection of the ulnar nerve at the elbow and sural grafting 6 months.

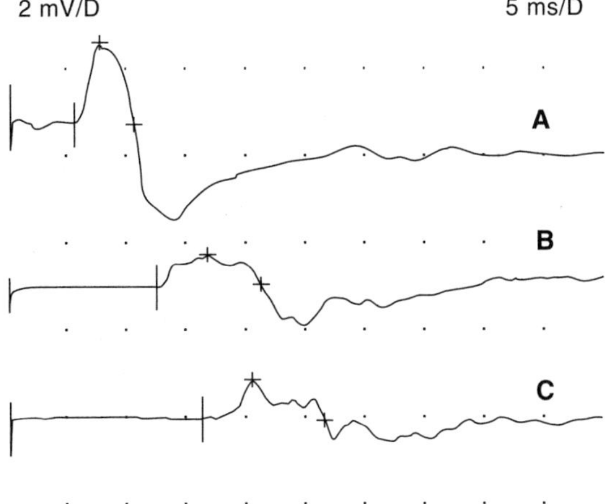

Figure 20.5. Ulnar motor nerve conduction study in a patient with complete transection of the ulnar nerve at the elbow and sural grafting 3 years earlier. (A = stimulation at the wrist, B = stimulation below the elbow, C = stimulation above the elbow). The compound muscle action potential is low in amplitude and shows significant dispersion and differential slowing. The conduction velocities for the below elbow to wrist and above elbow to below elbow segments are 30.9 and 33.3 m/sec, respectively.

Another form of aberrant regeneration occurs following partial injury to the C5 spinal root proximal to the branch to the phrenic nerve. Motor axons destined for the diaphragm may get misdirected to one or more shoulder muscles (biceps, deltoid, or spinati). As a result, the shoulder muscles fire in time with the respiratory cycle (breathing arm).[20,21] Similar phenomena were recently reported from obstetric brachial plexopathies involving the lower plexus and T1 cervical roots, resulting in aberrant reinnervation of hand muscles from axons destined for intercostal muscles (breathing hand).[3]

REFERENCES

1. Al Hakim M, Katirji MB: Femoral mononeuropathy induced by the lithotomy position: A report of 5 cases and a review of the literature. Muscle Nerve 16:891–895, 1993.
2. Chaudhry V, Cornblath DR: Wallerian degeneration in human nerves: Serial electrophysiologic studies. Muscle Nerve 15:687–693, 1992.
3. Friedenberg SM, Hermann RC: The breathing hand: Obstetric brachial plexopathy reinnervation from thoracic roots? J Neurol Neurosurg Psychiatry 75:158–160, 2004.
4. Gilliatt RW,Taylor JC: Electrical changes following section of the facial nerve. Proc R Soc Med 52:1080, 1959.
5. Gutierrez A, England JD: Peripheral nerve injuries. In: Katirji B, Kaminski HJ, Preston DC, Ruff RL, Shapiro EB (eds): Neuromuscular Disorders in Clinical Practice. Boston, Butterworth-Heinemann, 2002, pp 736–743.
6. Katirji B: The clinical electromyography examination. An overview. Neurol Clin North Am 20:291–303, 2002.
7. Katirji B: Clinical electromyography. In: Bradley WG, Daroff RB, Fenichel GM, Jankovic J (eds): Neurology in Clinical Practice, 4th ed. Boston, Butterworth-Heinemann, pp 491–520, 2004.
8. Kent KC, Moscussi M, Gallagher SG, et al: Neuropathy after cardiac catheterization: Incidence, clinical patterns and long term outcome. J Vasc Surg 19:1008–1012, 1994.
9. Kline DG: Surgical repair of peripheral nerve injury. Muscle Nerve 13:843–852, 1990.
10. Kline DG, Hackett ER: Reappraisal of timing for exploration of civilian peripheral nerve injuries. Surgery 78:54–65, 1975.
11. Miller RG: Injury to peripheral motor nerves. Muscle Nerve 10:698–710, 1987.
12. Noble J, Munro, CA, Prasad VSSV, et al: Analysis of upper and lower extremity peripheral nerve injuries in a population of patients with multiple injuries. J Trauma 45:116–122, 1998.
13. Robinson LR: Traumatic injury to peripheral nerves. Muscle Nerve 23:863–873, 2004.
14. Schmalzried TP, Amstutz HC, Dorey FJ: Nerve palsy associated with total hip replacement. Risk factors and prognosis. J Bone Joint Surg 73A:1074–1080, 1991.
15. Seddon HJ: Surgical Disorders of the Peripheral Nerves, 2nd ed. New York, Churchill Livingstone, 1975.
16. Seddon HJ, Medawar PB, Smith H: Rate of regeneration of peripheral nerves in man. J Physiol 102:191–215, 1943.
17. Spinner RJ, Kline DG: Surgery for peripheral nerve and brachial plexus injuries or other nerve lesions. Muscle Nerve 23:680–695, 2000.
18. Stone L, Keenan MA: Peripheral nerve injury in the adult with traumatic brain injury. Clin Orthop Relat Res 233: 136–144, 1988.
19. Sunderland S: Nerve Injuries and Their Repair: A Critical Appraisal. Edinburgh, Churchill Livingstone, 1991.
20. Swift TR:The breathing arm. Muscle Nerve 17:125–129, 1994.
21. Swift TR, Leshner RT, Gross JA: Arm-diaphragm synkinesis: Electrodiagnostic studies of aberrant regeneration of phrenic motor neurons. Neurology 30:339–344, 1980.
22. Watchmaker GP, Mackinnon SE: Advances in peripheral nerve repair. Clin Plast Surg 24:63–73, 1997.
23. Wilbourn AJ: Nerve conduction study changes in human nerves undergoing wallerian degeneration. Neurology 31:96, 1981.
24. Wilbourn AJ: Iatrogenic nerve injuries. Neurol Clin North Am 16:55–82, 1998.
25. Wilbourn AJ: Nerve conduction studies: Types, components, abnormalities and value in localization. Neurol Clin North Am 20:305–338, 2002.

Chapter 21

Surgery of the Injured Peripheral Nerve and Brachial Plexus

SHADEN MARZOUK,
H. BRUCE HAMILTON,
AND DAVID G. KLINE

Injury of the peripheral nervous system is common and often requires multiple treatment modalities. Surgical intervention is frequently a necessary step to ensure an optimal outcome in these patients. The neural response to injury, mechanisms, diagnosis, indications, and timing of surgical treatment, as well as some basic surgical options, are addressed in this chapter. A general treatment algorithm is constructed as a guide for the caregivers of these patients. An expanded discussion of injury to the brachial plexus is included, as these lesions are the most debilitating peripheral nerve lesions, the most challenging to manage, and the most frequent cause of questions directed to the peripheral nerve surgeon. The role and limitations of surgery in the successful care of the injured peripheral nerve completes our discussion of these traumatic lesions.

Neural Response to Injury

When a peripheral nerve is injured, a set of well-described events take place in the neuron and axon. The nerve cell body, which is located in the anterior horn of the spinal cord, in the dorsal root ganglion, or in a ganglion of the autonomic nervous system, reacts to injury by undergoing chromatolysis. The production and accumulation of RNA and associated proteins result in enlargement of the cell body,[60] a prelude to the regenerative process ahead.

The injured axon responds in three basic clinical ways: neurapraxia, axonotmesis, and neurotmesis.[61,67] In neurapraxic injuries, impulse conduction is blocked despite a minimal degree of wallerian degeneration. A concussive event is believed to be responsible for such lesions.[18] These injuries most commonly involve the larger, more heavily myelinated fibers serving motor activity, light touch, and position sense while sparing the finer fibers involved in pain and the autonomic system.[65] The relative sparing of these fine fibers often results in the presence of pain. With neurapraxic injuries, the axon and associated connective tissues are not seriously disrupted, allowing for the recovery of complete or near-complete function usually several days to 6 weeks after injury.

Axonotmesis is an axonal injury in which axonal and myelin continuity is disrupted while the connective tissues of the axon remain, for the most part, intact.[51] The process of wallerian degeneration follows. This injury involves both the sensory and motor fibers. Retrograde proximal degeneration is followed by the regeneration of fibers to the site of injury, across the lesion, and then to the distal nerve. At that point, regeneration may continue to the end organ, be it muscle or sensory organ. The relative maintenance of intact connective tissues allows for much recovery of function. Such recovery is limited by the rate of neural regeneration, as well as by the distance of regeneration required. Proximal lesions typically grow 2 to 3 mm/day, whereas more distal lesions grow 1 mm/day or less.[66] Regeneration through proximal lesions of the nerve that must travel far to reach significant end points is typically less effective.

Neurotmesis is typified by loss of continuity in both the axon and the connective tissues of the nerve. These lesions range from complete transection of the nerve to severe compressive and stretch injuries that fail to produce a loss in nerve continuity but destroy the internal anatomy of the nerve. All motor, sensory, and autonomic fibers are usually involved equally. Wallerian degeneration is inevitable and is followed by attempted regeneration. Regeneration and recovery of function are severely limited in these patients by the formation of a neuroma. A neuroma is a segment of nerve composed of very disorganized connective tissue intermixed with, for the most part, fine axons that have branched many times in an attempt to grow distally. When fibers are able to regenerate past the site of such injury, functional return is further inhibited by failure to return to preinjury destinations and by defective myelination within the damaged distal sheaths.[36]

In addition to the previous grading system popularized by Seddon, Sunderland devised a clinical grading system in which neuronal injury was divided into five grades.[61,67] Grade I injury is a pure neurapraxic injury in which a conduction block is created without the presence of physical disruption of the axonal or connective tissues. Grade II injury is that in which the fascicular and connective tissues are maintained but with a loss of axonal continuity, that is, a pure axonotmetic lesion. Grade III injuries are those in which the axon and endoneurium are disrupted while most of the remaining connective tissues of the fascicular structure are maintained. Adequate regeneration sometimes but not always occurs with such a lesion. Grade IV lesions occur when there is loss of axonal continuity, severe distortion of the endoneurial and perineurial structure, and usually complete disruption of fascicular structure. In Grade V injury, the nerve has been transected, with complete disruption of all neural elements. Whichever system one uses in determining the type and severity of injury, an accurate assessment of the extent of the nerve lesion is paramount in planning and instituting the treatment course to be undertaken.

Much basic science research has been done, providing some understanding of nerve injury on a molecular level. Current developments in the field of neural trauma are intimately involved with basic science research. Information regarding ion channels, cellular messengers, and regeneration promoters is key to understanding and treatment.

When nerves are injured, tumor necrosis factor-alpha and interleukin-one are released by macrophages during the inflammatory phase. These cytokines can make functional nerve regeneration difficult by stimulating kinases that encourage fibroblast and neuroma formation.[41] Sodium channels accumulate abnormally in neuromas, leading to the axonal hyperexcitability underlying post-traumatic pain and paresthesias.[14] Ankyrin G is a transmembrane protein of the axolemma. Overexpression of this protein can lead to sodium channel clustering and painful neuromas.[39] Painful neuromas have more pronounced clustering of sodium channels and ankyrin G than nonpainful neuromas.[38] In addition, abnormal clustering of potassium channels is found in neuromas.[15]

Avulsion injuries have a poorer outcome than more peripheral nerve damage. In the experimental setting, heavier weights lead to avulsion of more roots.[63] One explanation for the poorer outcomes of avulsion injuries is that nerve root avulsion from the spinal cord leads to increased and prolonged expression of c-*fos*. C-*fos* causes increased transcription of new messages for recovery, survival, or cell death.[72] GAP-43 and p75 are proteins that promote nerve regeneration. They are elevated for approximately the first year after nerve injury, then decrease. This finding offers support for earlier repair of peripheral nerves when indicated.[19]

The cortex also undergoes changes secondary

to peripheral nerve injury. A significant bilateral reduction in intracortical inhibition of the motor cortex developed in subjects after limb trauma.[59] This may explain some of the pain-related phenomena these patients experience.

Mechanisms of Nerve Injury

The mechanism of injury to peripheral nerve determines in large part the treatment required for the optimal recovery of function, the appropriate timing of surgical intervention when required, and ultimately the prognosis for functional recovery.

Transecting Injuries

Transection of peripheral nerves occurs in 30% of patients with severe or complete loss of function distal to the injury site.[12] In the remaining 70% of serious nerve injuries, there is a lesion in continuity where a variable degree of intraneural damage occurs without transection. Nearly 15% of the potentially transected nerves possess a variable amount of continuity.[36] Some of the loss in these cases is due to contusion and stretch rather than frank laceration. Spontaneous recovery in the transected nerve or transected portion of the nerve is very rare. However, partial recovery in these lesions may occur if the transection is incomplete and the remaining portion in continuity recovers function.

The mechanism of transection is the determining factor in the timing of surgery, as well as the surgical procedure required.[21] Sharp transections usually do not have a significant contusive component; that is, the injury is quite focal, with minimal damage in the nerve on either side of the injury site, and is a purely neurotmetic injury. If the sharply transected nerve is not repaired acutely, the amount of neuroma is limited, although the retracted ends will be invested in scar.

Blunt transections are associated with more extensive contusion than those due to a sharp mechanism and sometimes have intraneural hemorrhage proximal and distal to the site of transection. Large neuromas develop on both stumps of the transected nerve, with typically more severe retraction and scarring around the nerve as compared to that with sharp transecting injuries.[11]

In Continuity Injuries

The most common injury to peripheral nerve, which accounts for up to 70% of severe lesions, is that in which gross continuity of the nerve is maintained. Recovery in these lesions is much less predictable, but partial functional loss is more likely to improve spontaneously. Recovery in lesions with complete functional loss can range from near-complete spontaneous recovery to the total absence of recognizable functional recovery unless resection and repair are done. Determination of the potential for recovery can be complicated and imprecise with serious lesions in continuity.

Lesions in continuity can consist of a combination of neurapraxia, axonotmesis, and neurotmesis.[36,61,62,70] The more serious the injury and the greater the functional deficit, the more likely that axonotmesis and neurotmesis are involved and the less likely that spontaneous functional recovery will result. The amount of connective tissue damage within the nerve largely determines the amount of functional spontaneous recovery. This is because the regeneration of poorly organized connective tissue impedes and misdirects axonal regrowth into the distal stump. A neuroma in continuity (consisting of poorly organized connective tissues and misguided axons) is the result, with very few fibers of any maturity growing across the injury and fewer yet reaching the appropriate end organs.

Despite the above, the prognosis for recovery after these in continuity lesions is very difficult to determine. This is partly due to the wide range of injury severity as well as the length, and thus the proximal and distal extent, of these injuries. As a result, these lesions should be followed and reassessed for 2 to 5 months before surgical intervention and further intraoperative evaluation are indicated.

Burns, Radiation, and Injection Injury

While transection and in continuity injury are the two main categories of peripheral nerve injury, other mechanisms deserve mention. Burn victims can have peripheral nerve injuries because of direct trauma to the nervous tissue or because of secondary involvement due to compartment syndromes or escar.[56,58] The damage is usually from an open flame, but similar thermal injuries can be caused by high-voltage electricity or caustic chemicals.[56] The thermal energy released causes a focal area of nerve injury, but surrounding tissues are damaged as well, often needing a fasciotomy and escarotomy. Due to the extent of scar formation, these are difficult injuries to reverse.[71]

Radiation can also cause serious tissue damage to peripheral nerves. This can bear some resemblance to thermal injury, particularly with high radiation doses. Usually, with moderate doses, a typical sequence of acute, early, and late delayed changes will occur.[56,58]

Injection injuries of peripheral nerves most commonly affect the radial or sciatic nerves. The needle itself or its injection contents can harm the nerve. The blood–nerve barrier breaks down and intraneural fibrotic scarring occurs.[16] Axons cannot regenerate through this fibrotic tissue, and patients can have a neurological deficit as well as pain.

Diagnosis of Peripheral Nerve Injury

The mechanism of injury, the particular nerve and level involved, and the degree of functional loss are the key issues in determining the prognosis, optimal treatment, and timing of surgery (if needed). Mechanisms of injury are usually apparent through history taking. However, the specifics of involvement and the functional loss require careful physical and neurological examinations.[25,53] Detailed assessment of motor, sensory, and autonomic deficits is clearly the easiest and most readily accessible method of determining nerve injury and functional loss. The details of examination are not included in this chapter, as more complete works dedicated to peripheral nerve examination are available. Associated injuries, pain, overlap innervation for various functions, and compensatory movements can complicate the physical examination and result in an erroneous picture. Nonetheless, most peripheral nerve lesions can be localized accurately by a thorough physical examination.

After a good physical examination, the clinician uses an assortment of tests, including electrophysiological studies and radiological examinations, to verify and supplement the basic clinical findings. The electromyogram (EMG), a study with which most neurologists are familiar, is perhaps the most frequently used of the electrophysiological studies. The magnitude and extent of denervation can be determined by the third week postinjury, serving as a baseline for future studies to establish the presence or absence of regeneration. Evidence of reinnervation does not ensure that recovery of function will follow, but does establish that nerve fibers have indeed regenerated to the muscle being tested.[40] In general, the initial EMG is performed several weeks after injury and repeated every few months as determined by the estimate of time required to grow the distance to the denervated muscle. Remember, the regeneration of a peripheral nerve can be estimated to proceed at a rate of 1 mm/day, or 1 inch/month. More proximal lesions regenerate up to 3 mm/day, but as an estimate, 1 mm/day allows for the process of wallerian degeneration, axonal crossing of the site of injury, growth, and reinnervation of the end organs. Therefore, 1 mm/day is a good rule of thumb for estimating required regrowth time. If no evidence of regeneration has occurred in a timely fashion, surgical intervention can be considered.

Direct nerve stimulation studies, sensory nerve action potentials, and somatosensory evoked potentials can further localize the site of injury, estimate the degree of damage, and establish the presence of regeneration in injured nerves.[23,40] During surgical exposure of the nerves, direct recording of nerve action potentials along the nerve can not only localize the injury but more precisely direct the surgeon to resect or not resect the lesion in continuity. These studies are addressed more directly in our later discussion of brachial plexus lesions.

Radiographic studies allow for the assessment of secondary injury, as well as the assignment of some causes of nerve damage. Fracture of the long bones is frequently associated with peripheral nerve injury, whereas other fractures, such as those of ribs, clavicles, and scapula, provide a clue to the amount of force involved in the injury. Spine fractures may be associated with proximal injuries to the spinal nerve or roots.[4] Computed tomography (CT) and magnetic resonance imaging (MRI) exams can sometimes delineate the site and extent of injury. Fractures, dislocations, and tumorous masses compressing nerves can be seen on these images. Sometimes scans display meningoceles, commonly seen in root avulsion or near root avulsions with severe injuries of the brachial plexus. The myelogram is much more sensitive in detecting meningoceles and can provide further evidence of proximal injury by displaying the extravasation of contrast material through tears in the arachnoid and dura[26] (Figure 21.1).

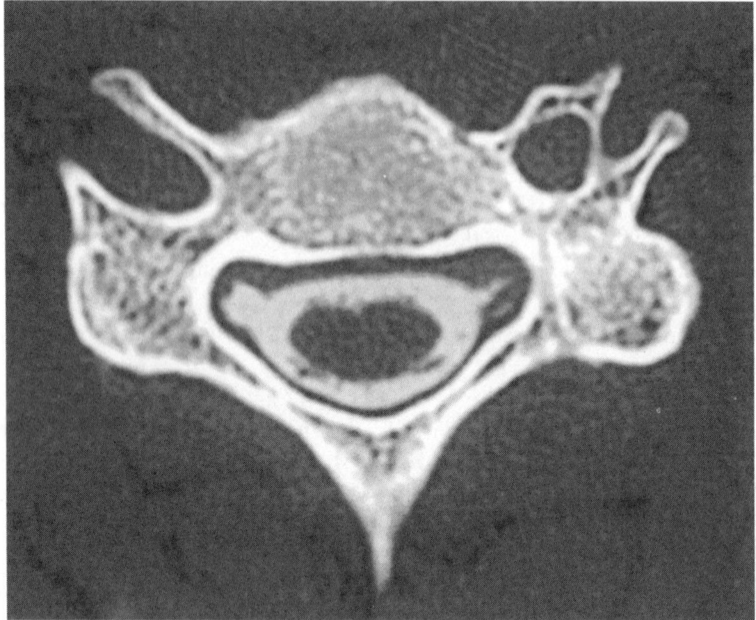

Figure 21.1. This axial CT myelogram of the cervical spine demonstrates the empty root sleeve.

Magnetic resonance imaging exams are capable of displaying some nerve roots, occasionally damage to these roots, and the subsequent degeneration of the neural elements, as well as trophic changes in the denervated musculature.[2] However, in our experience, a thorough myelogram provides the most information about stretch injuries when compared to CT or MRI. Magnetic resonance imaging of muscles distal to a nerve injury can provide the earliest evidence of denervation (5 to 6 days). On T_1 scars the denervated muscles will have a whitened appearance.

In discussing diagnosis of peripheral nerve injury, and later when discussing treatment and outcome, it is important to refer to a common grading scale. The authors prefer the Louisiana State University Medical Center Motor, Sensory, and Whole Nerve Injury scales developed by the senior author (DGK). These scales are described in Tables 21.1, 21.2, and 21.3.

Indications and Timing in the Surgical Intervention of the Injured Nerve

Magnification, the development of intraoperative electrophysiological equipment, and the expansion of surgical principles developed at around the time of the Second World War have led to modern techniques and refinements in the surgical treatment of nerve injury.[36] The requirement for, timing of, and prognosis of peripheral nerve surgery are largely dependent on the mechanism of injury. Therefore, transecting nerve lesions are addressed separately from the more common lesions in continuity.

Vascular lesions, such as expanding blood clots, traumatic pseudoaneurysms, arteriovenous fistulas, ischemic compartment syndromes, or the presence of intraneural foreign bodies, are examples of injuries that can further compromise the nerve and should usually be addressed by relatively early operative exploration.

Nerve Transection

Surgical repair of transected peripheral nerve can be divided into two categories, as determined by the type of the transecting injury. Primary or acute repair is undertaken at the time of initial wound exploration and closure, or within 72 hours of the injury. Secondary repair is performed after a delay of several weeks, when the full extent of the lesion can be assessed accurately.[36,42,43]

Acute (in the first 72 hours) repair of the transected peripheral nerve is indicated when the injury to the nerve is the result of a sharp, relatively

Table 21.1. Louisiana State University Medical Center Motor Scale

Grade	Description
0	No contraction
1	Trace contraction
2	Movement against gravity
3	Movement against gravity and some mild resistance
4	Movement against moderate resistance
5	Movement against maximal resistance

clean laceration, such as those common in knife wounds, scalpel transections, razor blade lacerations, and some glass injuries. Partial as well as complete transections in this group of sharp injuries should be primarily repaired. This early repair allows for identification of the nerve stumps without requiring excessive surgical exploration. Retraction and scarring are minimized, and there is less possibility that tension must be applied to the stumps to obtain reapproximation or that grafts will be required to span the gap due to retraction.

During surgical exposure of a potentially transected sharp injury, the nerve may be partially in continuity. Under these circumstances, the transected portion is acutely repaired and the portion in continuity is left alone. With time, if there is not significant recovery in the distribution of the in continuity portion, and if that loss is significant, then a secondary operation is needed. Common in any potential transecting lesion is an in continuity

Table 21.2. Louisiana State University Medical Center Sensory Scale*

Grade	Description
0	No response to touch, pin, or pressure
1	Testing produces hyperesthesia or paresthesia; deep pain recovery in autonomous zones
2	Sensory response sufficient for grip and slow protection; sensory stimuli mislocalized, with overresponse
3	Response to touch and pin in autonomous zones; sensation mislocalized and abnormal, with some overresponse
4	Response to touch and pin in autonomous zone; response localized but not normal; no overresponse
5	Normal response to touch and pin in entire field, including autonomous zone

*This system uses a comparison of touch and pinprick and the ability to localize stimuli.

Table 21.3. Louisiana State University Medical Center Whole Nerve Injury Scale

Grade	Description
0	No muscle contraction, absent sensation
1	Proximal muscles contract but not against gravity; sensory grade 1 or 0
2	Proximal muscles contract against gravity; distal muscles do not contract; sensory grade if applicable is usually 2 or lower
3	Proximal muscles contract against gravity and some resistance; some distal muscles contract against at least gravity; sensory grade is usually 3
4	All proximal and some distal muscles contract against gravity and some resistance; sensory grade is 3 or better
5	All muscle contract against moderate resistance; sensory grade is 4 or better

lesion. This lesion is damaged not by transection but by a variable degree of stretch, resulting in neurapraxia, axonotmesis, and neurotmesis. These lesions should then be treated like other lesions in continuity, with an appropriate delay for surgery. As previously reported by the senior author (DGK), in 75 cases of transected upper extremity nerves, including 29 radial, 27 median, and 19 ulnar nerves, grade 3 or better function was obtained in 79% acute end-to-end suture repairs, 70% secondary end-to-end suture repairs, and 64% secondary operations requiring grafts.[36]

In blunt transecting or high-velocity lacerating injuries, the surgical goal is to repair any associated injuries to structures other than the peripheral nerve. Also, the surgeon strives to prevent secondary manifestations of the injury from further damaging the remaining neural elements. Additionally important is the prevention of excessive retraction on severed nerve stumps, which can complicate a secondary repair—done 2 weeks to 1 month after injury.

In Continuity Injury

Compressive lesions, entrapments, and associated vascular lesions (such as pseudoaneurysm or clot) are the most common reasons for acute intervention with in continuity injury of peripheral nerves. Otherwise, acute intervention of the in continuity lesion is seldom needed. Surgical repair of in continuity lesions of the peripheral nerve should be considered only after a several-month delay.[20, 36,42,45] This deliberate delay allows time for spontaneous recovery of transient perturbations in nerve function, such as those occurring in partial or complete neurapraxic injuries. It also permits fibers damaged by axonotmesis to regenerate so that they can be documented through operative nerve action potential recording.

Although a delay in exploration of lesions in continuity is almost always indicated, prolonged delay can be detrimental to the chances for recovery. Optimal muscular function is obtained if reinnervation occurs by 24 to 30 months. Thereafter, muscular end-plate degeneration, atrophy, and fibrosis of denervated muscle, as well as the loss of functional muscle spindles, begin to diminish the potential for normal functional recovery, even if axons of sufficient number and size reach muscle. The maximum period of delay should be limited to optimize the possibility of maximal functional return. Relatively focal, isolated injuries, such as those resulting from fracture or high-velocity penetrating wounds, typically require a 2- to 3-month delay, whereas the more lengthy, diffuse lesions common after blunt contusive trauma and stretching injuries require delays of 4 to 5 months. Relating to these guidelines is the fact that the longer the regenerative distance required, the longer the period of time for reinnervation and the poorer the functional return. Thus, proximal nerve lesions and plexus element injuries need as early an operation as is feasible.

Baseline clinical and electrophysiological examinations should be used to delineate the nerve involved and the probable mechanism and severity of injury. If no clinical or electrical evidence of functional regeneration is identified on serial examination despite an appropriate delay, surgical exploration is indicated. Should functional recovery occur spontaneously, the electrical and clinical studies usually improve coincidentally. However, the presence or absence of electrical regenerative activity should not be used to either establish or refute the need for surgery, as the major goal in treating peripheral nerve injuries is to achieve functional recovery, not to obtain electrical evidence of regeneration. Nevertheless, EMG studies often aid in the decision on whether or not to surgically explore nerve injuries (Figure 21.2).

Results of operative repair of lesions in continuity are largely dependent on the type of surgical intervention required, as well as the nerve involved and the locus of the lesions. Lesions in which a nerve action potential is recorded across the site of injury intraoperatively usually require only neu-

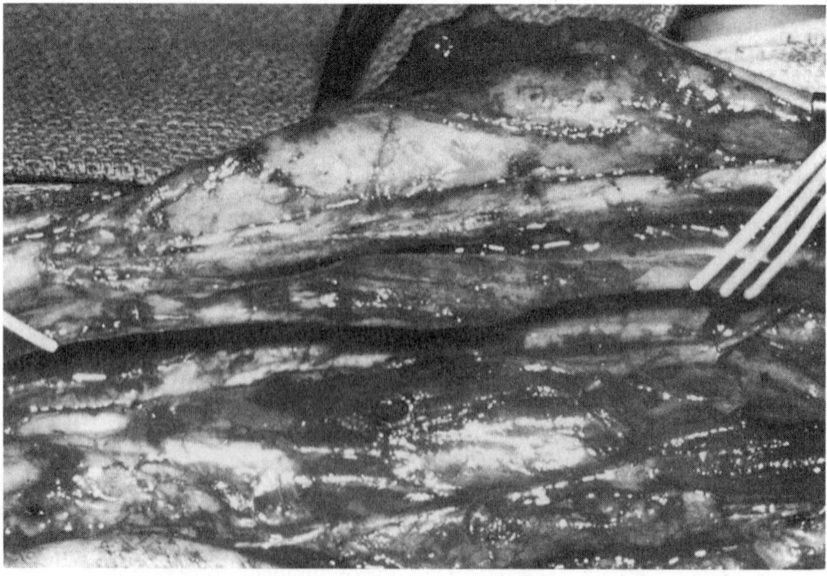

Figure 21.2. A contused swollen ulnar nerve associated with fracture of the humerus. NAPs were absent when electrical recordings were attempted across the lesion. Repair required resection of the neuroma and interfascicular grafts.

rolysis. In those nerves where a nerve action potential is present but one portion of the nerve is more seriously injured, internal neurolysis and a split graft repair may be indicated. In lesions where no nerve action potential is present across the site of injury, surgical transection and repair with suture alone or with grafts are required. In a review of cases of the senior author (DGK), grade 3 function or better was found in 90% of lesions in continuity when neurolysis based on nerve action potential recording was performed, 65% in those requiring surgical section and suture repair, and 50% in those requiring surgical section and grafts.[36]

Surgical Options and Common Procedures

Surgery of the peripheral nerve is performed by several specialties including neurosurgery, plastic surgery, and orthopedic surgery. Approaches taken by these specialties, as well as those followed by individual surgeons, vary significantly. The options and procedures that follow are those commonly used, and in some cases devised by the senior author (DGK) at Louisiana State University Medical Center (LSUMC) in New Orleans.

External Neurolysis

The initial step common to all surgical procedures on peripheral nerves is the isolation of the nerve from its surrounding tissues, which is called *external neurolysis*. In this step, all tissues surrounding the nerve are cleared away from the nerve over a length so that the nerve is completely mobilized 360° around for a distance both proximal and distal to the site of injury, as well as the injury site itself. With an injured nerve, external neurolysis entails removal of epineurial scar tissue, as well as any additional tissues that may be compressing the nerve. Dissection is continued proximally and distally until normal-appearing nerve free of obvious injury is encountered. An attempt is then made to record nerve action potentials (NAPs) across the area of injury so that the need for resection can be determined.

Nerve Action Potential Recording

As well as documenting intact function, NAP recording provides useful information regarding the regenerative potential of a damaged nerve long before that potential is clinically evident. This information is critical in the optimal management of nerve injuries.[69] Whenever possible, NAPs should be recordable proximal to the injury site to ensure that functional nerve exists there and to establish a baseline NAP waveform. The recording electrode is then advanced distally, first into the lesion, then through the lesion, and finally beyond it to determine the injury site and whether or not a potential is transmitted beyond the injury site. If an NAP is transmitted through the lesion, external neurolysis alone usually allows the regenerative process to continue. Such neurolysis may relieve pain, but this is variable. The major observation with NAP recording is whether a potential is present or not. The NAP amplitude and latency are of little importance unless one is recording 9 months or later postinjury[36] or dealing with a proximal plexus stretch injury where preganglionic injury is present.

Occasionally, a NAP is present but one portion of the cross section will appear worse than another. Then the injured portion can be split away and tested. If it does not transmit, it can be resected and repaired, sparing the portion that transmits. Failure of the NAP to be transmitted through a lesion necessitates surgical resection of the injury site and repair of the resulting nerve stumps. Where neurolysis was based on a recordable NAP across a lesion in continuity, 90% or more of patients recovered useful function (LSUMC grade 3 or better). Where resection of the lesion was based on absence of an NAP, the injury was, without exception, neurotmetic and/or one with poor potential for useful recovery without repair.[36]

Surgical Reanastomosis

Nerve that has been transected or nerve that remains in physical continuity but without the ability to transmit NAPs should be repaired. When the distance between the proximal and distal stumps allows, end-to-end repair is completed by suture reapproximation of the epineurium. Appropriate attempts to shorten the interstump distance (i.e., external neurolysis to free the stumps from surrounding scar and restrictive soft tissues), transposition of the nerve segments, and minor limb position adjustments should be completed before making the decision to use interposition grafts. The nerve repaired by end-to-end suture may be subjected to a small amount of tension, but this must be minimized to avoid potential separation at the repair site. When approximation of the nerve elements is not possible or when tension may lead to distraction, graft repair is required.

Interfascicular Grafts

Many patients with serious injury involving a length of nerve require grafts. The major reasons for the failure of end-to-end suture anastomosis are inadequate resection back to healthy fascicles and distraction. This makes the need for grafts more likely with serious injury. Interfascicular grafts are required to span the gap between the two stumps in nerves to be surgically repaired when direct anastomosis is impossible. An attempt is made to keep the length of the grafts at less than 5 cm when possible.

In the experimental setting, electrophysiological studies were used to evaluate neurological recovery in 14 rhesus monkeys with different nerve lesion lengths and graft lengths. After exposure of both sciatic nerves in each animal, baseline evoked nerve action potentials, muscle action potentials, and muscle strength values were determined for the posterior tibial nerves. Each nerve was then crushed over a measured distance. Three weeks later, the crushed segments were resected and the defects repaired with sural nerve grafts. In seven animals, 20 mm resection sites were repaired by 4 × 20 mm grafts in one leg and by 4 × 40 mm grafts contralaterally. In the other seven animals, the lengths of resection sites were 10 mm in one leg and 30 mm contralaterally; both nerve defects in these animals were repaired by 4 × 30 mm grafts. Electrophysiological studies were repeated at one interval of either 4, 7, or 12 months after repair. Postoperative electrophysiological values were compared to baseline values and described by their mean values and by percent recovery.[36]

Muscle strength recovery was significantly better in limbs with short lesions. In animals with identical lesion lengths, lesions repaired with shorter grafts (the same length as the defect) did significantly worse than did lesions repaired with longer grafts. This may suggest that any degree of tension at the graft repair site has a deleterious effect on functional nerve regeneration. Nevertheless, it was generally found that nerve lesion length had the greatest negative effect on functional nerve regeneration.[36]

Most graft material is obtained through harvest of the sural or antebrachial cutaneous nerves. This graft material is divided into segments slightly longer than the separation between proximal and distal stumps and sewn to proximal and distal groups of fascicles. This is termed an *interfascicular graft repair* (Fig. 21.3).

The efficacy of grafting is noted in the following study. Spinal nerve roots are often injured, and may be repaired if they can be exposed in their intraforaminal course. The posterior subscapular approach can offer that opportunity. Its main advantage is proximal exposure of the plexus spinal nerves, particularly at an intraforaminal level.[35] The technique should also be considered when prior operation, trauma, or irradiation to the neck or anterior chest wall makes a posterior exploration of the plexus easier than an anterior one. Anterior exposure of the plexus is the preferable approach for the majority of lesions needing an operation, but the posterior subscapular procedure can be useful in well-selected cases.[10]

Using the posterior subscapular approach in a series of *Macaca* rhesus monkeys, a 6 to 10 mm segment of spinal nerve not approachable by a more classic anterior operation was exposed. Sural grafts were placed from the dural exit of the spinal nerves to the cord level of the plexus. Nine surviving animals were followed for 36 to 54 months, and were observed for clinical evidence of return of function and given EMGs. The plexus was then reexposed, and intraoperative nerve action potentials were recorded across graft sites. Evoked muscle action potentials and cortical potentials were also recorded in six animals.[35]

Despite the proximal level of repair, adequate regeneration was shown by clinical, electrical, and histological studies. Functional return was best to the supraspinatus, biceps, wrist flexors, and finger flexors. Less clinical recovery was found for deltoid, wrist, and finger extensors and intrinsic muscles of the hand. Recovery of the infraspinatus muscle was poor. Despite the persistence of some denervational changes 3 years or more after injury and repair, reinnervational activity was recorded by EMG and evoked muscle action potential studies in most of the muscles studied.[36]

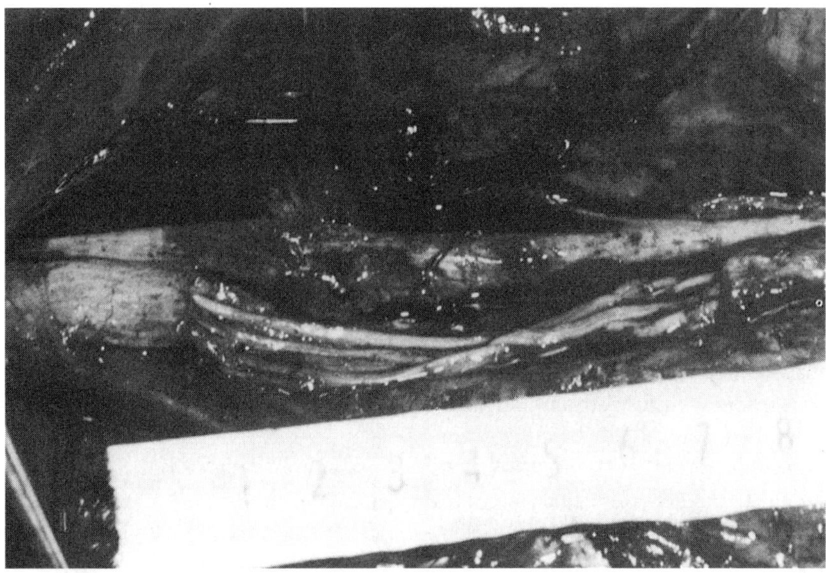

Figure 21.3. Split repair of a nerve injection injury requiring interfascicular nerve grafts. (From Kline DG, Hudson AR: Stretch injuries to the brachial plexus. In: Nerve Injuries: Operative Results for Major Nerve Injuries, Entrapments, and Tumors. Philadelphia, WB Saunders, 1995, p 174, with permission.)

Internal Neurolysis

Injury that is more severe in one portion of the cross section of the nerve or debilitating neuritic pain that is not responsive to conservative treatments are indications for internal neurolysis. The nerve is split into fascicular bundles that are then tested individually by NAP recording. Interfascicular repair with or without the use of interposition grafts is undertaken if the NAPs are absent from each individual fascicle or groups of fascicles. Fascicles that conduct NAPs through the site of injury are left in continuity, with all scar removed from around them, and allowed to continue regeneration. Fascicles that do not conduct NAPs are surgically transected back to normal-appearing fascicular structure and then repaired. In addressing partial nerve injuries in this fashion, the functional portion of the nerve is allowed to regenerate while only the damaged fascicles are repaired, giving the nerve maximal potential for functional recovery.

Internal neurolysis in patients with pain secondary to mild nerve injury and yet acceptable function may not lead to fascicular resection. At times, this can be an effective method for treating severe neuritic pain that has failed conservative treatment, although there is the risk of loss of some function.

Neurotization (Nerve Transfer)

In those injuries where proximal nerve fibers as lead outs for repair are not available, other nerves can sometimes be used as a source of proximal axons. Novel neural input, or neurotization, is most commonly used in stretch injury to the brachial plexus where nerve root damage is proximal to spinal nerves involving roots and they cannot be used as a source of axons or when frank avulsion has occurred. The intercostal nerves, medial pectoral nerves, and branches of accessory nerve are used as lead outs to distal plexus elements.

Whenever loss is confined to the proximal levels or C5 and C6 and is not directly repairable, medial pectoral branches from the medial cord can be transposed to distal musculocutaneous nerve to supply the biceps muscle, spinal accessory nerve can be anastomosed to the suprascapular nerve to initiate arm abduction, and the descending cervical plexus can be used as lead out to the posterior division of the upper trunk for possible deltoid function. The results of such procedures are quite variable, but in the situation where no other options exist, neurotization at least offers a chance of functional return.

Brachial Plexus Lesions

Injury of the brachial plexus occurs most commonly in the younger population and is one of the most debilitating nerve injuries.[22,24,45,55] As with other peripheral nerve lesions, evaluation of these injuries should be directed at determining the mechanism of injury and specific elements involved, as well as the extent of functional loss. Previously, it was thought that early amputation was the best way to manage severe combined vascular and neural injuries of the proximal upper extremity. A study by the senior author's group suggests that early amputation should not be performed unless there is massive tissue loss or an attempt at limb salvage might endanger life. Final outcomes cannot be predicted by the initial clinical presentation. As a group, the majority of these patients improve with aggressive intervention.[44] In addition, amputation does not usually help in the treatment of deafferentation pain, since it is of central origin.

The exact locus and distribution of plexus involvement should be established. Nerve root or spinal nerve, trunk, division, cord, and plexus to nerve level injuries display typical clinical manifestations during physical examination. The injury site largely determines the prognosis of these lesions. Upper nerve elements tend to have a better prognosis for recovery than lower nerve elements, and infraclavicular injuries recover more frequently than supraclavicular injuries. Injuries that involve long segments of the brachial plexus have a poorer prognosis than do the more focal injuries.

The mechanisms of brachial plexus injury can be divided into stretch injuries, gunshot wounds, lacerations, and iatrogenic damage. The three most common injuries are stretch injuries, which account for up to 70% of all serious plexus lesions, followed by gunshot wounds and lacerations. Each of these mechanisms is discussed individually in the following sections. Less frequent are iatrogenic injuries, including surgical and radiation complications, as well as birth injuries.

Management of brachial plexus lesions should follow the same rules as applied to other peripheral nerve lesions, with a few exceptions and areas requiring special emphasis. Sharp transection of the brachial plexus should be sutured end to end early, usually at the time of initial surgical exposure to allow for the distance and time required for these lengthy nerves to regenerate. Blunt transections should be observed for several weeks before surgical exploration and repair to permit accurate section beyond the areas of proximal and distal stump damage. Stretch and contusive injuries, as well as some gunshot wounds to the brachial plexus, should be observed over a period of 3 to 4 months with serial EMG and physical examinations to allow for spontaneous regeneration and recovery before consideration of surgery. Continued conservative care in the absence of regeneration should not exceed 6 months to allow for maximal recovery of function after repair. If repair is delayed too long, recovery is limited by the distance and time of the long regenerative process, as well as by progressive muscular atrophy and replacement by fibrosis and fat.

Surgical efficacy is demonstrated in the following two studies. Over a 30-year period, 1019 brachial plexus lesions underwent surgery at LSUMC, including 509 stretches/contusions, 118 gunshot wounds, and 71 lacerations. Injuries at the C5, C6, and C7 levels, the upper and middle trunk, the lateral cord to the musculocutaneous nerve, and the median and posterior cords to the axillary and radial nerves had the best results. Recoveries were poor for injuries at the C8 and T1 levels, and for lower trunk and medial cord lesions, with the exception of injuries of the medial cord to the median nerve. Favorable outcomes can be anticipated for appropriately selected patients.[27]

The epidemiology, preoperative management, operative findings, operative treatment, and postoperative results in 100 consecutive surgical patients with brachial plexus injuries at LSUMC were reviewed. The group included 81 males and 19 females ranging from 5 to 70 years of age. Illustrating the beneficial role of both graft repair and neurotization or nerve transfer, 78% of patients with open wounds recovered to a grade 3 or better level, as did 58% of patients with stretch injuries. One hundred percent of patients with C5-C6 stretch injuries recovered some useful arm function.[9]

Brachial Plexus Stretch Injuries

This most common injury to the brachial plexus is caused by stretch and contusion due to vehicular accidents and, less commonly, sporting injuries. Management of these lesions is a source of great debate despite the wide interest in and extensive writing about this type of injury. Most workers in the field believe that an initial period of conservative management is indicated during which serial physical examinations are used to establish regeneration and recovery. At LSUMC, such patients are followed for 4 months before surgical exploration is considered. Those with significant electrical evidence of regeneration or early recovery of function are followed further and not operated on. Those with persistent neurological deficits after this period of observation without evidence of regeneration are surgically explored, intraoperatively inspected, and tested with intraoperative NAP recordings. Evidence of regeneration of lack thereof can be established firmly, and resection with repair can be initiated if required.

A series of 204 operative patients with supraclavicular stretch injuries to the brachial plexus were followed for a minimum of 18 months at LSUMC.[36] Some recovery resulted from surgical repair. Thirty percent of patients with complete C5-6 injury (35 patients) regained significant spontaneous recovery. Those C5-C6 lesions that failed to recover usually had direct repair (although some needed nerve transfers) and recovered the greatest function of all of the operated plexus stretch lesions. Only 16% of patients with complete loss of C5-C7 (47 patients) achieved significant spontaneous recovery. These lesions had some direct repair, but this repair was frequently supplemented by neurotization or nerve transfers. Functional recovery was greatest in biceps and brachioradialis, with less effective deltoid recovery and even less triceps recovery.

Patients with flail arms involving all of the nerve roots of the brachial plexus, C5-T1 (106 patients), seldom regained significant spontaneous recovery (4%–5%). Repair consisted of direct graft repair of some elements and neurotization of others directed to salvage of the arm. In 40% of these surgically repaired plexus lesions, there was some return of shoulder abduction and biceps flexion. Only 30% of these patients regained triceps function. Recovery of hand function was quite rare. Other stretch injuries resulting in different patterns of plexus involvement were far less frequent (8%), but in general, elements derived from the upper plexus (C5-C7) experienced greater functional recovery with operation, whereas the lower elements (C8-T1) improved far less frequently.

A large series of infraclavicular plexus injuries were followed, and again, the major mechanism of injury was stretch and contusion.[36] Those patients requiring surgery because of persistent loss did best in the distribution of lateral cord to musculocutaneous and median nerves, and of posterior cord to axillary and some radial nerves. Medial cord to median nerve repair resulted in a surprisingly good recovery of function, whereas medial cord to ulnar nerve repair resulted in a lower grade of functional recovery. Axillary nerve injuries selected for operation had an overall recovery rate of 70% for a grade 3 LSUMC level or better recovery of deltoid.

Brachial Plexus Gunshot Wounds

Gunshot wounds are the second most common mechanism of injury to the brachial plexus in the United States.[36] In those lesions with complete loss distal to the injury site, a great majority of the elements remain in continuity, with a far lower incidence of physical disruption. Recovery of function is infrequent even in those elements that remain in continuity. Management of these lesions is initially conservative. Vascular compromise, other associated injuries necessitating surgical exploration, or debilitating persistent causalgia despite adequate conservative therapy are operative prompts. If early surgery is indicated, treatment of the wound itself should be directed to correction of associated injuries, debridement of the wound, and tacking down transected nerve elements to adjacent fascial structures to minimize retraction of the stumps.

Conservative management of gunshot wounds to the brachial plexus at LSUMC includes serial EMG and physical examinations to assess regeneration and functional recovery over a 2- to 5-month period before considering operative exploration. Absence of evidence of regeneration and functional recovery, evidence of vascular compression of the plexus elements, or debilitating pain indicates the need for lead surgery. Incomplete or complete loss of lower element function (C8 and T1) and excessive delay in referral after injury are relative contraindications for surgery. Operative exploration is designed to directly assess each element's functional status as determined by NAP recordings.

In a series of 141 gunshot wounds involving the brachial plexus reported by the senior author (DGK), 90 patients underwent operative exploration.[36] Persistent functional loss led to surgery in

79 patients, compression of plexus elements by pseudoaneurysms or clot in 6, and debilitating noncausalgic pain unresponsive to conservative management in the remaining 5 patients despite the presence of incomplete lesions. During operative exploration, it was found that of the 221 elements studied by NAP recordings, only 14 were transected, whereas the remaining 207 were lesions in continuity. The results of the NAP recordings in conjunction with visual inspection of the nerve determined the surgical approach for each specific element. When an NAP was recorded across the lesion (96 elements), the element was subjected to neurolysis, and in 4 of these elements a split repair was performed where a definite portion of the nerve was badly damaged with relative sparing of the remaining fascicular structure. No NAPs were recorded across the lesion in 125 of the elements studied, leading to resection and repair of these damaged elements. End-to-end anastomosis was possible in only 26 of these electrically silent elements, whereas 99 required graft interposition repair (Fig. 21.4).

As in the stretch injuries of the brachial plexus, the upper elements experience greater recovery after repair than do the lower elements. Supraspinatus, biceps, and brachioradialis recovered to a grade 3 or better level, whereas deltoid, triceps, and more distal muscles of the arm obtained lesser recovery. In the patients operated on for debilitating pain, roughly 50% obtained some degree of relief.

Brachial Plexus Lacerations

Lacerating injury is the third most common mechanism of injury to the brachial plexus and the most amenable to successful repair.[1,13,36] Management of these lesions is based on the assumption that lacerations to the tissues surrounding the plexus may also involve the neural elements of the plexus. When the neurological deficit is severe, these lesions should be explored at the time of surgical repair for associated injuries or within the first 72 hours if acute repair of associated injuries is not warranted. Sharp lacerations involving elements of the brachial plexus should be repaired acutely, as with other peripheral nerve lesions. A delay of 2 weeks or so is used for blunt transections of plexus elements to permit delineation of the proxi-

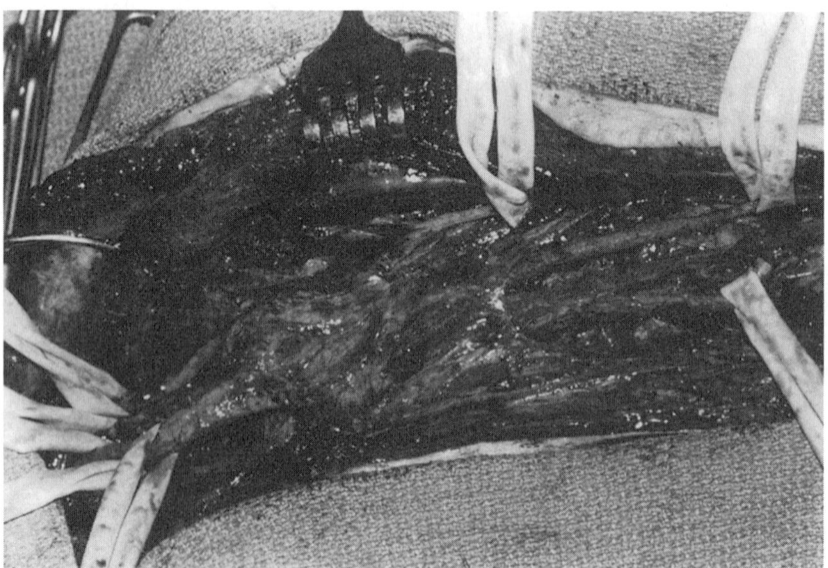

Figure 21.4. Infraclavicular gunshot wound with severe scar involving the cords of the plexus and axillary artery. Preoperative loss was complete in the lateral and posterior cord distribution and incomplete in that of the medial cord. Despite this, each of these plexus elements transmitted NAPs and were either regenerating well or partially injured to begin with thus requiring neurolysis alone. (From Kline DG, Hudson AR: Gunshot wounds to the brachial plexus. In: Nerve Injuries: Operative Results for Major Nerve Injuries, Entrapments, and Tumors. Philadelphia, WB Saunders, 1995, p 388, with permission.)

mal and distal extent of contusion. If acute exploration reveals a bluntly transected nerve, repair of the associated injuries, cleaning of the wound, and tacking of the proximal and distal stumps to fascial or muscular planes to maintain length should be performed. Definitive neural repair is then delayed for 2 to 4 weeks.

Of the 47 patients reported by Kline and Hudson[36] to have lacerating injuries of the brachial plexus, 142 elements were documented as seriously damaged by clinical and electrical examination. Operative exploration of these patients revealed that 60 neural elements were sharply transected, 52 were bluntly transected, and 30 remained in continuity with injury due to contusion and stretch despite a lacerating mechanism of injury.

In the sharp transecting injuries, 60 elements were found to be involved; 24 of these were repaired within 72 hours of injury with end-to-end suture repair, with the remaining 36 elements being repaired secondarily because of delayed referral. Interposition graft repair was required in 26 of the secondary repairs to overcome gaps due to retraction, with the remaining undergoing a secondary end-to-end repair. Blunt transections were found to involve 52 neural elements, with 47 requiring secondary interposition graft repair because proximal and distal stumps had to be trimmed back to normal fascicular structures. Only five such injuries could be secondarily repaired by end-to-end suture alone. Of the 30 lesions that were found to be in continuity despite a mechanism suggesting laceration, 10 transmitted NAPs through the injury site and had only neurolysis, whereas the remaining 20 required resection and repair; of these, 13 were repaired by interposition grafts and 7 had end-to-end suture.

Results were the best in the repair of transections when they were sharp, with grade 3 or better function being obtained in 63% of all sharp transections, whether done acutely or secondarily. Results were good in 75% of the acute suture repairs in this category, 70% of the secondary suture repairs, and 50% of the secondary repairs requiring interposition grafts. The blunt transecting injuries of the plexus had a somewhat poorer functional improvement, with 48% regaining grade 3 or better function. In these blunt injuries, 60% of the secondary end-to-end suture repairs and 47% of those requiring interposition grafts regained this level of function. Ninety percent of the lesions in continuity that transmitted NAPs and required neurolysis alone had return to a grade 3 level of function. Grade 3 recovery levels were achieved in 71% of patients with continuity lesions undergoing secondary end-to-end repair and in 77% of those who required grafts.

Obstetric Palsies

While a thorough discussion of obstetric palsies is beyond the scope of this chapter, they do merit a mention. Birth injuries are usually an upper brachial (Erb-Duchenne) plexus palsy, and less often a lower (Dejerine-Klumpke) palsy, and occur in 0.6–2.6 per 1000 births. The usual causes are maternal-fetal disproportion, prolonged labor, the need for forceps, and breech birth.[17,57] While controversy exists over when to stop expectant management and operate, at LSUMC the patients were between 9 and 26 months of age at the time of surgery. Favored, at LSUHSC if possible, is exploration at 9 to 12 months. Neuromas in continuity were the most common surgical finding.[36]

A meta-analysis compiled from Medline and Cochrane Library searches suggests that there is no conclusive evidence of a benefit of surgery over conservative management approaches in the treatment of patients with birth-related brachial plexus injuries. However, outcomes from surgical series are generally favorable (level III and V evidence). Direct comparison with the natural history could not be inferred from the series reviewed given the lack of controls. Surgery remains a valid practice option since there is level III and V evidence suggesting a possible benefit of surgery.[46]

Other Peripheral Nerves

While brachial plexus injuries are the most serious lesions a peripheral nerve surgeon deals with, surgical intervention is also performed for injuries of other nerves, including median, ulnar, radial, femoral, sciatic, and peroneal injuries. The aforementioned principles of evaluation and intervention apply. Several relatively recent clinical series have evaluated the treatment and outcome of peripheral nerve surgery on injured nerves and will be discussed in this section.

The femoral nerve can be injured during open or laparoscopic pelvic/abdominal procedures, as well as by gunshot, laceration, and stretch injury. At LSUMC, 78 traumatic injuries were seen in 94 patients with femoral neuropathies; 54 of these were operated on because of persistent complete functional loss and/or pain. Exploration and NAP recordings were done. Even with complete preoperative loss of function, 13 patients had recordable NAPs and underwent neurolysis, recovering to at least an LSUMC grade 3 level. Twenty-seven patients had sural graft repairs, and most recovered to grade 3 to 4 levels by 2 years postoperatively. Four of five patients with suture repairs recovered to grade 3 or better levels within 2 years postoperatively.[34]

Sciatic injuries are also amenable to surgery. Over a 24-year period, 380 patients with sciatic nerve injuries were evaluated.[37] Injection injury, gunshot wound, femur fracture, laceration, or contusion was seen. Twenty-three percent of injuries at the thigh level and almost 50% of those at the buttock level had partial deficits with significant spontaneous recovery, medically controlled pain, or late referral. Consequently, they were managed medically. Surgical intervention, with neurolysis, NAPs, graft, or suture repair, was required for more complete and persistent deficits or for severe pain not manageable medically. Overall, recovery was most notable in the tibial distribution; only 36% of patients who received suture or graft repairs of the peroneal division showed significant improvement. Regardless of the level or mechanism of injury, the tibial division of the sciatic nerve had a more favorable result than the peroneal division.

At the senior author's (DGK) institution, over a 21-year period, 302 patients with peroneal lesions were evaluated.[33] Traumatic lesions consisted of stretch injury with or without fracture, laceration, gunshot wound, compression, entrapment, and iatrogenic injury. Patients who did not experience spontaneous recovery by 4 to 6 months after injury had an operation. Seventy-five percent of patients with graft lengths of less than 5.5 cm recovered peroneal function to grade 3 or better and did not need an orthotic for ambulation. Thirty-five percent of those with graft lengths of 6 to 12 cm and only 14% of those with graft lengths of 13 to 20 cm recovered function to grade 3 or better. Eighty-two percent of end-to-end suture repair had grade 3 level function by 2 years, but these, by definition, were lesser injuries than those needing grafts. Eighty-nine percent of patients with transmittable nerve action potentials across lesions in continuity recovered peroneal ability even though the preoperative grade was poor.

Upper extremity injury has also been analyzed. A total of 167 patients with median nerve injury, such as laceration, fracture-associated stretch and contusion, gunshot wound, compression, and injection injuries, had surgery at LSUMC over a 30-year period.[32] For lesions in continuity, a functional recovery of grade 3 or better was seen in 95% of neurolysis patients, 86% of suture repair patients, and 75% of those with graft repairs. In lesions not in continuity, 91% of end-to-end suture repairs, 78% of secondary suture repairs, and 68% of graft repairs had grade 3 or better results.

A similar study was undertaken of the radial nerve in which 260 patients with injuries were evaluated. The most common mechanisms of injury were fracture of the humerus, laceration, blunt contusions, and gunshot wounds.[31] Sixty-nine percent of these patients underwent surgery, and 90% of them had à minimum of 1.5 years of follow-up. Recovery of motor function to grade 3 or better was observed in 91% of those with end-to-end suture repairs, 83% of those with secondary suture repairs, 80% of those who received graft repairs, and 98% of those who had neurolysis based on NAP recordings. Seventy-one percent of subjects with superficial sensory radial nerve injury achieved satisfactory pain relief after complete resection of a neuroma or neurolysis. Of interest, when dealing with patients at high risk for nonunion of humeral shaft fractures, transposition of the radial nerve at the time of plating is a useful adjunct.[52]

Thirty-two patients from the LSUMC pool of peripheral nerve patients had involvement of the posterior interosseous nerve exclusively.[6] Traumatic causes included laceration, fracture, compression, or contusion. In the operative series, all patients had recovery of function to LSUMC grade 3 or more after 4 years of follow-up.

Ulnar nerve injuries over a 30 year period included lacerations (12%), stretches/contusions (8%), fractures/dislocations (5%), gunshot wounds (2%), and injection-induced injuries (0.3%).[30] Functional recoveries of grade 3 or better were seen in 92% of patients who underwent neurolysis, 72% who received suture repair, and 67% who had graft repair. Nevertheless, fewer grade 4 or 5 recoveries were reached than in those patients with radial or median nerve injuries.

Pain and Nerve Trauma

The primary focus of brachial plexus or other peripheral nerve surgery is the restoration of function, as well as prevention of further loss. However, surgery on nerves can sometimes be used to treat pain. Working with pain and rehabilitation specialists can assist with this aspect of peripheral nerve injury. Posttraumatic pain can originate from the nervous system or from limb immobilization after peripheral nerve injury. Immobilization, even after surgery, should be minimal and never longer than 3 weeks.[68]

Neurogenic pain, whether denervational, regenerative, neuritic, or complex regional pain syndrome (which includes reflex sympathetic dystrophy and causalgia) or from a neuroma, has treatment options. Denervation pain will decrease with the plateauing of the atrophic process.[49] Regenerative pain occurs early in the regeneration process, and can be self-limited as the limb is used or managed with drugs like Elavil, Tegretol, or Neurontin.[50]

Neuritic pain occurs in the anatomical distribution of the injured nerve, and a Tinel's sign can be elicited. Medications can be tried, but surgical exploration usually demonstrates a surgically treatable condition such as a neuroma in continuity. If management of the in continuity lesion is not successful, dorsal root entry zone lesion placement of a stimulating electrode can be considered.[73]

The treatment of complex regional pain syndrome is beyond the scope of this chapter and is constantly evolving. Traditionally, sympathetic block followed by sympathectomy has been an option.[3] Neuroma pain is initially managed conservatively, with physical therapy, desensitization, pain medication, transcutaneous electrical nerve stimulation, or local steroid injection. If these modalities fail, surgery can be performed after a realistic discussion of the limitations of such management. Surgical management of the neuroma in continuity was discussed earlier in this chapter. If the neuroma is located at the end of a nerve stump, our preferred method is to inject an anesthetic in the nerve proximal to the site of section. Then the nerve is sectioned proximal to the neuroma, and the distal segment is removed whenever possible. The bipolar approach is used to seal the fascicles in the cut end, and this end is then placed under muscle.

Future Directions

A systematic approach to the surgical management of these neural lesions has evolved at our institution, based in part on experience with intraoperative recording of nerve action potentials and a resultant large number of referrals. Advanced microsurgical techniques including the use of grafts have expanded the scope of peripheral nerve surgery. These advances, coupled with intraoperative electrophysiological measurements, have improved the outcomes.[64]

What are the long-term subjective, employment, and functional outcomes following surgical treatment for brachial plexus injury? One study surveyed 32 such patients.[5] Their mean age was 37 years, and the mean postinjury time was 7 years. Twenty-five patients reported at least moderate satisfaction with overall life, and no patients reported extreme dissatisfaction. Ten patients reported that their injury greatly affected the quality of their lives, and only slightly more than half of the patients were employed at the time of the study. Workers compensation, litigation, pain, marital status, number of children, educational status, and degree of functional recovery did not affect the outcome. In general, during the first year after injury, most patients had a good quality of life and were employed.[5]

Developments in the field of muscle and tendon transfer have shown these procedures to be a useful adjuvant to nerve surgery and can offer additional hope for patients. By marrying anatomical knowledge, surgical judgment, and rehabilitative expertise, improvement in function can be dramatic.[48] On the other hand, an unsuccessful tendon transfer wastes a normal muscle-tendon unit and leaves the patient with less function than before.[54] Besides the hand, tendon and flexor muscle recession at the level of the elbow can sometimes restore flexion when the biceps is absent.[47] Tendon transfer procedures are also available for the lower extremity, particularly the foot.

Working with our plastic and orthopedic colleagues, we have developed more options for the peripheral nerve patient. For example, shoulder arthrodesis can help some patients. This places the shoulder in slight abduction, external rotation, and anterior elevation, and is useful for patients who have weakness in upper trunk innervated muscles with preservation of distal motor function.

Of course, prior to transfer and fixation procedures, the potential for nerve regeneration is the focus of treatment. One aspect of this field is the development of conduits. Rabbits have been used to study functional nerve regeneration through macropore, semipermeable, and nonpermeable collagen conduits.[29] The macropore–collagen tube group showed significantly greater functional recovery than the semipermeable or nonpermeable collagen tube groups, although more work in this area is needed.

Another study evaluated the ability of Schwann cell transplants in collagen tubes to enhance the recovery of function in injured nerves.[28] These results were compared to those achieved with sural nerve grafting after sciatic nerve injury. Physiological measurements showed that the Schwann cell implants induced return of function comparable to that of the sural nerve grafts, but there were greater numbers of myelinated axons in Schwann cell implants than in sural nerve grafts. At 4 months, prelabeled Schwann cells had migrated up to 30 mm away from the implant site.

An exciting development is the future possibility of allografts. The French have reported a double hand allograft placed by using conventional immunosuppression. Results were at least as good as those achieved in replanted upper extremities. However, longer follow-up will be necessary to demonstrate the final functional restoration.[7]

Summary

An algorithm for the treatment of the injured peripheral nerve and plexus is shown in Figure 21.5.[8] The selection of patients who will benefit from peripheral nerve surgery continues to evolve. The evaluation of patients with peripheral nerve problems, and the indications for and timing of surgery, were reviewed in this chapter. This includes patients with transections, lesions in continuity, entrapments, injection injuries, and birth palsies. The treatment outlined for patients with peripheral nerve and brachial plexus injuries is based on a comprehensive clinical and electrodiagnostic evaluation complemented by imaging studies.

While not all peripheral nerve surgery is done acutely, indications for acute surgery for peripheral nerve or brachial plexus dysfunction are sharp transections and extraneural injury requiring immediate repair to prevent further neurological loss. Examples include vascular lesions causing peripheral nerve compression (i.e., expanding hematoma, pseudoaneurysm) and compartment syndrome. If an injury affects an area where nerves can potentially be compressed, like the carpal tunnel, Guyon's canal, or the cubital tunnel, this area should be decompressed earlier rather than later.

The prognosis for in continuity lesions is difficult to quantitative preoperatively due to the variability of these injuries. These lesions should be followed and reassessed for several months before surgical intervention. Then, in the operating room, visual inspection and NAP recordings will dictate the further needed operative steps.

Delayed referral for surgical evaluation, particularly if a year or more has passed since the injury, can reduce the chances for a good surgical outcome from nerve repair. Denervation can be quantitated by the third week postinjury, and an EMG should be done then to serve as a baseline for future electrical and clinical studies. Electrical evidence of reinnervation does not ensure recovery of function, but does establish that nerve fibers have regenerated to a specific muscle. The EMG is repeated every few months, as determined by the estimated time required to grow the distance to the denervated muscle.

The decision to operate is based on lack of improvement in the early postinjury months. Secondary repair of all other injuries should be done in a timely fashion to allow the best environment for nerve regeneration. Burn, electrical, and obstetric injuries, as well as pain-related issues, often require a multispecialty team.

The period of delay for nerve repair should be limited to optimize the possibility of maximal functional return. Focal isolated injuries, such as those resulting from fracture or high-velocity penetrating wounds, typically require a 2- to 3-month delay, whereas the more lengthy, diffuse lesions common after blunt contusive trauma and stretching injuries requires delays of 4–5 months. Continued conservative care in the absence of regeneration should not exceed 6 months to allow for maximal recovery of function after repair. If repair is delayed too long, recovery is limited by the distance and time of the long regenerative process, as well as the subsequent muscular atrophy and replacement by fibrosis and fat.

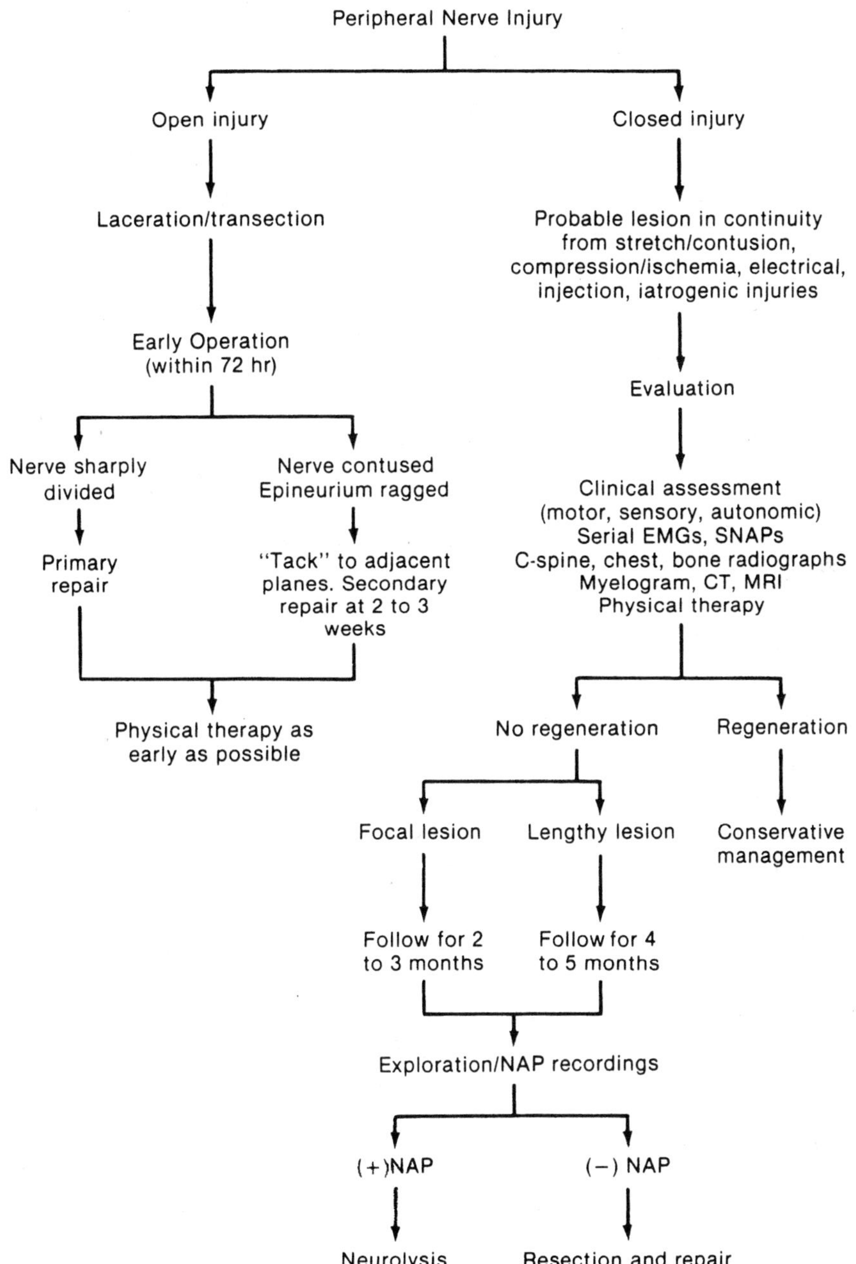

Figure 21.5. An algorithm for the treatment of nerve injuries. (From Dubuisson A, Kline DG: Indications for peripheral nerve and brachial plexus surgery. Neurol Clin 10:935–951, 1992, with permission.)

REFERENCES

1. Amine AR, Sugar O: Repair of severed brachial plexus: A plea to ER physicians. JAMA 239:1039, 1976.
2. Armington W, Harnsberger H, Osborn A, et al: Radiographic evaluation of brachial plexopathy. Am J Neuroradiol 8:361–367, 1987.
3. Atasoy E, Kleinert HE: Surgical sympathectomy and sympathetic blocks for the upper and lower extremities, and local and plexus levels. In: Omer GE Jr, Spinner M, Van Beek AL (eds): Management of Peripheral Nerve Problems, 2nd ed. Philadelphia, WB Saunders, 1998, pp 157–171.
4. Bateman JE: The Shoulder and Neck, 2nd ed. Philadelphia, WB Saunders, 1978, pp 656–676.
5. Choi PD, Novak CB, Mackinnon SE, Kline DG: Quality of life and functional outcome following brachial plexus injury. J Hand Surg 22:605–612, 1997.
6. Cravens G, Kline DG: Posterior interosseous nerve palsies. Neurosurgery 27:397–402, 1990.
7. Dubernard JM, Petruzzo P, Lanzetta M, Parmentier H, Martin X, Dawahra M, Hakim NS, Owen E: Functional results of the first human double-hand transplantation. Ann Surg 238:128–136, 2003.
8. Dubuisson A, Kline DG: Indications for peripheral nerve and brachial plexus surgery. Neurol Clin 10:935–951, 1992.
9. Dubuisson AS, Kline DG: Brachial plexus injury: A survey of 100 consecutive cases from a single service. Neurosurgery 51:673–682, 2002.
10. Dubuisson AS, Kline DG, Weinshel SS: Posterior subscapular approach to the brachial plexus. Report of 102 patients. J Neurosurg 79:319–330, 1993.
11. Ducker TB: Pathophysiology of peripheral nerve trauma. In: Omer GE, Spinner M (eds): Management of Peripheral Nerve Problems. Philadelphia, WB Saunders, 1980.
12. Ducker TB, Garrison W: Surgical aspects of peripheral nerve trauma. Curr Probl Surg 7:1–62, 1974.
13. Dunkerton MC, Boone RS: Stab wounds involving the brachial plexus. A review of operated cases. J Bone Joint Surg 70:566–570, 1988.
14. England JD, Happel LT, Kline DG, Gamboni F, Thouron CL, Liu ZP, Levinson SR: Sodium channel accumulation in humans with painful neuromas. Neurology 47:272–276, 1996.
15. England JD, Happel LT, Liu ZP, Thouron CL, Kline DG: Abnormal distributions of potassium channels in human neuromas. Neurosci Lett 255:37–40, 1998.
16. Gentili F, Hudson AR, Hunter D: Clinical and experimental aspects of injection injuries of peripheral nerves. Can J Neurol Sci 7:143–151, 1980.
17. Geutjens G, Gilbert A, Helsen K: Obstetrical brachial plexus palsy associated with breech delivery. A different pattern of injury. J Bone Joint Surg [Br] 78B:303–306, 1996.
18. Gilliatt RW, Ochoa J, Ridge P, Neary D: Cause of nerve damage in acute compression. Trans Am Neuroal Assoc 99:571–574, 1974.
19. Gilmer-Hill HS, Beuerman R, Ma Q, Jiang J, Tiel RL, Kline DG: Response of GAP-43 and p75 in human neuromas over time after traumatic injury. Neurosurgery 51:1229–1237, 2002.
20. Hentz VR, Narakas A: The results of microneurosurgical reconstruction in complete brachial plexus palsy. Assessing outcome and predicting results. Orthop Clin North Am 19:107–113, 1988.
21. Hudson AR, Hunter D: Timing of peripheral nerve repair: Important local neuropathologic factors. Clin Neurosurg 24:391–405, 1977.
22. Hudson AR, Trammer B: Brachial plexus injuries. In: Wilkins RG, Rengachary SS (eds): Neurosurgery, vol 2. Philadelphia, WB Saunders, 1985, pp 1817–1832.
23. Jones SJ: Diagnostic use of peripheral and spinal somatosensory evoked potentials in traction lesions of the brachial plexus. Clin Plast Surg 11:167–172, 1984.
24. Kanaya F, Gonzalez M, Park CM, et al: Improvement in motor function after brachial plexus surgery. J Hand Surg 15A:30–35, 1990.
25. Kaplan EB, Spinner MB: Normal and anomalous innervation patterns in the upper extremity. In: Omer G, Spinner M (eds): Management of Peripheral Nerve Problems. Philadelphia, WB Saunders, 1980.
26. Kewalramani L, Taylor R: Brachial plexus root avulsion: Role of myelography. J Trauma 15:603–608, 1975.
27. Kim DH, Cho YJ, Tiel RL, Kline DG: Outcomes of surgery in 1019 brachial plexus lesions treated at Louisiana State University Health Sciences Center. J Neurosurg 98:1005–1016, 2003.
28. Kim DH, Connolly SE, Kline DG, Voorhies RM, Smith A, Powell M, Yoes T, Daniloff JK: Labeled Schwann cell transplants versus sural nerve grafts in nerve repair. J Neurosurg 80:254–260, 1994.
29. Kim DH, Connolly SE, Zhao S, Beuerman RW, Voorhies RM, Kline DG: Comparison of macropore, semipermeable, and nonpermeable collagen conduits in nerve repair. J Reconstr Microsurg 9:415–420, 1993.
30. Kim DH, Han K, Tiel RL, Murovic JA, Kline DG: Surgical outcomes of 654 ulnar nerve lesions. J Neurosurg 98: 993–1004, 2003.
31. Kim DH, Kam AC, Chandika P, Tiel RL, Kline DG: Surgical management and outcome in patients with radial nerve lesions. J Neurosurg 95:573–583, 2001.
32. Kim DH, Kam AC, Chandika P, Tiel RL, Kline DG: Surgical management and outcomes in patients with median nerve lesions. J Neurosurg 95:584–594, 2001.
33. Kim DH, Kline DG: Management and results of peroneal nerve lesions. Neurosurgery 39:312–319, 1996.
34. Kim DH, Kline DG: Surgical outcome for intra- and extrapelvic femoral nerve lesions. J Neurosurg 83:783–790, 1995.
35. Kline DG, Donner TR, Happel L, Smith B, Richter HP: Intraforaminal repair of plexus spinal nerves by a posterior approach: An experimental study. J Neurosurg 76:459–470, 1992.
36. Kline DG, Hudson AR (eds): Nerve Injuries: Operative Results for Major Nerve Injuries, Entrapments, and Tumors. Philadelphia, WB Saunders, 1995.

37. Kline DG, Kim D, Midha R, Harsh C, Tiel R: Management and results of sciatic nerve injuries: A 24-year experience. J Neurosurg 89:13–23, 1998.
38. Kretschmer T, England JD, Happel LT, Liu ZP, Thouron CL, Nguyen DH, Beuerman RW, Kline DG: Ankyrin G and voltage gated sodium channels colocalize in human neuroma—key proteins of membrane remodeling after axonal injury. Neurosci Lett 323:151–155, 2002.
39. Kretschmer T, Nguyen DH, Beuerman RW, Happel LT, England JD, Tiel RL, Kline DG: Painful neuromas: A potential role for a structural transmembrane protein, ankyrin G. J Neurosurg 97:1424–1431, 2002.
40. Leffert RD: Clinical diagnosis, testing, and electromyographic study in brachial plexus traction injuries. Clin Orthop Rel Res 237:24–31, 1988.
41. Lu G, Beuerman RW, Zhao S, Sun G, Nguyen DH, Ma S, Kline DG: Tumor necrosis factor-alpha and interleukin-1 induce activation of MAP kinase and SAP kinase in human neuroma fibroblasts. Neurochem Int 30:401–410, 1997.
42. MacKinnon S, Dellon A: Surgery of the Peripheral Nerve. New York, Thieme, 1988.
43. Mailander P, Berger A, Schaller E, et al: Results of primary nerve repair in the upper extremity. Microsurgery 10:147–150, 1989.
44. Manord JD, Garrard CL, Kline DG, Sternbergh WC 3rd, Money SR: Management of severe proximal vascular and neural injury of the upper extremity. J Vasc Surg 27:43–47, 1998.
45. McGillicuddy JE: Clinical decision making in brachial plexus injuries. Neurosurg Clin North Am 2:175–185, 1991.
46. McNeely PD, Drake JM: A systematic review of brachial plexus surgery for birth-related brachial plexus injury. Pediatr Neurosurg 38:57–62, 2003.
47. Moneim MS, Omer GE: Latissimus dorsi muscle transfer for restoration of elbow flexion after brachial plexus disruption. J Hand Surg [Am] 11A:135–139, 1986.
48. Moran SL, Berger RA: Biomechanics and hand trauma: What you need. Hand Clin 19:17–31, 2003.
49. Noordenbos W: Pain. Amsterdam, Elsevier, 1959.
50. Ochoa J: Pain in local nerve lesions. In: Culp WJ, Ochoa J (eds): Abnormal Nerves and Muscles as Impulse Generators. New York, Oxford University Press, 1982, pp 568–587.
51. Ochoa J, Fowler RJ, Gilliatt RW: Anatomical changes in peripheral nerves compressed by a pneumatic tourniquet. J Anat 113:433–455, 1972.
52. Olarte CM, Darowish M, Ziran BH: Radial nerve transposition with humeral fracture fixation: Preliminary results. Clin Orthop, 413:170–174, 2003.
53. Prutkin L: Normal and anomalous innervation patterns in the lower extremities. In: Omer G, Spinner M (eds): Management of Peripheral Nerve Problems. Philadelphia, WB Saunders, 1980.
54. Richards RR: Tendon transfers for failed nerve reconstruction. Clin Plast Surg 30:223–245, 2003.
55. Rossom JW: Durability following closed traction lesions of the brachial plexus sustained in motorcycle accidents. J Hand Surg 12B:353–355, 1987.
56. Salisbury RE, Bevin AG, Lombardo AA: Burn-induced peripheral nerve injury. In: Omer GE, Spinner M, Van Beek AL (eds): Management of Peripheral Nerve Problems, 2nd ed. Philadelphia, WB Saunders, 1988, pp 623–639.
57. Salonen I, Uusitalo R: Birth injuries: Incidence and predisposing factors. Z Kinderchir 45:133–135, 1990.
58. Salzberg CA, Salisbury RE: Thermal injury of peripheral nerve. In: Gelberman RH (ed): Operative Nerve Repair and Reconstruction. Philadelphia, JB Lippincott, 1991, pp 671–678.
59. Schwenkreis P, Janssen F, Rommel O, Pleger B, Volker B, Hosbach I, Dertwinkel R, Maier C, Tegenthoff M: Bilateral motor cortex disinhibition in complex regional pain syndrome (CRPS) type I of the hand. Neurology 61:515–519, 2003.
60. Sears TA: Structural changes in motoneurons following axotomy. J Exp Biol 132:93–109, 1987.
61. Seddon H: Three types of nerve injury. Brain 66:237–288, 1943.
62. Seddon HJ (ed): Surgical Disorders of the Peripheral Nerves. Baltimore, Williams & Wilkins, 1972.
63. Spinner RJ, Khoobehi A, Kazmi S, Krumreich JA, Zhao S, Zhang Z, Kline DG, Beuerman RW: Model for avulsion injury in the rat brachial plexus using passive acceleration. Microsurgery 20:94–97, 2000.
64. Spinner RJ, Kline DG: Surgery for peripheral nerve and brachial plexus injuries or other nerve lesions. Muscle Nerve. 23(5):680–695, 2000.
65. Strain R, Olson W: Selective damage of large diameter peripheral nerve fibers by compression: An application of LaPlace's law. Exp Neurol 47:68–80, 1975.
66. Sunderland S: Rate of regeneration in human peripheral nerves. Arch Neurol Psychiatry 58:251–295, 1947.
67. Sunderland S: A classification of peripheral nerve injuries producing loss of function. Brain 74:491, 1951.
68. Tarlov IM: How long should an extremity be immobilized after a nerve suture? Ann Surg 126:366–376, 1947.
69. Tiel RL, Happel LT Jr, Kline DG: Nerve action potential recording method and equipment. Neurosurgery 39: 103–108, 1996.
70. Zachary RB, Roaf R: Lesions in continuity. In: Seddon HJ (ed): Peripheral Nerve Injuries: Medical Research Council Special Report Series No. 282. London, Her Majesty's Stationery Office, 1954.
71. Zelt RG, Daniel RK, Ballard PA, Brissette Y, Heroux P: High voltage electrical injury: Chronic wound evolution. Plast Reconstr Surg 82:1027–1041, 1988.
72. Zhao S, Pang Y, Beuerman RW, Thompson HW, Kline DG: Expression of c-Fos protein in the spinal cord after brachial plexus injury: Comparison of root avulsion and distal nerve transection. Neurosurgery 42:1357–1362, 1998.
73. Zorub DS, Nashold BS Jr, Cook WA Jr: Avulsion of the brachial plexus: A review with implications on the therapy of intractable pain. Surg Neurol 2:347–353, 1974.

Part IV

Posttraumatic Pain Syndromes

Chapter 22
Whiplash Injuries

RANDOLPH W. EVANS

The late comedian Rodney Dangerfield could have been the spokesman for whiplash injuries with his refrain, "I don't get no respect." Controversy is present among physicians[57] and the general public[4] about the pathology of the injury, cause of persistent symptoms, prognosis, medico-legal aspects, and treatment. As Fontanetta[207] notes:

> The term "whiplash," once introduced, quickly became a favorite of the legal profession and suit-conscious patient. To the orthopedic surgeon, "whiplash" connotes a lack of findings on physical and x-ray examination, an often profuse symptomatology, and prolonged disability. The ubiquitous cervical collar became socially acceptable, and colors other than white made their appearance on some pretty female neck.

Pearce[167] elaborates:

> Few topics provoke so much controversy or heated opinion, based on so little fact as whiplash injuries. In emergency departments, orthopaedic, neurological and rheumatological clinics, and not least in the Courts, this common syndrome is shrouded in mystery and creates clinical insecurity in those who attempt to explain its mechanism, its prognosis and treatment. These problems are compounded in medico-legal practice where the potential rewards of successful litigation may colour the clinical picture. . . . Most victims of whiplash injury have, however, sustained no more than a minor sprain to the soft tissues and unusually severe or protracted complaints may demand explanations which lie outside the fields of organic and psychiatric illness.

Porter,[176] however, counters, "Pain, suffering, and disability after acute neck sprains may be reduced by doctors recognizing that these injuries, especially those that occur after rearend impacts, may cause long term disability." The titles of articles over the years reflect this controversy: "The Enigma of Whiplash Injury,"[207] "Whiplash Injury of Neck—Fact or Fancy,"[22] and "Whiplash Syndrome: Fact or Fiction?"[92a] This chapter discusses the terminology, epidemiology, historical aspects, pathology, symptoms, prognosis, effect of litigation, and treatment of whiplash injuries.

Terminology

Whiplash describes the typical mechanism of the hyperextension followed by flexion of the neck that occurs when an occupant of a motor vehicle is hit from behind by another vehicle. Other types of collisions can also result in a whiplash-type injury with different sequences and combinations of flexion, extension, and lateral motion of the neck. Despite concern that the term is unscientific, *whiplash* has become well entrenched in the medical literature and the lay vocabulary. Interestingly, the definition of "whiplash injury" in *Webster's Third*

New International Dictionary is rather expansive: "injury of the cervical spine and cerebral concussion occurring in an automobile collision which causes forceful flexion or extension of the neck and violent oscillation of the head forward and backward or backward and forward."[78*]

Other terms used include *cervical sprain*, *cervical myofascial pain syndrome*, *acceleration-deceleration injuries*, and *hyperextension injury*. In some other languages, the term used for this injury is a literal translation of *whiplash*:[56] *latigazo* in Spanish (in Mexico and Chile), *chicotada* in Portuguese, and *colpo di frusta* in Italian. Other descriptive terms include *coup du lapin* in French, meaning "rabbit's blow," and *schleudertrauma* in German, meaning "slinging trauma."

In 1995, the Quebec Task Force proposed a classification system for whiplash injuries.[206] Grade 1 signifies neck complaints of pain, stiffness, or tenderness without physical signs. Grade 2 represents neck complaints and musculoskeletal signs including decreased range of motion and point tenderness. Grade 3 indicates neck complaints and neurological signs including decreased or absent deep tendon reflexes, muscle weakness, and sensory deficits. Grade 4 includes neck complaints and fracture or dislocation.

Epidemiology

According to an estimate of the National Safety Council, there were 10,900,000 motor vehicle accidents in the United States in 2004.[150] Of these, 3,330,000 were rear-end collisions. Although the precise number of whiplash injuries per year cannot be determined,[12] if Dolinis' finding that 35% of Australian drivers in rear-end collisions sustained whiplash injuries,[47] then more than 1 million persons in the United States may have whiplash injuries yearly. Dolinis also reported that a prior history of neck injury and female gender were independent risk factors for an acute whiplash injury from a cohort of 246 car drivers who were hit from behind.

Neck pain develops in 56% of patients involved in a front- or side-impact accident.[43] In a low-velocity rear-end collision, occupants of the vehicle being struck are more likely to develop neck pain than the occupants of the first vehicle, who sustain primarily a flexion-type injury.[129,198] Rear-end collisions are responsible for about 85% of all whiplash injuries.[42,93] In these collisions, the incidence of whiplash injuries decreases as crash severity increases (an 82% incidence of whiplash injuries in collisions in which the automobile is not towed away versus a 66% incidence in accidents in which the automobile is towed).[101]

Seventy-three percent of occupants wearing a seat belt develop neck pain compared to 53% not wearing seat belts.[43] Front-seat occupants not wearing a seat belt, however, may be propelled into the steering wheel, dashboard, or windshield or out of the car completely, sustaining more severe head and other trauma and avoiding the whiplash injury.

Head restraints for front seats have been required by the National Highway Traffic Safety Administration for all passenger cars sold in the United States after January 1, 1969. Proper use of headrests can reduce the incidence of neck pain in rear-end collisions by 24% to 28.3%.[148,154,235] Unfortunately, many people are uninformed about their proper use and consider the headrest a place to rest the head while waiting at red lights. The longer original term, *head restraint*, accurately describes the intended function. About 75% of adjustable restraints are left in the down position.[101] Adjustable restraints in the down or unextended position do not adequately protect a person of average height.[101,156] In one study, only 10% of drivers had headrests adjusted to the most favorable position to prevent neck extension.[235] If adjustable headrests are too low, the headrest can act as a fulcrum, resulting in a more severe hyperextension injury.[101] In a study of a self-aligning head restraint designed to move upward and forward by occupant motion in a rear-end crash providing earlier neck support even when the head restraint is positioned low, the incidence of whiplash injuries was reduced from 18% in a Saab with a standard restraint to 4% in a Saab with the self-aligning restraint.[236]

Center high-mounted stop lamps have been standard equipment on all new passenger cars sold in the United States since September 1, 1985, as required by Federal Motor Vehicle Safety Standard 108. Automobiles equipped with this lamp are

17% less likely to be struck in the rear while braking than automobiles without the lamp.[102]

Historical Aspects

Concepts of Disease

Do patients with chronic complaints after whiplash injuries have a disease? Jean-Martin Charcot wrote, "Disease is from old and nothing about it has changed. It is we who change as we learn to recognize what was formerly imperceptible." Concepts of what constitutes disease, however, change with the times. In the South during the 1850s, Cartwright described the disease "Drapetomania, the disease causing slaves to run away," and the disease "Dysaesthesia Aethiopis or hebetude of mind and obtuse sensibility of body-a disease peculiar to negroes-called by overseers 'rascality.'"[31]

Also during the nineteenth century, masturbation was considered a disease with many neurological sequelae, including epilepsy, blindness, vertigo, loss of hearing, headache, and loss of memory.[53] Occasionally, masturbation could be a virulent disease. Two such patients were admitted to Charity Hospital of Louisiana in New Orleans, one in 1872 and the other in 1887, for treatment of masturbation. Both died in the hospital, with the cause of death listed as masturbation.[53] Russell[190] performed an autopsy on a dead masturbator in Birmingham, England, and reported in 1863 that masturbation "seems to have acted upon the cord in the same manner as repeated small haemorrhages affect the brain, slowly sapping its energies, until it succumbed soon after the last application of the exhausting influence, probably through the instrumentality of an atrophic process previously induced, as evidenced by the diseased state of the minute vessels." (Current views on masturbation as a cause of neurotrauma are outside the scope of this book.) Conversely, neurological diseases such as many movement disorders (e.g., Gilles de la Tourette's syndrome and dystonia) and migraine, once considered functional, are now considered organic in origin.

From Railway Spine to the Whiplash

As symptoms persist for months or years after whiplash injuries, the argument is made that sprains should heal within a few weeks[168] and there must be another reason why patients still report symptoms. Nonorganic explanations advanced for persistent complaints include emotional problems;[151] a culturally conditioned and legally sanctioned illness or a man-made disease;[5,114] a result of social and peer copying;[123] and demanding explanations outside the fields of organic and psychiatric illness.[168] More than 100 years ago, similar issues were debated about the organicity of complaints after railway accidents known as the *railway spine*.[228] (This topic is discussed in more detail in Chapter 5.)

The whiplash mechanism of injury may have first been recognized in U.S. Navy pilots. According to McIntire:[136]

> Following World War I, the Navy instituted the launching of planes from the decks of battleships and cruisers by the catapult method. The mechanics of this is well understood now, but, in the earliest days, the pilot was not properly protected. Consequently, the violence to the cervical spine in catapulting was great enough to cause a blackout for a few seconds and accidents occurred that were undoubtedly due to the whiplash effect. Because this was recognized quickly, we were able to provide a protective headrest for the pilot, with adequate shoulder harness, so that no further damage to the neck and associated structures occurred and there were no further blackouts.

The automakers were not so quick to recognize this remedy and routinely install headrests and shoulder harnesses: 50 more years were required for routine use in the civilian sector.

In 1919, Marshall[132] reported on causes of mild neck injuries, including automobile accidents. Discussing the interpretation of cervical spine X-rays, he stated:

> Negative x-rays with severe ligamentous strain in [the] presence of existing hypertrophic bony changes do not necessarily signify a favorable prognosis. On the contrary, if hypertrophic changes represent serious wear and tear of past events and past time on the neck tissues, then the new trauma received is likely to start an increasing stiffness despite treatment.

Treatments discussed included orthopedic supports, exercises, manipulation, and physical therapy such as electricity, moist heat, and radiant heat. Marshall concluded, "'One-idea' diagnoses and treatments constitute an increasing menace to successful management of cases. . . ."

The first use of the term *whiplash* is not entirely certain. In a symposium in 1964, Crowe[36] stated:

> In 1928, presenting a report on eight cases of neck injuries resulting from traffic accidents before the Western Orthopedic Association in San Francisco, I used the unfortunate term whiplash. This expression was intended to be a description of motion, but it has been accepted by physicians, patients and attorneys as the name of a disease; and the misunderstanding has led to its misapplication by many physicians and others over the years.

The 1928 symposium, however, was not published.

The term *whiplash* first appears in the medical literature in a 1945 article by Davis:[40]

> Starting with the fact that the great majority of injuries of the cervical spine are in the nature of a "whip lash," and accepting the meaning of the term "whip lash" as a hyperflexion followed by spontaneous extensor recoil, the nature of a great variety of injuries of this section of the spinal column becomes understandable. . . . The common automobile street accident, falls from a height, diving accidents and blows striking the head sufficient to cause immediate disability and emergency rescue produce the usual obvious case.

The first use of the term *whiplash* in a book appeared in the fourth edition of *The Management of Fractures, Dislocations, and Sprains* by Key and Conwell in 1946[110] in a section written by Davis. He reported that automobile head-on collisions were the most common cause of cervical spine injuries in his experience.

During the 1950s, the term *whiplash* became widely used. In a 1953 article, Gay and Abbott[75] observed, "In our experience, most of the accidents that involved a whiplash injury of the neck were caused by a collision in which one vehicle was rammed from behind by another vehicle." The mechanism of the whiplash injury in a rear-end collision was incorrectly described as acute flexion followed by extension. Treatments discussed included "unusual personal attention, explanation, and reassurance"; analgesics; use of a cervical collar; physical therapy; and cervical traction. From serial follow-up of 50 patients, they concluded: "Characteristically, these patients were more disabled and remained handicapped for longer periods than was anticipated, considering the mild character of the accident."

Severy et al.,[198] in 1955, performed a pioneering series of staged rear-end collisions using humans and dummies, recording the events with high-speed photography and accelerometers. They correctly identified the sequence of hyperextension of the neck followed by flexion, which prior investigators had reversed. Severy et al. observed:

> The low-speed rear-end collision is one of the more common types of urban automobile accidents and it is probably the most misleading. Unlike most types of collisions, the rear-end collision frequently results in minor car damage with major bodily injury. Also, unlike most injury-producing accidents there is generally no visible sign of injury for the rear-end collision victim.

Myofascial Pain

Because most patients with whiplash injuries have injuries only to muscle, ligaments, and connective tissue, a myofascial injury, the history of this concept is briefly reviewed. During the 1930s, two landmark articles appeared. In 1934, Mixter and Barr[147] published their article "Rupture of the Intervertebral Disc with Involvement of the Spinal Canal." Since then, the surgical community has been fixated on disk disease. Some surgeons have been on search-and-destroy missions in treating patients with actual or possible disk disease complaining of neck and back pain.

Unfortunately, the equally important observations of Kellgren[107] in his 1938 article, "A Preliminary Account of Referred Pain Arising from Muscle," have been relatively overlooked. He had initially documented that injection of a 6% solution of sodium chloride (often using himself as a subject) into different muscles produced distinctive patterns of referred pain, whereas injection of fascia and tendon sheaths produced only sharply localized pain.[108] He described patients with neck and back pain both traumatically induced and occurring spontaneously with local "tender spots" and referred pain in the ipsilateral extremity. The local and referred pains were totally abolished with local infiltration of the tender spots with procaine (Novocain).

The concept of myofascial pain has evolved over the past 150 years.[227] In 1876, Helleday[88a] described a myalgic condition, chronic (rheumatic) myositis, characterized by pain and nodules in the affected muscles that could only be diagnosed with experience and a proper technique of palpation.

In 1904, Gowers[79] first used the term *fibrositis* by analogy with cellulitis to describe inflammation of the fibrous tissue. He stated:

> Another definite form of fibrositis is the traumatic, induced by sudden violent tension on tendinous and ligamentous structures, much less frequently by tension on the muscles. Examples of this are common in many situations. . . . A violent strain on the spinal ligaments may be followed by enduring susceptibility to pain on any tension, a condition often met with after railway accidents and other injuries. Like other subjective symptoms, it is open to forensic depreciation, but its peculiar relation to tension clearly establishes its genuine character.

Although one of his suggested treatments, deep hypodermic injection of cocaine, repeated daily for 2 or 3 weeks, is not recommended, his conclusions are still perfectly appropriate:

> At present we are without any direct evidence of the real nature of these affections, such as can only be furnished by the microscope and modern methods of discerning that which it reveals. We cannot wonder at our ignorance, still less complain of it, for it is only quite recently that the minute structure of the sensory elements of muscle and tendon has been clearly perceived, and much of the normal structure still seems obscure. It is one of the departments of pathology in which the recognition of the changes that attend disease has to come long after the full discernment of the normal structure. We must therefore be content to wait, and content also meanwhile to rely on the apparent meaning of the symptoms of disease, as far as that meaning can be made out.

To describe the tender area of the affected muscle, the term *tender zone* was used by Edeiken and Wolferth[50] in 1936 in a paper on persistent shoulder pain following myocardial infarction. In a paper read in 1939 on low back pain, Steindler[209] used the terms *trigger point* and *myofascial pain* for the first time. During the next 50 years, Travell[225–227] was a vigorous popularizer and proponent of myofascial pain syndromes with trigger points.

In 1938, Cyriax[39] used the term *rheumatic headache* to refer to headaches that could be referred to the eye or the ear from upper posterior or lateral cervical muscles and relieved by massage, passive stretching, active exercises, and infiltration of tender spots in the muscles with procaine. His brief historical review noted that this type of headache had been described repeatedly since 1615. In 1906, Peritz[171] treated this type of headache by muscular infiltration with saline both to elicit the pain and as a form of treatment. In 1940, Hadden[86] discussed occipital neuralgia, which he thought was a neglected subject.

Pathology

Structural damage from whiplash-type injuries has been demonstrated both in animal studies and in humans.[12] Experimentally caused acceleration/extension injuries in different species of monkeys have demonstrated injuries to multiple structures including muscle tears, avulsions, and hemorrhages; rupture of the anterior longitudinal and other ligaments, especially between C4 and C7; avulsions of disc from vertebral bodies and disc herniations; retropharyngeal hematoma; intralaryngeal and esophageal hemorrhage; cervical sympathetic nerve damage associated with damage to the longus colli; nerve root injury; cervical spinal cord contusions and hemorrhages; cerebral concussion; and gross hemorrhages and contusions over the surface of the cerebral hemispheres, brain stem, and cerebellum.[129,158,243] Vertebral fractures and dislocations were rare, although apophyseal joint injuries were often noted with tears of the capsular fibers, cartilage fissuring with subchondral bone fractures, and cartilage degeneration and regeneration.[243]

Some of these experimentally induced lesions have been described in human studies. A magnetic resonance imaging (MRI) study of selected patients within 4 months of whiplash injuries has demonstrated ruptures of the anterior longitudinal ligament, horizontal avulsion of the vertebral end plates, separation of the disc from the vertebral end plate, occult fractures of the anterior vertebral end plates, acute posterolateral cervical disc herniations, focal muscular injury of the longus colli muscle, posterior interspinous ligament injury, and prevertebral fluid collections.[41] In an MRI study of 92 chronic whiplash-injured patients, grade 2–3 lesions of the tectorial membranes were present in 27%, and were present in 17% of the posterior atlanto-occipital membranes compared to minor changes in controls.[116] These patients were also found to have abnormal alar[115] and transverse ligaments[117] compared to the controls. Autopsy series have demonstrated clefts in the cartilage plates of the intervertebral discs, posterior disc herniation through a damaged annulus fibrosis, and hemarthrosis in facet joints.[216–218]

Perforation of the esophagus and a descending mediastinitis have been reported, perhaps from impingement of the esophagus against an exostosis on the edge of a vertebral body or entrapment of the esophageal wall between the vertebral bodies in the recoil flexion phase.[121,212,223] Injury of the second cervical ganglion and nerve has been documented as a rare cause of unilateral neck and suboccipital area pain with decreased sensation in the C2 dermatome;[106] greater occipital neuralgia is probably the more common cause.

Other Proposed Etiologies

Physicians generally attribute symptoms of common whiplash within the first 3 months to soft tissue injuries. However, when symptoms persist, as discussed in the opening section of this chapter, the etiology of the chronic or late whiplash syndrome is controversial.[59] Nonorganic explanations advanced for persistent complaints include emotional problems, a culturally conditioned and legally sanctioned illness,[146] social and peer copying,[123] secondary gain and malingering,[32,193] and demands for an explanation outside the realm of organic psychiatry and neurology.[168] In addition, persistent complaints of those involved in low-speed rear-end collisions are not seen in volunteer subjects exposed velocity changes from 8.7 to 14.2 km/h.[33] However, in another study, approximately 29% and 38% of the subjects exposed to 4 km/h and 8 km/velocity changes, respectively, experienced symptoms, with cervical symptoms and headaches predominating.[23]

A study that retrospectively examined the incidence of chronic symptoms after rear-end motor vehicle accidents in Lithuania, where few people are covered by insurance, also challenged the organicity of chronic complaints.[155,195] Chronic pain and headaches were no more common in 202 accident victims than in controls. The authors concluded that expectation of disability, a family history, and attribution of preexisting symptoms to the trauma may be important determinants for those who develop chronic symptoms. Although the results are intriguing, the study is probably not valid because of significant sampling bias.[19,66] In addition, more than 4000 individuals in each group would be needed to discover with 80% probability a statistically significant difference in the occurrence of chronic neck complaints between subjects who had and had not been involved in a collision.[187]

Pobershin performed a similar study in the United Kingdom of 503 persons (66% female) ages 18 and over out of 1147 total who reported a rear end collision which did not involve a head injury to the Devon and Cornwall police (response rate of 44%).[174b] Of the respondents, 78% had neck pain lasting for more than a week and 52% still had pain at 1 year (the 1 year response rate was 80.5%). The most important predictors of pain at 1 year were the initial neck visual analogue scale score (1.03, 1.01–1.05) and the presence of a compensation claim (4.09, 1.62–10.32). There was no improvement in symptoms once the claim was settled. In fact, people who had settled their claim by 2 years seemed more likely to have neck pain of similar severity compared to those who had ongoing claims. Pobershin states, "This suggests that there is something about the stress and anxiety of the claim itself that tends to prolong symptoms in people seeking compensation." However, it is also possible that the subjects had persistent pain complaints because they were really injured and were not cured by a verdict. The low response rates and disproportionate percentage of female respondents may have biased the outcome of the study.

Despite the questions about these studies, the medico-legal setting is important. When the tort compensation system in Saskatchewan, Canada, was changed to a no-fault system without payments for pain and suffering, the number of claims decreased by about 25%.[32]

Central hyperexcitability or sensitization (sensitization of spinal cord neurons, which results in increased responsiveness to peripheral stimuli) is a possible mechanism for increased levels of pain subacutely and chronic pain. In a study of 80 subjects evaluated within 1 month of an accident, acute whiplash subjects with higher levels of pain and disability were distinguished by sensory hypersensitivity to a variety of stimuli suggestive of central nervous system sensitization.[211] These responses occurred independently of psychological distress. Spinal cord hypersensitivity was also suggested in a study of 29 patients with whiplash pain compared to controls, who had significantly lower reflex thresholds of the nociceptive withdrawal reflex on stimulation of the sural nerve.[9]

In a prospective study of 76 whiplash subjects evaluated within 1 month of injury and then 2, 3, and 6 months postinjury, whiplash groups demonstrated local mechanical hyperalgesia in the cervical spine at 1 month postinjury.[210] This hyperalgesia persisted in those with moderate/severe symptoms at 6 months but resolved by 2 months in those who had recovered or reported persistent mild symptoms. Only those with persistent moderate/severe symptoms at 6 months demonstrated generalized hypersensitivity on all sensory tests. These changes occurred within 1 month of injury and remained unchanged throughout the study period. These findings suggest that those with persistent moderate/severe symptoms at 6 months display, soon after injury, generalized hypersensitivity suggestive of changes in central pain processing mechanisms. This phenomenon did not occur in those who recovered or those with persistent mild symptoms.

Compared with controls, chronic whiplash patients had muscle hyperalgesia and large areas of referred pain after intramuscular injections of hypertonic saline both in the infraspinatus and anterior tibialis muscles, which suggests a generalized central hypersensitivity.[114] Similar findings in whiplash patients have also been reported with electrical cutaneous and intramuscular stimulation of both the neck and lower limb.[38] Finally, in a study of brain stem-mediated antinociceptive inhibitory reflexes of the temporalis muscle of 82 patients with acute posttraumatic headache following whiplash injury, abnormal durations and latencies were present compared to controls. This suggests a transient dysfunction of the brain stem-mediated reflex circuit mainly of the late polysynaptic pathways. The reflex abnormalities are considered a neurophysiological correlate of the posttraumatic (cervico)-cephalic pain syndrome and point to altered central pain control in acute posttraumatic headache due to whiplash injury.

Symptoms and Signs

Table 22.1 lists the sequelae of whiplash injuries.

Neck Pain

Following a motor vehicle accident, 62% of patients presenting to the emergency room complain of neck pain.[43] The onset of neck pain occurs in 65% of patients within 6 hours, within 24 hours in an additional 28%, and within 72 hours in the remaining 7%.[42,82]

Table 22.1. Sequelae of Whiplash Injuries

Neck and back injuries
Myofascial
Fractures and dislocations
Disc herniation
Spinal cord compression
Spondylosis
Radiculopathy
Facet joint
Increased development of spondylosis
Headaches
Tension type
Greater occipital neuralgia
Temporomandibular joint injury
Migraine
Third occipital
Dizziness
Vestibular dysfunction
Brain stem dysfunction
Cervical origin
Barre syndrome?
Hyperventilation syndrome
Paresthesias
Trigger points
Thoracic outlet syndrome
Brachial plexus injury
Cervical radiculopathy
Cervical myelopathy
Facet joint syndrome
Carpal tunnel syndrome
Ulnar neuropathy at the elbow
Weakness
Radiculopathy
Cervical myelopathy
Brachial plexopathy
Entrapment neuropathy
Reflex inhibition of muscle contraction by painful cutaneous stimulation
Cognitive, somatic, and psychologic
Memory, attention, and concentration impairment
Nervousness and irritability
Sleep disturbances
Fatigue
Depression
Personality change
Compensation neurosis
Visual symptoms
Convergence insufficiency
Oculomotor palsies
Abnormalities of smooth pursuit and saccades
Horner's syndrome
Vitreous detachment
Rare sequelae
Torticollis
Tremor
Transient global amnesia
Esophageal perforation and descending mediastinitis
Hypoglossal nerve palsy
Superior laryngeal nerve paralysis
Cervical epidural hematoma
Internal carotid and vertebral artery dissection

The vast majority of whiplash injuries result in cervical sprains, that is, myofascial injuries. Rarely, partial rupture of muscles such as the sternomastoid may occur.[65] Cervical disc herniations, cervical spine fractures, and dislocations are uncommon.[153] Upper cervical trauma to the atlas, axis, and associated ligaments is much less common than lower cervical injury.[202]

Cervical zygapophyseal (facet) joint injury[125] can produce referred pain over the upper back, posterior neck, and head. Using normal volunteers, Dwyer and colleagues injected contrast media into the zygapophyseal joints at different levels and produced characteristic patterns of referred pain over the occipital, posterior cervical, shoulder girdle, and scapular regions.[3,49] Injection at the C2-3 level caused pain located in the upper cervical region and extending at least onto the occiput and at times extending toward the ear, vertex, forehead, or eye. Although injection of the C1-2 joint was not performed in this study, based on patients with symptomatic disease at this level, the pain may be referred to the posterior auricular and mastoid area extending to the angle of the mandible.[120] Using medial branch blocks of the cervical dorsal rami for the diagnosis of cervical facet joint pain,[11] Barnsley and colleagues reported that the pain arises from at least one facet joint in 54% of patients with chronic pain from whiplash injuries.[13] Posttraumatic facet joint pain is reviewed in Chapter 17.

Injury of the soft tissues of the upper cervical spine may also be responsible for pain complaints. Kaale et al. performed cervical spine MRI studies on 92 subjects with chronic neck pain following whiplash injuries (whiplash associated disorder, grade 2 using the Quebec classification) and 30 random controls.[103b] Lesions of the alar ligaments showed the most pronounced association with the severity of neck pain and functional disability. There was a weaker association with lesions of the posterior atlanto-occipital membrane and transverse ligament.

Headaches

In a prospective study of 180 patients seen within 4 weeks of a whiplash injury, 82% complained of headaches, which were occipitally located in 46%, generalized in 34%, and in other locations in 20%.[7] Fifty percent of the patients had pain more than half of the time. At 12 weeks, the headache persisted in 73%, with one-third having pain more than half of the time.

In a study of 112 patients with chronic posttraumatic headaches for a mean period of 2.5 years after the injury, 37% had tension-type headaches, 27% had migraine, 18% had cervicogenic headache, and 18% did not fulfill criteria of a particular category using International Headache Society Criteria.[178] Neck pain was associated with the headache in 93% of the cases.

Headaches following whiplash injuries are usually of the tension or muscle contraction type, often associated with greater occipital neuralgia. Greater occipital neuralgia can be caused by a direct blow to the suboccipital region or by an entrapment by the semispinalis capitis. The distinction between referred pain from the superior trapezius, semispinalis capitis, semispinalis cervicis, rectus capitis posterior minor and major, and obliquus capitis superior and inferior muscles and greater occipital neuralgia can be difficult to make because the distribution of pain and reproduction of symptoms by suboccipital palpation can be similar.[80,227] Whiplash injuries can also traumatize the temporomandibular joint, resulting in internal derangement or a myofascial injury with associated jaw pain and headaches.[24,119,241]

Whiplash injuries can occasionally precipitate recurring common, classic, and basilar migraines de novo.[97,242,245] The headaches can begin immediately or within a few days after the injury. The greater the latency between the injury and the onset of migraine, the more tenuous is the causal link.

Headache may be referred from the C2-3 facet joint, innnervated by the third occipital nerve, which Bogduk and Marsland have called *third occipital headache*.[20] Tenderness may be present over the C2-3 facet joint. Using third occipital nerve blocks, Lord and coworkers[126] reported that the prevalence of this type of headache among patients with persistent headaches after whiplash injury is 38%.

There is a single report of two patients who developed generalized throbbing headaches, tenderness of the anterior neck, and unilateral ptosis following whiplash injuries.[111] Bilateral sympathetic dysfunction has been suggested as the cause because of evidence of supraorbital anhidrosis and bilateral postganglionic Horner's syndrome.

Dizziness

Dizziness and disequilibrium are frequent complaints after whiplash injuries. In one study of 262 patients with persistent neck pain and headaches for 4 months or longer after the injury, symptoms were reported as follows: vertigo, 50%; floating sensations, 35%; tinnitus, 14%; and hearing impairment, 5%.[160] Injuries of various structures have been postulated as causing dizziness, including dysfunction of the vestibular apparatus, brain stem, cervical sympathetics, vertebral insufficiency, and cervical proprioceptive system.[221] Hyperventilation syndrome frequently occurs in anxious patients who are in pain and may cause dizziness at times associated with paresthesias that can be symmetric and bilateral as well as unilateral.[57]

Toglia[221] reported abnormal vestibular tests in 309 patients with dizziness following whiplash injuries: latent nystagmus in 29% of the patients, abnormal calorics in 57%, and abnormal rotatory tests in 51%. Hinoki[91] reported abnormal equilibrium tests, suggesting that overexcitation of cervical and lumbar proprioceptors owing to hypertonicity of the soft supporting tissues may cause some cases of dizziness. He also reported abnormal optokinetic nystagmus in other patients, suggesting brain stem and cerebellar dysfunction. Chester[34] described posttraumatic dysfunction of the semicircular canals, otolith structures, and occasionally perilymph fistulas documented by a variety of tests including moving platform posturography and electronystagmography studies.

Oosterveld et al.[160] reported the following abnormalities consistent with peripheral and central pathology in patients with posttraumatic dizziness with a duration of 4 months or longer: spontaneous nystagmus, 63%; positional nystagmus, 42%; cervical nystagmus, 79%; unilateral gaze nystagmus, 6%; bilateral gaze nystagmus, 26%; abnormal visual suppression test indicating central pathology, 37%; disturbances in saccadic visual pursuit movements suggesting brain stem and cerebellar pathology, 43%; and a unilateral labyrinthine lesion on caloric testing, 5%. In 41 of the patients with abnormal vestibular tests 1 year after the accident, repeat testing 2 years after the accident revealed no significant improvement. Although these studies reporting central and peripheral dysfunction in neurotololgical testing are intriguing, further confirmation using matched controls is important to ensure that the abnormal findings have adequate specificity. For example, 82.5% of controls have some degree of positional nystagmus in at least one of five test positions (A.C. Coats, personal communication, 1992).

In 1926, Barre[15] reported the posterior cervical sympathetic syndrome, which has been suggested as a cause of dizziness after whiplash injuries.[221] Symptoms of dizziness, headache, neck pain, blurred vision, irritability, poor concentration, and tinnitus are supposedly caused by osteophytes irritating the sympathetic nerve plexus enveloping the vertebral arteries. This concept has not been widely accepted in North America.[51]

Tamura[215] has extended this concept in a report of patients with similar symptoms who were found to have disc protrusions and root sleeve defects at C3-4 perhaps irritating the communicating branch of postganglionic sympathetic fibers at the C4 root level. Anterior cervical discectomy and fusion at C3-4 completely relieved the symptoms in 19 of 20 patients evaluated at an average of 30 months postoperatively. By contrast, 19 patients who did not have surgery had persistent symptoms after follow-up at an average of 24 months. It will be of interest to see if these excellent surgical results can be duplicated.

Vertigo has been postulated to occur from lesions of the soft tissues of the neck. In an experimental confirmation, De Jong et al.[44] injected two subjects with 10 ml 1% lidocaine in the paravertebral tissues at the level C2-3 halfway between the mastoid process and the carotid tubercle. The injection produced a sensation of being drawn toward the injected side, true vertigo, past-pointing toward the injected side, a broad-based staggering gait, and hypotonia of the ipsilateral arm and leg. Chronic vertigo from lesions of the soft tissues of the neck, however, is considered unlikely because of the relatively small cervical afferent input to the vestibular nuclei and the capacity for compensation.[8]

Paresthesias

Patients frequently complain of paresthesias in the upper extremities after whiplash injuries. In one study, 33% of patients with symptoms but no objective findings complained of paresthesias acutely; 37% reported paresthesias after a mean follow-up of 19.7 months.[153] All patients with symptoms, a reduced range of cervical movement, and evidence of objective neurological loss complained of paresthesias acutely; after a mean follow-up of 24.7 months, 60% still reported paresthesias.

Paresthesias in the upper extremities following whiplash injuries can be caused by myofascial injuries with trigger points, brachial plexopathy including thoracic outlet syndrome, entrapment neuropathies such as carpal tunnel syndrome; and less often by cervical radiculopathy and spinal cord compression. Trigger points in multiple muscles can cause referred paresthesias in the upper extremities, including the middle trapezius; anterior, medius, and posterior scalenes; supraspinatus; infraspinatus; teres minor; latissimus dorsi; teres major; subscapularis; deltoid; coracobrachialis; serratus anterior and posterior; and pectoralis major and minor muscles.[227]

Whiplash injuries are a common cause of thoracic outlet syndrome.[29,30,103a] In a surgical series of 491 patients, 56% of the cases of thoracic outlet syndrome were due to whiplash injuries.[192] Because women more commonly develop symptoms after whiplash injuries,[6,93,167] and because thoracic outlet syndrome is four times more common in women,[175] the great majority of patients with thoracic outlet syndrome following whiplash injuries are women.

The *thoracic outlet syndrome* refers to variable compression of the subclavian artery, vein, and brachial plexus that can occur in the interscalene triangle, the costoclavicular triangle, and the subcoracoid space.[165] A variety of normal and pathological anatomical features can result in compression, including the scalene muscles, an anomalous first rib, anomalous fibrous bands, anomalous muscle insertions, anomalous vessels, and a midclavicular fracture. A variety of compression syndromes can develop, depending upon the structures compressed, including neurogenic, vasomotor, and vascular types. Subjective sensory symptoms are often the earliest complaint, with pain and paresthesias predominating in 95% of patients.[231]

The thoracic outlet syndrome has been controversial because at least 85% of cases are due to the nonspecific neurogenic type, which is a diagnosis of exclusion.[244] Patients have subjective complaints of headaches, neck pain, and paresthesias of the extremity often radiating down the ulnar arm and forearm into the fourth and fifth fingers, with no objective findings on examination or electromyogram (EMG) and nerve conduction velocity studies.[37] Electromyogram and nerve conduction velocity studies, however, are still essential to exclude cervical radiculopathy, carpal tunnel syndrome, and ulnar compression in the cubital tunnel. The nonspecific neurogenic type may result from a myofasical injury of the scalene muscles or pectoralis minor,[95] which causes referred paresthesias from trigger points rather than from neurogenic irritation.

During the physical examination, Adson's test is often not helpful since more than 50% of normal, asymptomatic people will have a positive test.[197] Medial supraclavicular palpation of the anterior scalene muscle and associated structures should be routinely done to see if the paresthesias are reproduced. The most worthwhile stress tests are the 90° abduction external rotation test (the arm is abducted to a right angle and externally rotated with the forearm flexed at 90°, while the head is turned to the opposite side), the exaggerated military maneuver (the patient is asked to brace the shoulders downward and backward forcefully, with the chest thrust forward and the chin slightly elevated), and the hyperabduction test (the arms are brought together above the head).[165] When symptoms are present, the scalene-relief test (the patient places the symptomatic arm across the forehead while raising and pulling the shoulder forward) may be worth trying.[227]

Not infrequently, after whiplash injuries, patients complain of hand numbness and tingling and are documented to have carpal tunnel syndrome on electrical studies. Carpal tunnel syndrome may develop immediately or within 2 weeks of the accident[85] due to hyperextension of the wrists while gripping the steering wheel or bracing the hands on the dashboard during the collision.[84,118] In addition, if the patient has a cervical radiculopathy or neurogenic thoracic outlet syndrome from the injury, a double crush syndrome resulting in carpal tunnel syndrome or cubital tunnel syndrome could develop.[161,214] If the patient has a vasomotor thoracic outlet syndrome with hand edema, carpal tunnel syndrome could also ensue.

Weakness

After whiplash injuries, patients frequently complain of weakness, heaviness, or fatigue when there is no evidence of cervical radiculopathy or myelopathy, brachial plexopathy, or entrapment neuropathy.

The nonspecific neurogenic type of thoracic outlet syndrome can produce these complaints. Alternatively, patients may have a sensation of weakness or heaviness because of reflex inhibition of muscle due to pain[2] that can be overcome by more central effort.[12]

Cognitive and Psychological Symptoms

In a study of patients with chronic symptoms following a whiplash injury, the following percentages endorsed various symptoms as follows: 67%, nervousness and irritability; 50%, cognitive disturbances; 44%, sleep disturbances; 40%, fatigability; 38%, disturbances of vision; 37%, symptoms of depression; 85%, headache; 100%, neck pain; 72%, vertigo; and 60%, brachialgia.[112] These symptoms are all common in postconcussion syndrome, chronic pain syndromes,[142] posttraumatic stress disorder,[134] and neurosis.

The concept that a whiplash injury without direct head trauma can result in a cerebral concussion has been controversial.[17] Various types of data have been reported to support the cerebral concussion hypothesis.[200] The study using monkeys as subjects by Ommaya and coworkers[158] demonstrated that acceleration/deceleration forces without direct head impact can result in cerebral concussion as well as gross hemorrhages over the surface of the brain and upper cervical spinal cord. Ommaya and Yarnell[159] also reported two people with subdural hematomas after whiplash injuries. Neurotological studies previously described have suggested central pathology in some patients with complaints of vertigo. Oculomotor dysfunction was documented in a group of patients with chronic symptoms from whiplash injuries suggesting brain stem lesions.[90] Single case reports of bilateral abducens nerve palsy[202] and amnesia with a duration of 72 hours after a whiplash injury[62] also support the concept of brain stem and cerebral dysfunction.

Abnormal electroencephalograms in moderately impaired patients with whiplash injuries, no direct head trauma, and brief or no loss of consciousness have been reported,[76,222] with 46% abnormal records in one study.[222] Problems with patient selection, preexisting abnormal studies, and adequate controls, however, are confounding factors. A more recent study has demonstrated minimal electroencephalogram abnormalities in a small percentage of patients.[98]

Some studies have demonstrated cognitive impairment in a small minority of patients sustaining whiplash injuries,[55,112,183,246] although another found equivocal abnormalities.[157] Deficits were noted in tests of attention, concentration, cognitive flexibility, and memory. In a prospective study, Radanov et al.[181] reported difficulties with complex attentional processing in patients tested about 7 days after the injury with improvement to normal at 6 months. The complex attentional processing difficulty was felt to be due, at least in part, to adverse effects of medication. Another prospective study of 39 patients found no evidence of cognitive deficits.[104]

Psychological factors are commonly cited as the cause of or a risk factor for persistent symptoms. Kivioja et al.[113] compared the results of the Structured Clinical Interview for DSM-IV for patients with chronic pain from whiplash injuries after 1 year to those of patients who had recovered. A history of psychiatric disease (most commonly depression) was more common in patients with chronic symptoms both before and after the accident. Richter et al.[186] performed a 6-month prospective study of 43 consecutive patients with grade 1 or 2 whiplash-associated disorders with a 74% follow-up rate. Psychological factors were more relevant than collision severity in predicting the duration and severity of symptoms.

However, Radanov et al.[179] performed a prospective study of 78 consecutive patients with whiplash injuries demonstrating that psychosocial factors, negative affectivity, and personality traits were not significant in predicting the duration of symptoms. Older age of patients, initial neck pain intensity, and injury-related cognitive impairment were significant factors predicting illness behavior. In another prospective study, Radanov et al.[180] provide evidence that cognitive and psychological symptoms may be due to somatic symptoms. In those with chronic neck pain due to a single painful facet joint following whiplash injuries, psychological distress resolved following successful radiofrequency neurotomy.[239] Based upon a comparison of the psychological profiles of those with whiplash-associated headaches to those with nontraumatic headaches and controls, patients with whiplash-associated headache suffer psychological distress secondary to chronic pain and not from tension headache and generalized psychological distress.[238] In a 3-year prospective study of 278 patients, Mayou and Bryant found no special psychiatric symptoms in patients with whiplash neck injury.[133] Psychological variables and consequences were important following whiplash in a similar manner to other types of injury. Compensation neurosis probably accounts for only a minority of patients with persistent complaints.[199]

Back Pain

Interscapular and low back pain are rather frequent complaints after whiplash injuries and are reported in 20% and 35%, respectively, of patients during the first months after the injury.[93] In my experience, most of the symptoms are due to myofascial injuries, although occasionally, thoracic and lumbar disk herniations and vertebral body compression fractures can result. One study reports a 25% incidence of persistent back pain after a mean follow-up of 2 years.[89]

Other Sequelae

Visual symptoms, especially blurred vision, are common and are usually due to convergence insufficiency.[25a] Oculomotor palsies, abnormalities of smooth pursuit and saccades, Horner's syndrome, and vitreous detachment are uncommon complications of whiplash injuries.[26,201] A sensory deficit in C2 and C3 dermatomes and in a trigeminal nerve distribution has been described.[45]

Torticollis has rarely been precipitated by whiplash injuries, with onset within 6 days of the trauma.[63,99,229] The pathophysiology of peripherally induced dystonia has been the subject of much speculation.[99,100,224] This topic is also discussed in Chapter 33. Other rare sequelae include esophageal perforation,[212] descending mediastinitis,[223] transient global amnesia,[62] and hypoglossal nerve palsy.[48]

Radiographic Findings

Although cervical spine X-rays are routinely obtained after whiplash injuries, the yield of significant abnormalities is quite low in patients who are alert and have no focal findings on exam. Algorithms have been suggested to safely decrease the number of cervical spine series obtained.[46]

In patients without radicular complaints, cervical MRI studies have a low yield. In a cohort of 29 patients, the only significant findings were spondylosis and loss of lordosis.[237] No significant changes were found on follow-up scans obtained 6 months later on 19 of the patients. However, recent studies have reported an increased percentage of posttraumatic lesions of the tectorial and posterior atlanto-occipital membranes and alar and transverse ligaments as compared to controls.[115–117]

In some cases, the interpretation of the significance of radiographic abnormalities after a whiplash injury is difficult unless recent prior films are available because of the significant incidence of preexisting asymptomatic findings. Cervical spondylosis occurs with increasing frequency with older age and is often asymptomatic. Between the ages of 20 and 29 years, 13% of men and 5% of women will have evidence of spondylosis; after the age of 70, 100% of men and 96% of women will be affected.[96a] Degenerative disc disease also occurs with increasing frequency with older age and is often asymptomatic. Changes are seen in 6% of patients between the ages of 30 and 40 years and in 75% of patients between the ages of 60 and 70 years.[70] The C5-6 and C6-7 levels are most frequently affected.

Cervical disc protrusions can also be asymptomatic. In a study of 100 patients referred for MRI examinations of the larynx without symptoms of cervical spine disease, disc protrusions were present in 20% of patients 45 to 54 years of age and in 57% of patients older than 64 years.[220] Posterolateral protrusions were seen in 9% of patients studied. Spinal cord impingement was noted in 16% of patients 45 to 64 years of age and in 26% of patients over the age of 64. Spinal cord compression occurred in 7% of cases solely due to disc protrusion, with a reduction of the spinal cord area up to 16%.

Most studies have reported that trauma and whiplash injuries can accelerate the development of cervical spondylosis with degenerative disk disease, although two retrospective reports did not find an increased incidence of degenerative disc disease.[166,188] People with a history of a serious head or neck injury and miners under the age of 40 have an increased incidence of spondylosis.[96a] In a 7-year follow-up study of patients with whiplash injuries, no degenerative changes, and a mean age of 30, 39% had developed degenerative disc disease at one or more levels compared to the expected incidence of 6%.[93] In a similar 7-year follow-up study of patients who had preexisting degenerative changes at the time of a whiplash injury, new degenerative changes occurred at another level in 55%.[94] In a 10-year follow-up study, degenerative spondylosis was more common at all ages in patients than in age- and sex-matched controls, particularly in the 30 to 40 age group, where spondylosis occurred in 33%[73] compared with 10% of controls.[240] Finally, the incidence of a previous whiplash injury in patients underging anterior cervical discectomy and fusion was twice that of a control population.[87]

Functional Imaging

Cerebral hypoperfusion and functional imaging abnormalities have been reported after whiplash injuries. In a study of six patients compared to 12 controls, positron emission tomography (PET) and single photon emission computed tomography (SPECT) evidence of parieto-occipital hypometabolism was reported.[163] One possible explanation is stimulation of pain-sensitive afferents in the cervicotrigeminal system, which could have widespread effects on local vasoactive peptides and the cranial vascular system.[162,163]

In another study of 20 chronic whiplash patients (most with cognitive complaints), 65% had brain perfusion abnormalities in one or more regions.[124] Eight out of 15 patients tested had abnormal P300 event related potential studies. There was no significant correlation between the SPECT findings or the P300 results and the scores of attention and working memory on neuropsychological testing. There was, however, close agreement between the SPECT and P300 findings. In a functional MRI study of five chronic whiplash patients, reduced responses during coherent dot motion compared to controls were present.[67]

However, in another functional imaging study of 21 patients with late whiplash syndrome, Radanov and colleagues found no significant correlations between regional perfusion or metabolism in any brain area on SPECT or PET studies and the scores of divided attention or working memory. There were significant relations between state anxiety and divided attention.[177] Although HmPAO and ECD brain SPECT studies in patients with late whiplash syndrome and cognitive complaints have demonstrated parieto-occipital hypoperfusion,[162,164] similar findings have also been seen in patients with nontraumatic chronic cervical pain.[164] Depression can also cause perfusion abnormalities and fluorodeoxyglucose-PET (FDG-PET) does not allow reliable diagnosis of metabolic disturbances for individual patients; therefore, FDG-PET and HmPAO SPECT should not be used as diagnostic tools in the routine evaluation of patients with late whiplash syndrome.[18]

Prognosis

Studies on the prognosis of whiplash injuries are difficult to compare because of multiple methodological differences including selection criteria of patients, prospective and retrospective designs, patient attrition rates, duration of follow-up, and treatment used.[12,35,58] Although the majority of patients probably have only soft tissue or myofascial injuries, testing such as MRI studies, computed tomography (CT) scans, and myelography have not been routinely done to exclude other types of pathology such as disc disease and radiculopathy.

Symptoms

Three features of accident mechanisms are associated with more severe symptoms: an unprepared occupant, a rear-end accident, and a rotated or inclined head position at the moment of impact.[213] Neck pain and headaches persist in significant numbers of patients, as documented by multiple studies (Table 22.2).[10] A well-designed prospective study reported the following percentages of patients with complaints of neck pain and headaches, respectively, at various times after the injury: 92%, 57%, 1 week; 38%, 35%, 3 months; 25%, 26%, 6 months; and 19%, 21%, 12 months.[184] In a retrospective study,[31] 26% still complained of neck pain 1 year after the accident. By comparison, 7.2% of a control population reported neck pain. After 2 years, one-third of patients were still symptomatic, with neck pain reported in 89%, neck stiffness in 40%, shoulder pain in 37%, headache in 26%, interscapular pain in 29%, and referred symptoms in 40%.[131] Symptoms present 2 years after injury are still present 10 years after the injury.[73]

In a prospective study of 278 consecutive patients presenting to the emergency room with a whiplash injury, moderate to severe pain was reported by 27% at 1 year and by 30% at 3 years.[133] In another prospective study with follow-up questionnaires at 1 year[144] (182 subjects for a 91%

Table 22.2. Percentage of Patients with Persistence of Neck Pain and Headaches After a Whiplash Injury

	1 Week	1 Month	2 Months	3 Months	6 Months	1 Year	2 Years	10 Years
Neck pain (%)	92[184] 88[90]	64[42]	63[82]	38[184] 51[42]	25[184] 43[42]	19[184] 26[42]	16[180] 29[89,131] 44[153]	74[73]
Headaches (%)	54[89] 57[184]	82[7]		35[184] 73[7]	26[184]	21[184]	9[131] 15[180] 37[153]	33[73]

response rate) and 3 years[143] (144 subjects for a 79% response rate), nearly 10% and 11.8% of participants, respectively, reported that injury symptoms had caused their health to deteriorate significantly compared with before the accident. Three years after the accident, 17% of respondents were still using health services regularly for treatment.

In a retrospective study of 100 patients, 90% were seen within 6 months and 3 years of the accident.[7] Eighty percent were still having headaches, which occurred once a week or more in 40% and were constant in more than half of the cases. Half of the patients awoke with headaches, and in two-thirds the headaches were more prominent in the morning.

Chronic neck pain may persist for many years for some patients. Bunketorp et al. evaluated 121 patients with whiplash injuries in 2 emergency rooms in Sweden in 1983.[25b] In questionnaires completed by 108 subjects (89% response rate) seventeen years later, 55% reported persistent neck pain with no gender difference. In the control group, 29% reported neck pain. The neck disability index was also significantly higher in the exposed group than in the controls.

Prognostic Variables

Older age of patients has been found to be prognostically significant with persistent symptoms in follow-up studies performed at various times after the injury including 6 months,[182,184] 12 months,[184] 2 years,[131] and 10 years.[73] The majority of patients who develop the chronic whiplash syndrome are between the ages of 21 and 50.[6]

Persistent neck pain after whiplash injuries is more common in the female gender, especially in the 20- to 40-year age group, by 70% to 30%.[6,89a,93,167] This greater susceptibility of women to whiplash injuries might be due to a narrower neck with less muscle mass supporting a head of roughly the same volume compared to men.[101] Viano has provided experimental evidence that stiff car seats produce greater early neck displacements in women than in men because of a higher ratio of seat stiffness to torso mass and is another reason to explain the higher whiplash rates in women.[234] Viano also believes that one explanation for an increase in whiplash injuries in the past two decades is the increased use of stiffer car seats, which cause more neck displacement than yielding seats.[233]

Other risk factors for a less favorable prognosis (Table 22.3) include a higher intensity of initial neck

Table 22.3. Risk Factors for Persistent Symptoms

Accident mechanisms
Inclined or rotated head position
Unpreparedness for impact
Car stationary when hit
Occupant's characteristics
Older age
Female gender
Stressful life events unrelated to the accident
Pre-morbid depression
Symptoms
Intensity of initial neck pain or headache
Occipital headache
Interscapular or upper back pain
Multiple symptoms or paraesthesias at presentation
Signs
Reduced range of movement of the cervical spine
Objective neurological deficit
Radiographic findings
Pre-existing degenerative osteoarthritic changes
Abnormal cervical spine curves
Narrow diameter of cervical spinal canal

Source: From Evans RW: Whiplash syndrome. In: Evans RW, Baskin DS, Yatsu FM (eds): Prognosis of Neurological Disorders, 2nd ed. New York, Oxford University Press, 2000, p 158, with permission.

pain,[89a,184] interscapular or upper back pain,[82,131] occipital headache,[131] multiple symptoms or paresthesias at presentation,[73,93,131,184] reduced range of movement of the cervical spine,[104,153] the presence of an objective neurological deficit,[131,153] and preexisting degenerative osteoarthritic changes.[145,153] Abnormal cervical spine curves have been variably reported as prognostic[153] and not prognostic[131] of a poor outcome. A previous history of head trauma and pretraumatic headache are predictive of delayed recovery after 12 months.[184] A prior history of headache and more severe complaints of neck pain from the injury increase the likelihood of persistent headaches 6 months after the accident.[184,185] Cervical stenosis is a risk factor for the development of myelopathy after whiplash injuries both with cervical spine fractures or dislocations[52] and without them.[54] Stressful life events unrelated to the accident may increase the risk of persistent pain complaints.[103a,205] Other psychological factors are discussed above.

Occupational categories and the type and severity of the collision are other important variables. Although one study reported that persons in upper-middle compared to lower and higher occupational categories have an increased incidence of symptoms persisting for more than 6 months,[6] another found no relationship between persisting symptoms and the type of vocational acitivty.[184] The duration of symptoms was similar in patients involved in rear-end collisions compared to other types of collisions.[170] There is only a minimal association of a poor prognosis with the speed or severity of the collision and the extent of vehicle damage.[109]

Return to Work and Chronic Disability

In a series of consecutive medico-legal cases, 79% of patients returned to work by 1 month, 86% by 3 months, 91% by 6 months, and 94% by l year.[167] Radanov et al.[184] reported that 5% of patients were disabled 1 year after the accident. Nygren[154] reported that permanent medical disability occurred in 9.6% of patients involved in rear-end collisions and 3.8% involved in front- or side-impact accidents. One year after injury, Kasch et al.[105] found that 7.8% of patients had not returned to their usual level of activity or work.

In a retrospective analysis of over 5000 cases of whiplash injury, 26% of patients were not able to return to their normal activities at 6 months.[6] In a retrospective study of 102 consecutive patients seen in the emergency department, patients in the good prognostic group (66% of the total) had an average time off work of 2 weeks, with a maximum of 16 weeks.[131] One-third of these patients had no time off at all. In the poorer prognostic group of patients, the average time off work was 6 weeks; 20% had no time off work, and 9% did not return to work by 2 years.

Litigation and Symptoms

The rate of litigation is very high after whiplash injuries. In one follow-up study of 144 patients presenting to the emergency room, 81% were claiming compensation.[134] The rate of litigation can be almost twice as great in patients with severe compared to mild symptoms.[153]

The vast majority of patients file claims because they are truly injured and wish compensation. In a system of tort law where another party is responsible for the whiplash injury, this is exactly the expected result. However, by becoming involved in litigation, victims can be further victimized by unsympathetic family members, physicians, employers, agents of insurance companies, and plaintiff attorneys, who each have their own agenda. Conversely, neurotic, histrionic, or sociopathic patients may thrive on the attention and endless treatments recommended by physicians and encouraged by plaintiff attorneys.

Secondary gain, exaggeration, and malingering should be considered in all patients seen with whiplash injuries. In one study of litigants, 88.7% were found to have inconsistent nongenuine abnormalities on examination.[172] Schmand and colleagues performed neuropsychological studies of patients with late whiplash syndrome reporting memory or concentration problems.[194] In the context of litigation, the prevalence of underperforming was 61%, as defined by a positive score on the malingering test. Overall, however, the evidence suggests that these psychological factors and malingering are responsible for only a minority of patients with persistent complaints.[141,142] Premorbid psychopathology can be accentuated by pain and further obscure the nature of the symptoms. Of course, neurotic and histrionic individuals are not immune to actual injuries.

If pending litigation is the main reason for persistent symptoms, it is curious to note that the recovery rate is similar when litigants are compared to nonlitigants,[93,170] and similar response rates have been found in the treatment for facet joint pain.[127,193] MacNab[130] noted that in patients with whiplash as well as other injuries, the broken wrist or sprained ankle would heal as expected and yet the neck pain would persist. "It is difficult to understand why the patients' traumatic neurosis should be confined solely to their necks and not be reflected in continuing disability in relation to other injuries sustained at the same time." In addition, initiation of a lawsuit within the first month after injury did not influence recovery.

Nine studies have examined the effect of settlement of litigation on symptoms (Table 22.4). The different studies have assorted flaws, including biased patient selection; small numbers of subjects; different interview techniques; defining the sequelae of whiplash injuries as a homogenous syndrome without subgroups based on symptoms and signs; employing various nonstandardized treatments; and various periods of follow-up. However, the Norris and Watt study[153] was a prospective one of consecutive emergency room presentations.

The length of time from the injury until settlement of litigation can be important. Patients who settle the litigation within 1 year of the injury may have less significant injuries and therefore recover sooner than those who settle later and have persistent complaints.[93,153] Conversely, a prolonged period of pending litigation may encourage exaggeration of symptoms and unnecessary treatment.

The evidence indicates that most patients who are still symptomatic when litigation is completed are not cured by a verdict.[140,199] The end of litigation does not signal the end of symptoms for many patients. The patients who exaggerate or malinger are in a distinct minority. The clinician should evaluate the merits of each case individually. The available evidence does not support bias against patients just because they have pending litigation.[16]

Treatment

Routine treatment for acute injuries often consists of pain medications, nonsteroidal anti-inflammatory medications, muscle relaxants, and the use of a cervical collar for 2–3 weeks.[219] Range-of-motion exercises, physical therapy with the use of various modalities, and cervical traction are frequently prescribed.[59] A systematic review found the current evidence for use of Galvanic current (direct or pulsed), iontophoresis, TENS, electrical muscle stimulation, high frequency pulsed electromagnetic field and permanent magnets is either lacking, limited, or conflicting.[117b] There are a few prospective, controlled studies of treatment.[232] Early mobilization of the neck using the Maitland technique followed by local heat and neck exercises produces more rapid improvement after acute injuries than the use of a cervical collar and rest[138] and is as effective as physical therapy[137] performed during the first 8 weeks after the injury. A prospective, randomized study showed no added benefit of intermittent halter traction twice a week and instruction in neck and shoulder exercises compared to exercises alone in both 6- to 8-week and 5-month surveys.[134] Another prospective, controlled study found significant benefit during the first 12 weeks after the accident from use of shortwave diathermy with the generator incorporated in a soft collar worn 8 hours daily.[64] In another study, the outcome was better for patients who were encouraged to continue engaging in their normal preinjury activities than it was for patients who took sick leave from work and were immobilized during the first 14 days after the injury.[21] In a small prospective, randomized study of patients with neck pain and musculoskeletal signs (75% of the study group) and others with additional neurological signs (25% of the study group), the administration of high-dose methylprednisolone within 8 hours of the injury prevented extensive sick leave compared to the placebo controls at 6 months.[173]

Treatment of pain arising from facet joint injury may be effective. A controlled, prospective study showed a lack of effect of intra-articular corticosteroid injections in the cervical facet joints for chronic pain after whiplash injuries.[14] Percutaneous radiofrequency neurotomy and lower cervical medial branch neurotomy may be effective for the treatment of chronic facet joint pain documented by anesthetic blocks. In a small study of patients with chronic facet joint pain confirmed with double-blind, placebo-controlled local anesthesia, percutaneous radiofrequency neurotomy with multiple lesions of target nerves provided at least 50% relief for a median duration of 263 days compared to similar relief for 8 days in the control group.[128] The same patients found relief from second neurotomies for at least 219 days.[135]

Table 22.4. Persistence of Neck Symptoms After Settlement of Litigation

Study	No. of Patients	Selection of Patients	Time from Injury to Settlement	Length of Follow-up After Settlement	Neck Complaints (%)
Gotten, 1956[77]; Memphis, TN	100	Neurosurgery office practice	Not reported	1–26 months	54 no "appreciable" symptoms 34 minor symptoms 12 severe symptoms
MacNab, 1964[129]; Toronto, Ontario	145	Orthopedic office practice	Not reported	2 or more years	83 most with minor symptoms
Schutt and Dohan, 1968[196a]; Newark, NJ	7, all women	Employees of Radio Corporation of America (RCA) plant	Not reported	Not reported Follow-up 6–26 months after injury	71
Hohl, 1974[93]; Los Angeles, CA	102, total not stated	Orthopedic office practice, patients without cervical degenerative changes	Within 6 months	4.5 + years	17
Norris and Watt, 1983[153]; Sheffield, England		Prospective study of consecutive emergency room presentations	After 18 months	3.5 + years	62
Symptoms, no signs	14		17.25 ± 11.9 months	35.8 ± 8.4 months	50 improved 50 no change
Symptoms: reduced range of motion	14		15.9 ± 11.2 months	43.4 ± 9.4 months	64 no change 36 improved
Symptoms: reduced range of cervical movement and objective neurological loss	8		27.6 ± 6.5 months	43 ± 10 months	50 no change 25 improved 25 worse
Maimaris et al., 1988[131]; Leicester, England	10	Retrospective study of consecutive emergency room presentations	Average 9 months	15–20 months	100
Robinson and Caesar-Pullicino, 1993[188]; Shropshire, England	21	Retrospective study of orthopedic office practice	Not reported	Mean follow-up 13.5 years after injury	86
Parmar and Raymakers, 1993[166]; Leicester, England	100, all in accidents	Retrospective study of orthopedic office practice	Not reported	Mean follow-up 8 years after injury	55 14 significant pain
Pobershin, 2005;[174a] Devon and Cornwall, England	70	Prospective study of persons reporting rear-end collision to police	Not reported	Not reported Follow-up 2 years after accident	70

Source: From Evans RW. Whiplash injuries. In: Evans RW, Baskin DS, Yatsu, FM (eds): Prognosis of Neurological Disorders, 2nd ed. New York. Oxford University Press, 2000, p 161, with permission.

Trigger point injections can be beneficial for acute and chronic myofascial neck injuries. Injections of saline, local anesthetics, steroids, and sterile water have all been proposed. Although the precise mechanism of action of trigger point injections is not known, a few studies suggest intriguing hypotheses. The mechanism may be similar to that of acupuncture since there is a 71% correspondence between trigger points and acupuncture points.[139] Fine et al.[61] reported that the effects of trigger point injections were reversible with the administration of naloxone, suggesting that an endogenous opioid system may be a mediator. Another possible mechanism is suggested by Frost's study[71] demonstrating that injection of diclofenac, a non-steroidal anti-inflammatory drug that inhibits cyclo-oxygenase and the development of prostaglandins, may be more effective than lidocaine.

Although a variety of agents are used for injection of trigger points, the most effective is not certain. Dry needling trigger points alone without any type of injection is very effective.[122] Dry needling in comparison with injection of local anesthetics and/or steroids and saline may be equally or more effective.[72,74] Treatment of trigger points with a 10-second spray of ethyl chloride followed by 20 seconds of acupressure using the needle guard of a 21-gauge needle may be just as effective as needling with or without injection of any agent.[74] Subcutaneous sterile water injection over trigger points may be beneficial for patients with chronic neck pain after whiplash injuries.[27,28] This type of injection may not be helpful for patients with posttraumatic headache.[191] A mixture of .5 ml of 1% lidocaine and 1.5 ml of sterile water may be less painful during the injection and produce a longer lasting response than injection of 2 ml of 1% lidocaine for trigger points.[96b]

There is some evidence to suggest that injection of botulinum toxin may be helpful for posttraumatic neck pain and headaches. A single case report describes cervicogenic headache relief for 3 months at a time with injections of botulinum toxin in a trapezius muscle tender area.[92b] Two small series have found a reduction in neck pain[68] and headache[69] following trigger point injections with botulinum toxin compared to the response of injections of the trigger points in the control group with saline. However, another study found no benefit of injection of cervical and thoracic trigger points with botulinum toxin type A as compared to injections with saline.[60]

Appropriate treatment for posttraumatic headaches, dizziness, paresthesias, and cerebral symptoms can be determined after first making as precise a diagnosis as possible based upon the history, examination, and testing as indicated. Treatment of the different headache types and cerebral symptoms is reviewed in Chapter 50, Thoracic outlet syndrome improves in 50% to 90% of cases with a daily program of thoracic outlet exercises that widen the costoclavicular space by increasing the tone of the suspensatory muscles of the acromioclavicular joint.[165,169] Surgical decompression of the thoracic outlet by a variety of techniques, including scalenotomy and first rib resection, is rarely indicated but can be successful with proper patient selection.[165,192] Alpar et al.[1] have proposed that chronic neck and shoulder pain in chronic whiplash syndrome is due to carpal tunnel syndrome with normal electrodiagnostic studies. In a series of 38 such patients, 90% were reported as improved. This study should certainly be replicated.

Patients with persistent symptoms undergo an astounding array of treatments that have been poorly studied in randomized, prospective studies. Patients desperate for pain relief seek treatment from both physicians and other healers who are unwitting partners in health care.[149] According to one estimate, 94% of patients with chronic whiplash symptoms see more than one specialist.[6]

In addition to the medications noted, tricyclic antidepressants are frequently prescribed. Chronic use of narcotics, benzodiazepines, and barbiturates should be sparingly used because of the potential for addiction. Surgery is sometimes recommended inappropriately for bulging discs and spondylosis. A multitude of physical therapy modalities are used, including heat, cold, traction, massage, ultrasound, stretch and spray, electrical stimulation, and acupressure. Transcutaneous electrical nerve stimulators may help reduce myofascial pain.[81,174a] Cervical epidural steroid injections may be beneficial for chronic pain,[208] particularly with radicular symptoms and signs,[60] but prospective, controlled data on patients with only whiplash injuries are not available. In a study of 15 patients with cervical spondylotic radicular pain after whiplash injuries, a mean of 3.7 therapeutic selective nerve roots blocks was not effective.[204] Acupuncture, osteopathic manipulation,[83] and chiropractic adjustments (occasionally under general anesthesia) are performed. A variety of psychological treatments are sometimes used, including psychotherapy, biofeedback, progressive relaxation techniques, and hypnosis.

These various treatments are often uncritically provided without allowing for the importance of placebo effects.[230] The efficacy, duration, and intensity of treatment, as well as guidelines for patient selection, are not well established. Although these treatments are usually provided by well-meaning practitioners trying to reduce pain and increase function, some providers are more motivated by financial interest. In addition, a small minority of plaintiffs and their attorneys encourage excessive treatment, attempting to magnify the alleged injury. Adequately controlled prospective studies of current treatments[152,189,196b] and more effective treatments for chronic pain are greatly needed.

REFERENCES

1. Alpar EK, Onuoha G, Killampalli VV, et al: Management of chronic pain in whiplash injury. J Bone Joint Surg [Br] 84:807–811, 2002.
2. Aniss AM, Gandevia SC, Milne RJ: Changes in perceived heaviness and motor commands produced by cutaneous reflexes in man. J Physiol 397:113–126, 1988.
3. Aprill C, Dwyer A, Bogduk N: Cervical zygapophysial joint pain patterns. 1: A clinical evaluation. Spine 15: 458–461, 1990.
4. Aubrey J, Dobbs AR, Rule BG: Laypersons' knowledge about the sequelae of minor head injury and whiplash. J Neurol Neurosurg Psychiatry 52:842–846, 1989.
5. Awerbuch MS: Whiplash in Australia: Illness or injury? Med J Aust 157:193–196, 1992.
6. Balla JI: The late whiplash syndrome. Aust NZ J Surg 50:610–614, 1980.
7. Balla JI, Karnaghan J: Whiplash headache. Clin Exp Neurol 23:179–182, 1987.
8. Baloh RW: Dizziness, Hearing Loss and Tinnitus: The Essentials of Neurotology. Philadelphia, FA Davis, 1984, p 152.
9. Banic B, Petersen-Felix S, Andersen OK, et al: Evidence for spinal cord hypersensitivity in chronic pain after whiplash injury and in fibromyalgia. Pain 107:7–15, 2004.
10. Bannister G, Gargan M: Prognosis of whiplash injuries: A review of the literature. Spine: State Art Rev 7:557–569, 1993.
11. Barnsley L, Lord SM, Bogduk N: Comparative local anaesthetic blocks in the diagnosis of cervical zygapophysial joint pain. Pain 55:99–106, 1993.
12. Barnsley L, Lord S, Bogduk N: Whiplash injury. Pain 58:283–307, 1994.
13. Barnsley L, Lord SM, Wallis, BJ, Bogduk N: Chronic cervical zygapophysial joint pain: A prospective prevalence study. Br J Rheumatol 32 (suppl 2):52, 1993.
14. Barnsley L, Lord SM, Wallis BJ, Bogduk N: Lack of effect of intraarticular corticosteroids for chronic pain in the cervical zygapophysial joints. N Engl J Med 330: 1047–1050, 1994.
15. Barre JA: Sur un syndrome sympathique cervical posterieur et sa cause frequente, l'arthrite cervicale. Rev Neurol (Paris) 33:1246–1248, 1926.
16. Benoist M: Natural evolution and resolution of the cervical whiplash syndrome. In: Gunzburg R, Szpalski M, (eds): Whiplash Injuries: Current Concepts in Prevention, Diagnosis, and Treatment of the Cervical Whiplash Syndrome. Philadelphia: Lippincott-Raven, 1998, pp 117–126.
17. Berry H: Psychological aspects of whiplash injury. In: Wilkins RH, Rengachary SS (eds): Neurosurgery, vol 2. New York, McGraw-Hill, 1985, pp 1716–1719.
18. Bicik I, Radanov BP, Schafer N, et al: PET with 18-fluorodeoxyglucose and hexamethylpropylene amine oxime SPECT in late whiplash syndrome. Neurology 51:345–350, 1998.
19. Bjorgen IA: Late whiplash syndrome. Lancet 348:124; author reply 125–126, 1996.
20. Bogduk N, Marsland A: On the concept of third occipital headache. J Neurol Neurosurg Psychiatry 49:775–780, 1986.
21. Borchgrevink GE, Kaasa A, McDonagh D, et al: Acute treatment of whiplash neck sprain injuries. A randomized trial of treatment during the first 14 days after a car accident. Spine 23:25–31, 1998.
22. Braaf MM, Rosner S: Whiplash injury of neck—fact or fancy. Int Surg 46:176–182, 1966.
23. Brault JR, Wheeler JB, Siegmund GP, Brault EJ: Clinical response of human subjects to rear-end automobile collisions. Arch Phys Med Rehabil 79:72–80, 1998.
24. Brooke RI, LaPointe, HJ: Temporomandibular joint disorders following whiplash. Spine: State Art Rev 7: 443–454, 1993.

25a. Brown S: Effect of whiplash injury on accommodation. Clin Exp Ophthalmol 31:424–429, 2003.

25b. Bunketorp L, Stener-Victorin E, Carlsson J: Neck pain and disability following motor vehicle accidents—a cohort study. Eur Spine J 14(1):84–89, 2005.

26. Burke JP, Orton HP, West J, Strachan IM, Hockey MS, Ferguson DG: Whiplash and its effect on the visual system. Graefe's Arch Clin Exp Ophthalmol 230:335–339, 1992.
27. Byrn C, Bornstein P, Linder L-E: Treatment of neck and shoulder pain in whip-lash syndrome patients with intracutaneous sterile water injections. Acta Anaesthesiol Scand 35:52–53, 1991.
28. Byrn C, Olsson I, Falkheden L, et al: Subcutaneous ster-

ile water injections for chronic neck and shoulder pain following whiplash injuries. Lancet 341:449–452, 1993.
29. Capistrant TD: Thoracic outlet syndrome in whiplash injury. Ann Surg 185:175–178, 1977.
30. Capistrant TD: Thoracic outlet syndrome in cervical strain injury. Minn Med 69:13–17, 1986.
31. Cartwright SA: Report on the diseases and physical peculiarities of the negro race. New Orleans Med Surg J 7:707–709, 1850–1851.
32. Cassidy JD, Carroll LJ, Cote P, et al: Effect of eliminating compensation for pain and suffering on the outcome of insurance claims for whiplash injury. N Engl J Med 342:1179–1186, 2000.
33. Castro WH, Schilgen M, Meyer S, et al: Do "whiplash injuries" occur in low-speed rear impacts? Eur Spine J 6:366–375, 1997.
34. Chester JB: Whiplash, postural control, and the inner ear. Spine 16:716–720, 1991.
35. Cote P, Cassidy JD, Carroll L, et al: A systematic review of the prognosis of acute whiplash and a new conceptual framework to synthesize the literature. Spine 26:E445–E458, 2001.
36. Crowe H: A new diagnostic sign in neck injuries. Calif Med 100:12–13, 1964.
37. Cuetter AC, Bartoszek DM: The thoracic outlet syndrome: Controversies, overdiagnosis, overtreatment, and recommendations for management. Muscle Nerve 12:410–419, 1989.
38. Curatolo M, Petersen-Felix S, Arendt-Nielsen L, et al: Central hypersensitivity in chronic pain after whiplash injury. Clin J Pain 17:306–315, 2001.
39. Cyriax J: Rheumatic headache. Br Med J 2:1367–1368, 1938.
40. Davis AG: Injuries of the cervical spine. JAMA 127: 149–156, 1945.
41. Davis SJ, Teresi LM, Bradley WG, Ziemba MA, Bloze AE: Cervical spine hyperextension injuries: MR findings. Radiology 180:245–251, 1991.
42. Deans GT, McGalliard JN, Kerr M, Rutherford WH: Neck sprain—a major cause of disability following car accidents. Injury 18:10–12, 1987.
43. Deans GT, McGalliard JN, Rutherford WH: Incidence and duration of neck pain among patients injured in car accidents. Br Med J 292:94–95, 1986.
44. de Jong PTVM, de Jong JMBV, Cohen B, et al: Ataxia and nystagmus induced by injection of local anesthetics in the neck. Ann Neurol 1:240–246, 1977.
45. Di Carlo V, Di Carlo J, Garner R: Neurotrauma from whiplash: Sensory deficit in C2 and C3 dermatomes and in trigeminal nerve distribution. Neurol 44(suppl 2): A201–A202, 1994.
46. Diliberti T, Lindsey RW: Evaluation of the cervical spine in the emergency setting: Who does not need an x-ray? Orthopedics 15:179–183, 1992.
47. Dolinis J: Risk factors for "whiplash" in drivers: A cohort study of rear-end traffic crashes. Injury 28:173–179, 1997.
48. Dukes IK, Bannerjee SK: Hypoglossal nerve palsy following hyperextension neck injury. Injury 24:133–134, 1993.
49. Dwyer A, Aprill C, Bogduk N: Cervical zygapophyseal joint pain patterns I: A study in normal volunteers. Spine 15:453–457, 1990.
50. Edeiken J, Wolferth CC: Persistent pain in the shoulder region following myocardial infarction. Am J Med Sci 191:201–210, 1936.
51. Edmeads J: The cervical spine and headache. Neurology 38:1874–1878, 1988.
52. Eismont FJ, Clifford S, Goldberg M, Green B: Cervical sagittal spinal canal size and spine injury. Spine 9:663–666, 1984.
53. Engelhardt HT: The disease of masturbation: Values and the concept of disease. Bull His Med 48:234–248, 1974.
54. Epstein N, Epstein JA, Benjamin V, Ransohoff J: Traumatic myelopathy in patients with cervical spinal stenosis without fractures or dislocation—methods of diagnosis, management, and prognosis. Spine 5:489–496, 1980.
55. Ettlin TM, Kischka U, Reichmann S, Radii EW, Heim S, Wengen D, Benson DF: Cerebral symptoms after whiplash injury of the neck: A prospective clinical and neuropsychological study of whiplash injury. J Neurol Neurosurg Psychiatry 55:943–948, 1992.
56. Evans RW: Whiplash around the world. Headache 35: 262–263, 1995.
57. Evans RW: Neurologic aspects of hyperventilation syndrome. Semin Neurol 15(2):115–125, 1995.
58. Evans RW: Whiplash syndrome. In: Evans RW, Baskin DS, Yatsu FM (eds): Prognosis of Neurological Disorders, 2nd ed. New York, Oxford University Press, 2000, pp 152–167.
59. Evans RW, Evans RI, Sharp, MJ: The physician survey on the post-concussion and whiplash syndromes. Headache 35:268–274, 1994.
60a. Ferrante FM, Bearn L, Rothrock R, King L: Evidence against trigger point injection technique for the treatment of cervicothoracic myofascial pain with botulinum toxin type A. Anesthesiology. 103(2):377–383, 2005.
60b. Ferrante FM, Wilson SP, Iacobo C, Orav EJ, Rocco AG, Lipson S: Clinical classification as a predictor of therapeutic outcome after cervical epidural steroid injection. Spine 18:730–736, 1993.
61. Fine PG, Milano R, Hare, BD: The effects of myofascial trigger point injections are naloxone reversible. Pain 32:15–20, 1988.
62. Fisher CM: Whiplash amnesia. Neurology 32:667–668, 1982.
63. Foley-Nolan D, Kinirons M, Coughlan RJ, et al: Post whiplash dystonia well controlled by transcutaneous nervous stimulation (TENS): Case report. J Trauma 30:909–910, 1990.
64. Foley-Nolan D, Moore K, Codd M, Barry C, O'Connor P, Coughlan RJ: Low energy high frequency pulsed electromagnetic therapy for acute whiplash injuries. A double blind randomized controlled study. Scand J Rehabil Med 24:51–59, 1992.

65. Frankel VH: Whiplash injuries to the neck. In: Hirsch C, Zotterman Y (eds): Cervical Pain. Oxford, Pergamon Press, 1972, pp 97–112.
66. Freeman MD, Croft AC, Rossignol AM, et al: A review and methodologic critique of the literature refuting whiplash syndrome. Spine 24:86–96, 1999.
67. Freitag P, Greenlee MW, Wachter K, et al: fMRI response during visual motion stimulation in patients with late whiplash syndrome. Neurorehabil Neural Repair 15:31–37, 2001.
68. Freund BJ, Schwartz M: Treatment of whiplash associated neck pain [corrected] with botulinum toxin-A: A pilot study. J Rheumatol 27:481–484, 2000.
69. Freund BJ, Schwartz M: Treatment of chronic cervical-associated headache with botulinum toxin A: A pilot study. Headache 40:231–236, 2000.
70. Friedenberg ZB, Miller WT: Degenerative disc disease of the cervical spine. A comparative study of asymptomatic and symptomatic patients. J Bone Joint Surg 45A: 1171–1178, 1963.
71. Frost A: Diclofenac versus lidocaine as injection therapy in myofascial pain. Scand J Rheumatol 15:153–156, 1986.
72. Frost FA, Jessen B, Siggaard-Anderson J: A controlled, double-blind comparison of mepivicaine injection versus saline injection for myofascial pain. Lancet 1:499–501, 1980.
73. Gargan MF, Bannister GC: Long term prognosis of soft tissue injuries of the neck. J Bone Joint Surg 72B:901–903, 1990.
74. Garvey TA, Marks MR, Wiesel SW: A prospective, randomized, double-blind evaluation of trigger-point injection therapy for low-back pain. Spine 14:962–964, 1989.
75. Gay JR, Abbott KH: Common whiplash injuries of the neck. JAMA 152:1698–1704, 1953.
76. Gibbs FA: Objective evidence of brain disorder in cases of whiplash injury. Clin Electroencephalogr 2:107–110, 1971.
77. Gotten N: Survey of 100 cases of whiplash injury after settlement of litigation. JAMA 162:865–867, 1956.
78. Gove PB (ed): Webster's Third New International Dictionary of the English Language Unabridged. Springfield, MA, Merriam-Webster, 1986.
79. Gowers WR: A lecture on lumbago: Its lessons and analogues. Br Med J 1:117–121, 1904.
80. Graff-Radford SB, Jaeger B, Reeves JL: Myofascial pain may present clinically as occipital neuralgia. Neurosurgery 19:610–613, 1986.
81. Graff-Radford SB, Reeves, JL, Baker, RL, et al: Effects of transcutaneous electrical nerve stimulation on myofascial pain and trigger point sensitivity. Pain 37:1–5, 1989.
82. Greenfield J, Ilfeld FW: Acute cervical strain: Evaluation and short term prognostic factors. Clin Orthop 122:196–200, 1977.
83. Greenman PE: Manual and manipulative therapy in whiplash injuries. Spine: State Art Rev 7:517–530, 1993.
84. Guyon MA, Honet JC: Carpal tunnel syndrome or trigger finger associated with neck injury in automobile accidents. Arch Phys Med Rehabil 58:325–327, 1977.
85. Haas DC, Nord SG, Borne MP: Carpal tunnel syndrome following automobile collisions. Arch Phys Med Rehabil 62:204–206, 1981.
86. Hadden SB: Neuralgic headache and facial pain. Arch Neurol Psychiatry 43:405–408, 1940.
87. Hamer AJ, Gargan MF, Bannister GC, Nelson RJ: Whiplash injury and surgically treated cervical disc disease. Injury 24:549–550, 1993.
88a. Helleday U: Om myitis chronica (rheumatica). Ett bidrag till dess diagnostik och behandling. Mord Med Ark 8: art 8, 1876.
88b. Hendrik EJ, Scholten-Peeters GG, van der Windt DA, et al: Prognostic factors for poor recovery in acute whiplash patients. Pain 114(3):408–416, 2005.
89. Hildingsson C, Toolanen G: Outcome after soft-tissue injury of the cervical spine. Acta Orthop Scand 61:357–359, 1990.
90. Hildingsson C, Wenngren BI, Bring G, et al: Oculomotor problems after cervical spine injury. Acta Orthop Scand 60:513–516, 1989.
91. Hinoki M: Vertigo due to whiplash injury: A neurotological approach. Acta Otolaryngol (Stockh) Suppl 419:9–29, 1985.
92a. Hirsch SA, Hirsch PJ, Hiramoto H, et al: Whiplash syndrome:. Fact or fiction? Orthop Clin North Am 19:791–795, 1988.
92b. Hobson DE, Gladish DF: Botulinum toxin injection for cervicogenic headache. Headache 37:253–255, 1997.
93. Hohl M: Soft tissue injuries of the neck in automobile accidents: Factors influencing prognosis. J Bone Joint Surg 56A:1675–1682, 1974.
94. Hohl M, Hopp E: Soft tissue injuries of the neck. II. Factors influencing prognosis (abstr). Orthop Transact 2:29, 1978.
95. Hong CZ, Simons DG: Response to treatment for pectoralis minor myofascial pain syndrome after whiplash. J Musculoskel Pain 1:89–129, 1993.
96a. Irvine DH, Fisher JB, Newell DJ, Klukvin BN: Prevalence of cervical spondylosis in a general practice. Lancet 1:1089–1092, 1965.
96b. Iwama H, Akama Y: The superiority of water-diluted 0.25% to neat 1% lidocaine for trigger-point injections in myofascial pain syndrome: a prospective, randomized, double-blinded trial. Anesth Analg 91(2):408–409, 2000.
97. Jacome DE: Basilar artery migraine after uncomplicated whiplash injuries. Headache 26:515–516, 1986.
98. Jacome DE: EEG in whiplash: A reappraisal. Clin Electroencephalogr 18:41–45, 1987.
99. Jankovic J: Post-traumatic movement disorders: Central and peripheral mechanisms. Neurology 44:2006–2014, 1994.
100. Jankovic J, Van Der Linden C: Dystonia and tremor induced by peripheral trauma: Predisposing factors. J Neurol Neurosurg Psychiatry 51:1512–1519, 1988.
101. Kahane CJ: An Evaluation of Head Restraints. U.S. De-

partment of Transportation, National Highway Traffic Safety Administration Technical Report DOT HS-806-108. Springfield, VA, National Technical Information Service, February 1982.

102. Kahane CJ: An Evaluation of Center High Mounted Stop Lamps Based on 1987 Data. U.S. Department of Transportation, National Highway Traffic Safety Administration Technical Report DOT HS 807 442. Springfield, VA, National Technical Information Service, July 1989.

103a. Kai Y, Oyama M, Kurose S, et al: Neurogenic thoracic outlet syndrome in whiplash injury. J Spinal Disord 14:487–493, 2001.

103b. Kaale BR, Krakenes J, Albrektsen G, Wester K: Whiplash-associated disorders impairment rating: Neck disability index score according to severity of MRI findings of ligaments and membranes in the upper cervical spine. J Neurotrauma 22(4):466–475, 2005.

104. Karlsborg M, Smed A, Jespersen H, et al: A prospective study of 39 patients with whiplash injury. Acta Neurol Scand 95:65–72, 1997.

105. Kasch H, Bach FW, Jensen TS: Handicap after acute whiplash injury: A 1-year prospective study of risk factors. Neurology 56:1637–1643, 2001.

106. Keith WS: "Whiplash"—Injury of the 2nd cervical ganglion and nerve. Can J Neurol Sci 13:133–137, 1986.

107. Kellgren JH: A preliminary account of referred pain arising from muscle. BMJ 1:325–327, 1938.

108. Kellgren JH: Observations on referred pain arising from muscle. Clin Sci 3:175–190, 1938.

109. Kenna C, Murtagh J: Whiplash. Aust Family Physician 16:727, 729, 733, 736, 1987.

110. Key JA, Conwell HE: The Management of Fractures, Dislocations, and Sprains. St. Louis, Mosby, 1946.

111. Khurana RK, Nirankari VS: Bilateral sympathetic dysfunction in post-traumatic headaches. Headache 26: 183–188, 1986.

112. Kischka U, Ettlin TH, Heim S, Schmid G. Cerebral symptoms following whiplash injury. Eur Neurol 31: 136–140, 1991.

113. Kivioja J, Sjalin M, Lindgren U: Psychiatric morbidity in patients with chronic whiplash-associated disorder. Spine 29:1235–1239, 2004.

114. Koelbaek Johansen M, Graven-Nielsen T, Schou Olesen A, et al: Generalised muscular hyperalgesia in chronic whiplash syndrome. Pain 83:229–234, 1999.

115. Krakenes J, Kaale BR, Moen G, et al: MRI assessment of the alar ligaments in the late stage of whiplash injury—a study of structural abnormalities and observer agreement. Neuroradiology 44:617–624, 2002.

116. Krakenes J, Kaale BR, Moen G, et al: MRI of the tectorial and posterior atlanto-occipital membranes in the late stage of whiplash injury. Neuroradiology 45:585–591, 2003.

117a. Krakenes J, Kaale BR, Nordli H, et al: MR analysis of the transverse ligament in the late stage of whiplash injury. Acta Radiol 44:637–644, 2003.

117b. Kroeling P, Gross A, Houghton PE: Electrotherapy for neck disorders. Cochrane Database Syst Rev 18(2): CD004251, 2005.

118. Label LS: Carpal tunnel syndrome resulting from steering wheel impact. Muscle Nerve 14:904, 1991.

119. Lader E: Cervical trauma as a factor in the development of TMJ dysfunction and facial pain. J Craniomandib Pract 1:88–90, 1983.

120. Lamer TJ: Ear pain due to cervical spine arthritis: Treatment with cervical facet injection. Headache 31:682–683, 1991.

121. La Rocca H: Cervical sprain syndrome. In: Frymoyer JW (ed): The Adult Spine: Principles and Practice. New York, Raven Press, 1991, p 1055.

122. Lewitt K: The needle effect in the relief of myofascial pain. Pain 6:83–90, 1979.

123. Livingston M: Whiplash injury and peer copying. J R Soc Med 86:535–536, 1993.

124. Lorberboym M, Gilad R, Gorin V, et al: Late whiplash syndrome: Correlation of brain SPECT with neuropsychological tests and P300 event-related potential. J Trauma 52:521–526, 2002.

125. Lord S, Barnsley L, Bogduk N: Cervical zygapophyseal joint pain in whiplash. Spine: State Art Rev 7:355–372, 1993.

126. Lord SM, Barnsley L, Wallis BJ, Bogduk N: Third occipital headache: A prevalence study. J Neurol Neurosurg Psychiatry 57:1187–1190, 1994.

127. Lord SM, Barnsley L, Wallis BJ, et al: Chronic cervical zygapophysial joint pain after whiplash. A placebo-controlled prevalence study. Spine 21:1737–1744; discussion 1744–1735, 1996.

128. Lord SM, Barnsley L, Wallis BJ, et al: Percutaneous radio-frequency neurotomy for chronic cervical zygapophyseal joint pain. N Engl J Med 335:1721–1726, 1996.

129. MacNab I: Acceleration injuries of the cervical spine. J Bone Joint Surg 46A:1797–1799, 1964.

130. MacNab I: The whiplash syndrome. Orthop Clin North Am 2:389–403, 1971.

131. Maimaris C, Barnes MR, Allen MJ: Whiplash injuries of the neck: A retrospective study. Injury 19:393–396, 1988.

132. Marshall H W: Neck injuries. Boston Med Surg J 180: 93–98, 1919.

133. Mayou R, Bryant B: Psychiatry of whiplash neck injury. Br J Psychiatry 180:441–448, 2002.

134. Mayou R, Bryant B, Duthie R: Psychiatric consequences of road traffic accidents. BMJ 307:647–651, 1993.

135. McDonald GJ, Lord SM, Bogduk N: Long-term follow-up of patients treated with cervical radiofrequency neurotomy for chronic neck pain. Neurosurgery 45:61–67; discussion 67–68, 1999.

136. McIntire RT: Opening remarks of the Symposium on Whiplash Injuries. Int Rec Med 169:2, 1956.

137. McKinney LA, Dornan JO, Ryan M: The role of physiotherapy in the management of acute neck sprains following road-traffic accidents. Arch Emerg Med 6:27–33, 1989.

138. Mealy K, Brennan H, Fenelon GCC: Early mobiliza-

tion of acute whiplash injuries. Br Med J 292:656–657, 1986.
139. Melzack R, Stillwell DM, Fox EJ: Trigger points and acupuncture points for pain: Correlations and implications. Pain 3:3–23, 1977.
140. Mendelson G: Not "cured by a verdict." Effect of legal settlement on compensation claimants. Med J Aust 2:132–134, 1982.
141. Merskey H: Psychiatry and the cervical sprain syndrome. Can Med Assoc J 130:1119–1121, 1984.
142. Merskey H: Psychological consequences of whiplash. Spine: State Art Rev 7:471–480, 1993.
143. Miettinen T, Leino E, Airaksinen O, et al: Whiplash injuries in Finland: The situation 3 years later. Eur Spine J 13:415–418, 2004.
144. Miettinen T, Lindgren KA, Airaksinen O, et al: Whiplash injuries in Finland: A prospective 1-year follow-up study. Clin Exp Rheumatol 20:399–402, 2002.
145. Miles KA, Maimaris C, Finlay D, Barnes MR: The incidence and prognostic significance of radiological abnormalities in soft tissue injuries to the cervical spine. Skeletal Radiol 17:493–496, 1988.
146. Mills H, Horne G: Whiplash—man-made disease? NZ Med J 99:373–374, 1986.
147. Mixter WJ, Barr JS: Rupture of the intervertebral disc with involvement of the spinal canal. N Engl J Med 211:210–216, 1934.
148. Morris F: Do head restraints protect the neck from whiplash injuries? Arch Emerg Med 6:17–21, 1989.
149. Murray RH, Rubel AJ: Physicians and healers—unwitting partners in health care. N Engl J Med 326:61–64, 1992.
150. National Safety Council: Accident facts. Itasca, IL, National Safety Council, 2006.
151. Neck injury and the mind (editorial). Lancet 338:728–729, 1991.
152. Newman PK: Whiplash injury. Long term prospective studies are needed and, meanwhile, pragmatic treatment. BMJ 301:2–3, 1990.
153. Norris SH, Watt I: The prognosis of neck injuries resulting from rear-end vehicle collision. J Bone Joint Surg 65B:608–611, 1983.
154. Nygren A: Injuries to car occupants: Some aspects of the interior safety of cars. Acta Otolaryngol Suppl (Stockh) 395:1–164, 1984.
155. Obelieniene D, Schrader H, Bovim G, et al: Pain after whiplash: A prospective controlled inception cohort study. J Neurol Neurosurg Psychiatry 66:279–283, 1999.
156. O'Neill B, Haddon W, Kelley AB, et al: Automobile head restraints—frequency of neck injury claims in relation to the presence of head restraints. Am J Public Health 62:403, 1972.
157. Olsnes BT: Neurobehavioral findings in whiplash patients with long-lasting symptoms. Acta Neurol Scand 80:584–588, 1989.
158. Ommaya AK, Faas F, Yarnell P: Whiplash injury and brain damage—an experimental study. JAMA 204:285–289, 1968.
159. Ommaya AK, Yarnell P: Subdural hematoma after whiplash injury. Lancet 2:237–239, 1969.
160. Oosterveld WJ, Kortschot HW, Kingma GG, et al: Electronystagmographic findings following cervical whiplash injuries. Acta Otolaryngol (Stockh) 111:201–205, 1991.
161. Osterman AL: The double crush syndrome. Orthop Clin North Am 19:147–155, 1988.
162. Otte A, Ettlin T, Fierz L, et al: Parieto-occipital hypoperfusion in late whiplash syndrome: First quantitative SPECT study using technetium-99m bicisate (ECD). Eur J Nucl Med 23:72–74, 1996.
163. Otte A, Ettlin TM, Nitzsche EU, et al: PET and SPECT in whiplash syndrome: A new approach to a forgotten brain. J Neurol Neurosurg Psychiatry 63:368–372, 1997.
164. Otte A, Mueller-Brand J, Fierz L: Brain SPECT findings in late whiplash syndrome. Lancet 345:1513, 1995.
165. Pang D, Wessel HB: Thoracic outlet syndrome. Neurosurgery 22:105–121, 1988.
166. Parmar HV, Raymakers R: Neck injuries from rear impact road traffic accidents: Prognosis in persons seeking compensation. Injury 24:75–78, 1993.
167. Pearce JMS: Whiplash injury: A re-appraisal. J Neurol Neurosurg Psychiatry 52:1329–1331, 1989.
168. Pearce JMS: Polemics of chronic whiplash injury. Neurology 44:1993–1997, 1994.
169. Peet RM, Henriksen JD, Anderson TP, et al: Thoracic outlet syndrome. Mayo Clin Proc Staff Meet 31:281–287, 1956.
170. Pennie BH, Agambar LJ: Whiplash injuries: A trial of early management. J Bone Joint Surg 72B:277–279, 1990.
171. Peritz G: Uber die Aetiologie und Therapie des neurasthenischen Kopfschmerzes, des neurasthenischen Schwindels und der Migräne. Med Klinik 2:1145, 1906.
172. Peterson DI: A study of 249 patients with litigated claims of injury. Neurologist 4:131–137, 1998.
173. Pettersson K, Toolanen G: High-dose methylprednisolone prevents extensive sick leave after whiplash injury. A prospective, randomized, double-blind study. Spine 23:984–989, 1998.
174a. Phero JC, Raj PP, McDonald JS: Transcutaneous electrical nerve stimulation and myoneural injection therapy for management of chronic myofascial pain. Dent Clin North Am 31:703–723, 1987.
174b. Pobereskin LH: Whiplash following rear end collisions: a prospective cohort study. J Neurol Neurosurg Psychiatry 76(8):1146–1151, 2005.
175. Pollack EW: Surgical anatomy of the thoracic outlet syndrome. Surg Gynecol Obstet 150:97–103, 1980.
176. Porter KM: Neck sprains after car accidents: A common cause of long term disability BMJ 298:973–974, 1989.
177. Radanov BP, Bicik I, Dvorak J, et al: Relation between neuropsychological and neuroimaging findings in patients with late whiplash syndrome. J Neurol Neurosurg Psychiatry 66:485–489, 1999.
178. Radanov BP, Di Stefano G, Augustiny KF: Symptomatic

approach to posttraumatic headache and its possible implications for treatment. Eur Spine J 10:403–407, 2001.
179. Radanov BP, Di Stefano G, Schnidrig A, Ballinari P: Role of psychosocial stress in recovery from common whiplash. Lancet 338:712–715, 1991.
180. Radanov BP, Di Stefano G, Schnidrig A, Sturzenegger M: Common whiplash: Psychosomatic or somatopsychic? J Neurol Neurosurg Psychiatry 57:486–490, 1994.
181. Radanov BP, Di Stefano G, Schnidrig A, Sturzenegger M, Augustiny KF: Cognitive functioning after common whiplash. A controlled follow-up study. Arch Neurol 50:87–91, 1993.
182. Radanov BP, Dvorak J, Valach L: Psychological changes following whiplash injury of the cervical vertebrae. Schweiz Med Wochenschr 119:536–543, 1989.
183. Radanov BP, Dvorak J, Valach L: Cognitive deficits in patients after soft tissue injury of the cervical spine. Spine 17:127–131, 1992.
184. Radanov BP, Sturzenegger M, Di Stefano G, Schnidrig A: Relationship between early somatic, radiological, cognitive and psychosocial findings and outcome during a one-year follow-up in 117 patients suffering from common whiplash. Br J Rheumatol 33:442–448, 1994.
185. Radanov BP, Sturzenegger M, Schnidrig A, Aljinovic M: Factors influencing recovery from headache after common whiplash. BMJ 307:652–655, 1993.
186. Richter M, Ferrari R, Otte D, et al: Correlation of clinical findings, collision parameters, and psychological factors in the outcome of whiplash associated disorders. J Neurol Neurosurg Psychiatry 75:758–764, 2004.
187. Rø M, Borchgrevink G, Daehli B, Finset A, Lilleås F, Laake K, et al: SMM Report 5/2000: Whiplash Injury—Diagnosis and Evaluation. Oslo: Senter for Medisinsk metodevurdering [Norwegian Centre for Health Technology Assessment]; 2000, pp. 44–46 (translation from original Norwegian).
188. Robinson DD, Cassar-Pullicino VN: Acute neck sprain after road traffic accident: A long-term clinical and radiological review. Injury 24:79–82, 1993.
189. Rodriquez AA, Barr KP, Burns SP: Whiplash: Pathophysiology, diagnosis, treatment, and prognosis. Muscle Nerve 29:768–781, 2004.
190. Russell J: Cases illustrating the influence of exhaustion of the spinal cord in inducing paraplegia. Med Times Gazette (Lond) 2:456, 1863.
191. Sand T, Bovim G, Helde G: Intracutaneous sterile water injections do not relieve pain in cervicogeneic headache. Acta Neurol Scand 86:526–528, 1992.
192. Sanders RJ, Pearce WH: The treatment of thoracic outlet syndrome: A comparison of different operations. J Vasc Surg 10:626–634, 1989.
193. Sapir DA, Gorup JM: Radiofrequency medial branch neurotomy in litigant and nonlitigant patients with cervical whiplash: A prospective study. Spine 26:E268–E273, 2001.
194. Schmand B, Lindeboom J, Schagen S, et al: Cognitive complaints in patients after whiplash injury: The impact of malingering. J Neurol Neurosurg Psychiatry 64:339–343, 1998.
195. Schrader H, Obelieniene D, Bovim G, et al: Natural evolution of late whiplash syndrome outside the medicolegal context. Lancet 347:1207–1211, 1996.
196a. Schutt CH, Dohan FC: Neck injury to women in auto accidents: A metropolitan plague. JAMA 206:2689–2692, 1968.
196b. Seferiadis A, Rosenfeld M, Gunnarsson R: A review of treatment interventions in whiplash-associated disorders. Eur Spine J 13(5):387–397, 2004.
197. Seike FW, Kelly TR: Thoracic outlet syndrome. Am J Surg 156:54–57, 1988.
198. Severy DM Mathewson JH, Bechtol CO: Controlled automobile rear-end collisions, an investigation of related engineering and medical phenomena. Can Serv Med J 11:727–759, 1955.
199. Shapiro AP, Roth RS: The effect of litigation on recovery from whiplash. Spine: State Art Rev 7:531–556, 1993.
200. Shapiro AP, Teasell RW, Steenhuis R: Mild traumatic brain injury following whiplash. Spine: State Art Rev 7:455–470, 1993.
201. Shifrin LZ: Bilateral abducens nerve palsy after cervical spine extension injury. A case report. Spine 16:374–375, 1991.
202. Shkrum MJ, Green RN, Nowak ES: Upper cervical trauma in motor vehicle collisions. J Forensic Sci 34: 381–390, 1989.
203. Simons DG: Myofascial pain syndromes: Where are we? Where are we going? Arch Phys Med Rehabil 69: 207–212, 1988.
204. Slipman CW, Lipetz JS, DePalma MJ, et al: Therapeutic selective nerve root block in the nonsurgical treatment of traumatically induced cervical spondylotic radicular pain. Am J Phys Med Rehabil 83:446–454, 2004.
205. Smed A: Cognitive function and distress after common whiplash injury. Acta Neurol Scand 95:73–80, 1997.
206. Spitzer WO, Skovron ML, Salmi LR, et al: Scientific monograph of the Quebec Task Force on Whiplash-Associated Disorders: redefining "whiplash" and its management. Spine 20:1S–73S, 1995.
207. States JD, Korn MW, Masengill JB: The enigma of whiplash injury. New York State J Med 70:2971–2978, 1970.
208. Stav A, Ovadia L, Sternberg A, Kaadan M, Weksler N: Cervical epidural steroid injection for cervicobrachialgia. Acta Anaesthesiol Scand 37:562–566, 1993.
209. Steindler A: The interpretation of sciatic radiation and the syndrome of low-back pain. J Bone Joint Surg 22: 28–34, 1939.
210. Sterling M, Jull G, Vicenzino B, et al: Sensory hypersensitivity occurs soon after whiplash injury and is associated with poor recovery. Pain 104:509–517, 2003.
211. Sterling M, Jull G, Vicenzino B, et al: Characterization of acute whiplash-associated disorders. Spine 29:182–188, 2004.
212. Stringer WL, Kelly DL, Johnston FR, et al: Hyperex-

tension injury of the cervical spine with esophageal perforation. J Neurosurg 53:541–543, 1980.
213. Sturzenegger M, DiStefano G, Radanov BP, Schnidrig A: Presenting symptoms and signs after whiplash injury: The influence of accident mechanisms. Neurology 44: 688–693, 1994.
214. Swensen RS: The "double crush syndrome." Neurol Chronicle 4(2):1–6, 1994.
215. Tamura T: Cranial symptoms after cervical injury. Aetiology and treatment of the Barre-Lieou syndrome. J Bone Joint Surg [Br] 71B:283–287, 1989.
216. Taylor JR, Finch PM: Neck sprain. Aust Fam Physician 22:1623–1629, 1993.
217. Taylor JR, Kakulas BA: Neck injuries. Lancet 338:1343, 1991.
218. Taylor JR, Twomey LT: Acute injuries to cervical joints. An autopsy study of neck sprain. Spine 18:1115–1122, 1993.
219. Teasell RW, Shapiro AP, Mailis A: Medical management of whiplash injuries: An overview. Spine: State Art Rev 7:481–500, 1993.
220. Teresi LM, Lufkin RB, Reicher MA, Moffit BJ, Vinuela FV, Wilson GM, Bentson JR, Hanafee WN: Asymptomatic degenerative disk disease and spondylosis of the cervical spine: MR imaging. Radiology 164:83–88, 1987.
221. Toglia JU: Acute flexion-extension injury of the neck. Electronystagmographic study of 309 patients. Neurology 26:808–814, 1976.
222. Torres F, Shapiro SK: Electroencephalograms in whiplash injury. Arch Neurol 5:28–35, 1961.
223. Totstein OD, Rhame FS, Molina E, et al: Mediastinitis after whiplash injury. Can J Surg 29:54–56, 1986.
224. Trauma and dystonia (editorial). Lancet 1:759–760, 1989.
225. Travell J, Rinzler SH: The myofascial genesis of pain. Postgrad Med 11:425–434, 1952.
226. Travell J, Rinzler SH, Herman M: Pain and disability of the shoulder and arm. Treatment by intramuscular infiltration with procaine hydrochloride. JAMA 120: 417–422, 1942.
227. Travell JG, Simons DG: Myofascial Pain and Dysfunction. The Trigger Point Manual. Baltimore, Williams & Wilkins, 1983.
228. Trimble MR: Post-Traumatic Neurosis. Chichester, UK, Wiley, 1981.
229. Truong DD, Dubinsky R, Hermanowicz N, et al: Posttraumatic torticollis. Arch Neurol 48:221–223, 1991.
230. Turner JA, Deyo RA, Loeser JD, Von Korff M, Fordyce WE: The importance of placebo effects in pain treatment and research. JAMA 271:1609–1614, 1994.
231. Urschel HC, Razzuk MA: Management of the thoracic outlet syndrome. N Engl J Med 286:1140–1143, 1972.
232. Verhagen AP, Scholten-Peeters GG, de Bie RA, Bierma-Zeinstra SM: Conservative treatments for whiplash. Cochrane Database Syst Rev (1):CD003338, 2004.
233. Viano DC: Seat properties affecting neck responses in rear crashes: A reason why whiplash has increased. Traffic Inj Prev 4:214–227, 2003.
234. Viano DC. Seat influences on female neck responses in rear crashes: A reason why women have higher whiplash rates. Traffic Inj Prev 4:228–239, 2003.
235. Viano DC, Gargan MF: Headrest position during normal driving: Implication to neck injury risk in rear crashes. Accid Anal Prev 28:665–674, 1996.
236. Viano DC, Olsen S: The effectiveness of active head restraint in preventing whiplash. J Trauma 51:959–969, 2001.
237. Voyvodic F, Dolinis J, Moore VM, et al: MRI of car occupants with whiplash injury. Neuroradiology 39:35–40, 1997.
238. Wallis BJ, Lord SM, Barnsley L, et al: The psychological profiles of patients with whiplash-associated headache. Cephalalgia 18:101–105; discussion 172–103, 1998.
239. Wallis BJ, Lord SM, Bogduk N: Resolution of psychological distress of whiplash patients following treatment by radiofrequency neurotomy: A randomised, double-blind, placebo-controlled trial. Pain 73:15–22, 1997.
240. Watkinson AF: Correspondence: Whiplash injury. BMJ 301:983, 1990.
241. Weinberg S, Lapointe H: Cervical extension-flexion injury (whiplash) and internal derangement of the temporomandibular joint. J Oral Maxillofac Surg 45:653–656, 1987.
242. Weiss HD, Stern BJ, Goldberg J: Post-traumatic migraine: Chronic migraine precipitated by minor head or neck trauma. Headache 31:451–456, 1991.
243. Wickstrom J, Martinez J, Rodriguez R: Cervical sprain syndrome and experimental acceleration injuries of the head and neck. In: Selzer ML, Gikas PW, Huelke DF (eds): Proceedings of the Prevention of Highway Accidents Symposium. University of Michigan, Ann Arbor, 1967, pp 182–187.
244. Wilbourn AJ: The thoracic outlet syndrome is overdiagnosed. Arch Neurol 47:328–330, 1990.
245. Winston K: Whiplash and its relationship to migraine. Headache 27:452–457, 1987.
246. Yarnell PR, Rossie GV: Minor whiplash head injury with major debilitation. Brain In 2:255–258, 1988.

Chapter 23
Myofascial Pain Disorders

CHARLES E. ARGOFF AND
ANTHONY H. WHEELER

Voluntary muscle is the largest human organ system. Muscular injury can occur when soft tissues are exposed to single or recurrent episodes of biomechanical overloading. Muscular pain is often attributed to a myofascial pain syndrome (MPS), a common condition originally described by Drs. Janet Travell and David Simons.[93] Among patients seeking treatment from a variety of medical specialists, myofascial pain (MP) has been reported to vary from 30% to 93%, depending on the subspecialty practice and setting; however, controversy exists among medical specialists regarding the diagnostic criteria for MP and the very existence of this disorder as a pathological entity.[9,10] Therefore, the mere acknowledgment and inclusion of this entity in a neurology textbook is controversial among neurologists. While challenges exist regarding the nosology, and no specific diagnostic tool is available to validate and accurately identify MPS, it is a common pain disorder that deserves recognition clinically. The purpose of this chapter in covering this subject is to arm the neurologist with the essential tools to understand, diagnose, and treat this condition. As with the management of migraine headache, a painful state that poses similar challenges, we should not confuse the lack of omniscience regarding MPS with the lack of need for assessment and treatment.

Muscle Pain

Muscular pain and injury occur when the musculotendinous contractual unit is exposed to single or recurrent episodes of biomechanical overloading. Acute muscular pain with a duration of less than 6 weeks can result when biomechanical overloading of the musculotendinous unit occurs during the active contraction or stretch phase.[72,111] Muscle spasm is increased muscle tension due to involuntary motor activity and is often found in injured or painful muscles.[72,111] Muscular contusions and lacerations are typically caused by macrotrauma, whereas delayed-onset muscular soreness and strain usually results from repetitive overloading.[72] Delayed-onset muscular pain is common, with the usual onset noticed several hours following physical overactivity and then gradually worsening, becoming maximal over 1–3 days.[72]

Musculoskeletal pain is designated as chronic after 12 weeks.[38,111,116] Chronic muscular injury may be caused by repetitive activities that cause cumulative overwork of specific musculotendinous groups. Muscles that brace or support working muscles are at risk for painful strain, as well as muscles which have reciprocal antagonist-agonist relationships within the kinetic chain.[111]

Definition

Myofascial pain is characterized by muscles that are in a shortened or contracted state with increased tone and stiffness and containing *trigger points* (TrPs).[1] These are tender, firm nodules 3–6 mm in size that are discovered by palpatory exam.[93] Palpation provokes radiating, aching-type pain into localized *reference zones.* These reference zones exist in an area distant from the TrP and may exhibit various sensory, motor, and autonomic effects.[93] Mechanical stimulation of a hyperirritable spot within the TrP termed the *taut band* by rapid transverse pressure or needle insertion will often elicit a *localized muscle twitch response*. Sometimes TrP palpation will elicit a *jump sign*, an involuntary reflex or flinching of the patient that is greater than would be expected based on the palpatory pressure applied.[93,111] A TrP can be *active* (symptomatic) or *latent* (asymptomatic); the natural history of active and asymptomatic TrPs is unknown.[93] An active TrP is painful at rest and with motion of the affected muscle. Full lengthening of the affected muscle is limited by pain and stiffness. In contrast, a latent Trp is painful only when palpated and is not necessarily associated with shortening of muscle fibers. Trigger points associated with MP and dysfunction may become symptomatic from direct or indirect trauma, exposure to cumulative and repetitive strain, postural dysfunction, and physical deconditioning.[111] Autonomic dysfunction often accompanies symptomatic TrPs.

Epidemiology

No large studies have been published to date that address the incidence and prevalence of MPS. The Nuprin Report, a 1985 publication addressing the prevalence of pain, provides the most widespread available data and suggests that 53% of Americans experience muscular pain.[88] Sola et al., in their examination of 200 otherwise healthy young adults, found latent TrPs in the shoulder girdle muscles of 54% of the females and 45% of the males studied.[96] In another study performed by Sola and Bonica, a survey of 1000 outpatients demonstrated that 32% of them met criteria for MPS, with a prevalence of 36% among the 598 women and of 26% among the 402 men studied.[95] Myofascial pain is estimated to account for 85% of muscular pain due to injury[34] and for 90% of patients treated in pain clinics.[42] A Danish study found that MP was present in 37% of the men and 65% of the women in a randomly selected population of 1504 people aged 30 to 60 years.[30] Over 44 million Americans are estimated to suffer from this condition at a cost of $47 billion per year.[13,62]

Background

There has been interest in muscle-related pain for centuries. One of the most vexing problems has been the difficulty of correlating the palpable abnormalities of muscle with any definable and consistent histopathological and/or neurophysiological changes. In addition, the use of multiple, perhaps overlapping, terms in describing these disorders has created further misunderstanding and miscommunication regarding MPS. For example, *muscular rheumatism*, *nonarticular rheumatism, idiopathic myalgia*, *muscular sciatica*, *fibrositis*, and *myalgia spots* are among the many terms that have been used historically to describe MPS.[93] This is similar to the classification of headache, which for years suffered from a plethora of overlapping nosologies for syndromes with similar descriptions or definitions. Although the term *myofascial pain syndrome* is currently widely used and accepted in the recent medical literature, older medical publications are frequently confusing because various synonymous terms are used to describe this disorder.

Pathophysiology

The pathogenesis of MP and TrPs remains unproven. Originally, they were thought to be caused by a local disturbance of muscle. However, histological studies of muscles with TrPs and with MP and dysfunction have not clearly demonstrated why their presence is associated with pain. One biopsy study led investigators to hypothesize that the development of TrPs might be caused by a primary muscular disturbance or by excessive muscle tension.[48] Biopsy samples from active TrPs revealed that adenosine triphosphate, phosphocreatine, and glycogen concentrations were reduced and lactate levels were normal. Other investigators, including Simons et al., have maintained that TrPs result from repeated microtrauma and biomechanical overloading of the musculotendinous unit.[93] Calliet has proposed that myofascial TrPs result from blood and other materials that are not completely degraded and reabsorbed following soft tissue damage.[18] Conversely, Gunn postulated that the hypersensitivity and pain associated with TrPs are caused by a neuropathy with aberrant neural input to the affected muscle.[44]

Extensive work by Mense demonstrated that peripheral nociception in skeletal muscle can lead rapidly to central sensitization. For example, Menses placed a microelectrode into the dorsal horn of the spinal cord and mapped the receptive field identified with a specific muscle. Immediately following a bradykinin injection into the muscle, the dorsal horn neuron responded to a painful stimulus normally; for example, the pain threshold for activation of the neuron was normal. However, within 15 minutes after the injection, he demonstrated that the receptive field expanded and the neuron responded to a weaker pain stimulus consistent with sensitization. In general, this sensitization process is similar to that seen in the sensory processing of chronic neuropathic pain.[66,92] Recently, a potential relationship between chronic muscle pain and the presence of intramuscular hypoperfusion with abnormalities of adrenergic receptors was identified in patients with MPS. However, the study results were not uniform. Therefore, data to support this general hypothesis are insufficient at this time.[43,60]

Other researchers have noted and suggested similar hypotheses regarding the pathogenesis of MPS. Zimmerman postulated that because the muscle fibers that "form" the myofascial TrP are contracted for an extended period of time, muscle fatigue and ischemic changes within the muscle may occur. This change in the local environment may lead to changes in the extracellular milieu of affected muscle fibers resulting in the release of neuropeptides, such as histamine, prostaglandins, and kinins, which can promote nociception. Ongoing motor activity may recruit or enhance sensory and autonomic input, resulting in pain. Zimmerman also emphasized the role of the central nervous system in facilitating this process.[121] In an attempt to develop a human model of myofascial pain, Mork and colleagues infused numerous endogenous algogenic substances such as bradykinin, serotonin, histamine, prostaglandin E, adenosine triphosphate and combinations of these into the trapezius muscle of normal humans to determine if any of them reproduce MP. They found that a combination of bradykinin, serotonin, histamine, and prostaglandin E in normal humans produced prolonged, moderately severe pain and muscle tenderness similar to that seen in MPS.[70] The same group used this model to see if prolonged muscle tenderness could be induced in patients with tension-type headache compared with controls. Infusion of the same combination of substances into patients with tension-type headaches produced a mild increase in muscle tenderness, but the difference was not statistically significant. The authors concluded from these results that afferent input from peripheral muscles with increased excitability might be an important pathophysiological mechanism of tension-type headache.[71] Mense and colleagues recently proposed that dysfunctional neuromuscular end plates may lead to increased acetylcholine release, which in turn may lead to abnormal muscle contraction and provide the basis for the formation of myofascial TrPs. They tested this hypothesis by lesioning rat skeletal muscle after small amounts of an acetlycholinesterase inhibitor were injected into the muscle and neuromuscular stimulation was completed for approximately 60 minutes. Only the fibers, which were injected with the acetlycholinesterase inhibitor, demonstrated tissue damage and concomitant abnormalities of contraction.[67]

Audette and his colleagues measured electromyographic activity in patients with MPS, and compared symptomatic muscles with TrPs to contralateral unaffected muscles, as well as those of age-matched controls, following the placement of an acupuncture needle into the taut band of an active myofascial TrP (dry needling). They observed electromyogrphic (EMG) reactivity in the muscles contralateral to the muscles undergoing dry needling of the TrPs; however, similar findings were not seen in controls. These observations led Audette et al. to conclude that the perpetuation of pain associated with an active myofascial TrP may not depend solely on factors located within the muscle, but also on changes that occur within the central nervous system, particularly within the dorsal horn of the spinal cord.[4] These findings together support the role of both the peripheral and central nervous systems in the development and maintenance of the factors that cause MPS.

In a 1993 study, Hubbard and Berkoff found increased spontaneous muscle activity and spike discharges in human TrPs examined by needle EMG.[51] They postulated that this EMG spike activity was generated by efferent sympathetically induced hyperactivity of the muscle spindle[50,51] recorded from intrafusal muscle fibers, as opposed to the assumption by most electromyographers that this activity was due to the firing of extrafusal muscle fibers in the sarcolemmal end plate and caused by needle irritation.[16,84] Pharmacological studies by Hubbard revealed that the alpha-adrenergic antagonist phentolamine temporarily reduced TrP electrical activity when injected intravenously or intramuscularly in the vicinity of the TrP.[50] Trigger points injected with another alpha-adrenergic antagonist, phenoxybenzamine, demonstrated a longer duration of pain reduction that lasted for up to 4 months after injection.[50] Although these studies seemed promising, some participants developed subcutaneous fat necrosis at the injection sites. Furthermore, to date, double-blind, controlled research that supports the use of phenoxybenzamine for MP treatment has not been published.

A recent review of the neurophysiology of MP cited anecdotal EMG findings supporting the idea that TrPs may represent an area of focal dystonia.[84] Animal studies show that TrPs can be abolished by transection of efferent motor nerves or infusion of lidocaine; however, spinal transection above the level of segmental innervation of a TrP-containing muscle does not alter the TrP response.[84] To date, research suggests that myofascial dysfunction with characteristic TrPs is a spinal segmental reflex disorder.[84]

Simons et al. postulate that abnormally increased production and excessive release of acetylcholine at the neuromuscular junction causes sustained depolarization of the postjunctional muscle cell membrane under resting conditions, with persistent shortening of sarcomeres.[93] The resultant muscle spasm may impair arterial inflow and with it the supply of oxygen, calcium, and other nutrients necessary to induce energy-dependent muscle relaxation and to meet the higher energy demands required by aberrantly sustained muscle contraction.[93] In addition, continued contractile unit shortening and spasm can cause distortion and damage of involved tissues, which may precipitate the synthesis and release of endogenous algogenic biochemical and inflammatory substances that enhance nociception.[26,76,87]

Transduction is the process whereby noxious afferent stimuli are converted from chemical to electrical neural messages leading to transmission, which is the transfer of afferent nociceptive information from the periphery into the networks of neural relays in the spinal cord that communicate cephalad to the brain stem, thalamus, and cerebral cortex.[78,100] Peripheral and central sensitization occurs through activation of *N*-methyl-D-aspartate (NMDA) receptor sites and release of substance P.[5,20,33,59,78,100]

Other consequences of ongoing noxious stimuli include activation of NMDA receptors by repetitive peripheral nerve stimulation that activates C-fibers, leading to increased discharges of second-order neurons in the spinal cord. Chronic nociception may also recruit sympathetically mediated influences that augment pain intensity and autonomic changes such as abnormal sweating or vasomotor instability.[110,116] Therefore, the intensity and character of pain that is initially generated from a primary muscle site can be influenced by multiple neurochemical mechanisms, which in turn cause more durable and enduring nociceptive activity. Ongoing and excessive acetylcholine release, occurring at the neuromuscular junction, generates sustained muscle contraction and a continuous reverberating cycle that has been postulated to result in painful and dysfunctional extrafusal muscle contraction that forms the TrP.[93]

Generalized musculotendinous pain can occur when biomechanical loads are shifted from painful structures to neighboring joints and muscles within the kinetic chain, causing pain secondary to compensatory overuse, for example, low back pain following an injury to the hip or knee.[110,111] Also, pain spread may result when agonist muscles are overexerted to compensate for the lack of assistance usually provided by another muscle group that shares a specific movement (e.g. mouth closure augmented by ipsilateral temporalis muscles to rest an inefficient, painful masseter muscle in spasm).[111] Fibromyalgia is a frequently diagnosed disorder characterized by diffuse somatic hyperalgesia affecting both contractile and noncontractile connective tissues, and diagnostic guidelines have been established by the American College of Rheumatology.[119] Myofascial pain syndrome frequently coexists with this disorder. In addition, multiple other chemical and neurophysiological influences have been discovered that support the spread of pain to other tissues and body areas.[5,20,33,59,78,100,110]

Guidelines for Clinical Evaluation

Medical examination of patients with MP first requires identification of the location and source of the soft tissue pain pertinent to the patient's symptoms and concerns and determining whether contractile or noncontractile elements are causative.[110,111] Although diagnostic guidelines for MPS are generally accepted as those defined by Travell and Simons, there is no published consensus among practicing physicians with evidence-based support. However, a survey of pain management practitioners who commonly see patients with MPS revealed data that showed general agreement regarding many of the signs and symptoms of this disorder.[46]

Myofascial pain may appear acutely following an identifiable incident of macro-trauma or may develop over a longer period of time in a more insidious manner due to recurrent or cumulative micro-traumatic injuries. Focal or regional pain in muscles that are described as weak and stiff are usual presenting symptoms of MPS. As discussed, the key sign of MPS is the presence of TrPs. Involved muscles with symptomatic TrPs may be described by the patient as more painful with movement, especially functional use. Myofascial pain with associated painful TrPs may become symptomatic during an illness (e.g., viral infection); during periods of increased emotional stress and anxiety; or when exposed to cold damp weather conditions. Myofascial pain due to TrPs may be reduced by a period of rest; by relaxation of the affected muscle; and by physical measures such as stretching, repetitive light exercise, and application of thermal therapies (heat or cold). Symptoms such as muscle stiffness and reduced range of motion tend to be increased after periods of inactivity (e.g. when arising in the morning). Patients with MPS may complain of muscle weakness that appears to be related to pain avoidance, rather than actual loss of muscle power as demonstrated by a manual muscle exam. Abnormalities of autonomic function including changes in skin temperature and sweating (hyperhidrosis) in an affected extremity have been reported in patients with MPS.[80,93]

The diagnosis of MPS requires a physician history and thorough general physical, neurological, and musculoskeletal examinations. The examiner must determine whether muscular symptoms are primary or secondary to another biomechanical, neurological, visceral, or referred source in order to formulate a treatment plan. In evaluating the patient with MPS, one must be careful to exclude a primary structural or systemic etiology of the disorder. Numerous structural (degenerative joint or disc disease), metabolic (electrolyte disturbance, hypothyroidism, connective tissue disease), and infectious etiologies exist that either may result in an MPS-like presentation or may exacerbate pain in patients with preexisting MPS.

Muscular dysfunction is described not only in terms of spasm, pain, and tenderness, but also in terms of reduced strength and flexibility.[110] Dr. James Cyriax developed examination methods for discriminating between contractile and noncontractile sources of pain.[19,25,61,110,111] Many physicians and physiotherapists advocate the Cyriax method of selective tissue tension as an adjunct to evaluation techniques described by Simons et al.[93] Using selective tissue tension, the examiner firmly immobilizes the joint proximally and distally so that the muscle under scrutiny can be tested within a range at about 50% into the muscle's movement arc. If a contractile element is at fault, then pain should be elicited by isometric contraction. Noncontractile tissues are suspect when pain is not elicited by isometric contraction. Although useful, the absence of symptom reproduction using this evaluation technique does not eliminate a musculotendinous cause.[110,111]

Travell and Simons have advocated the identification and palpation of tender muscular TrPs as the primary method for evaluating and identifying dysfunction within the contractile elements. However, this approach alone also has limitations because it does not address all associated and pertinent biomechanical factors that play a role in causation and chronicity.[110,111] Also, tenderness is frequently elicited when asymptomatic musculotendinous tissues are palpated and is commonly found in normal functioning muscles.[110,111]

Physical examination of MPS requires a search for symptomatic muscles containing TrPs. With the symptomatic muscle placed in an intermediate position as described above, palpation is performed perpendicular to the direction of the involved muscle fibers using a pincer or flat palpation. Although the index finger is most commonly used, the thumb may be the most sensitive digit for manual palpation. The examiner should feel an area of focal spasm within which a small

2–4 mm taut band is present. A transverse flicking movement across the band may elicit a twitch response or an involuntary jump sign. Palpation pressure can be applied consistently if the examiner uses enough pressure so that the nail bed of the palpating finger begins to blanch. The examiner may ask the patient to rate the tenderness from 0 to 10 (0 = no pain; 10 = the worst possible pain) and should question the patient regarding radiation of the pain pattern or any other sensations experienced.

The range of motion and strength (power) of the affected muscle should be determined. Also the patient should be examined for musculoskeletal and neurological abnormalities, which can lead to increased biomechanical stress including scoliosis, hemiparesis, and leg length or other limb length discrepancies.

Selective tissue tension testing and TrP palpation are most effective when used together.[110,111] Physicians should coordinate with physical therapists and other coproviders to develop a consistent evaluation and management style with concordant palpation techniques and nomenclature.[110,111]

General Treatment Strategies

Rational therapies can be selected by determining the relevant pathoanatomy and causal pain mechanisms. For instance, treatment would logically be directed at the site or cause of primary injury to muscle, an example of *nociceptive pain*, which is caused by potential or actual tissue damage. By contrast, therapeutic approaches would differ for treament of a neuropathic pain condition, which is caused by primary dysfunction or disease involving peripheral and/or central nervous systems.[110] Regardless of this distinction, medical treatments that influence neural processing can reduce nociceptive transmission or perception. Myofascial pain can occur not only at a localized site of tissue damage, but also from neuropathic disorders at sites where pain is referred. Muscles affected by neuropathic pain may be injured due to prolonged spasm, mechanical overload, or metabolic and nutritional shortfalls.[110] Furthermore, pathophysiological explanations for MP have focused on neural mechanisms.[110]

When injured muscle is the primary source of nociception, treatment should include consideration of therapies that eliminate ongoing biomechanical causes, even short-term rest, supplemented by pharmacological therapies aimed directly at the dysfunctional muscle to assist healing. Successful treament often depends upon cooperative patient behaviors such as exercise, stretching, or pacing. When MP is secondary to a neuropathic pain generator, medical therapies should probably be initiated at the causative neural lesion. Physical treatments of the involved muscle may provide adjunctive pain relief in these cases, and perhaps also prevent long-term changes that may induce a primary self-sustaining MPS by recruiting local and central neurophysiological mechanisms.[110]

In general, muscle pain caused by acute injury usually improves when causative or aggravating activities are restricted and when passively applied therapies to encourage soft tissue healing are added.[72,111] Commonly used treatments include short-term rest; thermal therapies such as ice for the first 24–48 hours and heat thereafter; compression to control associated swelling; and, in some cases, a corset or brace to provide support across affected joints.[72,111] Passively applied modalities, education, manual therapy, stretching, and exercise are commonly used to address injury and pain but do not necessarily shorten the illnesses' duration. Physiotherapy using ice or topical skin refrigerants (ethyl chloride) coupled with stretching techniques are described by Simons et al.[93] Similar stretching techniques may be augmented by injection therapy or dry needling. Cryotherapy, using ice or spraying a vapocoolant from origin to insertion along a painful muscle, probably enhances spinal segmental inhibitory mechanisms but also inhibits pain transmission, muscle spasm, and inflammation.[29,57,105] Simons et al. advocate cryotherapy followed by muscle stretching.[93] Also, musculotendinous stretching may be augmented by oral medications advocated for the treatment of musculoskeletal pain, which include nonsteroidal anti-inflammatory drugs (NSAIDs), opioid and nonopioid analgesics, muscle spasmolytics, and tricyclic antidepressants. Topical analgesics such as the 5% lidocaine patch have been studied and suggest possible benefit as treatment for MPS.[2]

As pain, tenderness, and any associated autonomic dysfunction are reduced, manual therapy including muscle energy techniques can be added to improve flexibility. Instruction regarding self-care of the injured area and a home flexibility and strengthening program are necessary to abort chronicity or prevent recurrence.[115]

When musculoskeletal pain due to injury persists for more than 6 weeks, responsibility for rehabilitation and recovery should be transferred from the therapist to the patient, if possible.[3,111,115] By this time, the patient should have received the necessary education to begin self-care. A patient-specific exercise protocol should be prescribed to optimize support, protection, and movement across the injured and dysfunctional sites within the kinetic chain. Treatment goals include improvement in strength, flexibility, and aerobic endurance. Therefore, patients may need to be guided to develop an independent home exercise program that includes additional activities such as supervised weight training, water therapy, and "land" aerobic exercise. Many patients require postural and ergonomic instruction and advice regarding modification of lifestyle activities and expectations. Tertiary treatment usually consists of a multidisciplinary evaluation to develop a care plan that addresses psychosocial, physical, medical, and disability-related issues. Understanding operant influences and identifying the patient's liabilities and assets for achieving successful treatment should be recognized and addressed.[53,115]

Oral Pharmacology

While numerous options exist for pharmacotherapeutic management, in general few medications have been studied specifically for the treatment of MPS. Furthermore, most published research aimed at evaluating medication efficacy for the treatment of MP has demonstrated faulty methodology and inadequate patient description.[28] In part, these flaws relate to the confusion and controversy among physicians regarding the definition and identification of MPSs. Therefore, patients with MP may be lumped together with patients who have been diagnosed with fibromyalgia or mechanical low back pain.[28] Nevertheless, anecdotal and research evidence has led most experts to recommend medication as an adjunctive treatment to injection and exercise therapy in acute and chronic musculoskeletal pain. Oral pharmacology for chronic MPS is usually directed at the same neurochemical and neurophysiological influences that comprise or accompany most chronic pain conditions, such as fibromyalgia, chronic daily headache, or osteoarthritis.

Nonsteroidal Anti-Inflammatory Drugs

Nonsteroidal anti-inflammatory agents, that is, nonselective or cox-2 specific drugs, are known to have multiple actions within the peripheral and central nervous systems. Although this group of medications has not been found to be specifically helpful to patients with MPS, their use is often advocated by experts for pain relief[69] and to ameliorate theorized inflammation.[72] Well-designed clinical trials have demonstrated NSAIDs to be useful as a treatment for pain. However, long-term use of NSAIDs should be discouraged due to the frequent occurrence of adverse renal and gastrointestinal side effects.[3,11,27,69,91] Furthermore, the effects of these medications in the management of chronic musculoskeletal pain remains unclear, and no studies have demonstrated their clear superiority over aspirin.[28] No research supports the use of a single or specific agent over others, and sometimes switching from an ineffective NSAID to another one that belongs to a different chemical family through sequential trials may provide benefit in some patients.[3,110]

Opioid Analgesics

Low-dose opioid medications may be useful for the treatment of MP, but long-term use may lead to aberrant behaviors such as drug abuse and addiction.[3,110] In some cases of chronic MPS, long-acting opioids can help activate an injured patient for participation in physical and psychological rehabilitation.[3,110] When treating chronic pain with opioids, physicians are encouraged to incorporate appropriate medication-use behaviors into a written agreement. This agreement should indicate that patients obtain scheduled medications only through one treating physician and that escalation of the dosage must be approved by the treating medical facility. We recommend that patients understand the definitions of terms associated with opioid use, have written and signed informed consent, and have a physician's statement of medical necessity in the record. Long-acting opioids have been shown to reduce pain, and therefore may improve physical functioning in some patients with chronic or severe MP when used as an adjunct to ongoing physical and cognitive behavioral therapies.[3,110]

Nonopiate analgesics such as acetaminophen are also often used. However, caution must be exercised in using this agent since long-term use of even recommended doses of acetaminophen can be associated with renal and hepatic toxicities.[22]

Muscle Spasmolytics

Muscle spasmolytics or *relaxants* are frequently used to treat painful musculoskeletal disorders. Despite being widely prescribed, few formal studies have been completed regarding the use of muscle relaxants for the treatment of MPS. In one recent randomized study, the combination of cyclobenzaprine with ibuprofen was compared to ibuprofen alone for the treatment of acute MP. No significant differences in analgesia were found.[99] Some muscle spasmolytics are also considered potentially addictive and have abuse potential, especially more traditional agents such as diazepam, butalbital, and phenobarbital.[110] Examples of commonly used muscle relaxants include cyclobenzaprine, carisoprodol, methocarbamol, chlorzoxazone, and metaxalone; however, sedative side effects sometimes limit their use to bedtime. Metaxalone is the least sedative spasmolytic of the group. Benzodiazepines may be appropriate for concurrent anxiety states, and in these cases clonazepam should be considered. Clonazepam is a benzodiazepine that operates via GABA-mediated mechanisms through internuncial neurons of the spinal cord to provide muscle relaxation. A 1991 double-blind, controlled study demonstrated that clonazepam was effective for the treatment of temperomandibular dysfunction.[47] Although baclofen (a GABA agonist) has been found effective for the treatment of trigeminal neuralgia, it is sometimes used empirically in cases of MP; however, no controlled research studies support its use.[36]

Tizanidine

Tizanidine is a central alpha$_2$-adrenoreceptor agonist that was developed for the management of spasticity but also has demonstrated efficacy when compared to other muscle spasmolytics.[102] Clinical trials have demonstrated that tizanidine is useful as an adjunctive treatment for a variety of painful conditions including headache and spinal pain.[102] According to the authors of several small studies, tizanidine appears to have some positive effect on the treatment of MPS.[1] The muscle spasmolytic effects of tizanidine are thought to relate primarily to centrally acting alpha$_2$-adrenergic activity at both the spinal cord and supraspinal levels.[101] Primary clinical efficacy to reduce muscle spasm occurs presynaptically at the spinal cord level, with resultant reduction in the effect of released excitatory transmitters that are thought to be responsible for increased muscle tone and spasticity.[68]

Tizanidine appears to inhibit alpha motoneurons of the spinal reflex arc, which may also explain its efficacy in the reduction of pain and spasm associated with acute musculoskeletal conditions of the neck and back.[117] In addition to its already described effects on muscle spasm, tizanidine exerts a dose-dependent antinociceptive effect through alpha-adrenergic receptors, which is thought to be largely due to inhibition of the release of aspartic and glutamic acids, as well as substance P.[74] Tizanidine has not been associated with dependence after long-term use in humans.[56]

Numerous clinical trials have demonstrated the clinical efficacy of tizanidine in the treatment of acute neck and back pain.[7,32] Although it has not been approved by the Food and Drug Administration (FDA) for pain treatment, controlled studies have demonstrated reduced analgesic use and muscle spasm in patients with acute neck and back pain.[7,32] Specifically, comparison studies have shown that tizanidine is as effective as diazepam and chlorzoxozene for treatment of these acute conditions.[37] Tizanidine exerts no significant effect on normal muscle tone; therefore, patients report muscle weakness less often as a side effect compared to diazepam or other muscle relaxants.[98] The onset of action of tizanidine is rapid, with peak plasma concentrations occurring at 1–2 hours following oral administration.[98] The elimination half-life of tizanidine is approximately 2.5 hours, with significant interpatient variability. Further investigation of tizanidine as a treatment for MPS is warranted due to its favorable characteristics, including its rapid onset of action and its muscle spasmolytic and antinociceptive properties.[98]

Neuropathic Analgesics

Because MP may be a spinal-mediated disorder and may occur in musculotendinous structures affected by neuropathic dysfunction, conventional treatments for neuropathic pain, including anticonvulsants, can be considered. A popularly prescribed anticonvulsant for chronic pain is gabapentin, which was shown to be effective for the treatment of MP and neuropathic pain.[85]

Antidepressants

Tricyclic antidepressants (TCAs) are commonly used for chronic pain treatment to alleviate insomnia, enhance endogenous pain suppression, reduce painful dysesthesia, and eliminate other painful disorders such as headaches.[3] Research supports the use of TCAs to treat both nociceptive and neuropathic pain syndromes.[12,17,27,40,52,54,58,64,65,75,77,81,83,94,103,104,110] The presumed mechanism of action is related to the TCAs' capacity to block serotonergic uptake, resulting in a potentiation of noradrenergic synaptic activity in the central nervous system brain stem-dorsal horn nociceptive-modulating system. Also, recent studies in animals suggest that TCAs may act as local anesthetics by sodium channel blockade where ectopic discharges are generated.[52,75] Evidence supporting the use of selective serotonin reuptake inhibitors (SSRIs) to attenuate pain intensity is less impressive, and recent studies have suggested that these agents are at best inconsistently effective for neuropathic pain.[12,52] Venlafaxine is a structurally novel antidepressant shown to produce strong uptake inhibition of both serotonin and norepinephrine, as well as anesthetic properties similar to those of the TCAs. An uncontrolled case series reported that venlafaxine provided pain relief in a variety of neuropathic pain disorders.[97]

However, the use of TCAs has become less popular, particularly in geriatric populations, due to cardiovascular effects such as tachycardia; anticholinergic side effects including dry mouth, increased intraocular pressure, and constipation; oversedation; and dizziness, including orthostatic hypotension. The SSRIs should be considered for symptoms commonly associated with chronic pain including reduced coping, depression, anxiety, and fatigue. Overall, SSRIs have fewer adverse side effects than TCAs. Side effects associated with SSRIs include anxiety, nervousness, and insomnia; drowsiness and fatigue; tremor; increased sweating; appetite and gastrointestinal dysfunction; and male sexual dysfunction. Many pain specialists consider TCAs as first-line pain medications for the treatment of persistent neuropathic pain, especially as an adjunct to peripheral therapies and to manage the adverse influences of chronic illness.

Therapeutic Injections

Historically, these injections have been given empirically, often resulting in variable or temporary benefit despite the risk and potential complications. Usually, therapeutic injections for treating MP are directed at the most symptomatic TrPs within the target muscle and then at other regionally symptomatic muscles that have a functional or structural relationship. Injection treatment strategies include blockade or inhibition of afferent and efferent neural pathways to induce muscular elongation. Common TrP injectates include local anesthetics, corticosteroids, and normal saline; less commonly, neurolytic agents or dry needling are used.[110]

Local Anesthetics

Several clinical characteristics should be considered when choosing a local anesthetic (LA) for soft tissue injections. The latency of onset of LA action depends on the concentration, total dose, distance between the injection site and the target, and relative penetrance of the compound.[14,108] The duration of the LA depends on its pharmacodynamic properties, concentration, total dose, and vascularity of the region under scrutiny.[14,15,108] All LAs have similar basic chemical structures with an aromatic and amino end joined by an intermediate chain.[14,15,108] The amino esters use an ester link between the aromatic and the intermediate chain.[14,15,108] Popular amino amides for treating MP include lidocaine, mepivacaine, and bupivacaine. Lidocaine is widely used due to its rapid onset, potency, and tissue penetration.[15] Injections of TrP using an LA combined with a corticosteroid have long been advocated; however, there are conflicting reports as to whether any therapeutic substance injected into a muscle provides more benefit than dry needling alone.[41]

Bupivacaine has a longer duration of action; however, it alters myocardial conduction more dramatically than lidocaine.[15,31,108] Therefore, its use for the treatment of patients with comorbid cardiac disease may require cardiorespiratory monitoring. Many experts limit the concentration of bupivicaine to 0.125% and that of lidocaine to 0.5% to avoid anaphylactic or other adverse reactions and because local anesthetics are myotoxic.[24,31] However, ablation of a chronically painful TrP may provide long-term benefit; therefore, I typically use a higher concentration of lidocaine (2%) without epinephrine and bupivicaine (0.5%) and limit the dosages of lidocaine to 4 cm^3 and of bupivicaine to 12 cm^3. The maximum dosage of bupivicaine to be used in a treatment session should not exceed 2.5 mg/kg or 300 mg lidocaine.[55,110]

Corticosteroids

Injectable corticosteroids have been advocated by many for the treatment of MP, unless contraindicated due to infection or skin breakdown at the target site or in patients with poorly controlled diabetes.[63] Continuous large doses of a corticosteroid adversely affect collagen synthesis and therefore connective tissue strength.[23,118] The frequency of injections must be monitored to prevent generalized or focal immune suppression, thereby causing infection or impaired tissue healing.[63]

Physician preference among commonly used injectable corticosteroids is often arbitrary. Corticosteroid esters have long been preferred due to their relative safety and efficacy. The relative solubility of these solutions is considered a factor when determining the appropriate injectate.[63] Highly soluble steroids such as betametasone sodium phosphate or betamethazone acetate are rapidly absorbed and therefore pose less risk for connective tissue injury such as tendon rupture, fat atrophy, and muscle wasting. Corticosteroids are frequently used in combination with LAs for TrP injections. The action by which corticosteroids ameliorate the pain or integrity of the TrP is unclear. It may be attributed to anti-inflammatory properties incurred by inhibition of phospholipase A_2, which interrupts inflammatory mediators in both the cyclooxygenase and lipoxygenase pathways.[63] Corticosteroids also inhibit prostaglandin synthesis and may stabilize neural membranes. Commonly experienced side effects or adverse reactions due to corticosteroids include lightheadedness, nervousness, facial flushing, insomnia, and increased appetite.[23] A flare-up of pain symptoms lasting for 24–48 hours may occur in 10% of patients[63] and is presumably related to a local inflammatory response to corticosteroid crystals. The propensity for flare-ups can be reduced by using a soluble rapidly absorbed corticosteroid. Rest and physical therapy are sometimes necessary in these cases. In addition, adverse reactions may occur in persons who have active peptic ulcer disease or infection, ulcerative colitis, hypertension, congestive heart failure, renal disease, and psychiatric illness.[31] Hyperglycemia in known diabetics warrants careful postprocedural monitoring. Other less serious side effects of corticosteroids include injection site hyperpigmentation, subcutaneous fat atrophy, peripheral edema, dyspepsia, and malaise.[31,63] Systemic responses frequently occur even with local injections of corticosteroids. Allergic reactions to systemic glucocorticoids in slow-release formulations have been reported to occur up to 1 week after injection.[31]

Neurolytic Agents

Neurolytic agents are commonly employed for destruction of a peripheral pain generator after it has been clearly identified by anesthetic blocking procedures. Both chemical and physical methods can be used for neurolysis. Physical methods include radiofrequency neurotomy and cryoneurolysis. Commonly used substances for chemical neurolysis include phenol, ethyl alcohol, propylene glycol, chlorocresol, glycerol, cold saline, hypertonic solutions, and hypotonic solutions.[31]

Phenol (carbolic acid) is gaining popularity for TrP injections and causes nonselective nerve destruction, muscle atrophy, and soft tissue necrosis within the injection site. Two to 6% concentrations of phenol are commonly used for TrP injections, sometimes mixed with equal parts of glycerin before dilution with normal saline.[31] Protection of the patient and medical personnel, especially the eyes and face, is mandatory since contact with phenol can cause erythema and necrosis.[31,110] We advocate using 0.5 to 1.5 cc of 3% to 6% phenol after a local anesthetic and corticosteroid to reduce postinjection soreness. Provocation of pain and careful aspiration confirm that the needle is safely placed within the target TrP. Generally, patients tolerate the procedure well, and localized postinjection pain occurs infrequently. Intravascular or central nervous system placement can result in serious complications which including cardiac dysrhythmia, hypertension, venous thrombosis, soft tissue and neural infarction, and chemical meningitis.[31]

Chemodenervation: Botulinum Toxin

Botulinum toxin (BTX) is a potent neurotoxin with seven serotypes (A, B, C_1, D, E, F, and G), which are produced by the gram-positive anaerobic bacterium *Clostridium botulinum* and act by blocking acetylcholine release at the neuromuscular junctions.[53] Two serotypes, botulinum toxin A (BTXA) and B (BTXB), are currently available for clinical use. Botulinum toxin A has been under investigation since 1968 and has been widely used for the treatment of focal muscle overactivity for more than 15 years.[53,106,110] It has been approved by the FDA for the treatment of strabismus, blepharospasm, and seventh nerve disorders in patients 12 years of age or older since 1989. Recently, the FDA has approved BTXA for cosmetic use and BTXB for cervical dystonia. Furthermore, clinical investigation supports the treatment of many focal dystonic and nondystonic disorders of muscle spasm with BTXA, which has not yet received FDA approval.[53,106] The therapeutic benefit of BTXA-induced neuromuscular blockade in humans usually lasts for 3 to 4 months and ranges from 2 to 6 months or more following an injection session.[53] The degree and duration of pain relief may be greater than the motor benefit observed.[45,114] Animal and human research suggests that BTX reduces pain by multiple mechanisms in muscle and the central nervous system. Peripheral benefits may result from neuromuscular blocking of extrafusal fiber overcontraction and inhibition of gamma-motor endings in muscle spindles.[45,109b] Central effects may be ascribed to BTX actions on spinal interneurons, as a substance P antagonist, and as an analgesic.[45,109b]

In the hands of physicians who are experienced in using BTX, treatment is usually safe, with few side effects. Some injections require EMG, ultrasonography, or radiology for guidance of needle placement into target muscles. Outside neural and vascular complications, potential problems posed by needle placement with BTX include excessive or adjacent unwanted muscle weakness. Discretion with BTX use is recommended for treatment of patients with potential or preexisting disorders of the neuromuscular junction, such as myasthenia gravis, Lambert-Eaton's syndrome, and motor neuron disease. Botulinum toxin should not be given to patients during pregnancy or lactation, or to patients taking aminoglycoside antibiotics or other drugs that interfere with neuromuscular transmission.[53,106]

Some studies have revealed potential benefit from BTX when used to treat common painful disorders[8] such as muscle tension headache,[73,82,89,122] muscular neck pain,[21,45,49,107,113,114,120] and MP.[21,35,49,79,86,107,112–114,120] Porta et al. compared the efficacy of BTXA versus methylprednisolone mixed with 0.5% bupivicaine for treatment of patients with chronic MP.[79] Improvement in the BTXA group was superior to that in the methylprednisolone group at 2 months when initial improvement in the comparison group waned. Porta stressed the importance of combining BTXA injections with physiotherapy.[79] A prospective, double-blind, randomized, controlled study revealed no statistically significant benefit from BTXA for the treatment of cervical MPs when using doses similar to those used to treat cervical dystonia and without adjunctive physiotherapy.[114] Some clinical studies demonstrating therapeutic benefit from BTXA for MP treatment have used weak measurement criteria[21] or patient data were compared across time rather than with those of a control group.[35]

Placement of the neurotoxin into symptomatic TrPs is consistent with theories and practices originally described by Simons et al.[93] In fact, the mechanism by which BTX may alleviate MP is unknown, and may be due primarily to peripheral- and central nervous system–mediated effects rather than to a purely neuromuscular junction effect.[109a,109b] Subdermal injection of BTX may be adequate to access active nociceptive pathways. Therefore, varied opinions exist regarding injection placement, dosing, and the number of injection sessions deemed most effective for the treatment of MP.[109] These technical aspects of BTX use must be studied to optimize and understand its benefit.

A recent observational study of BTXA treatment for cervical MP demonstrated a high incidence (28%) of postprocedure painful injection-site muscle spasm, which was alleviated by physical therapy using myofascial release techniques.[112] Manual myofascial release oriented along the working axis of the muscle was effective in alleviating this painful muscle spasm. These manual therapy techniques are theorized to work by destroying the presumed aberrant collagen crosslinks that are found in chronic muscle spasm. Other commonly reported BTX side effects include a short-lived flu-like syndrome and, more specifically with BTXB, dyspepsia and systemic anticholinergic effects such as dry mouth.

Conclusion

Most treatments for MP are empiric and aimed at the painful TrP with the purpose of ablating muscle spasm and restoring normal muscle length, function, and strength. Any benefit from oral pharmacology is adjunctive. Medications, in part, also help the physician and the treatment team address the multifactorial physiological and psychosocial aspects of pain. Consensus among researchers for defining and describing MP using concordant terminology and examination techniques is requisite. Multiple questions and other variables impeding research include study design, that is, exclusion/inclusion criteria, procedural methodology, and injection techniques. Botulinum toxin is a logical treatment choice in line with theories and treatments described by Simons et al.[93] as well as Hubbard.[50] It has demonstrated promise as a treatment for MP when used in lower doses than are typical for dystonia,[114] with one or two repeat injection sessions,[112,113] and when combined with physical therapy.[79,90,112]

REFERENCES

1. Argoff CE (ed.): The role of alpha-adrenergic agonists in the pain management. In: Abstract Review: Current Research and Expert Commentary 2002 Medical Education Network.
2. Argoff CE: Targeted topical peripheral analgesics in the management of pain. Curr Pain Headache Rep 7(1): 34–38, 2003.
3. Argoff CE, Wheeler AH: Spinal and radicular pain disorders. Neurol Clin 4:833–849, 1998.
4. Audette J, Wang F, Smith H. The electrophysiological characteristics of myofascial pain: Characteristics of the local twitch response in subjects with active myofascial pain of the neck compared to a control group with latent trigger points. NEPA J 7:10–14, 2002.
5. Bennett RM: Emerging concepts in the neurobiology of chronic pain; evidence of abnormal sensory processing in fibromyalgia. Mayo Clin Proc 74:385–398, 1999.
6. Berry H, Hutchinson DR: A multicenter placebo-controlled study in general practice to evaluate the safety and efficacy of tizanidine in acute low back pain. J Int Med Res 16:75–82, 1988.
7. Berry H, Hutchinson DR: Tizanidine and ibuprofen in acute low back pain: Results of a multicenter double-blind study in general practice. J Int Med Res 16:83–91, 1988.
8. Blasi J, Chapman ER, Link E, et al: Botulinum neurotoxin A selectively cleaves the synaptic protein SNAP-25. Nature 365:160–163, 1993.
9. Bohr TW: Fibromyalgia syndrome and myofascial pain syndrome. Do they exist? Neurol Clin 13(2):365–384, 1995.
10. Bohr TW: Problems with myofascial pain syndrome and fibromyalgia syndrome. Neurology 79:593–597, 1996.
11. Bombardier C, Laine L, Reicin A, et al: Comparison of upper gastrointestinal toxicity of roxecob and naproxen in patients with rheumatoid arthritis. N Engl J Med 343(21):1520–1528, 2000.
12. Bonezzi C, Demartini L: Treatment options in postherpetic neuralgia. Acta Neurol Scand Suppl 173:25–35; discussion 48–52, 1999.
13. Bonica JJ: The Management of Pain, vol 1, 2nd ed. Philadelphia, Lea & Febiger, 1990, pp 180–196.
14. Bonica JJ, Buckley FO: Regional anesthesia with local anesthetics. In: Bonica JJ (senior ed), Loeser JD, Chapman RC, Fordyce WE (eds): The Management of Pain, 2nd ed. Philadelphia, Lea & Febiger, 1990, pp 1980–2039.
15. Brown DL: Atlas of Regional Anesthesia. Philadelphia, WB Saunders, 1992.
16. Brown WF, Varkey GP: The origin of spontaneous electrical activity at the end-plate zone. Ann Neurol 10: 557–560, 1981.
17. Bardin M, Chantelauze C, Lavarenne J, Eschalier A: Study of the sensitivity of the diabetes-induced pain model in rats to a range of analgesics. Pain 57:153–160, 1994.
18. Calliet R: Soft Tissue Pain and Disability. Philadelphia, FA Davis, 1977.
19. Cantu RI, Grodin AJ: Myofascial Manipulation: Theory and Clinical Application. Gaithersburg, MD, Aspen, 1992.
20. Carlton SM, Zhou S, Coggeshal RE: Evidence for the interaction of glutamate and NK1 receptors in the periphery. Brain Res 83:160–169, 1998.
21. Cheshire WP, Abashjan SW, Mann JD: Botulinum toxin in the treatment of myofascial pain syndrome. Pain 59: 65–69, 1994.
22. Clissold SP: Paracetamol and phenacetin. Drugs 32(suppl 4):46–59, 1986.
23. Cohen IK, Diegelmann RF, Johnson ML: Effect of corticosteroids on collagen synthesis. Surgery 82:15–20, 1977.
24. Criscuolo CM: Interventional approaches to the management of myofascial pain syndrome. Curr Pain Head Rep 5:407–411, 2001.
25. Cyriax J: Textbook of Orthopaedic Medicine: Diagnosis of Soft Tissue Lesions, 8th ed. Baltimore, Williams & Wilkins, 1984.

26. Davidoff RA: Trigger points and myofascial pain: Toward understanding how they affect headaches. Cephalalgia 18:436–448, 1998.
27. Deyo RA: Drug therapy for back pain. Which drugs help which patients? Spine 21:2840–2850, 1996.
28. Deyo RA: Nonoperative treatment of low back disorders: Differentiated useful from useless therapy. In: Frymoyer JW (ed-in-chief), Ducker TB, Hadler NM, Kostuik JP, Weinstein JN, Whitecloud III (eds): The Adult Spine: Principles and Practice. Philadelphia, Lippincott-Raven, 1997, pp 1777–1793.
29. Downer AH: Physical Therapy Procedures. Springfield, IL, Charles C Thomas, 1970.
30. Drewes AM, Jennum P: Epidemiology of myofascial pain, low back pain, morning stiffness and sleep-related complaints in the general population [abstract]. J Muscoskel Pain 3(suppl 1):G8, 1995.
31. Dreyer SJ: Commonly used medications in pain procedures. In: Lennard JA (ed): Pain Procedures in Clinical Practice. Philadelphia, Hanley & Belfus, 2000, pp 1–9.
32. Felder M: Tizanidine in the treatment of neck and low back pain. Aids Int 1:9, 1990.
33. Fields HL: Pain. New York, McGraw-Hill, 1987.
34. Fishbain DA, Goldberg M, Meagher BR, et al: Male and female chronic pain patients' categories by DSM-III psychiatric diagnostic criteria. Pain 26:181–197, 1986.
35. Freund BJ, Schwartz M: Treatment of whiplash associated with neck pain with botulinum toxin-A: A pilot study. J Rheumatol 27:481–484, 2000.
36. Fromm GH, Terence CF, Chatta AS: Baclofen in the treatment of trigeminal neuralgia. Ann Neurol 15:240–247, 1984.
37. Fryda-Kaurimsky Z, Muller-Fassbender H: Tizanidine in the treatment of acute paravertebral spasms: A controlled trial comparing tizanidine with diazepam. J Int Med Res 9:501–505, 1981.
38. Frymoyer JW: Back pain and sciatica. N Engl J Med 318:291–300, 1988.
39. Galer BS, Dworkin RH: A Clinical Guide to Neuropathic Pain. Minneapolis, McGraw-Hill, 2000.
40. Garcia J, Altman RD: Chronic pain states: Pathophysiology and medical therapy. Semin Arthritis Rheum 27: 1–16, 1997.
41. Garvey TA, Marks MR, Wiesel SW:. A prospective, randomized double-blind evaluation of trigger-point injection therapy for low-back pain. Spine 14:962–964, 1989.
42. Gerwin RD: A study of 96 subjects examined both for fibromyalgia and myofascial pain [abstract]. J Musculoskel Pain 3(suppl 1):121, 1995.
43. Graven-Nielsen T, Arendt-Nielsen L: Is there a relation between intramuscular hypoperfusion and chronic muscle pain? T J Pain 3(4):261–263, 2002.
44. Gunn CC. Prespondylosis and some pain syndromes following denervation suprasensitivity. Spine 1980; 5: 185–192.
45. Guyer BA: Mechanism of botulinum toxin the in relief of chronic pain. Curr Rev Pain 3:427–431, 1993.
46. Harden RN, Bruehl SP, Fass S, et al: Signs and symptoms of the myofascial pain syndrome: A national survey of pain management providers. Clin J Pain 16:64–72, 2000.
47. Harkens S, Linford J, Cohen J, Kramer R, Cueva L: Administration of clonazepam in the treatment of TMD and associated myofascial pain: A double-blind pilot study. J Cranio Mandib Disord Facial Oral Pain 5:179–186, 1991.
48. Henriksson KG, Bengtsson A, Larsson J, et al: Muscle biopsy findings of possible diagnostic importance in primary fibromyalgia (fibrositis, myofascial syndrome) (letter). Lancet 2:1395, 1982.
49. Hobson D, Gladish D: Botulinum toxin injection for cervicogenic headache. Headache 36:253–255, 1997.
50. Hubbard DR: Chronic and recurrent muscle pain: Pathophysiology and treatment, and review of pharmacologic studies. J Musculoskel Pain 4:123–143, 1996.
51. Hubbard DR, Berkoff GM: Myofascial trigger points show spontaneous needle EMG activity. Spine 18:1803–1807, 1993.
52. Jacobson LO, Bley K, Hunter JC, et al: Anti-thermal hyperalgesic properties of antidepressants in a rat model of neuropathic pain Am Pain Soc [abstract] 1995.
53. Jankovic J, Brin JF: Therapeutic uses of botulinum toxin. N Engl J Med 342:1186–1194, 1991.
54. Jay GW: Chronic daily headache—pathophysiology and treatment. Pain Dig 16:851–868, 1994.
55. Lacy CF, Armstrong LL, Goldman MP, Lance LL: Drug Information Handbook. Hudson, OH: Lexi-comp, 1999.
56. Lataste X, Emre M, Davis C, et al: Comparative profile of tizanidine in the management of spasticity. Neurology 44:53–59, 1994.
57. Lee JM, Warren MP, Mason, SM: Effects of ice on nerve conduction velocity. Phys Ther 64:2, 1978.
58. Lipman AG: Analgesic drugs for neuropathic and sympathetically maintained pain. Clin Geriatr Med 12:501–515. 1996.
59. Liu H, Mantyh PW, Basbaum AI: NMDA-receptor regulation of substance P release from primary afferent nociceptors. Nature 386(6626):721–724, 1997.
60. Maekawa K, Clark GT, Kuboki T: Intramuscular hypoperfusion, adrenergic receptors, and chronic muscle pain. T J Pain 3(4):251–260, 2002.
61. Magee DJ: Orthopedic Physical Assessment, 2nd ed. Philadelphia, WB Saunders, 1992.
62. Magni G: The epidemiology of musculoskeletal pain. In: Voeroy H, Merskey H (eds): Progress in Fibromyalgia and Myofascial Pain. Amsterdam, Elsevier Science, 1993, pp 3–20.
63. Mayo NA, Fadale PD: The role of injectable corticosteroids in orthopedics. Orthopedics 24:400–405, 2001.
64. McCain GA: Fibromyalgia and myofascial pain syndromes. In: Wall PD, Melzack R (eds): Textbook of Pain, 3rd ed. New York: Churchill Livingstone, 1994, pp 475–493.
65. McQuay HJ, Moore RA, Eccleston C, Morley S, Williams AC: Systemic review of outpatient services for chronic pain control. Health Tech Assess 1:i–iv, 1–135, 1997.

66. Mense S: Nociception from skeletal muscle in relation to clinical muscle pain. Pain 54:241–289, 1993.
67. Mense S, Simons DG, Hoheisel U, et al: Lesions of rat skeletal muscle after local block of acetlycholinesterase and neuromuscular stimulation. J Appl Physiol 94(6): 2494–2501, 2003.
68. Milanov I, Georgiev D: Mechanisms of tizanidine in spasticity. Acta Neurol Scand 89:274–279, 1994.
69. Miyoshi HR: Systemic nonopioid analgesics. In: Loeser JL (ed): Bonica's Management of Pain, 3rd ed. Philadelphia, Lippincott Williams & Wilkins, 2001, pp 1667–1681.
70. Mork H, Ashina M, Bendtsen L, et al: Experimental muscle pain and tenderness following infusion of endogenous substances in humans. Eur J Pain 7(2):142–153, 2003.
71. Mork H, Ashina M, Bendtsen L, et al: Induction of prolonged tenderness in patients with tension-type headache by means of a new experimental model of myofascial pain. Eur J Neurol 10(3):249–256, 2003.
72. Noonan TJ, Garrett WE: Muscle strain injury: Diagnosis and treatment. J Am Acad Orthop Surg 7:262–269, 1999.
73. O'Brien CF: Clinical applications of botulinum toxin: Implications for pain management. Pain Dig 8:342–345, 1998.
74. Ono H, Mishima A, Ono S, et al: Inhibitory effects of clonidine and tizanidine on release of substance P. Neuropharmacology 30:585–589, 1991.
75. Pancrazio JJ, Kamatchi GL, Roscoe AK, Lynch C III: Inhibition of neuronal Na^+ channels by antidepressant drugs. J Pharmacol Exp Ther 284:208–214, 1998.
76. Pappagallo M: Aggressive pharmacologic treatment of pain. Rheum Dis Clin North Am 25:193–209, 1999.
77. Pettengill CA, Reisner-Keller L: The use of tricyclic antidepressants for the control of chronic orofacial pain. J Craniomandib Pract 15:53–56, 1997.
78. Pillemer SR, Bradley LA, Crofford LI, et al: The neuroscience and endocrinology of fibromyalgia. Arthritis Rheum 40:1703–1707, 1997.
79. Porta M: A comparative trial of botulinum toxin type A and methylprednisolone for the treatment of myofascial pain syndrome and pain from chronic muscle spasm. Pain 85:101–105, 2000.
80. Rashiq S, Galer BS: Proximal myofascial dysfunction in complex regional pain syndrome: A retrospective prevalence study. Clin J Pain 15(2):151–153, 1999.
81. Redillas C, Solomon S: Prophylactic pharmacological treatment of chronic daily headache. Headache 40:83–102, 2000.
82. Relja M: Treatment of tension-type headache by local injection of botulinum toxin. Eur J Neurol 4(suppl 2): S71–S73, 1997.
83. Reveille JD: Soft-tissue rheumatism: Diagnosis and treatment. Am J Med. 102(suppl 1A):23S-29S, 1997.
84. Rivner MH: The neurophysiology of myofascial pain syndrome. Curr Pain Headache Rep 5:432–440, 2000.
85. Rosenberg JM, Harrell C, Rishi H, Werner RA, deRosayro AM: The effect of gabapentin on neuropathic pain. Clin J Pain 13:251–255, 1997.
86. Royal MA, Gunyeu I, Bhatia B, et al: Botulinum toxin type A in the treatment of refractory myofascial pain [abstract]. Neurology 58(suppl 3):A350, 2001.
87. Russell IJ: Neurochemical pathogenesis of fibromyalgia syndrome. J Musculoskel Pain 4:61–92, 1996.
88. Russell IJ: Fibromyalgia syndrome. In: Loeser JD (ed): Bonica's Management of Pain. Philadelphia, Lippincott Williams & Wilkins, 2001, pp 543–556.
89. Schiavo G, Benfenati F, Poulain B, et al: Tetanus and botulinum-B neurotoxins block neurotransmitter release by proteolytic cleavage of synaptobrevin. Nature 359:832–835, 1992.
90. Schneider P, Mororu E, Bitttner C, et al: Physical therapy and botulinum toxin type A in patients with cervical associated headache according to IHS-criteria: Double-blind placebo-controlled study [abstract]. Neurology 58(suppl 3):A349, 2001.
91. Silverstein F, Faich G, Goldstein JL, et al: Gastrointestinal toxicity with celecoxib vs nonsteroidal anti-inflammatory drugs for osteoarthritis and rheumatoid arthritis. The class study: A randomized controlled trial. JAMA 284(10):1247–1255, 2000.
92. Simons DG, Mense S: Understanding and measurement of muscle tone as related to clinical muscle pain. Pain 75(1):1–17, 1998.
93. Simons DG, Travell JG, Simons LS: Myofascial Pain and Dysfunction: The Trigger Point Manual, 2nd ed. Baltimore, Williams & Wilkins, 1999.
94. Sindrup SH, Jensen TS: Efficacy of pharmacological treatments of neuropathic pain: An update and effect related to mechanism of drug action. Pain 83:389–400, 1999.
95. Sola AE, Bonica JJ: Myofascial pain syndromes. In: Loeser JD (ed): Bonica's Management of Pain. Philadelphia, Lippincott Williams & Wilkins, 2001, pp 530–542.
96. Sola AE, Rodenberger ML, Gettys BB: Incidence of hypersensitive areas in posterior shoulder muscles. Am J Phys Med 34:585–590, 1955.
97. Taylor K, Rowbotham MC: Venlafaxine for chronic pain. American Pain Society annual meeting [abstract]. 1995.
98. Tse FLS, Jaffe JM, Bhuta S: Pharmacokinetics of tizanidine in health volunteers. Fundam Clin Pharmacol 1:479–488, 1987.
99. Turturro MA, Frater CR, D'Amico FJ: Cyclobenzaprine with ibuprofen alone in acute myofascial strain: A randomized, double blind clinical trial. Ann Emerg Med 41(6):818–826, 2003.
100. Urban MO, Gebhart GF: Central mechanisms in pain. Med Clin North Am 83:585–596, 1999.
101. Wagstaff AJ, Bryson HM. Tizanidine: A review of pharmacology, clinical efficacy and tolerability in the management of spasticity associated with cerebral and spinal disorders. Drugs 53:436–451, 1997.
102. Waldman SD: Recent advances in analgesic therapy—tizanidine. Pain Digest 9:40–43, 1999.

103. Wasner G, Backonja M-M, Baron R: Traumatic neuralgias: Complex regional pain syndromes (reflex sympathetic dystrophy and causalgia): Clinical characteristics, pathophysiologic mechanisms and therapy. Neurol Clin 16:851–868, 1998.
104. Watson CP: The treatment of neuropathic pain: Antidepressants and opioids. Clin J Pain 16(2 suppl):S49–S55, 2000.
105. Waylonis GW: The physiological effects of ice massage. Arch Phys Med Rehabil 48:37, 1967.
106. Wheeler AH: The therapeutic uses of botulinum toxin. Am Fam Physician 55:541–545, 1997.
107. Wheeler AH: Botulinum toxin-A, adjunctive therapy for refractory headaches associated with pericranial muscle tension. Headache 38:468–471, 1998.
108. Wheeler AH: Therapeutic injections for pain management. In: Mendozabal J, Talavera F, Halsey JH, Benbadis SR, Lorenzo NY (eds): Neurology section of EMedicine [textbook online]. Updated 02/03/2000.
109a. Wheeler AH: Botulinum toxin injection technique for treatment of headaches. Aesthetic Surg J 22:65–68, 2002.
109b. Wheeler AH: Botulinum toxin A for the treatment of neuropathic pain. AJPM 14(4):151–156, 2004.
110. Wheeler AH: Myofascial pain disorders. Drugs 64(1): 45–62, 2004.
111. Wheeler AH, Aaron GW: Muscle pain due to injury. Curr Pain Headache Rep 5:441–446, 2001.
112. Wheeler AH, Goolkasian P: Open label assessment of botulinum toxin A for pain treatment in a private outpatient setting. J Musculoskel Pain 9:67–82, 2001.
113. Wheeler AH, Goolkasian P, Gretz SS: A randomized double-blind prospective pilot study of botulinum toxin injection for refractory, unilateral, cervicothoracic paraspinal, myofascial pain syndrome. Spine 23:1662–1667, 1998.
114. Wheeler AH, Goolkasian P, Gretz SS: Botulinum toxin A for the treatment of chronic neck pain. Pain 94:255–260, 2001.
115. Wheeler AH, Hanley EN: Nonoperative treatment of low back pain: Rest to restoration. Spine 20:375–378, 1995.
116. Wheeler AH, Murrey DB: Chronic lumbar spine and radicular pain: Pathophysiology and treatment. Curr Pain Headache Rep 6:97–105, 2002.
117. Wiesendanger M, Coboz M, Palmeri A, et al: Noradrenergic mechanisms involved in muscle relaxation: Significance for the treatment of spasticity. Schweiz Acta Neurol Psychiatry 142:132–134, 1991.
118. Wiggins ME, Fadale PD, Barrach H, Ehrlich MG, Walsh WR: Healing characteristics of a type I collagenous structure treated with corticosteroids. Am J Sports Med 22:279–288, 1994.
119. Wolfe F, Smythe HA, Yunus MB, et al: The American College of Rheumatology 1990 Criteria for the Classification of Fibromyalgia. Arthritis Rheum 33:160–172, 1990.
120. Yue SK: Initial experience in the use of botulinum toxin A for the treatment of myofascial related muscle dysfunction. J Musculoskel Pain 3(suppl 1):22, 1995.
121. Zimmerman M: Peripheral and central nervous system mechanisms of nociception, pain and pain therapy: Facts and hypotheses. In: Bonica JJ, Liebskind JC, Albe-Fessard DG (eds): Advances in Pain Research and Therapy, vol 3. New York, Raven Press, 1979, pp 3–32.
122. Zwart JA, Bovim G, Sand T, et al: Tension headache: Botulinum toxin paralysis of temporal muscles. Headache 34:458–462, 1994.

Chapter 24

Chronic Regional Pain Syndrome I/II

ROBERT J. SCHWARTZMAN
AND YAKOV VOROBEYCHIK

Complex Regional Pain Syndrome I/II

Intensive study of the complex regional pain syndrome I/II (CRPSI/II) over the past 10 years has demonstrated new clinical features in each of the main domains of the syndrome. These remain (1) pain, (2) autonomic dysregulation, (3) swelling, (4) movement disorders, and (5) atrophy and dystrophy.[37,88] It is clear that there are subcategories of patients that reflect different aspects and different degrees of dysfunction in some or all of these parameters.[11] Complete consensus and validation of the diagnostic criteria has not been achieved.[32] New diagnostic criteria are expected shortly.[18a]

It is clear that the process may be sympathetically maintained (usually early in the course), sympathetically independent, or never have many sympathetic signs or symptoms.[75] It frequently spreads contralaterally and may generalize to affect the entire body.[58] It may be dissociated in that a patient may have pain, autonomic and motor dysfunction, or any combination of signs ipsilaterally and only the movement disorder or autonomic dysregulation contralaterally.[87] The process clearly affects both the peripheral (PNS) and central nervous systems (CNS).[41] This has been demonstrated by changes in magnetic resonance imaging (MRI) magnetoencephalography, and quantitative sensory testing in both the CNS and PNS.[25,44] A sustaining nociceptive barrage appears to be necessary to maintain the abnormal state of central pain-projecting neurons.[37] Deep somatic and articular pain is frequently prominent. Some genetic evidence for susceptibility to the illness has been presented.[55,56] Patients are depressed due to their severe pain. They do not differ from other patients with chronic pain, and there is no psychological profile for these patients.[18]

Central sensitization is the most likely physiological phenomenon that underlies the clinical spectrum of pain phenomena seen in CRPSI/II.[85] This process induces (1) hypersensitivity at the site of injury (transformational changes in nociceptor transducer proteins and changes in their membrane excitability so that they fire more readily in response to mechanical, thermal, or chemical stimuli); (2) mechanical and thermal allodynia (an innocuous mechanical or thermal stimulus causes pain); (3) hyperalgesia (increased pain from a noxious stimulus); (4) hyperpathia (an increased pain threshold that, once exceeded, induces severe pain that reaches maximum intensity too rapidly and is not stimulus bound); and

(5) extraterritoriality (pain in a regional rather than a root or nerve distribution).[71,72]

Central sensitization is initiated by intense firing of unmyelinated C fibers and thinly myelinated A-delta fibers (50 to 200 Hz) that project to Rexed layers I, II, and V of the dorsal horn. The central pain-projecting neurons demonstrate slow excitatory postsynaptic potentials (EPSP) that may last for 20 seconds rather than the usual fast pain potentials that are in the millisecond range.[96] Further repetitive afferent nociceptor barrages cause temporal summation of these slow potentials, which releases the Mg^{2+} block of the *N*-methyl-D-aspartate (NMDA) receptor that, in turn, induces the *windup* phenomenon such that further C fiber and A-delta fiber afferent input causes repetitive firing of these central pain-projecting neurons (CPPN), which amplifies the pain response.[106] The gain of this neuronal response is controlled by an activity-dependent NMDA receptor.[22,66] Patients with CRPSI and II may also have decreased sensation in an area of injury.[79] At times, one part of an extremity demonstrates mechanical and thermal allodynia, hyperalgesia, and components of hyperpathia, while a more distal or proximal segment has increased thresholds to all sensory modalities. These phenomena are similar to long-term potentiation (LTP) and long-term depression (LTD), which have been extensively studied in regard to memory mechanisms.[89]

AMPA (α-amino-3-hydroxy-5-methyl-4-isoxaleproprionic acid) glutamate receptors mediate fast pain (that normally experienced following injury) and the rapid EPSC that occurs in pain neurons. Recent evidence suggests that the plasticity of synaptic transmission is due to the activity and number of AMPA receptors at the postsynaptic locus.[89] The induction of LTP or LTD, as studied in the hippocampus, is dependent on calcium influx through the NMDA receptor. These same mechanisms apply to dorsal horn (DH) CPPNs. The NMDA receptor is pivotal in the physiology that aggregates or disperses AMPA receptors at the postsynaptic membrane. The greater the number of AMPA receptors at postsynaptic sites, the greater the synaptic efficacy of transmission of EPSP. If the AMPA receptors are dispersed postsynaptically, LTD will be the consequence, with decreased synaptic firing (no pain).[89] The postsynaptic density (PSD) is a dynamic structure that anchors NMDA receptors in the postsynaptic membrane but also mediates many components of postsynaptic signaling. The PSD is dynamic in its interactions with its associated proteins, as well as in trafficing and stabilizing NMDA receptors.[16,89] Calcium influx through activated NMDA receptors (following removal of the Mg^{2+} block of its calcium channel) initiates several intracellular enzymatic cascades that change the excitability of the neuron. Calcium-calmodulin-dependent protein kinase II (Ca MKII) is consistently activated during this process and is critical for NMDA-dependent LTP.[13] It binds to the cytoplasmic domain of the NMDA receptor subunit NR2B, which locks it into an activated state that cannot be reversed by phosphatases. It binds AMPA receptors to the synapse by increasing their anchoring sites. The calcium influx through the NMDA channel activates several other important signaling cascades, two of which are the Ras-mitogen activated protein kinase (MAPK) and inositide 3-kinase pathways. These are complicated cascades with regulatory and enhancing proteins that are located in the PSD. Activation of these cascades is essential for learning as well as NMDA receptor-dependent LTP. The regulation of various transcription factors such as cyclic adenosine 5' monophosphate (cAMP) response element binding protein (CREB) by the RAS-MAPK cascade is important for gene expression.[43] As noted earlier, a sustained nociceptive barrage induces immediate early response genes to produce C-fos and C-Jun that have been shown to induce the synthesis of the pro stimulatory neuropeptide dynorphin in central pain-projecting neurons (CPPNs).[16,46] Activation of gene expression by persistent pathological pain induces the transcription of new sodium channels that are inserted into the damaged peripheral nerve twigs that change their firing characteristics.[9,20,53] Small guanosine triphosphatases (GTPases) (Rac, Rap) as well as nonreceptor tyrosine kinases are all fixed in the NMDA-PSD complex and contribute to the synaptic plasticity of the CPPN.

Phosphatases of the NMDA complex (PP2B and PP1) are thought to cause synaptic depression, possibly by inducing internalization of AMPA receptors of CPPNs that would decrease their firing.[16] AMPA receptor regulation is critical for synaptic efficacy. Direct Ca MKII phosphorylation of the glutamate 1 receptor (GluR1), increases single-channel conductance.[13] As noted earlier, synaptic delivery of GluR1-containing AMPA receptors to the synapse is induced by Ca MKII and activation of the NMDA receptor, both of which are critical for LTP. Delivery of AMPA receptors to the neuronal surface is also a mechanism of increasing synaptic efficacy and LTP. The opposite effect, internalization of AMPA receptors or their disposal from synaptic sites, is a mechanism of LTD.[91]

In summary, present evidence points to the critical contribution of the NMDA receptor on CPPNs of Rexed layers I, II and V of the DH for the inductance and maintenance of central sensitization. A maintained primarily C-fiber nociceptive barrage lifts the magnesium blockade of the calcium pore of the NMDA receptor because of cumulative depolarization by summated slow synaptic potentials. Enhanced NMDA gating causes increased intracellular calcium influx. The changes induced in the NMDA receptor that allow this influx are caused by (1) G protein–coupled neurokinin receptors (NK_1) and receptor tyrosine kinases, (2) phosphokinases, and (3) presynaptic NMDA receptors. This plasticity is maintained by a persistent nociceptive barrage from the periphery, calcium-dependent second messenger system cascades, and decreased DH inhibition.[67] It may also be enhanced by activation of A-delta primary afferent fibers that synapse on inhibitory L-aminobutyric acid (GABA)/glycinuric interneurons of the DH and initiate LTD of this inhibitory circuitry.[52]

There is an active dynamic interplay from the periphery to the DH and CNS structures that alters structural and activity characteristics of the CPPN.[105] At the site of peripheral nerve injury there is local increased production of growth factors from fibroblasts, macrophages, and lymphocytes that are retrogradely transported back to the dorsal root ganglion (DRG) and substantia gelatinosa.[17] These alter G protein–coupled receptors, transmitters, and synaptic modulators. In experimental pain models, following injury to peripheral nerves or their terminal twigs, there is a proliferation of DRG satellite cells and a change in their gene expression that is manifested by up-regulation of the p75 receptor, which may guide sympathetic fibers from blood vessels within the ganglion to specific cells. The neuroactive cytokine leukemia inhibitory factor (LIF) is induced at the site of injury and is retrogradely transported to the DRG, where it induces sympathetic sprouting. These sympathetic fibers form basket complexes around large-diameter touch neurons and may be associated with the mechanoallodynia seen in sympathetically maintained pain states.[41] Peripheral nerve injury also up-regulates constitutively expressed genes and induces novel genes that change the physiological characteristics of DRG nociceptive neurons.[59a] Ectopic firing of DRG nociceptive neurons is posited to cause spontaneous pain and occurs near the DRG. Induction and coexpression of abnormal combinations of several types of sodium channels may allow subthreshold membrane potential oscillations to initiate ectopic nerve firing at the DRG level and not at the peripheral site of injury.[102] Continued discharge of a damaged nerve can alter transcription in sensory neurons that changes their neurophysiological characteristics. The expression of novel genes is seen in the phenotypic switch of Aβ fibers, which begin to express substance P and brain derived neurotropic factor (BDNF) after sustained discharge. This may contribute to the ability of these low-threshold mechanoreceptors to induce central sensitization.[106]

There is some evidence that peripheral nerve injury with increased and continuous nociceptive barrage may induce loss of DH inhibitory neurons.[54,93] Recent evidence does not support the hypothesis that Aβ afferents gain the vacated terminals of C fibers in the DH.[35]

Central sensitization with both LTP and LTD is a dynamic and plastic process. Recent evidence suggests that the NR2B subunit of the NMDA receptor is particularly important for pain perception.[50a] Development of NR2B-selective compounds with tolerable side effect profiles and good efficacy may be an effective management strategy for neuropathic pain.[15] There is considerable evidence that ketamine, a noncompetitive antagonist of the NMDA receptor or Ca^{2+} channel pore, is effective in treating neuropathic pain. At clinically significant serum concentrations, ketamine blocks the phencyclidine (PcP) binding site that inhibits NMDA receptor activity only when the channel has been opened, which occurs in chronic pain states. Ketamine has been used successfully in anesthetic doses with intractable generalized CRPSI/II patients.[2,7,34,45]

Central Autonomic Dysregulation in Complex Regional Pain Syndrome I/II

Almost all patients with CRPSI/II have symptoms and signs that reflect central autonomic dysregulation. A warm, vasodilated limb is often seen in the initial stages of the disorder. Loss of cutaneous vasoconstrictor activity at the spinal level that leads to disturbances in skin microvasculature has been demonstrated in patients with warm limbs.[100] Resting sweat output, as well as thermoregulatory and axon reflex sweating, are increased in patients with CRPSI.[8,40] These actions have to be central in origin, as sweat glands do not develop denervation supersensitivity.[24] Studies of central sympathetic reflexes, as expressed by sympathetic vasoconstrictor extremity activity, have been performed using whole body warming and cooling and manipulation of respiratory reflexes. In early CRPSI/II (<6 months), central cooling and inspiratory reflexes do not activate spinal vasoconstrictor sympathetic neurons.[100] Norepinephrine concentrations in the venous effluent draining the affected arm are low.[23] An intermediate pattern was noted in which temperature and perfusion varied, depending on spinal cord sympathetic neuronal activity. In chronic pain patients with cold extremities, temperature, perfusion, and norepinephrine levels are low on the affected side.[101] In patients with acute CRPS (<20 months), the central vasomotor reflex abnormalities are fully reversible with successful treatment. Chronic CRPSI patients have cold, vasoconstricted skin possibly secondary to abnormalities of neurovascular transmission in vascular smooth muscle due to sustained decreased activity of spinal vasoconstrictor neurons.[28] There is an increased density of α-adrenoreceptors in the skin of CRPSII patients that may respond to circulating adrenal norepinephrine.[23] The location and nuclei involved in these central autonomic circuits are unknown. Animal experimental nerve lesions have demonstrated long-lasting changes in baroreceptor, chemoreceptor, and nociceptive reflexes after nerve injury but not in muscle vasoconstrictor neurons.[37,39] In animal models, cutaneous vasoconstrictor neurons demonstrate reflex activity identical to that of muscle vasoconstrictor neurons.

In many patients, sympathetic abnormalities are noted bilaterally and in apparently unaffected extremities even early in the illness.[87] Particularly important may be the early loss of the usual rhythmic variation in microcirculatory flow that suggests an abnormality of the spinal component of skin blood flow that is coordinated supraspinally (nucleus magnus raphe).[49] In patients undergoing deep ketamine anesthesia for intractable generalized CRPSI, rhythmic variations in microcirculatory flow returns during the third day.[68]

Edema and Inflammation

At some point during the progression of CRPSI/II, patients suffer edema of the affected area.[88] It may be extreme and often spreads proximally. It may acquire a reddened, brawny character. It is generally thought to represent neurogenic edema and often responds to sympathetic blockade. Sympathetic vasoconstrictor neurons innervate precapillary blood vessels (arterioles) and postcapillary veins. Venous plethysmography has demonstrated increased capillary hydrostatic pressure on the affected side of CRPS patients. The venous side of this network has a minimal sympathetic innervation to maintain intense vasoconstriction.[83] Recent evidence has demonstrated that substance P (SP) released from C fibers may cause leakage of plasma through the endothelium of arterioles, and the calcitonin gene-related peptide (CGRP) also released from C fibers paralyzes smooth muscle.[4,46] A sympathetic drive of these C afferents in the area of injury that releases these neuropeptides could directly affect the microcirculation, as well as stimulate macrophages to release inflammatory cytokines. Interleukin-6 (IL-6) and tumor necrosis factor alpha (TNF-α) have been demonstrated in the blister fluid of affected areas in CRPS patients.[36] These inflammatory cytokines directly depolarize C fibers.

There is solid evidence for an inflammatory process that occurs in the skin, deep somatic tissues, and bone in the affected areas of CRPSI patients. Radiolabeled immunoglobulins extravasate, with accompanying hypervascularity and neutrophil infiltration in affected areas.[65] Triple phase bone scintigraphy reveals periarticular uptake and pooling in late stages in approximately 30% of patients.[51] Microdialysis studies of the skin in affected areas support the concept of peptide-induced neuroinflammation and anoxia in affected areas.[103] Animal evidence has demonstrated oxygen-derived free radical increases in vascular permeability pain and soft tissue damage that is proposed as a mechanism in the early stages of CRPS.[29] A sympathetic blockade, ketamine, and lidocaine infusions diminish edema and aspects of this inflammatory response.

The role of the immune system in chronic pain is being actively explored and is giving insights into the interaction of the immune and pain components of both the peripheral and central nervous system.[1a,50b,59b]

Movement Disorder of Complex Regional Pain Syndrome I/II

The movement disorder of CRPS is seen in virtually all patients with this disorder and is often noted in the contralateral extremity that is not painful. It consists of six major components: (1) difficulty in initiating movements, (2) weakness, (3) dystonia, (4) decrease in joint mobility, (5) tremor, and (6) increased reflexes and spasms.[86,98] Patients frequently fall due to failure to sustain movement once initiated. The dystonia is frequently noted in the fourth and fifth fingers initially in the upper extremity. A plantar-flexed inverted foot is characteristic in the lower extremity. In some patients, the disorder may generalize to total body dystonia. Spasms and myoclonus are frequently severe problems.

Dystonia may be secondary to failure of GABAergic inhibitory mechanisms at the spinal level.[98] Alternatively, it may represent enhancement of nociceptor flexor withdrawal reflexes and decreased presynaptic inhibition.[57] The tremor is caused by an enhancement of the normal physiological tremor.[19] A neglect-like syndrome has been noted in the affected extremity.[26] Kinematic analysis of target reaching and grip force suggests dysfunction of sensorimotor integration in the parietal cortex.[82] These deficits were noted bilaterally. They have been partially corrected by use of a mirror to reflect the input from the moving unaffected limb that reestablishes normal sensory feedback and movement.[61]

Atrophy and Dystrophy in Complex Regional Pain Syndrome I/II

Early in the course of CRPS there is increased growth curliness and thickness of the hair on the affected side. The nails become thickened, ridged, and split. In the later stages of the illness, patients lose hair, the underlying muscle atrophies, and the integument vessel thickens and fibroses. Patients frequently lose their teeth from bone resorption of the jaw. Early cataracts occur. There have been no major studies that have elucidated mechanisms for the dystrophy and atrophy of CRPS, but lack of nutritive blood flow to affected areas may cause diffuse atrophy, and the inflammatory changes noted above are a likely mechanism.[68]

Treatment

Recent studies have shown reorganization and relocation of specific sodium channel subtypes following nerve injury. Type III tetrodotoxin (TTX)-S-(sensitive) sodium channels are expressed de novo by DRG cells. Sensory nerve–specific SNS/PN3 channels relocate from DRG to the nerve injury site, while sensory neuron specific sodium channel 2 (SNS2/NaN) and SNS/PN3 channels are down-regulated in the DRG. The normally silent type III (TTX)-S Na^{2+} channels play a role in ectopic firing of nociceptive afferent fibers that is pivotal for eliciting spontaneous pain.[9,53,80,102] The limited effectiveness of phenytoin, carbamazepine, lamotrigine, topiramate, and felbamate rests on their action as nonselective Na^+ channel blocking agents. Topiramate also blocks excitatory glutamate activity via AMPA and kainate receptors, and lamotrigine suppresses glutamate release from presynaptic neurons. Lidocaine and its analogues (mexiletine and tocainide) similarly block activity-dependent sodium channels. These agents, with the exception of lidocaine, have been minimally effective in treating CRPSI/II.[3,22,42]

Lidocaine infusion over 5 days to a dose of 3–5 mg/ml is effective in treating deafferentation and central pain. It also is effective in some patients with generalized CRPSI/II. It is a more selective Na^+ channel blocker. There is evidence that TTX-S channels are four times more sensitive to lidocaine than TTX-R (resistant) channels in DRG neurons, which correlates with decreased ectopic neuronal firing and mechanoallodynia. At therapeutic levels that suppress ectopic nerve afferent discharges, it does not block nerve conduction.[21] It has been recently demonstrated that IV lidocaine significantly decreases mechanical and thermal allodynia in CRPSI/II patients.[99] The usual side effects are lightheadedness, nausea, and somnolence. Bradycardia and seizures may occur if higher doses are utilized. If effective, mexiletine (150 mg BID) may maintain benefits for 3–6 months.

Calcium Channel Blockers

In animal models of nociceptive pain, the spinal N-type voltage-dependent calcium channel (VDCC) appears to be the predominant isoform involved in pre- and postsynaptic processing of nociceptor information. These channels are concentrated in laminae I and II of the DH at the site of nociceptive primary afferent synaptic terminals. Their activation causes Ca^{2+} influx and neurotransmitter release.[22] Messenger RNA and protein for the alpha$_2$delta subunit of VDDC are up-regulated in the DRG and spinal cord of rats with L4/L5 root ligation. Specific antagonists of N-type VDCC attenuate heat hyperalgesia, mechanical allodynia, and hyperalgesia in experimental studies.[104] Gabapentin may affect this channel by its ability to bind the alpha$_2$delta subunit of VDCC. Gabapentin has been shown to be partially effective in CRPSI/II patients at doses of 900–2400 mg/day.[63] Another novel N-type VDCC blocker, ziconotide, inhibits substance P release and is antinociceptive in experimental pain models. It was spectacularly effective when given intrathecally to a patient with intractable CRPS and phantom limb pain secondary to brachial plexus avulsion.[10] Its congener, cilnidipine, suppresses the sympathetic nerve stimulation–induced pressor response in rats.[95] The antisympathetic activity of this drug may prove to be of particular importance in the treatment of CRPSI/II due to the significant role of sympathetically augmented discharge of sensitized nociceptive afferents.

γ-Aminobutyric Acid Agonists

γ-Aminobutyric acid (GABA) is a major inhibitory transmitter that is found in nearly all layers of the spinal cord. Its receptors mediate depolarization of primary inhibitory interneurons that affect presynaptic inhibition of CPPN. The GABA antagonist bicuculline is associated with a dose-dependent allodynia in experimental pain models. Midazolam enhances GABAergic function and suppresses evoked responses after nerve injury.[47] It is posited that part of the mechanism of action of topiramate, gabapentin, valproate, and felbamate in blocking nociception is enhancement of GABAergic inhibition.

Activation of GABA B presynaptic receptors leads to a reduction of excitatory neurotransmitter release from primary nociceptive afferents that results in the inhibition of primary afferents to motor neurons.[57] In a double-blind, randomized, placebo-controlled crossover trial, van Hilten and colleagues demonstrated significant effects of intrathecal boluses of 50 and 75 μg of the GABA agonist baclofen on both dystonia and pain in six of seven CRPSI/II patients.[98]

Antidepressants and a_2-Adrenergic Agonists

Descending pathways from noradrenergic and serotonergic nuclei that include the dorsal raphe nuclei, the periaqueductal gray matter, and the locus ceruleus form part of the diffuse descending nociceptive inhibitory complex (DNIC) that modulates pain transmission in the DH. The effects of these descending systems are mediated in part by norepinephrine, which modulates inhibitory adrenoreceptors that are concentrated in the substantia gelatinosa and the superficial laminae of the DH.[64] Antidepressants act by inhibiting serotonin and or noradrenalin reuptake, which causes enhancement of descending monoaminergic inhibitory pathways.[60] Both a_2-adrenoreceptor and 5-hydroxytryptamine (5-HT) receptor antagonists inhibit antinociception by antidepressants.[30] Adenosine and opioid systems are implicated in mechanisms of analgesia following the systemic administration of some antidepressants.[81] Selective serotonin reuptake inhibitors are generally less effective than nonselective inhibitors, which suggests that increasing synaptic levels of both serotonin and noradrenalin are necessary for antinociception.[1b]

The α_2-adrenoreceptor plays an important role in pain modulation. Potent antinociceptive effects of spinally applied α_2-adrenoreceptor agonists have been demonstrated both behaviorally and electrophysiologically.[64] Clonidine is the most common α_2-receptor agonist currently available for clinical use. Due to the high density of α_2 receptors at the spinal cord level, epidural or intrathecal administration of clonidine is most effective.[77] Intrathecal clonidine has given significant pain relief in some patients. Sedation and hypotension limit its use as an analgesic. There are ongoing attempts to develop drugs with greater affinity for the α_{2a} (α subunit) that are more selective for pain modulation. Dexmedomidine, which has an α_{2a}: α_1 selectivity ratio of 1300:1, has been shown to be effective in neuropathic pain models as well as in initial human trials.[69]

Opioids

The doses of opioids necessary to obtain analgesic effects in chronic neuropathic pain are twice as high as those required in acute nociceptive pain.[5] In chronic neuropathic pain states, μ-opioid receptors are down-regulated in the DRG, while cholecystokinin RNA (cholecystokinin is an opioid antagonist) is up-regulated in both the DRG and the ventral medullary nucleus of the descending inhibitory system.[107] In the spinal cord, opioid receptors are localized on the presynaptic terminals of primary afferents in the DH. Degeneration of primary afferent neurons is observed in animal models of neuropathic pain, which suggests a mechanism for the observed decrease in μ-opioid receptor binding. Neuropathic pain and that of CRPSI/II does respond to dose escalations significantly higher than those needed in nociceptive pain states.[70] Intrathecal administration of morphine in the spinal nerve ligation model of neuropathic pain produces greater inhibition of noxious stimuli than systemically administered morphine, with fewer side effects than those produced by an equivalent peripherally administered dose.[94]

N-*Methyl*-D-*Aspartate Receptor Blockers*

In recent years, it has been shown that the activation of NMDA receptor is pivotal in the maintenance of central sensitization that underlies the pain and many of the clinical features of CRPSI/II.[85] Diverse NMDA blockers including MK801, AP-5, ketamine, memantine, and dextromethorphan prevent or reduce features of neuropathic pain in experimental models.[92] Recently, ketamine, a noncompetitive NMDA antagonist with moderate affinity (the most potent available for clinical use), has been shown to be tolerated by patients, with minimal side effects, and is effective in the treatment of various neuropathic pain states.[73] Kiefer and colleagues used IV ketamine at anesthetic doses (up to 7 mg/kg/hr for 5 days) in 10 patients who had failed all known treatments for CRPSI/II. All patients had initial compete pain relief.[45] They all remained pain free for 4–6 weeks and one for 3 years. Five of the 10 patients have had sustained pain relief for over 2 years. Mechanical and thermal allodynia as well as deep muscle hyperalgesia appear most responsive to treatment. Midazolam at a dose of 0.15–0.25 mg/kg/hr was administered concomitantly with ketamine to minimize psychiatric side effects. Two patients had episodes of anxiety for 2 months that were controlled with Ativan. No patient sustained serious side effects. Extensive neuropsychological testing revealed no deterioration in any sphere of cognitive function. An increase in skin blood flow in previously underperfused areas was demonstrated, which correlated with the resumption of normal sympathetic tone.[68] Harbut and Correll reported a 6-day constant infusion of subanesthetic doses of ketamine (30 mg/hr) to treat a patient with a 9-year history of CRPSI/II. No side effects were reported, and the patient remained pain-free for 7 months after the treatment.[31]

Preservation of the efficacy of high-affinity NMDA antagonists, while limiting side effects, may be possible with the synthesis of subtype receptor-selective drugs. Immunocytochemical studies have shown that the NR2B subunit of NMDA receptors has a restricted distribution with moderate labeling in the nociceptive terminal zone of the superficial DH. In animal studies, the NR2B-selective antagonists demonstrate significant antinociceptive effects with a greatly improved side effect profile compared with nonselective drugs of this class.[12]

Sympathetic Blockade

The sympathetic nervous system plays a very important role in pain pathogenesis in some CRPSI/II patients in early stages of the illness.[84] Experimental pain models show that abnormal connectivities develop between the sympathetic and sensory nervous systems following nerve injury. These may include (1) direct chemical coupling of neuronal terminals within peripheral effector sites; (2) ephaptic nerve coupling at the site of injury; (3) indirect coupling via peripheral sensitizing mechanisms involving the release of inflammatory mediators from sympathetic terminals that discharge primary pain afferents; and (4) direct coupling between the sympathetic and sensory nervous systems in the DRG.[9] McLachlan and colleagues described sprouting of noradrenergic perivascular sympathetic axons into the DRG after ligation of the sciatic nerve. These sympathetic fibers encase large sensory afferent neurons in a basket like arrangement.[62]

In a recent review article, Cepeda and colleagues summarized the effect of local anesthetic sympathetic blockade in CRPS, pooling the data from 29 studies that evaluated 1144 patients.[14] Twenty-nine percent of the patients were reported to have a full response, 41% had partial relief of pain, and 32% had no or a minimal response to sympathetic blockade. Reiestad and colleagues observed significant pain relief in upper extremity CRPSI/II patients after five daily injections of 0.5% bupivacaine through a catheter into the interpleural space. Three out of seven patients were pain-free for 4–10 months, and three patients had only minimal pain requiring no medication.[78] The authors explained that by proper positioning of the patient, the local anesthetic injected into the pleural space diffuses through the medial surface of the parietal pleura and blocks the cervical portion of the sympathetic chain and the stellate ganglion. Major but uncommon complications of intrapleural blocks are pneumothorax and infection. Continuous epidural analgesia with 0.1% bupivacaine is accompanied by significant sympathetic blockade and may be useful in lower extremity CRPSI/II treatment.[74]

Other Systemic Treatment

There are several case reports and clinical trials of successful treatment of CRPSI/II with different drugs. A 43-year-old woman with severe CRPSI/II pain was apparently cured after 1 month of thalidomide treatment at a dose of 400 mg/day. The authors hypothesized that the effect of the medication was related to its effect on efferent sympathetic nerves coupled with its anti-inflammatory properties.[76]

In a placebo-controlled study of 66 patients with CRPSI/II, Gobelet et al. reported significant improvement in pain, mobility, and ability to work with three daily doses (100 U/day) of intranasal calcitonin.[27] Unfortunately, the opposite results were demonstrated in a prospective, randomized, double-blind study where 400 IU of nasal calcitonin had no effect on CRPSI/II pain.[6]

Based on the evidence that adenosine receptors play an important inhibitory role in the development and maintenance of central sensitization of spinal DH neurons, Sollevi and colleagues infused 50–70 μg/kg/min of adenosine IV in two patients with peripheral neuropathic pain. In one patient, spontaneous pain, allodynia, and hyperalgesia were attenuated during the infusion, and the reported effects lasted for hours after termination of the infusion.[90] Studies demonstrating the analgesic effect of adenosine on CRPSI/II have not been done.

Zuurmond and colleagues studied the effect of 50% dimethylsulfoxide cream on 32 CRPSI/II patients in a placebo-controlled, double-blind study.[108] The results suggest partial antinociception of this agent in patients suffering from CRPSI/II. Unfortunately, the blinding procedure was not flawless, as the side effects differ distinctively between placebo and the actual treatment.

There are several reports that bisphosphonates (pamidronate, alendronate, and clodronate) may mitigate pain and lead to functional improvement in CRPSI/II patients.[48] Among the possible mechanisms of action are inhibition of release of substance P and CGRP from primary nociceptive afferents, decreased prostaglandin E2 production, and amelioration of bone resorption.

The central nicotinic cholinergic receptor agonist epibatidine has significant antinociceptive effect in rats, but its nicotinic side effect profile precludes its clinical use. Its synthetic congener, ABT-594, though less potent, is better tolerated and might emerge as a prospective medication for CRPSI/II pain.[97]

Conclusion

A great deal is now known about the mechanisms that underlie CRPSI/II. It is clearly a disease of both the PNS and, more importantly, the CNS. It appears to be reversible even in late stages. The influx of excessive calcium through the NMDA receptor initiates destructive cascades that alter the membrane characteristics of CPPNs, which is the basis of central sensitization.

Enough experimental and clinical evidence has been accrued to allow a mechanism-based approach to treatment that appears promising.

REFERENCES

1a. Alexander GM, van Rijn MA, van Hilten JJ, Perreault MJ, Schwartzman RJ: Changes in cerebrospinal fluid levels of pro-inflammatory cytokines in CRPS. Pain 116(3): 213–219, 2005.

1b. Ansari A: The efficacy of newer antidepressants in the treatment of chronic pain: A review of current literature. Harv Rev Psychiatry 7:257–277, 2000.

2. Arendt-Nielsen L, Petersen-Felix S, Fischer M, Bak P, Bjerring P, Zbinden AM: The effect of *N*-methyl-D-aspartate antagonist (ketamine) on single and repeated nociceptive stimuli: A placebo-controlled experimental human study. Anesth Analg 81(1):63–68, 1995.
3. Attal N: Pharmacologic treatment of neuropathic pain. Acta Neurol Belg 101:53–64, 2001.
4. Baluk P: Neurogenic inflammation in skin and airways. J Invest Dermatol Symp Proc 2:76–81, 1997.
5. Benedetti F, Vighetti S, Amanzio M, Casadio C, Oliaro A, Bergamasco B, Maggi G: Dose-response relationship of opioids in nociceptive and neuropathic postoperative pain. Pain 74:205–211, 1998.
6. Bickerstaff DR, Konis JA: The use of nasal calcitonin in the treatment of post traumatic algodystrophy. Br J Rheumtol 31:567–569, 1992.
7. Bion JF: Intrathecal ketamine for war surgery. A preliminary study under field conditions. Anaesthesia 9:1023–1028, 1984.
8. Birklein F, Sittl R, Spitzer A, Claus D, Neundorfer B, Handwerker HO: Sudomotor function in sympathetic reflex dystrophy. Pain 69:49–54, 1997.
9. Bridges D, Thompson SW, Rice AS: Mechanisms of neuropathic pain. Br J Anaesth 87:12–26, 2001.
10. Brose WG, Gutlove DP, Luther RR, Bowersox SS, McGuire D: Use of intrathecal SNX-111, a novel N-type, voltage-sensitive, calcium channel blocker, in the management of intractable brachial plexus avulsion pain. Clin J Pain 13:256–259, 1997.
11. Bruehl S, Harden RN, Galer BS, Saltz S, Backonja M, Stanton-Hicks M: Complex regional pain syndrome: Are there distinct subtypes and sequential stages of the syndrome? Pain 95:119–124, 2002.
12. Carpenter KJ, Dickenson AH: Amino acids are still as exciting as ever. Curr Opin Pharmacol 1:57–61, 2001.
13. Carroll RC, Zukin RS: NMDA-receptor trafficking and targeting: Implications for synaptic transmission and plasticity. Trends Neurosci 25(11):571–577, 2002.
14. Cepeda MS, Lau J, Carr DB: Defining the therapeutic role of local anesthetic sympathetic blockade in complex regional pain syndrome: A narrative and systematic review. Clin J Pain 18:216–233, 2002.
15. Chizh BA, Headley PM, Tzschentke TM: NMDA receptor antagonists as analgesics: Focus on the NR2B subtype. Trends Pharmacol Sci 22:636–642, 2001.
16. Choquet D, Triller A: The role of receptor diffusion in the organization of the postsynaptic membrane. Nat Rev Neurosci 4:251–265, 2003.
17. Chung K, Lee BH, Yoon YW, Chung JM: Sympathetic sprouting in the dorsal root ganglia of the injured peripheral nerve in a rat neuropathic pain model. J Comp Neurol 9(376):241–252, 1996.
18. Ciccone DS, Bandilla EB, Wu W: Psychological dysfunction in patients with reflex sympathetic dystrophy. Pain. 71:323–333, 1997.
18a. CRPS: Current diagnosis and therapy. In: Wilson PP, Stanton-Hicks M, Harden RN (eds): Progress in Pain Research and Management. Volume 32. Seattle, International Association for the Study of Pain Press, 2005.
19. Deuschl G, Blumberg H, Lucking CH: Tremor in reflex sympathetic dystrophy. Arch Neurol 48:1247–1252, 1991.
20. Devor M, Keller CH, Deerinck TJ, Levinson SR, Ellisman MH: Na^+ channel accumulation on axolemma of afferent endings in nerve end neuromas in *Apteronotus*. Neurosci Lett 31(102):149–154, 1989.
21. Devor M, Wall PD, Catalan N: Systemic lidocaine silences ectopic neuroma and DRG discharge without blocking nerve conduction. Pain 48:261–268, 1992.
22. Dickenson AH, Matthews EA, Suzuki R: Neurobiology of neuropathic pain: Mode of action of anticonvulsants. Eur J Pain 6(suppl A):51–60, 2002.
23. Drummond PD, Skipworth S, Finch PM: Alpha $_1$-adrenoceptors in normal and hyperalgesic human skin. Clin Sci (Lond) 91:73–77, 1996.
24. Fleming WW, Westfall DP: Adapative super sensitivity. In: Trendelen Surg U, Weiner N (eds): Handbook of Experimental Pharmacology, vol 90/I: Catecholamines. New York, Springer-Verlag, 1998; pp 509–559.
25. Fukumoto M, Ushida T, Zinchuk VS, Yamamoto H, Yoshida S: Contralateral thalamic perfusion in patients with reflex sympathetic dystrophy syndrome. Lancet 354:1790–1791, 1999.
26. Galer BS, Butler S, Jensen MP: Case reports and hypothesis: A neglect-like syndrome may be responsible for the motor disturbance in reflex sympathetic dystrophy (complex regional pain syndrome-1). J Pain Symptom Manage 10:385–391, 1995.
27. Gobelet C, Waldburger M, Meier JL: The effect of adding calcitonin to physical treatment on reflex sympathetic dystrophy. Pain 48:171–175, 1992.
28. Goldstein DS, Tack C, Li ST: Sympathetic innervation and function in reflex sympathetic dystrophy. Ann Neurol 48:49–59, 2000.
29. Goris RJ: Reflex sympathetic dystrophy: Model of a severe regional inflammatory response syndrome. World J Surg 22:197–202, 1998.
30. Gray AM, Pache DM, Sewell RD: Do alpha$_2$-adrenoceptors play an integral role in the antinociceptive mechanism of action of antidepressant compounds? Eur J Pharmacol. 378:161–168, 1999.
31. Harbut RE, Correll GE: Successful treatment of a nine-year case of complex regional pain syndrome type-I (reflex sympathetic dystrophy) with intravenous ketamine-infusion therapy in a warfarin-anticoagulated adult female patient. Pain Med 3:147–155, 2002.
32. Harden RN, Bruehl S, Galer BS, Saltz S, Bertram M, Backonja M, Gayles R, Rudin N, Bhugra MK, Stanton-Hicks M: Complex regional pain syndrome: Are the IASP diagnostic criteria valid and sufficiently comprehensive? Pain 83(2):211–219, 1999.
33. Harden RN, Duc TA, Williams TR, Coley D, Cate JC, Gracely RH: Norepinephrine and epinephrine levels in affected versus unaffected limbs in sympathetically maintained pain. Clin J Pain 10:324–330, 1994.
34. Hirota K, Lambert DG: Ketamine: Its mechanism(s) of

action and unusual clinical uses. Br J Anaesth 77(4):441–444, 1996.

35. Hughes DI, Scott DT, Todd AJ, Riddell JS: Lack of evidence for sprouting of Abeta afferents into the superficial laminas of the spinal cord dorsal horn after nerve section. J Neurosci 23(29):9491–9499, 2003.
36. Huygen FJ, De Bruijn AG, De Bruin MT, Groeneweg JG, Klein J, Zijistra FJ: Evidence for local inflammation in complex regional pain syndrome type 1. Mediators Inflamm 11:47–51, 2002.
37. Janig W, Baron R: Complex regional pain syndrome: Mystery explained? Lancet Neurol 2:687–697, 2003.
38. Janig W, Habler HJ: Neurophysiological analysis of target-related sympathetic pathways—from animal to human: Similarities and differences. Acta Physiol Scand 177:255–274, 2003.
39. Janig W, McLachlan EM: Characteristics of function-specific pathways in the sympathetic nervous system. Trends Neurosci 15:475–481, 1992.
40. Janig W, Levine JD, Michaelis M: Interactions of sympathetic and primary afferent neurons following nerve injury and tissue trauma. Prog Brain Res 113:161–184, 1996.
41. Janig W, McLachhan EM: Neurobiology of the autonomic nervous system. In: Mathias CJ, Bannister R (eds): Autonomic Failure, 4th ed. Oxford, Oxford University Press, pp 3–15, 1999.
42. Jensen TS: Anticonvulsants in neuropathic pain: Rationale and clinical evidence. Eur J Pain 6 (suppl A):61–68, 2002.
43. Ji RR, Baba H, Brenner GJ, Woolf CJ: Nociceptive-specific activation of ERK in spinal neurons contributes to pain hypersensitivity. Nat Neurosci 2:1114–1119, 1999.
44. Juottonen K, Gockel M, Silen T, Hurri H, Hari R, Forss N: Altered central sensorimotor processing in patients with complex regional pain syndrome. Pain 98:315–323, 2002.
45. Kiefer RT, Rohr P, Ploppa A, et al: Ketamine-midazolam anesthesia for intractable complex regional pain syndrome. Abstract ID:1210-P126. Tenth World Congress on Pain, San Diego, CA, August 17, 2002.
46. Kilo S, Harding-Rose C, Hargreaves KM, Flores CM: Peripheral CGRP release as a marker for neurogenic inflammation: A model system for the study of neuropeptide secretion in rat paw skin. Pain 73:201–207, 1997.
47. Kontinen VK, Dickenson AH: Effects of midazolam in the spinal nerve ligation model of neuropathic pain in rats. Pain 85:425–431, 2000.
48. Kubalek I, Fain O, Paries J, Kettaneh A, Thomas M: Treatment of reflex sympathetic dystrophy with pamidronate: 29 cases. Rheumatology (Oxford) 40:1394–1397, 2001.
49. Kurvers HA, Jacobs MJ, Beuk RJ, van den Wildenberg FA, Kitslaar PJ, Slaaf DW, Reneman RS: The spinal component to skin blood flow abnormalities in reflex sympathetic dystrophy. Arch Neurol 53:58–65, 1996.
50a. Laube B, Hirai H, Sturgess M, Betz H, Kuhse J: Molecular determinants of agonist discrimination by NMDA receptor subunits: Analysis of the glutamate binding site on the NR2B subunit. Neuron 18(3):493–503, 1997.
50b. Ledeboer A, Sloane EM, Milligan ED, Frank MG, Mahony JH, Maier SF, Watkins LR: Minocycline attenuates mechanical allodynia and proinflammaotyr cytokine expression in rate models of pain facilitation. Pain 115(1–2):71–83, 2005.
51. Leitha T, Korpan M, Staudenherz A, Wunderbaldinger P, Fialka V: Five phase bone scintigraphy supports the pathophysiological concept of a subclinical inflammatory process in reflex sympathetic dystrophy. Q J Nucl Med 40:188–193, 1996.
52. Lin Q, Peng Y, Willis WD: Glycine and GABAA antagonists reduce the inhibition of primate spinothalamic tract neurons produced by stimulation in periaqueductal gray. Brain Res 654:286–302, 1994.
53. Lyu YS, Park SK, Chung K, Chung JM: Low dose of tetrodotoxin reduces neuropathic pain behaviors in an animal model. Brain Res 14;871:98–103, 2001.
54. Ma QP, Woolf CJ: Progressive tactile hypersensitivity: An inflammation-induced incremental increase in the excitability of the spinal cord. Pain 67:97–106, 1996.
55. Mailis A, Wade J: Profile of Caucasian women with possible genetic predisposition to reflex sympathetic dystrophy: A pilot study. Clin J Pain 10:210–217, 1994.
56. Mailis A, Wade J: Genetic considerations in CRPS. In: Harden RN, Baron R, Janig W (eds): Complex Regional Pain Syndrome. Seattle, IASP Press, 2001, pp 227–238.
57. Malcangio M, Bowery NG: GABA and its receptors in the spinal cord. Trends Pharmacol Sci 17:457–462, 1996.
58. Maleki J, LeBel AA, Bennett GJ, Schwartzman RJ: Patterns of spread in complex regional pain syndrome, type I (reflex sympathetic dystrophy). Pain 1(88):259–266, 2000.
59a. Mannion RJ, Costigan M, Decosterd I, Amaya F, Ma QP, Holstege JC, Ji RR, Acheson A, Lindsay RM, Wilkinson GA, Woolf CJ: Neurotrophins: Peripherally and centrally acting modulators of tactile stimulus-induced inflammatory pain hypersensitivity. Proc Natl Acad Sci USA 3(96):9385–9390, 1999.
59b. Marchand F, Perretti M, McMahon SB: Role of the immune system in chronic pain. Nat Rev Neurosci 6(7): 521–532, 2005.
60. Max MB: Antidepressants as analgesics. In: Fields HL, Liebskind JC (eds): Progress in Pain Research and Therapy, vol I. Seattle, IASP Press, 1994, pp 229–246.
61. McCabe CS, Haigh RC, Ring EF, Halligan PW, Wall PD, Blake DR: A controlled pilot study of the utility of mirror visual feedback in the treatment of complex regional pain syndrome (type 1). Rheumatology (Oxford) 42:97–101, 2003.
62. McLachlan EM, Janig W, Devor M, Michaelis M: Peripheral nerve injury triggers noradrenergic sprouting within dorsal root ganglia. Nature 363:543–546, 1993.
63. Mellick GA, Mellick LB: Reflex sympathetic dystrophy treated with gabapentin. Arch Phys Med Rehabil 78:98–105, 1997.
64. Millan MJ: The induction of pain: An integrative review. Prog Neurobiol 57:1–164, 1999.

65. Oyen WJ, Arntz IE, Claessens RM, Van der Meer JW, Corstens FH, Goris RJ: Reflex sympathetic dystrophy of the hand: An excessive inflammatory response? Pain 55:151–157, 1993.
66. Parsons CG: NMDA receptors as targets for drug action in neuropathic pain. Eur J Pharmacol 19(429):71–78, 2001.
67. Petrenko AB, Yamakura T, Baba H, Shimoji K: The role of *N*-methyl-D-aspartate (NMDA) receptors in pain: A review. Anesth Analg 97:1108–1116, 2003.
68. Ploppa A, Kiefer RT, Nohe B, Rohr P, Grothusen J, Distler L, Dietrich HJ, Unertl K, Schwartzman RJ: Skin blood flow changes during ketamine/midazolam anesthesia for intractable CRPSI. Tenth Work Congress on Pain. San Diego, CA, August 17–22, 2002.
69. Poree LR, Guo TZ, Kingery WS, Maze M: The analgesic potency of dexmedetomidine is enhanced after nerve injury: A possible role for peripheral $alpha_2$-adrenoceptors. Anesth Analg 87:941–948, 1998.
70. Portenoy RK, Foley KM, Inturrisi CE: The nature of opioid responsiveness and its implications for neuropathic pain: New hypotheses derived from studies of opioid infusions. Pain 43:273–286, 1990.
71. Price DD, Bennett GJ, Rafii A: Psychophysical observations on patients with neuropathic pain relieved by a sympathetic block. Pain 36:273–288, 1989.
72. Price DD, Long S, Huitt C: Sensory testing of pathophysiological mechanisms of pain in patients with reflex sympathetic dystrophy. Pain 49(2):163–173, 1992.
73. Rabben T, Skjelbred P, Oye I: Prolonged analgesic effect of ketamine, an *N*-methyl-D-aspartate receptor inhibitor, in patients with chronic pain. J Pharmacol Exp Ther 289:1060–1066, 1999.
74. Raj PP, Anderson SR: Continuous regional analgesia. In: Waldman SD (ed): Interventional Pain Management. Philadelphia, WB Saunders, 2001, pp 423–433.
75. Raja SN, Treede RD, Davis KD, Campbell JN: Systemic alpha-adrenergic blockade with phentolamine: A diagnostic test for sympathetically maintained pain. Anesthesiology 74:691–698, 1991.
76. Rajkumar SV, Fonseca R, Witzig TE: Complete resolution of reflex sympathetic dystrophy with thalidomide treatment. Arch Intern Med 161:2502–2503, 2001.
77. Rauck RL, Eisenach JC, Jackson K, Young LD, Southern J: Epidural clonidine treatment for refractory reflex sympathetic dystrophy. Anesthesiology 79:1163–1169, 1993.
78. Reiestad F, McIlvaine WB, Kvalheim L, Stokke T, Pettersen B: Interpleural analgesia in treatment of upper extremity reflex sympathetic dystrophy. Anesth Analg 69:671–673, 1989.
79. Rommel O, Gehling M, Dertwinkel R, Witscher K, Zenz M, Malin JP, Janig W: Hemisensory impairment in patients with complex regional pain syndrome. Pain 80:95–101, 1999.
80. Roy ML, Narahashi T: Differential properties of tetrodotoxin-sensitive and tetrodotoxin-resistant sodium channels in rat dorsal root ganglion neurons. J Neurosci 12: 2104–2111, 1992.
81. Sawynok J, Esser MJ, Reid AR: Antidepressants as analgesics: An overview of central and peripheral mechanisms of action. J Psychiatry Neurosci 26:21–29, 2001.
82. Schattschneider J, Wenzelburger R, Deuschl G, Baron R: Kinematic analysis of the upper extremity in CRPS. In: Harden RN, Baron R, Janig W (eds): Complex Regional Pain Syndrome. Seattle, IASP Press, 2001, pp 119–128.
83. Schurmann M, Zaspel J, Gradl G, Wipfel A, Christ F: Assessment of the peripheral microcirculation using computer-assisted venous congestion plethysmography in post-traumatic complex regional pain syndrome type I. J Vasc Res 38:453–461, 2001.
84. Schwartzman RJ: New treatments for reflex sympathetic dystrophy. N Engl J Med 343:654–656, 2000.
85. Schwartzman RJ, Grothusen J, Kiefer TR, Rohr P: Neuropathic central pain: Epidemiology, etiology, and treatment options. Arch Neurol 58:1547–1550, 2001.
86. Schwartzman RJ, Kerrigan J: The movement disorder of reflex sympathetic dystrophy. Neurology 40:57–61, 1990.
87. Schwartzman RJ, McLellan TL: Reflex sympathetic dystrophy. A review. Arch Neurol 44(5):555–561, 1987.
88. Schwartzman RJ, Popescu A: Reflex sympathetic dystrophy. Curr Rheumatol Rep 4:165–169, 2002.
89. Sheng M, Kim MJ: Postsynaptic signaling and plasticity mechanisms. Science 25;298(5594):776–780, 2002.
90. Sollevi A, Belfrage M, Lundeberg T, Segerdahl M, Hansson P: Systemic adenosine infusion: A new treatment modality to alleviate neuropathic pain. Pain 61:155–158, 1995.
91. Song I, Huganir RL: Regulation of AMPA receptors during synaptic plasticity. Trends Neurosci 25:578–588, 2002.
92. Sotgiu ML, Biella G: Differential effects of MK-801, a *N*-methyl-D-aspartate non-competitive antagonist, on the dorsal horn neuron hyperactivity and hyperexcitability in neuropathic rats. Neurosci Lett 283:153–156, 2000.
93. Sugimoto T, Bennett GJ, Kajander KC: Transsynaptic degeneration in the superficial dorsal horn after sciatic nerve injury: Effects of a chronic constriction injury, transection, and strychnine. Pain 42(2):205–213, 1990.
94. Suzuki R, Chapman V, Dickenson AH: The effectiveness of spinal and systemic morphine on rat dorsal horn neuronal responses in the spinal nerve ligation model of neuropathic pain. Pain 80:215–228, 1999.
95. Takahara A, Koganei H, Takeda T, Iwata S: Antisympathetic and hemodynamic property of a dual L/N-type Ca(2+) channel blocker cilnidipine in rats. Eur J Pharmacol 434:43–47, 2002.
96. Thompson SW, King AE, Woolf CJ: Activity-dependent changes in rat ventral horn neurons in vitro: Summation of prolonged afferent evoked postsynaptic depolarizations produce ad-2-amino-5-phosphonovaleric acid sensitive windup. Eur J Neurosci 2:638–649, 1990.
97. Traynor JR: Epibatidine and pain. Br J Anaesth 81:69–76, 1998.
98. van Hilten BJ, van de Beek WJ, Hoff JI, Voormolen JH,

Delhaas EM: Intrathecal baclofen for the treatment of dystonia in patients with reflex sympathetic dystrophy. N Engl J Med 343:625–630, 2000.

99. Wallace MS, Ridgeway BM, Leung AY, Gerayli A, Yaksh TL: Concentration-effect relationship of intravenous lidocaine on the allodynia of complex regional pain syndrome types I and II. Anesthesiology 92:75–83, 2000.

100. Wasner G, Heckmann K, Maier C, Baron R: Vascular abnormalities in acute reflex sympathetic dystrophy (CRPS I): Complete inhibition of sympathetic nerve activity with recovery. Arch Neurol 56(5):613–620, 1999.

101. Wasner G, Schattschneider J, Heckmann K, Maier C, Baron R: Vascular abnormalities in reflex sympathetic dystrophy (CRPS I): Mechanisms and diagnostic value. Brain 124:587–599, 2001.

102. Waxman SG. The molecular pathophysiology of pain: Abnormal expression of sodium channel genes and its contributions to hyperexcitability of primary sensory neurons. Pain Suppl 6:S133–S140, 1999.

103. Weber M, Birklein F, Neundorfer B, Schmelz M: Facilitated neurogenic inflammation in complex regional pain syndrome. Pain 91:251–257, 2001.

104. White DM, Cousins MJ: Effect of subcutaneous administration of calcium channel blockers on nerve injury-induced hyperalgesia. Brain Res 801:50–58, 1998.

105. Woolf CJ, Costigan M: Transcriptional and posttranslational plasticity and the generation of inflammatory pain. Proc Natl Acad Sci USA 96:7723–7730, 1999.

106. Woolf CJ, Salter MW: Neuronal plasticity: Increasing the gain in pain. Science 288(5472):1765–1769, 2000.

107. Zhang X, Bao L, Shi TJ, Ju G, Elde R, Hokfelt T: Down-regulation of mu-opioid receptors in rat and monkey dorsal root ganglion neurons and spinal cord after peripheral axotomy. Neuroscience 82:223–240, 1998.

108. Zuurmond WW, Langendijk PN, Bezemer PD, Brink HE, de Lange JJ, van Loenen AC: Treatment of acute reflex sympathetic dystrophy with DMSO 50% in a fatty cream. Acta Anaesthesiol Scand 40:364–367, 1996.

Part V

Sports and Neurological Trauma

Chapter 25
Epidemiology of Sports Injuries

CORY TOTH

Injury to the nervous system may occur with essentially any sport and may involve multiple levels of the nervous system, including peripheral nerves, brachial and lumbar plexi, spinal roots, spinal cord, brain stem, and cerebrum. While particular sports can be associated with a high incidence of injury, such as football, boxing, and hockey, other sports are less commonly associated with nervous system injury. Many sports are associated with sport-specific forms of injury. Injuries may range from serious central nervous system (CNS) injury associated with great morbidity and even mortality to peripheral nervous system (PNS) injury with lengthy disability. Management of these problems is often the responsibility of a number of medical specialties, including neurologists, emergency room physicians, sports medicine physicians, surgeons, and general physicians. As concerns regarding concussion and other injuries mount, sports neurology will gain even greater importance. Improved assessment of injuries, such as the Canadian registry of hockey-related spinal injuries and recent National Football League (NFL) investigations into pathophysiologies of cerebral injury, will enhance our understanding of injury mechanisms. In all likelihood, these important measurements will lead the way to improved injury prevention schemes as well.

There are many considerations for documentation of sport exposure and its association with injury. First, the duration of exposure within a given sport (e.g., baseball) may be examined for a season of play, while another sport (e.g., boxing) may have exposure of only one bout over a year. Within individual sports, the time spent around the action may be dramatically different as well (e.g., a football quarterback vs. a place kicker). Calculation of injury risk is thus dependent upon athletic exposure and is best stated as injuries per season, per hour, or per exposure.

This chapter is designed to assist the physician in the assessment of sport-related injuries of the nervous system. In particular, the epidemiology of particular forms of injury within certain sports will be examined. Such relationships are often speculative in many sports, but certain sports have been extensively examined for the allocation and dynamics of neurological injuries. In some situations, association does not necessarily imply cause and effect. However, the absence of studies examining the removal of a supposed cause within sports is conspicuous, preventing strong association formation.

Injuries of the nervous system will be discussed by sport, with certain sports grouped due to similarity of the sport and mechanisms of injuries within those sports. Although comments about pathogenesis and prognosis have been included where known, this chapter will concentrate on providing an inventory of known neurological injuries within each sport. Sporting activities associated with neurological injury are listed in Table 25.1; neurological injuries occurring by sport are provided in Table 25.2; while individual sport-related neurological injuries by specific lesion localization are presented in Table 25.3. Sports in which injury rates per exposure may be calculated are presented in Table 25.4.

Archery

Mononeuropathies associated with the use of an archery bow include digital neuropathies,[71a] median neuropathy at the wrist and at the pronator teres intersection,[71a] and isolated long thoracic nerve palsy, perhaps due to repeated drawing of the bow and related hypertrophy of shoulder and periscapular muscles.

Table 25.1. Sporting Activities Associated with Nervous System Injury Categorized by Sport

All-terrain vehicle riding	Kickboxing
Archery	Lacrosse
Arm wrestling	Lawn darts
Australian rules football	Luge
Auto racing	Motorbiking
Ballet dancing	Mountain climbing
Baseball	Paragliding
Basketball	Racquetball
Bicycling	Rodeo
Bodybuilding	Running
Bowling	Rollerblading
Boxing	Rugby
Cheerleading	Scuba diving
Cricket	Shooting
Cross-country skiing	Skateboarding
Dancing	Skating
Darts	Skiing
Diving	Ski jumping
Equestrian sport	Sledding
Field hockey	Snowboarding
Figure skating	Snowmobiling
Football	Soccer
Frisbee	Softball
French boxing	Speed skating
Golf	Squash
Gymnastics	Surfing
Handball	Swimming
Hang gliding	Taekwandoe
Hiking	Tennis
Horse racing	Volleyball
Ice hockey	Weightlifting
In-line skating	Wheelchair basketball
Judo	Wrestling
Karate	

Arm Wrestling

Arm wrestling is associated with a relatively common complication of humeral shaft fractures, and in 23% of these cases, concurrent radial nerve palsy has occurred.[58]

Auto Racing

Over six seasons of racing at Indianapolis Raceway Park, less than 1% of all drivers were admitted to a hospital for head injury. While head trauma occurs in 29% of all injuries in professional auto racing, open head injuries comprise only 5% of these. Closed head injuries rarely include intracranial hemorrhage and diffuse axonal injury.[23] Heat stroke has been reported in one professional auto driver. Spinal injuries comprise 20% of all serious injuries suffered by professional auto drivers, most commonly associated with a vehicular rollover and with cervical spine injury.

The brachial plexus of race car drivers is at risk of injury due to the tight fastening of the arm to the helmet to prevent centrifugal force on auto drivers. In addition, the sciatic and peroneal nerves are subject to compression due to the small size of the car cockpit.[87]

Ballet and Other Professional Dancing

Repetitive, forceful movements of a dancer's arm with external rotation and abduction can produce both clinical and electrophysiological evidence of entrapment of the suprascapular nerve at the spinoglenoid notch. Femoral neuropathy can occur in dancers who perform repeated simultaneous hip extension and knee flexion (the *Horton Hinge*). Peroneal and sural neuropathies due to tight ribbons and elastic in dancing shoes have also been reported. Prolonged sitting on the dorsum of feet has been associated with dorsal cutaneous neuritis.[77] Like active runners, professional dancers occasionally present with a Morton's neuroma of the plantar nerves.

Table 25.2. Locations of Neurological Injuries by Sport

Archery

Digital nerve compression
Median neuropathy at the wrist
Median neuropathy at the pronator teres
Long thoracic nerve palsy

Arm Wrestling

Radial nerve palsy

Auto Racing

Closed head injuries
Open head injuries
Intracranial hemorrhage
Diffuse axonal brain injury
Heat stroke
Spinal cord injuries
Cervical cord injury
Brachial plexopathy
Sciatic neuropathy
Peroneal neuropathy

Ballet Dancing

Suprascapular neuropathy
Femoral neuropathy
Peroneal neuropathy
Sural neuropathy
Dorsal cutaneous neuropathy
Morton's neuroma

Baseball

Mild traumatic brain injury
Epidural hematoma
Cervical spinal cord injury
Concussion
Suprascapular neuropathy
Radial neuropathy
Ulnar neuropathy
Median neuropathy at the pronator teres
Thoracic outlet syndrome
Axillary neuropathy with quadrilateral space syndrome
Digital neuropathy at thumb
Brachial plexopathy ("pitcher's arm")

Basketball

Suprascapular neuropathy
Stinger
Median neuropathy at the wrist (wheelchair athletes)
Ulnar neuropathy at the wrist (wheelchair athletes)

Bicycling

Concussion
Ulnar neuropathy at Guyon's canal
Ulnar neuropathy at the elbow
Median neuropathy at the wrist
Pudendal neuropathy
Posterior cutaneous nerve of the thigh neuropathy
Sciatic nerve palsies (unicyclists)

Bodybuilding/Weightlifting

Benign exertional headache
Ulnar neuropathy at the deep motor branch
Ulnar neuropathy at the flexor carpi ulnaris
Ulnar neuropathy at the deep palmar branch
Ulnar neuropathy at the elbow
Posterior interosseous neuropathy
Medial pectoral neuropathy
Suprascapular neuropathy
Median neuropathy at the wrist
Long thoracic neuropathy
Lateral antebrachial cutaneous neuropathy
Musculocutaneous neuropathy
Femoral neuropathy
Thoracodorsal neuropathy
Dorsoscapular neuropathy
Stinger
Rectus abdominis syndrome with rhabdomyolysis

Bowling

Digital neuropathy of the thumb

Boxing

Concussion
Acute subdural hematoma
Chronic traumatic brain injury
Dementia pugilistica
Cervical spinal cord injury
Stinger

Cheerleading

Concussion
Closed head injury
Cervical spinal cord injury
Digital neuropathy
Median neuropathy at the palmar branch

Cricket

Intracranial hemorrhage
Closed head injury

Darts

Open head injury

Diving

Cervical spinal cord injury
Carotid artery dissection with stroke

(continued)

Table 25.2. Continued

Equestrian/Horse Racing

Closed head injury
Intracerebral hemorrhage
Cervical spinal cord injury

Field Hockey/Lacrosse

Closed head injury
Concussion
Epidural hematoma

Figure Skating

Concussion

Football

Concussion
Closed head injury
Posttraumatic headache
Chronic traumatic brain injury
Subdural hematoma
Cervical spinal cord injury
Transient quadriparesis
Stinger
Upper trunk brachial plexopathy
Radiculopathy of C5, C6, L5, or S1 roots
Axillary neuropathy with separated shoulder
Suprascapular neuropathy
Ulnar neuropathy at the elbow
Median neuropathy at the wrist
Long thoracic neuropathy
Radial neuropathy
Iliohypogastric neuropathy
Peroneal neuropathy with knee dislocation
Sciatic nerve (hamstring syndrome)

Golf

Vertebral artery dissection with stroke
"Yips"
Closed head injury (due to a golf cart, golf club, or golf ball)
Spinal cord injury (due to golf cart accidents)
Thoracic spinal cord injury due to osteoporotic fracture of vertebra or thoracic disc prolapse
Median neuropathy distal to wrist
Ulnar neuropathy at the flexor carpi ulnaris

Gymnastics

Cervical spinal cord injury
Spinal cord injury (trampoline and aeroball)
Vertebral artery dissection with stroke (trampoline)
Lateral femoral cutaneous neuropathy
Femoral neuropathy

Handball

Handball goalie's elbow

Hang Gliding/Paragliding

Spinal cord injury

Hockey

Concussion
Epidural hematoma
Subdural hematoma
Subarachnoid hemorrhage
Spinal cord injury
Stinger
Tibial neuropathy due to tarsal tunnel syndrome
Peroneal neuropathy

In-Line Skating, Rollerskating and Skateboarding

Closed head injury
Superfical peroneal neuropathy

Judo, Karate, Kickboxing, and Taekwondoe

Vertebral artery, carotid artery dissection with stroke
Cervical spinal cord injury due to disc herniation
Closed head injury
Subdural hematoma
Intracranial hemorrhages
Morton's neuroma of a plantar nerve
Ulnar neuropathy at a trauma site
Axillary neuropathy at a trauma site
Spinal accessory neuropathy at a trauma site
Long thoracic neuropathy at a trauma site
Peroneal neuropathy at a trauma site

Motorbiking

Closed head injury
Intracranial hemorrhages
Spinal cord injury

Mountain Climbing, Hiking

Acute mountain sickness with headache
Cerebral edema syndrome due to high elevation
Tarsal tunnel syndrome
Rucksack paralysis—brachial plexopathy (upper and middle trunks)
Suprascapular neuropathy
Axillary neuropathy
Long thoracic neuropathy

Rodeo Riding

Concussion
Closed head injury

(continued)

Table 25.2. Continued

Rubgy/Australian Rules Football

Cervical spinal cord injury
Transient quadriparesis
Concussion
Mild traumatic brain injury
Obturator neuropathy

Running

Peroneal neuropathy
Lateral femoral cutaneous neuropathy
Tibial neuropathy at the tarsal tunnel
Posterior tibial neuropathy
Morton's neuroma of a plantar nerve
Interdigital neuropathies
Plantar neuropathies
Calcaneal neuropathy
Sural neuropathy
Superficial peroneal neuropathy
Saphenous neuropathy
Rhabdomyolysis

Scuba Diving

Cerebral arterial oxygen bubble emboli with stroke and encephalopathy
Cerebral infarction related to cardiopulmonary shunt and paradoxical thromboembolism
Skip breathing headache
"Goggles headache"
Lateral femoral cutaneous neuropathy

Shooting

Long thoracic neuropathy

Skiing, Snowboarding, Sledding, and Ski Jumping

Spinal cord injury
  Thoracolumbar (skiing)
  Cervical (snowboarding)
  Cervical spinal epidural hematoma
Closed head injury
Concussion
Intracranial hemorrhages
Femoral neuropathy (cross-country skiing)
Ulnar neuropathy (cross-country skiing)

Snowmobiling and All-Terrain Vehicle Riding

Closed head injury
Spinal cord injury
Brachial plexopathy
Ulnar neuropathy at Guyon's canal

Soccer

Concussion
Closed head injury
Intracranial hemorrhages
Epidural hematoma
Acute subdural hematoma
Chronic subdural hematoma
Basal skull fracture with meningitis development
Mild traumatic brain injury
Peroneal neuropathy

Speed Skating

Concussion

Surfing

Common peroneal neuropathy
Saphenous neuropathy
Surfer's myelopathy

Tennis/Racquetball

Posterior interosseous neuropathy at the arcade of Frohse
Suprascapular neuropathy
Long thoracic neuropathy
Radial neuropathy secondary to fibrous arches at the lateral head of the triceps

Volleyball

Suprascapular neuropathy
Axillary neuropathy
Long thoracic neuropathy

Wrestling

Mild traumatic brain injury
Concussion
Closed head injury
Spinal cord injury
Transient quadriparesis
Vertebral artery territory stroke due to prolonged wrestling hold
Stinger
Brachial plexopathy
Axillary neuropathy
Ulnar neuropathy
Median neuropathy at the wrist
Long thoracic neuropathy
Suprascapular neuropathy

Table 25.3. Neurological Injuries of the Central Nervous System Due to Sport Classified by Anatomical Location and Injury Type

Spinal Cord

- Any location
  - Auto racing
  - Golf
  - Gymnastics
  - Hang gliding/paragliding
  - Hockey
  - Snowmobiling
  - All-terrain vehicle riding
  - Wrestling
- Cervical
  - Auto racing
  - Baseball
  - Boxing
  - Cheerleading
  - Diving
  - Equestrian sport
  - Football
  - Gymnastics
  - Rubgy
  - Snowboarding
- Thoracic
  - Skiing
  - Surfing
- Lumbar
  - Skiing
- Transient quadriparesis
  - Football
  - Rubgy
  - Wrestling
- Epidural hematoma
  - Snowboarding

Brain Stem

- Stroke
  - Golf
  - Gymnastics
  - Judo, karate, and kickboxing
  - Wrestling

Cerebrum

- Concussion
  - Auto racing
  - Baseball
  - Bicycling
  - Boxing
  - Cheerleading
  - Field hockey/lacrosse
  - Figure skating
  - Football
  - Hockey
  - Rodeo
  - Rubgy
  - Skiing
  - Snowboarding
  - Soccer
  - Speed skating
  - Wrestling
- Closed head injury
  - Auto racing
  - Boxing
  - Cheerleading
  - Cricket
  - Equestrian sport
  - Field hockey/lacrosse
  - Football
  - Golf
  - In-line skating, roller skating, and skateboarding
  - Judo, karate, and kickboxing
  - Motorbiking
  - Rodeo riding
  - Rubgy
  - Skiing
  - Snowboarding
  - Snowmobiling
  - All-terrain vehicle riding
  - Soccer
  - Wrestling
- Open head injury
  - Auto racing
  - Darts
- Stroke
  - Diving
  - Scuba diving
  - Judo, karate, and kickboxing
- Subdural hematoma
  - Auto racing
  - Boxing
  - Equestrian sport
  - Football
  - Hockey
  - Judo, karate, and kickboxing
  - Motorbiking
  - Skiing
  - Snowboarding
  - Soccer
- Epidural hematoma
  - Auto racing
  - Baseball
  - Cricket
  - Equestrian sport
  - Field hockey/lacrosse
  - Hockey
  - Soccer
- Subarachnoid hemorrhage
  - Hockey
  - Judo, karate, and kickboxing
  - Motorbiking
  - Skiing
  - Snowboarding
- Diffuse axonal injury
  - Auto racing
- Cerebral Edema
  - Mountain climbing
- Chronic traumatic brain injury
  - Boxing
  - Football
- Dementia pugilistica
  - Boxing
- Heat stroke
  - Auto Racing
- Headache
  - Bodybuilding/weightlifting
  - Scuba diving
  - Football
  - Mountain climbing
- Movement disorder
  - Golf

Peripheral Nerves

- Digital Nerves
  - Archery
  - Baseball
  - Bowling
  - Cheerleading
  - Tennis
- Median Nerve
  - Wrist
    - Archery
    - Basketball (wheelchair)
    - Bicycling
    - Bodybuilding/weightlifting
    - Football
    - Golf
    - Wrestling
  - Palmar branch
    - Cheerleading
    - Golf
  - Pronator teres
    - Archery
    - Baseball
- Ulnar Nerve
  - At the elbow
    - Baseball
    - Bicycling
    - Bodybuilding/weightlifting
    - Judo, karate, and kickboxing
    - Cross-country skiing
    - Wrestling
  - At the wrist
    - Basketball (wheelchair)
    - Bicycling
    - Football
    - Cross-country skiing
    - Snowmobiling
  - At the flexor carpi ulnaris
    - Bodybuilding/weightlifting
    - Golf
  - At the deep motor branch
    - Bodybuilding/Weightlifting
- Radial Nerve
  - Arm Wrestling
  - Baseball
  - Football
  - Tennis/racquetball
- Posterior Interosseous Neuropathy
  - Bodybuilding/weightlifting
  - Frisbee
  - Gymnastics
  - Tennis/racquetball
- Superficial Radial Nerve
  - Tennis/Racquetball
- Axillary nerve
  - Baseball
  - Football
  - Hiking
  - Hockey
  - Judo, karate, and kickboxing
  - Rugby
  - Volleyball
  - Wrestling
- Spinal accessory nerve
  - Judo, karate, and kickboxing
- Musculocutaneous nerve
  - Bodybuilding/weightlifting
- Lateral antebrachial cutaneous neuropathy
  - Bodybuilding/weightlifting
  - Tennis
- Thoracic outlet syndrome
  - Baseball

(continued)

Table 25.3. Continued

- Football
- Swimming
- Tennis

Long Thoracic Nerve
- Archery
- Bodybuilding/weightlifting
- Football
- Judo, karate, and kickboxing
- Hiking
- Shooting
- Tennis/racquetball
- Volleyball
- Wrestling

Thoracodorsal Neuropathy
- Bodybuilding/weightlifting

Dorsoscapular Nerve
- Bodybuilding/weightlifting

Suprascapular Nerve
- Ballet Dancing
- Baseball
- Basketball
- Bodybuilding/weightlifting
- Football
- Hiking
- Tennis/racquetball
- Volleyball
- Wrestling

Medial Pectoral Neuropathy
- Bodybuilding/weightlifting

Brachial Plexus
- Auto racing
- Baseball
- Football (upper trunk)
- Hiking (Upper, middle trunks)
- Snowmobiling
- Wrestling

Stinger
- Basketball
- Bodybuilding/weightlifting
- Boxing
- Football
- Hockey
- Wrestling

Cervical Radiculopathy
- Football

Femoral Nerve
- Ballet Dancing
- Bodybuilding/weightlifting
- Gymnastics
- Cross-country skiing

Obturator Nerve
- Rubgy/Australian rules football

Peroneal Nerve
- Auto racing
- Ballet dancing
- Football
- Hockey
- Judo, karate, and kickboxing
- Running
- Soccer
- Surfing

Pudendal nerve
- Bicycling

Iliohypogastric nerve
- Football

Sciatic nerve
- Auto racing
- Bicycling
- Football (hamstring syndrome)

Superficial peroneal nerve
- Running

Interdigital nerves of the foot
- Running

Tibial nerve
- At the tarsal tunnel
  - Hockey
  - Hiking
  - Running

Sural nerve
- Ballet dancing
- Running

Lateral femoral cutaneous nerve
- Gymnastics
- Running
- Scuba diving

Posterior cutaneous nerve of the thigh
- Bicycling

Superficial peroneal nerve
- Rollerskating
- Running

Saphenous nerve
- Surfing
- Running

Dorsal cutaneous nerve of the foot
- Ballet dancing

Lumbar radiculopathy
- Football

Morton's neuroma of the plantar nerve
- Ballet dancing
- Judo, karate, and kickboxing
- Running

Plantar nerves of the feet
- Running

Calcaneal neuropathy
- Running

Baseball

The most frequent mechanism (62%) of acute baseball-related injury is being hit by the ball. In one study of trauma center hospital assessments of 10- to 19-year olds, 55% of all baseball injuries involved ball or bat impact, often of the head.[10] The addition of a face guard on the batting helmet has led to relative injury reduction without adverse effects on player performance or player acceptability.

In children aged 7–13, the acute injury rate per 100 athlete exposures is 1.7 for baseball and 1.0 for softball. Most injuries were contusions, while concussion comprised about 1%.[70] The frequency of injury per team per season is 3.0 for baseball and 2.0 for softball.[70] In children aged 7–13, games are more likely than practice to lead to injury.[70] In Little Leaguers aged 7–18, an overall injury rate is .057 per 100 player-hours, with a severe injury rate of .008 per 100 player-hours, much lower than with other common sports.[61] The occurrence of mild traumatic brain injuries (MTBIs) in children's softball (2.1%) and baseball (1.2%) is quite limited relative to other sports.[67] The incidence of MTBI among high school baseball players is similarly low (0.23 per 100 player-seasons) and is 15 times less than that of football.[67] A retrospective study of baseball bat–related injuries revealed craniocerebral injury to be the most frequent cause of injury and death. One study of players struck in the head showed that 26% sustained an intracranial hemorrhage, with an epidural hematoma reported once.

Even rarer than severe head injury is spinal cord injury. One player suffered an acute central cervical spinal cord syndrome after a hyperextension injury.

The pitching arm is vulnerable to mononeuropathies, including suprascapular nerve injuries. Entrapment of the suprascapular nerve in pitchers may occur at the suprascapular or spinoglenoid notches.[45] Windmill pitching, used in softball, has

Table 25.4. Rate of Neurological Injuries in Major Sports

Sport	Acute Injury Rate per 100 Athlete-Exposures	Acute Injury Rate per 100 Athlete-Seasons	Frequency of Injury per Team per Season	Incidence of Mild Traumatic Brain Injury per 100 Player-Seasons
Baseball				
Aged 7–13 y	1.7		3.0	
Aged 7–18 y				0.2
Basketball				
Aged 13–18 y (male)		0.8		
Aged 13–18 y (female)		1.0		
Cross-Country Skiing		0.1		
Field Hockey		0.5		
Football				
Aged 7–13 y			14.0	
Aged 15–18 y		3.7		
Aged 18–23 y	1.5			6.1
Hockey				
Aged 14–18 y (male)	0.9	75		3.7
Aged 14–18 y (female)	0.8			
Aged 18–23 y (male)	0.5			4.2
Aged 20–36 y (male)	11.9			6.6
Luge		39		
Martial Arts				
Amateur	2.4			
Professional	0.7–2.8			
Aged 7–14 y	0.6			
taekwandoe	6.3			
Mountain Climbing	0.2			
Rodeo Riding	3.2			
Roller Hockey	13.9			
Skiing	0.2			
Ski Jumping	0.1–0.4	9.4		
Soccer				
Aged 14–18 y (male)		0.9		
Aged 14–18 y (female)		1.1		
Aged 18–23 y	2.1		3.0	
Softball				
Aged 7–13 y	1.0		2.0	
Volleyball		0.1		
Wrestling		1.6		

been associated with radial neuropathy at different anatomical sites.[82] Humeral shaft fracture in softball and baseball pitchers has been associated with radial nerve palsies in 16% of cases.[59] Ulnar neuropathy at the elbow is common among baseball pitchers. In one study of 72 professional baseball players undergoing arthroscopic or open elbow surgery, ulnar neuropathy was diagnosed in 15%. Adolescent players have developed cubital tunnel syndrome affecting the ulnar nerve with initial presentation as medial elbow pain. Surgical treatment with anterior subcutaneous transposition of the ulnar nerve can relieve symptoms for more than 3 postoperative years. At surgery, medial protrusion of the triceps irritating the ulnar nerve or fibrosis surrounding the ulnar nerve has appeared to be causative.[1c] Pronator syndrome may occur in the pitching arm with median nerve entrapment by fibrous bands of the pronator teres. Thoracic outlet syndrome presented as numbness in the fingers of the throwing hand of a college baseball player, with compression of the neurovascular bundle demonstrated using magnetic resonance angiography with the arm held in abduction. The quadrilateral space syndrome in the pitching arm of a baseball pitcher developed with compression of the distal axillary nerve and partial compression of the posterior humeral circumflex artery. Batters may be occasionally susceptible to a traumatic neuroma of the ulnar digital nerve of the thumb.

Electrodiagnostic testing has led to the notion of a *pitcher's arm*, which makes evaluation of potential neuropathy in the baseball pitcher difficult. Asymptomatic professional and amateur baseball pitchers have reduced sensory nerve action potentials in the throwing arm, although this does not appear to impact their performance. Pitcher's arm may be a repetitive use syndrome of the brachial plexus.[46] Recurrent trauma to the axillary artery in a pitching arm may lead to aneurysm and thrombus formation, which is rarely associated with distal extremity ischemia and stroke.

Basketball

While basketball injuries are relatively common, neurological injuries are relatively rare in basketball players. The incidence of MTBI in high school basketball players is lower than that of other organized sports such as football, wrestling, and soccer. The injury rates reported in an observational cohort study per 100 high school player-seasons were 1.04 for girls' basketball and 0.75 for boys' basketball.[67] Head injuries in basketball players aged 10–19 years are related to striking the basketball pole or rim, or being struck by a falling pole or backboard.

Suprascapular neuropathy may occur due to repeated nerve traction over the coracoid notch during dunking of the basketball. The burner, or stinger, has rarely been seen in basketball players. Compression neuropathies of the arms are common injuries in wheelchair basketball players; carpal tunnel syndrome (CTS) has been diagnosed clinically in 30% of world-class wheelchair basketball players, and 70% of these players had electrodiagnostic abnormalities on median nerve conduction studies.[7,32a] An additional 12% of wheelchair basketball players had abnormalities on ulnar nerve conduction studies at the wrist.[7,32a]

Bicycling

Head injuries and helmet use for bicyclists have become a common political topic. A Canadian study demonstrated that helmet use lowered the probability of hospital admission following overall injury, head and facial injury, and concussion. In California, bicycle safety helmet legislation has led to statistically significant reductions in head injuries among bicyclists aged 17 years and under, although there was no statistically significant change in injury outcomes for adult bicyclists.[43b] For children beginning cycling, injury rates are reduced if the age of first starting bicycling debut is delayed until 7 or 8 years instead of at 4 or 5 years.[26b] Children's helmet use has also led to a lower incidence of skull fractures and possible improvement in head injury mortality rates.

Bicycle motorcross (BMX)-style bike riders, while subject to injuries due to stunt performance, do not appear to have a different overall injury rate than those using standard bikes. Concussions may constitute 7% of all BMX bike-riding injuries. Off-road bicycle racing may have a smaller incidence of concussion (<1%), which is still about 40% less than that of other forms of cycling.[73] This low incidence may be due to the significantly higher rate of helmet usage in off-road bikers.[73] Interestingly, women appear to be much more likely than men to sustain a serious injury during off-road biking.

Bicycling accidents have been associated with cervical spinal cord injury in children, and with thoracic disc herniation leading to myelopathy in one female adult.

The most common form of nerve entrapment in bicyclists is ulnar nerve entrapment at the wrist within Guyon's canal, resulting in weakness of grip and numbness of the fourth and fifth digits,[29a,47] reported in as many as 30% of professional cyclists. Recovery from ulnar neuropathy may occur with avoidance of activity or via modification of hand grips on the bicycle handlebars. Besides the ulnar nerve, the median nerve may be abnormal in many (25%) cyclists, with 62% of symptomatic hands tested demonstrating abnormal median nerve conduction,[9] sometimes bilateral.[6]

Pudendal neuropathy is unique to the cyclist, as well as common (22% of professional cyclists) secondary to bicycle saddle pressure upon the perineum.[1a,91] Forty-five percent of racing cyclists report mild or transient perineal numbness, 10% report severe symptomatology, and 2% report requiring temporary breaks due to symptoms. Changes in bike saddle position and riding technique may lead to symptomatic improvement. Bicycle seat neuropathy is likely due to entrapment of the pudendal nerve passing through the Alcock canal enclosed by ischial bone and obturator internus. Symptoms may persist for weeks and may include transient impotence. Many cyclists with pudendal neuropathy may be more liable to nerve entrapment, as 85% of these cyclists also report hand numbness after cycling.[1a] Pudendal neuropathy is not exclusive to male cyclists, as 34% of female cyclists also report perineal numbness. Another neuropathy due to prolonged bicycle use is posterior cutaneous thigh neuropathy. A unique injury dubbed *pedal pusher's palsy*, with bilateral sciatic nerve palsies, can occur following prolonged unicycle riding.

Bodybuilding/Weightlifting

Repeated bench pressing has been associated with entrapment of the deep motor branch of the ulnar nerve and compression of the ulnar nerve between the heads of flexor carpi ulnaris. Power squats were suspected to be a cause of posterior interosseous neuropathy in a professional bodybuilder. A progressive bilateral medial pectoral neuropathy secondary to postulated pectoralis minor hypertrophy and subsequent intramuscular entrapment of the medial pectoral nerves was reported.[42] A compressive lesion of the deep palmar branch of the ulnar nerve was reported with an intensive program of push-ups on a hard floor. Other forms of mononeuropathy reported in bodybuilders include suprascapular neuropathy, CTS, ulnar neuropathy at the elbow, long thoracic neuropathy, lateral antebrachial cutaneous neuropathy, musculocutaneous neuropathy, thoracodorsal neuropathy, dorsoscapular neuropathy, femoral neuropathy, and entrapment of the terminal branch of the suprascapular nerve.[42] Brachial plexus injuries are rare in the bodybuilder, but stingers have rarely been reported in weightlifters.

Bowling

The repetitive nature of bowling may lead to injuries to the digital nerve of the thumb placed inside the 10 pin bowling ball holes.[90] Perineural fibrosis of the digital nerve of the thumb,[90] as well as a thumb neuroma, have both been reported as a result of chronic trauma due to bowling.

Boxing

The assessment of boxing-related neurological injuries requires two important considerations: first, acute neurological injuries need to be distinguished from chronic brain injuries; second, the level of competitive boxing, amateur or professional, will influence the nature of injuries. Amateur boxing differs from professional boxing in the duration of fights, rules and regulatory policies, degree of medical evaluation, and use of protective devices such as headgear. It is suspected that the incidence of serious acute head injury in amateur boxing is lower than in the professional ranks, perhaps due to greater regulation and headgear use.

Acute neurological injuries such as concussion, postconcussion syndrome, and intracranial hemorrhage are easily identified. In amateur ranks, serious head injuries comprised only 0.3% of all boxing-related injuries in a study of 60,000 participants.[75] Another study of amateur boxing found that 0.58% of participants suffered a severe concussion or multiple knockouts.[3] In professional boxers, most studies have occurred in New York

State and have demonstrated knockout rates of 3% per participant during the 1950s, compared with about three head injuries per 10 boxers over a 2-year period in the 1980s.[34] Differences in reporting and better definitions of concussion may play a role in these differences. The incidence of intracranial hemorrhage in boxers remains unknown, but acute subdural hematomas are probably the leading cause of boxing-related mortality.

The impact of boxing competition upon cognitive status has been widely studied. Acutely, computerized cognitive assessment in military cadet boxers demonstrates inferior performances on simple reaction time and continuous performance tests after boxing-induced concussion compared with baseline testing. Measures of more chronic effects of boxing and of neuropsychological and cognitive effects vary, with some studies demonstrating few limitations of cognition and physiological function. For example, a study of former Swedish amateur boxers identified only one task with impaired performance relative to other athletes: finger tapping. Similarly, electrophysiological testing, including electroencephalography and brain stem auditory evoked responses, has demonstrated little abnormality in long-term boxers. Chronic neurological injuries from boxing seem to start insidiously and often present after cessation of boxing.[33] Of ex-professional boxers who had participated in the sport for at least 3 years, 17% were found to have clinical evidence of cerebellar, extrapyramidal, and intellectual impairments felt to be attributable to boxing.[74a] The most severe form of postboxing encephalopathy has been termed *dementia pugilistica*. Besides cerebellar, extrapyramidal, and intellectual dysfunction, this disorder may include tremor, dysarthria, and psychiatric changes such as explosive behavior and paranoid and jealous delusions. Risk factors for CNS deficits after boxing include professional boxing (as opposed to amateur boxing), the number of punches taken, and lack of *scientific boxing ability*. In support of these findings, a small number of amateur boxers demonstrated no abnormalities on detailed neurologic examinations and with magnetic resonance imaging (MRI) of the brain. When professional boxers are scored on the Chronic Brain Injury (CBI) scale, greater impairment is significantly correlated with a greater number of bouts.

Possible markers for neurological deficit in boxers have been examined in recent years. Those boxers with an apolipoprotein E $\epsilon 4$ allele present also demonstrated a significantly greater tendency toward a CNS deficit.[35] While amateur boxers and controls do not demonstrate abnormalities in regional cerebral blood flow (rCBF) with inhalation of 133-xenon, professional boxers demonstrate diffuse reductions in rCBF, especially in the frontocentral regions. Neuropathological abnormalities documented in ex-professional boxers include scarring of cerebellar folia, loss of cerebellar Purkinje cells, degeneration of the substantia nigra, presence of neurofibrillary tangles in limbic gray matter, and cavum septum pellucidum.[13] In contrast, computed tomography (CT) scans of amateur boxers do not identify an increased incidence of cavum septum pellucidum. Neurofibrillary tangles in brains with dementia pugilistica are concentrated in superficial neocortical layers, in contrast to Alzheimer's disease, where they predominate in deep layers.[27] Studies on the molecular profile of tau pathology in patients with chronic traumatic injury, including boxers with dementia pugilistica, have demonstrated the same tau epitopes found in filamentous tau inclusions in brains with Alzheimer's disease. Thus, recurrent brain injury in boxers may activate pathological mechanisms similar to those seen in Alzheimer's disease. The level of the glial protein S-100B increases in serum after amateur boxing competitions. It is correlated significantly with the number and severity of blows to the head and may be related to the presence of cognitive deficits.

Cervical spine fractures are rare in boxers. A transient spinal cord injury occurred in a young male boxer who had an os odontoideum, possibly placing him at risk for such injury. Another boxer sustained a C6 vertebral body fracture and quadriplegia during a boxing match.

The lone PNS lesion known is the rarely reported burner or stinger.

Cheerleading

Major injuries in cheerleaders include cervical fractures or cervical ligament injuries leading to paralysis, as well as spinal cord contusions with transient symptoms. In high school cheerleaders, concussion rates are 9.36 per 100,000 athlete-exposures,[80b] with most injuries due to pyramid building. In one study of high school athlete concussion rates, cheerleading was unique as the only sport for which concussion rate was greater in practice than during the game.[80b] Severe head injuries including skull fractures, hematomas, or cerebral edema have occurred following accidents. Mortality at the time of or within days of a severe head injury has occurred in two cheerleaders.[5]

Median neuropathy within the palm, perhaps due to repeated baton tossing, has been reported in one cheerleader.

Cricket

Injuries in cricket appear to occur most commonly to the head, hands, and forearms, and are usually secondary to being struck by a ball in children playing cricket. Uncommonly, head injuries can be severe, with intracranial hemorrhage.[88]

Darts and Lawn Darts

The head is the most common body part to be injured by the dart, almost always in children. In particular, lawn darts have been associated with penetrating skull injuries, sometimes associated with development of a polymicrobial brain abscess. Neurological impairment occurs in up to 50% of lawn dart–associated head injuries.[83]

Diving

Diving is the predominant mechanism of injury associated with water activities, with cervical spinal cord injury (SCI) comprising 4.9% of all water-related accidents in children.[31] Among all sports, diving is the most common cause of SCI (21.6%) and most commonly affects males (88%) of young age (mean age of 28.5 years).[38a] Patients sustaining a cervical SCI are more likely to be in the early-mid teenage years (10–14 years in one study) and to be experienced divers.[31] The second most common group to suffer high cervical SCI due to diving is young adult male divers. Most SCIs related to diving (87%) occur in private or residential swimming pools. In approximately 50% of diving-associated SCIs, alcohol or a pool party was involved in a retrospective study. As expected, most diving-related SCIs (57%) occur in less than 4 feet of water. Absence of a lifeguard on duty was noted in 94% of cases in a retrospective study. Ordinary diving accounts for 70% of SCI cases, with unusual or trick dives less commonly associated with injury.[17] The type of dive determines the risk of injury; dives with a maximized flight distance and a low entry angle appear to be safest.

In older adults, rare reports of internal carotid artery occlusion and carotid dissection have occurred following a sports dive. At autopsy, gas emboli are detected in cerebral and spinal arteries.[60a]

Equestrian Sports and Horse Racing

Perhaps surprisingly, injuries in equestrian sports are very common, perhaps 20 times more common than those in motorcycling.[25] The majority of equestrian-related injuries (60%) are caused by falling from the horse, while a smaller percentage (40%) are due to being kicked by a horse, even as a bystander.[41] In one Canadian retrospective study, closed head injury was the most common cause of admission to a hospital after equestrian-related trauma. Closed head injuries of varying severity have been associated with fourth nerve palsy in 46% of patients and with loss of vision in 20%. Intracranial hematomas, sometimes fatal, have been reported with equestrian trauma, including pediatric cases.[41] Helmet use reduces the risk and severity of head injuries, including those in pediatric riders, and should be vigorously promoted, as most riders are helmetless.[41] Pediatric head injury due to an equestrian-related cause was second only to automobile-related accident head injuries in one study. Professional horse racing may have injury rates similar to those in equestrian activities, but this is understudied.

The incidence of degenerative changes of both the cervical and lumbar spine are higher in jockeys than in age-matched controls in a prospective study with both clinical and radiographic evaluation of the spine. Although not as common as head injuries, spinal injuries causing quadriplegia or paraplegia make up 30% of severe injuries.[41]

Field Hockey and Lacrosse

Injury rates in lacrosse and field hockey, despite the use of a hard ball and sticks used by aggressive players, tend to be much less than in other major sports. In high school players, the injury rate per 100 player-seasons was 0.46 for field hockey.[68] Overall, lacrosse-related trauma is more common among male players (81% of all cases in a male-dominated sport) and teenage players (mean age of 16.9 years).[18] Closed head injuries comprise 6% of all lacrosse-related injuries. Although most injuries occur in males, female players are more likely to suffer head or face injury (30% vs. 18% in males), perhaps due to the lesser likelihood of females to wear helmets.[18] The overall head and face injury rate is 0.71 per 1000 exposures (games and practices) and is usually due to ball contact.[18] In terms of sports leading to MTBIs, field hockey was the least likely sport studied to cause head injury (1.1% of all MTBIs).[67] The rate of concussion is less than 1 per 10,000 exposures,[53] with one case of epidural intracranial hematoma reported after the player was hit by a lacrosse stick.

Football

In most studies, football is reported as the sport most likely to be associated with injury, specifically neurological injury. The injury rate for college football players is estimated at 1.5 per 100 athlete exposures in games as well as practices.[70] High school football also was associated with the highest injury rate per 100 player-seasons (3.66) of all sports studied.[67] Contact with another player is the most frequent method of injury in football.[70] Of all injuries reported, 14% are considered serious (fracture, dislocation, or concussion).[70] The frequency of injuries per professional team per season is 14, more than three times that of all other team sports for children aged 7–13 years.[70]

Even with helmets, the high velocity and violent nature of football lead to many head injuries. Of 10 sports investigated, football accounted for 63% of MTBIs.[67] Concussions occurred in football at an estimated rate of 6.1 per 100 athlete-seasons in one study,[12] more than twice the incidence of other team sports. In high school football players, concussion rates are 33.09 per 100,000 athlete-exposures.[80b] The use of a helmet for protection can also lead to injuries, as 7% of all football injuries involve being struck by an opponent's helmet. The incidence of concussion in football has significant variation, partly due to overreporting of recalled episodes of concussion in teammates compared with self-reports and videotape analysis. High school football players self-report an incidence of concussion of 47% over one season, with 35% of all players reporting multiple concussions over one season. Another study of both high school and college football players reported that only 5% of players sustained one concussion, but 15% of those players sustained a second concussion during the same season. The most common specific diagnosis of injury in Canadian varsity players is concussion. A study of Canadian Football League professional players suggested a 45% concussion incidence rate over one season, with a 70% incidence of multiple concussions in players reporting at least one. An episode of concussion may triple or quadruple the risk for recurrence, which may also mean an increased risk of the recently popularized yet highly controversial second impact syndrome.[50] Players perhaps subject to an increased incidence of concussion, according to older studies, include offensive and defensive linemen, as well as special teams players. This may be due to blocking resulting in more concussions than tackling. A more recent study identified the players at greatest relative risk for concussions to be quarterbacks (1.62 concussions/100 game positions), wide receivers (1.23 concussions/100 game positions), tight ends (0.94 concussion/100 game positions), and defensive secondary backs (0.93 concussion/100 game positions).[62]

Fortunately, the majority of football-related concussions are mild (88%–95%). The use of artificial turf may play a role in the high incidence of concussion in football players. Suspected high rates of head injuries in football players during the 1960s and 1970s led to the development of a helmet with improved headform composed of synthetic materials, which led to improved impact performance. Significant reductions in youth football injuries followed, including a 65% reduction in cranial fractures, a 51% reduction in fatal head injuries, and a 35% reduction in concussions. Video analysis of professional football plays resulting in head injuries, as well as laboratory reconstructions using helmeted dummies, have determined that concussions are primarily related to translational acceleration at the time of impact, as well as significant acceleration or deceleration.[64] The majority of impacts (71%) leading to concussion are due to an opponent's helmet, arm, or shoulder pad striking the side of the player's helmet, and often these impacts are on the highest portion of the helmet.[63] The most common symptoms of MTBI in professional football players are headaches (55.0%), dizziness (41.8%), and blurred vision (16.3%),[62] with loss of consciousness occurring in 9.3% of cases.[62]

When high school and college football players are assessed immediately and 15 minutes after concussion, neurocognitive impairment is evident relative to a preseason baseline score. Players with a concussion and loss of consciousness (grade 3 concussion) were found to be the most severely impaired immediately after injury, allowing gradation of the effects of concussion on neurocognition. A neuropsychological study showed that college football players with prior concussion demonstrate learning disabilities. The presence of posttraumatic headache in football players after collisions is common (21%), particularly among offensive and defensive linemen and defensive backs, and is often unreported to trainers.

Although publicized in the past, the prevalence of second impact syndrome is difficult to calculate. This syndrome has been defined as a sustained head injury after an initial head injury, usually a concussion, where symptoms associated with the first injury have not fully cleared. It has been postulated that this second impact may lead to rapid development of cerebral vascular congestion and increased intracranial pressure, resulting in brain stem herniation and death.[50] Although some of the first reported patients with second impact syndrome were football players (also noted in ice hockey and boxing), skepticism about this entity exists. The absence of specific risk factors and the presence of only scattered case reports (17) make this syndrome and its postulated severe complications controversial and questionable.[50] Despite this, greater education is obviously required, as a recent study suggested that only 18%–23% of concussed college and professional football players realized they had suffered a concussion.[16a,16b] Similarly, the presence of chronic traumatic brain injury (CTBI), as seen in boxing, has been postulated in football, but without significant evidence. Occurrence of intracranial hemorrhage, particularly subdural hematoma, has rarely been reported in football. Players who tackle with the head down and use the head as a battering ram may be at increased risk for more severe forms of injuries to the head and neck.

Next to diving and skiing, football is the most common cause of sports-related SCI (13% of all sports-related SCIs). The most common mechanism of football-related SCI is axial loading of the cervical spine, as opposed to neck hyperextension or hyperflexion, using film analysis of plays with injuries. Transient quadriparesis, or cervical transient neurapraxia, seems to be most common in football secondary to a blow to the head with sudden neck flexion or extension. Clinically, the player experiences transient weakness and numbness to the extremities for a period of seconds to a few days. The incidence of this condition is one to six per 10,000 players. In children 7–15 years of age who develop cervical cord neurapraxia due to a football-related injury, the mobility of the pediatric spine rather than congenital cervical spinal stenosis may play a role, although this is controversial. In recent decades, changes in football including modifications of the penalty systems, emphasis upon tackling with the shoulders as opposed to using the head as a spear, and new design of helmets and protective equipment have led to a significant reduction of cervical spine injuries associated with quadriplegia in football since 1976.

In Canadian varsity football players, brachial plexus injury was the third most common specific diagnosis in football injuries,[51] while at two university centers it accounted for half of all injuries.[11] The incidence of plexus injury has been reported to be as high as 2.2 cases per 100 football players per season. The stinger, or burner, comprises approximately 36% of all neurological upper extremity injuries related to football. The stinger may be radiculopathic in nature or it may be due to dysfunction of the upper trunk of the brachial plexus. More persistent cervical plexus football injuries include upper trunk brachial plexopathies and C5 or C6 radiculopathies. Thoracic outlet syndrome was previously reported to affect the throwing shoulder of football quarterbacks.

Mononeuropathies reported in upper limbs of football players include axillary neuropathy, suprascapular neuropathy, ulnar neuropathy, median neuropathy at the carpal tunnel, long thoracic neuropathy, and radial neuropathy.[42] Axillary neuropathy can be associated with shoulder dislocation[40a,42] or can be due to direct trauma over the anterolateral deltoid region. *Footballer's hernia* with lower abdominal bulging may relate to an iliohypogastric neuropathy. Lower limb mononeuropathies in football players consist of peroneal neuropathy, particularly in cases where complete knee dislocation and ligamentous injury has occurred,[42] and sciatic neuropathy as part of the controversial *hamstring syndrome*. Lumbosacral radiculopathy may rarely be related to football injury.[42]

Frisbee Playing

One very active frisbee player has developed a posterior interosseuos nerve syndrome.[20b]

Golf

Many golf-related injuries to the CNS are actually due to golf cart accidents, which have led to rare SCIs[39] and head injuries including cerebral contusion, skull fracture, and extradural hematoma. Head injury due to a golf club (91% of all golf-related head injuries) or golf ball has been reported in children aged 3–13 years, predominantly males (78%), with 4% of these children suffering a compound depressed skull fracture.[48] There are no reports of adults being injured with golf clubs or balls. Golf may have led to vertebral artery dissection and Wallenberg syndrome in one case, perhaps due to torsion of the neck.

Thoracic spinal injuries including acute thoracic spinal disc prolapse following a golf swing has been recorded in a male with a decade-long history of L'hermitte's symptom,[32b] and thoracic spinal osteoporotic fractures in women have been noted.[19b]

Median neuropathy in the palm has occurred in a neophyte golfer.[29b] The relationship of golf to CTS is less clear, but repetitive gripping and sustained hyperflexion and hyperextension may contribute to median entrapment. Ulnar neuropathy with a focal conduction block in the distal forearm, perhaps due to enlargement of the flexor carpi ulnaris and subsequent compression of the adjacent ulnar nerve, has been noted.[8b]

Gymnastics

The spine and spinal cord are at particular risk for injury with gymnastics. Young female gymnasts demonstrate quite abnormal radiographic changes for their age in more than 50% of cases, including spondylolysis, spondylolisthesis, retrolisthesis, and scoliosis. In young adult gymnasts, the most common mechanism of injury may be failure to perform a technically adequate somersault.[57]

The number of injuries to the cervical spine among gymnasts in some studies is next to that of only football and wrestling. Gymnastics is also one of the sports in which high school and college participants are at greatest risk of death.

The trampoline has come under attack in recent years as a cause of overall injury, and of SCIs, which comprise 12% of all trampoline-related injuries. Trampolines were held responsible for more than 6500 pediatric cervical spine injuries in 1998 in the United States, a fivefold increase in incidence over the past 10 years. Neck injuries more commonly occur in younger trampoline users. As a result of these injury patterns, many authors have called for a ban on the use of trampolines. Aeroball, a sport played on a trampoline court, has been associated with rare cervical spinal injury as well. As well as SCIs, a trampoline injury was deemed responsible for a vertebral artery dissection in an 11-year-old boy.

Femoral neuropathy secondary to iliacus hematoma within the nerve sheath has been seen in gymnasts. Lateral femoral cutaneous neuropathy was attributed to an intensive program of jumping rope involving repetitive hip flexion and extension. Repetitive wrist dorsiflexion was held responsible for a distal posterior interosseous neuropathy in a gymnast.

Hang Gliding and Paragliding

As would be expected in hang gliding, the majority of injuries (60%) occur during landing.[43a] As in other sports, the majority of injuries reported occur in 20- to 40-year-olds. In particular, SCIs leading to paraplegia or tetraplegia have been reported following faulty landings, and spinal injuries comprise 36% of all injuries.[43a]

Hockey

Despite increasing public concern about the number of hockey injuries in both amateur and professional leagues, good epidemiological studies of injury rates and incidence are lacking in ice hockey. Known injury rates are high, including a total injury rate of 75 per 100 high school level player-seasons, or 5 injuries per 1000 hours of play.[24] A Danish study of adult hockey players found an equally high injury rate of 90 per 100 players per season, or 4.7 injuries per 1000 hours of exposure.[36] Injury rates increase with age and are much higher in males (9:1) under the age of 18 years.[28b] In American men's collegiate ice hockey, overall injury rates are 4.9 per 1000 athlete exposures (13.8 per 1000 game athlete exposures and 2.2 per 1000 practice athlete exposures), with higher injury rates occurring during games than during practices.[20c] In adult players, concussions accounted for 12%–14% of all injuries.[24,36] In studies where all injuries are considered, the incidence of injuries in ice hockey is astonishingly high: 36 to 66 per 1000 player-game hours.

Some of the risk factors for injury in ice hockey are distinct from those in other sports. The more experienced player is significantly more likely to sustain injury.[24] The older, taller, and heavier a player is, the greater the risk of injury as well.[24] Positions most likely to sustain injury are defensemen and wings.[24] As with other sports, the majority of injuries occur during competition.[24] Particular events associated with injury include forechecking and breakout plays (head injury) and backchecking.[24] Illegal activities in hockey such as elbowing and high sticking are responsible for 26% of injuries.[24]

Bodychecking remains the most common cause of overall injury in hockey, as child and teenage players in contact leagues are 4 times more likely to be injured and 12 times more likely to receive a fracture than players in noncontact leagues. Female and male hockey players have similar overall injury rates (9.19 per 1000 male athlete-exposures [AE] vs. 7.77 per 1000 female AE) despite the fact that intentional bodychecking is not allowed in women's hockey.[79] Women are more likely than men to be injured with contact with the boards, but women sustain less serious injuries.[79] Injuries to children playing hockey are predominantly due to checking (57%). In contrast to adult players, only 4% of children's injuries are due to illegal activity; however, in one survey,[71b] 32% of children stated that they would check illegally to win, and 6% said that they would purposely injure their opponent to win.

Most hockey injuries affect the head and neck. Peak accelerations inside the helmet are significantly higher for hockey players than for football players, which likely contributes to the risk of head injury. Every season, 10%–12% of minor league hockey players 9–17 years old suffer a head injury, usually concussive. In some studies, concussion is the most common ice hockey–related injury in adults. Concussions occur in hockey at an overall estimated rate of 3.7 per athlete-season, or 4.6–6.0 concussions per 1000 player-game hours. The annual risk of concussion related to professional ice hockey is about 5% per player.

As with spinal injuries in hockey, the frequency of concussion may be increasing, although increased attentiveness and improved diagnostic skills may bias this observation. The rate of concussion rises with the age of the player. Players 5–17 years old suffer 2.8 concussions per 1000 player-hours; university hockey players have a rate of 4.2; and elite amateur players have a rate of 6.6.[28a] This strong correlation with age is probably associated with greater rates of bodychecking. In the professional ranks, concussion rates are even higher, ranging from 20 to 30 concussions per player-hour. Of even more concern is the significant increase in concussion rates during recent seasons of professional ice hockey. While this increase may be due to increased recognition and reporting, larger and faster players as well as harder sideboards and glass may be contributing factors. Head injuries in ice hockey are most commonly associated with collision with another player (45%); other causes include hitting the boards (34%) or being hit by a stick (22%). Surprisingly, fighting does not appear to be a common cause of concussion. In contrast to other sports, the incidence of concussion increases with higher levels of play and with the experience of the player. The use of face shields was studied in Canadian university hockey players, with comparison of full and half face shields, which seem to reduce the severity of concussion. Other, more severe forms of brain injury, such as epidural and subdural hematoma, are rare. There are rare occurrences of mortality in an observer or participant secondary to the head being struck by a puck. Fatal rupture of a left vertebral artery berry aneurysm followed a hockey puck's striking the left mastoid region in one case.

Spinal injuries, although less common, are probably the most devastating form of ice hockey–related injury. A Canadian registry of hockey–related spinal injuries includes cases from 1966 to 1996 of any fracture or dislocation of the spine, with or without injury to the spinal cord or nerve roots, as well as cases of transient quadriplegia.[85] Since 1981, there has been an apparent rise in spinal injuries, although reporting bias, increasing populations of hockey players, and better diagnostic and reporting skills may play a role.[85] An average of 17 major spinal injuries occur annually in Canada,[86a] and there have been six deaths there due to spinal injury over the monitored period.[85] The great majority of male athletes suffering major spinal injuries, usually at the cervical spinal level (85%),[85] are aged 16–20 years.[86a] Most commonly, spinal injuries are due to pushing or checking into the back, which may or may not lead to impact with the boards (40%), while impact with the boards accounts for 77% of spinal injuries.[85] The injury suffered at impact with the boards is often a burst fracture of the cervical spine while the neck is slightly flexed. Approximately 50% of SCIs occur in the 16- to 20-year age group, with most occurring in competitive games.[85] New rules, such as the introduction of *checking from behind* rules, may be more effective in decreasing the number of severe spinal injuries in ice hockey, but these rules have been implemented in Canada over the past two decades without changing the number of injuries reported annually.

Although more common in football players, the stinger has also been reported in hockey players. Axillary neuropathy due to direct trauma without shoulder dislocation has been documented in two hockey players.[65a] Inflatable ice hockey skates were blamed for the development of tarsal tunnel syndrome in a male recreational hockey player, with remission after he stopped wearing the skates. Peroneal neuropathy may occur either with laceration of the nerve by a skate blade or with direct blunt nerve trauma.

In-Line Skating, Roller Hockey, and Skateboarding

Although less common than ice hockey, professional roller hockey, or in-line hockey, may actually be associated with more overall injuries than ice hockey, perhaps due to differences in playing surfaces or the difficulty in stopping on in-line skates. One study found similar overall injury rates between roller hockey (139 per 1000 AE) and ice hockey (119 per 1000 AE), and noted that the number of games lost due to injuries was greater in ice hockey (8.3 games in ice hockey vs. 6.5 in in-line hockey).[30] Roller hockey may have a smaller incidence of head and neck injuries as ice hockey.[30]

In-line skating injuries are more common in boys (61%) with a mean age of 12 years. Head and neck injuries comprise 16% of all injuries, with inexperience commonly to blame. However, head injuries with in-line skating (34%) are significantly less common than with skateboarding (51%), and the severity of injury is significantly less. Helmet usage has been advocated in all three sports.

The use of tight roller skates has been associated with an entrapment of the superficial peroneal nerve.

Judo/Karate/Kickboxing and Related Sports

The incidence of injuries occurring in each of these disciplines is roughly similar, at least among karate, taekwondo, and Muay Thai kickboxing.[21] Annual injury rates are estimated to be 2.43/1000 for amateurs and 2.79/1000 for professionals.[21] In young taekwondo athletes involved in tournaments, young male athletes had a higher total head and neck injury rate (21.42/1000 AE) than females (16.91/1000 AE).[66] Next to contusion, concussion was the most common form of head injury in both sexes.[66] Male adult full-contact taekwondo competitors have slightly higher rates (7.04/1000 AE) than child athletes, with the dominant injury mechanism at all ages being a blow to the head (6.46/1000 AE).[66] Of all martial arts, taekwondo is perhaps the most likely to produce injury (three times greater than in karate).[94] Professional taekwondo athletes have an overall rate of injuries of 62.9/1000 athlete-exposures,[38b] and a concussion rate of 6.9/1000 athlete exposures.[38b]

Vertebral artery dissection due to cervical trauma during karate has led to a *locked-in* syndrome. Strokes have also been reported in martial arts competitors secondary to carotid dissection after neck-holding maneuvers or blows to the head or neck, including persons involved with kickboxing and French boxing. Cervical trauma in judo was associated with an acute cervical disc herniation and cervical myelopathy, perhaps associated with congenital cervical canal stenosis. More serious judo injuries have included chronic subdural hematomas and other forms of intracranial hemorrhage.[16c,40b] The occurrence of dementia pugilistica or other chronic cognitive changes in participants of martial arts has not been reported.

Peripheral nerve injury may occur with direct trauma leading to a presumed nerve contusion affecting the ulnar, axillary, spinal accessory, long thoracic, and peroneal nerves. A Morton's neuroma in a karate participant was attributed to repeated irritation of the ball of the foot from fighting stances.

Motorbiking

Injuries to motorcycle racers are quite common and are often associated with mortality (9% of all injuries).[89] Of all injuries, 10%–30% are head injuries and 25% of these head injuries are severe, with associated intracranial hemorrhage or mortality.[89] Spinal fractures are uncommon, however, representing only 4% of all injuries.

Mountain Climbing/Hiking

Injury rates among climbers are estimated at 2 per 1000 climbers.[81] Obviously, head and spinal injuries are possible, but no medical literature information on this is available. Headache, perhaps due to cerebral edema, is a prominent feature of acute mountain sickness, as well as dyspnea, weakness, asthenia, and nausea. Headache may be secondary to intracranial vascular dilatation due to hypercapnia prior to the development of hyperventilation due to hypoxia. The headache is often clinically similar to migraine. Cerebral edema likely occurs only above 12,000 feet and generally requires 2–3 days to develop. The incidence of cerebral edema in all climbers above 12,000 feet may be as high as 1.8%, and it may occur even in experienced climbers. Vasogenic edema likely predominates early, followed by later development of cytotoxic edema. High-altitude cerebral edema is associated with MRI changes including reversible white matter edema, with a predilection for the splenium of the corpus callosum.

Tarsal tunnel syndrome due to repetitive dorsiflexion of the ankle has rarely been found in mountain climbers. The hiker's backpack has been associated with rucksack paralysis, a syndrome with injury of the brachial plexus at the upper and middle trunks, and occasionally of the suprascapular, axillary, and long thoracic nerves.[26a] Traction on the brachial plexus is the probable basis, with the use of a pack without waist support being a proposed predisposing factor.[26a]

Rodeo

Injury rates vary by rodeo event but are highest in bull riding, bareback riding, and saddle bronc events.[8a] Bull riding has a high injury rate of 32 injuries per 1000 competitor-exposures (CE),[8a] while the overall injury rate is 2.3 per 100 CE, lower than that of most contact sports. Concussions account for 9% of all reported rodeo injuries,[8a] second only to knee injuries. Head and neck injuries, including concussions, in rodeo most commonly occur during dismounting due to the violent motions of the animal. In contrast to other sporting events, experienced rough stock rodeo competitors have a higher rate of injury, and of severe injury, than inexperienced competitors.

Axillary neuropathies secondary to shoulder dislocation, as well as a radial neuropathy secondary to humeral fracture, have been witnessed in rodeo cowboys.

Rugby and Australian Rules Football

The majority of rugby-related injuries affect the head and neck, and injuries to the cervical spine can be among the most serious injuries. The most common mechanism of neck injury appears to be cervical spine hyperflexion, often during scrimmaging or tackling, producing fracture dislocations of C4–C5 or C5–C6. The number of serious spinal injuries has increased over the past decade despite change in rules to prevent injury.[78] Transient quadriparesis has been observed in rugby as well.[78]

Cerebral concussion is also a concern in both of these sports. As noted with ice hockey, the incidence of concussion appears to be rising in Australian rules football, from 2.2 to 4.7 concussions per 1000 player-hours between 1992 and 1996.[60a] Concussion rates are higher in junior rules football players than in more senior players. Video analysis reveals that concussions are most commonly due to direct head contact, usually in the temporoparietal region. As in American football players, neurocognitive difficulties in rugby players correlate with the presence of concussion. Despite rugby players' belief that headgear offers protection against concussion (62%), only a minority report use of headgear (27%) and only 24% feel that helmet use should be mandatory.

Australian rules football players are at risk for obturator neuropathies due to fascial entrapment of the obturator nerve at the short abductor muscle of the thigh. Direct trauma to the anterolateral deltoid without shoulder dislocation has caused axillary neuropathy in rugby players.

Running

In a detailed assessment of 25 long-distance runners, no signs of clinical neuropathy were found, although mild changes in quantitative sensory threshold amplitudes and nerve conduction velocities suggesting subclinical neuropathy were noted.[19a] The *runner's foot* may also include subclinical electrophysiological abnormalities of the medial plantar nerve. Peroneal entrapment neuropathies due to entrapment at the fibular neck have occurred in long-distance runners, in one case bilaterally. One cause of peroneal neuropathy or superficial peroneal neuropathy due to running is inversion ankle sprain. Meralgia paresthetica has also been attributed to jogging. Tarsal tunnel syndrome can result from repetitive dorsiflexion of the ankle in very active runners. The anterior calcaneal branch of the tibial nerve can become entrapped between the edges of the deep fascia of abductor hallucis and os calcis. Other neuropathies of the foot in runners may affect the interdigital nerves, posterior tibial nerve, superficial peroneal nerve, sural nerve, and saphenous nerve. Morton's neuroma can occur in runners, and must be differentiated from plantar fasciitis and metatarsal bursitis.

Scuba Diving

Cerebral arterial oxygen gas bubble emboli in scuba divers have been clinically associated with alterations of consciousness, seizures, and focal neurological deficits.[56] Cerebral infarction has been reported in professional breath-hold divers during repetitive dives, with MRI demonstrating multiple T2-weighted hyperintensities corresponding to their neurological deficit. Neurological decompression illness, both cerebral and spinal dysfunction, and the presence of a large cardiopulmonary shunt have a probable association with this disease.

Headaches reported in divers include *skip breathing* headache, with migraine-like features, possibly associated with carbon dioxide accumulation. Another headache presenting with faciotemporal steady discomfort in divers is due to an excessively tight face mask or goggles placing pressure on superficial cutaneous nerves or the supraorbital nerve.[65b]

The most sensitive, but nonspecific, diagnostic testing procedures for patients with neurological decompression illness are electroencephalography (EEG) and MRI, although there is controversy regarding the presence of significant differences from controls. In divers with arterial gas emboli, MRI of the brain identified ischemic cerebrovascular lesions in 75% of patients compared to focal hyperintensities in 25% of divers with decompression illness only.[72] Magnetic resonance imaging of the spinal cord is less sensitive in divers with decompression illness, with focal hyperintensities identified in only 14% of patients.[72] Somatosensory evoked potentials (SSEP) have identified latency abnormalities in 81% of patients with decompression illness affecting the spinal cord. Brain stem auditory evoked potentials (BAEP) have demonstrated prolonged cochleopontine and cochleomesencephalic transmission times after diving in patients with clinical symptoms and signs of vertigo, postural and intentional hand tremor, ataxia, and opsoclonus. These features have also been referred to as *otic barotrauma*.

Lateral femoral cutaneous neuropathy may occur in scuba divers due to compression by the diver's weight belt.

Shooting

A single report of a long thoracic neuropathy due to positional stress with repetitive shooting postures has been reported in a world-class marksman.[92]

Skiing, Snowboarding, Sledding, Skating, and Ski Jumping

Although many winter sport injuries are orthopedic, head and spinal injuries are the most commonly occurring serious maladies.[80a] The incidence of downhill skiing injuries is 2.05 per 1000 skier-days,[12b] and mortality rate is 1.6 per 1,000,000 skier-days. Older skiers have the highest skiing-related injury rates, greatest in 55–64 year old skiers (29.0 per 1000 participants), and less in 65+ year old skiers (21.7 per 1000 participants), and 45–54 year old skiers (15.5 per 1000 participants).[93b] Twenty-five percent of sports-related SCIs in Germany were due to downhill skiing accidents.[80a] Estimated incidences of spinal injury due to downhill skiing and snowboarding are 0.01 per 1000 skier-days and 0.04 per 1000 snowboarder-days, respectively.[84] The majority of spinal injuries (70%) caused by downhill skiing result from a simple fall followed by striking a tree.[94a] Of all winter sports–related injuries, spinal trauma comprised about 5%, with 82% of these due to skiing accidents. Of all skiing-related injuries, 1.4% are spinal.[94a] Those most affected by spinal trauma in winter sports are in the 15- to 25-year age group (40%). In contrast to spinal injury in other sports and recreational activities, most skiing-related spinal traumas occur in the thoracolumbar region (47%), followed by the cervical region (39%), and are usually compressive (38%). In contrast, serious injuries to the spinal canal in snowboarding-related injuries occur mostly at the cervical level, and 3% of all snowboard-related injuries are spinal.[94] Snowboard-related spinal injuries also differ from skiing-related injuries in having a significantly higher incidence of transverse process fractures.[94a] Cervical spinal epidural hematoma with delayed presentation occurred in a snowboarder after striking his occiput.

Beginner snowboarders are significantly more often subject to spinal injury than beginner skiers.[94a] In contrast, intermediate to expert snowboarders are more likely to be injured while attempting tricks or jumping,[94a] usually leading to a backward fall and striking the occiput or cervical area. Intentional jumping may be the cause of injury in as many as 77% of snowboarding-related injuries compared to only 20% of skiing injuries. More than half (53%) of all surgically treated winter sports–related spinal injuries showed some neurological impairment of the spinal cord, while 17% had evidence of a complete transverse lesion of the spinal cord.[22] Often, the presence of a spinal injury in these athletes heralds another second serious injury, such as craniocerebral trauma (36%).[22]

Head injuries, although not as well publicized as spinal injuries, are common in downhill skiing. The estimated incidence of head injury is 6.5 per 100,000 visits for snowboarders and 3.8 per 100,000 visits for skiers. As in spinal injuries,[94a] beginning snowboarders are significantly more likely than beginning skiers to suffer a head injury. Head and face injuries comprise 17%–22% of injuries in recreational skiers reporting injuries.[49a] Approximately 22% of these injuries are related to concussion, and this is the body region injured most frequently in male skiers.[49a] In one Canadian study, 60% of skiers presenting after trauma had suffered a head injury, with approximately 69% of these injuries being concussive.[44] However, 14% of these patients suffered severe brain injuries, with an overall mortality rate of 4% with a severe head injury.[44] Compared to other forms of skiing-related injury, collision with a tree or another skier is the mechanism of injury in 47% of skiing-related head injuries.[44] Collisions with trees are more likely to produce severe head injury and mortality.[44] The risk of head injury from skiing is greatest in males and in those <35 years old.[44] Snowboarders appear to have even higher rates of head injury, three times higher than those of skiers.[44] In fact, snowboarders are more likely to suffer intracranial hemorrhage with head injury (71%) than skiers (28%). Risk factors for snowboarding-related major head injuries include falling backward (68%), occipital impact (66%), a gentle-moderate ski slope (76%), and inertia (76%).[55] Of the cases involving inertia, contracoup injury occurred in 8% of patients.[55] Risk factors for acute subdural hematoma as a snowboarding-related injury include falling backward and occipital impact.[55] Risk factors for subcortical hemorrhagic contusion include falling during a jump, a temporal impact, or falling on a jump platform.[55] In particular, jumping is a much more frequent cause of head injury in snowboarders (30%) than in skiers (2.5%). These snowboarding-related injuries are related to the opposite-edge phenomenon, which results from a fall on a gentle or moderate slope leading to occipital impact.[55] Rarely, skiers and snowboarders can be trapped in an avalanche, which may be associated with closed head injury. Suggestions have been made for snowboarders to wear protective gear over the occipital region and for beginners to refrain from jumping.[55]

Ski jumping, despite jumps of close to 100 meters high, is not commonly associated with injury. One estimate of risk in experienced ski jumpers was 9.4 injuries per 100 participant-years.[93a] Injury rates for non–World Cup and World Cup competitions were estimated at 4.3 and 1.2 injuries per 1000 skier-days, respectively, roughly equivalent to injury rates due to alpine skiing. Neurological injuries are uncommon, with four patients reported to have closed head injuries, including concussions. Freestyle skiing is an evolving sport involving high-speed jumps, somersaults, and twists. One patient suffered from multiple concussions after striking her occiput with a maneuver called a *snap back*, in which the participant's head snaps forward after landing with the body backward extended at least 45°.

Injury in short-track speed skating is seldom reported, but 6% of elite-level speed skaters are subject to concussions due to accidents during competition.[69] Junior figure skaters can also incur head injuries, which comprise about 10% of the injuries occurring in pairs skating, but this has not been reported to occur in single figure skaters.

The risk of sustaining an injury in luge is 0.39 per person per year, with most injuries being musculoskeletal.[14] Concussions comprise 2% of all injuries, most of which are due to crashes.[14] Recreational sledding has overall injury rates comparable to those of skiing, but has a significantly higher incidence of head injuries (34%) and spinal injuries (3%).

Cross-country skiing has an injury rate of 0.72 per 1000 skier-days, with injuries often occurring in inexperienced skiers on a downhill slope. An isolated femoral neuropathy has been reported in a single cross-country skier with vigorous activity, and ulnar neuropathy has been reported in another, perhaps due to forceful poling.

Snowmobiling and All-Terrain Vehicle Riding

Participants injured using snowmobiles are usually males (85%–90%) and have an average age of 25–29 years.[2] Helmets are used sparingly (35%), and alcohol intake is present in 44% of cases.[2] Serious head injuries comprise 34% of all injuries, while spinal injuries comprise 18%.[2] Snowmobiling can be associated with a risk of avalanche, depending upon the setting, and closed head injuries have been reported as a result.

All-terrain vehicles (ATVs) are commonly associated with injury in pediatric populations, which comprise 65% of injured riders.[76] Patients as young as 2–4 years of age have been reported to suffer injury from ATV riding.[76] As with snowmobiling, the minority of injured riders do not wear a helmet. The most common mechanisms of injury are falling off the ATV to the ground, striking a tree, or flipping backward.[76] Next to orthopedic injuries, closed head injuries are most commonly reported. In terms of neurological injuries, cranial injuries comprise 64% of the total and spinal injuries 36%.[76] Helmet use has been suggested for ATV users.[76]

Brachial plexus injuries occur in 4.8% of snowmobile accident victims,[52] often are complete (67%), and often are associated with orthopedic shoulder injuries. Supraclavicular injuries are more common and more severe than infraclavicular injuries.[52] One patient developed bilateral ulnar neuropathies at Guyon's canal after a full day of snowmobiling with his hands secured to the handlebars with duct tape.

Soccer

Many of the injuries experienced by soccer players are musculoskeletal, affecting the lower extremities, but head and neck injuries can also occur. Injury rates in college soccer players are estimated at 2.1 per 100 AE during total events (games plus practices),[70] with 1% of all injuries considered serious.[70] The frequency of injuries per team per season (FITS) for soccer is three for total events, much less than in American football.[70] Of all injuries over a 3-year period, MTBIs in soccer accounted for 6.2% in both boys' and girls' soccer at the child and high school levels.[67] At the high school level, injury rates per 100 player-seasons were 1.14 for girls' soccer and 0.92 for boys' soccer.[67]

Head injuries account for 4%–22% of soccer injuries, with an incidence of 1.7 per 1000 player hours, and with a concussion rate of 0.5 per 1000 player hours.[1b] The most common actions to lead to head injury are heading duels (58%), while the body parts striking the injured player's head are the elbow/arm/hand (41%), head (32%), and foot (13%).[1b] Direct heading of the ball is unlikely to produce head injury (6%) when compared to other forms of contact.[65c] The action of heading the ball leads to high accelerational forces with significantly higher peak accelerations (160%–180%) compared to impacts occurring in football or hockey. Sixty-three percent of Canadian university soccer players self-reported symptoms of a concussion during the previous year, while only 20% of the concussed soccer players realized that they had suffered a concussion due to lack of recognition of symptoms.[16a] Of those soccer players experiencing concussion, multiple concussions were experienced by 82%, suggesting that particular players are more susceptible to head injury.[16a] A recognized risk factor for concussion is female sex.[16a] Of all soccer positions, goalies are the players most commonly affected by concussion, even though they rarely head the ball.[16a] Although heading the ball causes most reported concussions, goal post injuries have been reported as well. Serious acute head injuries are less commonly reported in soccer. Both chronic-subacute subdural hematomas and an epidural hematoma were reported after a soccer ball struck a player's head. A female patient suffered a concussion and a basal skull fracture after being struck by a soccer ball, followed by bacterial meningitis and subsequent fatality.

The presence of long-term neuropsychological dysfunction in soccer players is controversial. One study of former soccer players found 81% to have mild-moderate neuropsychological impairment. In a study of professional active soccer players, the number of headers occurring in one season was associated with poor results on attention and visual/verbal memory tests, while occurrence of soccer-related concussions was related to poor results on attention and visuoperceptual processing tests.[49b] In another study, comparison of soccer players with control athletes revealed that amateur soccer players exhibited impaired performance on tests of planning and memory, with the number of concussions incurred inversely related to the neuropsychological performance.[49c] However, neither participation in soccer nor a history of soccer-related concussions was found to be associated with impaired neurocognitive function in high-level soccer players or teenage players in other studies. Electrophysiological evidence of abnormalities due to heading is improbable. Nonspecific abnormalities on EEG were found in about 33% of former and active soccer players, although EEG changes seemed to be more prevalent among players who considered themselves *nonheaders* as compared to *headers*. A noncontrolled study suggested that 33% of former soccer players had mild central cerebral atrophy identified with CT scan of the brain.

Rarely, peroneal nerve compression at the fibular neck may be attributed to excessive soccer playing.

Swimming

Rarely, the controversial thoracic outlet syndrome may be seen in association with hypertrophied pectoralis minor muscles of a swimmer.

Surfing

Prolonged wave surfing has been associated with a common peroneal neuropathy or a saphenous neuropathy. Surfer's myelopathy is a nontraumatic spinal cord injury that occurs in inexperienced surfers, presenting with back pain, paraparesis, and urinary retention. While more than 50% of surfers have a complete recovery, some remain mildly impaired or even paraplegic. Abnormal magnetic resonance imaging signal change can be identified in the lower thoracic spinal cord in some patients.[86b]

Tennis and Other Racquet Sports

Posterior interosseous nerve entrapment at the arcade of Frohse appears to be common among tennis players.[37] Suprascapular neuropathy has also been reported in tennis players as being due to compression at the suprascapular or supraglenoid notches, as well as to a ganglion cyst.[15] Long thoracic neuropathy is rarely reported in the tennis player, as well as radial nerve palsy secondary to fibrous arches at the lateral head of the triceps. Compression of the lateral cutaneous nerve of the forearm has also been seen in an active tennis player. The use of a constrictive wrist band or racquetball strap has been associated with a superficial radial neuropathy. Digital nerve injuries have been seen in very active tennis players. Serving arm shoulder pain with radiation due to possible thoracic outlet syndrome may rarely occur in tennis players.

Volleyball

Volleyball's injury rate is only 0.14 per 100 volleyball player-seasons for high school student participants, the lowest of 10 sports examined in one study.[59] A frequent form of mononeuropathy is an isolated entrapment of the suprascapular nerve at the spinoglenoid notch in the dominant arm.[20a] In one study of international-level volleyball players, the overall prevalence of suprascapular neuropathy was surprisingly high, between 33% and 45%, based upon clinical and electrophysiological examination. Up to 12% of volleyball players may have subclinical suprascapular neuropathy.[20a] Isolated mononeuropathies of the axillary nerve and long thoracic nerve have also been reported in younger volleyball players, perhaps related to a quadrilateral space syndrome in the case of axillary mononeuropathy.

Wrestling

Injury rates in wrestling are second only to those in football among high school competitors, with an injury rate of 1.58 per 100 player-seasons.[67] Wrestling also accounts for the second highest rate (10.5%) of MTBIs in college athletes.[67] Severe injuries consisting of CNS trauma leading to disability in wrestlers have been estimated to occur at a rate of 1 per 100,000 participants, with the majority of severe injuries occurring during competitions (80%).[4] A higher rate of injuries in the low- and middle-weight classes has been noted.[4] Certain positions in wrestling have been more frequently associated with injury, including the defensive position during takedown maneuvers (74%), the down position (23%), and the lying position (3%). Severe injuries include cervical spinal fractures (77%), spinal cord contusions with transient quadriparesis (12%), severe closed head injury (8%), and acute lumbar disc herniation (3%), resulting in quadriplegia (33%), residual neurological deficits (20%), paraplegia (3%), and death due to head injury (3%).[4] Reports of SCI are not unusual in wrestling competitions. The majority of severe head injuries are secondary to head-to-head collision but also can be due to slams to the mat. The rate of concussion in wrestling has been estimated at 2.5 per athlete-season in one study.[12] A unique wrestling-related injury occurred with a vertebral artery territory stroke due to a prolonged half-Nelson, as reported in a single 17-year-old.[74b]

Brachial plexus injury is relatively common in wrestling compared to other sports, and occurs with holds that force the opposing wrestler's head into a direction opposite to one shoulder, such as with a full- or half-Nelson hold. The stinger accounts for 37% of all head and neck injuries in competitive wrestlers. Other neuropathies in wrestlers include axillary neuropathy, ulnar neuropathy, CTS, long thoracic neuropathy, and suprascapular neuropathy.[42]

Sports without Evidence of Neurological Injuries

Participants in and fans of the sports not listed in Table 25.1 can be reassured that there are no medical reports in the recent medical literature regarding injuries to the nervous system in those sports.

Conclusion

Injury to the nervous system can occur with almost any sport. Even seemingly benign sporting activities such as darts and driving a golf cart have been associated with neurological injury. Particular sports are associated with alarming rates of injury, such as trampoline use, boxing, football, and hockey. Obviously, although this chapter has been as thorough as possible, many injuries occur outside of the scope of this chapter, probably due to lack of reporting. As observation of sports-related neurological injuries becomes more vigilant, this important field will continue to grow.

REFERENCES

1a. Andersen KV, Bovim G: Impotence and nerve entrapment in long distance amateur cyclists. Acta Neurol Scand 95(4):233–240, 1997.

1b. Andersen TE, Arnason A, Engebretsen L, Bahr R: Mechanisms of head injuries in elite football. Br J Sports Med 38(6):690–696, 2004.

1c. Aoki M, Kanaya K, Aiki H, Wada T, Yamashita T, Ogiwara N: Cubital tunnel syndrome in adolescent baseball players: A report of six cases with 3- to 5-year follow-up. Arthroscopy. 21(6):758, 2005.

2. Beilman GJ, Brasel KJ, Dittrich K, Seatter S, Jacobs

DM, Croston JK: Risk factors and patterns of injury in snowmobile crashes. Wilderness Environ Med 10(4): 226–232, 1999.

3. Blonstein JL, Clarke E: Further observations on the medical aspects of amateur boxing. BMJ 1:362–364, 1957.
4. Boden BP, Lin W, Young M, Mueller FO: Catastrophic injuries in wrestlers. Am J Sports Med 30(6):791–795, 2002.
5. Boden BP, Tacchetti R, Mueller FO: Catastrophic cheerleading injuries. Am J Sports Med 31: 881–889, 2003.
6. Braithwaite IJ: Bilateral median nerve palsy in a cyclist. Br J Sports Med 26(1):27–28, 1992.
7. Burnham RS, Steadward RD: Upper extremity peripheral nerve entrapments among wheelchair athletes: Prevalence, location, and risk factors. Arch Phys Med Rehabil 75(5):519–524, 1994.

8a. Butterwick DJ, Hagel B, Nelson DS, LeFave MR, Meeuwisse WH: Epidemiologic analysis of injury in five years of Canadian professional rodeo. Am J Sports Med 30(2):193–198, 2002.

8b. Campbell WW: AEEM case report #18: Ulnar neuropathy in the distal forearm. Muscle Nerve 12(5):347–352, 1989.

9. Chan RC, Chiu JW, Chou CL, Chen JJ: [Median nerve lesions at wrist in cyclists] [in Chinese]. Zhonghua Yi Xue Za Zhi (Taipei) 48(2):121–124, 1991.
10. Chang TL, Fields CB, Brenner RA, Wright JL, Lomax T, Scheidt PC: Sports injuries: An important cause of morbidity in urban youth. District of Columbia Child/Adolescent Injury Research Network. Pediatrics 105(3): E32, 2000.
11. Clancy WG, Brand RL, and Bergfield JA: Upper trunk brachial plexus injuries in contact sports. Am J Sports Med 5: 209–216, 1977.

12a. Clarke KS: Prevention: An epidemiologic view. In: Torg JS (ed): Athletic Injuries to the Head, Neck and Face. Philadelphia, Lea and Febiger, 1982, pp 15–26.

12b. Corra, S, Conci A, Conforti G, Sacco G, De Giorgi F: Skiing and snowboarding injuries and their impact on the emergency care system in South Tyrol: A restrospective analysis for the winter season 2001–2002. Inj Control Saf Promot 11(4):281–285, 2004.

13. Corsellis JAN, Bruton CJ, Freeman-Browne D: The aftermath of boxing. Psychol Med 3:270–303, 1973.
14. Cummings RS Jr, Shurland AT, Prodoehl JA, Moody K, Sherk HH: Injuries in the sport of luge. Epidemiology and analysis. Am J Sports Med 25(4):508–513, 1997.
15. Daubinet G, Rodineau J: [Paralysis of the suprascapular nerve and tennis. Apropos of three groups of professional players]. Schwiez Z Sportmed 39:113–118, 1991.

16a. Delaney JS, Lacroix VJ, Leclerc S, Johnston KM: Concussions among university football and soccer players. Clin J Sport Med 12(6):331–338, 2002.

16b. Delaney JS, Lacroix VJ, Leclerc S, Johnston KM: Concussions during the 1997 Canadian Football League season. Clin J Sport Med 10(1):9–14, 2000.

16c. DeVera-Reyes JA: Three cases of chronic subdural hematoma caused by the practice of judo. Acta Luso Esp Neurol Psiquiatr 29:53–56, 1970.

17. DeVivo MJ, Sekar P: Prevention of spinal cord injuries that occur in swimming pools. Spinal Cord 35(8):509–515, 1997.
18. Diamond PT, Gale SD: Head injuries in men's and women's lacrosse: A 10 year analysis of the NEISS database. National Electronic Injury Surveillance System. Brain Inj 15(6):537–544, 2001.

19a. Dyck PJ, Classen SM, Stevens JC, O'Brien PC: Assessment of nerve damage in the feet of long-distance runners. Mayo Clin Proc 62:568, 1987.

19b. Ekin JA, Sinaki M: Vertebral compression fractures sustained during golfing. Mayo Clin Proc 68:566–570, 1993.

20a. Ferretti A, Cerullo G, Russo G: Suprascapular neuropathy in volley-ball players. J Bone Joint Surg [Am] 69:260–263, 1987.

20b. Fraim CJ, Peters BH: Unusual cause of nerve entrapment. JAMA 242(23):2557–2558, 1979.

20c. Flik K, Lyman S, Marx RG: American collegiate men's ice hockey: An analysis of injuries. Am J Sports Med 33(2):183–187, 2005.

21. Gartland S, Malik MH, Lovell ME: Injury and injury rates in Muay Thai kick boxing. Br J Sports Med 35(5): 308–313, 2001.
22. Genelin A, Kathrein A, Daniaux A, Lang T, Seykora P: [Current status of spinal injuries in winter sports]. Schweiz Z Med Traumatol (1):17–20, 1994.
23. Gennarelli TA: Cerebral concussions and diffuse brain injuries. In: Cooper PR (ed): Head Injury, 2nd ed. Baltimore, Wilkins & Wilkins, 1987, pp 108–124.
24. Gerberich SG, Finke R, Madden M, et al: An epidemiologic study of high school ice hockey injuries. Child Nerv Syst 3:59–64, 1987.
25. Gierup J, Larsson M, Lennquist S: Incidence and nature of horse-riding injuries. Acta Chirop Scand 142:57–61, 1976.

26a. Goodson JD: Brachial plexus injury from light tight backpack straps. N Engl J Med 305(9):524–525, 1981.

26b. Hansen KS, Eide GE, Omenaas E, Engesaeter LB, Viste A: Bicycle-related injuries among young children related to age at debut of cycling. Accid Anal Prev 37(1):71–75, 2005.

27. Hof PR, Bouras C, Buee L, Delacourte A, Perl DP, Morrison JH: Differential distribution of neurofibrillary tangles in the cerebral cortex of dementia pugilistica and Alzheimer's disease cases. Acta Neuropathol (Berl) 85(1):23–30, 1992.

28a. Honey CR: Brain injury in ice hockey. Clin J Sport Med 8(1):43–46, 1998.

28b. Hostetler SG, Xiang H, Smith GA: Characteristics of ice hockey-related injuries treated in US emergency departments, 2001–2002. Pediatrics 114(6):661–666, 2004.

29a. Howse C: Wrist injuries in sport. Sports Med 17(3):163–175, 1994.

29b. Hsu WC, Chen WH, Oware A, Chiu HC: Unusual entrapment neuropathy in a golf player. Neurology 59(4):646–647, 2002.

30. Hutchinson MR, Milhouse C, Gapski M: Comparison of injury patterns in elite hockey players using ice versus

in-line skates. Med Sci Sports Exerc 30(9):1371–1373, 1998.

31. Hwang V, Shofer FS, Durbin DR, Baren JM: Prevalence of traumatic injuries in drowning and near drowning in children and adolescents. Arch Pediatr Adolesc Med 157(1):50–53, 2003.

32a. Jackson DL, Hynninen BC, Caborn DN, McLean J: Electrodiagnostic study of carpal tunnel syndrome in wheelchair basketball players. Clin J Sport Med 6(1):27–31, 1996.

32b. Jamieson DR, Ballantyne JP: Unique presentation of a prolapsed thoracic disk: Lhermitte's symptom in a golf player. Neurology 45(6):1219–1221, 1995.

33. Jordan BD: Neurologic aspects of boxing. Arch Neurol 44(4):453–459, 1987.

34. Jordan BD, Campbell E: Acute boxing injuries among professional boxers in New York State: A two year survey. Phys Sports Med 12:53–67, 1988.

35. Jordan BD, Relkin NR, Ravdin LD, Jacobs AR, Bennett A, Gandy S: Apolipoprotein E epsilon4 associated with chronic traumatic brain injury in boxing. JAMA 278(2): 136–140, 1997.

36. Jorgensen V, Schmidt-Olsen S: The epidemiology of ice hockey injuries. Br J Sports Med 20:7–9, 1986.

37. Kaplan PE: Posterior interosseous neuropathies: Natural history. Arch Phys Med Rehabil 65(7):399–400, 1984.

38a. Katoh S, Shingu H, Ikata T, Iwatsubo E: Sports-related spinal cord injury in Japan (from the nationwide spinal cord injury registry between 1990 and 1992). Spinal Cord 34(7):416–421, 1996.

38b. Kazemi M, Pieter W: Injuries at the Canadian National Tae Kwon Do Championships: A prospective study. BMC Musculoskelet Disord 5(1):22, 2004.

39. Kelly EG: Major injuries occurring during use of a golf cart. Orthopedics 19(6):519–521, 1996.

40a. Kessler KJ, Uribe JW: Complete isolated axillary nerve palsy in college and professional football players: A report of six cases. Clin J Sports Med 4:272–274, 1994.

40b. Koiwai EK: Fatalities associated with judo. Phys Sportsmed 9:61–66, 1981.

41. Kriss TC, Kriss VM: Equine-related neurosurgical trauma: A prospective series of 30 patients. J Trauma 43(1):97–99, 1997.

42. Krivickas LS, Wilbourn AJ: Sports and peripheral nerve injuries: Report of 190 injuries evaluated in a single electromyography laboratory. Muscle Nerve 21(8):1092–1094, 1998.

43a. Lautenschlager S, Karli U, Matter P: [Paragliding accidents—a prospective analysis in Swiss mountain regions]. Z Unfallchir Versicherungsmed Suppl 1:55–65, 1993.

43b. Lee BH, Schofer JL, Koppelman FS: Bicycle safety helmet legislation and bicycle-related non-fatal injuries in California. Accid Anal Prev 37(1):93–102, 2005.

44. Levy AS, Hawkes AP, Hemminger LM, Knight S: An analysis of head injuries among skiers and snowboarders. J Trauma 53(4):695–704, 2002.

45. Liveson JA, Bronson MJ, Pollack MA: Suprascapular nerve lesions at the spinoglenoid notch: Report of three cases and review of the literature. J Neurol Neurosurg Psychiatry 54:241–243, 1991.

46. Long RR, Sargent JC, Pappas AM, Hammer K: Pitcher's arm: An electrodiagnostic enigma. Muscle Nerve 19(10): 1276–1281, 1996.

47. Lorei MP, Hershman EB: Peripheral nerve injuries in athletes. Treatment and prevention. Sports Med 16(2): 130–147, 1993.

48. Macgregor DM: Golf related head injuries in children. Emerg Med J 19(6):576–577, 2002.

49a. MacNab AJ, Cadman R: Demographics of alpine skiing and snowboarding injury: Lessons for prevention programs. Inj Prev 2(4):286–289, 1996.

49b. Matser JT, Kessels AG, Lezak MD, Troost J: A dose-response relation of headers and concussions with cognitive impairment in professional soccer players. J Clin Exp Neuropsychol 23(6):770–774, 2001.

49c. Matser EJ, Kessels AG, Lezak MD, Jordan BD, Troost J: Neuropsychological impairment in amateur soccer players. JAMA 282(10):971–973, 1999.

50. McCrory PR, Berkovic SF: Second impact syndrome. Neurology 50(3):677–683, 1998.

51. Meeuwisse WH, Hagel BE, Mohtadi NG, Butterwick DJ, Fick GH: The distribution of injuries in men's Canada West university football. A 5-year analysis. Am J Sports Med 28(4):516–523, 2000.

52. Midha R: Epidemiology of brachial plexus injuries in a multitrauma population. Neurosurgery 40(6):1182–1188, 1997.

53. Mueller FO, Blyth CS: A survey of 1981 college lacrosse injuries. Phys Sports Med 10:87–93, 1982.

54. Myles ST, Mohtadi NG, Schnittker J: Injuries to the nervous system and spine in downhill skiing. Can J Surg 35(6):643–648, 1992.

55. Nakaguchi H, Tsutsumi K: Mechanisms of snowboarding-related severe head injury: Shear strain induced by the opposite-edge phenomenon. J Neurosurg 97(3):542–548, 2002.

56. Newton HB: Neurologic complications of scuba diving. Am Fam Physician 63(11):2211–2218, 2001.

57. Noguchi T: A survey of spinal cord injuries resulting from sport. Paraplegia 32(3):170–173, 1994.

58. Ogawa K, Ui M: Humeral shaft fracture sustained during arm wrestling: Report on 30 cases and review of the literature. J Trauma 42(2):243–246, 1997.

59. Ogawa K, Yoshida A: Throwing fracture of the humeral shaft. An analysis of 90 patients. Am J Sports Med 26(2): 242–246, 1998.

60a. Orchard J: AFL 1996 Injury Report. Melbourne, Australian Football League Medical Officers Association, 1995, pp 7–8.

60b. Ozdoba C, Weis J, Plattner T, Dirnhofer R, Yen K: Fatal scuba diving incident with massive gas embolism in cerebral and spinal arteries. Neuroradiology 47(6):411–416, 2005.

61. Pasternack JS, Veenema KR, Callahan CM: Baseball injuries: A Little League survey. Pediatrics 98(3 pt 1):445–448, 1996.

62. Pellman EJ, Powell JW, Viano DC, Casson IR, Tucker AM, Feuer H, Lovell M, Waeckerle JF, Robertson DW: Concussion in professional football: Epidemiological features of game injuries and review of the literature—part 3. Neurosurgery 54(1):81–94, 2004.
63. Pellman EJ, Viano DC, Tucker AM, Casson IR, Committee on Mild Traumatic Brain Injury, National Football League: Concussion in professional football: Location and direction of helmet impacts—Part 2. Neurosurgery 53(6): 1328–1340, 2003.
64. Pellman EJ, Viano DC, Tucker AM, Casson IR, Waeckerle JF: Concussion in professional football: Reconstruction of game impacts and injuries. Neurosurgery 53(4):799–812; discussion 812–814, 2003.
65a. Perlmutter GS, Leffert RD, Zarins B: Direct injury to the axillary nerve in athletes playing contact sports. Am J Sports Med 25(1):65–68, 1997.
65b. Pestronk A, Pestronk S: Goggle migraine. N Engl J Med 308:226–227, 1983.
65c. Pickett W, Streight S, Simpson K, Brison RJ: Head injuries in youth soccer players presenting to the emergency department. Br J Sports Med 39(4):226–231, 2005.
66. Pieter W, Zemper ED: Head and neck injuries in young taekwondo athletes. J Sports Med Phys Fitness 39(2): 147–153, 1999.
67. Powell JW, Barber-Foss KD: Traumatic brain injury in high school athletes. JAMA 282(10):958–963, 1999.
68. Prabhu VC, Bailes JE: Chronic subdural hematoma complicating arachnoid cyst secondary to soccer-related head injury: Case report. Neurosurgery 50(1):195–197, 2002.
69. Prall JA, Winston KR, Brennan R: Spine and spinal cord injuries in downhill skiers. J Trauma 39(6):1115–1118, 1995.
70. Radelet MA, Lephart SM, Rubinstein EN, Myers JB: Survey of the injury rate for children in community sports. Pediatrics 110(3):e28, 2002.
71a. Rayan GM: Archery-related injuries of the hand, forearm, and elbow. South Med J 85(10):961–964, 1992.
71b. Reid SR, Losek JD: Factors associated with significant injuries in youth ice hockey players. Pediatr Emerg Care 15(5):310–313, 1999.
72. Reuter M, Tetzlaff K, Hutzelmann A, Fritsch G, Steffens JC, Bettinghausen E, Heller M: MR imaging of the central nervous system in diving-related decompression illness. Acta Radiol 38(6):940–964, 1997.
73. Rivara FP, Thompson DC, Thompson RS, Rebolledo V: Injuries involving off-road cycling. J Fam Pract 44(5):481–485, 1997.
74a. Roberts AH: Brain Damage in Boxers. London, Pittman Medical Scientific Publishing, 1969.
74b. Rogers L, Sweeney PJ: Stroke: A neurological complication of wrestling: A case of brainstem stroke in a 17-year-old athlete. Am J Sports Med 7:352–354, 1979.
75. Ross RT, Ochsner MG Jr: Acute intracranial boxing-related injuries in U.S. Marine Corps recruits: report of two cases. Mil Med 164(1):68–70, 1999.
76. Russell A, Boop FA, Cherny WB, Ligon BL: Neurologic injuries associated with all-terrain vehicles and recommendations for protective measures for the pediatric population. Pediatr Emerg Care 14(1):31–35, 1998.
77. Sammarco GL, Miller EH: Forefoot conditions in dancers: Part II. Foot Ankle 3(2):83–98, 1982.
78. Scher AT: Rugby injuries to the cervical spine and spinal cord: A 10-year review. Clin Sports Med 17(1):195–206, 1998.
79. Schick DM, Meeuwisse WH: Injury rates and profiles in female ice hockey players. Am J Sports Med 31(1):47–52, 2003.
80a. Schmitt H, Gerner HJ: Paralysis from sport and diving accidents. Clin J Sport Med 11(1):17–22, 2001.
80b. Schulz MR, Marshall SW, Mueller FO, Yang J, Weaver NL, Kalsbeek WD, Bowling JM: (2004) Incidence and risk factors for concussion in high school athletes, North Carolina, 1996–1999. Am J Epidemiol 160(10):937–944, 2004.
81. Schusman LC, Lutz LJ: Mountaineering and rock climbing accidents. Phys Sports Med 10:52–61, 1982.
82. Sinson G, Zager EL, Kline DG: Windmill pitcher's radial neuropathy. Neurosurgery 34(6):1087–1089, 1994.
83. Sotiropoulos SV, Jackson MA, Tremblay GF, Burry VF, Olson LC: Childhood lawn dart injuries. Summary of 75 patients and patient report. Am J Dis Child 144(9):980–982, 1990.
84. Tarazi F, Dvorak MF, Wing PC: Spinal injuries in skiers and snowboarders. Am J Sports Med 27(2):177–180, 1999.
85. Tator CH, Carson JD, Cushman R: Hockey injuries of the spine in Canada, 1966–1996. Can Med Assoc J 162(6): 787–788, 2000.
86a. Tator CH, Carson JD, Edmonds VE: New spinal injuries in hockey. Clin J Sport Med 7(1):17–21, 1997.
86b. Thompson TP, Pearce J, Chang G, Madamba J: Surfer's myelopathy. Spine 29(16):353–356, 2004.
87. Trammell TR, Olivary SE: Crash and injury statistics from Indy-Car racing 1985–1989. In: Association for Advancement of Automotive Medicine, Proceedings, 34th Annual Conference, Scottsdale, AZ, October 1–3, 1990. The Association, 1991, pp 329–335.
88. Upadhyay V, Tan A: Cricketing injuries in children: From the trivial to the severe. NZ Med J 113(1105):81–83, 2000.
89. Varley GW, Spencer-Jones R, Thomas P, Andrews D, Green AD, Stevens DB: Injury patterns in motorcycle road racers: Experience on the Isle of Man 1989–1991. Injury 24(7):443–446, 1993.
90. Viegas SF, Torres FG: Cherry pitter's thumb. Case report and review of the literature. Orthop Rev 18(3):336–338, 1989.
91. Weiss BD: Clinical syndromes associated with bicycle seats. Clin Sports Med 13(1):175–186, 1994.
92. Woodhead AB: Paralysis of the serratus anterior in a world class marksman. Am J Sports Med 13:359–362, 1985.

93a. Wright JR Jr, McIntyre L, Rand JJ, Hixson EG: Nordic ski jumping injuries. A survey of active American jumpers. Am J Sports Med 19(6):615–619, 1991.

93b. Xiang H, Kelleher K, Shields BJ, Brown KJ, Smith GA: Skiing- and snowboarding-related injuries treated in U.S. emergency departments, 2002. J Trauma 58(1):112–118, 2005.

94a. Yamakawa H, Murase S, Sakai H, Iwama T, Katada M, Niikawa S, Sumi Y, Nishimura Y, Sakai N: Spinal injuries in snowboarders: Risk of jumping as an integral part of snowboarding. J Trauma 50(6):1101–1105, 2001.

94b. Zetaruk MN, Violan MA, Zurakowski D, Micheli LJ: Injuries in martial arts: A comparison of five styles. Br J Sports Med 39(1):29–33, 2005.

Chapter 26
Athletic Head Injury

RICHARD S. POLIN AND NIDHI GUPTA

A ubiquitous feature of participation in organized or recreational athletics is the inherent risk of injury. Although most participants never consider the possibility of head injury, brain trauma remains a major cause of both severe and mild disability after athletic injury. In this chapter, the epidemiology of brain trauma in sports is defined, focusing on the well-established connection of these injuries with some high-profile athletic activities. The literature regarding head injury associated with boxing, football, and several other sports is then reviewed. We differentiate between the short- and long-term effects of athletic head injury, focusing on the neurological examination, neuroradiographic evaluation, and neuropsychological outcome parameters. Next, we discuss the prevention, management, assessment, and treatment of acute injuries, including new pharmacological interventions. A prospective study at our institution of clinical symptoms and neuropsychological deficits in athletes with mild head injury is considered. Finally, several controversies in sports neurotrauma are presented, including the timing of return to activity after head injury and the effect that recurrent mild trauma has on the risk of catastrophic injury and the second impact syndrome.

It is a common perception that clinicians in the neurological sciences have ignored the field of sports medicine. In the preface to *Athletic Injuries to the Head, Neck, and Face*, Torg[107] writes that, with rare exceptions, "the concern of the neurosurgical community with neurologic problems confronting those who participate in recreational and competitive athletics can be described as underwhelming. As one prominent neurosurgeon admitted, 'If it's not a brain tumor, we are not really interested.'" However, Dr. Robert Cantu, a past president of the American College of Sports Medicine, is a neurosurgeon, and well-attended seminars have become a constant feature at annual neurosurgical meetings. Perhaps a more telling statistic is Jorgensen and Schmidt-Olsen's[53] finding that, although 72% of knee injuries suffered in the Danish elite ice hockey leagues were managed by a physician, only 8% of head injuries in the same league were examined by a physician. Fortunately, the attention paid to these injuries is increasing. Greater cooperation from professional and college sports leagues and athletic organizations has resulted in better-quality studies and more scientifically based recommendations for athletes and trainers.

Epidemiology of Sports Head Injuries

Athletic head injury encompasses a spectrum from mold head injury, characterized by transient alteration in consciousness, to severe injuries causing major morbidity and mortality. Sequelae range from a transient inability to function to the extreme of dementia pugilistica. The incidence of mild head injury can be difficult to quantify accurately because complete documentation is impossible; however, a concerted effort to document severe cases has allowed a more accurate assessment of fatal and near-fatal traumatic brain injury.

Regional reports on the incidence of severe head injury in sports depend considerably on the activities undertaken in the particular area. For instance, in a 5-year study of 52 cases of athletic brain trauma (representing 2.7% of all head injury patients needing a hospital stay) requiring hospital admission in Glasgow, Lindsay et al.[63] reported that golf and horseback-riding injuries were most common. Among these 52 victims, 39 were male. There was one death and six cases of prolonged disability, with riding accidents associated with the highest frequency of coma on presentation and late disability. The same article claimed a higher percentage of athletic injuries among all head trauma cases compared to other series of head trauma (versus motor vehicle accidents, fall, etc.), with 11% of all brain trauma cases in 1974 in Scotland occurring during leisure activities.[63,97] Vigouroux et al.[112] recorded all athletic injuries occurring during a 10-year period in southern France and found that equestrian events and soccer accounted for the majority of severe cranial events. Lingard et al.[64] examined all athletic injuries occurring during winter in New Zealand. The overwhelming majority (103 of 123) of injuries involved rugby, with six soccer and six horseback-riding injuries tied for second place. Overall, athletic injuries accounted for 15% of all head traumas requiring hospital admission.

Carlsson[19] reported from a Swedish population study that the largest percentage of athletic injuries occurred, as would be expected, during the second to the fourth decades, with a peak of approximately 5000 accidents among 100,000 teenagers. Derek Bruce's series from the United States suggests a similar pattern.[8] The majority of American athletic participants, and therefore accident victims, in organized sports come from high school and college. The National Center for Catastrophic Sports Inury Research was established in 1982 at Chapel Hill, North Carolina, to compile and analyze national statistics. Football accounted for the majority of serious head injuries, with 34 fatalities resulting directly from brain trauma and 18 additional cases of severe brain injury occurring between the fall of 1982 and the spring of 1989. Wrestling accounted for 24 serious or fatal injuries in this interval, almost all involving the head or spine.[77] At least one death from brain stem ischemia resulting from vertebral artery injury after a hyperflexion neck injury has been reported.[92] The required use of protective headgear limited ice hockey injuries to one. Baseball, gymnastics, diving, and soccer each produced cases of brain injury at the high school and college levels during this period.[77] Acute injury from motor sports is not considered in this review, as the mechanism of injury is similar to that discussed in existing studies of series of brain trauma.

Boxing

No sport has garnered more adverse publicity because of its neurological sequelae than boxing. The debate over the risk of long-term neurological and neuropsychiatric deficits among ex-boxers and the concern generated by recent catastrophic injury in the ring have focused the attention of the medical community and the public on the risks of boxing.

Chronic Brain Injury from Boxing

Literature Review of Boxing Injury

In 1928, Harrison Martland[68] delivered a paper before the New York Pathological Society on the mannerisms of fighters after repeated blows to the head. He termed the condition *punch drunk* and stated that it developed most rapidly in sparring partners and poor technicians who absorbed the greatest number of blows to the head. Martland described the earliest symptoms as including "uncertainty in equilibrium," "very slight flopping of one foot or leg in walking," and "periods of slight mental confusion." As the disease progressed, Martland noted "a general slowing in muscular movements of the head." Finally, in the late stages of the disease, Martland remarked on a similarity in gait and facial expression to persons with Parkinson's disease, with severe truncal ataxia and often a coinciding degree of mental deterioration. Martland attributed this punch-drunk condition to a mild form of diffuse deep cerebral hemorrhages that he had observed in a series of autopsy examinations of trauma victims. Millspaugh later coined the term *dementia pugilistica* to describe the condition.[76]

Neuropathology and Neuroradiology

Speculation on the neuropathological changes in the brains of ex-fighters with dementia pugilistica was first advanced by Brandenberg and Hallervorder[5] in their report of a 51-year-old ex-boxer with parkinsonism and dementia who suffered a lethal intracerebral hemorrhage. They documented histology suggestive of Alzheimer's disease with amyloid vascular deposition. Grahmann and Ule[35] described a 46-year-old victim of dementia pugilistica with considerable cortical atrophy, a large cavum septum pellucidum, and neurofibrillary tangles found most extensively in the brain stem. The finding of cavum septum pellucidum was replicated by Spillane[102] in four of five ex-boxers undergoing air encephalography and by Mawdsley and Ferguson,[69] who found a cavum septum pellucidum and neurofibrillary changes of severe Alzheimer's disease in the midbrain of four ex-fighters. Constantinies and Tissot[24] described the brain of a former Swiss champion pugilist who had developed dementia, early parkinsonism, and epilepsy before his death at age 58. The patient not only had a cavum septum pellucidum and diffuse neurofibrillary changes of Alzheimer's disease in the mesial temporal gray matter, but also extensive gliosis and complete pigment loss in the substantia nigra, suggesting a direct cause-and-effect relationship for progressive parkinsonism in these patients. Payne[81] added the observation of small foci of degeneration scattered in the cerebral and cerebellar white matter.

The most extensive neuropathological examination to date is the Corsellis et al.[27] study of the brains of 15 ex-boxers with clinical symptoms of dementia pugilistica. Twelve of these 15 individuals had been professional boxers, and 2 were former world champions. The most striking abnormality was the presence of a fenestrated cavum septum pellucidum in 12 of 13 ex-boxers (2 ex-boxers who had this abnormality died of intraventricular hemorrhage and were excluded) compared to only 3% of 500 controls examined prospectively. Moreover, the fighters' abnormalities were on average three times as wide as those of the controls, and the septal leaves were more highly fenestrated. In the fighters, the fornix and corpus callosum were detached from each other and splayed. The researchers hypothesized that during repeated blows to the head, the thin dorsal septum pellucidum is stretched and detached from the more solid ventral septum, which is tethered by the fornix. The presence of vetriculomegaly further stretches the septum and accelerates cavum formation.

Isherwood and colleagues[46] performed the first systematic radiographic analysis of ex-boxers and found that 9 of 16 (56%) had a cavum septum pellucidum in communication with the ventricular system. With the advent of routine computed tomography (CT) for active fighters, some current pugilists have also been found to harbor a cavum septum pellucidum. After two such findings within the first 13 boxers tested, Macpherson and Teasdale[66] undertook a study of 1000 normal subjects and found the overall rate of the anomaly to be 5.5%. A cavum velum interpositum was discovered in 9.5% of these normal subjects and a cavum vergae in 0.5%. Bogdanoff and Natter[4] examined a series of 1914 consecutive adults undergoing CT scans and found 14 (0.73%) with a cavum septum pellucidum. Of these 14, 9 were male. Furthermore, of these nine, five were former boxers, and one had a history of repeated head trauma in adolescence. Three of the five former boxers demonstrated evidence of progressive dementia.

The septum pellucidum normally contains cerebrospinal fluid (CSF) in the fetus and at birth but seals off early in infancy. There is no evidence that the incidence of the anomaly of cavum septum pellucidum increases with age, with the incidence of dementia, or with the degree of cerebral atrophy. The average width of the cavum in former boxers is more than 5 mm compared to an average of between 1.6 and 2.5 mm in controls. Many authors, including Corsellis[26] and Casson et al.,[24] feel that the presence of a cavum abnormality in boxers represents the effects of chronic, repeated brain injury and will in time lead to dementia pugilistica. However, by examining all boxers, one will find that a certain percentage of young boxers, approximately 5%, will harbor this developmental anomaly independent of their fighting careers. The question of how to resolve this issue is a potentially important one since the growth pattern of a cavum septum pellucidum in fighters is not known.

We suggest that routine CT scanning be performed on all prospective pugilists, and then once every 2 years and after each knockout. The appearance of a new cavum anomaly should immediately disqualify the individual from further participation in boxing. If the fighter had a known cavum septum pellucidum before his career, he should be allowed to continue unless the space grows by more than 1 mm. In this way, the boxing federations could curtail chronic brain damage while not dismissing those who simply harbor a developmental anomaly.

Cerebellar damage might also be inferred from the characteristic wide-based gait of the ex-boxer. Corsellis and colleagues[27] uncovered evidence of Purkinje cell loss, thinning of the granule cell layer, gliosis, and cortical scarring on the inferior surface of the lateral lobes in the region of the cerebellar tonsils. Purkinje cell loss was marked compared to age-matched controls in 9 of 11 former fighters. It was felt that this damage, which was largely confined to the tonsils, might result from repetitive instances of transient tonsillar herniation from blows to the head. Transient vascular insufficiency to the vulnerable Purkinje cells might extend the damaged region.

Cortical damage had been more difficult to determine neuropathologically than septal cavum formation or tonsillar herniation. In Corsellis and colleagues'[27] investigation there was no clear pattern of damage in the brains of former boxers. They found patchy areas of demyelination, but these were neither localized nor consistent. Diffuse axonal injury is the most likely finding in a brain subjected to repeated trauma; however, no specific staining was performed to test for this condition. The only consistent pattern was the finding of neurofibrillary tangles without (except in one instance) senile plaques. Tokuda et al.[106] reexamined these brains with immunohistochemical markers for amyloid beta-protein and paired helical filaments (PHF)-related gamma-protein and found significant temporal lobe staining from both markers in areas with prominent neurofibrillary tangles. Furthermore, Roberts and colleagues[91] used antibody raised against the beta-protein present in Alzheimer's plaques to show the presence of these markers in boxers' brains, providing evidence of Alzheimer's plaques as well as tangles. Additionally, in three of eight patients, beta-protein deposits in leptomeningeal and cortical vessels were evident. Dale et al.[29] stained 16 boxers' brains for BF10, a monoclonal antibody directed against an epitope of an Alzheimer's-related neurofilament and ubiquitan, a protein found in neurofibrillary tangles. Staining of BF10 and ubiquitan was demonstrated in patients with clinical dementia pugilistica, though the former was a more sensitive marker. These changes indicate a final common pathway between Alzheimer's disease and dementia pugilistica, although the underlying cause may diverge.

The finding of amyloid protein deposition in cortical and leptomeningeal vessels suggests that these individuals may have a tendency toward cerebral hemorrhage. Adams and Bruton[1] examined the brains of 22 former fighters (including some studied by Corsellis) and found evidence of previous bleeding in 17. Four had suffered acute intracerebral hemorrhage, seven demonstrated previous perivascular hemorrhage, and seven showed evidence of subpial siderosis. In a control population, 11% of brains demonstrated previous perivascular hemorrhage, and 4% showed meningeal siderosis. Although it is unclear whether there is a tendency toward cerebral hemorrhage in dementia pugilistica or simply a high incidence of subclinical traumatic intracerebral and subarachnoid hemorrhage in fighters, the finding of amyloid angiopathy leads to the suspicion that these individuals would be at increased risk of cerebral hemorrhage.

The clinical similarities between dementia pugilistica and Parkinson's disease have prompted investigators to search for neuropathological similarities. Brandenberg and Hallervorder[5] observed a loss of pigmented neurons and Alzheimer's neurofibrillary changes in one ex-boxer, as did Graham and Ule[35] in a later case report. In Corsellis and colleagues' series,[27] intense pigment loss and neurofibrillary changes were found in the four patients who displayed the most parkinsonian features. Seven of the remaining 11 patients had some degree of nigral degeneration. The intermediate and lateral nuclear groups were most affected. Lewy bodies were absent, and the tissue was said to resemble postencephalitic parkinsonism more than the primary disease.

Neurology of Boxing Injury

The observations made by Martland in 1928[68] about the neurological condition of ex-boxers are still valid today. The publicity garnered by the disability of several well-known ex-champions has served to focus not only the medical community but also the general public on the potentially devastating sequelae of boxing.

Memory loss and dementia have been frequent findings in ex-fighters. The pathological correlation of this impairment may stem in part from mesial temporal neurofibrillary tangle formation, disruption of the fornix by caval septum formation, atrophy and gliosis of the mammillary bodies, or generalized cerebral atrophy. Corsellis and colleagues[27] interviewed the families of the boxers whose brains they examined. They found that individuals with the longest and most severe histories of memory loss had the most profound temporal lobe gliosis. In the four ex-pugilisits with the least clinical memory disturbance, minimal temporal lobe tangle formation was found. Only three of their subjects had no evidence of progressive dementia at the time of death. Casson et al.[22] examined 13 ex-fighters and reported an organic mental syndrome or some degree of memory loss in 4 of these individuals. As a whole, their subjects were younger and had suffered fewer knockdowns and amnestic episodes than the individuals in the Corsellis et al. series. Roberts[90] examined 224 former boxers and determined that 17% displayed signs of brain damage, with the number of fights correlating with the severity of impairment. Johnson[47] evaluated a series of former boxers who had fought at least 200 times. Approximately half of these individuals displayed signs of *traumatic encephalopathy*. Studies of current boxers have not demonstrated consistent evidence of neurological disease. In a study of six Finnish professional fighters, only one individual demonstrated mental slowness.[54]

Given the relationship between neurological dysfunction and professional boxing, there has been interest in analyzing the relationship between amateur boxing and chronic brain damage. Thomassen and colleagues[105] examined 53 former champion amateur boxers. Compared to controls (athletes in a noncontact sport), former boxers showed no increased evidence of memory disturbance or dementia. The boxers did fare statistically worse in a test of logical memory. Haglund et al.[39,40] completed a similar study in Sweden of 47 former amateur pugilists and found no neurological difference from controls. None of the ex-boxers displayed impairment of memory or cognitive function.

Motor impairment of former fighters has been apparent on both physical examination and provocative testing. The pathological correlation for motor dysfunction includes neuronal loss in the lateral substantia nigra and in the cerebral and cerebellar cortices. The prevalence of parkinsonian symptomatology and tremor is difficult to determine from the existing analyses. Clearly, the majority of individuals progressing to memory loss and dementia have coexisting motor effects of dementia pugilistica. Further research will be required to predict which ex-boxers will display tremor and dyskinesia, to characterize the progression of their disease, and to determine markers of early motor system damage.

Electroencephalogrpahy and Boxing Injury

Electroencephalography (EEG) has been used as a screening tool for the detection of neurological abnormalities in ex-boxers. The EEG recordings at the cortical surface would most likely detect cortical disease. Casson et al.[22] reported that 7 of 13 former fighters had abnormal EEGs, with the majority showing diffusely abnormal or bitemporal accentuation rhythms. Subjects with abnormal EEGs showed greater impairment on neuropsychological testing. Roberts[90] obtained EEGs on 168 former boxers and found that although abnormal studies were common, the EEG did not predict the degree of clinical impairment. In Thomassen and colleagues' study[105] of former amateur fighters there was no statistical difference between the ex-boxers and matched controls. Haglund et al.[38] found frequent (16 of 47) cases of minor abnormalities but no marked disturbances in the EEG pattern among ex-fighters. McLatchie et al.[73] examined 20 current amateur boxers and found EEG abnormalities ranging from mild bilateral slowing to markedly abnormal patterns in 40% (compared with 10% to 20% in a normal population). An EEG disturbance, however, did not predict neurological exam findings or reflect the number of bouts the fighter had waged. Older individuals displayed more abnormalities than younger ones. Sironi and colleagues[100] found a pathological EEG in 4 of 10 professional boxers. A one-time EEG may not have predictive value in dementia pugilistica; however, following changes on sequential EEGs may help identify early evidence of dementia pugilistica and prompt these athletes to take early retirement to prevent further damage.

Neuropsychological Testing of Boxers

Formal neuropsychological testing may elicit subtle deficits before they become clinically evident. Casson et al.[21] examined 15 former and current professional fighters and found multiple abnormalities in all. In particular, subjects performed poorly on the Wechsler Memory Test and the 5-s Bender Gestalt Test, suggesting symptoms of early dementia. Most subjects had abnormal results on at least half of the studies performed. Thomassen et al.[105] found greater impairment in former amateur boxers than in controls in tests of the left hand, three-dimensional visual orientation, logical memory, and phonetic synthesis of language. However, after correcting between the boxers and controls for educational level, only left hand dysfunction remained statistically significant. Conversely, in an investigation of former Swedish amateur boxers, Haglund and Persson[40] found no difference between controls and fighters in neuropsychological profile and brain stem evoked potentials. In Kaste and colleagues'[54] study of current and former boxers, only 2 of 14 showed definitive impairment, although on one test of organic brain damage, the Trail-Making test, 12 of the 14 performed poorly. In the same group, 6 of 13 had abnormal EEG findings.

Neuropsychological examination of active amateur fighters has been performed to assess for early brain damage. In McLatchie and colleagues'[73] investigation of 20 active amateurs, 15 had abnormal neuropsychological profiles; deficiencies of memory and attention were found most commonly. Boxers also had poorer reaction time compared to controls in a four-choice reaction test. Levin et al.[62] compared 13 pugilists to normal controls. The only test that elicited a significant difference in performance was a verbal learning task. Retesting the subjects 6 months later revealed no change. Porter performed a detailed analysis of 20 amateur fighters compared to normal controls. Over a 9-year period, he performed serial neuropsychiatric testing and found no significant difference between the fighters and the control population.[87]

Thorough investigation of former and current fighters has demonstrated progressive impairment on neurological and neuropsychological examination, EEG testing, and neuroimaging that seems to correlate roughly with the length of these individuals' careers and their number of fights; however, no evident pattern of progressive damage has been able to predict early dysfunction. It is clear that one-time testing in any of these modalities is inadequate to predict future dementia pugilistica. The determination of progressive impairment may provide an appropriate medical impetus to help boxing federations decide rationally when the continuation of a career risks further dysfunction; however, follow-up on the existing studies will ultimately be essential in modeling the pattern of progressive impairment, which may increase the safety of the sport. Unfortunately, many of the young boxers who have been tested in the existing series will progress to the recognized complex of dementia pugilistica.

Acute Brain Injury from Boxing

The possibility of devastating traumatic brain injury has been recognized as long as boxing has been considered a sport. In 1937, there were at least 300 reported fatalities in boxing in Great Britain. Over the same interval there were 25 deaths in Germany. Between 1945 and 1980 there were 335 documented fatalities in the ring. In the 1970s, 63 deaths were recorded, showing that the mortality rate remained fairly constant over this interval.[95,96] Between 1979 and 1983, 28 deaths were reported. McCunney and Russo[72] estimated the rate of annual boxing fatalities in 1984 to be 10 out of 78,000 participants, or 0.13 per 1000 participants. This rate is at least an order of magnitude lower than for horse racing, parachuting, hang gliding, mountaineering, or scuba diving and is somewhat lower than for college football. In a detailed examination of boxing injuries in the Royal Air Force between 1953 and 1966, Brennan and O'Conner[6] describe 139 head and neck injuries, with decreasing frequency from the early to the later years of the study. There were two deaths, both attributable to "brain laceration." Between 1918 and 1983, 190 of 645 boxing fatalities involved amateurs.[95,96]

Mild Head Injury in Boxing

Mild head injury typified by transient amnesia, brief loss of consciousness, and persistent headache or mild neurological signs is more difficult to document than severe or moderate head injury. In an analysis of 1165 bouts, Sercl and Jaros[99] found that 79% of boxers had momentary neurological signs, whereas 21% demonstrated deficits for at least 24 hours. Holzgraefe and colleagues[44] prospectively examined 13 amateur boxers for neurological symptomatology after bouts. Five had transient neurological findings, including amnesia in all five, ataxia in two, and visual impairment in one. A study done by Jordan[49] through the New York State Boxing Commission found 262 head and neck injuries among 3110 rounds of boxing between August 1982 and July 1984. Four patients required hospitalization, and one individual died of brain injury. In the Royal Army Medical Corps between 1969 and 1980, there were 296 hospital admissions for head injuries resulting from boxing. Of these, only two cases involved "cerebral laceration and contusion," and there were no deaths. Only one victim was discharged from the army because of injuries received while boxing. An estimation of injury frequency predicted one hospital admission for brain injury for every 9000 hours of boxing participation.[80]

Pathophysiology of Boxing Injury

The vast majority of boxing head injuries are mild. The implications and clinical course of mild athletic head injury are discussed in detail later in the chapter. Moderate and severe head injuries most frequently cause subdural hematoma, which accounts for 75% of all injuries and most fatalities. Subdural hematoma results from tearing of the bridging veins during an acceleration/deceleration injury to the brain. Less frequent pathophysiology includes epidural hematoma, diffuse axonal injury, and intercerebral hemorrhage. Cerebral contusion, which accelerates cerebral swelling, can complicate each entity. The pattern of multiple petechial hemorrhage can be particularly difficult to manage, as intracranial pressure is elevated in the absence of a surgically evacuable lesion. In this injury, small hemorrhages are seen commonly in the parasagittal cortex, corpus callosum, deep white matter, and cerebellar peduncles.

The forces needed to create traumatic brain injury in boxing are tremendous; most blows involve a combination of rotational and linear acceleration forces. On the basis of experimental study, it is thought that angular rotation of the skull carries a higher risk of severe head injury than linear movements, theoretically by creating greater tension on stretched blood vessels or brain tissue.[57,111] Striking the head on the ring floor with the knockout can provide an additional impetus for brain injury. The use of padded helmets in amateur boxing has lessened the impact of individual blows and reduced the severity of injury for a given level of mechanical force.

Radiographic Examination of Boxers

Neuroradiographic evaluation of fighters may document both evidence of acute injury and chronic brain damage. The CT scan is superior for demonstrating acute blood in the head, whereas magnetic resonance imaging (MRI) provides better information about chronic injury and diffuse axonal injury. Several investigators have used neuroimaging to assess brain damage in active boxers. Jordan and Zimmerman[51] obtained MRI studies on nine amateurs knocked out during Golden Gloves competition. All nine studies were normal. Holzgraefe et al.[44] imaged 13 amateurs with MRI before and after fights and again found no chronic or acute abnormalities. Computed tomography imaging by Sironi and colleagues[100] of 10 professional fighters showed two cases of atrophy out of proportion to age. Casson et al.[21] obtained CT scans on 10 professional boxers who had suffered knockouts and found cerebral atrophy inconsistent with age in 5. Levin et al.[62] found no abnormalities on MRI in a group of nine pugilists who had performed well on neuropsychological testing. Jordan and Zimmerman[52] obtained CT and MRI images on 20 current boxers and found that MRI was the more sensitive study. It uncovered a chronic subdural hematoma, one case of advanced periventricular white matter disease, and a left frontal lobe contusion not seen on head CT. Furthermore, several lesions seen on CT were shown to be artifactual. Seven patients demonstrated evidence of old trauma on MRI, with most of these changes being encephalomalacia.

Molecular Biology of Boxing Injuries

Mounting evidence points to molecular determinants of sensitivity to repetitive head blows in sports such as boxing. Based on the finding that apoprotein E polymorphism influences amyloid beta-protein deposition, Teasdale and coworkers prospectively analyzed the functional outcome in closed head injury based on the presence or absence of the apoprotein E-ϵ4 allele. They found a significantly poorer 6-month favorable outcome in individuals who harbored this allele.[104] Promoter polymorphisms were thought to be consistent with this effect.[61] The same group, however, found no evidence of chronic brain injury or increased Alzheimer's disease risk in individuals with this allele 15 to 25 years after closed head injury.[75]

Jordan and associates examined volunteer former boxers for the apoprotein E-ϵ4 allele and attempted to correlate apoprotein polymorphism with cognitive abnormalities. Jordan found that all boxers with sever impairment had at least 1 apoprotein E-ϵ4 allele. Overall, the risk of severe impairment was predicted by a history of high exposure (at least 12 professional fights) and the presence of the apoprotein E-ϵ4 allele.[50]

Other Organized Sports

Brain Injury in Football

Perhaps no sport has attempted to document head injury as diligently as American football.[109] In the early days of the sport, violence was the dominant theme: a total of 18 individuals were killed in the 1905 season alone. President Theodore Roosevelt was among many who demanded rule changes if the game was to continue.[78] Since 1931, the American Football Coaches Association has compiled data on catastrophic head injuries in the sport. A total of 433 fatalities from brain injury were recorded between 1945 and 1984.[78] Subdural hematoma was the major injury in 337 cases. The majority of injuries were related to high school athletics (73.7%), and most occurred in games as opposed to practice (62% versus 38%). Between 1945 and 1974 the number of brain injury fatalities increased with each decade to a maximum of 162 between 1965 and 1974. In the next decade, rules standardizing protective equipment and curtailing spearing helped reduce this number to 69. Over this period, 87% of fatalities involved subdural hematoma, and 83% occurred during high school participation. After subdural hematoma, brain contusion ranked second. Most severe head injuries resulted from tackling or other collisions on the field.[78] Cantu and Mueller updated these data in 2003, tabulating brain injury–related deaths from football up to 1999. Overall, the death rate continued to decline to a record low of 9 between 1990 and 1994.[18]

There is also a considerable incidence of mild head injury. In a study of Minnesota high school football players, Gerberich and colleagues[33] reported that 19 per 100 players had experienced a mild head injury characterized by transient amnesia, disorientation, or loss of consciousness. Almost 70% of players returned to play the same day after suffering a loss of consciousness. These results concur with Brooks and Young's[7] previous report of approximately 14 head injuries per 100 participants. Players with a prior history of closed head injury carried a four times greater risk of suffering a subsequent episode. Six of these individuals experienced permanent disability from their injuries. The players reported that the most common long-term sequelae from these mild injuries were headache and dizziness. Disorientation, blurred vision, and diplopia lingered infrequently. Buckley[10] studied an average of 49 collegiate teams per season from 1975 to 1982 for the incidence of concussion. He found 1005 game-related and 2124 overall concussions out of a total of 36,000 athlete-seasons. Mild concussion occurred at a rate of 5.3 cases per 100 athletes. There were 208 injuries requiring a cessation of participation of at least a week. The highest risk of concussion involved running backs and defenders being blocked on running plays. The neuropsychological consequences of football-induced head injuries are considered later in the chapter.

Brain Injury in Rugby and Australian Rules Football

Rugby, like American football, features collisions and tackling that can potentially cause head injuries. Unlike football, the sport is not centralized, and no reports exist that provide an overall rate of injury. Roy[94] reported that approximately 2% of rugby injuries in South Africa involved concussion with no consistent standard of care for these injuries. Gibbs[34] reported that only 5.7% of rugby injuries in an Australian professional rugby league involved the head, with the majority of these classified as concussions. Only one player suffered recurrent episodes requiring cessation of participation. Athletes were not polled on long-term postconcussive symptomatology. Australian rules football led to concussion in approximately 1% of 1253 participants during the 1992 season. Three players suffered a loss of consciousness, and none of the injuries was considered serious. No long-term follow-up was performed.[74]

Brain Injury in Ice Hockey

Ice hockey injuries commonly involve the central nervous system. Jorgensen and Schmidt[53] reported the incidence in a series of elite Danish ice hockey players and found that 14% of their injuries involved concussion. Although the majority involved disability of less than a week, five patients demonstrated continued impairment 1 month after injury. Only 8% of players with brain injuries were managed by a physician compared to 72% of those with knee injuries. Gerberich et al.[32] found nine head injuries characterized by loss of consciousness or awareness per 100 high school hockey players between 1976 and 1983. Of the brain injury victims, 27% had experienced a previous loss of consciousness, with a resultant odds ratio of 1.8 for subsequent head injury. Up to 35% complained at some point during the season of dizziness or headache. Blurred vision, diplopia, nausea, and tinnitus were less frequent.

Brain Injury in Soccer

Soccer players may receive multiple repeated blows to the cranium in the course of heading the ball. Schneider and Lichte[98] estimate that a ball kicked with full power from 10 m carries a force of 116 kPa. The speed of the delivered ball, according to Tysvaer and Storli,[110] can reach 120 km/hr. Therefore, the risk for acute or chronic neurological injury is not negligible. Sortland and Tysvaer[101] reviewed 33 former Norwegian national team players and found that one-third had cerebral atrophy. Two of the players had abnormalities of the cavum septum pellucidum. Tysvaer and Storli conducted examinations and performed EEGs on 69 current Norwegian club players and found a higher incidence of EEG abnormalities in athletes versus age-matched controls.[110]

Summary on Organized Sports

Clearly, organized sports with a focus on violence have a high incidence of head injury, and individual players who suffer a mild head injury will have an increased incidence of future events. The continuous occurrence of these incidents in an individual should trigger a neurological workup including a neuroimaging study, a neurological examination, and neuropsychological testing. Although there are no studies demonstrating definite pathological changes in football players, hockey or soccer goalies, or rugby players, it is clear that these individuals may carry a risk for traumatic encephalopathy. Therefore, although there is no clear evidence that catastrophic injury occurs more frequently in these individuals, concussion in a football player should at least be associated with a period of nonparticipation.

Brain Injuries in Recreational Sports

Many nonorganized recreational athletic activities carry the potential for serious head trauma; these include hang gliding,[85] scuba diving,[58] mountaineering,[89] horseback riding,[28,36] and skiing.[59] In organized team sports such as football and hockey, the risk of brain damage is inherent in the violence of the game; however, inexperience, poor technique, and equipment failure are causative factors in recreational injuries. Furthermore, because these activities tend to develop in locales removed from traditional avenues of medical supervision, care, and transport, minor head injury is seldom reported, and a large percentage of potentially curable serious injuries become fatalities.

Most series of these injuries are generated from regional reports in which a particular sport predominates. Strohecker and colleagues[103] reported a total of 33 severe brain injuries from skiing during a single winter, accounting for approximately one-fifth of all severe head trauma seen over this interval at their center: four patients died, three survived with significant disability, and seven patients required neurosurgical intervention. At least one comprehensive series of sledding injuries has been reported, detailing an incidence of 8% head injuries with no mortality.[41] Penschuck[85] analyzed a series of injuries associated with hang gliding and found a surprisingly small (less than 10%) incidence of head injury, with three injuries over 2½ years. Reid et al.[89] performed autopsies on 42 victims of mountaineering accidents in Scotland and determined that head injury was the major cause of death in 21 (50%). Among 34 patients with evidence of brain trauma, 17 sustained skull fractures, with the majority involving both the cranial vault and the skull base; 28 individuals had evidence of focal brain injury with 10 focal bleeds and 18 hemorrhagic contusions, and 17 victims displayed evidence of diffuse brain damage or increased intracranial pressure (ICP) without a clear mass lesion. Only five of the subjects were wearing safety helmets at the time of their injuries. In many cases, several days elapsed between injury and discovery of the victim.

Scuba Diving

Scuba diving accidents involve an interesting dual mechanism of injury (see Chapter 30). The risk of traditional direct head impact is low; however, decompression sickness, or *the bends*, may have several neurological sequelae. In this syndrome, excessively rapid ascent causes solubilization of gas in the diver's bloodstream, causing the equivalent of an air embolus. Common neurological symptoms may mimic brain stem stroke and include ophthalmoplegia, transient visual disturbance, and lower cranial nerve signs. True air embolism, thought to result from breathholding during ascent that causes rupture of lung tissue due to increased pulmonary pressure, can result as well. Improper breathing systems may cause nitrogen narcosis, carbon monoxide or carbon dioxide toxicity, or anoxia.[58] As in mountaineering accidents, these victims suffer from medical inaccessibility in the acute stages of brain injury.

Equestrian Sports

In many rural regions, horseback-riding injuries are the most frequent cause of athletic brain trauma. A 1-year study from May 1972 to April 1973 in Sweden revealed 174 total injuries, with 44% involving the central nervous system. There were 20 isolated cases of mild or moderate head injury and 10 more severe multisystem traumas including one death.[30] Ilgren and colleagues[45] examined the brains of six victims of horseback-riding fatalities (of 23 fatalities over a 3-year period in seven British counties) and found significant coup or contrecoup contusions in five; three had neurosurgical intervention before death. The authors concluded that inadequate head protection played a role in each injury. Professional or expert riders had a significantly lower rate of injury than amateurs (4% versus 16%). This association of head injuries with improperly helmeted amateurs was also seen in a study of 72 horseback-riding injuries at the University of Virginia Health Sciences Center reported by Grossman et al. in 1978.[36] D'Abreu[28] reported that although proper helmeting reduced the annual incidence of head injuries among National Hunt Club jockeys from 46 to 27, overall horseback riding–associated injuries were still the most common cause of athletic brain injury in England, followed by rugby and soccer.

Multiple falls among professional jockeys may predispose these individuals to a traumatic encephalopathy similar to that seen in boxers. Foster et al.[31] compiled five cases of early neurological deterioration in National Hunt Club jockeys in Great Britain. Each man had a history of repeated falls. Two subjects had new onset of temporal lobe seizures; one individual suffered a fatal riding accident at age 26 with pathological evidence of acute hemorrhage in the midbrain, with hemorrhagic contusion of the left temporal lobe and right basal ganglia, and inferior cerebellar Purkinje cell loss and atrophy similar to that seen in boxers.

Many athletic pursuits such as these carry a small risk of preventable head injury. The key to reducing this risk is increasing medical access to accident victims, recognizing the importance of cerebral protection, and properly supervising amateurs who are attempting dangerous activities. Foster and colleagues' report of traumatic encephalopathy in jockeys indicates further that any activity carrying the risk of chronic low-level brain injury can initiate long-term neurological sequelae.[31]

Prevention, Management, Assessment, and Treatment of Sports-Induced Brain Injuries

Prevention

The ability to adapt existing regulation of equipment and rules of play in the interest of safety makes athletic brain injury particularly amenable to preventive interventions. Many examples of changes in injury rates based on the introduction of new legislation are available. The introduction of required headgear and the three-round limit in amateur boxing have certainly generated fewer acute injuries and a smaller rate of chronic encephalopathy than in the professional sport. In football, the elimination of spearing and the development of standards for helmets helped reduce brain trauma fatalities by 57% (162 versus 69) between the periods 1965 to 1974 and 1975 to 1984.[78] Introduction of the helmet and face shield had a similar effect in ice hockey.[95,96] Standardization of the riding helmet reduced the annual incidence of head injuries among National Hunt Club jockeys from 46 to 27.[28] Recreational sports such as diving, hang gliding, mountaineering, horseback riding, skiing, and skydiving all carry a tangible risk that is minimized by the appropriate training of participants, improvement in safety equipment, and recognition of safety precautions.[60] Given the probable increased risk of repeated head injuries, teams should endeavor to keep records of the number of mild injuries that each individual suffers. For instance, if one athlete has more than two episodes in a particular season, neurological, neuropsychological, and neuroradiographic evaluation may be warranted before a return to competition.

Management

Victims of athletic head trauma often have a significant advantage over trauma victims in general, namely, the presence at the scene of injuries of team physicians, athletic trainers, and other persons trained in basic life support. Furthermore, many organized activities have planned sequences for rapid triage in cases of severe injury requiring urgent intervention.

Cantu[14–16] divides concussion into three grades: grade 2 injuries involve loss of consciousness of less than 5 minutes or posttraumatic amnesia of more than 30 minutes but less than 24 hours (Table 26.1). These cases with documented loss of consciousness should receive medical attention. A course of 24 hours of observation or a head CT scan is appropriate in patients without residual findings. Computed tomography must be performed in individuals with neurological deficits. In grade 1 concussion there is no loss of consciousness, and posttraumatic amnesia lasts for less than 30 minutes. Transient disorientation or amnesia should necessitate abstinence from further athletic participation on the day of injury and close observation on an outpatient basis for 24 hours. Grade 3 injuries involving prolonged loss of consciousness and prolonged posttraumatic amnesia are treated according to advanced trauma life support (ATLS) guidelines: establishing a functioning airway and then ensuring adequate breathing and circulation are the first priorities. While moving victims, immobilization of the cervical spine is also essential.[88] In severe injury, the Glasgow Coma Scale (GCS) score should be obtained in the field to allow comparison over time. The neurosurgical team will need to know the mechanism of the injury and the sequence of deterioration. The pupillary exam also should be documented. In cases of suspected severe injury without concomitant systemic hypotension, the patient should be transported in a reverse Trendelenburg position to reduce intracranial pressure. Headgear should not be removed until adequate personnel are available for rigid neck immobilization.[88] When the patient arrives in the emergency department, more detailed neurological and general examinations should be performed, with rapid acquisition of a head CT scan.

Assessment

In the acute phase, assessment of the severely head-injured athlete consists of serial neurological examinations and a CT scan. Computed tomography demonstrates skull fracture, bleeding, and

Table 26.1. Grading Scales for Athletic Concussion

	Mild—Grade 1	Moderate—Grade 2	Severe—Grade 3
Cantu	No LOC or PTA <1 hr	LOC <5 min or PTA of 1–24 hr	<5 min or PTA of >24 hr
Torg	Grades I and II: no LOC, no amnesia (or PTA only)	Grades III and IV: LOC <few minutes PTA or retrograde amnesia	Grades V and VI: LOC (coma) Confusion with amnesia
Colorado	No LOC Confusion without amnesia	No LOC Confusion with amnesia	LOC

LOC, level of consciousness; PTA, posttraumatic amnesia.

cerebral swelling, and at most institutions can be performed directly on presentation to the emergency department. Magnetic resonance imaging provides superior visualization of the posterior fossa and can more reliably discern shear injury of the corpus callosum or brain stem.

Chronic brain injury may be attributable to the traumatic encephalopathy of boxing, the result of repetitive blows over a long period of time (discussed elsewhere in this chapter), or a postconcussive syndrome may be attributable to a single incident. In patients with severe postconcussive syndrome, posttraumatic epilepsy, or progressive deficits, a CT scan may reveal a chronic subdural hematoma or hygroma or hydrocephalus.[42]

Postconcussive syndrome encompasses myriad symptoms experienced in the interval after head injury. Typical complaints include headache, dizziness, tinnitus, confused thinking, and difficulty concentrating. Although this syndrome is common during recovery from severe brain injury, its incidence in victims of mild head injury is surprisingly high. Wilberger[113] found that over half of high school football players complained of fatigue, difficulty concentrating, memory disturbance, and dizziness after mild head injury. He studied 62 high school football players who suffered two concussions in a single season and found that at 1 month, 47% of them demonstrated persistent deficiencies on tests of attention and concentration such as the Paced Auditory Serial Addition Test (PASAT). These abnormalities persisted at 3 months postinjury in 26%; postconcussive symptoms remained prevalent in these patients. Cook[25] reported that rugby players suffering mild head injury had a shorter duration of headache and less time off from work than controls, which he attributed to a high motivation for recovery. Carlsson et al.[20] examined all victims of head injury and found that postconcussive symptoms persisted longer in patients with a history of previous brain trauma.

To document specific neuropsychological impairment after mild head injury, a 4-year prospective study of football players was undertaken at our institution. Players from 10 university football teams were evaluated before the season and then serially retested if they developed a grade 1 or 2 concussion. In 4 years, 2300 players were evaluated, of whom nearly 200 sustained head injuries. Control tests were obtained from normal students and from team members with orthopedic injuries. Testing consisted of a neurobehavioral test protocol and a brief psychosocial assessment protocol. The first set of tests included Reitan's Trail-Making tests, Smith's Symbol Digit Test, Gronwall's PASAT, and Ammon's Quick Test. The second battery consisted of a psychiatric research epidemiology interview and a review of subjective complaints.[2]

A total of 183 individuals sustained 196 head injuries. Only nine (4.7%) suffered a significant episode of loss of consciousness, none for longer than 5 minutes. Virtually every patient suffered a brief period of disorientation, with this clouding of consciousness lasting for less than 5 minutes in half of the patients. Disorientation persisted for more than 1 hour in 14% of individuals. The head-injured players had significantly more complaints of headache, dizziness, and memory deficits at 1 and 5 days after injury, with an increase in memory complaints persisting at 10 days (Figs. 26.1 and 26.2). Posttraumatic performance on the neuropsychological battery was impaired compared to that of controls, and this impairment persisted until the postconcussive complaints resolved. The final tests to normalize and symptoms to resolve involved attention and concentration.[2] Most improvement was seen between days 1 and 5 after injury, although significant improvement also occurred

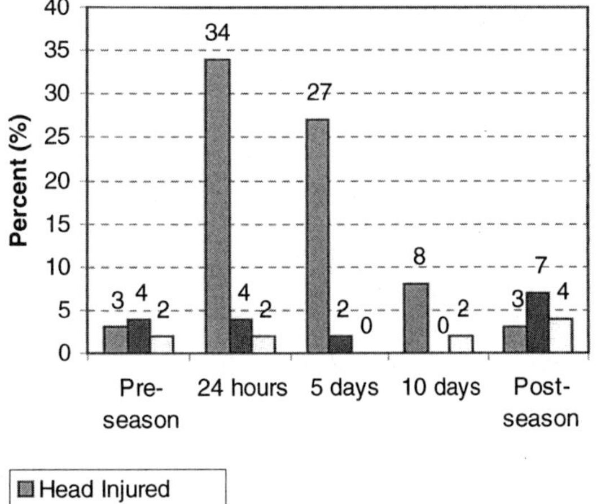

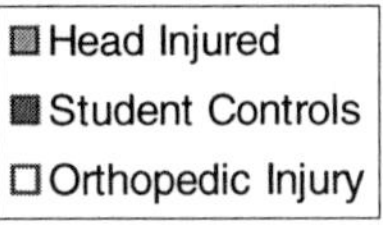

Figure 26.1. Memory disturbance complaints. (Adapted from Alves WM: Football-induced mild head injury. In Torg JS (ed): Athletic Injuries to the Head, Neck, and Face. St. Louisa, Mosby Year Book, 1991, pp 283–304, with permission.)

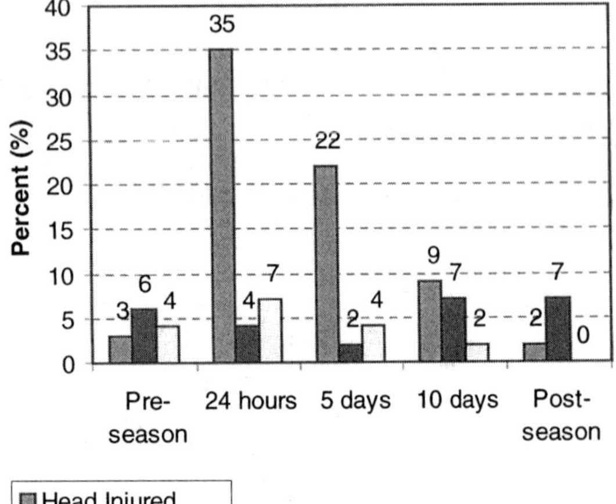

Figure 26.2. Complaints of dizziness. (Adapted from Alves WM: Football-induced mild head injury. In Torg JS (ed): Athletic Injuries to the Head, Neck, and Face. St. Louisa, Mosby Year Book, 1991, pp 283–304, with permission.)

between days 5 and 10. Most players returned to competition by day 5.[65]

McCrea and associates undertook a similar study of 1631 college football players over three seasons. Ninety-four of these individuals suffered concussions. The players were then tested 3 hours, 1 day, 2 days, 3 days, 5 days, 7 days, and 90 days after their injury. The athletes had higher concussion severity scores, more cognitive impairment, and more balance problems than nonconcussed controls. However, these differences were largely resolved by 7 days in all categories and were entirely resolved by 90 days.[70] In this population, 6.3% of players suffered a concussion and 6.5% of these individuals suffered a second concussion in the same season. Players with a history of at least three previous concussions had a three times greater frequency of concussion. Patients with previous concussions also had twice the rate of symptoms progressing for more than 1 week (30% versus 15%).[37]

Collins and coworkers performed neuropsychiatric assessments of 16 college football players who suffered concussion as part of a prospective cohort. Testing compared to controls revealed slower recovery to baseline in the concussed patients. Individuals with a history of learning disability and multiple concussions demonstrated further impairment.[23]

Professional football has also granted greater access to concussion researchers. Pellman and colleagues studied National Football League (NFL) concussions over the 6-year period from 1996 to 2001. During this period there were 787 reported concussions in the NFL for an average of .41 concussions per game. Quarterbacks were the most likely players to suffer concussions. The majority of injuries were due to helmet impacts. Symptoms charted in the postconcussive phase included headache (55%), dizziness (42%), difficulty with recall (26%), retrograde amnesia (18%), impaired cognition (17.5%), and blurry vision (16%). Only 9.3% of these injuries involved loss of consciousness and only 2.4% required hospitalization. Ninety-two percent of these athletes returned to practice within 7 days.[82] More detailed impact reconstructions were used to help guide further improvements in helmet design and understand injury biomechanics.[83,84]

Treatment

Serious brain trauma associated with athletics most often involves subdural hematoma. The neurosurgical treatment of subdural as well as epidural and intracerebral hemorrhage is well documented and noncontroversial. However, a significant percentage of athletic brain injury is related to the so-called second impact syndrome.[16,97] These cases involve individuals with a previous history of mild head injury who suffer an apparently rapid decline, with CT evidence of massive cerebral edema without a mass lesion despite an apparently minor impact. Traditional neurosurgical management of these patients has involved ICP monitoring (either subarachnoid or intraventricular), elevation of the head, hyperventilation, diuretics, and mannitol to control cerebral edema. Decompressive bifrontal craniectomy has been effective at our institution in relieving pathologically elevated ICP in head trauma victims. Furthermore, if patients whose injuries are refractory to conventional medical management of elevated ICP undergo surgery within 48 hours of the time of injury and ICP does not become sustained over 40 cm H_2O, they have more favorable outcomes than GCS-matched controls.[86]

Current Controversies in Head Injury of Athletes

Return to Competition

Most mild head injury in athletics never receives medical attention; however, symptomatology, as measured by subjective complaints and neuropsychological impairment, may persist for weeks after injury. In this interval of recovery, athletic performance will certainly be substandard. Additionally, it is postulated that an individual may be at risk for severe brain injury during this period. Therefore, guidelines on the conditions of return to participation, although inexact, are necessary to ensure the safety of the head-injured athlete. Factors to consider in formulating these regulations include severity of the insult, frequency and timing of previous incidents, and the presence of postconcussive syndrome.[3,9,48,79]

To define factors regulating the return to athletic competition, one must first define a scale detailing the severity of concussion. Most existing grading systems use loss of consciousness and posttraumatic amnesia as guidelines. Three widely applied and similar scales are detailed in Table 26.1. In general, amnesia and loss of consciousness are used to differentiate mild from moderate and severe concussion.

Reinstatement has traditionally been based upon the severity of injury and the history of previous injury. Cantu[12–15,17] has developed a comprehensive set of guidelines based upon his classification of head injury. His algorithm demands termination of participation with a third injury or a second severe concussion. His recommendations are summarized in Table 26.2. The University of Colorado group[55] suggests a minimum of 20 minutes of asymptomatic observation for grade 1 (confusion without amnesia) injuries. They require patients with grade 2 concussion (confusion with amnesia, no loss of consciousness) to undergo serial neurological examination for 24 hours, with reinstatement only after a week-long asymptomatic interval. Finally, patients with loss of consciousness must be evaluated in a hospital setting, with reinstatement after 2 symptom-free weeks. With more elite athletes, the level of contact is much higher, and standards for return should therefore be even more strict.

Kelly and Rosenburg's[56] guidelines for concussion grade and return to activity have also been widely adapted. These American Academy of Neurology guidelines define grade 1 concussion as involving no loss of consciousness, transient confusion, and concussion symptoms or mental status abnormality that resolve in <15 minutes. Grade 2 concussion involves no loss of consciousness and only transient confusion. Concussion symptoms or mental status abnormality resolve in less than 15 minutes. Grade 3 concussion is defined by any loss of consciousness, either brief or prolonged. Individuals suffering a grade 1 concussion should be removed from the contest and examined immediately and every 5 minutes thereafter for development of mental status abnormalities or postconcussive symptoms at rest and with exertion. The guidelines allow these athletes to return to the contest if the examination is normal and no symptoms develop for at least 12 minutes. Patients with grade 2 concussion are removed from the contest and may not return. They should be examined frequently for signs of evolving intracranial pathology and reexamined daily. They may return to practice only after 1 full week without symptoms both at rest and with exertion. Athletes suffering a

Table 26.2. Return to Competition Guidelines of Cantu

Concussion Grade	First Concussion	Second Concussion	Third Concussion
Grade 1—mild	May return when asymptomatic	May return in 2 weeks if asymptomatic for 1 week	Terminate season
Grade 2—moderate	May return when asymptomatic for 1 week	May return in 1 month if asymptomatic for 1 week	Terminate season
Grade 3—severe	May return in 1 month if asymptomatic for 1 week	Terminate season	

Source: Adapted from reference 12.

grade 3 concussion should be transported from the field to the nearest hospital emergency department by ambulance if they are still unconscious or if worrisome signs are detected, with cervical spine immobilization if indicated. A thorough neurological evaluation should be performed emergently, including a CT or MRI scan when appropriate. The athlete is typically barred from contact sports for 1 month after a grade 3 concussion. Return to play before 1 month is allowed only if the athlete has been asymptomatic at rest and with exertion for at least 2 weeks.[56]

Newer methods for concussion assessment have introduced sideline neuropsychiatric testing to confirm and quantitate concussion. McCrea and colleagues used the sideline assessment of concussion (SAC) in 91 athletes within 15 minutes of concussion. Over 95% of these athletes showed decline from preinjury scores on the SAC. More prolonged recovery periods were seen in more severely impaired athletes.[71] Maroon and associates have described an alternative method of sideline assessment, the immediate measurement of performance and cognitive testing (IMPACT).[67]

Unfortunately, simple reliance on concussion severity to judge the ability to return to competition may be flawed. Hinter-Bayre and Geffen examined 21 rugby players after concussion with neuropsychological testing. Test performance was not influenced by concussion grade, regardless of which conventional concussion scale was used.[43]

Prescreening for Competition

In general, prescreening of athletes before participation in contact sports has traditionally involved the patient's history and a neurological examination, which often may be cursory. A history of headache, ataxia, diplopia, tinnitus, or memory disturbance should prompt investigation before participation. The neurological examination should include a funduscopic examination for signs of papilledema, a detailed cranial nerve examination, evaluation for truncal and extremity ataxia, and a mini-mental status examination. Because boxing carries a known risk, we suggest that professional fighters be prescreened with a CT scan. Individuals demonstrating a large cavum septum pellucidum or atrophy inappropriate for age should be excluded from competition. Subsequent scans obtained at 2-year intervals or after a knockout could prevent second impact injuries.

Important issues in sports neurology are the workup of headache in the athlete that seems to be temporally unrelated to physical contact and the prescreening of athletes for contact sports to detect factors or conditions that may predispose the player to injury. Athletes are just as prone to migraine headaches as the general population and may be more liable to develop exertional or stress headaches. A certain number of sports participants with headache will harbor intracranial pathology that explains their symptoms. Furthermore, a chronic subdural hematoma may present with headache far removed from any actual traumatic episode. The evaluation of headache in the athlete therefore must recognize that although typical causes of headache occur most frequently, any pattern of change in headache merits thorough investigation.[11]

When interviewing an athlete in a contact sport who has headaches, the most important task for the clinician is deciphering the pattern of the headache and pinpointing factors that induce change. An athlete who continues to have once-a-week migraines months after a mild head injury is less worrisome than one with the same complaint whose pain was initiated by a precise event or one whose headache has progressed over several months. Physical examination is likewise essential, with attention to evidence of neck or eye strain that may initiate headache.

In patients whose headache dates clearly from the time of an injury, CT evaluation of chronic pain is a valuable first step. A CT scan will distinguish hydrocephalus from previous traumatic subarachnoid hemorrhage, chronic subdural hematoma, and most cortical contusions. An MRI scan will evaluate shear injury of the brain stem or corpus callosum more completely, but these conditions are not treatable. If headache persists after a negative CT scan, MRI imaging would be indicated. As previously mentioned, participation in contact sports is contraindicated while this pain persists.

In athletes with progressive headache independent of known injury, MRI may provide a better primary evaluation than CT. Rooke[93] studied 103 patients with presumed benign tension headache; among 10 patients found to harbor an underlying disease process, 7 had lesions visualized significantly better on MRI than on CT (three Chiari 1 abnormalities, two cases of platybasia, one basilar impression, and one cerebellar hemangioblastoma). Magnetic resonance imaging is superior to CT in demonstrating tumors, vascular lesions, and any brain stem or skull base pathology. Again, athletes with progressive headaches should be withdrawn from contact sports until a thorough neurological evaluation and the pertinent imaging analysis are performed.[93]

Second Impact Syndrome

Many isolated case reports detailing malignant brain edema resulting from relatively mild head trauma that occurred after a recent concussion have been published.[97] These incidents have been attributed to second impact syndrome in which persistent subclinical brain swelling from a traumatic insult makes the brain more susceptible to further injury. Acccording to Cantu,[16] the National Center for Catastrophic Sports Injury Research identified 29 such cases between 1980 and 1991 among football players alone. The pathophysiology is believed to involve loss of the brain's autoregulatory capacity and consequent elevated ICP from vascular congestion and markedly poor intracranial compliance; while this condition persists, the athlete experiences symptoms of the postconcussive syndrome. This markedly poor compliance leads to rapid deterioration after a relatively mild second impact. Torg and associates[108] have described several cases of malignant cerebral edema occurring after relatively mild injuries in athletes who had mononucleosis with encephalitis. This condition can also lead to vasomotor dysfunction, relatively increased ICP, and poor brain compliance after a second insult. Because these victims are not hospitalized at the time of second injury, there is no direct ICP evidence for the existence of the syndrome. However, pathological evidence of subacute contusions has been consistently found in these athletes. The syndrome underscores the necessity to monitor athletes carefully to ensure absence of postconcussive symptomatology for a significant length of time before return to competition.

Treatment of second impact syndrome is a particular problem in that the patients already have severe intracranial hypertension at presentation. The need for skilled personnel to perform rapid intubation and mild hyperventilation and to initiate treatment of elevated ICP with mannitol is paramount. These patients will seldom have surgically correctable lesions; therefore, monitoring and maintenance of an ICP above 20 cm H_2O demands additional treatment, including pharmacological management with barbiturates or bifrontal decompressive craniectomy. Experimental pharmacological agents, as mentioned previously, are now in trial. As in many other areas of neurological sports injury, however, prevention is the key in second impact syndrome. Adherence to one of the existing sets of standards for the return to participation potentially can make this entity extremely rare.

Conclusion

Athletic head injuries provide unique models of brain trauma due to the often repetitive nature of the insults, the lack of medical management in many of the episodes, and the ability to assess rapidly the effect of the use of particular safety standards. Boxing stands virtually alone as being assailed by the medical community as a sport in which the stated goal is to pummel the opponent, with the head as the likely target. Although the amateur sport has been reformed to a certain degree, professional boxing continues to produce unfortunate cases of chronic brain injury. Whether boxing survives will largely remain an economic issue; however, the guidelines we suggest based on available studies of the neuropathological, neuroradiological, neurological, and neuropsychological assessment of boxers' brains provide a rational framework for limiting the participation of individuals with a high risk of chronic injury.

Many sports have reduced the rate of head injury through the use of improved protective equipment; football, ice hockey, and equestrian events have all demonstrated the potential for intervention. Still, the lack of universally applied standards for an athlete's return to participation in contact sports and the remarkably low rate of medical attention that mild head injuries in these sports receive highlight the need for further improvement. We have proposed a rational scheme for the classification of mild head injury in athletes and have devised guidelines for return to participation based on measurable grades and the potential danger of second impact syndrome. Criteria not obvious to the team physician or trainer at the time of injury have intentionally been deemphasized. The plan does assume a knowledge of the GCS that most trained support personnel would be expected to have. Of course, like the many similar schemes that have preceded ours, the Virginia Neurological Institute's severity of mild head injury scale and guidelines for athletic reinstatement are based less on hard data than on common sense and actual experience with head injury.

REFERENCES

1. Adams CWM, Bruton CJ: The cerebral vasculature in dementia pugilistica. J Neurol Neurosurg Psychiatry 52: 600–604, 1989.
2. Alves WM: Football-induced mild head injury. In: Torg JS (ed): Athletic Injuries to the Head, Neck, and Face. St. Louis, Mosby Year Book, 1991, pp 283–304.
3. Bailes JE, Cantu RC: Head Injury in Athletes. Neurosurgery 48(1):26–45, 2001.
4. Bogdanoff B, Natter HM: Incidence of cavum septum pelluciduin in adults: A sign of boxer's encephalopathy. Neurology 39:991–992. 1989.
5. Brandenburg W, Hallervorden J: Dementia Puglistica mit Anatomischem Befund. Virchows Arch 325:680–709, 1954.
6. Brennan TNN, O'Connor PJ: Incidence of boxing injuries in the Royal Air Force in the United Kingdom 1953–66. Br J Industr Med 25:326–329, 1968.
7. Brooks WH, Young AB: High school football injuries: Prevention of injury to the central nervous system. South Med J 69:1258–1260, 1976.
8. Bruce DA, Schut L, Sutton LN: Brain and cervical spine injuries occurring during organized sports activities in children and adolescents. Clin Sports Med 1:495–513, 1982.
9. Bruno LA, Gennerelli TA, Torg JS: Management guidelines for head injuries in athletics. Clin Sports Med 6:17–29, 1987.
10. Buckley WE: Concussions in college football. A multivariate analysis. Am J Sports Med 16:51–56, 1988.
11. Caccayorin ED, Petro GR, Hochhauser L: Headache in the athlete and radiographic evaluation. Clin Sports Med 6:739–749, 1987.
12. Cantu RC: Guidelines for return to contact sports after a cerebral concussion. Physician Sportsmed 14:75–83, 1986.
13. Cantu RC: Head and spine injuries in the young athlete. Clin Sports Med 7:459–472, 1988.
14. Cantu RC: Head and neck injuries. In: Mueller FO, Ryan AJ (eds): Prevention of Athletic Injuries: The Role of the Sports Medicine Team. Philadelphia, FA Davis, 1991, pp 201–212.
15. Cantu RC: Criteria for return to competition after a closed head injury. In: Torg JS (ed): Athletic Injuries to the Head, Neck, and Face. St. Louis, Mosby Year Book, 1991, pp 323–330.
16. Cantu RC: Second impact syndrome. Immediate management. Physician Sportsmed 20:55–66, 1992.
17. Cantu RC: Athletic head injuries. Clin Sports Med 16(3): 531–543, 1997.
18. Cantu RC, Mueller FO: Brain injury–related fatalities in American football, 1945–1999. Neurosurgery 52:846–853, 2003.
19. Carlsson GS: Head injuries in a population study. Acta Neurochir 36(suppl):13–15, 1986.
20. Carlsson GS, Svardsodd K, Welm L: Long-term effects of head injury sustained during life in three male populations. J Neurosurg 67:197–205, 1987.
21. Casson IR, Sham R, Campbell EA, et al: Neurological and CT evaluation of knocked-out boxers. J Neurol Neurosurg Psychiatry 45:170–174, 1982.
22. Casson IR, Siegel 0, Sham R, et al: Brain damage in modern boxers. JAMA 251:2663–2667, 1984.
23. Collins MW, Grindel SH, Lovell MR, et al: Relationship between concussion and neuropsychological performance in college football Players. JAMA 282:964–970, 1999.
24. Constantinides J, Tissot R: Lesions Neuro-fibrillaires d'Alzheimer generalisees sans plaques Seniles. Arch Suisse Neurol Neurochir Psychiatry 100:117–130, 1967.
25. Cook JB: The effects of minor head injury sustained in sport and the post-concussional syndrome. In: Walker AE, et al (eds): Late Effects of Head Injury. Springfield, IL, Charles C Thomas, 1969, pp 408–413.
26. Corsellis JAN: Boxing and the brain. BMJ 298:105–109, 1989.
27. Corsellis JAN, Bruton CJ, Freeman-Browne D: The aftermath of boxing. Psychol Med 3:270–303, 1973.
28. D'Abreu F: Brain damage in jockeys. Lancet 1:1241, 1976.
29. Dale CE, Leigh PN, Luthert P, et al: Neurofibrillary tangles in dementia pugilistica are ubiquinated. J Neurol Neurosurg Psychiatry 54:116–118, 1991.
30. Danielsson LG, Westlin NE: Riding accidents. Acta Orthop Scand 44:597–603, 1973.
31. Foster JB, Leiguardia R, Tilley PJB: Brain damage in National Hunt jockeys. Lancet 1(7967):981–983, 1976.
32. Gerberich SG, Finke R, Madden M, et al: An epidemiological study of high school ice hockey injuries. Childs Nerv Syst 3:59–64, 1987.
33. Gerberich SG, Priest JD, Boen JR, et al: Concussion incidences and severity in secondary school varsity football players. Am J Public Health 73:1370–1375, 1983.
34. Gibbs N: Injuries in professional rugby league. A three-year prospective study of the South Sydney Professional Rugby League Football Club. Am Sports Med 21:696–700, 1993.
35. Grahmann H, Ule G: Beitrag zur Kenntnis der Chronischen Cerebralen Krankheitsbilder bei Boxern. Psychiatry Neurol 134:261–283, 1957.

36. Grossman JA, Kuland DN, Miller CW, et al: Equestrian injuries—results of a prospective study. JAMA 240:1881–1882, 1978.
37. Guskiewicz KM, McCrea M, Marshall SW, et al: Cumulative effects associated with recurrent concussion in collegiate football players: The NCAA Concussion Study. JAMA 290:2549–2553, 2003.
38. Haglund Y, Edman G, Murelius O, et al: Does Swedish amateur boxing lead to chronic brain damage? 1. A retrospective medical, neurological, and personality trait study. Acta Neurol Scand 82:245–252, 1990.
39. Haglund Y, Eriksson E: Does amateur boxing lead to chronic brain damage? Am J Sports Med 21:97–109, 1993.
40. Haglund Y, Persson HE: Does Swedish amateur boxing lead to chronic brain damage? 3. A retrospective clinical neurophysiological study. Acta Neurol Scand 82:353–360, 1990.
41. Hedges J, Greenberg M: Sledding injuries. Ann Emerg Med 9:131–133, 1980.
42. Henderson JM, Browning DG: Head trauma in young athletes. Med Clin North Am 78:289–303, 1994.
43. Hinton-Bayre AD, Geffen G: Severity of sports-related concussion and neuropsychological test performance. Neurology 59:1068–1070, 2002.
44. Holzgraefe M, Lemme W, Funke W, et al: The significance of diagnostic imaging in acute and chronic brain damage in boxing. Int J Sports Med 13:616–620, 1992.
45. Ilgren EB, Teddy PJ, Vafadis J, et al: Clinical and pathological studies of brain injuries in horse-riding accidents: A description of cases and review with warning to the unhelmeted. Clin Neuropathol 3:253–259, 1984.
46. Isherwood I, Maudsley C, Ferguson FR: Pneumoencephalographic changes in boxers. Acta Radiol 5:654–661, 1966.
47. Johnson J: Organic psychosyndrome due to boxing. Br J Psychiatry 115:45–53, 1969.
48. Johnson KN, Lassonade M, Ptito A: A contemporary neurosurgical approach to sports-related head injury: The McGill Concussion Protocol. J Am Coll Surg 192(4): 515–525, 2001.
49. Jordan BD: Neurologic aspects of boxing. Arch Neurol 44:453–459, 1987.
50. Jordan BD, Relkin NR, Ravdin LD, et al: Apolipoprotein E epsilon 4 associated with chronic traumatic brain injury in boxing. JAMA 278:136–140, 1997.
51. Jordan BD, Zimmerman RD: Magnetic resonance imaging in amateur boxers. Arch Neurol 45:1207–1208, 1988.
52. Jordan BD, Zimmerman RD: Computed tomography and magnetic resonance imaging comparisons in boxers. JAMA 263:1670–1674, 1990.
53. Jørgensen U, Schmidt-Olsen S: The epidemiology of ice hockey injuries. Br J Sports Med 20:7–9, 1986.
54. Kaste M, Vilkki J, Sainio K, et al: Is chronic brain damage in boxing a hazard of the past? Lancet 2:1186–1188, 1982.
55. Kelly JP, Nichols JS, Filley CM, et al: Concussion in sports. Guidelines for the prevention of catastrophic outcome. JAMA 266:2867–2869, 1991.
56. Kelly JP, Rosenburg JH: Diagnosis and management of concussion in sports. Neurology 48:575–580, 1997.
57. Lampert PW, Hardman JM: Morphological changes in brains of boxers. JAMA 251:2676–2679, 1984.
58. Lehman LB: Scuba and other sports diving. Nervous system complications. Postgrad Med 80:68–70, 1986.
59. Lehman LB: Neurologic injuries from winter sporting accidents. Postgrad Med 80:88–98, 1986.
60. Lehman LB: Sports-related CNS injuries in children and adolescents. Postgrad Med 82:141–142, 1987.
61. Lendon CL, Harris JM, Pritchard AL, et al: Genetic variation of the *APOE* promoter and outcome after head injury Neurology 61:683–685, 2003.
62. Levin HS, Lippold SC, Goldman A, et al: Neurobehavioral functioning and magnetic resonance imaging findings in young boxers. J Neurosurg 67:657–667, 1987.
63. Lindsay KW, McLatchie G, Jennett B: Serious head injury in sport. BMJ 281:789–791, 1980.
64. Lingard DA, Sharrock NE, Salmond CE: Risk factors of sports injuries in winter. NZ Med J 83:69–73, 1976.
65. Macciocchi SN, Barth JT, Alves W, et al: Neuropsychological functioning and recovery after mild head injury in collegiate athletes. Neurosurgery 39:510–514, 1996.
66. Macpherson P, Teasdale E: CT Demonstration of a fifth ventricle-a finding to KO boxers? Neuroradiology 30:506–510, 1988.
67. Maroon JC, Lovell MR, Norwig J, et al: Cerebral concussion in athletes: Evaluation and neuropsychological testing. Neurosurgery 47:659–672, 2000.
68. Martland HS: Punch drunk. JAMA 91:1103–1107, 1928.
69. Mawdsley C, Ferguson FR: Neurological disease in boxers. Lancet 2:795–801, 1963.
70. McCrea M, Guskiewicz KM, Marshall SW, et al: Acute effects and recovery time following concussion in collegiate football players: The NCAA Concussion Study. JAMA 290:2556–2563, 2003.
71. McCrea M, Kelly JP, Randolph C, et al: Immediate neurocognitive effects of concussion. Neurosurgery 50:1032–1042, 2002.
72. McCunney RJ, Russo PK: Brain injuries in boxers. Physician Sportsmed 12:53–67, 1984.
73. McLatchie G, Brooks N, Galbreath S, et al: Clinical neurological examination, neuropsychology, electroencephalography and computed tomographic head scanning in active amateur boxers. J Neurol Neurosurg Psychiatry 50:96–99, 1987.
74. McMahon KA, Nolan T, Bennett CM, et al: Australian rules football injuries in children and adolescents Med J Aust 159:301–306, 1993.
75. Millar K, Nicoll JAR, Thornhill S, et al: Long term neuropsychological outcome after head injury: Relation to APOE genotype. J Neurol Neurosurg Psychol 74:1047–1052, 2003.
76. Millspaugh JA: Dementia pugilistica. US Navy Med Bull 35:297–303, 1937.
77. Mueller FO: Catastrophic sport injuries. In: Mueller FO,

Ryan AJ (eds): Prevention of Athletic Injuries: The Role of the Sports Medicine Team. Philadelphia, FA Davis, 1991, pp 26–34.

78. Mueller FO, Blyth CS: Fatalities from head and cervical spine injuries occurring in tackle football: 40 years' experience. Clin Sports Med 6:185–196, 1987.
79. Nelson WE, Jane JA, Gieck JH: Minor head injury in sports: A new system of classification and management. Physician Sportsmed 12:103–107, 1984.
80. Oleman B, Rose C, Arlow K: Boxing injuries in the Army. J R Army Med Corps 129:22–27 1983.
81. Payne EE: Brains of boxers. Neurochirurgia 11:173–188, 1968.
82. Pellman EJ, Powell JW, Viano DC, et al: Concussion in professional football: Epidemiological features of game injuries and review of the literature—Part 3. Neurosurgery 54:81–96, 2004.
83. Pellman EJ, Viano DC, Tucker AM, Casson IR: Concussion in professional football: Location and direction of helmet impacts—Part 2. Neurosurgery 53:1328–1341, 2003.
84. Pellman EJ, Viano DC, Tucker AM, et al: Concussion in professional football: Reconstruction of game impacts and injuries. Neurosurgery 53:799–814, 2003.
85. Penschuck C: Verletzungsursachen beim Drachenfliegan. Chirurgie 51:336–340, 1980.
86. Polin RS, Shaffrey MS, Tisdale N, et al: The efficacy of bifrontal decompressive craniectomy in the management of severe refractory post-traumatic cerebral edema. Neurosurgery 41:84–95, 1997.
87. Porter MD: A 9-year controlled prospective neuropsychologic assessment of amateur boxing. Clin J Sport Med 13(6):339–352, 2003.
88. Reid SE, Reid SEJ: Head and Neck Injuries in Sports. Springfield, IL, Charles C Thomas, 1984.
89. Reid WA, Doyle D, Richmond HG, et al: Necropsy study of mountaineering accidents in Scotland. J Clin Pathol 39:1217–1220, 1986.
90. Roberts AH: Brain Damage in Boxers. London, Pitman Medical Scientific Publishing, 1969.
91. Roberts GW, Allsop D, Bruton CJ: The occult aftermath of boxing. J Neurol Neurosurg Psychiatry 53:373–378, 1990.
92. Rontoyannis GP, Pahtas G, Dinas D, et al: Sudden death of a young wrestler in competition. Int J Sports Med 9:353–355, 1988.
93. Rooke ED: Benign exertional headache. Med Clin North Am 52:801–808, 1968.
94. Roy SP: The nature and frequency of rugby injuries. S Afr Med J 48:2321–2327, 1974.
95. Ryan AJ: Protecting the sportsman's brain (concussion in sport). Br J Sports Med 25:81–86, 1991.
96. Ryan AJ: Intracranial injuries resulting from boxing. In: Torg JS (ed): Athletic Injuries to the Head, Neck, and Face. St. Louis, MosbyYear Book, 1991, pp 55–71.
97. Saunders RL, Harbaugh RE: The second impact in catastrophic contact—sports head trauma, JAMA 252:538–539, 1984.
98. Schneider Von PG, Lichte H: Untersuchungen zur Grobe der Krafteinwirkung beim Kopfballspeil des Fubballers. Sportarzt Sportmed 26:222–223, 1975.
99. Sercl M, Jaros O: The mechanisms of cerebral concussion in boxing and their consequences. World Neurol 3:351–357, 1962.
100. Sironi VA, Scotti G, Ravagnati L, et al: CT-scan and EEG findings in professional pugilists: Early detection of cerebral atrophy in young boxers. J Neurosurg Sci 26:165–168, 1982.
101. Sortland O, Tysvaer AT: Brain damage in former association football players. Neuroradiology 31:44–48, 1989.
102. Spillane JD: Five boxers. BMJ 2:1205–1210, 1962.
103. Strohecker J, Furst A, Kollman H, et al: Craniocerebral injuries from skiing. Wien Med Wochenschr 134:11–13, 1984.
104. Teasdale GM, Nicoll JA, Murray G, Fiddes M: Association of apolipoprotein E polymorphism with outcome after head injury. Lancet. 350:1069–1071, 1997.
105. Thomassen A, Juul-Jensen P, De Fine Olivarius B, et al: Neurological, electroencephalographic and neuropsychological examination of 53 former amateur boxers. Acta Neurol Scand 60:352–362, 1979.
106. Tokuda T, Ikeda S, Yanagisawa N, et al: Re-examination of ex-boxers' brains using immunohistochemistry with antibodies to amyloid °-protein and Tau protein. Acta Neuropathol 82:280–285, 1991.
107. Torg JS: Preface. In: Torg J (ed): Athletic Injuries to the Head, Neck, and Face. St Louis, Mosby Year Book, 1991, pp xi–xii.
108. Torg JS, Beer LA, Begso J: Head trauma in football players with infectious mononucleosis. Physician Sportsmed 8:107–110, 1980.
109. Torg JS, Truex RJ, Quedenfeld TC, et al: The National Football Head and Neck Injury Registry. Report and conclusions 1978. JAMA 241:1477–1479, 1979.
110. Tysvaer AT, Storli O: Soccer injuries to the brain. Am J Sports Med 17:573–578, 1989.
111. Unterharnscheidt F: About boxing: Review of historical and medical aspects. Tex Rep Biol Med 28:421–495, 1970.
112. Vigouroux RP, Guillermain P, Verrando R: Neurotraumatology of sportive origin. Neurochirurgie 24:247–250, 1978.
113. Wilberger JE: Minor head injuries in American football. Prevention of long term sequelae. Sports Med 15:338–343, 1993.

Chapter 27
Athletic Spine Injury

S. TAYLOR JARRELL,
ANDREW CHENELLE,
JOSHUA M. AMMERMAN,
AND RICHARD S. POLIN

Injuries to the spine from athletic activities frequently come to the attention of the medical practitioner. Because the majority of spine injuries resulting from athletic participation involve the cervical spine, that region is the focus of this chapter. However, injuries to the thoracic and lumbar regions also occur and are mentioned when appropriate. This chapter reviews the epidemiology, diagnosis and evaluation, management, and prognosis of a variety of sports-related spine injuries. By necessity, it focuses only on the highlights, as entire books have been written on the subject of athletic injury.[77]

Epidemiology

There are variations in the estimated percentage of spinal injuries and spinal cord injuries (SCIs) attributable to sporting activity. In Toronto, Tator and colleagues found that 22.9% of patients with SCIs admitted to their center from 1974 to 1981 were sports-related.[71] The National Spinal Cord Injury Statistical Center (NSCISC) at the University of Alabama–Birmingham found that sporting activity was the cause of 8% of SCI in its 1996 database, while Bailes's 1991 study lists only 2% of 3200 studied SCI cases as sports-related.[7,55] More recently, Berkowitz et al. estimated sports and recreation as the cause of SCI in 18% of cases.[10] The NSCISC estimates that in the United States, there are 32 new SCIs per million population per year, or about 7800 cases per year. It cautions that this is likely a gross underestimate, stating that an additional 20 patients per million die before reaching the hospital.[55] Other estimates of the annual incidence, in developed countries, of acute SCI vary from 11.5 to 53.4 per million.[31,41–43] If one combines these data and estimates that approximately 10% of catastrophic SCIs occur as a result of athletics, a rough estimate of the incidence of SCI as a result of sports participation varies from one to five per million population.

The six sporting activities most frequently resulting in catastrophic SCI are diving, motor sports, hockey, snowmobiling, waterskiing, and horseback riding.[72] In one series, over half of sports-related catastrophic SCIs resulted from diving accidents.[72] Not surprising are the facts that the majority of SCIs resulting from diving occur in unsupervised or nonsponsored activities and that alcohol is often implicated.[37,67] American football, gymnastics, and ice hockey were the team sports most often implicated in SCI.[21] American football, often thought of as a dangerous sport from the perspective of SCI, was the cause of injury in only 2.2% of patients in Tator and Edmonds's series.[72] Fifty-eight percent of the athletes in the Bailes et al. study developed permanent neurological deficits as a result of their cervical spine injuries.[7]

Even though very few data exist on the overall incidence of SCI in athletic activities, some very good data exist for individual sports. There are good epidemiological reports for American football, rugby, swimming and diving, cheerleading, and gymnastics.

American Football

Schneider and colleagues in 1961 first highlighted the risk of neck injury in football.[65] They stated that serious neurological damage could result from violent hyperextension of the neck while tackling or falling. Excellent data on athletic SCI have been compiled at the National Center for Catastrophic Sports Injury Research (NCCSIR), located since 1980 in Chapel Hill, North Carolina. A recent report lists 223 football players with catastrophic cervical SCI since 1977.[22] High school football players accounted for 82% of the injuries. They estimated an incidence rate of catastrophic SCI per 100,000 athletes to be 0.52 in high school, 1.55 in college, and 14 in professional football, perhaps a reflection of the increased speed and violence of higher levels of play.[22] Most injuries occurred in games rather than practice, and defensive players, particularly defensive backs and linebackers, were found to be most prone to sustaining SCI, accounting for 71% of the total injuries.[22]

A disturbing trend seen in the late 1970s was a drop in the number of serious head injuries due to better helmet designs but an increase in the number of catastrophic cervical spine injuries due to the use of these newer helmets as weapons.[7] The incidence of cervical spine injuries has now fallen due to improved coaching of tackling techniques and the outlawing of the spear tackle in 1976, in which contact is first made with the helmet. Over the years 1993 to 2002, there were an average of 7.1 cervical cord injuries with incomplete neurological recovery in football, including 6 in 2002.[53] This represents a dramatic decrease compared to the data published on the 1971 to 1975 seasons, when permanent quadriplegia from neck injuries involved an average of 35 cases annually.[51,52] Alarming, however, is that in one study of freshman collegiate football players at the University of Iowa, 32% had radiographic evidence of an old cervical spine injury.[4]

Most catastrophic cervical spine injuries in football occur with the neck in flexion.[44,48] However, because of the multiplicity of directional forces in football, hyperextension, lateral flexion, compressive, and rotational forces may produce cervical fractures.[7,48] The neck is placed in a position of weakness when the head is lowered to block or tackle, and thus is vulnerable to fracture/dislocation with severe SCI.[48]

Fifty-two percent of quadriplegic injuries studied by Torg et al. were found to be the result of direct-compression, head-on injuries in which initial contact was made with the top of the helmet.[83] Cantu and Mueller found 69% of the injured players to be in the act of tackling, 25% of those documented as tackling incorrectly and illegally, with the head down.[22] The football face mask can also be a source of injury to the neck in that it can be grabbed by an opponent and a twisting force applied to the neck, a maneuver outlawed in football. Because the face mask gives the tackler a sense of security, as the vulnerable facial structures are protected, contact during a tackle can be made with the head without fear of broken noses or lost teeth, but with an increased risk of neck injury compared with a block or tackle that is initiated properly with the shoulder.

The NCCSIR recorded no incidence of catastrophic injury to the thoracic or lumbar regions from 1977 to 2001. Disc herniations and facet fractures secondary to repetitive trauma, however, are not uncommon injuries in football players.

Rugby Football

Another sport with well-characterized spinal injury statistics is rugby football. A study performed in Wales found a drastic increase in cervical spine injuries in rugby beginning in the 1980s.[88,89] Scher, in a 1998 10-year review of SCIs due to rugby accidents, described 87 players admitted to the Spinal Cord Injury Centre in Cape Town, South Africa, an increase of 61% over the 54 players admitted during the previous 10 years.[64] One study shows the risk of catastrophic cervical injury to be 4.5 per 100,000 players per year.[17] Though Torg et al. suggested a higher risk of spinal injury in school-age players, Kew et al. found that 69% of SCIs occurred in adults, despite far greater numbers of schoolboy players.[36,81]

There are two major mechanisms of injury in rugby football: twisting injury due to high tackles and hyperflexion injuries caused by collapsing scrums. Most injuries in rugby appear to occur in the scrum. Taylor and Coolican found that 62% of catastrophic cervical spine injuries occurred during initial contact in, or collapse of, the scrum.[75] In this formation, players are locked in a tight group with their heads in a position of flexion. When the ball is put into play, the row of players pushes forward, often collapsing, with the front-line players at risk of striking the ground forehead first, producing a hyperflexion injury. Most commonly this mechanism, plus the weight of an entire team, results in midcervical unilateral or bilateral locked facets with severe SCI.

Open field tackling can also produce spinal injuries, especially the high tackle, which can produce a variety of extension/rotation injuries to the spine, including odontoid fractures.

The position played is relevant to the risk of cervical injury. Forwards are at high risk due to their exposure in scrums.[87] In fact, in one study, twice as many injuries were sustained by forwards as by backs.[18] The player at maximal risk is the hooker, who is at the center of the scrum.[75]

International rugby laws have responded with effective rules changes, such as outlawing rushing the scrum, to prevent scrum collapse. Far fewer cervical injuries occurred in New Zealand than expected after the rules were revised in 1980 to modify mauls and scrums.[17]

An excellent comprehensive review of cervical spine injuries and SCI among rugby players has recently been published by Quarrie et al.[58]

Ice Hockey

Spinal injuries in ice hockey have also been well studied, beginning in 1981 with the establishment of the Committee on Prevention of Spinal Cord Injuries Due to Hockey and its successor, SportSmart Canada. It first reported on 42 cases of catastrophic spinal injury in 1984. By 1993, SportSmart Canada had recorded 241 cases, with 22 injuries in 1990, the highest number in 1 year in the 27 years of the registry.[69,73]

Most injuries occurred during organized game play, with 52% of injured players being between the ages of 16 and 20.[70] Cervical injuries constituted 89% of cases, with injuries at the thoracic, thoracolumbar, and lumbosacral levels accounting about equally for the remainder of injuries.[70] Injuries at the C5-6 level accounted for 40 of the 241 reported cases in the registry.[70]

A push or check from behind was the inciting event in 36% of the cases.[70] In 70% of instances the injury occurred when a player's head struck the boards, a mechanism akin to that of a spear tackle in American football.[70] Many players suffered a midcervical burst fracture or fracture-dislocation. The recent increase in spinal injuries in hockey is thought to be due to the same phenomenon experienced in American football: with the addition of a helmet and face mask, players are likely to become more aggressive and to use their head as a weapon.[29]

Prevention of spinal injuries in hockey has centered on conditioning and coaching techniques and, most importantly, rules changes. For example, in 1985, the Canadian Amateur Hockey Association moved to outlaw the check or push from behind, and in 1994 USA Hockey made it illegal for a player to check an opponent after he is no longer in control of the puck. Many recreational leagues have a no-check rule, significant in that checking is involved in the great majority of injuries of all types.

Diving

The majority of sports-related cervical spine traumas result from diving accidents.[66] Up to 10% of catastrophic SCIs are caused by diving accidents.[72] As with most SCIs, the majority of patients are male.[74] From 60% to 100% of diving injuries occur outside the realm of supervision.[67] The majority of these injuries occur in oceans, lakes, or rivers rather than in swimming pools. The predominant injury is a compression or burst fracture that results from the head striking the bottom of the pool, lake, or river.[62,63] However, ligamentous instability without fracture can occur with improper water entry.[6]

Water depth is one of the most important factors in diving injuries. Shields et al. reported that the average depth in which the injuries in their series occurred was 5 feet.[66] A diver's velocity is not dissipated until a depth of 12 feet is reached.[3] Public education, however, has lowered the incidence of diving-related cervical trauma in recent years.

Other Sports

A sporting activity that less commonly results in spine injuries is wrestling. Three such cases were reported in 1985 and four in 1990.[1,90] These injuries resulted from throws in which the wrestler landed on the head or neck and from an illegal hold, the full Nelson.

Equestrian sports can also be a source of spinal trauma. Twenty spinal injuries were reported from Alberta in 1993.[32] The location of injuries was about evenly divided among cervical, thoracic, and lumbar levels. The relatively high incidence of thoracolumbar fractures is unique to equestrian sports. These injuries occur when the rider is thrown from the horse and lands on the buttocks, with subsequent burst fracture of a lower thoracic or lumbar vertebral body.[14] The much-publicized injury to Christopher Reeve, of *Superman* fame, was a type II odontoid fracture after the actor landed perpendicularly on his helmet during an equestrian competition in May 1995.[49]

Gymnasts are at risk for both acute and chronic injury to the spinal column. Most catastrophic SCIs result from falls during dismounts.[9] It is clear that the trampoline and mini-trampoline are major causes of injury, with 32 of 50 cases reported to the National Spinal Cord Injury Data Research Center in its 1982 report resulting from trampoline accidents. A 2001 Consumer Product Safety Commission report stated that trampoline injuries resulted in 83,000 visits to emergency rooms in 1996, most as a result of backyard accidents.[24] Furnival et al. reported in 1999 on 86 spinal injuries due to trampoline accidents. Six patients had spinal cord contusions, and seven children developed cervical or thoracic fractures.[28] The American Academy of Pediatrics in 1977 recognized the trampoline as a cause of paraplegia and even attempted to ban it in schools.

Chronic axial loading resulting in fracture of the pars interarticularis is a common problem in gymnasts, and anterior and middle column injuries, consisting of premature degenerative disc disease and compression fractures, have been reported.[2,35] A 1991 study by Sward et al. found a 75% prevalence of disc degenerative disease in 24 male gymnasts (aged 19–29), selected without regard to symptoms, compared to 31% in a control group of nonathletes.[68] These chronic injuries are more likely to result in back pain than neurological deficit, and rarely require surgical intervention, but clearly may be disabling enough to prevent further competition.

Scuba diving and windsurfing also cause unique injuries to the spine. Decompression sickness, otherwise known as the *bends*, can cause cord ischemia and paraplegia. If recognized, it usually resolves with hyperbaric oxygen therapy.[27] Cases of acute thoracic pain have been reported in windsurfers.[57] This pain is likely due to the unique strain put on the thoracic spine by the act of holding the sail upright against a strong wind; vascular compression/ischemia or herniated discs result from this strain.

Spinal injuries have also been reported in such activities as martial arts and cricket.[40,59]

Mechanism of Injury

Depending on the sport, all types of cervical, thoracic, and lumbar fractures can be encountered. The common types, etiological mechanisms, and associated sports are discussed in this section. For an additional review, an excellent paper on the biomechanics of spinal injury has been written by Sances et al.[61] Injury of the spinal cord without fracture in the form of the central cord syndrome will also be addressed.

Cervical Spine

The cervical spine is the most frequently injured region of the spine in sporting activities. It is composed of seven vertebrae. Half of flexion-extension and rotation occurs at the occiput-C1 and C1-C2 junctions, respectively.[34] Each vertebral body has two facet joints that allow maximum flexion, extension, lateral flexion, and rotation. The total amount of flexion-extension is 100 degrees, the total rotation is 80 degrees to either side, and the total lateral flexion is 30–50 degrees to either side.[34] The cervical vertebrae are separated by intervertebral discs that support and cushion the vertebral bodies. They are stabilized by the anterior and posterior longitudinal ligaments, the ligamentum flavum, the interspinous, intertransverse, and supraspinous ligaments, and the paravertebral musculature. Eight pairs of cervical nerve roots are associated with the cervical spine, each exiting laterally above the pedicle of the corresponding vertebral level.

Fractures of the upper cervical spine are quite rare but may occur from flexion, extension, axial loading, or rotational forces. Flexion may cause odontoid fracture, or rupture of the transverse ligament. Hyperextension may also result in odontoid fracture. Axial loading is the mechanism responsible for the Jefferson fracture. Rotational forces may result in rotatory C1-C2 subluxation.[30] Upper cervical spine injuries, if they do not cause death via spinal cord compression, are usually not associated with neurological injury due to the large diameter of the spinal canal at this level.

Most athletic lower cervical spine injuries occur when the neck is in a position of flexion. Flexion of the cervical spine removes the protection afforded by its natural lordosis, reducing its ability to absorb axial loads. An axial load of 500–750 pounds, which can commonly occur in sporting impacts, has been shown to induce fracture-dislocation of the cervical spine when it is in modest flexion.[26] Burst fractures are caused by axial loading to the vertex of the head and often compromise the cervical canal with a retropulsed fragment, usually resulting in severe SCI. This mechanism is responsible for many diving injuries and for football spear tackler injuries.[46] On the other hand, a simple anterior wedge compression fracture, with intact posterior elements and without violation of the spinal canal, usually causes no neurological injury. If an axial load is applied to a flexed and rotated neck, a unilateral facet dislocation can occur. In this case, a unilateral nerve root entrapment or some degree of SCI often occurs. When the neck is loaded in, or forced into, extreme flexion, bilateral facet dislocations can result, with a high incidence of total cord injury.

Bony injury as the result of hyperextension is a rare occurrence in the young, healthy athlete. However, hyperextension can result in a central cord syndrome, usually due to a hypertrophied anterior bony spur or thickened ligamentum flavum compressing the spinal cord when the neck is in hyperextension. In this syndrome there is motor damage, which, due to the somatotopic arrangement of upper extremity motor fibers more medially in the corticospinal tract, causes a motor loss that is more severe in the arms than the legs. Typically, there is disruption of the crossing spinothalamic tract at the anterior commissure of the spinal cord, resulting in some degree of pain and temperature loss below the level of injury. Dorsal column function classically is spared. The prognosis is good for at least some degree of return of function in central cord syndrome. Most athletes are too young to have significant anterior osteophyte formation, but a congenitally narrow spinal canal can predispose to this injury. The consensus definition of a narrow cervical spinal canal is 14 mm or less or a canal diameter/vertebral body diameter ratio (Torg ratio) of less than 0.80.[33,81]

A common injury sustained in football is the stinger, or burner. This is usually attributed to stretch injury of the brachial plexus in extreme lateral flexion of the neck in combination with violent depression of the shoulder. A stinger presents as dysesthetic pain in a single shoulder and arm.[38] Up to 50% of collegiate football players are estimated to experience a stinger during the course of a season.[8] Page and Guy reported that at the University of South Carolina, football players with a Torg ratio of less than 0.80 were four times more likely to suffer a stinger.[56] It is usually a transient phenomenon, unassociated with radiographic abnormalities, and signs of spinal cord involvement are absent.

To be distinguished from the stinger is the so-called burning hands syndrome, which is a milder form of the central cord syndrome and is characterized by its bilaterality of sensory and motor findings.[47] Recognition of this syndrome as an SCI is important and may have implications for the player's return to action.

In addition, Torg et al. estimated that 1.3 athletes per 10,000 participants in college football experience more serious transient neurapraxia and quadriparesis.[81]

Thoracic Spine

The thoracic spine is composed of 12 vertebrae separated by intervertebral discs. The stability of the thoracic spine is enhanced by the presence of its articulations with the rib cage. Thoracic spine injuries in athletes are largely anterior wedge compression fractures and burst fractures. These occur when the spine is violently flexed around a fixed pivot point, as happens in automobile crashes when the body is rotated around a seat belt. Axial loading can result in burst fracture. Thoracic fractures are rare but are seen in equestrian sports. If retropulsed fragments in a burst fracture compromise the narrow spinal canal in the thoracic region, SCI of varying degrees can result.

Lumbar Spine

The lumbar spine is composed of five vertebrae separated by interarticular discs. The spinal cord ends before the lumbar spine at T12-L1. Thus, if injuries to the lumbar spine occur that compromise the thecal sac, paraplegia is rarely the result. However, a variety of radiculopathies can occur. The most common types of injuries to the lumbar spine, other than muscle strains, are fractures of the pars interarticularis with spondylolisthesis and herniated discs.[5] Most athletic injuries to the lumbar spine are a result of repeated trauma.

Fractures of the weak pars interarticularis are due to repeated stress caused by hyperextension of the lumbar spine.[5] These injuries are common in gymnasts. Occasionally, bilateral pars fractures can result in spondylolisthesis.

Herniated lumbar discs occur frequently in weight lifters and football players due to chronic sustained axial loading of the lumbar spine.

Damage and Outcomes

The NSCISC estimates that SCI costs the United States $9.7 billion per year in medical care, equipment, and disability support.[55] If it is assumed that 10% of injuries are sports-related, then it can be estimated that the yearly cost of caring for athletic SCI is approximately $1 billion, making this a major societal problem in addition to the costs to the individual patient.

The lifetime cost of caring for a 25-year-old low quadriplegic, excluding lost wages, averages $1,235,841 (in 1999 dollars).[55] This is an especially troubling figure, given that the majority of catastrophic sporting injuries produce quadriplegia and that the mean age of this group of patients is 17.6.[7] In addition, only 52% of SCI patients are covered by private insurance at the time of injury.[55]

Given the young age of most SCI patients, many productive years are lost. Even in cases of less severe injury to the spinal cord, the effect on the athlete can be great. Often, an athlete is prevented from continuing in a sport that is a part of his or her identity, and an entire life can be disrupted.

Though the life expectancy for survivors of SCI is improving, it does not yet approach that of the non-SCI population, and long-term complications are common. Though renal failure and urosepsis in the past was the most common cause of death in SCI, the conditions now most often implicated are pneumonia, pulmonary emboli, and sepsis, according to the NSCISC.[55] Pressure sores are a major problem and alone are estimated to cost $1.2 billion annually.[19] In addition, many patients require operative stabilization of the fractured spine to provide support for an upright wheelchair-bound posture and for a posture more conducive to good respiratory function.

Prevention

As the road to recovery from SCI is typically long and difficult, and as many productive years are lost by young people suffering such injuries from athletic activity, preventing these injuries is key. Public education about diving into shallow water, such as the "Look Before You Leap" program, has done much to reduce the incidence of SCI caused by diving into shallow lakes, rivers, and pools. Appropriate signage around public pools and beaches warning against diving into shallow water has been recommended.[73] This public information effort is one of the best ways to prevent injuries in unsupervised swimming and diving areas.

Carter has written an excellent review of the steps needed to prevent injuries in competitive divers.[23] He recommends designing diving pools so that the shallow end does not slope into the deeper diving area of the pool. Teaching children with adequate professional instruction from the outset and the use of spotting belts are also recommended. Presently, competitive swimmers are using a deeper dive at the start of races than previously. Thus, it is imperative that the pool under the starting platform be deep enough to accommodate these deeper dives.[51]

Much of the effort to limit the incidence of SCI in American football involves redesigning the rules of the game. Indeed, in the Points of Emphasis section of its rulebook, the National Collegiate Athletic Association (NCAA) specifically cites the importance of "protection of the defenseless player," including kick receivers, quarterbacks, kickers and punters, and wide receivers.[54] Recent rules changes in the NCAA and the National Football League have included adoption of the halo rule for punt returners, and have imposed stricter penalties for unnecessary roughness and late hits on the quarterback. The outlawing of the spear tackle in 1976 is credited with having the most impact in drastically reducing the incidence of cervical spine injuries in football.

Violent collisions are an unavoidable part of football, but proper coaching techniques with emphasis on avoidance of the spear tackle and face masking are critical to the prevention of spinal injuries. Coaches should instruct players not to use the helmet as a battering ram and to keep their necks in the strongest and most stable position when making contact, that is, neutral or 10 degrees of extension.[44] Flexion of the neck during contact should be avoided, and players caught spearing during practice or games should be removed. Rather, Torg advocates the face in the numbers technique as a safer and still effective way of subduing an opponent.[76] Adequate neck conditioning and the use of isometric exercises are thought to be critical to the prevention of neck injuries.[44] Several types of cervical orthoses are available to football players, often as an attachment to the shoulder pads. These include neck rolls, cowboy collars, and butterfly restrictors and are designed to limit excessive, but not normal, range of motion of the neck. The goal of these designs is prevention of brachial plexus or stinger-type injuries caused by violent hyperextension and lateral flexion of the neck.[25]

Prevention of SCI in rugby has also been approached through rules changes. Deliberate collapsing of the scrum is now illegal.[16] Specific rules change in hockey to prevent spearing and cross-checking from behind are being sought.[76] In wrestling, illegal takedowns that involve the head and neck are to be avoided, and penalties are severe. Again, in these violent sports, adequate conditioning may help to avoid catastrophic injury in combination with the use of proper athletic techniques.

To prevent injuries in gymnastics, proper coaching techniques should be used, spotting should be maximized when learning new maneuvers, and the use of the trampoline and mini-trampoline should be avoided.

Cheerleading, a particularly hazardous sporting activity underwent several rules changes in the 1990s designed to prevent serious injuries.[11] These include a limit on pyramid height to 2 levels in high school and 2.5 body lengths in college, spotters for each person above shoulder level, and a limit of four throwers on the basket toss. In addition, no complex stunts are allowed while the game is in play or if the floor is wet. Boden et al. also recommend improved spotter training and certification for cheerleading coaches.[11]

Diagnosis, Evaluation, and Management

An important step in the management of SCI is preactivity screening of sports participants. As part of the routine preparticipation physical examination, questions should be asked about previous spinal trauma. Those with a history of transient neurological symptoms should be screened with cervical spine X-rays, and those with spinal stenosis along with a history of transient quadriparesis should be excluded from contact sports, as recommended by Torg et al.[81] Others and we agree.[60] The difficult issue is deciding whether to allow participation by players in whom an episode of transient quadriparesis occurs and a normal spine is found on radiographic studies. According to Torg et al., an episode of transient quadriparesis does not predispose a player to later permanent SCI, and if the spine radiographs are normal, the individual should not be barred from participating in contact sports, though a 56% chance of recurrence was found.[78] Others feel that an episode of transient quadriparesis is an absolute contraindication to participation in contact sports with or without associated bony abnormalities.[15] We feel that repeated episodes of transient neurological symptoms should certainly be criteria for exclusion from play in contact sports.

In the evaluation of an athlete seeking clearance to play in a contact sport, it is our policy to obtain a single lateral C-spine X-ray to evaluate for congenital lesions of the cervical spine that are potentially unstable. Such lesions would include os odontoideum, atlanto-occipital fusion, and types I and II but not type III Klippel-Feil abnormalities.[79] Common congenital conditions that offer no contraindication to contact sports include spina bifida occulta and idiopathic scoliosis with a curvature of less than 20 degrees with no radiographic progression, as documented before and after the season or at 3- to 4-month intervals during training. With increasing participation in Special Olympics sports, more high-risk individuals are coming to the attention of spine specialists. Down syndrome is associated with ligamentous laxity and occipito-cervical and atlanto-axial instability, and flexion-extension X-rays of the cervical spine are warranted prior to competition.

In order to minimize injury and retain maximal neurological function in an injured player, coaches, trainers, and team physicians must be prepared to manage spinal injuries during games and on the practice field. Coaches should be encouraged to attend American Red Cross first aid and American Heart Association cardiopulmonary resuscitation (CPR) courses. Spine boards, cervical collars, and airway management equipment should be readily available at all games and practice sessions. Players and coaches should be instructed not to raise an injured player to a standing position without prior evaluation by the team physician or trainer.[44]

When a player is injured, the assessment must begin with the ABCs: airway, breathing, and circulation. The player's neurological status should be quickly assessed, and if spinal instability or SCI is suspected, it should be assumed until proven otherwise. Trainers and coaches should be taught by the team physician to perform a basic screening neurological examination. Simple knowledge of the dermatomal distribution of paresthesias and numbness, as well as how to evaluate muscle power, would aid trainers and coaches in evaluating potential injuries.

Removal of helmets and shoulder pads should be avoided, which requires a large pair of bolt cutters to be available to cut away face masks in order to establish an airway. Guidelines established in 1999 by the Inter-Association Task Force for the Appropriate Care of the Spine-Injured Athlete give only four instances in which the helmet should be removed: (1) if the helmet and chin strap do not hold the head securely, such that immobilization of the helmet does not also immobilize the head; (2) if the design of the helmet is such that even after removal of the face mask the airway cannot be controlled or ventilation provided; (3) if the face mask cannot be removed after a reasonable period of time; and (4) if the helmet prevents immobilization for transport in an appropriate position.[39] The face mask, however, should always be removed prior to transportation, regardless of the player's current respiratory status.[39]

Immobilization of the cervical spine with a cervical collar and log-rolling onto a backboard are key to the management of these athletes to prevent further injury. One person should stabilize the neck while six others log-roll the patient onto the spine board.[39]

An excellent short review of emergency procedures for management of on-field injuries is presented by Walters.[85]

In the ambulatory patient without neurological complaints, neck pain and weakness can be tip-offs to more severe injuries. When evaluating a player for weakness, one should keep in mind that athletes are stronger than the general population and that subtle weakness can be missed.[8] Marks et al. emphasize that a player must have a full, painless range of motion before returning to the field of play.[45] Otherwise, players with neck pain and weakness should be immobilized and sent to a medical center for further evaluation.

On arrival at the emergency room, it is standard practice to obtain plain films of the cervical spine to elucidate the nature of a spine fracture. Computed tomography (CT) is often helpful in better defining the bony anatomy and extent of a fracture. Myelograms can show compression of the spinal cord, but in a patient with suspected SCI, emergent magnetic resonance imaging (MRI) is indicated to examine sites of compression of the cord, traumatic herniated discs, soft tissue and ligamentous injury, and damage to the spinal cord itself.

Acute management of SCI includes the institution of the so-called Bracken Protocol of administration of methylprednisolone.[12] In this protocol, 30 mg/kg of methylprednisolone is given over 15 minutes and then 5.4 mg/kg/hr for 23 hours if started within 3 hours of injury or 47 hours if started within 8 hours. This has been shown to improve the outcome in both complete and incomplete injuries at 1 year if administered within the specified time frames.[13] In addition, it is currently our and others' policy to use volume expansion and pressors if necessary to raise the mean arterial pressure to 85 mm Hg or above in order to maximize perfusion of the injured spinal cord.[84] This we continue for a minimum of 72 hours after injury.

Cervical subluxations should be reduced by cervical traction as soon as possible. It is our practice to do an MRI scan on patients with incomplete injuries and subluxations before reduction. It is important to rule out a herniated disc as the cause of neurological compromise before reduction because reduction could worsen the compression caused by the disc, possibly turning an incomplete injury into a complete one. If significant compression is due to a herniated disc, emergent anterior decompression, reduction, and fusion are undertaken.

Operative decompression and stabilization should proceed as soon as the diagnostic workup is complete. Complete injuries are stabilized as soon as the patient is stable enough to undergo surgery, as the earlier a patient can assume an upright posture, the lower the risk of pulmonary complications.

We attempt to transfer these injured athletes to a comprehensive rehabilitation center as soon as they are medically stable. Injured athletes are a highly motivated group, and frustration with the therapy services available in the acute hospital setting frequently develops.

Return to Play

One of the most controversial issues in the treatment of athletes is when to permit the return to play or participation in athletics after the diagnosis of cervical stenosis. We feel that cervical stenosis alone does not contraindicate participation in contact sports; however, the athlete and his or her parents must be counseled about the theoretically increased risk of participation. If neurological symptoms develop in the athlete with a congenitally narrowed spine, one must recommend discontinuation of the sport. However, even the diagnosis of cervical stenosis is not so simple in athletes. Given the large body habitus of many athletes, correspondingly large vertebral bodies can produce an abnormal Torg ratio in asymptomatic individuals without a truly narrow spinal canal. Torg himself confirmed the high sensitivity but low specificity and low positive predictive value of the Torg ratio in football players.[80] Others have written that functional spinal stenosis, as defined by loss of cerebrospinal fluid space around the cervical cord on MRI, rather than the ratio method of Torg, should be used to evaluate cervical stenosis in athletes.[20] Cantu argues that if functional spinal stenosis exists, the athlete should be barred from contact sports.[20] In contrast, we feel that functional spinal stenosis is a very strong contraindication, but not an absolute contraindication, to participation in contact sports. Therefore, the athlete must be counseled about the much increased risk of catastrophic neck injury.

Torg coined the term *spear tackler's spine* in 1993.[82] In this study, radiological findings of loss of cervical lordosis, cervical stenosis, and posttraumatic degenerative changes were related to the documented use of spear-tackling techniques in 15 players. Four of the players in Torg et al.'s study experienced permanent neurological deficits, prompting them to pronounce this constellation of findings an absolute contraindication to participation in contact sports. Certainly the spear tackler's spine is a more complicated and more advanced condition than simple cervical stenosis, and we support Torg et al. in prohibiting this subgroup of athletes from engaging in contact sports.

Marks and colleagues have developed a modification of the classification scheme originally developed by Watkins for assessment of the risk of further injury after return to contact sports following cervical spine injury.[45,86] They classify risk as mild, moderate, high, or severe. A mild degree of risk is reserved for instances, such as cervical sprain, in which there is "very little degree of increased risk of severe injury with continued participation as compared with the risk inherent in the activity itself."[45] A moderate risk is assumed if there is a reasonable risk of symptom recurrence but a small chance of catastrophic injury. Examples include healed cervical fractures without instability, asymptomatic disc herniations, one-level anterior cervical fusion, C1–C2 posterior fusion, and two-level posterior cervical fusion. If the risk of permanent or catastrophic injury is higher, such as in a healed fracture with instability or canal compromise, a symptomatic disc with mild canal impingement, or an episode of neurapraxia with cervical stenosis, then the patient is placed in the high-risk category. A severe degree of risk would be presumed for unhealed cervical fractures, instability, and symptomatic discs with a high degree of canal stenosis.[45,86] As a general rule, Marks et al. do not allow injured athletes to return to contact sports if they fit into the high-risk or severe-risk categories.[46]

Bailes and Maroon have classified athletic SCI into three types with appropriate return-to-play recommendations.[8] Type I athletic injuries to the cervical spine are those that cause neurological injury. This group would include those who sustain permanent injury, as well as having MRI evidence of injury to the spinal cord. Patients with type I injuries are not allowed further participation in contact sports. Type II injuries consist of transient neurological deficits without radiographic evidence of abnormalities; these injuries do not prohibit further participation in contact sports unless they become repetitive. An episode of transient neurapraxia and burning hands syndrome would be categorized as type II injuries. Type III injuries are those that cause radiological abnormalities alone, and for these there is a mixed group of recommendations. Athletes with type III injuries that involve a significant structural component of the vertebral column, ligamentous instability, spinal cord contusion, or congenital cervical stenosis should not return to competitive contact sports. Other radiological abnormalities, such as congenital fusion, ligamentous ruptures, degenerative spinal disease, and herniated discs, require individual consideration.[7]

In spite of the numerous guidelines published in the literature regarding return to play after spine injury, adherence among practitioners is meager as best. Of 105 respondents in a survey of athletic spinal injury, only 49% reported using accepted guidelines in their decision-making process for return to play in athletic competition.[50] It is the responsibility of the spine specialist to understand and apply the published guidelines in his or her individual practice.

Back surgery in the athlete is controversial. Fortunately, the most common operative lesions that we are asked to evaluate as neurosurgeons are herniated cervical or lumbar discs, most of which will resolve with rest and physical therapy. We feel that this conservative approach is wisest with athletes, just as it is with the general population. We recommend that an athlete with a cervical herniated disc stop playing and undergo intensive physical therapy and often traction. With a season of rest and physical therapy, most symptomatic discs resolve, and play can be continued the following year.

If a herniated lumbar disc must be removed surgically, a limited laminotomy and microscopic discectomy can be performed in the standard fashion. Alternatively, newer endoscopic techniques have emerged that allow for minimal muscle dissection, little discomfort, and a much earlier return to play. We allow athletes undergoing lumbar discectomies to return to play in as little as 4 to 6 weeks postoperatively.

In the cervical spine, a laterally situated disc herniation can often be approached posteriorly with the aid of a microendoscope. We keep our cervical discectomy patients away from contact sports for 2 to 3 months in order to allow for full reconditioning of the neck muscles. If an anterior approach is used in the case of a more midline herniation, we keep the player out of contact sports for at least 1 year and ensure that significant bony fusion has occurred before allowing the return to contact sports.

It is generally felt that anything more than a one-level fusion in the cervical spine is an absolute contraindication for participation in contact sports. Marks et al. and Watkins have classified a patient undergoing a two-level or more anterior cervical discectomy and fusion as being at high risk for catastrophic injury.[45,86] It remains to be seen, however, whether technology has outpaced that assessment. With recent improvement in cervical plating systems, the fusions that we are achieving are becoming more solid and consistent. In select cases in which a solid two-level anterior cervical fusion is obtained, we would consider allowing an athlete to return to competition.

Summary

Sports-related SCIs account for up to 1000 cases per year in the United States alone, or about 10% of all SCIs. Most of the victims are young and healthy, which magnifies the financial and emotional strain that such an injury creates. Football, diving, motor sports, snow sports, and hockey are often implicated, and there are very good epidemiological data for many sports, especially football. There has been a decrease in the number of football injuries over the past 20 years owing to rules changes, and many sports, such as gymnastics and hockey, have followed suit with good results.

Given its mobility requirements, the cervical spine is relatively vulnerable to injury and is the part of the spine most often injured, despite its ligamentous attachments. While most catastrophic cervical spine injuries occur when a compressive force is applied to the vertex with the neck in a relatively weak position of flexion, spine injuries have been recorded from extension, lateral flexion, and rotatory forces as well. A congenitally narrowed spinal canal, defined most commonly by the Torg ratio, may predispose the spinal cord to injury. The thoracic and lumbar spines are less commonly injured in sports, though chronic trauma in weightlifting and gymnastics may cause injury to the intervertebral disc or pars interarticularis.

Prevention of athletic spine injury remains key. Public education, improved training and conditioning, and enforcement of safety rules are just a few of the steps that have been taken to curb the incidence of these potentially devastating injuries. Perhaps the most controversial issue in athletic SCI is if, and when, the spine specialist should allow the patient to return to athletic activity. Published guidelines are available to help the clinician make the decision together with the athlete and family.

REFERENCES

1. Acikgoz B, Ozgen T, Erbengi A, et al: Wrestling causing paraplegia. Paraplegia 28:265–268, 1990.
2. Akau CK, Press JM, Gooch JL: Sports medicine. 4. Spine and head injuries. Arch Phys Med Rehabil 74:443–446, 1993.
3. Albrand ON, Walter J: Underwater deceleration curves in relation to injuries from diving. Surg Neurol 4:461–464, 1975.
4. Albright JP, Moses JM, Feldrick HG, et al: Nonfatal cervical spine injuries in interscholastic football. JAMA 236: 1243–1245, 1976.
5. Alexander MJL: Biomechanical aspects of lumbar spine injuries in athletes: A review. Can J Appl Sport Sci 10:1–20, 1985.
6. Badman BL, Rechtine GR: Spinal injury considerations in the competitive diver: A case report and review of the literature. Spine J 4:584–590, 2004.
7. Bailes JE, Hadley MN, Quigley MR, et al: Management of athletic injuries of the cervical spine and spinal cord. Neurosurgery 29:491–497, 1991.
8. Bailes JE, Maroon JC: Management of cervical spine injuries in athletes. Clin Sports Med 8:43–58, 1989.
9. Bailes JE, Maroon JC: Spinal cord injuries in athletes. NY State J Med 91:44–45, 1991.
10. Berkowitz M, O'Leary P, Kruse D, et al: Spinal Cord Injury: An Analysis of Medical and Social Costs. New York, Demos Medical, 1998.
11. Boden BP, Tacchetti R, Mueller FO: Catastrophic cheerleading injuries. Am J Sport Med 31(6):881–888, 2003.
12. Bracken MB, Shepard MJ, Collins WF, et al: A randomized controlled trial of methylprednisolone or nalaxone in the treatment of acute spinal cord injury. N Engl J Med 322:1405–1411, 1990.
13. Bracken MB, Shepard MJ, Holford TR, et al: Administration of methylprednisolone for 24 or 48 hours or tirilazad mesylate for 48 hours in the treatment of acute spinal cord injury. Results of the Third National Acute Spinal Cord Injury Randomized Controlled Trial. National Acute Spinal Cord Injury Study. JAMA. 277(20):1597–1604, 1997.
14. Brooks WH, Bixby-Hammett D: Head and spinal injuries associated with equestrian sports: Mechanisms and prevention. In: Torg JS (ed): Athletic Injuries to the Head, Neck, and Face. St Louis, Mosby Year Book, 1991, pp 133–141.
15. Brooks WH, Young AB: High school football injuries: Prevention of injury to the central nervous system. South Med J 69:1258–1260, 1976.
16. Bruce DA, Schut L, Sutton LN: Brain and cervical spine injuries occurring during organized sports activities in children and adolescents. Clin Sports Med 1:495–514, 1982.
17. Burry HC, Calcinai CJ: The need to make rugby safer. Br J Med 296:149–150, 1988.
18. Burry HC, Gowland H: Cervical injury in rugby football—a New Zealand survey. Br J Sports Med 15:56–59, 1981.
19. Byrne DW, Salzberg CA: Major risk factors for pressure ulcers in the spinal cord disabled: A literature review. Spinal Cord 34:255–263, 1996.
20. Cantu RC: Functional cervical spinal stenosis: A contraindication to participation in contact sports. Med Sci Sports Exerc 8:316–317, 1993.
21. Cantu RC, Mueller FO: Catastrophic spine injuries in football (1977–1989). J Spinal Disord 3:227–231, 1990.
22. Cantu RC, Mueller FO: Catastrophic spine injuries in American football, 1977–2001. Neurosurgery 53(2):358–363, 2002.
23. Carter RL: Prevention of springboard and platform diving injuries. Clin Sports Med 5:185–194, 1986.
24. Consumer Product Safety Commission: Trampoline Safety Alert. Bethesda, MD, CPSC, 2001.
25. Cross KM, Serenelli C: Training and equipment to prevent athletic head and neck injuries. Clin Sport Med 22:639–667, 2003.
26. Davis PM, McKelvey MK: Medicolegal aspects of athletic cervical spine injury. Clin Sports Med 17:147–154, 1998.
27. DiLibero R, Pilmanis A: Spinal cord injury resulting from scuba diving. Am J Sports Med 11:29–33, 1983.
28. Furnival RA, Street KA, Schunk JE: Too many pediatric trampoline injuries. Pediatrics 103(5):e57, 1999.
29. Gererich SG, Finke R, Madden M, et al: An epidemiological study of high school ice hockey injuries. Child's Nerv Syst 3:59–64, 1987.
30. Ghiselli G, Schaadt G, McAllister DR: On-the-field evaluation of an athlete with a head or neck injury. Clin Sports Med 22:445–465, 2003.
31. Gjone R, Nordlie L: Incidence of posttraumatic paraplegia and tetraplegia in Norway: A statistical survey of the years 1974 and 1975. Paraplegia 16:88–93, 1978.
32. Hamilton MG, Trammer BI: Nervous system injuries in horseback-riding accidents. J Trauma 34:227–232, 1993.

33. Hashimoto I, Tak YK: The true sagittal diameter of the cervical spinal canal and its diagnostic significance in cervical myelopathy. J Neurosurg 47:912–916, 1977.
34. Jackson DW, Lohr FT: Cervical spine injuries. Clin Sports Med 5:373–380, 1986.
35. Katz DA, Scerpella TA: Anterior and middle column thoracolumbar spine injuries in young female gymnasts. Am J Sports Med 31(4):611–616, 2003.
36. Kew T, Noakes TD, Scher AT, et al: A retrospective study of spinal cord injuries in Cape Province rugby players, 1963–1989. S Afr Med J 80:127–133, 1991.
37. Kewelramani LS, Taylor RG: Injuries to the cervical spine from diving accidents. J Trauma 15:130–142, 1975.
38. Kim DH, Vaccaro AR, Berta SC: Acute sports-related spinal cord injury: Contemporary management principles. Clin Sports Med 22:501–512, 2003.
39. Kleiner DM, Almquist JL, Bailes JE, et al: Prehospital Care of the Spine-Injured Athlete: A document from the Inter-Association Task Force for the Appropriate Care of the Spine-Injured Athlete. Dallas, National Athletic Trainers' Association, 2001.
40. Kochhar T, Back DL, Mann B, et al: Risk of cervical injuries in mixed martial arts. Br J Sports Med 39:444–447, 2005.
41. Krause JF: Injury of the head and spinal cord. The epidemiological relevance of the medical literature published from 1960 to 1978. J Neurosurg 53:S3–S10, 1980.
42. Krause JF, Franti CE, Riggens RS, et al.: Incidence of traumatic spinal cord lesions. J Chronic Dis 28:471–492, 1975.
43. Kurtzke JF: Epidemiology of spinal cord injury. Exp Neurol 48:163–236, 1975.
44. Leidholt JD: Spinal injuries in athletes: Be prepared. Orthop Clin North Am 4:691–706, 1973.
45. Marks MR, Bell GR, Boumphrey FR: Cervical spine fractures in athletes. Clin Sport Med 9(1):13–29, 1990.
46. Marks MR, Bell GR, Boumphrey FR: Cervical spine injuries and their neurologic implications. Clin Sports Med 9:263–279, 1990.
47. Maroon JC: "Burning hands" in football spinal cord injuries. JAMA 238:2049–2051, 1977.
48. Maroon JC, Steele PB, Berlin R: Football head and neck injuries—an update. Clin Neurosurg 27:414–429, 1980.
49. McDonald JW, Becker D, Sadowski CL, et al: Late recovery following spinal cord injury—Case report and review of the literature. J Neurosurg-Spine 97(2):252–265, 2002.
50. Morganti C, Sweeney CA, Albanese SA, et al: Return to play after cervical spine injury. Spine 26(10):1131–1136, 2001.
51. Mueller FO, Blyth C: Epidemiology of sports injuries in children. Clin Sports Med 1:343–353, 1982.
52. Mueller FO, Cantu RC: Catastrophic injuries and fatalities in high school and college sports, fall 1982–spring 1988. Med Sci Sports Exerc 22:737–741, 1980.
53. Mueller FO, Cantu RC: National Center for Catastrophic Sport Injury Research, Annual Survey of Catastrophic Football Injuries 1977–2002. Available at http://www.unc.edu/depts/nccsi.
54. National Collegiate Athletic Association: Football 2003 Rules and Interpretations, Indianapolis, IN, May 2003. Available at http://www.ncaa.org/library/rules/2003/2003_football_rules.pdf.
55. National Spinal Cord Injury Association Resource Center Fact Sheet #2. Birmingham: National Spinal Cord Injury Association, University of Alabama-Birmingham, 1996.
56. Page S, Guy JA: Neurapraxia, "stingers," and spinal stenosis in athletes. South Med J 97(8):766–769, 2004.
57. Patel MK, Abbott RJ, Marshall WJ: Spinal cord injury during windsurfing. Paraplegia 24:191–193, 1986.
58. Quarrie KL, Cantu RC, Chalmers DJ: Rugby union injuries to the cervical spine and spinal cord. Sports Med 32(10):633–653, 2002.
59. Ranson CA, Kerslake RW, Burnett AF, et al: Magnetic resonance imaging of the lumbar spine in asymptomatic professional fast bowlers in cricket. J Bone Joint Surg 87–B(8):1111–1116, 2005.
60. Rathbone D, Johnson G, Letts M: Spinal cord concussion in pediatric athletes. J Pediatr Orthop 12:616–620, 1992.
61. Sances A, Mykleburst JB, Maiman DJ, et al.: The biomechanics of spinal injuries. CRC Crit Rev Biomed Eng 11:1–75, 1984.
62. Scher AT: Spinal cord injuries due to diving accidents. J Sports Med 18:67–70, 1978.
63. Scher AT: Diving injuries to the cervical spinal cord. S Afr Med J 59:603–605, 1981.
64. Scher AT: Rugby injuries to the cervical spine and spinal cord: A 10-year review. Clin Sports Med 17(1):196–206, 1998.
65. Schneider RC, Reifel E, Chrisler HO, et al: Serious and fatal football injuries involving the head and spinal cord. JAMA 192:613–614, 1965.
66. Shields CL, Fox JM, Stouffer ES: Cervical cord injuries in sports. Physicians Sports Med 6:71–76, 1978.
67. Steinbruch K, Paelsack V: Analysis of 139 spinal cord injuries due to accidents in water sports. Paraplegia 18:86–93, 1980.
68. Sward L, Hellstrom M, Jacobsson B, et al: Disc degeneration and associated abnormalities of the spine in elite gymnasts: A magnetic resonance imaging study. Spine 16:437–443, 1991.
69. Tator CH, Carson JD, Edmonds VE: New spinal injuries in hockey. J Clin Sport Med 7:17–21, 1997.
70. Tator CH, Carson JD, Edmonds VE: Spinal injuries in ice hockey. Clin Sports Med 17(1):183–194, 1998.
71. Tator CH, Duncan EG, Edmonds VE, et al: Changes in epidemiology of acute spinal cord injury from 1947 to 1981. Surg Neurol 40:207–215, 1993.
72. Tator CH, Edmonds VE: Acute spinal cord injury: Analysis of epidemiologic factors. Can J Surg 22:575–578, 1979.
73. Tator CH, Edmonds VE: National survey of spinal injuries in hockey players. Can Med Assoc J 130:875–880, 1984.
74. Tator CH, Edmonds VE, New ML: Diving: A frequent and potentially preventable cause of spinal cord injury. Can Med Assoc J 124:1323–1324, 1981.
75. Taylor TKF, Coolican MRJ: Spinal cord injuries in Aus-

tralian footballers, 1960–85. Med J Aust 147:112–118, 1987.
76. Torg JS: Epidemiology, pathomechanics, and prevention of athletic injuries to the cervical spine. Med Sci Sports Exerc 17:295–303, 1985.
77. Torg JS: Athletic Injuries to the Head, Neck, and Face. St Louis, Mosby Year Book, 1991.
78. Torg JS, Corcoran TA, Thibault LE, et al: Cervical cord neurapraxia: Classification, pathomechanics, morbidity, and management guidelines. J Neurosurg 87(6):843–850, 1997.
79. Torg JS, Glasgow SG: Criteria for return in contact activities after cervical spine injury. In: Torg JS (ed): Athletic Injuries to the Head, Neck, and Face. St Louis, Mosby Year Book, 1991, pp 589–608.
80. Torg JS, Naranja RJ, Pavlov H, et al: The relationship of developmental narrowing of the cervical spinal canal to reversible and irreversible injury of the cervical spinal cord in football players. J Bone Joint Surg [Am] 78(9): 1308–1314, 1996.
81. Torg JS, Pavlov H, Gennario SE, et al: Neuropraxia of the cervical spinal cord with transient quadriplegia. J Bone Joint Surg 68A:1354–1370, 1986.
82. Torg JS, Sennett B, Pavlov H, et al: Spear tackler's spine. Am J Sports Med 21(5):640–649, 1993.
83. Torg JS, Truex R, Quedenfeld TC, et al: The national football head and neck injury registry. JAMA 241:1477–1479, 1979.
84. Vale FL, Burns J, Jackson AB, et al: Combined medical and surgical treatment after acute spinal cord injury: Results of a prospective pilot study to assess the merits of aggressive medical resuscitation and blood pressure management. J Neurosurg 87(2):239–246, 1997.
85. Walters R: Management of the critically injured athlete: Packaging of head and cervical spine injuries. South Med J 97(9):843–846, 2004.
86. Watkins RG: Neck injuries in football players. Clin Sports Med 5:215–246, 1986.
87. Wigglesworth EC: Spinal injuries and football. Med J Aust 147:109–110, 1987.
88. Williams JPR, McKibbin B: Cervical spinal injuries in rugby football. Br Med J 2:17–47, 1978.
89. Williams P, McKibbin B: Unstable cervical spine injuries in rugby—a 20 year review. Injury 18:329–332, 1987.
90. Wu WQ, Lewis RC: Injuries of the cervical spine in high school wrestling. Surg Neurol 23:143–147. 1985.

Part VI

Environmental Trauma

Chapter 28
High-Altitude Neurology

RALF W. BAUMGARTNER

In the past decades, the number of persons who choose to spend time at high altitude for leisure activities has considerably increased. Ascent of unacclimatized persons to high altitude may lead to neurological dysfunctions such as high-altitude headache (HAH), acute mountain sickness (AMS), high-altitude cerebral edema (HACE), and ataxia of stance. High-altitude headache and AMS are common complications and have become public health problems. In contrast, HACE is rare, but potentially fatal.

In this chapter, diagnosis, characteristics, epidemiology, pathogenesis, prevention, and therapy of AMS, HAH, HACE, and ataxia of stance will be discussed.

Acute Mountain Sickness

Diagnosis and Clinical Characteristics

Acute mountain sickness consists of nonspecific symptoms, which may develop in an unacclimatized subject within 6–12 hours after he has reached an altitude above 2500 m. A recent study suggests that AMS may also occur at altitudes between 1500 and 2500 m.[35] The symptoms of AMS include headache and at least one of the following: insomnia, dizziness, lassitude, fatigue, or gastrointestinal symptoms such as anorexia, nausea, or vomiting.[89] A recent study showed impaired speech control during exposure to simulated altitude, which was correlated with AMS severity.[26] Diagnostic signs of AMS are absent, and the presence of abnormal neurological or respiratory signs suggests progression to high-altitude pulmonary edema (HAPE) or HACE. The nonspecific symptoms of AMS can be confounded with those of other disorders, such as dehydration, exhaustion, hypothermia, alcohol hangover, and migraine.

Epidemiology

The incidence of AMS rises with increasing altitude.[28] It is 22% in mountaineers examined at altitudes of 1850–2750 m,[58] 42% at an altitude of 3000 m,[28] and about 50% at altitudes higher than 4000 m.[48,49] Risk factors for AMS include a history of AMS, residence at an altitude below 900 m, the rate of ascent, the altitude reached, physical exercise, obesity, and individual susceptibility.[47,58,88,92] Subjects over 50 years of age are somewhat less susceptible to AMS than younger subjects,[49,58,90] whereas children and younger adults appear to be equally affected.[82,103] Some studies found that women were just as susceptible to AMS as men,[49,58] whereas other investigations reported a higher incidence of this altitude illness in women.[66,76,78]

Respiratory tract infection[77] and neck irradiation or surgery[9] are potential risk factors for AMS that warrant further study. Physical fitness is not protective against AMS.[74] Arterial hypertension, diabetes, coronary artery disease and mild chronic obstructive pulmonary disease do not increase susceptibility to AMS.[47,90]

Pathogenesis

The pathogenesis of AMS is unknown. Hypoxia might activate the trigeminovascular system and cause headache associated with AMS (see the section about HAH). Hypobaria and exercise might further activate or sensitize the trigeminovascular system, since Roach et al. have shown an increased severity of AMS during hypobaric hypoxia compared to hypoxia alone[91] and during exercise.[92]

Hypoxia dilates the cerebral resistance vessels, which increases cerebral blood flow (CBF) and volume (CBV).[45,83] Some authors speculate that the resulting rise of CBV, alone or in combination with the hypothesized development of brain edema, increases intracranial pressure (ICP) and lead to AMS. However, the majority of available data suggest that (1) changes in CBF and CBV at high altitude are not important for the development of AMS, (2) there is no or at best minimal, clinically irrelevant brain edema in AMS, and (3) ICP is essentially normal in AMS. Decompression chamber[17,85] and field[61] studies have shown that CBF may increase up to 52%, remain unchanged, or decrease up to 32% compared to baseline values during the first 6 hours at high altitude.[17,61,85] Cerebral blood flow increases of 20%–27% were reported in field studies 12–24 hours after arrival at high altitude.[14,61,63,81,97] However, no study found a correlation between CBF and the incidence or severity of AMS.[14,17,61,63,70,85] or the incidence of HAH.[85] Furthermore, therapeutic trials reported successful treatment of AMS in spite of increased, stable, or decreased CBF.[5,50,55,63,85] Recent magnetic resonance imaging (MRI) studies found no signs of intra- or intracellular brain edema 6–10 hours at simulated high altitude in subjects with and without AMS[6,33] and only a small brain volume increase of 0.6%–2.7% after 16–32 hours' exposure to simulated high altitude.[6,75] No MRI study found a correlation between brain swelling, brain water content or cerebrospinal fluid (CSF) volume with AMS.[6,33,75] Intracranial pressure values were normal in subjects with and without AMS decompressed to simulated high altitude[6,54,95,102] and may transiently increase during exercise and periodic breathing.[104]

Arterial PO_2 is well known to be lower in subjects with than without AMS. This suggests that tissue oxygenation or hypoxia-dependent yet unknown factors are important for the development of AMS.

Prevention

The best strategy for prevention of AMS is a gradual ascent to endorse acclimatization.[51] Hackett et al. stated that above an altitude of 2500 m, the sleeping altitude should not be increased by more than 600 m in 24 hours, and that an extra day for acclimatization should be added for every increase of 600 to 1200 m at this altitude.[51] Furthermore, oral administration of acetazolamide (alternative, dexamethasone) for prevention of AMS was recommended for subjects who plan an ascent from sea level to a sleeping altitude of more than 3000 m in 1 day and for those with a history of AMS.[51] Acetazolamide and dexamethasone are both effective,[30,43,49,52,64,87] but the combination is more effective than either alone.[18] Most authors recommend 500 mg/day acetazolamide,[11,51] although a meta-analysis advised 750 mg/day.[29] A recent controlled study performed in 197 mountaineers showed that a low dose of acetazolamide (125 mg twice a day) reduced the incidence of AMS by 51%.[10] Oral ginkgo biloba reduced the incidence[71,93] and severity[36,71,93] of AMS in three controlled trials, although different doses and schemes of drug administration were used. In the first study, a dose of 80 mg twice daily prevented AMS in all subjects during an ascent from 1800 to 5200 m over 10 days.[93] In the second study, gingko 120 mg twice daily taken for 5 days before an abrupt ascent to 4100 m reduced the incidence and severity of AMS by 50%.[71] In the third study, gingko 60 mg three times daily, started 1 day before a rapid ascent from sea level to 4205 m, reduced the severity but not the incidence of AMS.[36] In contrast, gingko was no better than placebo in preventing AMS in an unpublished study.[11] Prophylactic aspirin (325 mg every 4 hours for a total of three doses) reduced the incidence of HAH from 50% to 7%.[22] A small-scale study has demonstrated that enteral antioxidant vitamin supplementation (four capsules/day, each capsule containing 250 mg L-ascorbic acid, 100 IU dl-α-tocopherol acetate, and 150 mg alpha-lipoic acid) started for 3 weeks at sea level before the ascent and during a 10-day ascent to 5180 m reduced the severity of AMS.[2] The vitamins were assumed to antagonize free radical–mediated damage to the blood–brain barrier, a presumed mechanism of AMS.[2] However, a recent study found no free radical–mediated neuronal damage in the peripheral circulation.[3] Thus, further study evaluating the preventive efficacy of antioxidant vitamins is needed. In two controlled studies, medroxyprogesterone given at high altitude did not prevent the development of AMS.[101]

Therapy

Patients who suffer from AMS should (1) avoid further ascent until the symptoms have resolved, (2) descend if there is no improvement or if symptoms worsen, and (3) descend immediately in the presence of signs of HACE or HAPE.[11,47] Mild AMS is treated with rest, and analgesics or antiemetics may be added.[47] Moderate or severe AMS is treated with supplementary oxygen, and the patients should descend.[47] The symptoms of AMS generally resolve after a descent of 500–1000 m.[47] Portable hyperbaric chambers are a useful alternative, especially when the patients are in remote places.[8,65,67] When supplementary oxygen is not accessible or descent is impossible, medical therapy becomes important. Oral acetazolamide reduced the severity of AMS by 74% in a controlled small-scale study.[44] Dexamethasone has been as effective as or superior to acetazolamide in several controlled studies.[32,52,67,68] It is unclear whether the combination of acetazolamide and dexamethasone is superior to either agent alone. The effect of sumatriptan on AMS and HAH was evaluated in three controlled studies.[7,24,100] It showed a persistent[7] or transient[100] minor benefit in two studies, and no effect[24] in the third study.

High-Altitude Headache

Diagnosis and Clinical Characteristics

High-altitude headache is defined by the International Headache Society (IHS) as a headache that develops "within 24 hours after sudden ascent to altitudes above 3000 m" and is "associated with at least one other symptom typical of high-altitude including (A) Cheyne-Stokes respiration at night, (B) a desire to overbreathe and (C) exertional dyspnoea."[56] A recent study reported the clinical features of HAH by analyzing 138 headaches experienced by 69 persons.[98] Most headaches were bilateral, commonly frontal, diffuse, or temporal, and about one-third were pulsatile. Nausea was associated in 16%, sensitivity to light and sound in 11%. Headaches were worsened by movement in about 50% and forced the subject to lie down or rest in 33%. Two persons each described visual and sensory symptoms associated with their headaches. Persons with a history of migraine had sensitivity to noise more often than those without such a history. In 43% of headaches, no accompanying IHS symptoms were recorded, whereas in 52% of headaches, there were no accompanying symptoms of AMS. Half of the headaches were associated with AMS. Common aggravating factors were exercise or effort in 44%, movement in 38%, bending in 21%, and coughing or sneezing in 18%.

Epidemiology

High-altitude headache occurred in 83% of subjects who ascended gradually from low altitude.[98] Younger age was the only risk factor for HAH in a recent study, whereas sex, the presence or absence of headaches in daily life, and previous headaches or headaches at high altitude were not risk factors.[98] Women reported headaches of greater severity (5 to 10 points on a scale of 0 to 10, where 0 was pain-free and 10 the worst pain of one's life) and a greater frequency of headaches; age and previous headaches at altitude were not associated with an increase in headache frequency. These differences between the sexes are probably caused by a combination of differences in the reporting of pain between men and women and physiological differences between men and women.[56] At low altitude, the incidence of most headache disorders is higher in women compared to men, suggesting that women may be more susceptible to HAH.[98] It has not been investigated whether other AMS risk factors such as the rate of ascent and the altitude reached also increase the chance of developing HAH.

Pathogenesis

The pain-sensitive fibers of the ophthalmic division of the trigeminal nerve (V1) and the nerve roots of the second cervical nerve (C2) innervate the meninges, and the meningeal and pial vessels, and establish the trigeminovascular system.[31,80] When stimulated experimentally in humans, large dural and pial vessels generate throbbing ipsilateral migraine-like pain.[84] In nonhuman primates, stimulation activates neurons of the trigeminal nucleus caudalis (TNC) and the dorsal horns of C1 and C2 (trigeminocervical complex).[40,41,59] V1 and C2 sensory fibers overlap in the trigemiocervical complex, which explains the distribution of HAH over frontotemporal as well as other cranial and cervical regions. Thus, activation of the trigeminovascular system, which is the suspected cause of headache in migraine,[42] might also underlie HAH.[94] Cortical metabolic activity at high altitude may release potassium and hydrogen ions, neurotransmitters, and metabolites (e.g., nitric oxide, adenosine, arachinodate) into the perivascular and extracellular spaces, which may lead to activation or sensitization of perivascular V1 afferents.[19,94] An increase in prostaglandins during acute exposure to high altitude is discussed as a pain-generating mechanism,[86] because cyclooxygenase inhibitors are effective in the treatment of HAH.[20,22,24] An altered perception of trigeminovascular input might cause painful sensations from stimuli that are usually not painful.[21,73] Correspondingly, Noel-Jorand et al. reported a 30% decrease in pain threshold at high-altitude compared to controls.[79]

Prevention and Therapy

Prevention and therapy of AMS and HAH are identical, because most patients with AMS also have headache.[49] Prophylactic intake of oral aspirin (1 g) reduced the incidence of headache when exercising during high-altitude exposure (active group, 56%; placebo group, 93%) in a placebo-controlled, randomized trial.[23] Flunarizine, an approved drug for prevention of migraine attacks,[4,57,69,72] was unable to prevent HAH in a small randomized, placebo-controlled study.[16] Oral ibuprofen (400 or 600 mg/day) reduced[20] or resolved[24] HAH. Acetaminophen was as effective as ibuprofen in relieving HAH in a randomized, controlled trial; no case of HAPE or HACE was noted.[53]

High-Altitude Cerebral Edema

Diagnosis and Characteristics

High-altitude cerebral edema is defined as the onset of ataxia, altered consciousness, or both in a subject with AMS or HAPE.[51] Associated signs include papilledema, retinal hemorrhage, encephalopathy, cranial nerve palsy, focal neurological deficits, and, rarely, seizures.[51] Lumbar puncture shows increased pressure.[99] Magnetic resonance imaging revealed signs of a vasogenic edema of the supratentorial water matter that especially affected the splenium of the callosal body in seven patients investigated 16–132 hours after the onset of symptoms.[46] All MRI changes resolved completely at follow-up.[52] Autopsy shows generalized brain edema, intracerebral hemorrhages that are predominantly petechial or lobar, thrombosis, and infarcts.[49,60] Compared to AMS, the incidence of HACE and HAPE is in the range of 0.1–4.0%.[11]

Pathogenesis

The cause of HACE is assumed to be vasogenic edema, whereas the pathogenesis of the edema is unclear. Elevated capillary pressure in the presence of impaired cerebral autoregulation due to hypoxic vasodilation may lead to brain edema when mean arterial pressure exceeds the upper limit of autoregulation.[52,62] Animal studies have shown that hypoxia induces permeability in the endothelium of brain microvessels via vascular endothelial growth factor (VEGF) and nitric oxide (NO).[25,34,96] Thus, increased expression of VEGF and NO synthase during hypoxia might be an important mechanism of HACE.

Prevention and Therapy

Prevention of HACE includes the same measures as the prevention of AMS (see above). The treatment for HACE is immediate descent in conjunction with supplementation of oxygen and the administration of dexamethasone.[11]

Postural Ataxia at High Altitude

The development of ataxia in a person affected by AMS is assumed to represent the transition to

HACE.[51] Nevertheless, mild to moderate ataxia (1 to 2 points on a 4-point scale) may occur in subjects with and without AMS.[13,15] Two posturography studies confirmed that the deterioration in the stability of stance at high altitude was similar in healthy subjects and those affected by AMS.[15,27] The pathogenesis of ataxia of stance at high altitude is unknown. Selective vulnerability of Purkinje cells and/or neurotransmitters to hypoxia might be a possible mechanism.[1,12,37–39] In contrast to the symptoms of AMS, those of postural ataxia did not regress after inhalation of 3 l/min oxygen for at least 10 minutes.[13]

REFERENCES

1. Aikayama Y, Koshimura K, Ohue T: Effects of hypoxia on the activity of the dopaminergic neuron system in the rat striatum as studied by in vivo brain microdialysis. J Neurochem 57:997–1002, 1992.
2. Bailey DM, Davies B: Acute mountain sickness; prophylactic benefits of antioxidant vitamin supplementation at high altitude. High Alt Med Biol 2:21–29, 2001.
3. Bailey DM, Kleger G-R, Holzgraefe M, Ballmer PE, Bärtsch P: Pathophysiological significance of peroxidative stress, neuronal damage, and membrane permeability in acute mountain sickness. J Appl Physiol 96: 1459–1463, 2004.
4. Baker C: A double-blind evaluation of flunarizine and placebo in the prophylactic treatment of migraine. Headache 21:288–292, 1987.
5. Bärtsch P, Baumgartner RW, Waber U, Maggiorini M, Oelz O: Comparison of carbon-dioxide-enriched, oxygen-enriched, and normal air in treatment of acute mountain sickness. Lancet 336:772–775, 1990.
6. Bärtsch P, Berger M, Bailey D, Baumgartner RW: Acute mountain sickness—controversies and advances. High Alt Med Biol 5:110–124, 2004.
7. Bärtsch P, Maggi S, Kleger G-R, Ballmer PE, Baumgartner RW: Sumatriptan for high-altitude headache. Lancet 344:1445, 1994.
8. Bärtsch P, Merki B, Hofstetter D, Maggiorini M, Kayser B, Oelz O: Treatment of acute mountain sickness by simulated descent: a randomised controlled trial. BMJ 306:1098–1101, 1993.
9. Basnyat B: Neck irradiation or surgery may predispose to severe acute mountain sickness. J Travel Med 9:105, 2002.
10. Basnyat B, Gertsch JH, Johnson EW, Castro-Marin F, Inoue Y, Yeh C: Efficacy of low-dose acetazolamide (125 mg BID) for the prophylaxis of acute mountain sickness: A prospective, double-blind, randomized, placebo-controlled trial. High Alt Med Biol 4:45–52, 2003.
11. Basnyat B, Murdoch DR: High-altitude illness. Lancet 361:1967–1974, 2003.
12. Baumgartner RW: The Brain at High Altitude. Barcelona: Universitat de Barcelona, 2003.
13. Baumgartner RW, Bärtsch P: Ataxia in acute mountain sickness does not improve with short-term oxygen inhalation. High Alt Med Biol 3:283–292, 2002.
14. Baumgartner RW, Bärtsch P, Maggiorini M, Waber U, Oelz O: Enhanced cerebral blood flow in acute mountain sickness. Aviat Space Environ Med 65:726–729, 1994.
15. Baumgartner RW, Eichenberger U, Bärtsch P: Postural ataxia at high altitude is not related to mild-to-moderate severity of acute mountain sickness. Eur J Appl Physiol 56:322–326, 2002.
16. Baumgartner RW, Keller S, Regard M, Bärtsch P: Flunarizine in prevention of headache, ataxia and memory deficits during decompression to 4559 m. High Alt Med Biol 4:333–339, 2003.
17. Baumgartner RW, Spyridopoulos I, Bärtsch P, Maggiorini M, Oelz O: Acute mountain sickness is not related to cerebral blood flow. A decompression chamber study. J Appl Physiol 86:1578–1582, 1999.
18. Bernhard WN, Schalick LM, Delaney PA, Bernhard TM, Barnas GM: Acetazolamide plus low-dose dexamethasone is better than acetazolamide alone to ameliorate symptoms of acute mountain sickness. Aviat Space Environ Med 69:883–886, 1998.
19. Bolay H, Reuter U, Dunn AK, Huang Z, Boas DA, Moskowitz MA: Intrinsic brain activity triggers trigeminal meningeal afferents in a rodent model. Nature Med 8:136–141, 2002.
20. Broome JR, Stoneham MD, Beeley JM, Milledge JS, Hughes AS: High altitude headache: Treatment with ibuprofen. Aviat Space Environ Med 65:19–20, 1994.
21. Burstein R, Yarnitsky D, Goor-Aryeh I, Ransil BJ, Bajwa ZH: An association between migraine and cutaneous allodynia. Ann Neurol 47:614–624, 2000.
22. Burtscher M, Likar R, Nachbauer W, Philadelphy M: Aspirin for prophylaxis against headache at high altitudes: Randomised, double blind, placebo controlled trial. BMJ 316:1057–1058, 1998.
23. Burtscher M, Likar R, Nachbauer W, Philadelphy M, Pühringer M, Lämmle T: Effects of aspirin during exercise on the incidence of high-altitude headache: A randomized, double-blind, placebo-controlled trial. Headache 41:542–545, 2001.
24. Burtscher M, Likar R, Nachbauer W, Schaffert W, Philadelphy M: Ibuprofen versus sumatriptan for high-altitude headache. Lancet 346:254–255, 1995.
25. Clark IA, Awburn MM, Cowden WB, Rockett KA: Can excessive iNOS induction explain much of the illness of acute mountain sickness? In: Roach RC, Wagner PD, Hackett PH (eds): Advances in Experimental Medicine and Biology, vol 474. New York, Kluwer Academic/Plenum, 1999, p 373 (abstract).
26. Cymerman A, Lieberman P, Hochstadt J, Rock PB, Butterfield GE, Moore LG: Speech motor control and acute mountain sickness. Aviat Space Environ Med 73:766–772, 2002.

27. Cymerman A, Muza SR, Beidleman BA, Ditzler DT, Fulco CS: Postural instability and acute mountain sickness during exposure to 24 hours of simulated altitude (4300 m). High Alt Med Biol 2:509–514, 2001.
28. Dean AG, Yip R, Hoffmann RE: High incidence of mild acute mountain sickness in conference attendees at 10,000 foot altitude. J Wilderness Med 1:86–92, 1990.
29. Dumont L, Mardirosoff C, Tramer MR: Efficacy and harm of pharmacological prevention of acute mountain sickness: Quantitative systematic review. BMJ 321:267–272, 2000.
30. Ellsworth AJ, Meyer EF, Larson EB: Acetazolamide or dexamethasone use versus placebo to prevent acute mountain sickness on Mount Rainier. West J Med 154:289–293, 1991.
31. Feindel W, Penfield W, MacNaughton F: The tentorial nerves and localization of intracranial pain in man. Neurology 10:555–563, 1960.
32. Ferrazzini G, Maggiorini M, Kriemler S, Bärtsch P, Oelz O: Successful treatment of acute mountain sickness with dexamethasone. BMJ 294:1380–1382, 1987.
33. Fischer R, Vollmar C, Thiere M, Born C, Leitl M, Pfluger T, et al: No evidence of cerebral oedema in severe acute mountain sickness. Cephalalgia 24:66–71, 2004.
34. Fischer S, Clauss M, Wiesnet M, Renz D, Schaper W, Karliczek GF: Hypoxia induces permeability in brain microvessel endothelial cells via VEGF and NO. Am J Physiol 276:C812–C820, 1999.
35. Gabry AL, Ledoux X, Mozziconacci M, Martin C: High-altitude pulmonary edema at moderate altitude (<2400 m; 7870 feet): A series of 52 patients. Chest 123:49–53, 2003.
36. Gertsch JH, Seto TB, Mor J, Onopa J: Gingko biloba for the prevention of severe acute mountain sickness (AMS) starting one day before rapid ascent. High Alt Med Biol 3:29–37, 2002.
37. Gibson GE, Duffy TE: Impaired synthesis of acetylcholine by mild hypoxic hypoxia or nitrous oxide. J Neurochem 36:28–33, 1981.
38. Gibson GE, Peterson C, Sansone J: Decreases in amino acid and acetylcholine metabolism during hypoxia. J Neurochem 37:192–201, 1981.
39. Gibson GE, Pulsinelli W, Blass JP, Duffy TE: Brain dysfunction in mild to moderate hypoxia. Am J Med 70:1247–1254, 1981.
40. Goadsby PJ, Hoskin KL: The distribution of trigeminovascular afferents in the nonhuman primate brain *Macaca nemestrina*: A c-*fos* cytochemical study. J Anat 190:367–375, 1997.
41. Goadsby PJ, Knight YE, Hoskin KL: Stimulation of the greater occipital nerve increases metabolic activity in the trigeminal nucleus caudalis and cervical dorsal horn of the cat. Pain 73:23–28, 1997.
42. Goadsby PJ, Lipton RB, Ferrari MD: Migraine—current understanding and treatment. N Engl J Med 346:257–270, 2002.
43. Greene MK, Keer AM, McIntosh IB, Prescott RJ: Acetazolamide in prevention of acute mountain sickness: A double blind controlled cross-over study. BMJ 283: 811–813, 1981.
44. Grissom CK, Roach RC, Sarnquist FH, Hackett PH: Acetazolamide in the treatment of acute mountain sickness: Clinical efficacy and effect on gas exchange. Ann Intern Med 116:461–465, 1992.
45. Grubb RL, Raichle ME, Eichling JO, Ter-Pogossian MM: The effect of changes in PaCO2 on cerebral blood volume, blood flow and vascular mean transit time. Stroke 5:630–639, 1974.
46. Hackett P, Yarnell PR, Hill R, Reynard K, Heit J, McCormick J. High-altitude cerebral edema evaluated with magnetic resonance imaging. JAMA 280:1920–1925, 1998.
47. Hackett PH: High altitude and common medical conditions. In: Hornbein TF, Schoene RB, (eds): High Altitude: An Exploration of Human Adaptation. New York, Marcel Dekker, 2001, pp 1–37.
48. Hackett PH, Rennie D: Rales, peripheral edema, retinal hemorrhage and acute mountain sickness. Am J Med 67:214–218, 1979.
49. Hackett PH, Rennie ID, Levine HD: The incidence, importance, and prophylaxis of acute mountain sickness. Lancet 2:1149–1154, 1976.
50. Hackett PH, Roach RC: Oxygenation, But Not Increased Cerebral Blood Flow, Improves High Altitude Headache. Toronto, C Decker, 1990.
51. Hackett PH, Roach RC: High-altitude illness. N Engl J Med 345:107–114, 2001.
52. Hackett PH, Roach RC, Wood RA, Foutch RG, Meehan RT, Rennie D, et al: Dexamethasone for prevention and treatment of acute mountain sickness. Aviat Space Environ Med 59:950–954, 1988.
53. Harris NS, Wenzel RP, Thomas SH: High altitude headache: Efficacy of acetaminophen vs. ibuprofen in a randomized, controlled trial. J Emerg Med 24:383–387, 2003.
54. Hartig GS, Hackett PH: Cerebral Spinal Fluid Pressure and Cerebral Blood Velocity in Acute Mountain Sickness. Oxford, Pergammon Press, 1992.
55. Harvey TC, Raichle ME, Winterborn MH, Jensen J, Lassen NA, Richardson NV, et al: Effect of carbon dioxide in acute mountain sickness: A rediscovery. Lancet 2:639–641, 1988.
56. Headache Classification Committee of the International Headache Society: Classification and diagnostic criteria for headache disorders, cranial neuralgias and facial pain. Cephalalgia 7(suppl 7):1–96, 1988.
57. Holroyd KA, Penzien DB, Rokicki LA, Cordingley GE: Flunarizine versus propranolol: A meta-analysis of clinical trials. Headache 32:256–261, 1992.
58. Honigman B, Theis MK, Koziol-McLain J, Roach RC, Yip R, Houston C, et al: Acute mountain sickness in a general tourist population at moderate altitudes. Ann Intern Med 118:587–592, 1993.
59. Hoskin KL, Zagami A, Goadsby PJ: Stimulation of the middle meningeal artery leads to bilateral Fos expres-

sion in the trigeminocervical nucleus: A comparative study of monkey and cat. J Anat 194:579–588, 1999.
60. Houston CC, Dickinson J: Cerebral form of high altitude illness. Lancet 2:758–761, 1975.
61. Huang SY, Moore LG, McCullough RE, McCullough RG, Micco AJ, Fulco C, et al: Internal carotid and vertebral arterial flow velocity in men at high altitude. J Appl Physiol 63:395–400, 1987.
62. Jensen JB, Sperling B, Severinghaus JW, Lassen NA: Augmented hypoxic cerebral vasodilation in men during 5 days at 3810 m altitude. J Appl Physiol 80:1214–1218, 1996.
63. Jensen JB, Wright AD, Lassen NA, Harvey T-C, Winterborn MH, Raichle ME, et al: Cerebral blood flow in acute mountain sickness. J Appl Physiol 69:430–433, 1990.
64. Johnson TS, Rock PB, Fulco CS, Trad LA, Spark RF, Maher JT: Prevention of acute mountain sickness by dexamethasone. N Engl J Med 310:683–686, 1984.
65. Kasic JF, Yaron M, Nicholas RA, Lickeig JA, Roach R: Treatment of acute mountain sickness: hyperbaric versus oxygen therapy. Ann Emerg Med 20:1109–1112, 1991.
66. Kayser B: Acute mountain sickness in western tourists around the Thorong pass (5400 m) in Nepal. J Wilderness Med 2:110–117, 1991.
67. Keller HR, Maggiorini M, Bärtsch P, Oelz O: Simulated descent versus dexamethasone in treatment of acute mountain sickness: A randomised trial. BMJ 310:1232–1235, 1995.
68. Levine BD, Yoshimura K, Kobayashi T, Fukushima M, Shibamoto T, Ueda G: Dexamethasone in the treatment of acute mountain sickness. N Engl J Med 321:1707–1713, 1989.
69. Lücking CH, Oestreich W, Schmidt R, Soyka D: Flunarizine vs propranolol in the prophylaxis of migraine: Two double-blind comparative studies in more than 400 patients. Cephalalgia 8(suppl 8):15–20, 1988.
70. Lysakowski W, Von Elm E, Dumont L, Junod J-D, Tassony E, Kayser B, et al: Effect of magnesium, high altitude and acute mountain sickness on blood flow velocity in the middle cerebral artery. Clin Sci 106:279–285, 2004.
71. Maakestad K, Leadbetter G, Olson S, Hackett PH: Ginkgo biloba reduces incidence and severity of acute mountain sickness (abstract). Wilderness Environ Med 12:51, 2001.
72. Martinez-Lage JM: Flunarizine (sibelium) in the prophylaxis of migraine. An open, long-term, multicenter trial. Cephalagia 8(suppl 8):15–20, 1988.
73. May A, Buchel C, Turner R, Goadsby PJ: Magnetic resonance angiography in facial and other pain: Neurovascular mechanisms of trigeminal sensation. J Cereb Blood Flow Metab 21:1171–1176, 2001.
74. Milledge JS, Beeley JM, Broome J, Luff N, Pelling M, Smith D: Acute mountain sickness susceptibility, fitness and hypoxic ventilatory response. Eur Respir J 4:1000–1003, 1991.
75. Mórocz IA, Zientara GP, Gudbjartsson H, Muza S, Lyons T, Rock PB, et al: Volumetric quantification of brain swelling after hypobaric hypoxia exposure. Exp Neurol 168:96–104, 2001.
76. Murdoch DR: Altitude illness among tourists flying to 3740 meters elevation in the Nepal Himalayas. J Travel Med 2:255–256, 1995.
77. Murdoch DR: Symptoms of infection and altitude illness among hikers in the Mount Everest region of Nepal. Aviat Space Environ Med 66:148–151, 1995.
78. Murdoch DR, Curry C: Acute mountain sickness in the southern Alps of New Zealand. NZ Med J 111:168–169, 1998.
79. Noel-Jorand MC, Bragard D, Plaghki L: Pain perception under chronic high-altitude hypoxia. Eur J Neurosci 8:2075–2079, 1996.
80. O' Connor TP, Van der Kooy D: Pattern of intracranial and extracranial projections of trigeminal ganglion cells. J Neurosci 6:2200–2207, 1986.
81. Otis SM, Rossmann ME, Schneider PA, Rush MP, Ringelstein EB: Relationship of cerebral blood flow regulation to acute mountain sickness. J Ultrasound Med 8:143–148, 1989.
82. Pollard AJ, Niermeyer S, Barry P, Bärtsch P, Berghold F, Bishop RA, et al: Children at high altitude: An international consensus statement by an ad hoc committee of the International Society for Mountain Medicine, March 12, 2001. High Alt Med Biol 2:389–403, 2001.
83. Poulin MJ, Robbins PA: Indexes of flow and cross-sectional area of the middle cerebral artery using Doppler ultrasound during hypoxia and hypercapnia in humans. Stroke 27:2244–2250, 1996.
84. Ray B, Wolff H: Experimental studies on headache pain: Pain sensitive structures of the head and their significance in headache. Arch Surg 41:813–856, 1940.
85. Reeves JT, Moore LG, McCullough RE, McCullough RG, Harrison G, Tranmer BI, et al: Headache at high altitude is not related to internal carotid arterial blood velocity. J Appl Physiol 59:909–915, 1985.
86. Richalet JP, Hornych A, Rathat C, Aumont J, Larmignat P, Rémy P: Plasma prostaglandins, leukotrienes and thromboxane in acute high altitude hypoxia. Respir Physiol 85:205–215, 1991.
87. Ried LD, Carter KA, Ellsworth A: Acetazolamide or dexamethasone for prevention of acute mountain sickness: A meta-analysis. J Wilderness Med 5:34–48, 1994.
88. Ri-Li G, Chase PJ, Witkowski S, Wyrick BL, Stone JA, Levine BD, et al: Obesity: Associations with acute mountain sickness. Ann Intern Med 139:253–257, 2003.
89. Roach RC, Bärtsch P, Hackett PH, Oelz O: The Lake Louise AMS Scoring Consensus Committee. The Lake Louise Acute Mountain Sickness Scoring System. Burlington: Queen City Printers, 1993.
90. Roach RC, Houston CS, Honigman B, Nicholas RA, Yaron M, Grissom CK, et al: How well do older persons tolerate moderate altitude? West J Med 162:32–36, 1995.
91. Roach RC, Loeppky JA, Icenogle MV: Acute mountain sickness: Increased severity during simulated altitude

compared to hypoxia alone. J Appl Physiol 81:1908–1910, 1996.

92. Roach RC, Maes D, Sandoval D, Robergs RA, Icenogle M, Hinghofer-Szalkay H, et al: Exercise exacerbates acute mountain sickness at simulated high altitude. J Appl Physiol 88:581–585, 2000.
93. Roncin JP, Schwartz F, D'Arbigny P: EGb 761 in control of acute mountain sickness and vascular reactivity to cold exposure. Aviat Space Environ Med 67:445–452, 1996.
94. Sanchez del Rio M, Moskowitz M: High altitude headache: Lessons from headaches at sea level. In: Roach R, Wagner P, Hackett P, (eds): Hypoxia: Into the Next Millenium, vol 474. New York, Kluwer Academic/Plenum, 1999, pp 145–153.
95. Schaltenbrand G: Atmospheric pressure, circulation, respiration and cerebrospinal fluid pressure. Acta Aerophysiol 1:65–78, 1933.
96. Schoch HJ, Fischer S, Marti HH: Hypoxia-induced vascular endothelial growth factor expression causes vascular leakage in the brain. Brain 125:2549–2557, 2002.
97. Severinghaus JW, Chidi H, Eger EI, Brandstater B, Hornbein TF: Cerebral blood flow in man at high altitude: Role of cerebrospinal fluid pH in normalization of flow in chronic hypocapnia. Circ Res 19:274–282, 1966.
98. Silber E, Sonnenberg P, Collier DJ, Pollard AJ, Murdoch DR, Goadsby PJ: Clinical features of headache at altitude. A prospective study. Neurology 60:1167–1171, 2003.
99. Singh I, Khanna PK, Cardiology DM, Srivastava MC, Lal M, Roy SB, et al: Acute mountain sickness. N Engl J Med 280:175–184, 1969.
100. Utiger D, Eichenberger U, Bernasch D, Baumgartner RW, Bärtsch P: Transient minor improvement of high-altitude headache by sumatriptan. High Alt Med Biol 3:387–393, 2002.
101. Wright AD, Beazley MF, Bradwell AR, Chesner IM, Clayton RN, Forster PJ, et al: Medroxyprogesterone at high altitude. The effects on blood gases, cerebral regional oxygenation, and acute mountain sickness. Wilderness Environ Med 15:25–31, 2004.
102. Wright AD, Imray CHE, Morissey MSC, Marchbanks RJ, Bradwell AR: Intracranial pressure at high altitude and acute mountain sickness. Clin Sci Colch 89:201–204, 1995.
103. Yaron M, Waldman N, Niermeyer S, Nicholas R, Honigman B: The diagnosis of acute mountain sickness in preverbal children. Arch Pediatr Adolesc Med 152:683–687, 1998.
104. Zavasky D, Hackett P: Cerebral etiology of acute mountain sickness. MRI findings (abstract). Wilderness Env Med 6:229–230, 1995.

Chapter 29
Neurological Injury from Undersea Diving

E. WAYNE MASSEY

Scuba diving is becoming an increasingly popular sport. Data have been kept through the Diver's Alert Network (DAN) for years and can be evaluated to suggest the epidemiological characteristics of diving accidents. Although injured divers are not necessarily comparable to a normal diving population, injury occurrences are continuously being assessed by DAN. There are approximately 3 million certified divers in the United States.[9] There are approximately 1000 to 1200 injuries yearly (see Fig. 29.1 comparing 1987–2002).

The following information is based on the 2004 *DAN Report on Decompression Illness, Diving Fatalities and Project Dive Exploration*.[46] Epidemiological characteristics include several areas. The number of diving cases has increased yearly since 1987 (Fig. 29.1) Although there were about 600 cases in 1989, there were about 1100 cases in 2002. Many more people are scuba diving as a sport.

Among the many symptoms reported to DAN as problems from diving in 2002 (Fig. 29.2), the ones of most concern to neurologists involve the nervous system. Cases with motor symptoms or signs increased from 1998 to 2002 (Fig. 29.3). Bladder problems and altered consciousness remain a smaller percentage of all cases. Lower extremity involvement is most frequently seen (Fig. 29.4).

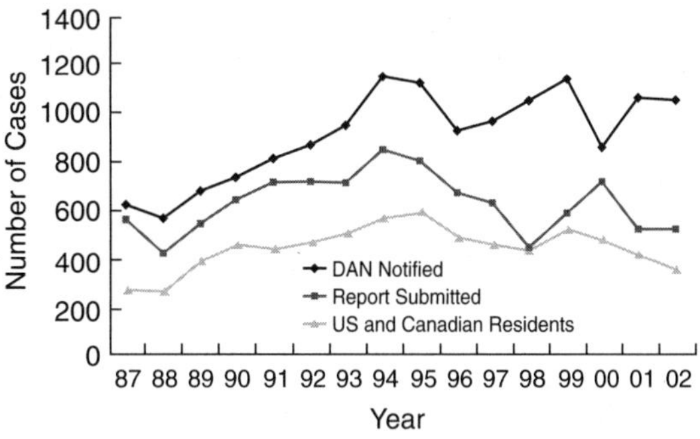

Figure 29.1. Annual record of dive injury cases.

Injured divers are more often male than female (Fig. 29.5). Of course, many more males do scuba diving than females, but behavior patterns could also be a factor.

Pain and numbness also are frequent complaints in scuba divers. Interestingly, pain is much more frequent in the upper extremities as are numbness and tingling, while weakness is more often found in the lower extremities (Fig. 29.6).

About fifty percent of injured divers were at beginning certification levels.[46] Forty-five percent were trained at advanced levels. Among the fatalities, it is difficult to obtain the exact number of

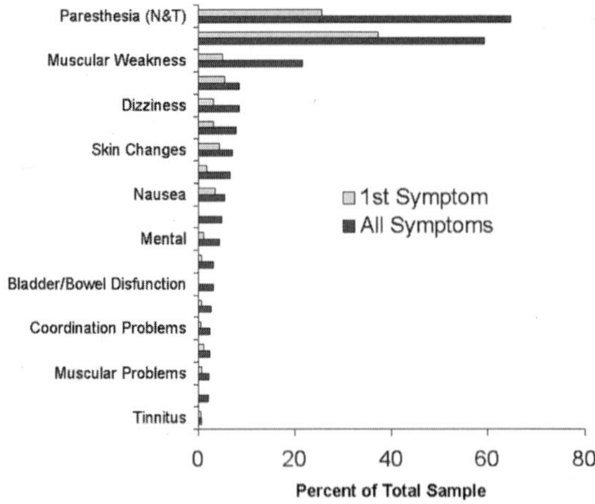

Figure 29.2. Symptoms in divers, 1998–2002.

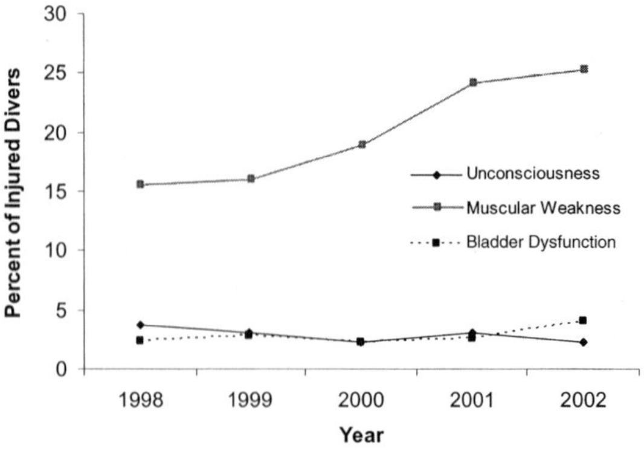

Figure 29.3. Percentage of dive injury cases involving unconsciousness, muscular weakness, or bladder dysfunction during 1998–2002.

dives and years the individual had been diving. The analysis is based on the number of dives reported to have been made by each individual. Nearly 60% of all fatalities occurred in divers who made 20 or fewer dives in their entire diving career. Initially, some divers at the intermediate and experienced levels were infrequent divers who used scuba only once yearly. Therefore, most accidents occurred in inexperienced divers. Additionally, the greatest proportion of diving was done by individuals who pursued the sport for only a short period of time.[13]

Other attributes of diving also have an effect. The 2004 DAN report summarizes some of them.[46] This report can be obtained on a yearly basis. Injuries and fatalities are categorized by geographic location, as well as by the clinical attributes of age, sex, diving experience, and clinical symptoms.

Decompression Sickness

Decompression sickness (DCS) (the bends, caisson disease) occurs when inert gas taken up during a dive comes out of solution, forming bubbles. The likelihood of bubble formation increases as a function of depth, time, and ascent rate. As the diver descends, pressure increases rapidly. The ambient pressure at 33 feet under the sea is twice that at the surface, and at 66 feet it is three times that at the surface. The partial pressure of the gases

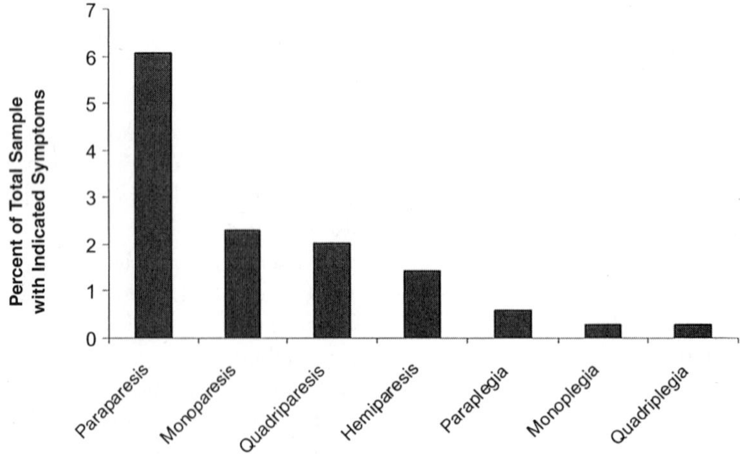

Figure 29.4. Distribution of muscular weakness.

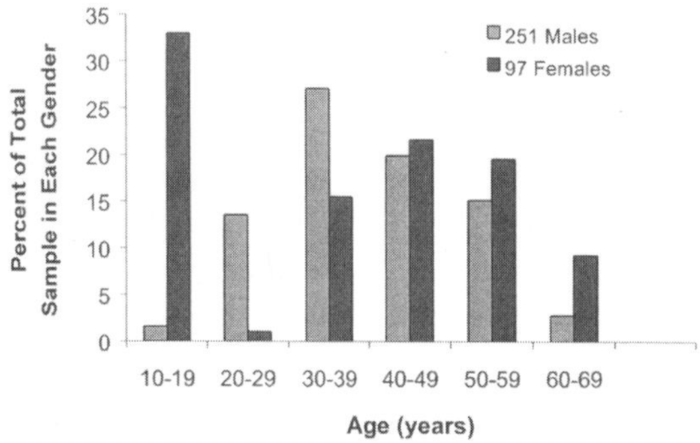

Figure 29.5. Age of injured divers by gender ($N = 348$).

breathed by the diver increases proportionately in accordance with Dalton's law. Thus, at 100 feet, the diver's tissues are exposed to a fourfold increase in gas pressure compared with sea level. Although oxygen is actively metabolized, nitrogen is essentially inert. The tissues soak it up and after a time become saturated. When the diver ascends, the reverse process takes place, gas moving from tissues to lower partial pressures in the blood and then being exhausted from the lungs. Trouble begins when the ascent is too rapid and the tissues are relatively supersaturated. The dissolved gas changes to free gas, creating bubbles in body tissues. The extent of this gas phase (bubbles) depends on the depth and duration of the dive and the rate of ascent.[36] The likelihood of injury is dose-related. A few bubbles seem to cause only a few symptoms, whereas a great shower may cause crippling or fatal disease.[2] Decompression sickness, a systemic disease, has characteristics of two types, which include the following:

DCS type I. Mild; peripheral pain, nonneurological. Type I is characterized only by itching of the skin, along with the pain in joints and limbs.

DCS type II. Serious; neurological. Type II is characterized by neurological problems including weakness, loss of sensation, ataxia, vertigo, disturbance of consciousness, disturbance of vision and mentation, and disturbance of bowel and bladder control. The majority of divers with type II DCS have symptoms referable to the thoracic spinal cord. The onset of girdle or pelvic pain and dysesthesia accompanied by sensory loss, weakness, and loss of bowel or bladder control is characteristic. The frequency of type II DCS varies from 26% to 61% of all cases. Cerebral involvement occurs in 30% of these cases. Objective complaints such as lethargy, mental cloudiness, confusion, and a feeling of illness may be much more common.

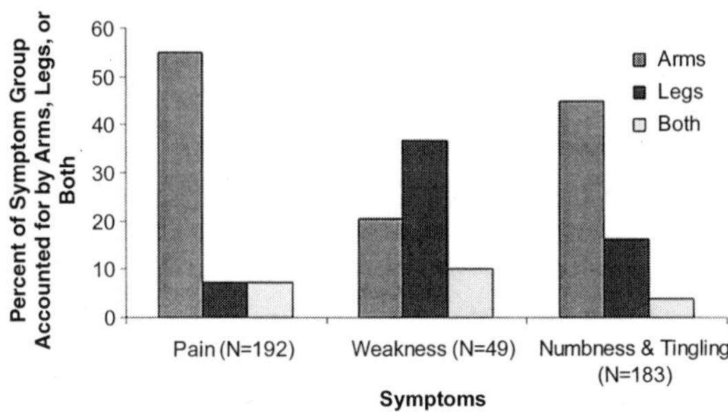

Figure 29.6. Distribution of pain, numbness and tingling, and muscular weakness by limb.

Bubbles may spread in any tissue and produce varied symptoms. With small gas loads, symptoms may be restricted to pain in a single joint (type I or pain only) or to itching in the skin (*niggles*). If the bubble load is larger, many systems may suffer. Most often the target organ is the spinal cord.[19]

The vascular anatomy of the spinal cord provides an opportunity for bubbles produced in the paravertebral veins (Batson's plexus) to collect in a stagnant froth, where they move to and fro with changes in intrathoracic pressure, creating stasis and venous infarction in the spinal cord. Patients commonly complain of pain or dysesthesia in the trunk and abdomen, and then develop weakness, sensory loss, and bladder dysfunction as the disease progresses. Symptoms usually begin within an hour of surfacing but may be delayed for many hours. The greater the gas load, the earlier the symptoms appear and the more ominous they are.[20]

Type II DCS (serious or neurological) produces neurological injury (Fig. 29.7). Although the spinal cord is most often involved, the brain may suffer as well. Divers with DCS frequently complain of fatigue, malaise, difficulty concentrating, and occasionally more specific cortical symptoms such as visual loss and dysphasia. Most commonly, DCS affects the spinal cord.[10,17]

Divers endeavor to protect themselves from DCS by observing decompression schedules established by the U.S. Navy and other agencies.[46] These schedules are based on both theoretical calculation

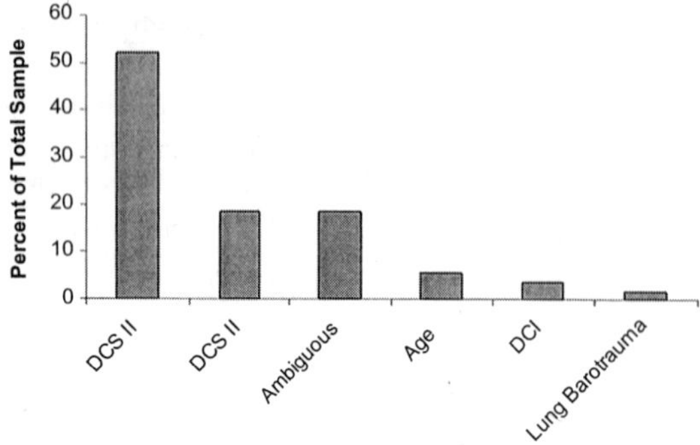

Figure 29.7. Distribution of cases according to reviewed diagnosis (N = 348).

and experience and are generally successful. Decompression sickness may occur in a small percentage of divers despite careful compliance with these schedules. Less than perfect compliance, particularly with rapid ascent, carries an increased likelihood of DCS. The greater the violation, the greater the likelihood of injury. Many divers use decompression computers, which provide real-time simulation of body inert gas uptake. Nevertheless, even careful divers may develops DCS.

Arterial Gas Embolism

Arterial gas embolism (AGE; air embolism, GAGE or cerebral gas embolism) results when a diver ascends without venting air from the lungs. As pressure decreases, volume increases in direct compliance with Boyle's law. A diver at the bottom of an 8-foot swimming pool who takes a full breath from a scuba tank, holds it, and ascends to the surface has a high likelihood of lung rupture. The alveoli can be ruptured with internal overpressure of as little as 90 cm of water.[3]

The characteristics of AGE include the following:

It is a serious consequence of pulmonary overinflation. Symptoms of pulmonary overinflation and AGE occur immediately during ascent or shortly after surfacing. Pain and respiratory distress are common, with coughing and hemoptysis. Headache is a common complaint, and unconsciousness may follow. The patient may experience aphasia or hemiparesis or become cortically blind. Quadriplegia and respiratory and cardiac arrest are sudden severe results.

It produces cortical and brain stem events; spinal cord lesions are rare.

It may be associated with atrial or ventricular paten ovale defect. Symptoms occur on ascent to the surface, and any diver found unconscious should be assumed to have cerebral AGE.

It most commonly occurs among untrained and newly trained divers. Free ascent and buoyant ascent exercises and buddy breathing drills are implicated frequently. Panic, particularly when the diver runs out of air at depth, is an important cause of AGE. Obstructive pulmonary disease, particularly asthma, is an important factor that often goes unrecognized.

When alveolar rupture occurs, air may dissect into the pleural space, causing pneumothorax; into the mediastinum, causing metastinal and subcutaneous emphysema in the supraclavicular space; or into the pericardium, causing pneumopericardium. All of these conditions may have clinical significance. A more serious event occurs when air dissects into the pulmonary-capillary system, is carried to the left atrium, and is then pumped into the arterial circulation. The bubbles are systemically distributed. Many bubbles are directed to the brain, causing sudden stroke-like events, which occur within a few minutes of reaching the surface. Patients may have a convulsion, suffer cardiorespiratory arrest, or have cortical blindness, hemiplegia, and aphasia. If the diver has taken up a significant amount of inert gas before the embolism, however, symptoms and signs more characteristic of DCS (i.e., affecting the spinal cord) may result.

Also, in contrast to DCS, AGE is neither time nor depth related. It may occur in the first minute of a dive and from shallow depth. The bubbles that reach the brain are forced into relatively small (50 μm) vessels and may conform to the vessels, causing occlusions 1 to 300 μm in length. They may be distributed to both hemispheres and to the posterior circulation as well.[16]

TREATMENT

Definitive treatment of DCS combines high partial pressure of oxygen and increased ambient pressure.

The two illnesses described earlier may coexist, and sometimes one cannot distinguish between them. Common to both DCS and AGE are nitrogen bubbles within tissue that occlude vessels, causing ischemia and acting as space-occupying lesions.

Increasing ambient pressure, by recompressing in a chamber, makes the bubble smaller. Doubling the pressure decreases the bubble volume by half. This can be expected to allow the bubble to move downstream, reducing the area of ischemia and in other tissues simply reducing the size of the lesion. There are limits to this mode. Enormous pressure is required to redissolve the bubble, far greater than can be achieved by practical recompression techniques. High air pressures also allow further nitrogen to be absorbed. As a practical matter, recompression to 165 feet of sea water (FsW) (6 absolute atmosphere [ATA]) brief periods is the highest therapeutic pressure used for AGE.

Oxygen is used to increase the rate of nitrogen removal. Assume that the offending tissue bubbles are purely nitrogen and that air in the alveoli is 80% nitrogen. At sea level, P_{N2} in the bubble is 760 torr and in the lungs it is about 600 torr. This leaves a nitrogen gradient of about 160 torr. These calculations exclude vapor pressure and P_{CO2} but serve to illustrate that a small natural gradient exists that tends to eliminate nitrogen bubbles from tissue. When the patient breathes pure oxygen and alveolar P_{N2} approaches zero, the off-gassing gradient is sharply increased. This principle (*oxygen window*) is the basis of oxygen treatment for dysbaric illness.[34]

It is obvious that an even greater advantage can be achieved by breathing oxygen under pressure. For instance, at 60 FsW (2.8 ATA), P_{N2} in the bubble is 2120 torr, P_{N2} in the alveoli is zero, and the off-gassing gradient therefore exceeds 2000 torr. This combination of increased ambient pressure and high partial pressure of oxygen is the basic treatment of dysbaric illness.

Just as there are limits to the use of pressure, there are limits to the use of oxygen. Under pressure and for prolonged periods, oxygen causes both cerebral and pulmonary toxicity. Inspired oxygen partial pressures above 3 ATA commonly cause convulsions. Moderately high oxygen pressures for prolonged periods cause pulmonary irritation, coughing, and, finally, loss of compliance.

Most commonly used treatment schedules have been established by the U.S. Navy, although similar schedules are published by other agencies. For example, DCS is usually treated on a U.S. Navy Table 6 schedule. The patient is recompressed to 60 FsW, breathing oxygen. Brief periods of air breathing are interposed to ameliorate the effects of oxygen toxicity. After 1¼ hours, the patient is gradually decompressed to 30 FsW, when additional oxygen breathing periods are employed. The total treatment takes 4¾ hours. If symptoms and findings do not resolve, the treatment may be extended to as long as 12 or 13 hours. More complex treatment schedules are employed in serious cases.

Other ancillary and supportive measures may be required. Dysbaric accidents may be complicated by near drowning, with its pulmonary implications.[7,12] Cardiopulmonary resuscitation may be required. Severely ill patients need intravenous fluids, catheterization, and treatment for shock. Adjunctive medications such as aspirin, steroids, or mannitol are sometimes used, although their role is unclear.[15]

Field Management

Decompression sickness occurs suddenly, evolves rapidly, and requires emergent treatment. The diagnosis depends on familiarity with diving physiology, observation, and physical examination. A physician being rarely on the scene, the assessment is usually made by a dive master, diving supervisor, or companion. In order of importance, management requires:

1. Prompt recognition. (Obviously, a temporal profile is helpful.)
2. Availability of oxygen with a mask and reservoir that will provide high fraction of inspired oxygen (FI_{O2}) and in quantities sufficient to continue treatment until the patient is delivered to a recompression chamber.
3. Resuscitation, if required, for respiratory compromise.
4. Transportation to a competent recompression chamber for definitive treatment.

There are several pitfalls here. These accidents often occur far from shore and hours away from a recompression chamber. The success of recompression treatment is time-dependent. If the leader of the dive party does not have a contingency plan or does not know the location of the nearest recompression chamber, valuable hours may be lost. Help with evacuation can often be obtained from the Coast Guard, Sheriff's Department, or Highway Patrol. A call to DAN will provide the location of the nearest recompression facility.

Diving-Related Illnesses

Decompression sickness is a problem among sport divers (few casualties occur in the commercial sector). Paying close attention to diving times and methods is important in the prevention of DCS.[29]

Arterial gas embolism occurs most commonly among untrained and newly trained divers. Free ascent and buoyant ascent exercises and buddy breathing drills are frequently implicated. Panic, particularly when the diver runs out of air at depth, is an important cause. Obstructive pulmonary disease, particularly asthma, is an important factor that often goes unrecognized.[32]

Among medical illnesses that increase the risks in diving individuals, the most common is pulmonary dysfunction.[32] Asthma is a relatively absolute contraindication to diving. It is best to follow the recommendations of the physician and to have a thorough evaluation if one has asthma. Likewise, any form of obstructive pulmonary disease, smoking history, or history of spontaneous pneumothorax (blebs) or similar pulmonary dysfunction should discourage an individual from active diving.

Preexisting neurological diseases (epilepsy, spinal surgery, migraine, cerebral palsy, paraplegia, multiple sclerosis, muscular dystrophy) may complicate the effort of diving.[33]

Previous episodes of loss of consciousness (seizure, or syncope) are a contraindication to diving.[18] In the case of syncope, the exact cause and potential recurrence are the major issues.[35] Cardiac arrhythmias are serious but can often be treated. Some syncope occurs in young women with migraine, and later recurrence is quite unlikely. If cardiac arrhythmia is suspected, however, recurrent spells of unconsciousness can occur. More importantly, a history of seizures with or without treatment with anticonvulsant medication is a contraindication to diving. Obviously, individual cases, such as a person with a previous single seizure who is receiving no treatment, must be determined without data because no adequate study of this situation exists.

Traumatic head injury is a relative contraindication unless the physician determines that there is no residual cerebral damage. Continued headaches, altered mental capacity, and mental lapses are contraindications to diving. In the case of back injuries the situation is less clear, but there is evidence that individuals with previous lumbar surgical procedures may have an increased risk of developing DCS. Other problems, such as neuropathy and myopathy, must be considered on an individual basis. However, if a patient is weak, such conditions will obviously increase the workload.

Diagnostic Studies

The diagnosis of diving-related neurological illness can and should be made by a clinical examination in the field. The history, including the history of the dive itself, and the neurological examination, including a mental status examination, virtually always provide a good understanding of the nature and extent of the injury. Laboratory studies add little to the diagnosis and seldom add to the direction of treatment.

Echocardiography

There is a particular place for echocardiography in patients with severe or repetitive episodes of DCS. A certain number of individuals develop dysbaric illness without breaking the rules. They dive neither too deeply nor too long but nevertheless sustain injury. This may be the result of bubble passage from the right to the left side of the heart through a patent foramen ovale. It is known that a diver can produce a few bubbles during decompression, perhaps quite a few without suffering DCS. It probably takes somewhat of a critical mass before symptoms develop. Many tiny bubbles are effectively screened out by the lungs. If there is a hole between the two sides of the heart, however, the small bubbles can be arterialized. A significantly increased incidence of patent foramen ovale has been demonstrated in divers with DCS. The whole role of patent foramen ovale in paradoxical embolic disease is not clear at this point. Echocardiography, enhanced with microbubble injection, is important.[35]

Neuropsychological Evaluation

Peters et al.[39] studied commercial and recreational divers with neurological examination and neuropsychological testing. These studies suggested that neuropsychological testing was at least as sensitive as and probably more sensitive than the clinical examination. Vaernes and Eidsvik[45] compared divers with a history of accidents and divers who had no such history using the Halstead Battery, Wechsler Intelligence Scale, Wechsler Memory Scale, Minnesota Multi-Phasic Personality Inventory, and skin conductance measurements. They discovered that these tests were no more sensitive in detecting abnormalities than was the clinical history.

Neuropsychological testing has to be in a form available for the evaluating physician. Diving-related degrees of abnormality are difficult to interpret without the presence of pre-dive controls. Aarli et al.[1] studied pre-dive and post-dive evaluations in 23 divers and found that neurological and neuropsychological abnormalities showed a small magnitude of change, possibly of minor clinical significance. Curley[8] administered a comprehensive neuropsychological battery before and after dives but did not observe significant changes in the neuropsychological test findings.

Neuroimaging

Kizer[27] described computed tomography (CT) scanning in two patients with diving accidents. One patient showed evidence of an embolic infarct in the left parietal lobe, and the other showed two nonenhancing low-density areas in the right frontal and parietal lobes compatible with embolic infarct. Subsequent experience, however, showed that CT scanning is relatively insensitive in detecting structural abnormalities associated with AGE or cerebral DCS. Occasionally, intravascular air has been seen after iatrogenic AGE, but the radiographic image has not affected the diagnosis or treatment.[12]

Magnetic resonance imaging (MRI) improved the sensitivity of intracranial pathology detection as well as imaging of the spinal cord. Warren et al.[47] reported studies in 21 patients with brain MRI studies as well as spinal cord regional imaging. In this small series, only 56% of intracranial abnormalities were demonstrated based on clinical symptoms, and only 33% of the cord abnormalities were demonstrated based on clinical symptoms. Levin et al.[28] reported two patients with cerebral symptoms post-dive, both of whom had abnormal MRI and neuropsychological test findings.

A difficulty here relates to unidentified bright objects that occur in MRI scans of normal individuals.[4,5] Because these may be age dependent, it is essential that possible abnormalities seen on MRI scans in diving accident victims must be interpreted as a function of AGE.[24]

Magnetic resonance imaging scanning is more sensitive than other imaging methods in the detection of AGE or DCS. These abnormalities may be seen in the absence of clinical signs. Intravenous injection of gadolinium-diethylene-triamine-penta-acetic acid (Gd-DTPA)[25] produces contrast enhancement of vascular structures analogous to that of contrast-enhanced CT. This clearly increases the sensitivity of MRI scanning in cerebral infarction, but its use in DCS or AGE remains unproved.

Cerebral perfusion studies that use single photon emission computed tomography after injection of radioisotope (SPECT/HMPAO) have not been of great value in the study of dysbaric illness.[21,23,28] Promising initial results were not borne out by case control studies of the same population.[22,40,48]

Electrophysiological Studies

Electroencephalography (EEG) is a nonspecific marker of structural brain damage. Sipinen and Halonen[43] reported EEG responses in 15 sport and professional divers who had had a diving accident with symptoms of DCS or AGE in the previous 10 years compared with healthy Navy divers. Electroencephalographic abnormalities were more than twice as common in the accident group. Gorman et al.[17] reported 88 divers with dysbaric injury, and within 1 week, 22 of 46 divers (47.7%) had an abnormal record. However, EEG clearly lacks specificity, as it does in most central nervous system diseases.

Electronystagmography (ENG) is useful in inner ear DCS.[14] The nystagmus associated with this disorder is suppressed by visual fixation. Therefore, ENG with the eyes closed can be quantified and is the diagnostic method of choice to complement a clinical examination. Caloric stimulation can also register the ocular motor response. This demonstrates an injury to the vestibular apparatus nerve or nucleus. Audiometry is useful in cochlear DCS and can assist in the assessment of middle ear or inner ear barotrauma.

Evoked potential studies evaluating sensory physiology include brain stem auditory evoked responses (BAERs), somatosensory evoked potentials (SSEPs), and visual evoked potentials (VEPs).[37] Motor response and motor pathways can be assessed by magnetic stimulation.[6] Generally, SSEPs are less sensitive than neurological examination in detecting abnormalities due to spinal cord DCS.[31]

Long-Term Neurological Consequences of Diving Injuries

Patients who survive AGE usually make an excellent recovery. Most are young and healthy, with an intact circulation and a firm brain, which presumably works in their favor. The symptoms most commonly reported by patients in the months after AGE are difficulties with short-term memory and concentration.[42] They are similar in that respect to the problems of patients with moderate head injury or brief hypoxic events.[41] Nevertheless, there is some pathological evidence of cerebral neuronal loss in such patients.

In 1976, Palmer[38] reported a neuropathological study of a diver who had survived significant spinal cord DCS, made a modest recovery, and returned to work, only to be killed in an unrelated accident. Section of the spinal cord demonstrated a remarkable degree of axonal loss. Since then, Palmer has been collecting neuropathological material from divers throughout Western Europe[38] in an effort to enlighten the issue of long-term neurologic risk.

Rather less certain is the issue of neurological damage from asymptomatic diving. That is to say, does a diver who never suffers clinical dysbaric illness nevertheless run a risk of developing occult neurological injury? Todnum et al.[44] approached this question by studying a large series of professional divers versus matched controls. These subjects were interviewed and examined for neurological symptoms and signs, and each earned a total score. The authors then carried out a multivariate analysis and demonstrated that the divers had significantly more neurological symptoms and neurological findings than the nondivers. The most important symptoms were difficulties with concentration, long-term and short-term memory, and the most prominent abnormal findings: distal spinal cord and nerve root dysfunction. These abnormalities were independently correlated significantly with diving exposure and prevalence of diving accidents. In other words, the patients who had recognized DCS had an expectedly higher incidence of symptoms and findings.[42] Nevertheless, if these patients were excluded by multivariate analysis, the patients who had not had symptomatic DCS nevertheless had a higher score.

Although this study does suggest that diving as a profession may be hazardous to a diver's health, even if the diver does not suffer recognized injury, it should be noted that none of these people were significantly disabled. The evidence of damage, if any, was subtle.

Rehabilitation of the Injured Diver

For the most part, neurological rehabilitation of patients suffering from AGE or DCS is related to the neurological disease entities. Several deficits need to be evaluated thoroughly and limited cognitive retraining efforts made, as with any other spinal cord–injured patient, including physical therapy, occupational therapy, nursing, and urological reports.[30]

Attempts have been made to assess the specific rehabilitation needs of these patients. A potentially unique factor is that patients with DCS may continue to improve over a longer period of time than those with other causes of spinal cord damage. Therefore, it is essential that these patients continue to receive therapy over a prolonged period of time, and rehabilitation efforts should be instituted even while chamber therapy is continuing.

Underwater diving may cause several unique neurological injuries because of exposure to rapid changes in pressure and volume. Decompression sickness, which results from extended deep dives and too rapid ascent, is a systemic disease that frequently causes spinal cord injury but may involve other organs as well. Arterial gas embolism results from pulmonary overpressure on ascent, with extravasation of air into the arterial system, and causes stroke-like brain injury. Both conditions are sudden in onset, progress rapidly, and require urgent attention. Definitive treatment includes administration of oxygen and recompression in a chamber. Permanent neurological injury may result.

Divers with Spinal Cord Injury

Since 1981, the Handicapped Scuba Association has attempted to help handicapped individuals enjoy sport diving. This can be accomplished.[7] However, spinal cord problems with thermoregulation, respiratory difficulty, urological dysfunction, autonomic dysreflexia (above T5), sensory loss and wound issues must be addressed.

ACKNOWLEDGMENT

I would like to thank Dr. Hugh Greer (deceased) for his contributions to the previous chapter and his wonderful inspiration as a friend and neurologist.

REFERENCES

1. Aarli JA, Vaernes R, Brubakk AO, et al: Central nervous dysfunction associated with deep sea diving. Acta Neurol Scand 71:2–10, 1985.
2. Adkisson GH, Hodgson M, Smith F, et al: Cerebral perfusion deficits in dysbaric illness. Lancet 2:119–122, 1989.
3. Air Decompression and Chamber Operator's Manual. Panama City, FL, Hydroquip Corp., 1976.
4. Awad IA, Johnson PC, Spetzler RF, et al: Incidental subcortical lesions identified on magnetic resonance imaging in the elderly. II. Postmortem pathological correlations. Stroke 17:1090–1097, 1986.
5. Awad IA, Spetzler RF, Hodak JA, et al: Incidental subcortical lesions identified on magnetic resonance imaging in the elderly. I. Correlation with age and cerebrovascular risk factors. Stroke 17:1084–1089, 1986.
6. Barker AT, Jalinous R, Freeston IL: Non-invasive magnetic stimulation of the human motor cortex. Lancet 1: 1106–1107, 1985.
7. Bove AA (ed). Diving Medicine, 4th ed. Philadelphia, WB Saunders, 2004.
8. Curley MD: U.S. Navy saturation diving and diver neuropsychologic status. Undersea Biomed Res 15:39–50, 1988.
9. Denoble PJ, Ugucciono D, Forbes R, Vann RD: The incidence of decompression illness in recreational divers is not homogeneous. Undersea Hyperbaric Med 30(3):208, 2003.
10. Dick APK, Massey EW: Neurologic presentation of decompression sickness and air embolism in sport divers. Neurology 35(5):667–671, 1985.
11. Drayer BP: Functional applications of CT of the central nervous system. AJNR 2:495–510, 1981.
12. Elliott DH, Kindwall EP: Manifestations of the decompression disorders. In: Bennett PB, Elliott DH (eds): Physiology and Medicine of Diving, 4th ed. Philadelphia, WB Saunders, 1993, pp 311–326.
13. Elliott DH, Moon RE: Manifestations of the decompression disorders. In: Bennett PB, Elliott DH (eds): The Physiology and Medicine of Diving. Carson, CA, Best Bookbinders, 1993, pp 481–505.
14. Farmer JC Jr: Otologic and paranasal sinus problems in diving. In: Bennett PB, Elliott DH (eds): The Physiology and Medicine of Diving. Carson, CA, Best Bookbinders, 1993, pp 507–536.
15. Francis TJR, Dutka AJ, Clark JB: An evaluation of dexamethhasone in the treatment of acute experimental decompression sickness. Ninth International Symposium on Underwater and Hyperbaric Physiology. Undersea Medical Society, Bethesda, MD, 1987, p 999.
16. Gorman DF, Browning DM, Parsons DW, et al: Distribution of arterial gas embolism in the pial circulation. SPUMS J 17:101, 1987.
17. Gorman DF, Edmonds CW, Parsons DW, et al: Neurological sequelae of decompression sickness: A clinical report. Ninth International Symposium on Underwater and Hyperbaric Physiology, Undersea and Medical Society. Bethesda, MD, 1987, pp 993–998.
18. Greer HD: Epilepsy in diving. Pressure 21:2–5, 1992.
19. Hallenbeck JM: Cinephoto-micrography of dog spinal vessels during cord damage in decompression sickness. Neurology 26(2):190, 1976.
20. Hallenbeck JM, Bove AA, Elliott DH: Mechanisms underlying spinal cord damage in decompression sickness. Neurology (Minn) 25:308–316, 1975.
21. Hodgson M, Smith DJ, et al: Case control study of cerebral perfusion deficits in divers using 99 TC^{m} HMPAO. Undersea Biomed Res 18:421, 1991.
22. Holman BL, Tumeh SS: Single-photon emission computed tomography (SPECT). JAMA 263:561–564, 1990.
23. Hughes RL, Yonas H, Greer D, et al: Cerebral blood flow determination within the first 8 hours of cerebral infarction using stable xenon-enhanced computed tomography. Stroke 20:754–760, 1989.
24. Hunt AL, Orrison WW, Yeo RA, et al: Clinical significance of MRI white matter lesions in the elderly. Neurology 39:1470–1474, 1989.
25. Imakita S, Nishimura T, Naito H, et al: Magnetic resonance imaging of human cerebral infarction: Enhancement with Gd-DTPA. Neuroradiology 29:422–429, 1987.
26. Kizer KW: The role of computerized tomography in the management of dysbaric diving accidents. Radiology 140: 705–707, 1981.
27. Levin HS, Goldstein FC, Norcross K, et al: Neurobehavioral and magnetic resonance imaging in two cases of decompression sickness. Aviat Space Environ Med 60:1204–1210, 1989.
28. Macleod MA, Adkisson GH, Fox MJ: $^{99\text{-}m}$Tc-HMPAO single photon emission tomography in the diagnosis of cerebral barotrauma. Br J Radiol 61:1106–1109, 1988.
29. Melamed Y, Shupak A: Medical problems associated with underwater diving. N Engl J Med 326:30, 1992.
30. Miller JN (ed): Rehabilitation of the Paralyzed Diver. Mobile, University of South Alabama, Undersea Medical Society, NOAA, 1985.
31. Moon RE (ed): Adjunctive therapy for decompression illness. Proceedings of the 53rd Workshop of Undersea and Hyperbaric Medical Society. Kensington, MD, Undersea and Hyperbaric Medical Society, 2003, pp
32. Moon RE, Bove A: Diving and asthma. Pressure 20:3–6, 1991.

33. Moon RE, Camporesi EM, Kisslo JA: Patent foramen ovale and decompression illness in divers. Lancet 1:513–514, 1989.
34. Moon RE, Gorman D: Treatment of the decompression disorders. In: Bennett PB, Elliott DH (eds): The Physiology and Medicine of Diving. Philadelphia, WB Saunders, 1993, pp 506–541.
35. Moon RE, Kisslo JA, Massey EW, et al: Patent foramen ovale (PFO) and decompression illness. Undersea Biomed Res 18(suppl):15, 1991.
36. NOAA Diving Manual. Washington, DC, Superintendent of Documents, U.S. Government Printing Office, 1980.
37. Overlock R, Dutka A, Farm F Jr, et al: Somatosensory evoked potentials measured in divers with a history of spinal cord decompression sickness. Undersea Biomed Res 16(suppl):89, 1989.
38. Palmer, AC: Neuropathology of brain in decompression sickness: European Underwater Biology Society Proceedings, Palermo, September, 1987. (presentation).
39. Peters BH, Levin HS, Kelly PJ: Neurologic and psychologic manifestations of decompression illness in divers. Neurology 27:125–127, 1977.
40. Phelps ME, Mazziotta JC: Positron emission tomography: Human brain function and biochemistry. Science 228: 799–809, 1985.
41. Robinson HJ Jr, Hartlebern PD, Lund G, et al: Evaluation of magnetic resonance imaging in the diagnosis of osteonecrosis of the femoral head. Accuracy compared with radiographs, core biopsy and intraosseous pressure measurements. J Bone Joint Surg [Am] 71:650–663, 1989.
42. Robinson JD, Reed WL, Freiberger JJ, Pollock NW: Perceived quality of life among previously injured recreational divers: A pilot study. Undersea Hyperbaric Med 30(3):212–213, 2003.
43. Sipinen SS, Halonen J-P: Effects of recompression treatment on EEG in diving accidents. Ninth International Symposium on Underwater and Hyperbaric Physiology, Bethesda, MD, Undersea Medical Society, 1987, pp 887–892.
44. Todnem K, Nyland H, Kambeetad BK, et al: Influence of occupational diving upon the nervous system. Br J Intern Med 47:708, 1990.
45. Vaernes RJ, Eidsvik S: Central nervous dysfunction after near-miss accidents in diving. Aviat Space Environ Med 53:803–807, 1982.
46. Vann R, Denoble P, Uguccioni D, et al: DAN Report on Decompression Illness, Diving Fatalities and Project Dive Exploration, 2004 ed. Durham, NC, Divers Alert Network, 2004.
47. Warren LP Jr, Djang WT, Moon RE, et al: Neuroimaging of scuba diving injuries to the CNS. Am J Radiol 151: 1003–1008, 1988.
48. Yamamoto YI, Thompson CJ, Diksic M, et al: Positron emission tomography. Neurosurg Rev 7:233–251, 1984.

Chapter 30
Lightning Injuries

MICHAEL CHERINGTON

Lightning is one of nature's powerful traumatic forces. Cloud-to-ground lightning flashes have peak currents of 20,000 to 40,000 amps at hundreds of millions of volts and can reach temperatures as high as 60,000°F.[33a,34] Researchers in the early twenty-first century have provided evidence that lightning is associated with the intense release of X-rays, electrons, and gamma rays.[30] With its enormous energy, extreme temperatures, electromagnetic clout, and explosive blast effects, it is not surprising that lightning is responsible for much human, environmental, and property damage. According to data from the National Oceanic and Atmospheric Administration, between 1959 to 1994 lightning was responsible for over 3000 deaths and 10,000 casualties.[25] The actual numbers are very likely to be higher because over 50% of lightning casualties go unreported.[14,35]

Clinical Manifestations of Lightning Injuries

Most people struck by lightning survive. Approximately 10% of lightning strike cases are fatal. Fatalities are usually the result of cardiac arrest. Many survivors have serious long-term neurological signs and symptoms.

Neurological complications of lightning strikes vary from transient benign symptoms to permanent disability. According to the current classification, neurological complications after lightning strikes can be divided into four groups:[10a]

1. *Immediate, transient, and usually benign.* These symptoms are often dramatic but short-lived. They include brief loss of consciousness (75% of patients), amnesia, confusion, headache, paresthesia, and limb weakness.[10a,22,24] Many patients experience a temporary paralysis of the limbs accompanied by sensory loss, pallor, and vasoconstriction. The lower limbs are affected more than the upper limbs. This temporary paralytic state is specific to lightning and has been termed *keraunoparalysis* (discussed below).
2. *Immediate and prolonged or permanent.* The great majority of these complications involve the central nervous system as opposed to the peripheral nervous system. These lesions, often seen on imaging studies, can be the cause of severe disability.
   a. Posthypoxic encephalopathy frequently ends tragically with death or serious permanent cognitive deficits. As in other cases of out-of-hospital cardiac arrest, the

prognosis for many of these lightning strike patients is poor. However, there are cases with brighter outcomes.[48] Magnetic resonance imaging (MRI) and computed tomography (CT) scan images are often consistent with cerebral edema.

b. Cerebral infarction is an uncommon sequela. This is surprising because blood vessels and nervous tissue are selectively damaged by lightning.[24] There is only one reported case of cerebral infarction evident on MRI.[18]

c. Intracranial hemorrhages include subarachnoid and intracerebral hemorrhages. The location of intracerebral hemorrhages in lightning strike patients often differs from the location seen in blunt trauma patients. The susceptible locations in lightning strike patients are the basal ganglia and the brain stem.[41] One explanation for the selective vulnerability of these sites is that current travels a path toward the basal ganglia and brain stem in patients who suffer direct strikes to the head.[2] Computed tomography scans are especially useful in localizing intracranial hematomas.[36,49,50]

d. Cerebellar syndrome is an uncommon complication. Fortunately, the symptoms are usually temporary.[17]

e. Myelopathy is an uncommon but devastating complication of lightning strikes. Patients usually have permanent disability.[12,45] Postmortem examination of the spinal cord reveals degeneration of myelin without inflammation.[27]

f. Peripheral nerve lesions are uncommon in lightning strike patients. By contrast, they are common in those with generated electrical trauma. In those instances, peripheral nerve damage is usually, but not always, associated with severe burns.[47] Lightning-related cranial nerve palsy has been reported.[20]

g. Autonomic nervous system disorders following lightning have rarely been reported.[21,54] Cold temperature insensitivity is a symptom reported by some lightning survivors. The pathophysiology of this symptom has not yet been elucidated. It may be due to hypothalamic damage (discussed below).

h. A large group of survivors suffer from neuropsychological and behavioral problems. This serious complication is discussed in greater detail below.

3. *Delayed and progressive*. Delayed neurological disorders attributed to lightning include motor neuron disease and movement disorders.[8,15,32,39] These sequelae follow lightning strikes by days to months to years[8] However, the cause–effect relationship between lightning and subsequent delayed neurological complications is open to question.

4. *Lightning-linked conditions second to trauma due to falls and blasts*. Patients may sustain serious head and neck damage when they are propelled or thrown down by explosive blast effects. Subdural and extradural hematomas are serious complications that can result from such trauma.

Neuropsychological and Behavioral Problems

Many lightning survivors are beset with enduring neuropsychological and behavioral problems. These can begin immediately or days or weeks after the lightning strike. Cognitive deficits resemble those seem in traumatic brain injury and posttraumatic stress disorder. The symptoms include memory deficit, sleep disturbances, pain syndromes, headache, attention deficit, fatigue, irritability, and depression.[29,42a,42b]

Who Is Likely to Be Struck by Lightning?

Demographic data from Colorado and elsewhere show that the typical victim is a previously healthy man in his mid-30s.[9] Male victims outnumber females by 4:5 to 1. Characteristically, the subject is engaged in outdoor recreational activities during summer months and during the late morning, afternoon, and early evening hours.

Mechanism of Damage by Lightning

Lightning current can reach a person by one of three paths: direct strike; side flash from a nearby object such as a tree; or via current traveling along the ground. Injury and death can result from any of these routes. Direct lightning strikes to the head are very serious, resulting in death or severe brain dysfunction.[55] We have offered the hypothesis that a fourth route can account for two known but unexplained lightning injury phenomena. Approximately 10% of patients with lightning-related cardiac arrest have no signs of electrical burns. Why? The second mystery relates to the situation in which lightning is fatal to one individual when other nearby people are not seriously hurt. We have postulated that magnetic field changes associated with lightning may induce a loop current within the human torso.[13] If this induced current occurs during the repolarization phase of the cardiac cycle, it could cause asystole or ventricular fibrillation. This hypothesis would explain the absence of skin burns because the lightning flash did not touch the patient. It would also explain why the induced current causes cardiac arrest in one person and not in another nearby person.

How does lightning damage tissues and organs? Mechanisms include thermal effects, electrical effects, induced currents, blast effects, and injuries related to falls. Electric fields can damage the structural integrity of nerve and muscle membranes. The electrical process that damages lipid bilayer membranes is termed *electroporation*.[34] Persons in the vicinity of the explosive waves of thunder may suffer tympanic membrane rupture, as well as pulmonary and intracranial hemorrhages.[37,40]

Distinct Clinical Features Found in Lightning Strike Patients

Four clinical features are distinctive to lightning-injured patients and are seldom, if ever, found in patients who suffer trauma from other causes. These four conditions are ball lightning encephalopathy, keraunoparalysis, Lichtenberg figures, and cold tolerance.

Ball Lightning-Coronal Discharge Encephalopathy

Ball lightning (BL) is an incompletely understood meteorological phenomenon that occurs in association with lightning storms. Several centers have recently proposed models to explain the physics of BL. One model suggests that BL has a core of clouds of electrons and ions.[46] Another theory is that BL represents burning particles of silicon.[1]

Ball lightning is a mobile, luminous, spheroidal, floating or bouncing ball of plasma that lasts for a few seconds before suddenly vanishing or exploding. These glowing spheres have been seen to float in the air, follow telephone and power lines, and travel down the aisles of airplanes. Coronal discharge (CD), another induced electrical event associated with lightning storms, remains fixed on a conductor and does not move like BL.

Since there are few comprehensive case reports in the medical literature, the spectrum of BL neurological complications is yet to be fully described. There are rare case reports in the literature of BL-CD encephalopathy.[16,19,28] The literature also contains reports of BL-CD skin burns.[44] Although some suggest that BL can be lethal, I have found no convincing fatal case reports in a Pub Med literature search.

Keraunoparalysis

Keraunoparalysis (KP) is a transient paralytic state that occurs in some lightning strike patients. In most cases, the lower limbs are weaker than the upper limbs. Associated symptoms include numbness and pallor of the extremities. According to many authorities on the medical aspects of lightning, J. M. Charcot was the first person to use the term *keraunoparalysis*, and the first to describe this unusual condition.[23,51] However, a review of Charcot's articles reveals that he did not use the term keraunoparalysis.[6,7] In 1890, Charcot did, in fact, describe a temporary paralysis of the lower limbs in lightning patients. Interestingly, James Parkinson described the same condition nearly 100 years earlier.[10b,10c] In 1932, Critchley may have been the first physician to use the term kerunoparalysis.[23]

Lichtenberg Figures

The Lichtenberg figure (LF), also known as a *ferning pattern*, is a pathognomonic sign that is found only in victims of lightning strikes. Lichtenberg figures are transient skin patterns. In 1777, Georg Lichtenberg, while performing experiments with static electricity, described similar figures on a cake of resin.[11] Lichtenberg figures on skin appear within 1 hour of the lightning strike and usually fade within 24 to 36 hours. Biopsy specimens reveal no pathological changes in epidermis, dermis, or collagen.[43] Ten Duis et al. asserted that LFs are fractal patterns caused by positive charges over the skin.[52]

Cold Tolerance

There are a few anecdotal cases of people who, after being struck by lightning, can tolerate cold temperatures without the need for warm clothing. There is almost no discussion in the literature of this unusual complication. The site of the lesion is unknown, but the hypothalamus is a likely location. Body temperature regulation occurs in the hypothalamus with input from thermoreceptors along the internal carotid artery, the posterior hypothalamus, and skin receptors.[4,53] This curious condition, cold tolerance in lightning patients, exists in contrast to hypothermia with impaired shivering responses seen in many trauma patients.[53] Both situations reflect some abnormality of the processes that control thermoregulatory responses in humans.

PREVENTION

Lightning fatalities and devastating neurological sequelae are especially tragic because they usually involve healthy young people engaged in sports or recreation. People should be familiar with lightning safety recommendations and take prudent precautions to reduce their risk of becoming lightning casualties. It is imperative that adults in charge of children, such as teachers, coaches, and lifeguards, know and implement lightning safety guidelines.

The old proverb "An ounce of prevention is worth a pound of cure" has been attributed to Lord Edward Coke, as well as to Benjamin Franklin. The message has remained true and applies to much of medicine, and especially to lightning injuries. The prudent person should have a lightning safety action plan before initiating an outdoor sports or recreation activity. That plan should include knowledge about the weather patterns of the location. For example, Rocky Mountain climbers should know that high-density lightning flash hours increase after late morning and continue during the afternoon and evening. Therefore, mountain climbers should begin early in the morning and be off the mountain by 11:00 A.M.[9]

Lightning safety recommendations have been drafted by the Lightning Safety Group (LSG). The guidelines for personal safety are available at several sites, including articles in the literature and on the Internet.[57] Although no place is absolutely safe, there are places of low risk. To lower the risk of being struck by lightning, one should seek shelter in a large structure (school, office building, house, etc.) that has plumbing and electrical wiring. However, when in such a building, one should avoid contact with plumbing and electrical equipment such as showers, bathtubs, and telephones. A fully enclosed metal vehicle is a relatively safe place. By contrast, standing near or leaning on the outside of a car or another vehicle is dangerous. Other high-risk places to avoid include isolated trees, flag poles, open fields, swimming pools, beaches, rivers, and metal fences. Golf carts, bicycles, and motorcycles are unsafe during lightning storms (Table 30.1).

The LSG warns that lightning danger may persist for 30 minutes after the last evidence of thunder or lightning. Therefore, it is prudent to remain in a safe shelter for at least 30 minutes before returning to the outdoor activity.

Interestingly, much of the sound advice on lightning safety of the twenty-first century was available over 60 years ago. Bellaschchi gave the following recommendations in 1942:[3]

> The moment a thunderstorm threatens, get into the house, preferably into a large house. . . . Stay away from windows, open doors, stoves, pipes, chimney, and fireplace. . . . Keep away from tall isolated trees, wire fences, poles, tractors, and other metal objects. Get away from beaches, swimming pools, and fishing ponds. Make for depressions, valleys or dense woods. If you are in your car it is the safest place. . . . Steel topped buses and trains are equally safe.

Table 30.1. What to Avoid During Lightning Storms

Open spaces
Isolated trees
Golf courses
Swimming pools
Beaches, lakes, rivers, and oceans
Metal fences
Ball fields and bleachers
Bicycles, motorcycles, and golf carts
Leaning against the outside of automobiles and other vehicles
Open picnic shelters and gazebos
Bathtubs, showers, and sinks
Indoor telephones
Computers and electrical appliances

TREATMENT

Treatment approaches for lightning strike patients depend on when the patient is brought to the neurologist's attention. Most often the neurologist is called to see a patient who presents with neurological complications. However, a neurologist, like anyone, might be in the vicinity of an immediate and emergency situation.

The rules of resuscitation for patients at the scene of the lightning strike are similar to those for other unconscious patients. One should assess airway, breathing, and circulation (ABC assessment). If the patient is apneic and has no pulse, cardiopulmonary resuscitation should be instituted immediately.[57] These patients may have suffered asystole from cardiac arrest and/or respiratory arrest with ventricular fibrillation. If a mobile phone is available, emergency services should be summoned. There are several factors specific to lightning that the rescuing party should realize. First, rescuers should avoid additional casualties by not putting themselves at risk if the lightning storm continues. Second, a lightning victim is not *charged* and therefore can be touched without receiving an electrical shock. This differs from the condition of some patients with electrical trauma who may still be connected to the power line or other energized source of electricity. In the latter case, the source of the electricity must be turned off or safely removed from the patient before resuscitation efforts begin. Third, rescue efforts should be directed at patients who may have suffered a cardiac or respiratory arrest. Most victims of lightning who are not unconscious and who have not had a cardiac arrest will survive.

Patients with hypoxic encephalopathy, cerebral infarction, and spinal cord injury (SCI) often require early evaluation and treatment in an intensive care unit until their condition is stabilized.[56] Patients with catastrophic brain damage need elaborate measures similar to those used in other severe brain trauma situations. Predicting long-term recovery is often difficult. A protracted comatose state and myoclonic seizures unresponsive to antiepileptic drugs (AEDs) are indicators of a poor outcome. For those patients with improving mental status, a comprehensive rehabilitation plan (including physical, speech, and occupational therapies) should be considered.

The risk of chronic epilepsy after lightning appears to be small. Those patients who do develop seizures require AED treatment. If long-term AED therapy is used, screening is useful in reducing adverse effects.[31] In contrast with lightning encephalopathy patients, more information is available regarding traumatic brain injury (TBI) and late seizures. Late seizures are not infrequent after TBI. A quality standards committee of the American Academy of Neurology concluded that in adults with severe TBI, AED prophylaxis is probably ineffective in decreasing the risk of late posttraumatic seizures.[5]

Category 4 patients who have lightning-linked or secondary complications from falling, blast effects, or trauma from flying debris may need surgical attention to treat intracranial hematomas.

Early rehabilitation is essential for SCI patients.[33b] These patients confront myriad problems or potential problems including neurogenic bladder, skin sores, deep vein thrombosis, and spasticity.[38] The management plan of lightning-related SCI is the same as that for other traumatic SCI patients. Standardized protocols for assessment of the outcome after SCI are being developed with the aim of monitoring the effects of new therapies as they become available.[26]

A large number of lightning survivors are plagued with neuropsychological and behavioral problems. Their symptoms (including impaired concentrations, sleep disturbances, depression, chronic pain, and fatigability) can begin immediately, or after a few days or weeks, and may persist for months or years. Their problems can interfere with employment and family life. Patients may improve with time, especially with assistance from concerned physicians, psychological counseling, and an understanding support group.

REFERENCES

1. Abrahamson J, Dinniss J: Ball lightning caused by oxidation of nanoparticle networks from normal lightning strikes on soil. Nature 403:519–521, 2000.
2. Andrews C: Structural changes after lightning strike, with special emphasis on special sense orifices as portals of entry. Semin Neurol 15:296–303, 1995.
3. Bellaschchi PL: How to dodge lightning. Clin Med 49: 167, 1942.
4. Blumberg MS: Body Heat. Cambridge, MA, Harvard University Press, 2002.
5. Chang BS, Lowenstein DH: Practice parameter: Antiepileptic drug prophylaxis in severe traumatic brain injury. Report of the Quality Standards Subcommittee of

the American Academy of Neurology. Neurology 60:10–16, 2003.

6. Charcot JM: Des accidents nerveux provoques par la foudre. Bull Med (Paris) 3:1323–1326, 1889.
7. Charcot JM: Wirkung des blitzschlages auf das nervensystem. Wien Med Wochenschr 40:10, 58, 105, 1890.
8. Cherington M: Central nervous system complications of lightning and electrical injuries. Semin Neurol 15:233–240, 1995.
9. Cherington M: Lightning injuries in sports: Situations to avoid. Sports Med 31:301–308, 2001.

10a. Cherington M: Neurologic manifestations of lightning strikes. Neurology 60:182–185, 2003.

10b. Cherington M: James Parkinson: Links to Charcot, Lichtenberg, and lightning. Arch Neurol 61:977, 2004.

10c. Cherington M: History of keraunoparalysis—a medical mystery. http://www.icolse.org/Abstracts/KMGeneral/CHERINGTON_History-of-Keraunoparalysis.doc (accessed September 2005).

11. Cherington M, Olson S, Yarnell PR: Lightning and Lichtenberg figures. Injury 34:367–371, 2003.
12. Cherington M, Vervalin C: Lightning injuries—who is at greatest risk? Physician Sportsmed 18:58–61, 1990.
13. Cherington M, Wachtel H, Yarnell PR: Could lightning injury be magnetically induced? Lancet 351:1788, 1998.
14. Cherington M, Walker J, Boyson M, Glancy R, Hedegaard H, Clark S: Closing the gap on the actual numbers of lightning casualties and deaths. Eleventh Conference of Applied Climatology, January 10–15, 1999. Dallas, American Meteorological Society, 1999, pp 379–380.
15. Cherington M, Yarnell PR: Lighting-related involuntary movement disorders. Neurology 58:A138, 2002.
16. Cherington M, Yarnell PR: Ball lightning encephalopathy. J Burn Care Rehabil 24:175, 2003.
17. Cherington M, Yarnell P, Hallmark D: MRI in lightning encephalopathy. Neurology 43:1437–1438, 1993.
18. Cherington M, Yarnell P, Lammereste D: Lightning strikes: Nature of neurological damage in patients evaluated in hospital emergency departments. Ann Emerg Med 21:575–578, 1999.
19. Cherington M, Yarnell PR, Lane J, Anderson L, Lines G: Lightning-induced injury on an airplane: Coronal discharge and ball lightning. J Trauma 52:579–581, 2002.
20. Cherington M, Yarnell PR, London SF: Neurologic complications of lighting injuries. West J Med 162:413–417, 1995.
21. Cohen JA: Autonomic nervous system disorders and reflex sympathetic dystrophy in lightning and electrical injuries. Semin Neurol 15:387–390, 1995.
22. Cooper MA: Lightning injuries: Prognostic signs for death. Ann Emerg Med 9:134–138, 1980.
23. Critchley M: The effects of lightning with especial reference to the nervous system. Bristol Med Surg J 49:285–300, 1932.
24. Critchley M: Neurological effects of lightning and electricity. Lancet 1:68–72, 1934.
25. Curran EB, Holle RL, Lopez RE: Lightning fatalities, injuries and damage reports in the United States, 1959–1994. NOAA Technical Memorandum NWS SR-193. Fort Worth, TX, National Weather Service 1–64, 1997.
26. Curt A, Schwab ME, Dietz V: Providing the clinical basis for new interventional therapies: Refined diagnosis and assessment of recovery after spinal cord injury. Spinal Cord 42:1–6, 2004.
27. Davidson GS, Deck JH: Delayed myelopathy following lightning strike: A demyelinating process. Acta Neuropathol 77:104–108, 1988.
28. Dmitriev MT, Lakshin AM, Morozov SS: Specific features of ball lightning injuries. Ortop Travmatol Protez 11:66–67, 1986.
29. Duff K, McCaffrey JR: Electrical injury and lightning injury: A review of their mechanisms and neuropsychological, psychiatric and neurological sequelae. Neuropsychol Rev 11:101–116, 2001.
30. Dwyer JR, Uman MA, Rassoul HK, Al-Dayeh M, Caraway L, Jerauld J, Rakov VA, Jordan DM, Rambo KJ, Corbin V, Wright B: Energetic radiation produced during rocket-triggered lightning. Science 299:694–697, 2003.
31. Gilliam FG, Fessler AJ, Baker G, Vable V, Carter J, Attarian H: Systematic screening allows reduction of adverse antiepileptic drug effects. A randomized trial. Neurology 62:23–27, 2004.
32. Jafari H, Couratier P, Camu W: Motor neuron disease after electric injury. J Neurol Neurosurg Psychiatry 71: 265–267, 2001.

33a. Krider EP, Uman MA: Cloud-to-ground lightning: Mechanisms of damage and methods of protection. Semin Neurol 15:227–232, 1995.

33b. Lammertse KP: Neurorehabilitation of spinal cord injuries following lightning and electrical trauma. NeuroRehabilitation 20:9–14, 2005.

34. Lee RC, Zhang D, Hannig J: Biophysical injury mechanisms in electrical shock trauma. Annu Rev Biomed Eng 2:477–509, 2000.
35. Lopez RE, Holle RL, Heitkamp TA, Boyson M, Cherington M, Langford K: The underreporting of lightning injuries and deaths in Colorado. Bull Am Meteor Soc 74: 2171–2178, 1993.
36. Mann H, Zellimir K, Boulos MI: CT of lightning injury. AJNR 4:976–977, 1983.
37. Morton RL, Jain S, Eid NS: Pulmonary sequelae of pediatr lightning injury. Ped Res 53:576A, 2003.
38. New PW, Rawicki HB, Bailey MJ: Nontraumatic spinal cord injury rehabilitation: Pressure ulcer patterns, prediction, and impact. Arch Phys Med Rehabil 85:87–93, 2004.
39. O"Brien CF: Involuntary movement disorders following lightning and electrical injuries. Semin Neurol 15:263–267, 1995.
40. Ohashi M, Yasuhiro H, Fujishiro Y, Tuyuki A, Kikuchi K, Obara H, Kitagawa N, Ishikawa T: Lightning injury as a blast injury of skull, brain and visceral lesions: Clinical and experimental evidences. Keio J Med 50:257–262, 2001.
41. Ozgun B, Castillo M: Basal ganglia hemorrhage related to lightning strike. AJNR 16:1370–1371, 1995.

42a. Primeau M: Neurorehabilitation of behavioral disorders following lightning and electrical trauma. NeuroRehabilitation 20:25–33, 2005.
42b. Primeau M, Englestatter GH, Bares KK: Behavioral consequences of lightning and electrical injury. Semin Neurol 15:279–285, 1995.
43. Resnik BI, Wetli CV: Lichtenberg figures. Am J Forensic Med Pathol 17:99–102, 1996.
44. Selvaggi G, Monstrey S, von Heimburg D, Hamdi M, Landuyt KV, Blondeel P: Ball lightning burn. Ann Plast Surg 50:541–544, 2003.
45. Sharma M, Smith A: Paraplegia as a result of lightning injury. BMJ 2:1464–1465, 1978.
46. Shmatov ML: New model and estimation of the danger of ball lightning. J Plasma Physics 69:507–527, 2003.
47. Smith MA, Muehlberger T, Dellon AL: Peripheral nerve compression associated with low-voltage electrical injury without associated significant cutaneous burn: Plast Reconstr Surg 109:137–145, 2002.
48. Soo LH, Gray D, Young T, Huff N, Skene A, Hampton JR: Resuscitation from out-of-hospital cardiac arrest: Is survival dependent on who is available at the scene? Heart 81:47–52, 1999.
49. Stanley LD, Suss RA: Intracerebral hematoma secondary to lightning stroke: Case report and review of the literature. Neurosurgery 16:686–688, 1985.
50. Steinbaum S, Harviel JD, Jaffin JH, Jordan MH: Lightning strike to the head: Case report. J Trauma 36:113–115, 1994.
51. Ten Duis HJ, Klasen JH: Keraunoparalysis, a "specific" lighting injury. Burns 12:54–57, 1986.
52. Ten Duis HJ, Klasen HJ, Nijsten MWN: Superficial lightning injuries: Their fractal shape and origin. Burns 13:141–146, 1987.
53. Tsuei BJ, Kearney PA: Hypothermia in the trauma patient. Injury 35:7–15, 2004.
54. Weeramanthri TS, Puddy IB, Beilin IJ: Lightning strike and autonomic failure—coincidence or causally related? J R Soc Med 84:687–688, 1991.
55. Yarnell PR, Cherington M: Lightning strikes to the head. Ann Neurol 38:347–348, 1995.
56. Yarnell PR, Lammertse DP: Neurorehabilitation of lightning and electrical injuries. Semin Neurol 15:391–396, 1995.
57. Zimmermann C, Cooper MA, Holle RL: Lightning safety guidelines. Ann Emerg Med 39:660–664, 2002.

Chapter 31
Electrical Injuries

MARY CAPELLI-SCHELLPFEFFER

With power in the extra-low frequency (ELF) 50–60 Hz range, the generation, transmission, and distribution of energy in industrial and public systems support virtually every aspect of daily living. Electricity is pervasive in modern environments and can be simply defined as "any effect resulting from the existence of stationary or moving electric charges."[32] Charge is an inherent property of electrons (negatively charged) and protons (positively charged). The motion of charge through a conductor is called *electrical current*.[35] Electrical current is described by the units volts (electrical force), amperes (electrical flow), and ohms (electrical resistance).

With engineering technology to control moving electrical charges, or current, diverse applications are possible across the electromagnetic spectrum, including ultralow frequencies such as AM/FM radio and television, short waves, microwaves, infrared radiation, visible light, ultraviolet radiation, hard and soft X-rays, and gamma rays.

As Haddon suggested in the 1970s, unintentional injuries and fatalities share an energy damage process.[28] In a fatality, the event has resulted in sufficient energy transfer, in such ways and amounts, from the environment to the person—via electrical, mechanical, radiation, acoustic, or pressure exposure—to result in an irreversible destructive effect.[15] Nonfatal events result from sublethal exposures.

Haddon's observation is illustrated graphically for the case of industrial electrical exposure in Figure 31.1 and staged under laboratory conditions as shown in Figure 31.2. At 50–60 Hz power frequencies, supraphysiological energy transfer from a power source to the victim is necessary to provoke an electrical injury response.

Nonoccupational and Occupational Injuries

Nonoccupational electrical injuries are sustained in common settings, including households, medical, civil justice, and educational/recreational areas (Table 31.1). Nonoccupational electrical injury and fatality statistics are not collected routinely, limiting injury and fatality estimates.

Statistics are more widely available for occupational or workplace electrical injuries. Published U.S. National Institute of Occupational Safety and Health (NIOSH) analyses of the U.S. Department of Labor (DOL) Bureau of Labor Statistics (BLS) data by Cawley and Homce on electrical incidents show from 1992 to 1998, in the United States, that 2267 people died because of an occupational contact exposure to power frequency electrical energy.[12] Cawley and Homce further analyzed 623 fatalities, and found that the incident voltage in 87% of the reports was noted as 15,000 V or less,

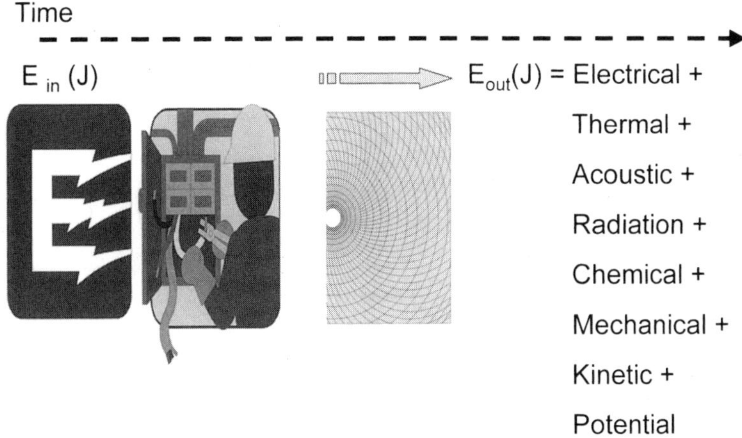

Figure 31.1. Industrial scenario with electrical energy input to a wall panel box while a worker is standing nearby. At the moment of the electrical incident event, electrical energy transformation occurs. Uncontrolled energy release follows, resulting in the transfer of electrical and other energy forms to the space and the nearby worker.[7]

with 32% of the fatalities noted during work on 0–600 V (Table 31.2). Overhead power lines were an electrical source in about 40% of the deaths.

From 1980 to 1995, electrocution accounted for 7.1% of occupational deaths in men and 0.7% in women.[50] Among young workers, electrocution was the cause of 12% of all workplace deaths and the third leading cause of work-related deaths among 16- and 17-year-olds after motor vehicle deaths and workplace homicide.[11] While comprising only about 7% of the U.S. workforce, construction workers sustained 44% of electrical fatalities.[12] Figure 31.3 illustrates possible electrical exposure hazards on a construction worksite with a haul truck and an overhead power line nearby.[13] In the illustration, electrical current flows from the power line through the truck to contacts between the truck tires and earth, and between the truck and worker, while the worker is standing on the earth.

As electrical events unfold, physics, environmental factors, and individual traits can combine to result in nonuniform electrical exposures. Alternatively, the combination of electrical event, physics, environmental factors, and individual traits can result in nonuniform electrical exposures complicated by coincident energy exposures, including thermal, radiation, acoustic, and mechanical energy released from an industrial or commercial

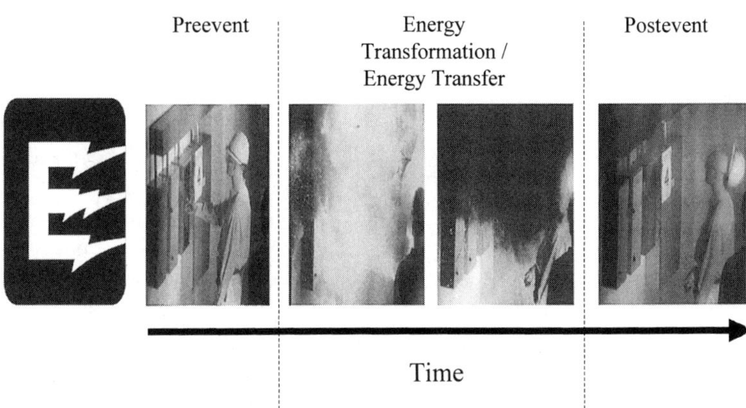

Figure 31.2. Staged test with a mannequin industrial worker standing near a panel box. Under high-voltage laboratory conditions with 480 V and approximately 22,000 A, electrical failure is staged to reproduce workplace conditions. (Adapted source video footage collected for Jones et al.[34])

Table 31.1. Common Sources of Nonoccupational Electrical Injuries and Fatalities

Setting	Source	Injury Example
Households	Receptacles	3900 injuries annually, with 33% affecting young children inserting metal objects[17]
Medical	Iatrogenic	Pectoral muscle damage after defibrillation[57]
Civil Justice	Stun guns	Associated with more than 50 fatalities since 2000[1]
Educational/recreational	Swimming pools	Electrocutions and electric shocks[16]
	Vending machines	Electrocutions, shocks[18]

power source with the electrical event. Consequently, when an electrical injury survivor has been exposed to an electrical source, neurological trauma evaluation may identify multifocal findings causally related to exposure to electrical and other forms of energy transfer.

Accidental injury results from exogenous exposure to supraphysiological conditions. With neurotoxins generally, the dose and duration of neural exposure influence the extent of injury.[45] By extension, the dose and duration of energy exposure influence the injury extent in an electrical event. Electrical exposures across the electromagnetic spectrum are described by the source energy form, frequency, and wavelength. Exposure duration is described in seconds.

Medical Consequences of Electrical Injury

The bioelectrical characteristics of human tissues under physiological conditions have been characterized.[3,20,21,24,25,29] Human tissues vary in their vulnerability to electrical forces, as suggested by the characteristics of conductivity (Table 31.4), impedance, and resistivity, affecting tissue responsiveness.

The remainder of this chapter focuses on the electrical effects of injuries from power frequency electrical sources. The complexity of patients' clinical presentation reflects the fundamental nature of electrical injury events: these are typically high-speed, multihazard incidents.[34,36,38] The clinical spectrum of electrical injury ranges from the absence of any external physical signs to severe multiple trauma requiring extensive surgical care.[6,33,40,52,55]

Table 31.2. Source Voltages Recorded in 623 Occupational Fatality Narratives[12]

% of Cases	No. of Deaths	Source Voltages
32%	198	0–600 V
	50	480 V
	18	440 V
	24	277 V
	36	220/240 V
	42	110/120 V
8%	50	601–5,000 V
35%	215	5,001–10,000 V
13%	81	10,001–15,000 V
13%	79	Over 15,001 V

Death from Electrical Shock

Fatal electrical shock is referred to as *electrocution*. The earliest electrocution in an occupational fatality dates to 1879 in a theater, while intentional electrical fatality as a form of capital punishment dates to the first electric chair execution in 1890.[58]

Table 31.3 illustrates current exposures under 600 V associated with cardiac conduction interference effects resulting in cardiac fibrillation, respiratory arrest, and death. In higher-voltage scenarios, less current over a shorter time period may result in fatal burns dominating the physical effects.

Local Effects of Electrical Exposure

When electromechanical and electrochemical coupling between a power energy source and a victim are sufficient to provide a supraphysiological applied electrical field, effects may be purely electrical, as in electroporation of cellular membranes with resulting metabolic exhaustion of cells, cell death, and tissue necrosis;[36–38,41] ohmic or joule heating of cells and tissues within the path of the applied electric field, with resulting burns;[30b,42] and/or induced electrical effects from the mag-

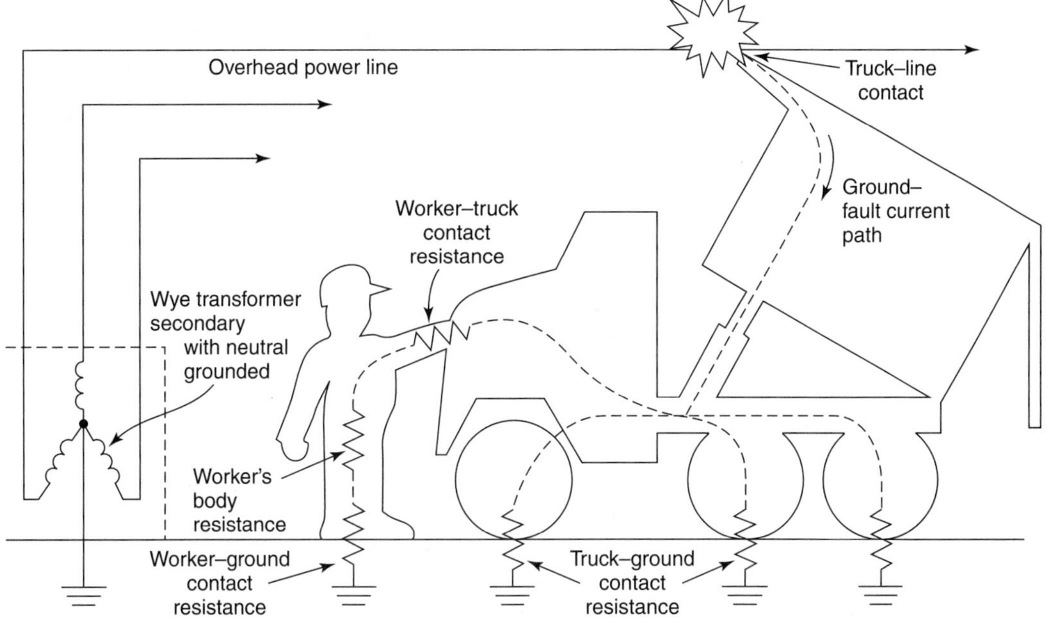

Figure 31.3. Electrical exposure of a worker to an overhead power line in a construction scenario with a haul truck contacting the power line. Overhead power lines account for about 40% of U.S. occupational electrical fatalities.[13] (Courtesy of James Cawley, National Institute of Occupational Safety and Health.)

netic field secondary to the electrical current flow.[2]

In the ELF electrical energy range relevant to commercially available power sources, the body's dissociated ions are the most important charge carriers, and passage of current during an electrical shock is mediated at the source–body interface by electrochemical reactions.[40]

Complications and Sequelae

The clinical course of electrical incident survivors can vary. Opinions differ about the nature and cause of patient symptoms and the relationship between symptoms and factors such as trauma severity, litigation, or premorbid personality. Not all survivors develop physical, cognitive, and/or emotional difficulties. No consistent relationship has been established between characteristics such as age, injury-related characteristics (e.g., voltage, current source, work error), and neuropsychological test performance.[30a,47,51]

As suggested by multiple case reviews, the clinical presentation of electrical injury patients may be specifically neurological, as with loss of consciousness; tinnitus and deafness; paraplegia; hemiplegia; aphasia; headache; memory disturbance; epilepsy; or progressive muscle atrophy. Or their presentation may be diffusely physical, including general fatigue or exhaustion; weakness in joints; muscle aches, spasm, cramps, or twitches; or extreme physical sensitivity.[19,44,47,54,56]

Neuropsychological symptoms may include increased emotional sensitivity; insomnia or other sleep disorders; unusual anxiety; reduced attention span/loss of concentration; personality changes; fear of electricity; and inability to cope.[47]

Electrical trauma survival can be associated with significant functional impairment. In their landmark retrospective study of employees of a national electrical energy company, Gourbiere et al. reviewed the electrical trauma survival experience during 1970–1989 for a workforce between 100,000 and 120,000. Electrical burns affected 2080 workers. Of these, 515 patients, or 25%, were noted to have postinjury complications, including 63% burn related, with amputations in 5%; 18% neuropsychiatric; 12% sensory; 5% orthopedic; and 1% cardiovascular. Sense organ disorders included vision-related changes due to conjunctivitis, keratitis, and cataracts; auditory sequelae, with conduc-

Table 31.3. Effects of Electrical Current on the Body for Source Currents of Less Than 600 V

Source Current	Human Response
1 mA	Perception of faint tingling
5 mA	Perception of slight shock, which may be disturbing but not painful. At this exposure, most people can "let go" or voluntarily relax a forceful hand grip. An involuntary startle response to this level of exposure may cause loss of balance during work, contact with nearby equipment, or other secondary injury.
6–12 mA (F) 9–30 mA (M)	Painful shock associated with loss of muscular control. Within this range of current, it may not be possible for the victim to voluntarily release a forceful grip or relax contracted muscles.
50–150 mA	Perception of an extremely painful shock, respiratory paralysis, and severe muscle contractions. Asymmetry in flexor and extensor muscle contractions can result in unpredictable spasmodic movement. Death is possible.
1000–4300 mA (1–4.3 A)	Ventricular fibrillation due to interference from an extraphysiological electrical source with cardiac conduction, muscle contraction, and neural damage. Death is likely.
10,000 mA (10 A)	Cardiac arrest and severe burns occur. Death is probable.
15,000 mA (15 A)	Lowest over current at which a typical electrical circuit protector (fuse, breaker) will operate.

Note: Differences in female (F) and male (M) responses are related to average differences in total body muscle and fat content. One milliamp (1 mA) is 1/1000th of one ampere (1 A). For example, household electrical sources are typically wired at 110–220 V with 200 A available current.

Source: Adapted from NIOSH[50] and DOL[23] based on research by Dalziel[20,21] and the presentation by Lee.[43]

Table 31.4. Summary of Human Tissue Conductivity σ [S/m]

Marrow bone	8.51e –01
Cancellous bone	8.21e –01
Blood	7.00e –01
Brain, white matter	6.55e –01
Eye, sclera wall	5.08e –01
Eye, cornea	4.28e –01
Eye, lens	3.33e –01
Muscle	3.34e –01
Blood vessel	3.11e –01
Cortical bone	2.03e –01
Skin, dermis	2.01e –01
Eye, aqueous	1.50e –01
Body fluid	1.50e –01
Brain, gray matter	1.07e –01

Source: Adapted from work done at Brooks Air Force Base as cited by Nadeem et al.[48]

tive or sensorineural hearing loss, tinnitus, and vertigo; and anosmia. In 59 of the 515 patients, disability was considered serious, with impairment rating from 31% to 100%.[26]

Because of the frequent occupational nature of injury scenarios,[9a] use of at least one hand in the task prior to injury is not uncommon, with possible median nerve and carpal tunnel involvement.[8,22,46] Peripheral nerve disorders, as described by Wilbourn[58] and others,[5,59] can complicate rehabilitation.

Treatment of Electrical Injury

The treatment of electrical injury depends on the patient's presentation and clinical history. Sometimes the injured person can "walk away" from the electrical event. However, this immediate post-incident behavior may be deceptive, given that the medical consequences of electrical trauma may unfold over minutes to hours to days following an electrical exposure.[6,14,27,31,44]

In the emergency or first response period, American Burn Association (ABA) Advanced Burn Life Support guidelines outline triage, initial resuscitation, and emergency transport protocols. On admission to the emergency room, physical examination, laboratory studies, and diagnostic radiology evaluation are prioritized, depending on the patient's clinical course.

Neurological evaluation of the central nervous system, audition, vision, and peripheral sensorimotor function can be managed intercurrently with stabilization of cardiorespiratory status and wounds.

When there is evidence or suspicion of exposure and electromechanical contact with an electrical source of more than 200 V potential and capable of more than 200 mA, hospital admission is warranted even in the absence of physical findings.[10]

Additional indications for hospital admission are a history of cardiopulmonary resuscitation or cardiac findings, including refractory cardiac arrhythmias; a history of loss of consciousness or disorientation; a history of a fall from a height; associated thermal injury to more than 15% of the body surface area, including burns to the hands, feet, face, or groin; suspicion of smoke/vapor inhalation or respiratory distress; spine fractures; serum electrolyte derangements; and compartment syndromes.[4,10,39,53]

Nonelectrical Effects in Electrical Events

The electrical system is evolving. As power density increases across more compact spaces, more fault energy is available in electrical installations. With installations designed to be compact, there are smaller spatial cushions and consequently less physical or spatial barrier protection emerging in innovative designs. The result is that there may be less time and less physical distance through which an unintentional release of energy can be dissipated during an electrical incident. With higher power density and smaller, more compact spaces, there is an increase risk of collateral damage from electrical incident effects.

High power density in a compact space has bomb-like potential, with characteristics of closed blast.[9b] For example, the potential ignition of 1 MW is roughly equivalent to the potential ignition of one stick of dynamite. One stick of dynamite is roughly 1/3 lb of TNT equivalent. So, a 100 MW scenario can be represented as loaded with 100 sticks of dynamite and a 300 MW scenario can be represented as loaded with 100 lb of TNT. A scenario in a closed space creates the possibility of closed blast effects; at a pole top in a vacant field, the space is more like an open area in a free blast scenario. A blast can result in tissue destruction from shrapnel, confined-space air contamination, acoustic or pressure effects and acceleration/deceleration forces. When a patient's neurological presentation is consistent with blunt force or blast injury after an electrical event, a high energy electrical explosion scenario complicating an electrical shock may contribute to the patient's condition.

REFERENCES

1. Andrews W: TASER Danger? Reported by CBS News, 2004. Retrieved in print format from www.cbsnews.com/stories/main648859.shtml
2. Bailey WH: Dealing with uncertainty in formulating occupational and public exposure limits. Health Physics 83(3):402–408, 2002.
3. Baker L: Principles of the impedance technique. IEEE EMBS 8(1):11–13, 1989.
4. Baxter CR: Present concepts in the management of major electrical injury. Surg Clin North Am 50(6):1401–1418, 1970.
5. Blom S, Ugland OM: Peripheral nerve injuries in electrical burns. Scand J Plast Reconstruct Surg 2(suppl): 68–74, 1967.
6. Bongard O, Fagrell B: Delayed arterial thrombosis following an apparently trivial low-voltage electrical injury. VASA 18:162–166, 1989.
7. Bowen JE, Wactor MW, Miller GW, Capelli-Schellpfeffer M: Catch the wave. IEEE Indust Applic Mag 10(4):59–67, July–August 2004.
8. Butler ED, Grant TD. Electrical injuries with special reference to the upper extremities. Am J Surg 134:95–99, 1977.

9a. Capelli-Schellpfeffer M: Roadblocks to return to work after electrical trauma. NeuroRehabilitation 20(1):49–52, 2005.

9b. Capelli-Schellpfeffer M, Miller GH, Humilier M: Thermo-acoustic energy effects in electrical arcs. Ann NY Acad Sci 888:19–32, 1999.

10. Capelli-Schellpfeffer M, Toner M, Lee RC, Astumian RD: Advances in the evaluation and treatment of electrical and thermal injury emergencies. IEEE Trans Indust Applic 31(5):1147–1195, 1995.
11. Castillo DN: NIOSH Alert: Preventing Death and Injuries of Adolescent Workers. DHHS (NIOSH) Pub. No. 95–125. Cincinnati: U.S. Department of Health and Human Services, Public Health Service, Centers for Disease Control and Prevention, National Institute for Occupational Safety and Health, 1995.
12. Cawley J, Homce G: Overview of electrical injuries, 1992–1998, and recommendations for future research. J Safety Res 34:241–248, 2003.
13. Cawley J, Homce GT, Sacks HK, Yencheck MR: Protecting workers from electrocution caused by contact of cranes, haul trucks, and drill rigs with overhead powerlines: A new approach. H3.4, Pittsburgh. Abstracts of the National Occupational Injury Research Symposium (NOIRS), 2000.
14. Christensen JA, Sherman RT, Balis GA, Wuamatt JP: Delayed neurologic injury secondary to high voltage current with recovery. J Trauma 20(2):166–168, 1980.
15. Christoffel T, Gallagher SS: Injury Prevention and Public Health. Gaithersburg, MD, Aspen, 1999.
16. Consumer Product Safety Commission: Don't swim with shocks: Electrical safety in and around pools, hot tubs, and spas. www.cpsc.gov/cpscpub.pubs/519.pdf, May 13, 2003.
17. Consumer Product Safety Commission: Electrical receptacle outlet injuries. CPSC document #524. URL: www.cpsc.gov/cpscpub/pubs/524.html, 2004.
18. Consumer Product Safety Commission. Standard submission to prevent electrocutions and non fatal electri-

cal shocks in vending machines based on CPSC 7 investigations of fatal and non-fatal serious injuries. www.cpsc.gov/volstd/gfci/422.xx.pdf, 2004.
19. Critchley M: Neurologic effects of lightning and electricity. Lancet 1:68–72, 1934.
20. Dalziel CF: Effect of frequency on let-go currents. Trans Am Inst Elect Engr 62:745–750, 1943.
21. Dalziel CF: Threshold 60-cycle fibrillating currents. AIEE Trans III Power Apparatus Syst 79:667–673, 1960.
22. Danielson JR, Capelli-Schellpfeffer M, Lee RC: Upper extremity electrical injury. Hand Clin 16(2):225–234, 2000.
23. Department of Labor: Controlling Electrical Hazards. Washington, DC, U.S. Department of Labor, Occupational Safety and Health Administration, 1997.
24. Freiberger H: The electrical resistance of the human body to DC and AC currents. Elecrtrizitatswirtschaft (Berl) 32(2):442–446; 32(17):373–375, 1933.
25. Geddes LA, Baker LE: The specific resistance of biological material—a compendium of data for the biomedical engineer and physiologist. Med Biol Eng 5:271–293, 1967.
26. Gourbiere E, Corbut J-P, Bazin Y: Functional consequence of electrical injury. Ann NY Acad Sci, 720:259–271, 1994.
27. Grube BJ, Heimbach DM: Neurological sequelae of electrical injury. In: Lee RC (ed): Electrical Trauma: The Pathophysiology, Manifestations, and Clinical Management. Cambridge: Cambridge University Press, 1992, pp 133–152.
28. Haddon W Jr: Energy damage and the ten countermeasure strategies. J Trauma 13(4):321–331, 1973.
29. Hammam MS: A range of body impedance values for low voltage, low source impedance systems of 60 Hz. IEEE Trans Power Apparatus Syst PAS-102 5:1097–1105, 1983.
30a. Hendler N: Overlooked diagnosis in chronic pain: Analysis of survivors of electric shock and lightning strike. JOEM 47(8):796–805, 2005.
30b. Hunt JL, Mason AD, Masterson TS, Pruitt BA: The pathophysiology of acute electrical injuries. J Trauma 16:335–340, 1976.
31. Hunt JL, Sato RM, Baxter CR: Acute electrical burns: Current diagnostic and therapeutic approaches to management. Arch Surg 115:434–438, 1980.
32. Isaacs A (ed): A Concise Dictionary of Physics. New York, Oxford University Press, 1990, p 77.
33. Jaffe RH: Electropathology: A review of the pathologic change produced by electrical currents. Arch Pathol 5: 839–869, 1928.
34. Jones R, Liggett DP, Capelli-Schellpfeffer M, Downey RE, Jamil S, Macalady T, McClung LB, Saporita VJ, Saunders LF, Smith A: Staged tests increase awareness of arc-flash hazards in electrical equipment. IEEE Trans Industry Applic Soc 36(2):659–667, 2000.
35. Knight R: Physics for Scientists and Engineers. San Francisco, Pearson Addison Wesley, 2004.
36. Lee RC: Physical mechanisms of tissue injury in electrical trauma. IEEE Trans Ed 34:223–230, 1992.
37. Lee RC: Tissue injury from exposure to power frequency fields. In: Lin JC (ed): Advances in Electromagnetic Fields in Living Systems, vol. 1. New York: Plenum, 1994, pp 81–127.
38. Lee RC, Aarsvold JN, Chen W, Astumian RD, Capelli-Schellpfeffer M, Kelley KM, Pliskin NH: Biophysical mechanisms of cell membrane damage in electrical shock. Semin Neurol 14(4):330–349, 1995.
39. Lee RC, Capelli-Schellpfeffer M: Electrical and lightning injuries. In: Cameron JC (ed): Current Surgical Therapy, 6th ed. St. Louis, Mosby, 1997, pp. 1021–1023.
40. Lee RC, Dougherty W: Electrical injury: Mechanisms, manifestations, and therapy. IEEE Trans Dielectr Electr Insulation 10(5):810–819, 2003.
41. Lee RC, Kolodney MS: Electrical injury mechanisms: Electrical breakdown of cell membranes. Plast Reconstr Surg, 80:672–679, 1987.
42. Lee RC, Tropea BI: Thermal injury kinetics in electrical trauma. J Biomech Eng 114:241–250, 1992.
43. Lee RL: Electrical safety in industrial plants. Am Soc Safety Eng J 18(9):36–42, 1973.
44. Levine NS, Atkins A, McKeel DW, Peck SD, Pruitt BA: Spinal cord injury following electrical accidents with case reports. J Trauma 15(5):459–463, 1975.
45. Manzo L: Cellular response to injury by neurotoxicants. In: Bleecker ML (ed): Neurotoxicology Clinics in Occupational and Environmental Medicine, vol. 1, part 3. Philadelphia, WB Saunders, 2001, pp 463–488.
46. Morse MS: A study of carpal tunnel injury following electrical trauma. Chicago, IEEE Proceedings of the 22nd Annual EMBS International Conference, July 23–28, 2000, pp 1417–1420.
47. Morse MS, Berg JS, TenWolde RL: Diffuse electrical injury: A study of 89 subjects reporting long-term symptomatology that is remove to the theoretical pathway. IEEE Trans Biomed Eng 51(8):1449–1459, 2004
48. Nadeem M, Thorlin T, Gandhi OP, Persson M: Computation of electric and magnetic stimulation in the human head using the 3-D impedance method. IEEE Trans Biomed Eng 50(7):900–907, 2003.
49. National Institute for Occupational Safety and Health: Worker Health Chartbook. DHHS (NIOSH) Pub. No. 2000-127. NIOSH, Atlanta, September 2000, Figure 2–6, p 33.
50. National Institute for Occupational Safety and Health: Electrical Safety: Safety and Health in Electrical Trades—Student Manual. DHHS (NIOSH) Pub No 2002-123. NIOSH, Cincinnati January 2002.
51. Pliskin NH, Capelli-Schellpfeffer M, Law RT, Malina AC, Law R, Kelley KM, Lee RC: Neuropsychologic symptom presentation after electrical injury. J Trauma 44:709–715, 1998.
52. Rosenburg DB: Neurologic sequelae of minor electric burns. Arch Phys Med Rehabil 70:914–915, 1989.
53. Salisbury RE, Hunt JL, Warden GD, Pruitt BA: Management of electrical burns of the upper extremity. Plast Reconstr Surg 51:648–652, 1973.

54. Silversides J: The neurologic sequelae of electrical injury. Can Med Assoc J 91:195–204, 1964.
55. Skoog T: Electrical injuries. J Trauma 10:816–830, 1970.
56. Varghese T, Mari MM, Redford JB: Spinal cord injuries following electrical accidents. Paraplegia 24:159–166, 1986.
57. Vogel U, Wanner T, Bultmann B: Extensive pectoral muscle necrosis after defibrillation: Nonthermal skeletal muscle damage caused by electroporation. Intens Care Med 24:743–745, 1998.
58. Wilbourn AJ: Peripheral nerve disorders in electrical and lightning injuries. Semin Neurol 15(3):241–255, 1995.
59. Wilkinson C, Wood M: High voltage electrical injury. Am J Surg 136:693–696, 1978.

Chapter 32
Neurology of Microgravity and Space Travel

MAVIS D. FUJII

The environment of space is toxic to humans and most other forms of life that have evolved on this planet. The toxicity occurs because space lacks gravity, a radiation shield, an atmosphere, warmth, food, water, and other humans—in short, all those things that ensure survival and provide physical and psychological happiness (Table 32.1). After a discussion of the methodological limitations of space science and a history of the exploration of space, this chapter reviews the environment of spaceflight in terms of the major effects of space, particularly of microgravity, on the nervous system and on those systems that have an impact on the nervous system.

Table 32.1. Hazards of Space

Weightlessness
Penetrating ionizing radiation
Vacuum
Meteorites
Stresses of acceleration and deceleration
Vastness, desolation, and silence
Temperature extremes
Equipment failure
Toxic fumes

Methodological Limitations

Our knowledge about space is in its infancy because of the limited opportunities for study of orbital flight, the small sample sizes of personnel involved, limited experimental protocols because of operational conditions and tasks that have been assigned higher priorities, and the extensive use of countermeasures, including drugs and exercises, without standard protocols or proper controls. Any conclusions based on studies to date therefore must be tentative and considered based on incomplete, inadequate, and possibly even inaccurate or erroneous data. It is hoped that as the era of exploration ends and the space station era begins, the unique environmental conditions of space—the foremost of these being microgravity—will be subjected to scientifically controlled, reproducible experiments that reach definite, firm conclusions furthering our understanding of fundamentals in biology and medicine that cannot be achieved by any other means.

History

The human adventure in space began on April 21, 1961, when Cosmonaut Yuri Gagarin aboard

Vostok 1, a spacecraft weighing 10,419 pounds, flew the first orbital mission, circling Earth in 1 hour and 48 minutes.[75] Four months later, Gorman Titov, during a similar orbital flight, gave the first report of neurological symptoms, complaining of dizziness, anorexia, vomiting, and disorientation, which were relieved by keeping his head and body relatively immobile. Titov was also the first human to sleep in space and was the first to exercise autonomous control of a spacecraft. Subsequently the Soviet Union, a space-faring nation second to none, amassed most of the early records, including the first woman in space, Valentina Tereshkova (June 16, 1963), and the first known death, of Vladimir Komarov, who in April 1967, aboard Soyuz 1, tried to abort the mission on the 18th orbit and, becoming tangled in parachute cords, crashed to earth. Boris Yegorov, a cosmonaut-physician, performed the first medical examination on October 12, 1964, and Aleksey Leonov performed the first extravehicular activity (EVA) in March 1965.

The first manned Apollo flight was scheduled for February 1967 but had to be postponed because on January 27, 1967, during a countdown rehearsal, a fire broke out in the cabin, which at the time was filled with pure oxygen at atmospheric pressure.[50,55a] Astronauts Virgil Grissom, Edward White, and Roger Chaffee died. Despite this inauspicious beginning, men finally did land on the moon on July 21, 1969. The Apollo project, from 1968 to 1970, involved 24 astronauts, landing 12 on the lunar surface who logged a total time of 160 man-hours there. Strangely, the crew of Apollo 8 were the first American astronauts to experience space motion sickness (SMS), even though their counterparts in the Soviet Union had been reporting SMS symptoms for at least 7 years. Perhaps the difference in reporting frequency was due to the fact that Soviet spacecraft were much larger than American spacecraft, providing more room for the cosmonauts to move around. Because of SMS, a planned EVA of Apollo 9 was rescheduled, being the first mission modification caused by a medical disorder. The historic Apollo 11 flight, which carried two astronauts to the moon's surface, had the first case of decompression sickness. Ventricular bigeminies, premature atrial contractions, and premature ventricular contractions occurred in the Apollo 15 astronauts during their moon walks and return flight, possibly owing to low serum potassium levels and fatigue from extensive work schedules. One episode of severe bradycardia occurred during sleep in one crew member.

The Skylab project, consisting of three missions, followed the Apollo flights, with an emphasis on the study of habitability in space and physiological adaptation to microgravity.[24,25,81] Skylab 2 had the first American physician on board, Joseph Kerwin, who, with Pete Conrad, conducted an unscheduled 4-hour EVA to release a solar array that had not deployed properly.

Extensive metabolic studies were performed on the crew during their 28-day mission. During the next Skylab mission of 59 days, crew members experienced severe SMS, in contrast to no cases occurring in the crew of the first Skylab mission. The astronauts of Skylab 4, with a space stay of 84 days, took anti–motion sickness medications and performed acrobatic maneuvers before launch to help prevent SMS. These measures were not completely effective because two members developed SMS. The Skylab project provided valuable information on the physiology of a human exposed to long stays in microgravity. Valuable information about orthostatic intolerance, muscle weakness, exercise effects, bone demineralization, electrolyte balance, and hormonal changes laid the foundation for the Soviet Union's extended flights in microgravity.[31]

While the United States was pursuing the Apollo and Skylab projects, the Soviets flew the Soyuz project, assessing the feasibility of a space station and longer stays in microgravity.[81] They experimented with docking spacecraft with EVA procedures and studied musculoskeletal and cardiovascular disorders with various therapeutic interventions. The Soviets tested antigravity suits similar to MAST (military antishock trousers) suits, consisting of inflatable bladders to compress the legs and lower abdomen to increase venous return to the heart, loading suits, and bungee-cord exercises. They also studied circulation rheography, showing increased blood flow to the brain, liver, and lungs.

The Apollo-Soyuz project, a joint space project between the United States and the Soviet Union, tested the ability of the two countries to conduct joint space rescue missions.[81] In addition to the rendezvous and docking of Apollo and Soyuz spacecraft, the five-man crew completed additional scientific and technical experiments. On reentry, the astronauts, who were accidentally exposed to nitrous tetroxide, a toxic gas used as a propellant in retrorockets for attitude adjustments, developed chemical pneumonitis. Intensive treatment prevented scheduled postflight medical studies.

The Soviets developed their space station program, Salyut, in the late 1960s, with the first crew inhabiting the craft in April 1971.[81] Owing to a delay caused by an accident that resulted in the deaths of three cosmonauts from rapid decompression, the Soviet space station Salyut-3 went into orbit in June 1974, followed by another Salyut station in April 1982.

Mission durations were longer, extending up to 185 days. After a 96-day flight, cosmonauts exhibited severe cardiovascular deconditioning, including orthostatic hypotension. Symptoms of SMS and other vestibular symptoms were found in cosmonauts during their 175-day flight and also postflight. The medical results of the Mir year-long mission have recently been published: compared with former flights, no new or qualitatively different changes were noted[32] (Table 32.2).

In contrast to the Soviets' space station program, the National Aeronautics and Space Administration (NASA) focused on a reusable space craft, the Space Transportation System (STS), commonly known as the Shuttle, for short-duration missions to conduct experiments and for launching and servicing satellites.[81] In April 1981, Bob Crippen and John Young made the first human-piloted hypersonic Shuttle flight and runway landing. Shuttle flights continued, with crews launching and repairing satellites and conducting biomedical and physical science experiments until the 1985 explosion of the Challenger, when seven astronauts died. This halted the American program for 3 years until September 1988, when STS-26 was launched. Onboard the Shuttle, biomedical experiments have been performed, investigating SMS, orthostatic hypotension, heart dimensions and function, erythrocyte function, hormonal and electrolyte dynamics, intraocular pressure, and pharmacokinetics. Treatments for orthostatic hypotension and SMS have been developed, and more effective therapies are being sought. Spacelab, a specialized modular element dedicated to biomedical research that fits into the payload bay, has greatly enhanced the ability to conduct medical research in space.

Joint efforts by NASA and the Soviet Union were later made, allowing astronauts to fly onboard Mir, the Russian space station, and cosmonauts to fly onboard the Shuttle.

Table 32.2. Some Medical Data from 366 Days Aboard MIR

Radiation dose
12.2–14.0 rem or 7.6–8.7 rad total were absorbed per person.

Space diet
Freeze-dried foodstuffs (65%) and canned items provided about 3000 kcal/day.

Daily routine
8.5 hours of work, 8–9 hours of sleep. Crew members worked for 5 days, then were off for 2 days. Toward the end of the mission, owing to fatigue and psychological problems, crew members required additional time off.

Countermeasures
Bicycle ergometer, treadmill, bungee cords, and "penguin" suits daily for 8 hours. At the end of the trip, crew members trained with a lower body negative pressure device. On the last flight day, crew members consumed water-salt supplements, and during reentry and immediately after landing wore anti-G suits.

Flight observations
All crew members noted fluid shift to the head, facial puffiness, and a nasal voice on insertion. One crew member had sensory illusions.

Postflight
Marked autonomic instability with orthostatic hypotension was reported in all astronauts. Sensory illusions were present in one.

Muscle
Leg circumference decreased 20%, whereas arm and forearm circumference remained unchanged. Anterior tibial muscle force losses were in the range of 23% to 50%, and the work capacity of calf muscles decreased fourfold. The usual past-pointing and severe changes of gaze fixation were present. Hypogravitational ataxia continued in cosmonauts for more than 2 weeks after return but was less severe than in the 170-day flight.

Heart
Echocardiography indicated a decrease in cardiac output, hyperkinesia of the septum, and a moderate increase in right ventricle anteroposterior size. Electrocardiogram showed minor changes of no importance.

Bone
Bone mineral losses averaged 10% (L1-3).

Source: Data from Grigoriev AI, Bugrov SA, Bogomolov VV, et al: Medical results of the Mir year-long mission. Medispace 3:31–41, 1991.

Exchange programs allowed cosmonauts to learn American and Shuttle procedures and American astronauts to learn Russian Mir operations. This short-lived program was followed by the development of the International Space Station.

The International Space Station resulted from an agreement between NASA, the Russian space agency, the European Space Agency (ESA), and the National Space Development Agency of Japan (NASDA) to fly cooperative missions and maintain a permanent presence in space. Both astronauts and cosmonauts have been and are currently onboard. Visitors from Canada and Japan have conducted experiments onboard. The first flight was STS 88, which was launched in December 1998 to attach the first two modules of the space station together. The shuttle with the Unity Module rendezvoused with the already launched Zarya Control Module. The Zarya provided propulsion, power, communications, and the capability for automated rendezvous. Three spacebars completed the construction project. Subsequent flights provided equipment and exchanged battery recharge controller modules. Solar arrays that quintupled the station's electrical power were deployed next. Subsequent flights followed that included flights to install solar panel arrays for energy, mating adapters to allow further expansion, trusses, airlocks, supplies, and other devices to facilitate and provide ongoing communication, power, and data transfer. STS-106 astronauts installed a toilet and a treadmill, along with battery converters and supplies. Astronauts aboard STS-108, launched December, 2001, released almost 6000 small U.S. flags into orbit to honor those killed in the September 11 terrorist attacks. They also launched Starshine Satellite 2, an ongoing program to release beach ball–sized, mirror-covered satellites into orbit, each lasting about 8 months, which can be seen in the early morning and evening twilight hours with the naked eye. Destiny, a laboratory, was attached to the space station during flight STS-98 in early 2001. During each of these flights, crew members were exchanged and those who had remained in space were brought back to Earth. Robotic arms and external handrails and foot grips were installed. With STS-111, a landmark stay in space of 198 days was made by the Expedition Four crew.

However, an impressive schedule of flights to the International Space Station ended abruptly when STS-107 exploded upon reentry. A number of physics and biological experiments had been completed by the seven-member crew of Columbia, some of these performed for student investigators. Upon liftoff, a large piece of insulating foam from the external fuel tank became dislodged and broke off several carbon heat tiles from the leading edge of the wing. Upon reentry, superheated gases leaked underneath the carbon tiles and melted the wing, thus destroying the control surfaces and allowing the Shuttle to burn up over Texas. An extensive investigation followed, with crew transfers and supply deliveries to the space station being performed by Russian spacecraft. Return to flight is anticipated in 2006 after foam debris from the external fuel tank fell off the shuttle launched in 2005.

Neurological Complications of Space Travel

Space Adaptation Syndrome

Space adaptation syndrome (SAS), another name for SMS, afflicts up to 67% of astronauts.[24] Symptoms include headache, malaise, nausea, vomiting, and sensitivity to body and head movements, especially in the pitch axis.[22,90,104,105,116,139] Usually SAS begins within minutes of obtaining orbit, peaks in 1 to 2 days, usually stops by day 4, and may recur after landing. Rarely, SAS lasts for the entire flight, 10 or even 14 days. It affects men more often than women: 65% of career male astronauts have experienced SAS symptoms compared with only 38% of career female astronauts. Sweating and pallor are not part of the symptom complex. Some investigators include perceptual illusions in SAS because position and motion illusions have been reported with other SAS symptoms by the Skylab, Apollo-Soyuz, and Space Transportation System (Shuttle) astronauts and Soviet cosmonauts.

The prognosis for SAS is excellent; no long-term effects have been documented. The mainstay of prevention is medication: scopolamine-Dexedrine or promethazine.[24,58] The scopolamine (0.4 mg)–Dexedrine (5.0 mg) combination, if taken shortly before launch or insertion into orbit, may inhibit the development of SAS. Promethazine, 25 mg self-administered intramuscularly, has been shown to be highly effective if there is uncertainty about oral absorption of medications or if symptoms are severe.[34] Astronauts with a history of SAS or no previous flight experience take medications before launch or about 10 minutes after orbital insertion (first in-flight orbital correction maneuver).[47] Experienced crew members with no history of SAS are not required to take antisickness drugs. Once taken, anti-SMS agents should be continued for at least the first 48 hours in microgravity lest symptoms occur.

The incidence of SAS varies with the flight program. No problems with SAS were reported for the Mercury or Gemini programs, in contrast to the Apollo, Skylab, and STS (Shuttle) programs,[24,34,45,86,128] perhaps because of the larger habitable volume of the more modern spacecraft, which allowed for more head and body movements.[45,47] Of the 33 Apollo astronauts, 11 experienced SAS.[40,98,99] Six had mild symptoms of only stomach awareness, but two had moderate symptoms of stomach awareness, nausea, and vomiting. In STS, 67% of astronauts experienced SAS: 46% of these had one to several mild transition symptoms, such as one episode of retching or vomiting, with resolution in 2 days; and 35% had moderate SAS, which included several persistent symptoms in addition to anorexia, malaise, lethargy, nausea, and one vomiting episode.[24] All symptoms resolved within 3 days. In comparison, 19% of Shuttle astronauts developed severe SAS lasting for more than 3 days such that they kept the head voluntarily immobile, more than two episodes of vomiting occurred, and performance became impaired.

Previous experience in microgravity seems to reduce the severity of SAS. Thirty-five percent of repeat flyers had less severe symptoms on their next flights, 57% had no change, and 8% had worse symptoms.[24,63,124] The susceptibility to SAS does not correlate with the susceptibility to motion sickness caused by ships, acrobatic maneuvers, rotating chairs, or parabolic flight.[34,47] The Soviet cosmonauts have experienced a similar incidence of SAS. The following are percentages of cosmonauts exhibiting symptoms in each flight project: Vostok, 15%; Voskhod, 60%; Soyuz/Salyut, 65%; ASTP, 0%; Salyut 6, 50%; and Salyut 7, 45%.[47]

Several theories have been advanced to explain SAS: sensory conflict, otolith tilt reinterpretation, vestibular hydrops, increased intracranial pressure, and cervical vertigo.[45,66,80,92,96,97,103,104,119,126,127] The most popular theory, the sensory conflict theory, also explains other forms of motion sickness, such as sea sickness and rotating chair sickness. Simply stated, a conflict occurs between the currently sensed spatial environment and that retained in memory based on previous experience.[119] The current spatial environment has an unnatural motion element to which the spatial senses—vestibular, visual, proprioceptive, and kinesthetic—respond. These signals do not correspond with a previously learned and remembered situation. A sensory conflict results, producing autonomic symptoms, The conflict may originate within the vestibular apparatus, such as between disparate signals from the semicircular canals and otoliths, or may stem from differing signals sent by the vestibular, visual, proprioceptive, or kinesthetic senses.[45,122] The central nervous system cannot integrate these differing signals initially, resulting in autonomic arousal. With continued exposure to the abnormal motion environment, the central nervous system adapts gradually, probably by ignoring or reducing the influence of one sensory system in favor of the remaining senses (compensation) or by reinterpreting the signals from the differing sense organ (reinterpretation).[96]

The sensory conflict theory helps explain the symptoms and signs exhibited by astronauts exposed to microgravity and when they return to Earth. The source of this sensory conflict may arise only within the vestibular system or may include all the spatial sensory systems.

With absent gravitational forces, the otolith organs respond only to inertial changes in head movement and not to changes in head position relative to the gravity vector.[94,95,96,137] In 1 *g* (terrestrial environment), otoliths respond to either body motion. When the head and body move in one direction, the sensory hairs bend in the opposite direction. The visual scene moves in the opposite direction to body movement. When the head tilts to one side, the otoconia hair cells signal in the same direction as the head tilt. In microgravity with no gravitational vector, however, otoliths respond only to inertial movements. All otoconia signals are interpreted as representing linear motion in the opposite direction. Therefore, if the head is tilted, the visual scene shifts, but there is no associated otolith signal, as would occur in 1 *g*. This creates a conflict situation that somehow, by mechanisms still unknown, precipitates the autonomic symptoms. Input from proprioceptive organs may also be in disagreement, with that from the vestibular and visual organs. The response to these contradictory signals results in SAS.[45,48,121,122]

The otolith reinterpretation theory narrows the sensory conflict to involving primarily the otolith organs and the visual system. Ocular counterrolling, which is exhibited post-flight, supports this theory.[96] A similar theory focuses the pathology on a mismatch between otolith and semicircular canal inputs to the central nervous system.[138]

Supportive evidence for the otolith translation theory rests with a study conducted by Markham and Diamond[75] and other investigators. Thirteen astronauts who had previously flown were studied during parabolic flight. Those astronauts who had a high degree of ocular torsional disconjugate gaze had the higher incidence of in-flight SMS. Those who had a lower degree of torsional disconjugancy had experienced SMS. This suggests that those individuals who had an anatomical or physiological otolith asymmetry had compensated for these differences under Earth's gravity but decompensated when exposed to microgravity. Vestibular canal stimulation or a visual phenomenon may have worsened the symptoms. Previous exposure to microgravity also affected the responses to outside perturbations.[93] Using a modified computerized dynamic petrography system, it was found that veteran fliers had better adaptive motor responses to perturbations to them than did first-time fliers. Sensory feedback and accurate internal models are also important for successful acclimation to microgravity and readaptation to 1 g.

Neuromuscular Fatigue and Weakness

Astronauts experience fatigue on returning to Earth even after only a few days in microgravity. Longer exposures tend to produce greater sensations of tiredness that require longer recovery times after flight.[26,36,63–65] Weakness, especially in the lower extremities, always occurs with flights longer than 4 weeks.[63–65,79,129] Complaints include the inability to lift a specific weight and shortened endurance for walking postflight. Diagnosis is made by measurement of strength, endurance, and estimation of muscle mass, all of which may be decreased. The surface electromyographic (EMG) signal from astronauts returning after 59 days of flight is altered, suggesting abnormal electrical activation of muscle.[4,5,67] Muscles atrophy in space, in particular the leg and back muscles.[61–65,129] Strength loss of up to 20% of preflight values occurs in the leg extensors and flexors.[124] In the biceps and other arm flexors, the decrement is up to 10% of control values after less than 3 months in microgravity. Similar trends occur in the triceps and other arm extensors. In a cosmonaut exposed to microgravity for 140 days, isometric strength of the gastrocnemius decreased by approximately 19%; the only isokinetic strength lost was 4% at 60 degrees/second.[60,62,64,65] In contrast, the tibialis anterior lost roughly 15% of maximum isometric strength, and under isokinetic conditions, approximately 17% loss occurred at 60 and 120 degrees/second. However, at higher velocities, such as 180 degrees/second, no strength loss was observed. Cervical muscles of cosmonauts in space for 185 days lost 30% of their strength, measured either isometrically or isokinetically. Pooled data from 17 cosmonauts, however, showed that leg extensor strength decreased 20% to 30% for both isometric and isokinetic strength.[62] Soviet studies suggest that the most significant loss of muscle strength occurs within the first 3 months of spaceflight.

Only one study to date has evaluated human muscle tissue.[41,52] Vastus lateralis samples were taken by needle biopsy from eight astronauts (five men and three women) before and after flights ranging from 5 to 11 days, in which preflight and in-flight exercise regimens were highly variable. Despite measuring cross-sectional area, adenosine triphosphatase (ATPase) activity, succinic dehydrogenase activity, glycerophosphate dehydrogenase activity, and their ratios, no definite conclusions could be reached. The cross-sectional areas of all fibers seemed to decrease in most of the subjects, but the variability was great. There also seemed to be a shift in fiber type from type I fibers to type II fibers in some, but not all, of the astronauts, which was supported by myosin heavy chain analysis. The authors also felt that the number of capillaries decreased but that mitochondrial and glycolytic enzyme activities remained unchanged. Ohira et al. studied the beta-adrenoceptor mitochondria enzyme activities and fiber type composition in rats flown for 14 days.[89] They found that the beta-hydroxyacyl coenzyme A (CoA) dehydrogenase activity did not change but that the activity of succinct dehydrogenase declined. The binding capacity of the beta-adrenoceptor was decreased and was associated with a lower activity of succinic dehydrogenase, an inner mitochondria membrane enzyme, but not that of a matrix enzyme, beta-hydroxyacyl CoA dehydrogenase. This experiment suggests selective changes within the cell in response to microgravity. A definitive study remains to be performed on human tissue that must standardize preflight and in-flight exercise regimens of the participants, in-flight drugs used, and flight time and should employ open muscle biopsy techniques to ensure adequate specimens.

Better-controlled studies on muscle pathology have been conducted on rats flown on American and Russian spacecraft—in particular, the Spacelab, Space and Life Sciences I, and Cosmos flights.[13,28,73,78,87,109,110,112,116,118] The slow-twitch soleus and extensor digitorum longus (EDL) of rats flown for 7 days onboard Spacelab 3 demonstrated a marked loss in mean fiber area, decreasing 35.8% and 24.9%, respectively.[110] Within the soleus muscle, slow-twitch fibers showed a 40% decrease in cross-sectional area (CSA) compared with a 30% decrease in CSA in fast-twitch fibers.[118] However, the EDL showed significant loss only in the CSA of fast-twitch fibers. The antigravity vastus intermedius displayed a 22% loss in muscle weight compared to a loss of only 15% in the fast-twitch vastus lateralis after 9 days of microgravity.[7] Furthermore, the change in functional characteristics, absolute maximal tension, and unit maximal tension depended on muscle function rather than on the degree of atrophy or fiber composition.[121] The soleus showed a decrease in absolute maximal tension but not in unit maximal tension. The gastrocnemius showed a decrease in both absolute and unit maximal tension. The EDL did not atrophy during weightlessness. The soleus fibers showed an increase in their contraction kinetics, but no changes were found for the gastrocnemius or EDL. These data imply that the effects of microgravity on muscle depend upon muscle function and fiber type.

Changes in muscle composition occur with a shift from slow-twitch, oxidative fiber types to fast-twitch glycolytic or fast-twitch glycolytic-oxidative fiber types or from type I fibers to type IIa and IIb fibers.[6,42,88] Approximately 15% more fibers in a slow-twitch muscle, such as the soleus, will express fast myosin after spaceflight lasting only as long as 1 week.[88] In the vastus intermedius, there was a 12% decrease in slow myosin heavy chain with a concomitant increase in type IIb myosin heavy chain.[6] These changes are associated with changes in enzymes. Pyruvate kinase, glycerol-3-phosphate dehydrogenase, and I-phosphofructokinase were elevated in fast-twitch soleus fibers. These enzymes are important for glycolysis.[14] Hexokinase was higher in both fiber types in both the soleus (slow-twitch muscle) and the tibialis anterior (fast-twitch muscle). In addition, there seemed to be a reduction in lipid oxidation. The pyruvate oxidative capacity was reduced in both fast- and slow-twitch muscles after spaceflight, but after 9 days of gravity the ability to oxidize lipids returned.[6,8]

In addition, the distribution of mitochondria and succinic dehydrogenase (SDH) within a muscle changes with microgravity exposure.[8] The number of subsarcolemmal mitochondria and SDH activity are reduced, whereas the intermyofibrillar mitochondrial number remains unchanged in the soleus fibers.[9,108] These changes may reflect spaceflight muscle atrophy, as subsarcolemmal mitochondria are involved in protein synthesis, whereas the intermyofibrillar mitochondria are involved in the relative maintenance of contraction/relaxation and cytoplasmic calcium homeostasis. However, the rate of force development after 5 to 7 days of microgravity increased in the soleus but decreased in the fast-twitch gastrocnemius.[44] This finding supports the idea of a shift in fiber types in specific muscles and contractility, regardless of mitochondrial number and activity.

Riley et al. have studied rats flown for various times.[108,112] In rats flown for 12.5 days aboard a Cosmos biosatellite, the antigravity adductor longus, soleus, and plantaris atrophied much more than the non-weight-bearing EDL. Furthermore, the CSA of slow-twitch myofibrils decreased more than that of fast-twitch myofibrils. Landing trauma also affected the muscles: there was increased interstitial edema and disruption of myofibril architecture. There were decreased numbers of capillaries and extravagated red blood cells. About 17% of flight adductor longus end plates showed total or partial denervation. The authors conclude that muscle weakness results from both muscle fiber atrophy and postflight segmental necrosis, denervation, and impaired microcirculation.[108,112]

Caiozzo et al. also found similar findings.[12] Rats flown for 14 days showed changes in the contractility of the antigravity muscles that were based on changes in the myosin heavy chain phenotype and decreased muscle mass. The mRNA levels were changed, but these changes were not reflected in the protein levels. Further studies need to focus on the various steps from DNA encoding to its end product of muscle proteins.

Once again, the response of a specific organ or tissue to microgravity appears to be time-dependent. For up to 5 days of spaceflight, adaptation consists primarily of changes in the regulation of a contraction. This appears to result from lower effectiveness of the excitation-contraction coupling mechanism due to losses of myofibril proteins as well as decreased calcium affinity.[31] After 2 to 3 weeks of flight, there are changes in the myofibril protein composition, as indicated from the rat data. The major initiating factor is loss of the biomechanical force, gravity.

Narici et al. studied four astronauts after 17 days of spaceflight.[83] Measurements of muscle twitch characteristics, ankle joint angle-twitch torque, and fatigability were assessed during all phases of this flight. Using a constant current electrical muscle stimulator and a torque-velocity dynamometer, the triceps surae was stimulated and the torque measurements were recorded. Muscle mass was determined anthropometrically from circumferential measurements after subtraction of subcutaneous fat. The authors found a decrease in muscle strength that was three times greater than the decrease in muscle size. There was also a decrease in torque per unit of muscle CSA, implying that postflight muscle was weaker and more fatigable. Based on findings concerning the frequency–torque relationship, the authors felt that there was similar atrophy in both the type 1 and type 2 fibers, which is different from that found in rat studies. The muscles fatigued faster, suggesting that there was a shift from aerobic metabolism using lipids to anaerobic metabolism using glycogen. This is supported by the finding of increased glycogen deposits in rat myofibrils and hepatocytes.[102]

Marked muscle tissue damage and microthrombosis occur within 48 hours after less than 2 weeks of spaceflight.[108] The adductor longus of rats showed a breakdown of myofibrillar proteins and eccentric-like lesions, such as tearing of the supporting connective tissue, hyperextension of sarcomeres with A- and Z-band filaments pulled apart and fragmented, extensive muscle necrosis, microhemorrhages, and edema in 44% of flight myofibrils. The formation of thrombi increased in the postcapillary venules and capillaries, leading to edema within 12 hours after landing. Another study showed a decrease or absence of synaptic vesicles that were replaced by microtubules and neurofilaments in the alpha motoneurons, degeneration of axon terminals, axonal spaces, and alterations of axonal sprouting suggestive of muscle denervation and regeneration, myofibrillar disruption and necrosis, and synaptic remodeling at the neuromuscular junction.[21] Presumably this damage is related to either the 2-g reentry forces or to eccentric reloading of an atrophied muscle.

Microgravity appears to alter gene expression. Kano et al. identified six genes that were up-regulated and three genes that were down-regulated in the gastrocnemius muscle of spaceflight rats after just 16 days of spaceflight.[55b] The up-regulated genes included those coding for insulin growth factor binding protein-1, titin, and mitrochondrial gene *16 S rRNA*. Those down regulated encoded for RNA polymerase II elongation factor-like protein and NADH dehydrogenase. These genes are those responsible for cellular metabolism.

No consistent hormonal abnormalities explain the muscle pathology associated with space travel.[1,49,60,64] Serum potassium may be increased or decreased, depending on the total body store. Urinary excretion of magnesium, phosphorus, calcium, and potassium is increased despite adequate dietary intake.[49,69] Blood urea nitrogen, creatine phosphokinase, and lactate dehydrogenase are elevated. In-flight, cortisol and adrenocorticotropic hormone (ACTH) may be either increased or decreased, growth hormone is increased, and insulin and catecholamines are decreased. Urinary catecholamines and cortisol are excreted to a greater extent than before flight. Postflight thyroxine, thyroid-stimulating hormone, cortisol, ACTH, and insulin are increased. Urinary cortisol and catecholamines are also increased. Exercise seems to ameliorate some of the strength loss in flight.[129,135] Treadmill walking and running with bungee cords for a minimum of 10 minutes daily seem to reduce the muscle loss in longer flights. A resistance device for the arms and legs is also beneficial. Cosmonauts spend 21/2 hours on a treadmill and on a resistance device for 3 consecutive days, with 1 day of no exercise.[135] During their flight, they wear a "penguin suit" for 16 hours a day. The suit consists of overalls with bungee cords attached at various intervals along the suit providing longitudinal forces or resistance parallel to the muscles, in particular the postural muscles.

Central Nervous System Alterations

Recent animal studies conducted on both American and Russian spaceflights reveal alterations in hormonal secretions and neuronal structure in the central nervous system (CNS).[71,72] Measured directly after landing, the norepinephrine content in the locus ceruleus decreased in rats exposed to microgravity for 9 days, but normalized in less than 2 weeks.[29] The vasopressin content increased in the posterior pituitary but decreased in the hypothalamus. These changes were thought to reflect an acute stress reaction that clouded the actual inflight central endocrine changes. However, contrary to this finding, other investigators measured decreases in posterior pituitary vasopressin and oxytocin ranging from 20% to 33%.[56]

Hormonal release from the hypothalamus is impaired under microgravity conditions. Reduced immunostaining for growth hormone (GH) and somatostatin (SS) occurred in the median eminences in hypothalami of flight rats.[115] The hypophysiotropic cells in the arcuate nucleus expressing pre-pro-growth hormone releasing factor decreased by 46% to 50% in number and signal intensity. Growth hormone–specific cytoplasmic staining intensity and cytoplasmic areas where the hormone was located increased.[51] There seems to be impaired GH secretion due to a lack of releasing factors and impaired release of GH, accounting for low levels of GH noted in other flight animal investigations.

Muscarinic cholinergic receptors in the CNS change as a result of spaceflight. In the corpus striatum the density of muscarinic cholinergic receptors decreased, possibly reflecting the functional changes in motor activity during microgravity exposure.[50]

The density of gamma-aminobenzoic acid-A (GABA-A) or benzodiazepine receptors was not altered. However, glutamate decarboxylase activity in the hippocampal areas averaged 30% higher in flight rats than in their controls.[65] Average GABA transaminase activity increased by 8% to 35% in all hippocampal areas studied, supporting the idea that GABA activity is significantly increased in certain regions of the brain during microgravity exposure.

Changes in hormonal binding sites of the choroid plexus could lead to impaired cerebrospinal fluid (CSF) dynamics.[42] The number of 125I-rANP (atrial natriuretic peptide) binding sites, as expressed by B_{max} values, was significantly increased in the choroid plexus of the lateral and third ventricles of spaceflown rats. Based on kilodalton values, there were no changes in the binding affinity. The fourth ventricle choroid plexus showed no alterations in binding capacity or affinity. In contrast, the meninges demonstrated a significant increase in kilodalton values but not in the number of binding sites, suggesting a reduced affinity of meningeal ANP receptors after space exposure. Atrial natriuretic reptide may reduce CSF production by inhibiting amiloride-sensitive sodium transport, but since ANP levels in the CSF are low, ANP receptors probably are not totally responsible for the regulation of CSF production. However, ANP, a natriuretic factor, by altering the fluid and electrolyte fluxes, in part could modify the volume, ion, or pressure balance of CSF dynamics. These responses could be a means of adjusting to any increased intracranial pressure that might result from cerebral vessel engorgement secondary to the headward fluid shift occurring under microgravity conditions.

Since a close relationship exists between alpha motoneurons and the myofibrils comprising the motor unit, it is not surprising that alpha motoneurons in the lumbosacral ventral horns displayed changes consistent with the shift of myofibrils to fast-twitch types. Although no significant differences in mean CSA and SDH were found in the flight versus control rats, the population distributions of both shifted by significant amounts.[53] The population of motoneurons from flight rats showed smaller CSAs and higher SDH activity and, in addition, showed a higher percentage of small cells with high SDH activities. Unfortunately, individual populations of neurons could not be identified, but further experiments have been planned to investigate this phenomenon.

In support of these changes, motoneurons taken from the lumbar enlargements in the spinal cords of rats flown in space by Soviet investigators showed a 12% decrease in the nucleolus volume and a 33% decrease in the number of perineuronal glial cells.[99] This finding probably reflected the lack of motor activity of the involved leg muscles. It is unclear whether the changes in the alpha motoneuron determined myofibril characteristics, such as fiber types and enzyme concentrations, or whether the functional requirements placed on the muscles elicit CNS alterations that then regulate any changes in fiber types and enzyme concentrations during and after spaceflight.[71]

Significant morphological changes in the lumbar intervertebral ganglia neurons were found by

Russian investigators.[99] The volume of the soma decreased by 31%, of the nucleus by 25%, and of the nucleolus by 13% after only 2 weeks of spaceflight. The number of capsular glia decreased by 27%, and the alkaline phosphatase activity declined. However, only the volume of the medium-sized neurons decreased. No changes in nociceptive neurons were detected. The investigators felt that these findings reflected diminished afferent input into the CNS.

Actual neuron and myofibril functioning in microgravity is unknown. An interesting study evaluated properties of embryonic spinal neurons and myocytes in a horizontal clinostat that provided a "vector-free" gravity environment to the cells.[38] Numerous large swellings appeared along the neuritic shafts when exposed to this environment. A logical question is: Is the normal axonal flow of nutrients and chemicals dependent upon the gravity vector, and if so, what effect does the lack of gravity have on neuron functioning?

Postural Disturbances and Ataxia

In-flight, astronauts assume a fetal position.[15–20,57,85,95,127,136] The typical posture involves a flexed spine, with loss of the normal thoracolumbar curve and the normal cervical curvature remaining, so that the head is flexed forward. Flexion occurs at the major joints except at the ankles, where the feet are plantar flexed. Even with visual references, astronauts may not be able to maintain an erect posture. The reason for this difficulty is not entirely clear, but it could relate to abnormal otolith and proprioceptive afferent inputs.[15–20,70] If vision is partially occluded, the body adopts a greater flexed attitude resembling a fetus in shape. The posture assumed in space may depend on past exposure to weightlessness because the hip and knee are more flexed in astronauts with previous flight experience.[17,19] The volume within the spacecraft also influences the development of a fetal-like posture: the Gemini and Mercury spacecraft had considerably less volume than did the Apollo, Skylab, and Shuttle craft, and astronauts showed no fetal posturing.[86] The duration of exposure to microgravity is not a factor because posture becomes flexed immediately on insertion into orbit.[15,17] With longer exposure, posture is not altered dramatically; however, muscle atrophy then becomes a problem, especially in the major postural muscles, which could eventually lead to greater flexion deformities.[45,47,133,134,136,139]

Ataxia and gait disturbances commonly occur postflight. Astronauts exhibit a wide-based gait.[57] They are unable to stand straight without visual cues even when asked to maintain an erect posture.[15,17,47] Further, they exhibit difficulty walking around corners, often falling out of a turn, and may exhibit flexion of the spine.[15,45,46,57] When released to fall from a ceiling-suspended harness, they are unsteady and have an unbalanced landing, being unaware of their foot position.[100,133,136] Some even have difficulty getting out of their seats immediately after landing.[40] Large individual differences exist in the time required to recover from these instabilities. Recovery may occur within the first 24 hours of landing or may require up to 4 to 6 days.[104,105,136,137] The length of time seems to depend on three factors: the initial severity of the response to microgravity, mission duration, and inflight exercise regimens.[32,135]

Postural Changes

Postflight gait disturbances last longer and are more severe in those astronauts who showed greater vestibular disturbances in microgravity and who spent longer times in space.[68,69,99,104] After several months in space, returning cosmonauts are found to be ataxic for weeks after exposures to 0 g for several months.[43–45,47,48] These flight-related abnormalities are evident on simple observation of space travelers, yet most of them do not realize they have any problem and may specifically deny that difficulties exist.[13,15,20,32,33] Postural readaptation, after spaceflights lasting for less than 2 weeks, is a biphasic process, beginning immediately upon landing and continuing rapidly for the first 10 to 12 hours.[93] Thereafter, there is a slower adaptation, usually extending over the next 2 to 4 days after preflight stability levels are achieved.

The primary cause of these disorders seems to reside in the vestibular or proprioceptive inputs into the CNS.[15–20,32,51,61,62,65,104,105,133,136] In 1 g, posture and gait rely on information from vestibular signals (otolith and semicircular canals), kinesthesia, vision, and touch. Disturbances in any or all of these sensory modalities could lead to the fetal posturing and ataxia associated with spaceflight.

Vision plays a major role in supplying information for balance posture, thus counteracting anormal vestibular and proprioceptive inputs.[46,57,136,137,139] Kenyon and Young evaluated balance, the stretch reflex, and the otolith-spinal reflex of four astronauts using the sharpened Romberg test and posture platform with and without vision. The sharpened Romberg test consisted of standing or walking on two rails of different widths, 0.75 inch and 2.25 inches, with or without vision. All four astronauts exhibited marked imbalance after 10 days in microgravity, which was especially pronounced when their eyes were closed.[57] Postflight, the astronauts did not stand on the rails as long as they did preflight when tested without visual input. For one astronaut, the time spent standing on the rails with his eyes closed was 14% and 21% of the preflight times for the landing day and the first postflight day, respectively. Time walking on the rails without falling decreased by 20% after flight. Similar changes were found for the three other astronauts. Again, ataxia was evident despite subjective impressions that no problem existed.

Illusions

About 80% of space travelers experience one or more illusions during and after flight.[59] A common illusion, concerning the perceived orientation of the body in three dimensions, probably relates to altered otolith function. For instance, vertical movements may be interpreted not as a fall, but as sudden, unpleasant movement of the environment as though "the floor came up to meet me."[15,107,133] An astronaut doing a pushup might experience the illusion that it is the floor, not he or she, that moves up and down. With any acceleration or deceleration, the space traveler may think that the environment moves or that he or she is pushed to one side or feels lateral acceleration.[57] On transfer from one spacecraft to another, the inversion illusion, the sensation that one has turned upside down, is not unusual.[135] Another illusion consists of an inaccurate perception of weights and masses, including one's own weight, a perception arising from decreased input from peripheral pressure and proprioceptive receptors.[113,114]

Back on Earth, astronauts feel extremely heavy and again experience abnormal subjective movements of either their environment or themselves.[15,95–97,109,114,136,139] They often feel pushed to the side, experiencing the illusion of lateral acceleration, or as though they are tumbling head over heels or moving sideways while standing or turning corners.[15,57,137] For the first few nights, some feel levitated above their beds and become comfortable only when adequate touch sensation is provided.[6] Sometimes getting out of bed may be a problem because of a kind of motor apraxia in which the correct procedure of putting the feet out and planting them firmly on the floor must be relearned; otherwise, they fall out of bed and may get hurt. Most perceptual illusions, fortunately, disappear within several days after landing.

Visual Disturbances

Abnormal vestibulo-ocular reflexes and optokinetic nystagmus have been found in astronauts and cosmonauts after spaceflight.[37,96,97,131] A few people demonstrate changes in contrast sensitivity and stereopsis.[33,85,123] Acuity, eye dominance, and flicker fusion frequency remain unaltered in microgravity.[33,85] Flashes of light are seen when astronauts are dark adapted, presumably resulting from high-energy heavy cosmic particles striking the retina.[43,91] As expected, the frequency and intensity of retinal flashes are greater in high Earth or polar orbit, the South Atlantic anomaly, or in deep space en route to the moon.

Postflight, part of the visual field can be constricted, and visual acuity can be slightly decreased. Several crew members have had constricted retinal arteries, veins, or both.[41] Changes in vision may relate to the increase in intraocular pressure that occurs in space. In Skylab, submarine eye, a difficulty in focusing at infinity first described among men on submarine duty, became a problem. Submarine eye responds to practice in focusing at a distance. Age, gender, and stress seem not to influence visual abnormalities. Recovery to normal after adequate rest and time in 1 g is expected.

Medical Problems of Space

Loss of Pressure

Several deaths have occurred in the Soviet space program due to the extreme vacuum of space, where the pressure is only 10 to 14 mm Hg.[131] Any unprotected exposure to this lack of pressure will result in ebullition (vaporization of blood) and death. Less severe losses of pressure result in hypoxia, the bends, chokes, and palsies, just as in deep-sea diving.

Radiation

During the pioneering era of manned spaceflight, when the hazards to astronauts were secondary to technical failure, the radiation environment was assessed mainly in terms of its possible interference with operational capacity during the mission.[132] Because of the altitudes and inclinations of the orbits chosen, along with the restricted mission durations and the fortunate absence of extraordinary solar particle events, all radiation exposures incurred so far by astronauts have remained well below levels at which, according to current knowledge, operational capacity or health would be affected. Exposures of 3.6 to 107.8 mirad/day, about 100 times or more of the terrestrial background radiation, with the higher levels associated with greater distances from Earth, are common.[103] In the South Atlantic radiation anomaly (0 to 60 degrees west longitude and 20 to 50 degrees south latitude), where the Van Allen belt hangs low to altitudes of 200 km, exposures are greater, and an EVA could result in a lethal dose of radiation if conducted during a solar particle event. If a space station were at an altitude of 463 km and an inclination of 28.5 degrees, the South Atlantic anomaly could account for the dominant fraction of total exposure, although traversing the anomaly will take less than about 15 minutes and occupy less than 10% of the total time in orbit. However, with a geosynchronous orbiting space station, solar flares could present a problem with radiation exposure. Retinal flashes observed with the eyes opened or closed, first reported by John Glenn, are thought to be due to radiation-induced depolarization of retinal neurons.

Sleeping, Eating, Waste Disposal, and Personal Hygiene

Sleep problems and fatigue were common until the 14-day Gemini mission in 1966, when strict attention to diurnal sleep patterns was enforced by synchronizing sleep to Cape Canaveral time. Owing to noise, excitement, and the lack of day-night clues, all astronauts have trouble adapting to the environment of space, and 20% take sleeping pills. Electroencephalography (EEG) studies show normal findings, except for a fourfold increase in rapid eye movement (REM) duration. No problems exist in chewing or swallowing, but questions remain regarding digestion. Daily calorie requirements average about 3000 kcal. Adequate personal waste disposal with good toilet facilities that continue to work throughout the flight can still be a problem, and there is a lack of privacy. Cutting hair or shaving in space takes time, and sweat remains layered on the body unless shaken or rubbed off. During Skylab missions, most astronauts showered once a week in a cylindrical cloth bag because to shower, remove the water, and dry out the cloth bag took up a considerable portion of the day.[54]

Bone Demineralization

Both weight-bearing and non-weight-bearing bones suffer loss during microgravity exposure. This appears to be dependent upon the length of time exposed to microgravity.[117,130] Two cosmonauts were studied after 1 and 6 months in space: bone loss was found at the tibia, evaluated by computerized tomo-densitometry and broadband attenuation, and at the calcareous, evaluated by broadband attenuation. By contrast, no changes were found in the radius.[21,130] Similar results have been reported by Schneider et al.[116] The density of the radius and ulna remains normal, whereas tibia and calcaneus bone show losses of up to 20%.[116] In rats, radial bone growth in the humerus was unchanged during a 4-day flight but decreased during a 10-day flight.[3] Activity in the biceps, calvarial eriostemon, and long-bone eriostemon was unchanged after spaceflight, as measured by expression of mRNA. Osteocalcin chain of type 1 precollagen in the 10-day flight mRNA levels decreased in long bone and calvarial eriostemon after exposure to microgravity. These findings suggest decreased expression of bone-specific genes and decreased bone formation.

Further experiments confirm the findings of bone loss. The fractional excretion of calcium increased in two astronauts who flew for over 1 week.[74] There was a negative calcium balance with an increase in urinary calcium. The bone mineral density of the lumbar spine at L2-4 decreased by 3%. Bone resorption was increased, as indicated by elevated urinary pyridino links and plasma acid phosphate activity. A bone formation marker, bone specific alkaline phosphate, was elevated, whereas intact osteocalcin was not. These changes occurred within the context of a loss in CSA of the leg muscles. The changes are due in part to a transient increased resorption and sustained decrease in bone formation.[130] It also appears that the time to recovery of bone mass is greater than the mission length. Further studies are needed to determine the exact nature of the hormonal and enzymatic changes that occur during and after spaceflight to further define and explain these changes, as it appears that overall parathyroid hormone, 1-alpha, 25-dihydroxycalciferol, and calcitonin are almost normal.[49,120]

Cardiovascular Adjustments to Microgravity

Right after insertion into orbit, fluid shifts from the lower to the upper body.[127] This shift does not relate to an increase in central venous pressure but is probably due to the loss of hydrostatic forces in general, so filtration pressures increase in regions above the heart and decrease in regions below it. The resulting shift of 1.5 to 2 L causes neck vein distention, headaches, stuffy nose, nasal voice, thickened and swollen eyelids, diuresis, decreased plasma volume, and severe orthostatic hypotension on return to Earth. Wearing positive-g (antigravity) suits and ingesting 1 to 2 g NaCI tablets with 8 ounces of water every hour for 4 hours before de-orbiting decreases the severity and frequency of orthostatic hypotension.[10]

Significant changes occur in the heart and blood vessels during and after exposure to low Earth orbit. Astronauts and cosmonauts were studied after 6 to 25 days and 6 months of space flight.[2] Left ventricular diastolic volume was decreased after just 1 week of microgravity. The ejection fraction remained unchanged, but the heartrate increased 5% to 10%. Mean blood pressure tended to decrease. Changes demonstrated a moderate and stable hypovolemia. Although there was no change in cerebral perfusion, a decrease in cerebral artery resistance was found after 2 to 3 weeks but not initially, suggesting that this change was not due to the headward fluid shifts. However, these changes were hypothesized to result from fluid transfer from the vascular to the interstitial brain compartment and/or to other factors modifying cerebral vascular resistance.

Changes in the cardiovascular system appear to be time sensitive, with the adaptation period lasting for at least 3 months but varying up to 6 months. In long-duration missions, the beat-to-beat interval increased by an average of 82 ms in the first 30 days of spaceflight. This corresponded to a 10% decrease in heart rate. During the seventh month, the average beat-to-beat interval was 94 ms.[39] The major change in heart rate appeared to occur during non-REM sleep, where the parasympathetic nervous system plays a larger role in regulating heart rate.

Stroke volume also depends upon the length of space exposure. In crew members flying for 4 to 17 days, the left ventricular systolic volume decreased and the ejection fraction increased, whereas in those who flew for 129 to 144 days there was an increase in left ventricular systolic volume and a decrease in ejection fraction.[76] The left systolic volume changed from –12% to 29% and the ejection fraction from 6% to –10.5%. In addition, the stroke volume decreased in longer-duration missions from –5% to –17.4%. Cardiac output also followed a similar trend: –2.3% to –12.2%. Mean circumferential shortening of the left ventricle increased from 8% in short-duration flight subjects compared to –11% in long-duration subjects. The researchers concluded that the cardiac differences—that is, changes in the ejection fraction and fractional shortening in short-duration versus long-duration exposure subjects—resulted from significant changes in the left ventricular systolic chamber size. Similar results were obtained by Perhonen et al.[98] Magnetic resonance imaging (MRI) data revealed that the left ventricular mass decreased after only 10 days of spaceflight. The left ventricular diastolic volume and stroke volume increased after 2 weeks, although central venous pressure was near 0 mm Hg. The authors hypothesized that there was an increase in cardiac filling due to a larger reduction in pericardial pressure from removing the gravity restraints on the chest wall. Taken in conjunction with measures of left ventricular compliance, the decrease in cardiac function after spaceflight is time-dependent, so any further studies must account not only for microgravity effects but also for the length of exposure. Studies differ on the reacclimation time needed. Mulvagh et al. suggest that return to a 1–g state required only 2 days after 4 to 5 days of microgravity.[76,81] However, 1 to 2 weeks were needed to return to baseline after 1 to 2 weeks of flight.[10,76] Therefore, it appears that any further research must take into account both the duration of spaceflight and the time of recovery, as any changes appear to occur at differing rates during each of these conditions.

Summers et al. found that decrements in left ventricular mass may be due to dehydration rather than to cardiovascular alterations in response to microgravity.[121b] Echocardiographic measurements of LV mass in astronauts decreased by 9.1% immedicately after spaceflight but returned to normal preflight values within 3 days. These results were similar to those produced by bedrest subjects in whom dehydration was thought to be the cause of temporary loss in left ventricular mass.

Orthostatic hypotension remains a mission concern. Astronauts exhibited significant drops in systolic blood pressure after 1 to 2 weeks in space from −1 mm Hg preflight to −10 mm Hg on landing day.[10,30] Two of 16 subjects walked off the Shuttle with difficulty and the stand test 1 to 2 hours postlanding was not completed by another two subjects; thus, 25% of astronauts have difficulty with orthostasis postflight. The plasma adrenalin and noradrenalin levels were increased, and the responses of the carotid baroreceptor cardiac reflex were altered.[30,134] Plasma noradrenalin concentrations increased 34% and adrenalin concentrations increased 65% postflight. Standing increased the values to 65% and 91% for plasma noradrenalin and adrenalin, respectively, on landing day. Supine heart rate and systolic blood pressures also increased 38% and 19%, respectively. However, the stroke volume was decreased 26% on landing day during standing. Some of these changes were due to volume depletion, but lowering of the parasympathetic drive and increases in sympathetic input may have influenced the response to reintroduction to Earth's gravity.

During exposure to microgravity, there are changes in the regulation of the autonomic nervous system. Mano, using microneurography which measures the sympathetic neural activity leading to skeletal muscles, recorded from human peripheral nerves.[74b] Two different groups of responses are possible to stressors: low and high responders to orthostatic stress seen in clinically significant orthostatic hypotension. The muscle sympathetic nerve activity was increased during the 12th and 13th days of spaceflight and immediately postflight. The astronaut responses to head-up tilt were preserved in those who were not orthostatic. Simulated microgravity studies showed that orthostatic intolerance was related to reduced muscle sympathetic nerve activity with impaired baroreflex activity. It appears that sympathetic neural control is lowered when exposed to short-term spaceflight but is increased after longer exposures to microgravity. Orthostatic intolerance results from an absence of the enhanced sympathetic neural response to orthostatic stress, rather than from directly from dehydration, although presumably this factor would also play a role.

Psychological Factors

Besides the isolation and removal from Earth of the astronauts, the dynamics of small-group interaction may become a problem not only between crew members but also between the fliers and ground control.[84] For the initial spaceflights such as the Apollo, Skylab, and Gemini missions, astronauts were taken primarily from the test pilot pool. These individuals acted in a single decision-making mode, being very disciplined and motivated. Future crews inhabiting the International Space Station will be different. They will consist of other professionals and crew members of different ethnic and cultural backgrounds for much longer time periods. The tasks will be more varied, and this will increase the complexity of interaction. Teamwork will be essential for surviving and completing their jobs. Currently, selection focuses on choosing the brightest and the best but does not focus on interpersonal or team skills. Interpersonal problems can occur on longer missions and compromise group performance. Poor communication, coordination, and decision making can doom a flight, particularly in an emergency, but preparation so that the members know what the team is doing and how it is doing its job, while the job is being done, can help prevent catastrophic errors.

Immunology

Astronauts and cosmonauts get sick during spaceflight, typically with viral infections that cause upper respiratory infections, influenza, pharyngitis, dermatitis, viral gastroenteritis, and rhinitis.[41,122,125] Immunological studies performed both in rats and in humans demonstrate alterations in immune function. The number of saprophytes decreases and the relative percentage of potentially pathogenic microorganisms increases. Yeast and filamentous fungi proliferate within the cabins, and there is cross-contamination between crew members. Lymphoid organs became hypoplastic and show decreased mitogen-induced blastogenesis.[27,125] Postflight there is a lymphopenia associated with an impaired ability of these cells to respond to mitogenic stimulation as well as a shift toward T4 cells. The number of monocytes varies, depending upon the study. Some studies have shown a decrease in monocytes resulting from impaired blastogenesis, whereas a study of 30 Shuttle astronauts found a 52% increase after flight thought to be related to neuroendocrine changes and sampling times.[125] The absolute neutrophil count doubled, associated with a drop in eosinophils. Gamma interferon was reduced but not interleukin-3 production in spleen cells.[119] Production of interleukin-2 was increased in some flyers postfight, whereas the ability to express interleukin-2 receptor was impaired 1 day after landing in two cosmonauts.[74] These studies suggest that the immune responses are complex and depend not only on the length of time exposed to microgravity but also on concurrent stress and other hormonal conditions.

Using the Merieux Multi test CMI system, cell-mediated immunity and delayed-type hypersensitivity were evaluated.[27,125] These tests evaluated responses to tetanus, diphtheria, streptococcus, proteus, and tuberculin, among other antigens. After flights of various lengths, all but one astronaut responded to fewer antigens in-flight than preflight, suggesting that hypoergy increases with flight duration up to about 10 days but that an adjustment occurs with longer spaceflights.

Pharmacology

Astronauts use drugs in space, primarily to counteract the effects of SMS and gastroenteritis. The drug use of astronauts flying 79 U.S. Shuttle missions was evaluated.[100] The drugs available were Afrin, zolpidem, aspirin, flurazepam, promethazine/dextroamphetamine, promethazine, diazepam, pseudoephedrine, thiethylperazine, bisacodyl, phenylephrine/phenylpropanolamine, simethicone, and acetaminophen. Ninety-four percent used a medication during flight; 45% were for SMS and 45% for insomnia, and other uses included the treatment of headaches, backaches, and sinus congestion. Eighty percent of the doses taken were effective, with the most reports of ineffectiveness occurring during the first in-flight day. Promethazine was the most often used drug, with the intramuscular route being most effective and having the fewest side effects. Drugs for insomnia were used throughout the missions. Pain medications were typically taken during the first 4 days of flight.

Putcha and Cintron measured drug absorption using saliva and urine sampling techniques.[101] Changes in the absorption phase were greater than in the elimination phase. The absorption of acetaminophen decreased, as shown by an increased time to maximum concentration. The maximum saliva concentrations were less than preflight values and were also more variable within a subject on different flight days. The authors hypothesize that pharmacokinetics in microgravity vary among individuals, since the intersubject variability preflight was minimal, as well as the length of the mission when the drug was taken.

Summary

Exposure to microgravity and space travel produces several neurological changes, including SAS, neuromuscular weakness and fatigue, ataxia, postural disturbances, and perceptual illusions. Inflight SAS, perceptual illusions, and ocular changes are more important. After landing, however, ataxia, neuromuscular weakness, fatigue, and perceptual illusions play greater roles in astronaut health and readaptation to a terrestrial environment. Cardiovascular adjustments to microgravity, bone demineralization, and possible decompression sickness and excessive radiation exposure contribute further to the medical problems of astronauts in space.

REFERENCES

1. Alexander WC, Leach CS, Fisher CL: Clinical biochemistry. In: Johnston RS, Dietlein LF, Berry CA (eds): Biomedical Results of Apollo. NASA SP-368. Washington, DC, NASA, 1975, pp 323–340.
2. Arbeille P, Fomina G, Roumy J, et al: Adaptation of the left heart, cerebral and femoral arteries, and jugular and femoral veins during short- and long-term head-down tilt and space flights. Eur J Appl Physiol 86(2):157–168, 2001.
3. Backup P, Westerlind K, Harris S, et al: Spaceflight results in reduced mRNA levels for tissue-specific pro-

teins in the musculoskeletal system. Am J Physiol 266: E567–E573, 1994.

4. Baker JT, Nicogossian AE, Hoffler GW, et al: Changes in the Achilles tendon reflexes following Skylab missions. In: Johnston RS, Dietlein LF, Berry CA (eds): Biomedical Results of Apollo. NASA SP-368. Washington, DC, NASA, 1975, pp 131–135.
5. Baker JT, Nicogossian AE, Hoffler GW, et al: Measurement of a single tendon reflex in conjunction with a myogram: The second manned Skylab mission. Aviat Space Environ Med 47:400–402, 1976.
6. Baldwin KM: Effects of zero gravity on biochemical and metabolic properties of skeletal muscle fiber types. In: Nicogossian AE (ed): Spacelab Life Sciences—I. 180-Day Preliminary Results. Washington, DC, NASA Special Publication, 1992, pp 3.4.2-1-11.
7. Baldwin KM, Herrick RE, Ilyina-Kakueva E, et al: Effects of zero gravity on myofibril content and isomyosin distribution in rodent skeletal muscle. FASEB J 4:79–83, 1990.
8. Baldwin KM, Herrick RE, McCue SA: Substrate oxidation capacity in rodent skeletal muscle: Effects of exposure to zero gravity. J Appl Physiol 75:2466–2470, 1983.
9. Bell GJ, Martin TP, Ilyina-Kakueva EI, Ogano VS, et al: Altered distribution of mitochondria in rat soleus muscle fibers after spaceflight. J Appl Physiol 73:493–497, 1992.
10. Bungo MW, Charles JB, Johnson PC: Cardiovascular deconditioning during space flight and the use of saline as a countermeasure to orthostatic intolerance. Aviat Space Environ Med 56:985–990, 1985.
11. Bungo MW, Goldwater DJ, Popp RL, Sandler H: Echocardiographic evaluation of space shuttle crew members. J Appl Physiol 62:278–283, 1987.
12. Caiozzo VJ, Haddad F, Baker MJ, et al: Microgravity-induced transformations of myosin isoforms and contractile properties of skeletal muscle. J Appl Physiol 81(1):123–132, 1996.
13. Castleman KR, Chui LA, Vandermeulen JP: Spaceflight effects on muscle fibers. In: Rosenzweig SN. Souza KA (eds): Final Reports of U.S. Experiments Flown on Soviet Satellite Cosmos 936. NASA TM-78526. Houston, NASA, 1978.
14. Chi MM, Choksi R, Nemeth P, et al: Effects of microgravity and tail suspension on enzymes of individual soleus and tibialis anterior fibers. J Appl Physiol 73(2 suppl):66S–73S, 1992.
15. Clement G, Berthoz A, Lestienne F: Adaptive changes in perception of body orientation and mental image rotation in microgravity. Aviat Space Environ Med 58(suppl): AI59–A163, 1987.
16. Clement G, Gurfinkel VS, Lestienne F, et al: A study of mechanisms of posture maintenance in the weightless state. Physiologist 26(suppl):S86–S89, 1983.
17. Clement G, Gurfinkel VS, Lestienne F, et al: Adaptation of postural control to weightlessness. Exp Brain Res 57:61–72, 1984.
18. Clement G, Gurfinkel VS, Lestienne F, et al: Changes of posture during transient perturbations in microgravity. Aviat Space Environ Med 56:666–671, 1985.
19. Clement G, Lestienne F: Adaptive modifications of postural attitude in conditions of weightlessness. Exp Brain Res 72:381–389, 1988.
20. Clement G, Vievile T, Lestienne F, et al: Modifications of gain asymmetry and beating field of vertical optokinetic nystagmus in microgravity. Neurosci Lett 63:271–274, 1986.
21. Collet P, Uebelhart D, Vico L, et al: Effects of 1- and 6-month space flight on bone mass and biochemistry in two humans. Bone [AM]20(6):547–551, 1997.
22. D'Amelio F, Daunton NG: Effects of spaceflight in the adductor longus muscle of rats flown in the Soviet Biosatellite COSMOS 2044. A study employing neural cell adhesion molecule (N-CAM) immunocytochemistry and conventional morphological techniques (light and electron microscopy). J Neuropathol Exp Neurol 51: 415–431, 1992.
23. Davis JR, Jennings RT, Beck BG, et al: Treatment efficacy of intramuscular promethazine for space motion sickness. Aviat Space Environ Med 64(3 pt 1):230–233, 1993.
24. Davis JR, Vanderploeg JM, Santy PA, et al: Space motion sickness during 24 flights of the space shuttle. Aviat Space Environ Med 59:1185–1189, 1988.
25. Dietlein LF: Skylab: A beginning. In: Johnston RS, Dietlein LF (eds): Biomedical Results from Skylab. NASA SP-377. Washington, DC, NASA, 1977, pp 408–418.
26. Draeger J, Wirt H, Schwartz R: Tonometry under microgravity conditions. In: Sahm PR, Jansen R, Keller MH (eds): Nordenerney Symposium on Scientific Results of the German Spacelab Mission D1. Nordenerney, Germany, 1986, pp 503–509.
27. Durnova GN, Kaplansky AS, Portuglov VV: Effect on a 22-day space flight on the lymphoid organs of rats. Aviat Space Environ Med 47:588–591, 1976.
28. Edgerton VR, Saltin B, Gollnick P: Adaptation of Human Muscle to Short Duration Spaceflight. Final Report for DSO 475. Houston, NASA Special Publication, 1992.
29. Fareh J, Cottet-Emard JM, Pequignot JM, et al: Norepinephrine content in discrete brain areas and neurohypophyseal vasopressin in rats after a 90d spaceflight (SLS-1). Aviat Space Environ Med 64:507–511, 1993.
30. Fritsch-Yelle JM, Charles JB, Jones MM, et al: Spaceflight alters autonomic regulation of arterial pressure in humans. J Appl Physiol 77(4):1776–1783, 1994.
31. Gazenko OG: Functional plasticity of skeletal muscles of mammals in space flight. Mater Med Pol (Poland) 22(4):251–254, 1990.
32. Gazenko OG, Genin AM, Egorov AD: Summary of medical investigations in the USSR manned space missions. Acta Astron 8(9–10):907–917, 1981.
33. Ginsberg AP, Vanderploeg J: Vision in space: Nearvision acuity and contrast sensitivity. In: Bungo MW,

Bagian TM, Bowman JA, Levitan BM (eds): Results of the Life Sciences DSOs Conducted Aboard the Space Shuttle 1981–1986. Houston, Space Biomedical Research Institute, NASA, 1987, pp 179–182.

34. Graybiel A, Miller EF, Billingham J, et al: Vestibular experiments in Gemini flights V and VII. Aerospace Med 38:360–370, 1967.
35. Grigoriev AI, Bugrov SA, Bogomolov VV, et al: Medical results of the Mir year-long mission (21.12.1987–21.12.1988). Medispace 3:31–41, 1991.
36. Grigoriev RA: USSR Delegation Presents Spaceflight Data from Mir. Houston, Medical Sciences Division, NASA, 1991.
37. Grigoriev RA, Gazenko OG, Kozlovskaya lB, et al: The vestibulo-cerebellar regulation of oculomotor reactions in micro gravitational conditions. In: Keller T, Zee D (eds): Adaptive Processes in Visual and Oculomotor Systems. New York, Pergamon, 1986, pp 42–58.
38. Gruener R, Hoeger G: Vector-averaged gravity alters myocyte and neuron properties in cell culture. Aviat Space Environ Med 62:1159–1165, 1991.
39. Gundel A, Dreswcher J, Spatenko YA, et al: Changes in basal heart rate in spaceflights up to 438 days. Aviat Space Environ Med 73:17–21, 2002.
40. Haddad F, Herrick RE, Adams GR, et al: Myosin heavy chain expression in rodent skeletal muscle: Effects of exposure to zero gravity. J Appl Physiol 75:2471–2477, 1993.
41. Hawkins WR, Zieglschmid JF: Clinical aspects of crew health. In: Johnston RS, Dietlein LF, Berry CA (eds): Biomedical Results of Apollo. NASA SP-368. Washington, DC, NASA, 1975, pp 43–81.
42. Herbute S, Oliver J, Davet J, et al: ANP binding sites are increased in choroid plexus of SLS-1 rats after 9 days of spaceflight. Aviat Space Environ Med 65:134–138, 1994.
43. Hoffman RA, Pinsky LS, Ashborne WZ, et al: Visual light flash observations on Skylab 4. In: Johnston RS, Dietlein LF, Berry CA (eds): Biomedical Results of Skylab. NASA SP-377. Washington, DC, NASA, 1977, pp 127–130.
44. Holy X, Mounier Y: Effects of short spaceflights on mechanical characteristics of rat muscles. Muscle Nerve 14:70–78, 1991.
45. Homick JL, Miller EF: Apollo flight crew vestibular assessment. In: Johnston RS, Dietlein LF, Berry CA (eds): Biomedical Results of Apollo. NASA SP-368. Washington, DC, NASA, 1975, pp 323–340.
46. Homick JL, Reschke MF: Postural equilibrium following exposure to weightless space flight. Acta Otolaryngol 83:455–464, 1977.
47. Homick JL, Reschke MF, Vanderploeg JM: Space adaptation syndrome: Incidence and operational implications for the Space Transportation System program. In: AGARD Conference Proceedings (CP-372) on Motion Sickness: Mechanisms. Prediction, Prevention, and Treatment. Williamsburg, VA, 1984, pp 36-1–36-6.
48. Homick JL, Vanderploeg JM: The neurovestibular system. In: Nicogossian AE, Huntoon CL, Pool SL (eds): Space Physiology and Medicine, 2nd ed. Philadelphia, Lea & Febiger, 1989, pp 154–166.
49. Huntoon CL, Johnson PC, Cintron NM: Hematology, immunology, endocrinology, and biochemistry. In: Nicogossian AE, Huntoon CL, Pool SL (eds): Space Physiology and Medicine, 2nd ed. Philadelphia, Lea & Febiger, 1989, pp 222–239.
50. Hyde TM, Wu LC, Krasnov IB, et al: Quantitative autoradiographic analysis of muscarinic cholinergic and GABA-A (benzodiazepine) receptors in the forebrain of rats flown on the Soviet Biosatellite COSMOS 2044. Brain Res 593:291–294, 1992.
51. Hymer WC, Grindeland R, Krasnov I, et al: Effects of spaceflight on rat pituitary cell function. J Appl Physiol 73(2 suppl):151S–157S, 1992.
52. Jiang B, Ohira Y, Roy RR, et al: Adaptation of fibers in fast-twitch muscles of rats to spaceflight and hindlimb suspension. J Appl Physiol 73 (2 suppl):58S–65S, 1992.
53. Jiang B, Roy RR, Polyakov IV, et al: Ventral horn-cell responses to spaceflight and hindlimb suspension. J Appl Physiol 73(2 suppl):1O7S–111S, 1992.
54. Johnston RS: Skylab medical program overview. In: Johnston RS, Dietlein LF (eds): Biomedical Results from Skylab. NASA SP-377. Washington, DC, NASA, 1977, pp 3–19.
55a. Johnston RS, Hull WE: Apollo missions. In: Johnston RS, Dietlein LF, Berry CA (eds): Biomedical Results of Apollo. NASA SP-368. Washington, DC, NASA, 1975, pp 9–40.
55b. Kano M, Kitano T, Ikemoto M, et al: Isolation and characterization of a novel gene sfig in rat skeletal muscle up-regulated by spaceflight (STS-90). J Med Invest Feb; 50(1–2):39–47, 2003.
56. Keil L, Evan J, Grindeland R, et al: Pituitary oxytocin and vasopressin content of rats flow on COSMOS 2044. J Appl Physiol 73(suppl):166S-168S, 1992.
57. Kenyon RV, Young LR: MIT/Canadian vestibular experiments on the Spacelab-1 mission: 5. Postural responses following exposure to weightlessness. Exp Brain Res 64:335–346, 1986.
58. Kohl RL, MacDonald S: New pharmacologic approaches to the prevention of space/motion sickness. J Clin Pharmacol 31:934–946, 1991.
59. Komilova LN, Yakovleva IY, Tarasov IK, Gorgiladze GI: Vestibular dysfunction in cosmonauts during adaptation to zero-g and readaptation to 1 g. Physiologist 26(suppl):S35–S36, 1983.
60. Kozerenko OP, Grigoriev AI, Egorov AD: Results of investigations of weightlessness effects during prolonged manned space flights onboard Salyut 6. Physiologist 24(6):S49–S54, 1981.
61. Kozlovskaya IB, Aslanova IF, Barmin VA, et al: The nature and characteristics of a gravitational ataxia. Physiologist 26(suppl):S37–S38, 1983.
62. Kozlovskaya IB, Aslanova IF, Grigorieva LS, et al: Experimental analysis of motor effects of weightlessness. Physiologist 25(suppl):S49–S52, 1982.

63. Kozlovskaya IB, Babaev BM, Barmin VA, et al: The effect of weightlessness on motor and vestibulo motor reactions. Physiologist 27(suppl):S111–S114, 1984.
64. Kozlovskaya IB, Kreidich YV, Oganov VS, et al: Pathophysiology of motor functions in prolonged manned space flights. Acta Astron 8:1059–1072, 1981.
65. Kozlovskaya lB, Kreidich YV, Rakhmanov AS: Mechanisms of the effects of weightlessness on the motor system of man. Physiologist 24(suppl):S59–S63, 1981.
66. Lackner JR, Graybiel A: Illusions of postural, visual, and aircraft motion elicited by deep knee bends in the increased gravito-inertial force phase of parabolic flight. Exp Brain Res 44:312–316, 1986.
67. LaFevers EV, Nicogossian AE, Hoffler GW, et al: Spectral Analysis of Skeletal Muscle Changes Resulting from 59 Days of Weightlessness in Skylab III. JSC 09996 NASA TM X58171. Houston, NASA, 1975.
68. Leach CS, Alexander WC, Johnson PC: Endocrine, electrolyte, and fluid volume changes associated with Apollo missions. In: Johnston RS, Dietlein LF, Berry CA (eds): Biomedical Results of Apollo. NASA SP-368. Washington, DC, NASA, 1975, pp 163–184.
69. Leach CS, Rambaut PC: Biochemical responses of the Skylab crewmen: An overview. In: Johnston RS, Dietlein LF (eds): Biomedical Results from Skylab. NASA SP-377. Washington, DC, NASA, 1977, pp 204–216.
70. Lestienne FG, Gurfinkel VS: Postural control in weightlessness: A dual process underlying adaptation to an unusual environment. TINS 11:359–363, 1988.
71. Lowry 0, McDougal D, Chi MM, et al: Effects of Microgravity on 1) Metabolic Enzymes of Type I and Type II Muscle Fibers and on 2) Metabolic Enzymes, Neurotransmitter Amino Acids, and Neurotransmitter Associated Enzymes in Motorand Somatosensory Cerebral Cortex. Houston, NASA Special Publication N90–26474, 1990.
72. Mader TH: Intraocular pressure in microgravity. J Clin Pharmacol 31:947–950, 1991.
73. Manchester JK, Chi MMY, Norris B, et al: Effect of microgravity on metabolic enzymes of individual muscle fibers. FASEB J 4:55–63, 1990.
74a. Manie S, Konstantinova I, Breittmayer JP, et al: Effects of long duration space flight on human T lymphocyte and monocyte activity. Aviat Space Environ Med 62: 1153–1158, 1991.
74b. Mano T: Autonomic neural function in space. Curr Pharm Biotechnol Aug;6(4):319–324, 2005.
75. Markham CH, Diamond SG: Space motion sickness. Aviat Space Environ Med 66(1):86–87, 1995
76. Martin DS, South DA, Wood ML, et al: Comparison of echocardiographic changes after short- and long-duration space flight. Aviat Space Environ Med 73:532–536, 2002.
77. Martin TP, Edgerton VR, Grindeland RE: Influence of spaceflight on rat skeletal muscle. J Appl Physiol 65: 2318–2325, 1988.
78. Miu B, Martin TP, Roy RR, et al: Metabolic and morphologic properties of single muscle fibers in the rat after spaceflight, Cosmos 1887. FASEB J 4:64–72, 1990.
79. Miyamoto A, Shigematsu T, Fukunaga T, et al: Medical baseline data collection on bone and muscle change with space flight. Bone 22(5 suppl):79S-82S, 1998.
80. Money KE, Watt DG, Oman CM: Preflight and postflight motion sickness testing of the Spacelab 1 crew. In: AGARD, Conference Proceeding (CP372) on Motion Sickness: Mechanisms, Prediction, Prevention, and Treatment. Williamsburg, VA, 1984, pp 33–1–33–8.
81. Mulvagh SL, Charles JB, Riddle JM, et al: Echocardiographic evaluation of the cardiovascular effects of short-duration space flight. J Clin Pharmacol 31:1024–1026, 1991.
82. Musacchia XJ, Steffen JM, Fell RD, et al: Skeletal muscle response to spaceflight, whole body suspension, and recovery in rats. J Appl Physiol 69: 2248–2258, 1990.
83. Narici M, Kayser B, Barattini P, Cerretelli P: Effects of 17-day space flight on electrically evoked torque and cross-sectional area of the human triceps surae. Eur J Appl Physiol 90:275–282, 2003.
84. Nicholas JM: Small groups in orbit: Group interaction and crew performance on space station. Aviat Space Environ Med 58:1009–1013, 1987.
85. Nicogossian AE: Overall physiological response to space flight. In: Nicogossian AE, Huntoon CL, Pool SL (eds): Space Physiology and Medicine, 2nd ed. Philadelphia, Lea & Febiger, 1989, pp 139–153.
86. Nicogossian AE, Garshnek V: Historical perspectives. In: Nicogossian AE, Huntoon CL, Pool SL (eds): Space Physiology and Medicine, 2nd ed. Philadelphia, Lea & Febiger, 1989, pp 3–44.
87. Oganov VS: Results of biosatellite studies of gravity-dependent changes in the musculoskeletal system of mammals. Physiologist 24(6):S55–S58, 1981.
88. Ohira Y, Jiang B, Roy RR, et al: Rat soleus muscle fiber responses to 14 days of spaceflight and hindlimb suspension. J Appl Physiol 73(2 suppl):51S–57S, 1992.
89. Ohira Y, Yasui W, Kariya F, et al: Spaceflight effects on beta-adrenoceptor and metabolic properties in rat lantaris. J Appl Physiol 81(1):152–155, 1996.
90. Oman CM, Lichtenberg BK, Money KE, McCoy RKL: M.I.T./Canadian vestibular experiments on the Spacelab-1 mission: 4. Space motion sickness: Symptoms, stimuli, and predictability. Exp Brain Res 64(2):316–334, 1986.
91. Osborne WZ, Pinsky LS, Bailey JV: Apollo light flash investigations. In: Johnston RS, Dietlein LF, Berry CA (eds): Biomedical Results of Apollo. NASA SP-368. Washington, DC, NASA, 1975, pp 355–365.
92. Paloski WH: Vestibulospinal adaptation to micro gravity. Otolaryngol Head Neck Surg 118(3 pt 2):S39–S44, 1998.
93. Paloski WH, Reschke MF, Black FO, et al: Recovery of postural equilibrium control following space flight. Ann NY Acad Sci 656:747–754, 1992.
94. Parker DE: Human vestibular function and weightlessness. J Clin Pharmacol 31:904–910, 1991.

95. Parker DE, Reschke MF, Aldrich NG: Performance. In: Nicogossian SE, Huntoon CL, Pool SL (eds): Space Physiology and Medicine, 2nd ed. Philadelphia, Lea & Febiger, 1989, pp 167–178.
96. Parker DE, Reschke MF, Arrott AP, et al: Otolith tilt-translation reinterpretation following prolonged weightlessness: Implications for preflight training. Aviat Space Environ Med 56:601–606, 1985.
97. Parker DE, Reschke MF, Ouyang L, et al: Vestibulo-ocular reflex changes following weightlessness and reflight adaptation training. In: Keller T, Zee D (eds): Adaptive Process in Visual and Oculomotor Systems. *New* York, Pergamon, 1986, pp 103–109.
98. Perhonen JA, Franco F, Lane LD, et al: Cardiac atrophy after bed rest and space flight. J Appl Physiol 91: 645–653, 2001.
99. Polyakov IV, Drobyshev VI, Krasnov IB: Morphological changes in the spinal cord and intervertebral ganglia of rats exposed to different gravity levels. Physiologist 34(1 suppl):S187–S188, 1991.
100. Putcha L, Berens KL, Marshburn TH: Pharmaceutical use by U.S. astronauts on space shuttle missions. Aviat Space Environ Med 70:705–708, 1999.
101. Putcha L, Cintron NM: Pharmokinetic consequences of spaceflight. Ann NY Acad Sci 618:615–618, 1991.
102. Racine RN, Cormier SM: Effect of space flight on rat hepatocytes: A morphometric study. J Appl Phyiol 73(2 suppl):136S-141S, 1992.
103. Reitz G, Facius R, Bucker H: Radiation biology. In: Oser H, Battrick B (eds): Life Sciences Research in Space. Paris, European Space Agency, ESA SP105, 1989, pp 65–79.
104. Reschke MF, Anderson DJ, Homick JL: Vestibulospinal reflexes as a function of microgravity. Science 225: 212–214, 1984.
105. Reschke MF, Anderson DJ, Homick JL: Vestibulospinal response modification as determined with the H-reflex during the Spacelab-1 flight. Exp Brain Res 64: 367–379, 1986.
106. Reschke MF, Parker DE: Effects of prolonged weightlessness on self-motion perception and eye movements evoked by roll and pitch. Aviat Space Environ Med 58(suppl):A153–A158, 1987.
107. Reschke MF, Parker DE, Homick JL, et al: Reinterpretation of otolith input as a primary factor in space motion sickness. In: Results of Space Experiments in Physiology and Medicine and Informal Briefings by the F-16 Medical Working Group. Aerospace Medical Panel Symposium. AGARD-CP-377. Istanbul, 1984, pp 3–1–3-18.
108. Riley DA: Effects of microgravity on the electron microscopy, histochemistry, and protease activities of rat hindlimb muscle. In: Nicogossian AE (ed): Spacelab Life Sciences 1 180-Day Preliminary Results. Houston, NASA Special Publication, 1992.
109. Riley DA, Ellis S, Giometti CS, et al: Muscle sarcomere lesions and thrombosis after spaceflight and suspension unloading. J Appl Physiol 37(2 suppl):33S–43S, 1992
110. Riley DA, Ellis S, Slocum GR, et al: Morphological and biochemical changes in soleus and extensor digitorum longus muscles of rats orbited in Spacelab 3. Physiologist 23:S207–S208, 1985.
111. Riley DA, Ellis S, Slocum GR, et al: In-flight and postfight changes in skeletal muscles of SLS-1 and SLS-2 space flown rats. J Appl Physiol 81(1):133–144, 1996.
112. Riley DA, Ilyina-Kakueva EI, Ellis S, et al: Skeletal muscle fiber, nerve, and blood vessel breakdown in space-flown rats. FASEB J 4(1):84–91, 1990.
113. Ross HE, Brodie EE, Benson AJ: Mass-discrimination in weightlessness and readaption to earth's gravity. Exp Brain Res 64:358–366, 1986.
114. Ross HE, Schwartz E, Emmerson P: The nature of sensorimotor adaptation to altered g-levels: Evidence from mass discrimination. Aviat Space Environ Med 58(suppl):A148–A152, 1987.
115. Sawchenko PE, Arias C, Krasnov I, et al: Effects of spaceflight on hypothalamic peptide systems controlling pituitary growth hormone dynamics. J Appl Physiol 73(2 suppl):154S–158S, 1992.
116. Schneider VS, Leblanc A, Rambaut PC: Bone and mineral metabolism. In: Nicogossian AE, Huntoon CL, Pool SL (eds): Space Physiology and Medicine, 2nd ed. Philadelphia, Lea & Febiger, 1989, pp 214–221.
117. Schneider VS, Oganov VA, Leblanc A, et al: Spaceflight bone loss and change in fat and lean body mass (abstract). J Bone Miner Res 7:S122, 1992.
118. Shipov AA, Sirota MG, Beloozerova IN, et al: Results of tests on the primate vestibulo-visual motor reactions in Biocosmos experiments. In: Keller T, Zee D (eds): Adaptive Processes in Visual and Oculomotor Systems. New York, Pergamon, 1986, pp 129–132.
119. Sonnenfeld G: The immune system in space and micro gravity. Med Sci Sports Exerc 34(12):2021–2027, 2002.
120. Stein TP, Schulter MD, Moldawer LI: Endocrine relationships during human space flight. Am J Physiol 276(1 pt 1):E155–E162, 1999.
121a. Stevens L, Mounier Y, Holy X: Functional adaptation of different rat skeletal muscles to weightlessness. Am J Physiol 264(4 pt 2):R770–R776, 1993.
121b. Summers RL, Martin DS, Meck JV, Coleman TG: Mechanisms of spaceflight-induced changes in left ventricular mass. Am J Cardiol May 1;95(9):1128–30, 2005.
122. Talbot JM (ed): Research Opportunities in Space Motion Sickness. NASA Contractor Report 3708. Washington, DC, NASA, 1983.
123. Task HL, Genco LV: Effects of short-term space flight on several visual functions. In: Bungo MW, Bagian TM, Bowman MA, Levitan BM (eds): Results of the Life Sciences DSOs Conducted Aboard the Space Shuttle 1981–1986. Houston, Space Biomedical Research Institute, NASA, 1987, pp 173–178.
124. Taylor GR: Space microbiology. Annu Rev Microbiol 28:121–137, 1974.
125. Taylor GR: Immune changes during short-duration missions. J Leukocyte Biol 54:202–208, 1993.

126. Thornton WE, Biggers WP, Thomas WG, et al: Electronystagmography and audio potentials in space flight. Laryngoscope 95:924–932, 1985.
127. Thornton WE, Hoffler GW, Rummel JA: Anthropometric changes and fluid shifts. In: Johnston RS, Dietlein LF (eds): Biomedical Results from Skylab. NASA SP-377. Washington, DC, NASA, 1977, pp 330–338.
128. Thornton WE, Moore TP, Pool SL, et al: Clinical characterization and etiology of space motion sickness. Aviat Space Environ Med 58(suppl):AI-A8, 1987.
129. Thornton WE, Rummel JA: Muscular deconditioning and its prevention in space flight. In: Johnston RS, Dietlein LF (eds): Biomedical Results from Skylab. NASA SP-377. Washington, DC, NASA, 1977, pp 191–197.
130. Vico L, Lafage-Proust MH, Alexandre C: Effects of gravitational changes on the bone system in vitro and in vivo. Bone 22(5 suppl):95S-100S, 1998.
131. Vieville T, Clement G, Lestienne F, et al: Adaptive modifications of the optokinetic and vestibulo-ocular reflexes in microgravity. In: Keller T, Zee D (eds): Adaptive Processes in Visual and Oculomotor Systems. New York, Pergamon, 1986, pp 111–119.
132. Waligora JM, Sauer RL, Bredt JH: Spacecraft life support systems. In: Nicogossian AE, Huntoon CL, Pool SL (eds): Space Physiology and Medicine, 2nd ed. Philadelphia, Lea & Febiger, 1989, pp 104–120.
133. Watt DGD, Money KE, Tomi LM: MIT/Canadian vestibular experiments on the Spacelab-1 mission: 3. Effects of prolonged weightlessness on a human otolith-spinal reflex. Exp Brain Res 64:308–315, 1986.
134. Whitson PA, Charles JB, Williams WJ, Cintron NM: Changes in sympathoadrenal response to standing in humans after space flight. J Appl Physiol 78(2):428–433, 1995.
135. Yegorov AD: Results of Medical Research During the 175-Day Flight of the Third Main Crew on the Salyut-6-Soyuz Orbital Complex. NASA TM-76450. Washington, DC, NASA, 1981.
136. Young LR, Oman CM, Watt DGD, et al: Spatial orientation in weightlessness and readaptation in weightlessness and readaptation to earth's gravity. Science 225:205–208, 1984.
137. Young LR, Shelhamer M: Microgravity enhances the relative contribution of visually-induced motion sensation. Aviat Space Environ Med 61:525–530, 1990.
138. Young LR, Sinha P: Spaceflight influences on ocular counter rolling and other neurovestibular reactions. Otolaryngol Head Neck Surg 118(3 pt 2):S31–S34, 1998.
139. Young LR, Watt DGD, Oman CM, et al: Spatial orientation in weightlessness and readaptation to earth's gravity. In: Results of Space Experiments in Physiology and Medicine and Informal Briefings by the F-16 Medical Working Group. AGARD-CP-377. Istanbul, Turkey, 1948, pp 2-1–2-5.

Part VII

Posttraumatic Sequelae and Medicolegal Aspects

Chapter 33

Movement Disorders: Posttraumatic Syndromes

CHRISTOPHER G. GOETZ
AND ILIA ITIN

For more than a century, physical trauma has been considered as an influence on the character and clinical outcome of various movement disorders. Parkinson,[127] Charcot,[29a] and Gowers[64] all alluded to an association between injuries and involuntary movements. In defining trauma, we restrict our definition to occupational accidents and physical injuries and do not emphasize movement disorders related to situations such as

- Emotional trauma, or stress
- Birth trauma, or injury that is usually considered under the discussions of anoxic, postanoxic, or metabolic encephalopathies
- Overuse syndromes increasingly described in professional athletes and musicians
- Psychogenic movement disorders often found in the context of a prior accident or litigious context

We will focus on two types of trauma, central and peripheral nervous system injury, and review a number of movement disorders including parkinsonism, tremors, dystonia, chorea, and myoclonus. Although the pathophysiology of all movement disorders relates primarily to dysfunction of subcortical nuclei and their axonal connections, the interplay between these basal ganglia structures and the cortex as well as the peripheral nervous system is becoming increasingly appreciated. We will mention instances in which nonnervous system injury can cause disorders that may resemble neurologically based movement disorders and emphasize that these orthopedic, muscular, or inflammatory conditions should be considered before a true movement disorder is diagnosed and putatively treated.

The primary questions of focus are:

- Does trauma cause movement disorders?
- Does trauma cause movement disorders that are clinically distinct from movement disorders otherwise considered idiopathic?
- Does trauma exacerbate or hasten the progression of already established idiopathic movement disorders?

There are implicit epidemiological and methodological limitations to a scientific analysis of trauma in the clinical situation. First, the actual frequency of trauma in the modern world is unknown; cases without sequelae are not regularly reported or followed. Furthermore, in spite of advances in the assessment of the frequency of the various movement disorders, accurate community-based prevalence figures for each disorder remain unknown. Therefore, current researchers have not established with certainty that trauma actually increases the likelihood of any movement disorder that would otherwise be considered idiopathic. There are a number of well-established posttraumatic syndromes that involve abnormal movements. In their classical form, these syndromes are distinctive in their clinical, neuroimaging, and temporal development patterns and do not resemble most primary movement disorders. The time frame of trauma-related influences is not completely understood. When a movement disorder occurs within hours or days of the trauma, inferences are more solidly confirmed, but when clinical dysfunction develops months or even years after the trauma, direct relationships become less obvious. On the other hand, if such disorders relate to aberrant healing, ephaptic transmission after injury, remyelinization, or late inflammatory changes, a longer time frame may be reasonable. An added limitation is the lack of accurate clinical data predating the trauma; since most patients are evaluated for the first time with expert neurological examinations after injury, the pretrauma data are almost always only historical. Mild movement disorders that were present but not problematic prior to trauma can be lost in the analysis. A litigious environment adds motivation to suppress dysfunction that predated trauma and place full emphasis on the injury as causal. Finally, there are no well-established scales for trauma evaluation; how is one accident or injury compared to another, and is there a threshold that is different for causation compared to that necessary for aggravating an already present disorder? In this discussion, we summarize reports that attempt to address these issues and highlight the areas that still require important investigation.

Pathophysiology

The pathophysiological mechanisms that underlie trauma-induced basal ganglia dysfunction are unknown. Structural damage to subcortical and substantia nigral neurons can occur acutely from direct penetration wounds, or from ischemic or hemorrhagic vascular lesions.[147] Late inflammatory changes, aberrant ephaptic transmission, and central synaptic reorganization have been proposed to play roles in the generation of involuntary movements seen in the months after trauma.[169] Recent evidence that tissue damage generates excessive hydroxyl radicals and other oxidants is of particular interest to the study of movement disorders because similar mechanisms have been suggested to play a possible role in the pathogenesis of idiopathic Parkinson's disease and Huntington's disease.[30,66] Recent developments provide further support for this hypothesis. The pattern of alpha-synuclein aggregation in the brains of the aged mice is influenced by experimental traumatic brain injury (TBI).[175] Researchers observed not only a transient increase in alpha-synuclein aggregation in the striatum but also the co-occurrence of conformationally different forms of alpha-synuclein and increased expression of nitric oxide synthase. Trauma-induced oxidative/nitrative stress has been posited as a contributing factor in the pathogenesis of Parkinson's disease developing after injuries.[17] Focal peripheral nervous system trauma may influence the development of movement disorders through alterations in afferent neuronal input to the spinal cord and secondarily affect higher brain stem and subcortical centers.[144]

Following deafferentation of the spinal cord, there is neuronal hyperexcitability that spreads beyond the involved spinal segment. Cortical representation of an injured body area also spreads to occupy broader topographic regions.[89] Several forms of brain plasticity, including changes in neuronal sprouting and diaschisis, have been suggested to occur in motor systems in response to trauma.[13] In whiplash injuries, additional muscle, soft tissue, and bony alterations can influence head posture and body postions.[161] Blood–brain barrier interruption after trauma, with resultant chronic seepage of unknown toxins into the central nervous system (CNS), has been suggested as a putative mechanism to explain sequelae of trauma occurring years after injury.[160] Neuronal reorganization after peripheral trauma associated with complex regional pain syndromes or reflex sympathetic dystrophy may also underlie some movement disorders, especially dystonia, that can be seen after injury to a limb, the face, or the neck (see the the section "Dystonia" below).

Neurochemically, the major neurotransmitter/receptor systems studied in trauma have been those involving acetylcholine/muscarinic and glutamate/*N*-methyl-D-aspartate (NMDA) activity.[90] The basal ganglia have dense interactions with these systems, although the animal models studied to date have focused most directly on cortex and spinal cord rather than subcortical anatomy.[2] The added impact of emotional stress with alterations in catecholaminergic and endorphin function may also be important to basal ganglia activity after trauma.[174] In this context, psychological factors may also play a physiological role in some cases of movement disorders after trauma. Intense psychotherapy has been associated with improvement or resolution of motor alterations in some cases, and both conscious and unconscious secondary gain may underlie these examples.[102,122a]

Parkinsonism/Parkinson's Disease

Parkinsonism is the clinical situation in which a patient has signs that include combinations of resting tremor, bradykinesia, rigidity, and postural instability. The prototype is Parkinson's disease (PD), in which a specific and localized degeneration of dopaminergic cells in the substantia nigra occurs, leading to nigrostriatal system dopaminergic underactivitiy.[9] Drug-induced parkinsonism, seen in patients who ingest antidopaminergic drugs, specifically neuroleptics or reserpine, causes dopaminergic underactivity in the nigrostriatal system, and though it is reversible, its signs are clinically indistinguishable from those of PD.[60] Other non-PD parkinsonian syndromes may have nigrostriatal system damage, but this degeneration occurs in the context of wider diffuse or multifocal anatomical alterations, and the parkinsonism is only one of several other accompanying neurological signs. This clinical and pathological distinction is important to a discussion of trauma-induced parkinsonism and the separate question of whether trauma-induced PD exists. Although James Parkinson himself alluded to a past history of trauma in his early report of the disease that bears his name, and although Jean-Martin Charcot recounted how one patient in his clinic had been injured with a thorn in the foot prior to his tremor onset in the same extremity, the suggestion that trauma causes PD has been widely questioned.[1,65,70,90,147] Schwab and England reviewed literature through 1965, including a large body of post–World War I and II studies, and concluded that unless there was definite evidence of trauma-induced midbrain damage, "one is on the most uncertain ground in establishing any causal relationship here.[147] Factor and colleagues reviewed more recent studies and likewise concluded that trauma does not cause PD.[49] A recent population analysis of 821 patients extended the neurological perspective to evaluate amyotrophic lateral sclerosis and Alzheimer's disease as well as PD. Head injury with presumed brain involvement was found to be an unlikely risk factor for any of them.[186]

If trauma itself does not cause PD, can it play a role as a risk factor in its eventual development? Some epidemiological studies have found a greater prevalence of head trauma in PD subjects than in controls.[63,183] In a questionnaire study completed by PD patients and spouse controls, more patients than spouses reported trauma, although the significance reached only $p < .05$, and injury occurred 32.3 years (mean) before PD onset.[50] A similar study of patients with onset of PD at a young age (before 40) demonstrated an odds ratio of 4.5 and a lag time after injury and before the appearance of symptoms of 14 years.[171] Conclusions from such studies are compromised by recall bias and a litigious environment. Recent studies have attempted to overcome this bias. Maher et al.[110] looked at siblings with PD as a part of the GenePD Study. Head trauma was linked to a 3.3-year younger age at onset. Differential recall is unlikely to have affected these data, because all siblings had PD. A study by Bower et al.[12] attempted to eliminate bias by conducting a population-based case-control study with controls nested within a cohort and by using recorded information regarding the head trauma. This study revealed that the overall chance of developing PD was much higher in cases than in controls (odds ratio of 4.3). Subjects with mild head injury without loss of consciousness did not have an elevated risk of developing PD, while subjects with severe head trauma accompanied by loss of consciousness had an odds ratio of 11. Because of the often long interval between trauma and PD, Stern suggested that trauma might alter blood–brain barrier protection, permit toxins to seep into the brain, and begin a process that could take several years or even decades to progress to clinical significance.[160] As a group, these studies leave open the question of trauma as a risk factor for later development of PD, but the relatively consistent patterns suggest that trauma may play a role in lowering the threshold for disease and possibly hastening the date of clinical onset. Even if proven to be a risk factor, a history of trauma is uncommon among subjects with PD (estimated at 5%),[12] so its direct role would still be considered as one among many factors.

Goetz and Stebbins[61] studied the effect of head trauma related to motor vehicle accidents in 10 patients with PD and compared their PD disability over 1 year with that of a control group of matched PD patients without head trauma. Because they regularly collected objective and subjective scores as part of routine care, they were able to compare pre- and posttrauma function in their patients. Objective and subjective disability increased immediately after the trauma, and parkinsonism scores were worse for all patients, both those with and without loss of consciousness at the time of trauma. The clinical decline in function was short-lived, with a significant increase in disability still present at 1- and 2-week evaluations. By 4 weeks, disability remained worse than baseline, but there was no longer a statistically significantly difference compared to pretrauma function. Thereafter, mean scores improved further, and by 12 weeks baseline function was reestablished. At 1 year, the cases and controls were equally impaired. This study suggests that trauma adversely affects parkinsonism immediately after head trauma but has no lasting impact, as measured at 1 year.

Recently, this clinical observation was buttressed by basic science data. Alpha-synuclein aggregation into insoluble fibrils and accumulation in Lewy bodies has been implicated in the pathogenesis of both sporadic and hereditary PD. Traumatic brain injury, especially severe trauma from acceleration/deceleration, results in diffuse axonal injury that causes disruption of fast axonal transport and abnormal protein accumulation, including synuclein. Uryu et al.[175] examined the relationship between brain trauma and synuclein accumulation. The accumulation of α-synuclein in the brains of aged, young, and alpha-synuclein knockout mice was traced over several weeks after TBI. The aged mice demonstrated an increase in alpha-synuclein immunoreactivity in the cortical, striatal and hippocampal neuropil after a brain trauma. Further, there was an increase in immunoreactivity labeling of the striatal axonal bundles with antibodies against nitrated or conformationally changed alpha-synuclein as well as against inducible nitric oxide synthase. These changes peaked after 1 week but returned to baseline after 16 weeks.[175] These findings may help to explain the initial worsening and subsequent return to baseline after 12 weeks in PD patients after head injury. The long-term subclinical sequelae of such injury remain to be studied in the laboratory. Some investigators have suggested that TBI may play a part in the pathogenesis of PD by increasing oxidative stress, as highlighted by the accumulation of conformationally changed and nitrated alpha-synuclein.[17,155]

In contrast to PD, however, parkinsonism occurring in the context of other neurological signs can clearly occur after two types of CNS trauma: severe and usually one-time head injury associated with well-circumscribed brain stem lesions and less severe but repeated closed head trauma, as seen with the widely publicized boxer's or pugilist encephalopathy. Dramatic cases of bullet and knife wounds that penetrate the brain stem show convincingly that parkinsonism can occur in this context.[65,147] Rondot et al. reported on a parkinsonian patient who suffered a midbrain bullet wound from a suicide attempt. His rest tremor, 4–6 Hz, had features typical of parkinsonism, but there was also a kinetic component and a poor response to levodopa. Additional neurological findings included hemiparesis, hemidystonia, and partial third nerve palsy. The clinical picture did not suggest typical PD but rather a mixed syndrome with parkinsonism as one feature.[135] Hemorrhagic circumscribed lesions after head injury may also precipitate parkinsonism. Bhatt et al.[11] reported three cases of *akinetic-rigid syndrome* developing several months after severe trauma; all patients had evidence of discrete basal ganglia (putamen, substantia nigra, and subpallidal region) damage on neuroimaging that was performed at the time of trauma or shortly thereafter. Two of the three patients had a good response to levodopa. In addition to features of typical parkinsonism, other signs included hemidystonia, extensor toe reflexes, and dysarthria. Doder et al.[42] described a case of unilateral levodopa-resistent parkinsonism that developed 6 weeks after severe head injury with loss of consciousness for 24 hours. The magnetic resonance imaging (MRI) scan disclosed a left caudate and lentiform nucleus infarction. In such cases, patients generally develop parkinsonism after long vegetative or comatose states, and parkinsonism usually emerges along with mental, ocular, and motor signs.[33,65,85] Although well documented, cases of posttraumatic parkinsonism from a single event appear to be remarkably rare. In Jellinger's extensive neuropathological studies including 520 cases of parkinsonism, he found only three cases (0.6%) in which parkinsonism occurred in this context.[84] The diagnostic evaluation of such patients revealed regular evidence of brain stem lesions usually in the form of hematomas or infarctions.[124]

The second category of CNS posttraumatic parkinsonism is the pugilist encephalopathy. In these cases, repeated blunt trauma is associated with the gradual development of motor, behavioral, and mental changes that can have parkinsonism as part of the more extensive clinical spectrum of signs. Scans and autopsy examinations show severe brain atrophy with cystic lesions in the hemispheres and cerebellum, sometimes with rupture of the septum pellucidum. Histologically, there may be neurofibrillary tangles in the cortex. Importantly, the time frame of this syndrome's evolution is typically very slow, with the first motor signs developing decades after the last cerebral insult.[55]

A pure striatal *punch-drunk syndrome* may be difficult to distinguish from idiopathic parkinsonism, especially if it develops years after the cessation of boxing.[106] In most of these cases, however, early speech deficits and extensor toe signs occur, features atypical of idiopathic PD. In a study by Turjanski et al.,[173] five former boxers and one steeplechase jockey, all with repeated head trauma in the past, developed parkinsonism and were investigated using F18 positron emission tomography (PET). They were compared to normal controls and age-matched PD patients without a history of trauma. In the idiopathic PD patients, F18–PET demonstrated a typical differential pattern of nigrostriatal involvement with much more pronounced putaminal terminal loss compared with the caudate.[22] In contrast, the patients with pure striatal form of pugilist encephalopathy showed uniform reduction in nigrostriatal uptake,[173] suggesting a different anatomical involvement in dopaminergic loss between the two patient groups. Parkinsonism in the context of other neurological dysfunction has also occurred after trauma to the peripheral nervous system. Schott identified patients whose trauma preceded parkinsonian symptoms by 1 month and whose symptoms coincided anatomically with the area of body injury.[145] He drew direct analogies to causalgia. Cardoso and Jankovic studied 28 patients who fit relatively rigorous criteria for a posttraumatic tremor condition: injury was severe enough to cause local symptoms lasting for at least 2 weeks and required acute medical attention; the movement disorder occurred within 1 year of the trauma; and the movement disorder began in the anatomical area of physical injury.[27] Eleven patients had parkinsonian features, and six of these had rest tremor in isolation. All patients had postural or kinetic tremors. The number of patients who would have been diagnosed with idiopathic PD if there were no trauma history was not indicated. There was a high prevalence of a family history of essential tremor in this group, as well as frequent dystonia and myoclonus as accompanying movement disorders. High-dose levodopa modestly ameliorated parkinsonian symptoms in 6/10 patients.[79] Fluorodopa PET scans showed decreased striatal uptake that in similar to PD in three patients and resembled normal values in one patient. Without refering to PD itself, the authors suggested that peripheral trauma can be associated with parkinsonism.

As a group, these studies do not resolve the question of a direct relationship between peripheral trauma and parkinsonism. It is possible that early parkinsonism was already present in the involved body area, causing that limb to be more prone to injury. It is also possible that patients' natural inclination to explain causes for illness heightened their recollection of trauma. However, it is also possible that trauma causes oxidative stress or injury either locally or by feedback to CNS nuclei that allows functional or anatomical impairments in the dopaminergic system.[156] These issues remain unresolved and await better animal model experiments.

Other Tremors

Tremors are defined as rhythmic to-and-fro oscillations and are named for the body position in which they are most prominent (*rest* when the tremor is maximal at repose; *postural* when the tremor develops as a patient maintains a position; and *kinetic* when the tremor develops as a patient carries out a movement). Additionally, rhythmic to-and-fro movements that occur in association with a particular type of activity have been described. These task-specific tremors include primary writing tremor, vocal tremor, and orthostatic tremor. Nonparkinsonian tremors related to trauma are generally postural, kinetic, or mixed in character.[54,99] In many cases, such tremors emerge in the context of posttraumatic hemiparesis due to underlying pyramidal-subcortical deficits or to cerebellar dysfunction and involvement of the dentato-rubral-thalamic circuit.[75] Krauss et al.[98] provided MRI evidence for the role of dentatothalamic derangement in the pathogenesis of the posttraumatic tremor. In a series of 19 patients with postural or kinetic tremors and in 14 patients with resting tremor, all showed evidence of diffuse axonal injury and dentatothalamic pathway lesions. These types of tremors typically develop following head, neck, or extremity trauma with or without loss of consciousness. Andrew et al. described eight patients with head injury and coma that lasted between 1 and 20 weeks who developed tremor that began 1 to 18 months after awakening.[3] In five, tremor occurred as hemiplegia abated. In all, tremor was kinetic, with a postural component in seven and a resting component in three. Myoclonic jerks were variably superimposed. Neurological imaging revealed no focal abnormalities, but thalamotomy ameliorated the postural-kinetic component by 50% in seven cases and abolished the rest component and myoclonus in all. Positron emission tomography was performed in one patient who developed a combined postural and rest tremor of the left hand after awakening from coma due to a right posttraumatic peduncular hematoma. A marked decrease in 18F fluorodopa uptake along with a normal 76Br bromolisuride uptake scan in the right striatum suggested to the authors that the posttraumatic mesencephalic-based tremor was related in part to dopaminergic striatal denervation.[37] Investigation of six patients with midbrain lesions and peduncular or rubral tremors further supported the dopaminergic hypothesis of such mixed tremors since all the patients had similar imaging data.[132] Notably, only two of these patients had trauma-related tremor; the rest developed their movement disorder after cerebrovascular strokes. All patients in this series responded to levodopa therapy at least modestly.

Zijlmans et al.[191] reported a case of a 19-year-old man who developed left kinetic and postural tremor several years after a severe head injury that led to 2 weeks of a comatose state. Single photon emission computed tomography (SPECT) imaging of the postsynaptic and presynaptic dopaminergic terminals revealed an analogous pattern to the finding reported above. However, unlike the patients in the series of Remy, this patient had marked absence of hypokinesia and rigidity. The authors postulated that absence of parkinsonian features in this patient may have been due to the right subthalamic nucleus hemosiderin deposit seen on MRI, indicating previous hemorrhage to this nucleus.

Adults and children with posttraumatic postural/kinetic tremors[46,164] have responded to propranolol with and without valproate therapy. Other treatments of posttraumatic tremors include l-tryptophan, levodopa/carbidopa, carbamezepine, and glutethimide.[1,67,133,140] Jacob et al.[77] described a 28-year-old man who sustained a head injury with 1 month of coma and presented with tremor 4 years later. His computed tomography (CT) scan demonstrated hematoma involving his left midbrain, thalamus, and medial temporal lobe. He tremor was characterized by a combination of right resting, postural, and kinetic components. The MRI scan revealed left lesions in the red nucleus and decussation of the superior cerebellar peduncles and the dorsomedial thalamus. The patient failed a clinical trial of levodopa/carbidopa and valproic acid but responded well to clonazepam.

Additional patients with apparently asymptomatic congenital anomalies have developed tremors after trauma. Vanhatalo et al.[178] reported a case of a 13-year-old boy with a type 2 Arnold-Chiari malformation who, after trauma, developed severe bilateral postural and kinetic tremors that prevented him from ambulating or using his hands. He had sustained only a very mild back and head injury with reported loss of consciousness for 10 seconds. The Arnold-Chiari malformation, though evident on the MRI scan, was not associated with brain stem compression, tissue damage, or spinal cord tethering. The symptoms persisted for 4 months despite numerous pharmacological trials and psychiatric interventions. Finally, the posterior fossa was decompressed surgically, and an unstable posterior arch of the C1, due either to trauma or to the primary congenital anomaly, was surgically removed. The patient's tremor gradually abated after the surgery. The authors postulated that the heretofore asymptomatic Arnold-Chiari malformation was sufficiently displaced by the trauma to cause midbrain herniation and stretching, with resultant functional lesions that could not be detected by conventional imaging.

Biary et al.[14] reported on seven patients with trauma-related tremor whose neurological examinations were otherwise normal, without signs or a history of hemiparesis or cerebellar dysfunction. These patients had no history of familial tremor, and their head trauma usually was mild, without loss of consciousness. The patients developed postural/kinetic tremors of the arms, legs, or head within weeks of their accidents. Superimposed large-amplitude myoclonic jerks occurred in most patients and responded to clonazepam. Krauss et al.[93,96] reported a large series of consecutive patients with severe (Glasgow Coma Scale score <8) and mild head injury and concentrated on those who subsequently developed movement disorders. Posttraumatic tremors were found in 42 of 221 (19%) movement disorder patients; 10% had transient tremors, and 9% had persistent ones. High-frequency postural and intention tremors occurred days and weeks after the injury, while low-frequency kinetic tremors had a latency of 2 weeks to 6 months. Several patients had simultaneous resting, postural, and kinetic tremors of the midbrain type. Focal rhythmic tongue movements occurred in two young adults with evidence of pontine injury after head and neck injury. These were short-lived and resolved in 4 months without therapy.[35] A single case of posttraumatic orthostatic tremor was reported that occurred 2 weeks after an elderly woman sustained a blow to the back of the skull.[141] The abnormal movement consisted of a 14–15 Hz asynchronous tremor that developed in the gastrocnemius, tibialis anterior, hamstrings, quadriceps, and paraspinals only upon standing. Athough the patient had not lost consciousness and had no other neurological sequelae, her head MRI scan showed ischemic-gliottic changes in the periventricular subcortical white matter, pons, and cerebellum. The tremor was not ameliorated by the administration of clonazepam, levodopa/carbidopa, alprazolam, valproic acid, or phenobarbital.

Other reports of trauma-related tremors include patients experiencing extremity injuries, including wrist fracture with immobilization[31] and fifth metacarpal fracture with external fixation,[69] who subsequently developed a 7 Hz intermittent postural/kinetic tremor after removal of the cast. These tremors occurred with writing, and no improvement occurred with propranolol or mysoline. Similarly, in a review of 3500 patients with various movement disorders, Jankovic described seven patients who developed tremor without other neurological abnormalities within 4 months following trauma to the extremities (six patients) or to the neck (one patient). Five had possible predisposing factors including a family history of tremor, drug exposure, or systemic illnesses that have been associated with tremors. These cases suggest that the trauma may have precipitated tremor in a susceptible or early case.[80] Ellis[45] reported a group of six patients who developed a variety of tremors after whiplash injury related to motor vehicle accidents with latency varying from immediate onset to 6 months. Hashimoto et al.[68] reported a case of a 55-year-old man who developed a coarse postural tremor 7 days after an injury to his neck. The patient had evidence of ulnar radiculopathy in the affected extremity. The authors considered the tremor to be an enhanced physiological tremor further augmented by the peripheral neuropathy. While some posttraumatic tremors spontaneously remit or are partially drug responsive, the majority remain refractory to standard medical treatment.[56] When cerebellar or brain stem involvement with dyssynergia and/or ataxia is concomitantly present in patients with posttraumatic tremor, individual case reports suggest improvement following ventrolateral cryothalamectomies.[24,54] Large retrospective surgical studies, however, are difficult to interpret due to the grouping of many cases into series with tremors of other etiologies.[62] Furthermore, long-term efficacy has not been addressed, as follow-up periods have seldomly exceeded 1 year. In one report, long-term results of stereotactic surgery for posttraumatic limb tremor in 35 young individuals (age, range, 3–29 years) were described.[94] Thirty-three patients developed tremor after "severe" head trauma, though alterations in consciousness were not reported. Postural, kinetic, or mixed bilateral[14] or unilateral[37] limb tremors of 2.5–4 Hz were noted. Nearly all patients had additional neurological findings including psychological/cognitive alterations (91%), dysarthria (86%), ataxia (91%), hemiparesis/tetraparesis (94%), and other movement disorders (46%). Forty-two surgeries were performed, with two patients receiving bilateral procedures and five unilateral reoperations. These procedures consisted of contralateral zona incerta lesions in 12 patients, while the ventrolateral thalamus was additionally targeted in the remaining 23. Long-term follow-up (mean period of 10.5 years) demonstrated persistent improvement in 88% of patients, with 65% experiencing a continued marked reduction or total absence of their tremor. Immediate postoperative side effects including worsened dysarthria, increased dysphagia, hemiparesis, truncal ataxia, and altered mentation occurred in 71% of patients and persisted in 38% of cases.

High-frequency thalamic stimulation has also been beneficial in isolated cases of posttraumatic tremor and is usually associated with limited perioperative morbidity.[8,131] Further carefully conducted long-term studies, however, are required to properly evaluate the role of this alternative treatment modality. Finally, botulinum toxin injections, although not specifically investigated in posttraumatic tremor, have been reported to improve tremors of various etiologies.[80,83]

In summary, an extensive literature suggests that although very uncommon, tremor may result from trauma either to the head or to the body. This relationship is best established when CT or MRI findings of CNS damage exist or when accompanying hemiparetic or cerebellar signs occur. When isolated posttraumatic tremor occurs without other neurological findings, reports have emphasized the frequent myoclonic elements and atypical medication responses that differ from those of traditional essential tremor. These features may be helpful in attempting to determine whether a case is likely due to trauma or not. Among movement disorders of psychogenic origin, most studies report tremor as the most frequent presentation, so that when the neurological examination is otherwise normal, this diagnosis should also be kept in mind by the astute clinician.

Dystonia

Dystonia is a slow muscle contortion that causes an abnormal, sustained body posture, frequently with a twisting character. Numerous reports document the close association between severe head trauma and resultant dystonia. The clearest instances are cases of focal dystonia or hemidystonia that occur in the days or weeks following severe trauma with loss of consciousness and are accompanied by contralateral basal ganglia lesions on scans.[74,113,130] The link between trauma and dystonia is usually only suggestive when minor head trauma without loss of consciousness occurs, when symptoms do not develop for months or years after the trauma, when there is no structural abnormality on scans, or when the dystonia is multifocal or diffuse in distribution.[25,119,139] One epidemiological study demonstrated that after severe head injury (Glasgow Coma Scale score <8), 4.1% of patients developed either focal dystonia or hemidystonia, with latency ranging between 2 months and 2 years after trauma A. Low Glasgow Coma Scale score on hospital admission and CT findings of brain edema were predictive of a higher risk of dystonia.[96] In mild to moderate brain injury (Glasgow Coma Scale score ≥9) there were no instances of dystonia over the 2-year follow-up period.[97] Physiological investigations like PET scans have been reported to be abnormal in some cases of posttraumatic dystonia without structural evidence of disease, although whether these findings reflect the cause or effects of the dystonic posturing is unclear.[129] The anatomical focus of almost all instances of trauma-related dystonia is the basal ganglia. Most cases of well-accepted posttraumatic dystonia related to severe head trauma have well-circumscribed lesions in the contralateral caudate nucleus and putamen. Less frequently, pallidal or thalamic lesions are found.[93] The interplay between cortical regions and the basal ganglia is extensive, and the reversibility of cases of torticollis after resection of frontal cortical scar tissue suggests that posttraumatic sequelae involving cortical lesions can potentially be associated with movement disorders.[34]

In contrast to other movement disorders suggested to result from CNS traumatic injury, posttraumatic dystonia has a more widely variable delay in onset, ranging in Lee et al.'s series from 1 month to 9 years after trauma.[105] In that study, dystonia began focally but spread in almost all instances to become segmental dystonia, hemidystonia, or generalized dystonia. The authors suggested dysfunction of the lenticulothalamic circuitry as the foundation of these posttraumatic dystonias. Other authors have also described a delayed-onset dystonia that may relate pathophysiologically to aberrant neuronal sprouting, late denervation hypersensitivity, or ephaptic transmission.[94,138] After combined injury to pyramidal and extrapyramidal systems, prominent hemiparesis and dystonia persist; this variant is termed *spastic dystonia*.[79] Another variant of posttraumatic hemidystonia is paroxysmal nocturnal dystonia, which can improve with acetazolamide.[15] Pathophysiologically, this form of dystonia may relate to aberrant myelination, similar to paroxysmal dystonias of multiple sclerosis that also respond to acetozolamide.[148] Paroxysmal nocturnal dystonia may also be potentially caused by a cortical lesion. Lombroso[109] described a case of paroxysmal nocturnal dystonia associated with focal cortical dysplasia; the dystonic symptoms relented after surgical excision of the dysplastic cortex. Like the instances cited above regarding cortical resection and torticollis, this observation suggests that trauma-related cortical lesions may play a role in the pathophysiology of dystonic syndromes.

The treatment of posttraumatic focal dystonia or hemidystonia after severe head injury has been a difficult pharmacological challenge. When spasticity accompanies the dystonia, oral baclofen or baclofen intrathecal pumps have been used.[120,128] Anticholinergic agents and botulinum toxin injections to the most involved body regions have also been used with modest success.[81] More promising, stereotaxic surgery has been used, with short-term reported successes.[93] The targets for hemidystonia are generally the contralateral ventrolateral thalamus, the globus pallidus internal segement, and the subthalamic nucleus.[95,126] Whereas most experience has focused on lesions, deep brain stimulation has been used in some reports with short-term success.[149]

An increasing emphasis has been placed on local trauma to a body part that subsequently develops dystonic posturing. Gowers described a local neck injury that led to torticollis and noted that a patient with writer's cramp had previously sprained his thumb.[64] In a literature review of torticollis and other forms of focal dystonia, Sheehy and Marsden found that 9% of patients had preceding local neck injuries. In some cases, the trauma was very minor and predated the first complaints of torticollis by years.[151] Other examples of peripherally induced dystonia are cases of oromandibular spasms that develop after facial trauma, dental manipulations or oral surgeries. In one report, restricted to cases developing within one year after such events, the mean time of onset of dystonia occurred after 65 days with a range of one day to one year. 37% of these patients had predisposing conditions for the development of oromandibular dystonia such as family history, exposure to neuroleptics or dystonia in other anatomical areas.[142] This issue of predisposing factors echoes other reports suggesting that trauma can precipitate dystonia in a predisposed person or may induce the spread of clinical dysfunction.[20] One case history described a subject who developed foot dystonia at age 38 after local trauma. Foot dystonia is a sign typical of childhood-onset DTY1 generalized dystonia but is a very rare clinical problem in adults.[19] Though previously asymptomatic, the patient progressed in disability and developed spasmodic dysphonia in addition to his foot dystonia. On genetic testing, the DYT 1 mutation was found and other family members were found to be affected by early-onset dystonia.[44]

Fletcher and colleagues found that among 104 patients with idiopathic generalized torsion dystonia, 16.4% had a history of exacerbation or precipitation of dystonia after peripheral injuries that included surgery, lacerations, fractures, and contusions.[53] If trauma preceded the first sign of dystonia, the posttraumatic dystonic movements appeared first in the injured area of the body and started within 1 year of the trauma. One report focused on different patterns of cervical dystonia that developed with short or long latencies after injury. In the group that developed symptoms immediately after trauma, local pain, marked limitation of neck and shoulder range of motion, abnormal neck postures without phasic compensatory movements, prominent shoulder elevation, and marked trapezius hypertropy occurred. Other muscles were not generally involved in dystonic spasms, no *geste antagoniste* was found, no increase in dystonia with activation occurred, and the pain persisted even after botulinum toxin treatment. There was usually no evidence of radiculopathy or myelopathy on neuroimaging or electromyography (EMG). In contrast, among the patients whose posttraumatic cervical dystonia occurred with a latency of more than 3 months, the clinical presentation was indistinguishable from that of idiopathic cervical dystonia, where onset was gradual, pain was less marked, multiple muscles were involved, and botulinum toxin, when used, was effective.[72,166,167,189]

The posttraumatic shoulder elevation dystonia syndrome has been a controversial topic. Tarsy[166] noted that all patients with shoulder elevation dystonia were involved either in worker's compensation or personal injury litigation. Sa et al.[136] investigated 16 patients with shoulder elevation dystonia and found features suggestive of psychogenic etiology: intravenous sodium amytal not only improved the posture and normalized pain in the majority of patients but also demonstrated absence of trapezius hypertrophy. This report concluded that all patients had psychological conflicts and considered them externalized into somatic manifestations. Further, although the patients reported that dystonia did not improve while sleeping, independent monitoring during sleep often revealed improved posture. Sa et al.[136] proposed classifying this disorder as *posttraumatic painful torticollis* rather than dystonia until more precise information and pathophysiological studies are available.

The pathophysiology of dystonia induced by peripheral nervous system trauma remains inadequately delineated, and studies of the phenomenon are limited by the absence of a good animal model of focal dystonia. Schott has suggested that spinal cord sensory inputs that are organized at the segmental level may be aberrant after injury.[145] The prominent feature of pain in trauma-induced dystonia also calls attention to the sensory system as a potential pathophysiological key.

Reflex sympathetic dystrophy, currently referred to as *complex regional pain syndrome* (CRPS), has been reported to occur in up to 35% of patients with peripheral nerve injuries and fractures.[182] A separate discussion of this topic is included in this volume (see Chapter 24). In addition to the boring pain of causalgia and the trophic skin changes that are classic manifestations of this syndrome, numerous motor aberrations have also been reported.[10,177] Since sometimes these motor signs include typical forms of movement disorders, the possibility of a link between physiological sympathetic nervous dysfunction and movement disorders has been suggested. Recent developments substantiate the connection between CRPS and movement disorders, especially dystonia. Van Hilten et al.[181] reported a series of 26 patients who developed CRPS (10 patients after peripheral injury or surgery), with subsequent multifocal and generalized tonic dystonia. These patients had common clinical features: most were young women (mean age 35, mean disease duration 11 years), the limb posture was flexor, and the patients had significant autonomic disturbances. In addition, there was a statistically significant association with human leukocyte antigen (HLA) type DR13.[180] Further, a genetic marker was identified that may differentiate between the patients who develop dystonia and CRPS after injury and spontaneously.[176] On the other hand, the patients in the same cohort had nonanatomical sensory deficits and elevated Minnesota Multiphasic Personality Inventory-2 (MMPI-2) scores (although in a nonspecific pattern common to other chronic diseases) evoke concerns about a significant psychogenic component in several of these cases.[177,179,181]

Abnormal postures that resemble dystonia can also occur after trauma and relate to peripheral nerve or nonneurological injury. Scherokman et al. reported cases of peripheral neuropathies and entrapment syndromes that presented as abnormal postures of apparently dystonic character; the clear abnormalities on EMG studies and the accompanying weakness of peripheral nerve origin distinguished these cases.[143] Extraocular palsy, specifically involving the fourth cranial nerve, can cause a head tilt that resembles torticollis. Although diplopia is the cardinal feature of the syndrome, the posture of the neck may suggest a primary movement disorder. Similarly, posttraumatic occipital lobe lesions that cause hemianopsia may cause secondary head turning to maximize the visual fields. The patient's consciousness of the visual field defect will depend largely on the degree of macular involvement of the hemianopsia.

Of nonneurological origin, atlantoaxial dislocation or subluxation (Grissell's syndrome) after neck injuries, often whiplash car accidents, will provoke a tilted neck posture and should be recognized by the fixed posture and lack of resolution during sleep. This syndrome is felt to be due to tearing and invagination of capsular ligaments about the atlantoaxial synovial joints.[162] Radiological evaluations will define the bony deformations of the clinical syndrome. Severe local injury can tear muscles and lead to unopposed contraction by antagonist muscles with resultant posturing of the injured body part. This syndrome is associated with extreme pain, evidence of soft tissue injury, and CT evidence of late formation of fibrosis.[29b] Treatment may necessitate surgical ligation of fibrotic bands with rehabilitative physical therapy.[146] Importantly, often airway or otorhinilaryngological infection in children with high fever can precipitate Grisell's syndrome.[18] In a series of 13 children presenting within 48 hours of the development of torticollis in this context, only 3 had the radiological evidence of atlantoaxial sublaxation The authors postulated that rotational deformity is the first stage in the development of Grisell's syndrome and, if left untreated, will progress to atlantoaxial subluxation. Early recognition and treatment of acute torticollis presenting in the setting of a febrile illness in children can prevent the development of Grisell's syndrome.[121]

Chorea, Choreoathetosis, and Ballismus

Chorea is a rapid, unpredictable body movement that generally spreads from one muscle group to another. When twisted movements accompany the rapid jerk, the term *choreoathetosis* is used. Ballismus involves large-amplitude and proximal, rather than distal, movements of the same character. The neuroanatomical areas of interest for chorea, choreoathetosis, and ballismus include the striatum, subthalamic nucleus, and anterior thalamus[39,73,89,114,152] Most cases of these posttraumatic hyperkinesias have involved blunt head trauma without direct, obvious injury to subcortical structures. Body injury has not been regularly hypothesized to play a role, although an elderly patient fell several meters, landed on his feet without head injury, and developed immediate hemiballismus.[114] With this latter notable exception, most cases of chorea, choreoathetosis, and ballismus in association with trauma have occurred days, weeks, or months after injury.

Chandra[28] described a 9-year-old boy who fell approximately 36 feet, became comatose, and showed signs of left cerebral damage. During the next 4 months, he developed choreoathetoid movements of his right arm in addition to right-sided spastic hemiplegia. Computed tomography revealed a large, hypodense lesion within the left hemisphere with ventricular dilatation. Electroencephalographic activity did not coincide with the choreic movements. Whereas phenytoin and phenobarbital treatment had no effect, the involuntary movements resolved within 12 hours of valproate therapy. Lodder and Ballard[108] described a patient who experienced mild head trauma without signs of concussion and developed involuntary ballistic movements of the left arm over 3 days. Two days later, all four extremities, the head, and the trunk became choreic and ballistic. Although both subthalamic nuclei were normal, CT scans showed bilateral hyperdensities in the head of the caudate nucleus and thalamus. Haloperidol ameliorated the movements, which did not return following discontinuation of the medication.

Additionally, chorea has rarely been associated with reports of subdural hematomas following blunt head trauma, although these cases were complicated by other medical conditions. Kotagal et al.[90] reported an elderly man with known frequent falling and head injury who developed bilateral proximal and distal upper extremity choreoathetosis and intermittent tongue undulations in association with bilateral subdural hematomas. All movements diminished during sleep. Computed tomography showed no additional abnormalities of basal ganglia structures, and all movements ceased following surgical drainage. Although the investigators suggested that obstruction of cerebral blood flow to motor cortex or the diencephalon occurred by external compression, the patient also had diabetes, and small vessel cerebrovascular disease could have played a role in the chorea.[90] Choreic movements occurred in another patient with a past history of subdural hematoma associated with head injury, although the movement disorder developed after the hematoma was drained.[43] Martin alluded to cases of subdural hematomas and contralateral chorea but gave no specific details.[114]

Trauma has been linked to paroxysmal choreoathetosis in which sudden and intermittent involuntary movements develop spontaneously or when patients volitionally move. A 33-year-old physician suffered multiple injuries following ejection from an aircraft and was unconscious for 20 minutes. Eight months later, when rising to a standing position, he experienced sudden choreoathetotic postures with involuntary adduction and internal rotation of the left upper extremity with flexion at the elbow. These movements lasted for 5–10 seconds and were preceded by poorly characterized paresthesias. Phenobarbital suppressed the movements, which later resolved without further treatment. One case of a penetrating wound to the frontal cortex also caused a similar action-induced involuntary posture of the contralateral body lasting for a few seconds.[133] Other cases involved paroxysmal movements of similar character lasting for several minutes and not specifically action-induced.[43] The pathophysiology of paroxysmal dyskinesia is controversial, and investigators are not certain whether this condition is an unusual form of epilepsy or a primary movement disorder related to putative aberrant ephaptic transmission involving basal ganglia structures.

Choreoathetosis may occur not only in the setting of cranial injury but also after spinal trauma. Tan et al.[165] described a 62-year-old woman who developed bilateral dystonic posturing at rest and choreoathetoid movements while extending her hands. The patient was found to have spinal cervical cord compression due to C3-C4 disc herniation. Three months after surgery the patient's choreoathetoid movements resolved. Syringomyelia is a common sequaela of spinal injury, occurring in up to 25% of patients.[21] Involuntary movements are common in patients with syringomyelia. Nogues et al.[125] described a series of 100 patients with a syrinx confirmed by MRI, although only 5 patients had posttraumatic syringomyelia. Twenty-percent of the patients had a variety of involuntary movements on examination consisting of segmental spinal myoclonus, propriospinal myoclonus, and dystonic athetoid limb posturing in one patient. Hill et al.[71] described a patient who developed right-hand choreoathetoid movements due to congenital syrinx, and Ghika and Bogousslavsky[57] reported bilateral athetosis in a patient with syrinx due to intramedullary tumor. The common motif was resolution of symptoms after drainage of the cavity and reappearance of symptoms upon cavity reaccumulation. The dysfunction of spinal gray matter interneurons activated by aberrant sensory stimuli was postulated to be a possible mechanism of choreoathetoid movements in syringomyelia patients.[71] Alternatively, Ghika and Bogousslavsky[57] suggested that lack of striatal sensory input due to spinal pathway interruption may be responsible for the "spinal pseudoathetosis."

Tics and Gilles de la Tourette Syndrome

A few case reports and anecdotes about trauma and tics exist.[47,51,93,153,154] In most instances, these concern adults who have developed unusual tics after head trauma ranging from mild to severe, with prolonged loss of consciousness. The tics have developed within months of the trauma. Most are cases of new tics, although exacerbation of existing tics has been reported.[89] Recently, Krauss and Jankovic[92] described three adult patients who developed complex tic disorder following craniocerebral trauma sustained in motor vehicle accidents. The latency varied from 1 day to several months. One patient had preceding tics (*sniffing*) and developed vocal and multifocal motor tics immediately following head trauma with brief loss of consciousness. Another patient developed multifocal motor tics and vocalizations within 1 day after a mild head injury without loss of consciousness. Of note, this patient had had a hemiatrophy and mild left hemiparesis since birth. The third patient was involved in two motor vehicle accidents (5 years apart), with subsequent prolonged loss of consciousness. In addition to multifocal motor and vocal tics, this patient exhibited obsessive-compulsive traits and cognitive difficulties commensurate with bifrontal damage. The MRI scan demonstrated cortical atrophy and extensive periventricular and subcortical leukoencephalopathy that was especially pronounced on the right-hand side but no involvement of the basal ganglia. Similarly, two recent reports from the pediatric literature describe patients who developed tics after sustaining cortical or subcortical damage. Yochelson and David[190] described a 16-year-old right-handed boy with left frontal arteriovenous malformation (AVM) who sustained left frontal intraparenchimal and subdural hemorrhage following resection of the AVM. The mechanism of insult may be similar to posttraumatic changes (hemorrhage), although this patient did not sustain the injury per se. The patient developed vocalizations and complex motor tics in the immediate postoperative period that were thought to be complex partial seizures. The patient's EEG revealed left temporal slowing but no epileptiform activity. The patient failed carbamazepine therapy but responded well to clonidine. He reported the urge to perform the tics, and he had supressibility. Majumdar and Appleton[111] described a 7-year-old girl who developed a tic disorder 15 months after severe head injury (Glasgow Coma Scale score of 4). She remained comatose for 7 days. The immediate damage consisted of left intraventricular and left internal capsule hemorrhage. The patient had mild right hemiparesis, ataxic gait, dysarthric speech, and behavioral problems. Twenty-four-hour video EEG monitoring revealed slowing in the left frontotemporal area but no epileptiform activity after the onset of tics. The MRI scan performed 16 months after the initial injury revealed an infarct encompassing the left putamen, globus pallidus, head of the caudate, and internal capsule. The left frontotemporal cortex was thinned. The child responded well to haloperidol, so much so that it was gradually withdrawn after 12 months. These cases illustrate the hypothesis that tic disorders may be caused by cortical lesions or derangements in the cortico-pallido-thalamocortical connections, as postulated by Leckman et al.[103]

Tics, like other movement disorders, can be associated with peripheral injury. Factor and Molho[48] presented two adult patients who developed focal tics subsequent to focal body injury, with tics arising in the injured body area. The latency varied from several days to several months. One patient had a family history of tics, suggesting that the patient was at genetic risk for a tic disorder and that the trauma precipitated or brought attention to previously inconsequential tics. Whereas some patients with peripheral trauma had both vocalizations and motor tics, only Ericksson and Persson and Fahn's cases fulfilled diagnostic criteria for Gilles de la Tourette syndrome.[47,51] Since tics are a frequent neurological feature in the general population, the actual causal role of trauma is difficult to assess from these case histories. Sometimes the relationship between trauma and tics is reversed and there are reported cases of violent complex tics, especially involving the head and neck, that cause sufficient neck trauma to induce cervical myelopathy.[41,59,91]

Myoclonus

Myoclonus is less well characterized than the other movement disorders, and the term is used to describe brief, lightning-like involuntary jerks sufficient in amplitude to move joints.[184] These movements may be focal or generalized, rhythmic or arrhythmic. In further characterizing myoclonus, Marsden has proposed the classification based on the neuroanatomical location of the causative dysfunction: cortical, reticular (brain stem), including pallidal, or spinal.[112,158] Trauma has been linked as a possible etiology to all categories. Although usually of central origin, myoclonus has also been reported in isolated reports with trauma of the peripheral nerves[137] and brachial plexus.[5] Recent case reports have described myoclonic-like activity developing in the wrist and foot after 1 month and 18 months after the initial insult, respectively. The common motif is damage to a peripheral nerve causing myoclonic activity in the distribution of another branch without an anatomical connection, thus implicating the central relay mechanism.[4,58,117] Myoclonic jerks can also be seen in the context of epilepsy (myoclonic epilepsy and epilepsy partialis continua) and anoxia,[52,101] but these conditions, even if associated with a past history of trauma, are not considered in this discussion.

Patients with trauma-induced cortical myoclonus without anoxia or epilepsy may demonstrate action myoclonus with body and extremity jerks that occur or increase when the patient attempts to move. Such movements are similar to those seen in postanoxic myoclonus and often cause patients to drop or involuntarily throw objects and fall due to jerking leg movements. A special form of myoclonus is palatal myoclonus, a rare movement disorder characterized by continuous, rhythmic contractions of the soft palate, usually persisting during sleep.[78,118,150,172] In a review by Deuschl et al. of 287 patients with rhythmic palatal myoclonus, 210 were of known causes, and of these, 23 related to various head and neck injuries. The latency of onset from the inciting event varied from immediate to longer than 2 years.[38] These movements are usually refractory to pharmacological therapy. Few anatomical studies have been performed. A 60-year-old patient who had a motor vehicle accident with loss of consciousness, left hemiparesis, and a Glasgow Coma Scale score of 6, showed T2 hyperintensities in the right midbrain and the right frontoparietal region, as well as hypertrophy of the bilateral inferior olivary nuclei on MRI. When he awoke, he developed postural and intention tremor in the left upper extremity, and later in the right one, and had symptomatic bilateral palatal myoclonus.[6] Thalamic lesions may also produce segmental myoclonus. Jacob and Chad[76] described a patient who sustained a right posterolateral thalamic hemorrhage following a motor vehicle accident and loss of consciousness for 15 days. The patient had action-induced myoclonic activity of the contralateral left lower extremity and, to a lesser extent, the left upper extremity. Birbamer et al. have reported three young adult patients who developed segmental myoclonus following motor vehicle accidents with severe head trauma.[16] All patients were acutely comatose and thereafter remained in an *apallic* state with concomitant hemiparesis or tetraparesis. Ten to 18 months after the trauma, rhythmic segmental myoclonus involving the palate, pharynx, and perioral muscles developed. Two patients additionally demonstrated synchronous involuntary myoclonic movements of the upper extremities.

Brain MRI scans revealed a consistent bilateral enlargement and increased signal intensity of the inferior olives on T2-weighted images. The authors suggested that the neuroimaging findings and the delay in onset of the myoclonus were related in part to inferior olivary nucleus denervation hypersensitivity with a heightened response to normal levels of circulating neurotransmitters.

Spinal myoclonus, although rare, has been associated with trauma.[188] Typically, these patients experience myoclonic jerks in muscle groups supplied by one or more segments of the cord contiguous to the lesion. Less commonly, myoclonus in muscle supplied by levels of the spinal cord well below the lesion has been described.[107] Bussel et al. reported a case of a 23-year-old man with MRI-proven complete transection of the cord at the C6-7 level. Fifteen months after the injury, rhythmic extension movements of the trunk and lower limbs developed. These movements occurred spontaneously or with external stimulation. Treatment with carbamazepine or valproate abolished the myoclonus.[26] Posttraumatic lingular myoclonus has also been described.[170]

Other Movement Disorders

Painful legs and moving toes syndrome, first described by Spillane et al., is characterized by persistent, involuntary, and irregular movements of the toes and feet, usually preceded by a deep, burning pain. In the initial description, trauma was alluded to as a possible underlying cause, and subsequent reports have reinforced this observation.[123,144,157] The injuries sustained by patients are seemingly inconsequential and have included minor lacerations,[123] sprained Achilles tendon, and traumatic hematomas of the foot.[144] The latency of onset after trauma is variable, ranging from 3 months to 10 years after injury. Presently, this condition is called *restless legs syndrome*, and an effective treatment with dopamine agonists is available.[32] There were several reports of restless legs syndrome/periodic limb movements developing after spinal cord injury, although some cases were due to malignancy or multiple sclerosis rather than trauma per se.[23] The symptoms were responsive to dopaminergic medication.[36,104,187] Tings et al.[168] suggested impairment of the sensory spinal pathways as a possible etiology. Hemifacial spasm, a syndrome characterized by brief, involuntary, episodic clonic jerks or twitches of muscles innervated by the seventh cranial nerve, has been rarely associated with trauma. Martinelli et al. described two patients who developed symptoms typical of hemifacial spasm 1 year following minor lacerations of the face.[115] Later, they described four more cases of hemifacial spasm occurring within 1 year after peripheral laceration of the facial nerve.[116] These cases, however are distinctly uncommon, and in a series of 1688 patients with hemifacial spasms, only 2 cases were attributable to trauma.[40]

Painful jumping dyskinesias of amputation stumps were first described during the Civil War period and have been attributed to trauma of various types.[134,159,185] The dyskinesias involve rapid jerking movements of the stump and are associated with pain and often with the perception of a sustained dystonic posture of the phantom limb.[82] The origin of observed and phantom limb dyskinesias is not fully understood, but may relate to aberrant healing and ephaptic transmission between somatic nerve circuits, possibly involving sympathetic fibers.[7] In this context, there may be overlap with reflex sympathetic dystrophy, in which involuntary movements have also been described after trauma.[163] Patients with muscle spasms and jumpy amputation stumps, yet without neuropathic pain or phantom sensations, have also been reported.[100]

Conclusions and Future Perspectives

Trauma can be cited as a cause of several movement disorders, but this association is rare and the resultant syndromes usually include additional signs that are not typical of the idiopathic movement disorders. Most instances of confirmed trauma-induced or -exacerbated movement disorders show lesions on CT or MRI scans of cerebral or basal ganglia structures. The role of trauma in movement disorders will be more clearly delineated as good animal models of human conditions are developed. Since complete nervous system evaluations are not routinely included in general screening physical examinations, baseline neurological function that precedes trauma is rarely known. More comprehensive and standardized well-patient examinations of children and adults could correct this limitation and provide important baseline information for future assessments. In this capacity, health maintenance organizations, the military, and other centralized health systems could potentially play leadership roles.

ACKNOWLEDGMENTS

This work was supported in part by the Parkinson's Disease Foundation.

REFERENCES

1. Aisen ML, Holzer M, Rosen M, Dietz M, et al: Glutethimide treatment of disabling action tremor in patients with multiple sclerosis and traumatic brain injury. Arch Neurol 48(5):513–515, 1991.
2. Anderson TE, Lighthall JW: An evaluation of experimental brain injury models: Need for continuing development. In: Hoff J, Anderson T, Cole T (eds): Mild to Moderate Head Injury. Boston, Blackwell Scientific, 1989, p 77.
3. Andrew J, Fowler CJ, Harrision MJG: Tremor after head injury and its treatment by stereotaxic surgery. J Neurol Neurosurg Psychiatry 45:815–819, 1982.
4 Assal F, Magistris MR, Vingerhoets FJ. Post-traumatic stimulus suppressible myoclonus of peripheral origin. J Neurol Neurosurg Psychiatry 64(5):673–675, 1998.
5. Banks G, Nielsen VK, Short MP, et al: Brachial plexus myoclonus. J Neurol Neurosurg Psychiatry 48:582–584, 1985.
6. Bansal B, Singh P, Shukla R. Palatal myoclonus following head injury (letter to the editor). Neurol India 50(2): 222–223, 2002.
7. Beacham WS, Pearl ER: Characteristics of a spinal sympathetic reflex. J Physiol (Lond) 173:431–448, 1964.
8. Benabid A, Pollak P, Gervason C, et al: Long-term suppression of tremor by chronic stimulation of the ventral intermediate thalamic nucleus. Lancet 337:403, 1991.
9. Bernheimer H, Birkmayer W, Hornykiewicz O, et al: Brain dopamine and the syndromes of Parkinson and Huntington. Clinical, morphological and neurochemical correlations. J Neurol Sci 20:415–455, 1973.
10 Bhatia KP, Bhatt MH, Marsden CD: Causalgia-dystonia syndrome. Brain 116:843–851, 1993.
11. Bhatt M, Desai J, Mankodi A, Elias M, Wadia N: Post-traumatic akinetic-rigid syndrome resembling Parkinson's disease: A report on three patients. Mov Disord 15(2):313–317, 2000.
12. Bower JH, Maraganore DM, Peterson BJ, McDonnell SK, Ahlskog JE, Rocca WA: Head trauma preceding PD: A case-control study. Neurology 60(10):1610–1615, 2003.
13. Boyeson MG, Jones JL, Harmon RL: Sparing of motor function after cortical injury. Arch Neurol 54:405–414, 1995.
14. Biary N, Cleeves L, Findley L, et al: Post-traumatic tremor. Neurology 39:103–106, 1989.
15. Biary N, Singh B, Bahou Y, AlDeeb SM, Sharif H: Posttraumatic paroxysmal nocturnalhemidystonia. Mov Disord 9:98–99, 1994.
16. Birbamer G, Gerstenbrand F, Kofler M, Buchberger W, Felber S, Aichner F: Post-traumatic segmental myoclonus associated with bilateral olivary hypertrophy. Acta Neurol Scand 87:505, 1993.
17. Bramlett HM, Dietrich WD: Synuclein aggregation: Possible role in traumatic brain injury. Exp Neurol 184(1):27–30, 2003.
18. Bredenkamp JK, Maceri DR: Inflammatory torticollis in children. Arch Otolaryngol Head Neck Surg 116(3): 310–313, 1990.
19. Bressman SB: Dystonia: Phenotypes and genotypes. Rev Neurol (Paris) 159(10 pt 1):849–856, 2003.
20. Brin MP, Fahn S, Bressman SB, Burke RE: Dystonia precipitated by peripheral trauma. Neurology 36(suppl 1):119, 1986.
21. Brodbelt AR, Stoodley MA: Post-traumatic syringomyelia: A review. J Clin Neurosci 10(4):401–408, 2003.
22. Brooks DJ, Ibanez V, Sawle GV, Quinn N, Lees AJ, Mathias CJ, et al: Differing patterns of striatal 18F-dopa uptake in Parkinson's disease, multiple system atrophy, and progressive supranuclear palsy. Ann Neurol 28(4): 547–555, 1990.
23. Brown LK, Heffner JE, Obbens EA: Transverse myelitis associated with restless legs syndrome and periodic movements of sleep responsive to an oral dopaminergic agent but not to intrathecal baclofen. Sleep 23(5):591–594, 2000.
24. Bucy PC: Relation to abnormal involuntary movements. In: Bucy PC (ed): The Precentral Motor Cortex, 2nd ed. Urbana, University of Illinois Press, 1949, p 395.
25. Burke RE, Fahn S, Gold AD: Delayed onset dystonia in patients with "static" encephalopathy. J Neurol Neurosurg Psychiatry 43:489–497, 1980.
26. Bussel B, Roby-Brami A, Azouvi P, Biraben A, Yakovleff A, Held JP: Myoclonus in a patient with spinal cord transection. Possible involvement of the spinal stepping generator. Brain; 111(pt 5):1235–1245, 1988.
27. Cardoso F, Jankovic J: Peripherally induced tremor and parkinsonism. Arch Neurol 52(3):263–270, 1995.
28. Chandra V: Treatment of post-traumatic choreoathetosis with sodium valproate. J Neurol Neurosurg Psychiatry 46:963–965, 1983.
29a. Charcot J-M: Lecon 5. De la paralysie agitante. In: Oeuvres Complètes, vol. 1, Paris, Bureaux du Progrès Mèdical, 1892, pp 155–189. (In English: On paralysis agitans. In: Sigerson G [trans]: Lectures on Diseases of the Nervous System. Philadelphia, H.C. Lea and Company, 1879, pp. 105–127.
29b. Chiapparini 1, Zorzi 6, deSimone T, et al: Persistent fixed torticollis due to atlanto-axial rotarory fixation. Neuropediatrics 36:45–49, 2005.

30. Cohen G, Dembiec D, Mytilineou C, et al: Oxygen radicals and the integrity of the nigrostrital tract. In: Birkmayer W, Hornykiewicz O (eds): Advances in Parkinsonism. Basle, Editions Roche, 1975, pp 251–257.
31. Cole JD, Illis LS, Sedgewick EM: Unilateral essential tremor after wrist immobilization: A case report. J Neurol Neurosurg Psychiatry 52:286–287, 1989.
32. Comella CL: Restless legs syndrome: Treatment with dopaminergic agents. Neurology 58(4 suppl 1):S87–S92, 2002.
33. Crouzon O, Justin-Besaucow L: Le parkinsonisme traumatique. Presse Med 37:1325–1327, 1929.
34. David M, Hecaen H, Constans T: Torticollis spasmodique consecutif à une lesion certicule traumatique discussion de resultant favorable obtenu excision de la lesion corticale. Rev Neurol 86:57–61, 1952.
35. Deane JR: Galloping tongue: Post-traumatic, episodic, rhythmic movements. Neurology 34:251–252, 1984.
36. de Mello MT, Poyares DL, Tufik S: Treatment of periodic leg movements with a dopaminergic agonist in subjects with total spinal cord lesions. Spinal Cord 37(9): 634–637, 1999.
37. de Recondo A, Rondot P, Loch C, et al: Unilateral post-traumatic mesencephalic tremor: A PET study of striatal dopaminergic innervation. Rev Neurol 149:46, 1993.
38. Deuschl G, Mischke G, Schenck E, Schulte-Monting J, Lucking CH: Symptomatic and essential rhythmic palatal myoclonus. Brain 113(pt 6):1645–1672, 1990.
39. Diersen G, Bergman LL, Gioino G, et al: Hemiballismus following surgery for Parkinson disease. Arch Neurol Psychiatry 5:627–637, 1961.
40. Digre K, Corbett JJ: Hemifacial spasm: Differential diagnosis, mechanism, and treatment. Adv Neurol 49: 151–176, 1988.
41. Dobbs M, Berger JR: Cervical myelopathy secondary to violent tics of Tourette's syndrome. Neurology 60(11): 1862–1863, 2003.
42. Doder M, Jahanshahi M, Turjanski N, Moseley IF, Lees AJ: Parkinson's syndrome after closed head injury: A single case report. J Neurol Neurosurg Psychiatry 66(3):380–385, 1999.
43. Drake ME, Jackson RD, Miller CH: Paroxysmal choreoathetosis after head injury J Neurol Neurosurg Psychiatry 49:837–843, 1986.
44. Edwards M, Wood N, Bhatia K: Unusual phenotypes in DYT1 dystonia: A report of five cases and a review of the literature. Mov Disord 18(6):706–711, 2003.
45. Ellis SJ: Tremor and other movement disorders after whiplash type injuries. J Neurol Neurosurg Psychiatry 63(1):110–112, 1997.
46. Ellison PH: Propranolol for severe post-head injry action tremor. Neurology 28:197–199, 1978.
47. Eriksson B, Persson T: Gilles de la Tourette's syndrome: Two cases with an organic brain injury. Br J Psychiatry 115:351–353, 1969.
48. Factor SA, Molho ES: Adult-onset tics associated with peripheral injury. Mov Disord 12(6):1052–1055, 1997.
49. Factor SA, Sanchez-Ramos J, Weiner WJ: Trauma as an etiology of parkinsonism: A historical review of the concept. Mov Disord 3:30–36, 1988.
50. Factor SA, Weiner WJ: Prior history of head trauma in Parkinson's disease. Mov Disord 6(3):225–229, 1991.
51. Fahn S: The clinical spectrum of motor tics. In: Friedhoff AJ, Chanse TN (eds): Gilles de la Tourette Syndrome (Advances in Neurology, vol 35). New York, Raven Press, 1982, pp 341–344.
52. Fahn S: Post-hypoxic action myoclonus: Literature review update. Adv Neurol 43:157–169, 1986.
53. Fletcher NA, Harding AE, Marsden CD: The relationship between trauma and idiopathic torsion dystonia. J Neurol Neurosurg Psychiatry 54:713–717, 1991.
54. Fox JL, Kurtzke JL: Trauma-induced intention tremor relieved by stereotaxic thalamotomy. Arch Neurol 15:247, 1966.
55. Friedman JH: Progressive parkinsonism in boxers. South Med J 82(no. 5):543–546, 1989.
56. Gerstenbrand F, Lucking CH, Peters G, et al: Cerebellar symptoms as sequelae of traumatic lesions of upper brain stem and cerebellum. Int J Neurol 7:271, 1970.
57. Ghika J, Bogousslavsky J: Spinal pseudoathetosis: A rare, forgotten syndrome, with a review of old and recent descriptions. Neurology 49(2):432–437, 1997.
58. Glocker FX, Deuschl G, Volk B, Hasse J, Lucking CH: Bilateral myoclonus of the trapezius muscles after distal lesion of an accessory nerve. Mov Disord 11(5):571–575, 1996.
59. Goetz CG, Klawans HL: Gilles de la Tourette syndrome and compressive neuropathies. Ann Neurol 8(4):453, 1980.
60. Goetz CG, Klawans HL, Tanner CM: Movement disorders induced by neuroleptic drugs. In: Shah RS (ed): Neuroleptic Drugs. New York, Grune and Stratton, 1986, pp 302–320.
61. Goetz CG, Stebbins GT: Effects of head trauma from motor vehicle accidents on Parkinson's disease. Ann Neurol 29:191–193, 1991.
62. Goldman MS, Kelley PJ: Symptomatic and functional outcome of stereotactic ventralis lateralis thalamotomy for intention tremor. J Neurosurg 77:223, 1992.
63. Goodwin-Austen RB, Lee DN, Marmot MG, et al: Smoking and Parkinson's disease. J Neurol Neurosurg Psychiatry 44:577–581, 1982.
64. Gowers WR: Manual of Diseases of the Nervous System, vol II. Darien, CT, Hofner, 1893.
65. Grimberg L: Paralysis agitans and trauma. J Nerv Ment Dis 79:14–42, 1934.
66. Halliwell B: Oxidants and the central nervous system: Some fundamental questions. Is oxidant damage relevant to Parkinson's disease, Alzheimer's disease, traumatic injury or stroke? Acta Neurol Scand Suppl 126: 23–33, 1989.
67. Harmon RL, Long DF, Shirtz J: Treatment of post-traumatic midbrain resting kinetic tremor with combined levodopa/carbidopa and carbamazepine. Brain Inj 5(2):213–218, 1991.
68. Hashimoto T, Sato H, Shindo M, Hayashi R, Ikeda S:

Peripheral mechanisms in tremor after traumatic neck injury. J Neurol Neurosurg Psychiatry 73(5):585–587, 2002.
69. Herbaut AG, Soeur M: Two other cases of unilateral essential tremor induced by peripheral trauma. J Neurol Neurosurg Psychiatry 52:1213, 1989.
70. Heyde W: Zur Frage des traumatischen Parkinsonismus, zugleich ein Beitrag zur kenntnis extrapyramidalmotorischer Störungen nach Hirnverletzungen. Arch Psychiatr 97:600–643, 1932.
71. Hill MD, Kumar R, Lozano A, Tator CH, Ashby P, Lang AE: Syringomyelic dystonia and athetosis. Mov Disord 14(4):684–688, 1999.
72. Hollinger P, Burgunder J: Posttraumatic focal dystonia of the shoulder. Eur Neurol 44(3):153–155, 2000.
73. Hughes B: Involuntary movements following stereotactic operations. J Neurol Neurosurg Psychiatry 28:291–303, 1965.
74. Isaac K, Cohen JA: Post-traumatic torticollis. Neurology 39:1642–1643, 1989.
75. Iwadate Y, Saeki N, Namba H, et al: Post-traumatic intention tremor: Clinical features and CT findings. Neurosurg Rev 12(suppl 1):500–507, 1989.
76. Jacob PC, Chand RP: A posttraumatic thalamic lesion associated with contralateral action myoclonus. Mov Disord 14(3):512–514, 1999.
77. Jacob PC, Pratap Chand R: Posttraumatic rubral tremor responsive to clonazepam. Mov Disord 13(6):977–978, 1998.
78. Jacobson MP, Garman VI: Palatal myoclonus and primary nystagmus following trauma. Arch Neurol Psychiatry 62:798–801, 1949.
79. Jankovic J: Posttraumatic movement disorders. In: Jankovic J (ed): Movement Disorders. Minneapolis, American Academy of Neurology Publications, 1994, pp 19–35.
80. Jankovic J: Post-traumatic movement disorders: Central and peripheral mechanisms. Neurology 44:2006–2014, 1994.
81. Jancovic J, Brin M: Therapeutic uses of botulinum toxin. N Engl J Med 324:1186–1194, 1991.
82. Jankovic J, Glass JP: Metoclopramide-induced phantom dyskinesia. Neurology 35:432–435, 1985.
83. Jankovic J, Schwartz K: Botulinum toxin treatment of tremors. Neurology 41:1185, 1991.
84. Jellinger K, Seitelberger F: Protracted posttraumatic encephalopathy, pathology and clinical observations. In: Walker AE, Caveness WF, Critchley M (eds): The Late Effects of Head Injury. Springfield, IL, Charles C. Thomas, 1969, pp 118–132.
85. Jenkins LW, Lyeth BG, Hayes RL: The role of agonist–receptor interactions in the pathophysiology of mild and moderate head injury. In: Hoff J, Anderson T, Cole T (eds): Mild to Moderate Head Injury. Boston, Blackwell Scientific, 1989, p 47.
86. Jenkins WM, Merzenich MM, Recanzone G: Neocortical representational dynamics in adult primates. Neurospsychologia 28:573–584, 1990.
87. Klempel K: Gilles de la Tourette's symptoms induced by L-dopa. S Afr Med J 48:1379–1380, 1974.
88. Koller WC, Nausieda PA, Weiner WJ, et al: The pharmacology of ballismus. Clin Neuropharm 4:157–174, 1979.
89. Koller WC, Wong GF, Lang A: Posttraumatic movement disorders: A review. Mov Disord 4:20–36, 1989.
90. Kotagal S, Shuter E, Horenstein S: Chorea as a manifestation of bilateral subdural hematoma in an elderly man. Arch Neurol 38:195, 1981.
91. Krauss JK, Jankovic J: Severe motor tics causing cervical myelopathy in Tourette's syndrome. Mov Disord 11(5):563–566, 1996.
92. Krauss JK, Jankovic J: Tics secondary to craniocerebral trauma. Mov Disord 12(5):776–782, 1997.
93. Krauss JK, Jankovic J: Head injury and posttraumatic movement disorders. Neurosurgery 50(5):927–939; discussion 939–940, 2002.
94. Krauss JK, Mohadjer M, Nobbe F, Mundinger F: The treatment of posttraumatic tremor by stereotactic surgery: Symptomatic and functional outcome in a series of 35 patients. J Neurosurg 80:810, 1994.
95. Krauss JK, Mohadjer M, Braus DF, Wakhloo AK, Nobbe F, Mundinger F: Dystonia following head trauma: A report of nine patients and review of the literature. Mov Disord 7(3):263–272, 1992.
96. Krauss JK, Trankle R, Kopp KH: Post-traumatic movement disorders in survivors of severe head injury. Neurology 47(6):1488–1492, 1996.
97. Krauss JK, Trankle R, Kopp KH: Posttraumatic movement disorders after moderate or mild head injury. Mov Disord 12(3):428–431, 1997.
98. Krauss JK, Wakhloo AK, Nobbe F, Trankle R, Mundinger F, Seeger W: Lesion of dentatothalamic pathways in severe post-traumatic tremor. Neurol Res 17(6):409–416, 1995.
99. Kremer M, Russell R, Smythe GE: A midbrain syndome following head injury. J Neurol Neurosurg Psychiatry 10:49–60, 1947.
100. Kulisevsky J, Marti-Fabregas J, Grau JM: Spasms of amputation stumps. J Neurol Neurosurg Psychiatry 55:626, 1992.
101. Lance JW, Adams RD: The syndrome of intention or action myoclonus as a sequel to hypoxic encephalopathy. Brain 86:111–130, 1963.
102. Lang A, Fahn S: Movement disorder of RSD. Neurology 40:1476–1477, 1990.
103. Leckman JF, Cohen DJ, Goetz CG, Jankovic J: Tourette syndrome: Pieces of the puzzle. Adv Neurol 85:369–390, 2001.
104. Lee MS, Choi YC, Lee SH, Lee SB: Sleep-related periodic leg movements associated with spinal cord lesions. Mov Disord 11(6):719–722, 1996.
105. Lee MS, Rinne JO, Ceballos-Baumann A, Thompson PD, Marsden CD: Dystonia after head trauma. *Neurology* 44:1374–1378, 1994.
106. Lees AJ: Trauma and Parkinson disease. Rev Neurol (Paris) 153(10):541–546, 1997.

107. Lhermitte JJ: LA section totale de la Moelle Dorsale. Bourges, Tardy Pigelet, 1919.
108. Lodder J, Baard WC: Paraballism caused by bilateral hemorrhagic infarction in basal ganglia. Neurology (NY) 31:494–496, 1981.
109. Lombroso CT: Nocturnal paroxysmal dystonia due to a subfrontal cortical dysplasia. Epileptic Disord 2(1): 15–20, 2000.
110. Maher NE, Golbe LI, Lazzarini AM, Mark MH, Currie LJ, Wooten GF, et al: Epidemiologic study of 203 sibling pairs with Parkinson's disease: The GenePD study. Neurology 58(1):79–84, 2002.
111. Majumdar A, Appleton RE: Delayed and severe but transient Tourette syndrome after head injury. Pediatr Neurol 27(4):314–317, 2002.
112. Marsden CD, Obeso JA, Traub MM, et al: Muscle spasms associated with Sudeck's atrophy after injury. BMJ 288:173–176, 1984.
113. Marsden CD, Obeso JA, Zarran JJ, et al: The anatomical basis of hemidystonia. Brain 108:463–483, 1980.
114. Martin JP: Choreatic syndromes. In: Vinken PJ, Bruyn GW (eds): Handbook of Clinical Neurology, vol 6. Amsterdam: North-Holland, 1968, pp 435–439.
115. Martinelli P, Gabellini AS, Lugaresi E: Facial nucleus involvement in post-paralytic hemifacial spasm. J Neurol Neurosurg Psychiatry 46:586–587, 1983.
116. Martinelli P, Giuliani S, Ippoliti M: Hemifacial spasm due to peripheral injury of facial nerve: A nuclear syndrome? Mov Disord 7(2):181–184, 1992.
117. Martinez MS, Fontoira M, Celester G, Castro del Rio M, Permuy J, Iglesias A: Myoclonus of peripheral origin: Case secondary to a digital nerve lesion. Mov Disord 16(5):970–974, 2001.
118. Matsuo F, Ajax ET: Palatal myoclonus and denervation supersensitivity in the central nervous system. Ann Neurol 5(1):72–78, 1979.
119. Messimy R, Diebler C, Metzger J: Dystonic de torsion du membre saperieur gauche probablement consecutive á eur traumatisme cransin. Rev Neurol 133:199–206, 1977.
120. Meythaler JM, Guin-Renfroe S, Grabb P, Hadley MN: Long-term continuously infused intrathecal baclofen for spastic-dystonic hypertonia in traumatic brain injury: 1-year experience. Arch Phys Med Rehabil 80(1): 13–19, 1999.
121. Mezue WC, Taha ZM, Bashir EM: Fever and acquired torticollis in hospitalized children. J Laryngol Otol 116(4):280–284, 2002.
122a. Monday K, Jankovic J: Psychogenic myoclonus. Neurology 43:349–352, 1993.
122b. Mukhida K, Kobayashi NR, Mendez I: A novel role for parkin in trauma-induced CNS secondary injury. Med Hypotheses 64:1120–1123, 2005.
123. Nathan PW: Painful legs and moving toes: Evidence on the site of the lesion. J Neurol Neurosurg Psychiatry 41:934–939, 1978.
124. Nayernouri T: Posttraumatic parkinsonism. Surg Neurol 24(3):263–264, 1985.
125. Nogues MA, Leiguarda RC, Rivero AD, Salvat F, Manes F: Involuntary movements and abnormal spontaneous EMG activity in syringomyelia and syringobulbia. Neurology 52(4):823–834, 1999.
126. Ondo WG, Desaloms JM, Jankovic J, Grossman RG: Pallidotomy for generalized dystonia. Mov Disord 13(4): 693–698, 1998.
127. Parkinson J: Essay on the Shaking Palsy. London, Sherwood, Neely and Jones, 1817.
128. Penn RD, Gianino JM, York MM: Intrathecal baclofen for motor disorders. Mov Disord 10(5):675–677, 1995.
129. Perlmutter JS, Raichle ME: Pure hemidystonia with basal ganglion abnormalities on positron emission tomography. Ann Neurol 15:228–333, 1984.
130. Pettigrew IC, Jankovic J: Hemidystonia: A report of 22 patients and a review of the literature. J Neurol Neurosurg Psychiatry 48:650–657, 1981.
131. Pollak P, Benabid AL, Gervason CL, et al: Interest of chronic VIM thalamic stimulation in the therapeutical and pathophysiological approach of tremors. Mov Disord 7(suppl 1):158, 1992.
132. Remy P, de Recondo A, Defer G, Loc'h C, Amarenco P, Plante-Bordeneuve V, et al: Peduncular "rubral" tremor and dopaminergic denervation: A PET study. Neurology 45(3 pt 1):472–477, 1995.
133. Richardson JC, Homes JC, Alimski MJ, et al: Kinesiogenic choreoathetosis due to brain injury. Can J Neurol Sci 14:626–628, 1987.
134. Ritchie RW: Neurological sequelae of amputation. Br J Hosp Med 6:607–609, 1970.
135. Rondot P, Bathien N, De Recondo J, Gueguen B: Dystonia-parkinsonism syndrome resulting from a bullet injury in the midbrain. J Neurol, Neurosurg Psychiatry 57:658–659, 1994.
136. Sa DS, Mailis-Gagnon A, Nicholson K, Lang AE: Posttraumatic painful torticollis. Mov Disord 18(12):1482–1491, 2003.
137. Said S, Bathien N: Myoclonies rythmees du quadriceps en relation aves un envahissement sarcombteux du nerf crural. Rev Neurol (Paris) 133 (3): 191–198, 1977.
138. Saint-Hilaire M-H, Burke RE, Bressman SB: Delayed onset dystonia due to perinatal or early childhood asphyxia. Neurology 41:216–222, 1991.
139. Samii A, Pal PK, Schulzer M, Mak E, Tsui JK: Posttraumatic cervical dystonia: A distinct entity? Can J Neurol Sci 27(1):55–59, 2000.
140. Sandyk R, Iacono RP, Fisher H: Posttraumatic cerebellar syndrome: response to L-tryptophan. Int J Neurosci 47(3–4):301–302, 1989.
141. Sanitate SS, Meerschaert JR: Orthostatic tremor: Delayed onset following head trauma. Arch Phys Med Rehabil 74:886, 1993.
142. Sankhla C, Lai EC, Jankovic J: Peripherally induced oromandibular dystonia. J Neurol Neurosurg Psychiatry 65(5):722–728, 1998.
143. Scherokman B, Husain F, Cuetter A, et al: Peripheral dystonia. Arch Neurol 43:830–832, 1986.
144. Schott GD: Painful legs and moving toes: The role of

trauma. J Neurol Neurosurg Psychiatry 44:344–346, 1981.

145. Schott GD: The relationship of peripheral trauma and pain to dystonia. J Neurol Neurosurg Psychiatry 48(7): 698–701, 1985.

146. Schuyler-Hacker H, Green R, Wingate L, et al: Acute torticollis secondary to rupture of the sternocleidomastoid. Arch Phys Med Rehabil 70(12):851–853, 1989.

147. Schwab RS, England AC Jr: Parkinson syndromes due to various specific causes. In: Vinken PJ, Bruyn GW (ed.): Hanbook of Clinical Neurology: Diseases of the Basal Ganglia, vol 6. Amsterdam, North-Holland, 1986, pp 227–247.

148. Sethi KD, Hess DC, Huffingale VH, Adams RJ: Acetazolamide treatment of paroxysmal dystonia in central demylinating disease. Neruology 42:919–921, 1992.

149. Sellal F, Hirsch E, Barth P, Blond S, Marescaux C: A case of symptomatic hemidystonia improved by ventroposterolateral thalamic electrostimulation. Mov Disord 8(4):515–518, 1993.

150. Shaddock SH, Shaddock LB, Black SPW: Palatal myoclonus following head injury. J Trauma 12:353–357, 1972.

151. Sheehy MD, Marsden CD: Trauma and pain in spasmodic torticollis. Lancet, 1:777–780, 1980.

152. Shoulson I: On chorea. Clin Neuropharm 9:585–599, 1986.

153. Siemers E: Posttraumatic tic disorder [letter]. Mov Disord 5(2):183, 1990.

154. Singer C, Sanchez-Ramos J, Weiner WJ: A case of posttraumatic tic disorder. Mov Disord 4(4):342–344, 1989.

155. Smith DH, Uryu K, Saatman KE, Trojanowski JQ, McIntosh TK: Protein accumulation in traumatic brain injury. Neuromol Med 4(1–2):59–72, 2003.

156. Snyder AM, Stricker EM, Zigmond MJ: Stress-induced neurological impairments in an animal model of parkinsonism. Ann Neurol 18(5):544–551, 1985.

157. Spillane JD, Nathan PW, Kelly RE, et al: Painful legs and moving toes. Brain 94:541–556, 1971.

158. Starosta-Rubinstein S, Bjork R, Snyder BD, Tulloch JW: Posttraumatic intention myoclonus. Surg Neurol 20:131, 1983.

159. Steiner JL, DeJesus PV, Mancall EL: Painful jumping amputation stumps: Pathophysiology of a "sore circuit." Trans Am Neurol Assoc 99:252–255, 1974.

160. Stern MB: Head trauma as a risk factor for Parkinson's disease. Mov Disord (no. 2) 6:95–97, 1991.

161. Sterzenegger M, DiStefano G, Radanov BP, Schnidrig A: Presenting symptoms and signs after whiplash injury. Neurology 44:688–693, 1994.

162. Suchowersky O, Calne DB: Non-dystonic causes of torticollis In: Fahn S, Marsden CD, Calne DB (eds): Advances in Neurology (Dytonia 2, vol. 50). New York, Raven Press, 1988, pp 501–515.

163. Swartzman RJ, Kerrigan J: The movement disorder of reflex sympathetic dystrophy. Neurology 40:57–61, 1990.

164. Szelozynska K, Znamirowski R: Extrapyramidal syndrome in post-traumatic hemiparesis in children. Neurol Neurochir Pol 8:167–170, 1974.

165. Tan EK, Lo YL, Chan LL, See SJ, Hong A, Wong MC: Cervical disc prolapse with cord compression presenting with choreoathetosis and dystonia. Neurology 58(4): 661–662, 2002.

166. Tarsy D: Comparison of acute- and delayed-onset posttraumatic cervical dystonia: Mov Disord 13(3):481–485, 1998.

167. Thyagarajan D, Kompoliti K, Ford B: Post-traumatic shoulder "dystonia:" Persistent abnormal postures of the shoulder after minor trauma. Neurology 51(4):1205–1207, 1998.

168. Tings T, Baier PC, Paulus W, Trenkwalder C: Restless legs syndrome induced by impairment of sensory spinal pathways. J Neurol 250(4):499–500, 2003.

169. Trauma and dystonia. Lancet, 1:759–760, 1989.

170. Troupin AS, Kamm RF: Lingual myoclonus: Case report and review. Dis Nerv Syst 35:378–380, 1974.

171. Tsai CH, Lo SK, See LC, Chen HZ, Chen RS, Weng YH, et al: Environmental risk factors of young onset Parkinson's disease: A case-control study. Clin Neurol Neurosurg 104(4):328–333, 2002.

172. Turazzi S, Alexandre A, Bricolm A, et al: Opsoclonus and palatal myoclonus during prolonged posttraumatic coma: A clinico-pathologic study. Eur Neurol 15:257–263, 1977.

173. Turjanski N, Lees AJ, Brooks DJ: Dopaminergic function in patients with posttraumatic parkinsonism: An 18F-dopa PET study. Neurology 49(1):183–189, 1997.

174. Urakami K, Masaki N, Shimoda K, et al: Increase of striatal dopamine turnover by stress in MPTP-treated mice. Clin Neuropharmacol 11:360–368, 1988.

175. Uryu K, Giasson BI, Longhi L, Martinez D, Murray I, Conte V, et al: Age-dependent synuclein pathology following traumatic brain injury in mice. Exp Neurol 184(1):214–224, 2003.

176. van de Beek WJ, Roep BO, van der Slik AR, Giphart MJ, van Hilten BJ: Susceptibility loci for complex regional pain syndrome. Pain 103(1–2):93–97, 2003.

177. van de Beek WJ, Vein A, Hilgevoord AA, van Dijk JG, van Hilten BJ: Neurophysiologic aspects of patients with generalized or multifocal tonic dystonia of reflex sympathetic dystrophy. J Clin Neurophysiol 19(1):77–83, 2002.

178. Vanhatalo S, Paetau R, Mustonen K, Hernesniemi J, Riikonen R: Posttraumatic tremor and Arnold Chiari malformation: No sign of compression, but cure after surgical decompression. Mov Disord 15(3):581–583, 2000.

179. van Hilten BJ, van de Beek WJ, Hoff JI, Voormolen JH, Delhaas EM: Intrathecal baclofen for the treatment of dystonia in patients with reflex sympathetic dystrophy. N Engl J Med 343(9):625–630, 2000.

180. van Hilten JJ, van de Beek WJ, Roep BO: Multifocal or generalized tonic dystonia of complex regional pain syndrome: A distinct clinical entity associated with HLA-DR13. Ann Neurol 48(1):113–116, 2000.

181. van Hilten JJ, van de Beek WJ, Vein AA, van Dijk JG, Middelkoop HA: Clinical aspects of multifocal or generalized tonic dystonia in reflex sympathetic dystrophy. Neurology 56(12):1762–1765, 2001.
182. Veldman PHJ, Reynen HM, Arntz IE, Goris RJA: Signs and symptoms of reflex sympathetic dystropy. Lancet 342:1012–1015, 1993.
183. Ward CD, Duvoisin RC, Ince SE, et al: Parkinson's disease in 65 pairs of twins and in a set of quadruplets. Neurology 33:815–824, 1983.
184. Weiner WJ, Lang AE: Movement Disorders: A Comprehensive Survey. Mount Kisco, NY, Futura, 1989, pp 457–529.
185. Weir MS: Injuries of Nerves and Their Consequences. New York: Dover, 1977, pp 363–368.
186. Williams DB, Annegers JF, Kokmen E, et al: Brain injury and neurologic sequelae. Neurology 41:1554–1557, 1991.
187. Winkelmann J, Wetter TC, Trenkwalder C, Auer DP: Periodic limb movements in syringomyelia and syringobulbia. Mov Disord 15(4):752–753, 2000.
188. Woo CC: Traumatic spinal myoclonus. J Manip Physiol Ther 12(6):478–481, 1989.
189. Wright RA, Ahlskog JE: Focal shoulder-elevation dystonia. Mov Disord 2000;15(4):709–713, 2000.
190. Yochelson MR, David RG: New-onset tic disorder following acute hemorrhage of an arteriovenous malformation. J Child Neurol 15(11):769–771, 2000.
191. Zijlmans J, Booij J, Valk J, Lees A, Horstink M: Posttraumatic tremor without parkinsonism in a patient with complete contralateral loss of the nigrostriatal pathway. Mov Disord 17(5):1086–1088, 2002.

Chapter 34

Psychiatric Aspects of the Neurology of Trauma

HAROLD MERSKEY

The cognitive effects of neural trauma frequently run side by side or are intermingled with emotional changes. This chapter deals with the psychiatric aspects of trauma other than changes in cognitive function. The recognition of psychological and neurological responses to trauma is discussed first. Some of the emotional changes that can occur in reaction to physical lesions, including neurological lesions, are then considered. Lastly, specific changes in personality or mental state that can result directly from brain damage are reviewed.

Posttraumatic Stress Disorders

Frightening experiences, or those that are very unpleasant or give rise to protracted distress, leave their mark on most people. Individuals who see or are involved in accidents frequently develop psychological symptoms related to those experiences. Even the common rear-end collision with subsequent cervical hyperextension flexion injury (whiplash) is often associated with subsequent fears of automobiles or of driving on busy streets.[10] Kuch et al.[37] described 33 patients with chronic pain from motor vehicle injuries, 23 (70%) of whom had such complaints. Individuals who have been injured in accidents and assaults have also been found to have quite marked short-term psychological reactions, which may reflect a long-term loss of self-confidence.[66a] If the disorder is severe or protracted, the individual will be frightened of driving or being driven, uneasy at the place where the accident occurred, and subject to recurring thoughts about it. Depression and associated difficulties with concentration, attention, sleep, irritability, and even self-blame complicate the worse cases.

Similar problems have often been observed in whole groups of people subject to the same catastrophe, such as French naval ships that blew up, with much loss of life,[28] mass deaths in a nightclub,[13] earthquakes, and a variety of natural and industrial phenomena. Disasters in civilian life have often been accompanied by automatic behavior and confusion, as well as overt panic, anger, and guilt.[14] Defensive reactions with hysterical dissociation are likewise recognized.[35]

A substantial literature has developed about posttraumatic stress disorder (PTSD). Many of the above-mentioned symptoms were observed in Vietnam veterans,[21] and the American Psychiatric Association produced formal criteria for the disorder in the *Diagnostic and Statistical Manual* (DSM-III)[3] on. The revised features in DSM-IV[4] include the following. The person has experienced an event that involves actual or threatened death or serious injury or witnessing an event that involves death, injury, or a threat to the physical integrity of another person; or learning about unexpected or violent death, serious harm, or threat of death or injury experienced by a family member or another close associate. The person's response must involve intense fear, helplessness, or horror. The characteristic symptoms resulting from exposure to such extreme trauma include persistent reexperiencing of the traumatic event, persistent avoidance of stimuli associated with the trauma, numbing of general responsiveness, and persistent symptoms of increased arousal. The relevant traumatic events may be, but are not limited to, military combat, violent personal assault (including sexual assault), being kidnapped or taken hostage, terrorist attack, torture, incarceration as a prisoner of war or in a concentration camp, natural or man-made disasters, severe automobile accidents, or being diagnosed with a life-threatening illness. Witnessed events include, but are not limited to, observing the serious injury or unnatural death of another person or unexpectedly seeing a dead body or body parts.

Reports are now available detailing the emotional and physical symptoms sustained by those who have been through a variety of events, including individual torture and coercive interrogation in most of the countries of the world.[2,63a,78a]

Difficulties in distinguishing between neurological and psychological symptoms have often appeared. There was a substantial controversy in the nineteenth century between those who thought that "concussion of the spine" was a physical illness produced by railway accidents[18,19,57] and their opponents.[30,58,62,74]

With hindsight, we can now recognize that the so-called concussion of the spine did not greatly affect neurons in the spinal cord, but probably had a significant relationship to cervical sprain and low-back sprain injuries. Erichsen[18,19] incidentally noted that the travelers in railway carriages who sustained the worst injuries were those who had their backs in the direction of the impact.

The differential diagnosis of neurological disorder from anxiety conditions and hysterical symptoms became exceptionally important during World War I. This is exemplified in discussions of *shell shock*, a term developed in Britain at the end of 1914 or the beginning of 1915 and abandoned officially in 1917.[50] In World War I, the stress of trench warfare on soldiers affected larger numbers than in any previous war. Most officers in regular combat for 6 weeks were expected to break down with nervous symptoms.[24a] Men died in enormous numbers fighting for a few yards of ground between trenches. In 4 months in 1916, the battle of the Somme cost the British 420,000 casualties, the French 194,000, the Germans 40,000. It is hardly surprising that cases of shell shock rose to a peak of 16,138 in the British forces from July to December 1916.

The prominent symptoms that marked this nervousness resulting from combat included tremor, fatigue, anxiety, and also probable hysterical complaints such as amnesia, blindness, deafness, and paralyses. Some very striking unusual complaints, such as camptocormia (extreme bent back), were found. Military and medical authorities did not wish to stigmatize as cowards men who had fought bravely and whose nerve had given way. Some of them had received the highest decorations for bravery. With an army of conscripts, elected governments also did not relish the anger of the relatives of such men in civilian life.

As in other wars, new technology in World War I presented new medical problems. In the past, the simple round ball from a cannon killed where it hit. Twentieth-century shells packed with high explosives caused blast damage far more widely. Men were known to have been blown some distance by shells, left unconscious, and then recovered without detectable external signs of injury. This led to the idea that subsequent symptoms might be due to minute hemorrhages in the lungs, spinal cord, and nerve roots, such as were demonstrated with experimental shock in rabbits[43a] and occasionally in postmortem examinations.[54] In the end, however, it was recognized that symptoms hardly ever occurred among war prisoners, could occur without actual explosions within the vicinity, and could be much influenced by suggestion and by psychological management. Since then, such symptoms have been recognized as largely due to anxiety or to so-called *hysterical dissociation*. Where the symptoms affect the body, rather than such psychological processes as amnesia, they are now conventionally known as *conversion symptoms*.

The lessons of World War I were remembered in World War II, and psychiatric management of soldiers and civilians became more available to both groups in the English-speaking countries; acute and chronic stress disorders were readily recognized as based primarily on anxiety and treated accordingly.[25,65] As well, fewer combatants but more civilians were killed.[51a]

The diagnostic category of PTSD—essentially an anxiety disorder—was formulated only in (DSM-IV) in 1994[4] and in the International Classification of Diseases in its 10th revision (ICD-10) in 1992.[31] Curiously, according to Allan Young,[79] an anthropologist, the formulation of PTSD was first put forward by Veterans' Administration psychiatrists who wished to create a category for individuals who had suffered in consequence of themselves causing suffering to others in Vietnam (i.e., torturers). The diagnosis gained immediate popularity for a wide variety of other patients and has given rise to concern over the frequency with which it is used. Since *recovered memories* lost respectability[40,56,59] it has been applied increasingly to individuals who were said to have childhood abuse, but for whom it was becoming inadmissible to make the diagnosis of multiple personality disorder, which has suffered a serious decline.[60]

These issues are increasingly distant from the direct neurology of trauma but lead to other complications. The diagnosis of PTSD is an alternative to the so-called *Gulf War syndrome*, which from a number of studies[73a,76] appears to be responsive to psychological circumstances. Thus, more memories of the past have appeared with time since the Gulf War,[69,73a] but not following traumatic experiences by peacekeepers in Bosnia.[76] When memories recur, such fluctuations appear to be related to concern over health.[76]

While wartime events have provided a clear model and much information about stress reactions, the most common cause of PTSD in peacetime appears to be motor vehicle collisions, and PTSD is a known sequela of such accidents.

Mayou and Bryant[44a] provide quite representative figures from a follow-up of a hospital emergency department series. Among 278 whiplash patients referred to an emergency department, moderate to severe pain was still reported at 1 year by 27% and at 3 years by 30%. Psychiatric sequelae were common. Posttraumatic stress disorder was diagnosed in 24% of the total at 3 months and in 17% at 3 years. Thus, prolonged pain from whiplash injuries is likely to be accompanied by PTSD. Phobic travel anxiety (therefore not full-scale PTSD) affected 21% at 3 months, 16% at 1 year, and 19% at 3 years. Other psychological conditions affected 37% of those with whiplash injury at 3 months and 35% at 1 year and 3 years. Interestingly, in the study by Mayou and Bryant, there was a similar rate of emotional problems in the 6 months before injury; they had been present in 20% of those with whiplash injury, 22% with other soft tissue injury, 21% with no injury, and 22% with bony injury—figures strikingly similar to those in groups that had been held to have different psychological patterns. Nevertheless, whiplash patients tended to show a higher rate of anxiety (46%) that was moderate or extreme after the injury compared with 36%, 35%, and 39% in the other three groups, respectively.[44a] When PTSD was examined 3 years after the injury, it was found to affect 24% of those with whiplash compared with 7%, 10%, and 12%, respectively, in the other three groups.

Anxiety and depression, according to the Hospital Anxiety and Depression Scale, affected rather similar percentages of persons at all stages and showed no significant difference among the groups. The same was true for phobic anxiety but the figures were less overall at 3 years than at 1 year, down to 19%, 13%, 10%, and 14%, respectively, in the four groups mentioned.

These figures indicate the importance of comparative analysis of data, since without them, support could be given to the notion—which is not validated by Mayou and Bryant's study—that whiplash has psychological causes.

Mayou and Bryant themselves considered that their findings show "that there is no special psychiatry of whiplash." Psychiatric outcomes were found to be comparable to those following other types of road traffic accident, and predictors of pain generally were very similar to those identified after other types of injury.

Although psychosocial variables complicate, or enter into, chronic pain, the evidence suggests that the greater proportion of them appears only after pain has been present for some time, as can be seen in the study by Mayou and Bryant, where individuals who made a legal claim by 3 months postinjury did worse, whether because of the severity of their original injury or because of a preference manifesting itself early for litigious involvement. There is no good reason, however, to adopt the pejorative explanation without evidence, as is apparently often the case at present.

It has also been alleged with great assiduity that psychosocial variables underlie pain following whiplash injury.[12a] This point of view, published in the *New England Journal of Medicine*, was based upon a remarkable treatment of the data, in which no less than 27% of potentially relevant data in patients who had insurance claims that were reopened were jettisoned by the investigators on dubious grounds. The justification for dropping the data was presented on one occasion as being "to maintain internal validity"[12a] and on another occasion, when challenged, as being to maintain confidentiality or because allegedly the insurance company that funded the work in question was unable to trace data adequately once it had closed a case[11] and then reopened it. This seems unsound scientifically, and the alleged inability of the insurance company to obtain data was roundly denied by a retired adjuster, who said it had become very easy to get data on her computer in the years just preceding the *New England Journal of Medicine* study.[36] This situation has led to an examination of pain in relation to insurance,[53] and it is suggested that there is evidence that many doctors may unreasonably favor insurance companies both historically and currently.

With respect to the treatment of PTSD, McNally et al.[45] have recently shown that early psychological intervention tends not to promote recovery from PTSD. In other words, the results of early psychological debriefing have been disappointing, so that although the majority of debriefed survivors describe the experience as helpful, there is no convincing evidence that it reduces the incidence of PTSD, and some control studies suggest that it may impede natural recovery from trauma.

Symptoms of Whiplash

The idea that the symptoms of whiplash were either malingered or hysterical has long been abandoned in most respectable neurological and psychiatric circles. When issues of possible conversion or dissociative symptoms occur after head injury, the differential diagnosis follows the usual lines of neurological practice. First, the symptom and the response to physical examination should indicate a pattern that corresponds to an idea in the patient's mind rather than to known neuroanatomical or neurological pathways. This approach is frequently effective but has some drawbacks. There are several symptoms, especially with sensory complaints such as pain, that may be regional but can occur on a physiological basis;[48] in any case, the diagnosis of hysteria according to several of the traditional criteria is notoriously unreliable.[22,47,68] Accordingly, not only should neurological evidence indicate the likelihood of the symptom being hysterical, but also it should be confirmed by subsequent inquiry and by evidence on the psychiatric side that there is sufficient change in the individual's mental state and life to account for the symptoms.

One of the common strong motives that have been put forward with respect to the detection of hysterical symptoms in civilian life is financial compensation. This is not reliable inasmuch as many individuals with chronic pain continue to experience it long after any chance of securing financial benefits arising from their pain has ended.[46]

It is worth emphasizing that although there are several psychological symptoms that require differential diagnosis from neurological ones, hysterical complaints that might be confused with neurological ones are relatively rare in civilian life except in neurological practice. This has given rise to discussion of the idea that neurological disease may predispose to hysterical symptoms.[52,68]

Concentration Camp Syndrome

Nazi concentration camps have been responsible for a large quota of individuals suffering from lifelong posttraumatic symptoms. Eighteen percent of concentration camp survivors have been found to have persistent emotional distress almost three decades later.[38] Their symptoms may be as slight as chronic agoraphobia with increased arousal at reports of war or potential international conflicts or as severe as a chronic paranoid delusional state, which has affected a number of the people who suffered most.[15] A bibliography in this field by Eitinger et al.[16] is available, and further review of research on this topic is provided by Weisaeth and Eitinger.[75] It proved difficult in many of these cases to disentangle the effects of physical ill treatment from the psychological stresses, as many who were threatened with death were also starved and subjected to malnutrition. Cachexia and edema were frequently found among the survivors[17] and may have contributed somewhat to cerebral impairment, which in turn may have been a factor in possible neurological complaints. The discrimination has been made, however, not only by Eitinger and Strom,[17] but also by Norwegian investigators[5,6,67] examining sailors with the so-called *war sailor syndrome*, which afflicted many Norwegian sailors. These were merchant sailors who undertook the most dangerous voyages throughout World War II and had a high casualty rate. Some suffered physical deprivation in the course of their service. Studies by Askevold et al.[5,6,67] have indicated that many developed a pseudodementia.

Neurologists examining patients with possible PTSD should probably look for answers on the following matters. First, they should seek evidence that a significant stress occurred and continues. Money is often not a sufficient explanation but can sometimes be relevant. Concomitant emotional stress, such as bereavement or a difficult marriage, ought to be noted. Sometimes additional stress follows from the initial one; for example, chronic pain causing loss of employment leads to financial change, a loss of the sense of self-worth, and impaired marriages. Second, in addition to taking a little time to consider the probable psychological evidence, the usual process of examination for possible conversion or dissociative symptoms is necessary. Third, psychiatric treatment may be required for confirmation, as already indicated.

Emotional Effects of Peripheral Lesions

Perhaps one of the most important stressors that the neurologist should be prepared to recognize is a physical illness itself. Presumed dissociative fits occurring in individuals rather than in groups almost always appear in individuals who have had epilepsy themselves or seen someone else in an epileptic fit. The former is more frequent among those who have such fits. Likewise, merely to be ill with a paralysis or chronic pain can be enough to cause significant emotional changes.[49] Severe psychological stress is well recognized as a cause of psychological and physical complaints, as noted earlier. It is common sense that physical conditions give rise to emotional responses and that this is part of the regular experience of physicians. Curiously, there seems to have been a tendency to underemphasize this basic sequence. It is more exciting to see how the mind affects the body than to recognize the humdrum impact of physical discomfort on the mind. Thus, for several decades, there was extensive writing on psychosomatic illness, that is, illness in which psychological factors contributed to produce such physical changes as peptic ulcer, irritable bowel syndrome, asthma, and even cancer.

Publications on the psychological effects of chronic physical illness and the issues of rehabilitation were less common previously but have now begun to appear more often. This situation is often confused by the pattern of selection that influences medical practice. Given the same number of physical problems, individuals who have a premorbid inclination to seek medical care will appear more often in medical clinics than those who shy away from physicians. Illnesses that threaten life or are recognized as having a large treatable physical component tend most often to lead to consultation with physicians. Many illnesses that are the focus of medical attention, however, are more protracted and less dangerous, so individuals can decide whether to tolerate them with or without the help of physicians. Persons with headaches, common colds, intermittent diarrhea, and even epilepsy are all known to show a selection pattern in the way in which they present for medical care, and this selection pattern is influenced by psychological factors.[7,61] Thus, in any neurological service, particularly the outpatient department, there will always be patients who seek advice by preference rather than necessity. In consequence, such conditions as migraines are thought to be liable to psychological problems, whereas the correct position is that those who present with them more often have psychological problems.

In addition to the influence of personality on seeking help, the consequences of an illness frequently affect the state of a patient. This is easily seen with chronic pain. Patients with intractable complex regional pain syndrome (type I) (reflex sympathetic dystrophy) before treatment frequently show significant emotional change.[8] There is no particular reason to think that this emotional change contributes to the origin of the illness. It frequently clears up if adequate relief can be provided for the patient, who then ceases to be depressed and irritable. Approximately 8% to 9% of the general population is liable to suffer from depression or dysthymia over a 6-month period,[55] and it has long been suspected that there is an increased rate of depression among patients with chronic pain. The figures range, however, from 10% to 100%, depending on the sample.[64] An epidemiological survey[41] demonstrated from findings with the Center for Epidemiologic Studies' self-report scale of depression (CES-D) that individuals free of chronic musculoskeletal pain had a rate of depression of 8.8%, whereas those with chronic pain had a rate of depression of 18.3%. In another study, the odds ratio on developing depression for those who start with chronic pain was 2.85 after an average of 8 years.[42] Those who began with depression without pain had an odds ratio of 2.15 of having pain as well after 8 years. Each seems likely to cause the other, with a slight effect in favor of musculoskeletal pain promoting depression more than depression promoting musculoskeletal pain. However, what looked like a strength in the study—namely, its long follow-up period—is probably a weakness since prospective studies of the interactions of pain and depression may show clearer evidence of which relationship was stronger if they last only 1 to 2 years.

Neurologists who see patients with chronic pain or other chronic physical conditions will naturally be aware of the possibility that physical causes may promote emotional change. This emotional change, in turn, may give rise to a pattern of hysterical conversion symptoms or other dissociative symptoms. Merskey and Buhrich[52] found, for example, that 12% of patients with hysterical symptoms seemed to have them as an emotional response to their physical illness and not in consequence of any other emotional cause. This happens more often with damage to the nervous system than with any other condition and can be expected after head injury or injury to the spinal cord. It was briefly indicated earlier that not all symptoms that have a regional distribution pattern are necessarily hysterical. Hypoesthesia to light touch or pin prick and regional syndromes of pain overlapping the boundaries of dermatomes or the distributions of nerves may be pathophysiological in origin.[48] The evidence for this comes directly from physiological experiments that show changes in receptor fields as a consequence of discrete lesions where the change in sensitivity extends well beyond the boundaries of local nerve territories.

Sometimes we also encounter surprising neurological lesions in association with what may be thought to be nonneurological disorders. Basilar migraine has been described after uncomplicated whiplash injuries.[32] Greater occipital nerve lesions after cervical spine injuries are well recognized, and thoracic outlet effects occur as well. Oculomotor problems after cervical spine injury have been described,[29] and, indeed, most of those who have seen individuals with neck injuries have also heard accounts of oculomotor difficulties, such as blurring of vision and double vision. Bilateral sympathetic dysfunction has been demonstrated in posttraumatic headaches.[34] Transient global amnesia may be triggered by mild head trauma,[27] and this should not be confused with hysteria.

Psychiatric Sequelae of Brain Damage

The postconcussion syndrome and cognitive changes from brain damage are not discussed in this chapter because they are covered elsewhere in this volume. Several other psychiatric or neuropsychiatric syndromes may result from brain damage and are outlined briefly here. They include schizophreniform illness, mania, depression, and obsessional illness. Protracted delirious states (i.e., conditions with impaired consciousness, often marked by delusions or hallucinations) may also be found in association with varying degrees of dementia. Lishman[39a] has provided an extensive discussion of these topics. A wide spectrum of psychiatric disabilities can be found in patients with penetrating injuries of the brain, including intellectual, affective, and behavioral changes and also persistent somatic complaints for which no physical basis could be discovered. Relevant etiological factors include the amount and location of brain damage, the development of epilepsy, the response to intellectual impairment, and the contribution of environmental factors, compensation, and litigation, as well as the emotional impact and emotional repercussions of injury and the original personality.

Achte et al.,[71] in a classic follow-up of brain-injured veterans from the Finnish wars of 1939 through 1945, observed psychoses in 8.9% of the veterans, a higher figure than was previously reported. Among the psychotic patients, 38.5% had suffered severe injuries compared with 19.4% in the rest of the veterans ($P < .0001$). Basal injuries showed a strong association with the development of psychosis. The most common psychoses were schizophrenic and paranoid, and they were more frequent than among the general population. Apart from the link with basal lesions, which were associated with dementias and the Korsakoff syndrome, no particular psychosis showed an association with particular areas of brain damage.

Work on schizophrenia[79] suggests that several areas of the brain are affected in schizophrenic illness. They include the left frontal areas, both temporal and parietal areas, and the basal ganglia. Hence schizophreniform illnesses would seem to be more likely to appear a priori after moderately severe brain damage. Fahy et al.[20] showed that among patients who had had amnesia lasting longer than 3 days, almost all were affected in some fashion, either physically or psychologically, after severe closed head injury. Thus, only one-third of patients examined were without neurological signs, electroencephalographic abnormalities occurred in more than two-thirds, and only 5 of 22 patients assessed were judged free of psychiatric sequelae at follow-up. Six had disabling symptoms short of dementia, such as forgetfulness; 2 had paranoid delusions; 1 had sudden modes of depression or disinhibition; 11 were demented; and some of the last-mentioned were epileptic and subject to violent paranoid and hallucinatory episodes.

There is little dispute that moderately severe or severe head injury will provoke schizophrenic types of illness in individuals who were not previously subject to such disorders. Grant and Alves[23] suggest that it is hard to determine if the prevalence of schizophrenia increases after head injury, and they are probably right if a narrow definition is used with the notion of *process schizophrenia.* The schizophreniform illnesses, however, are more common than ordinary episodes. Grant and Alves described brief reactive psychoses on the basis of the DSM-III category for this diagnosis, which is appropriate only if there are no coexisting signs of delirium or dementia. In such a condition, psychotic symptoms appear immediately after a recognizable psychosocial stressor, and the clinical picture involves incoherence, delusions, hallucinations, or disorganized or catatonic behavior. The illness lasts less than 2 weeks. The DSM-III also allows us to diagnose organic delusional syndromes, with delusions as a predominant clinical feature, no clouding of consciousness, significant loss of intellectual abilities, and no other relevant syndrome.[3] In DSM-IV this is called *psychotic disorder due to a general medical condition*.[4] Recognizable organic factors, such as a head injury, must be present. After severe head injury, there will usually be indications of dementia if some of these other concomitant phenomena are observed.

In addition, DSM-III and DSM-IV recognize depression and mania owing to head injury.[3,4] In DSM-IV these come under the heading of *mood disorder due to a general medical condition*. Varying degrees of depression are common in individuals who have suffered head injury with severe side effects. Guttmann observed that the great majority of depressive reactions among his patients were clearly reactive.[26] The organic depressive syndrome would be diagnosed only after head injury if, in addition to the overt signs of depression and enough symptoms to satisfy the criteria, there was no significant organic impairment and probably some other justification for attaching the diagnosis to the organic head injury rather than to the psychological consequences. Depression may be more likely in someone who has an anterior cerebral lesion particularly affecting the anterior portions of the frontal lobes of the brain.[71,72] The view that this is more likely in someone with left-sided lesions does not appear to have been sustained. If the psychological circumstances, however, were themselves sufficiently severe to be likely to provoke a depressive illness, one would be more disposed to attribute the depression to those psychological stresses, such as injury elsewhere in the body, chronic pain, and difficulty in rehabilitation, rather than to the organic disorder. In either case, antidepressant medication is relevant and can be extremely helpful. The diagnosis of Pain Disorder, as presented in DSM-IV is rarely justified because it should not be made if the condition is better accounted for by physical illness or a mood or anxiety disorder.

Mania is less frequent, and when it occurs after head injury, the chance of it being attributable to the organic effects are higher. Starkstein et al.[72] have suggested that lesions that involve the right frontal area (no matter how far back they extend) are related to mania after stroke, and it is appropriate to suppose that they would be similarly relevant to head injury. An elevated, expansive, or irritable mood is the precondition for the diagnosis of mania. The usual phenomena of mania include at least three of the following symptoms: increase in activity or physical restlessness, more talkativeness, or pressure to keep talking; flight of ideas or subjective experience of thoughts racing; inflated self-esteem, which may be so great that it is delusional; reduced need for sleep; distractability; and excessive involvement in poorly controlled external activities, such as buying sprees, sexual indiscretions, reckless driving, or foolish business investments. Several reports of mania after head injury have appeared, including those of Khanna and Srinath,[33] Whitlock,[77] Clark and Davison,[12b] Yatham et al.,[78b] Riess et al.,[63b] Shukla et al.,[66b] and Starkstein et al.[70] In the groups studied most carefully with respect to regional cerebral localization,[71,72] 8 of 11 patients had lesions involving limbic areas and frontal lesions occurred in the majority. In addition to focal brain injury, mean values for bifrontal and third ventricle brain ratios of manic patients were significantly increased. The authors conclude that certain specific factors may contribute to the production of a manic illness. These include the confluence of anterior subcortical atrophy with a focal lesion of a limbic region or with a region connected to the limbic system in the frontal regions, or genetic loading. The rare occurrence of both of these sets of phenomena accounts for the rarity of the disorder after head injury, although the nature and location of the lesions are of obvious interest in appreciating disturbances of brain function.

Obsessional symptoms are now well known to respond to serotoninergic antidepressants such as clomipramine or fluoxetine. Organic explanations for their occurrence have long been supported, particularly by their development after encephalitis lethargica.[73b] Grimshaw[24b] found that 19.4% of his patients with primary obsessional disorder had a previous important neurological disorder. Lishman[39b] found that only 1.4% of those with severe head injuries in his series developed obsessive-compulsive neurosis. Occasional cases may well be attributable to head injury, and McKeon et al.[44b] report four cases. One of their patients was unconscious for 10 days, but two were unconscious for only a few minutes each, although they had several hours or more of posttraumatic amnesia. One patient also was not really unconscious and had been struck by her mother. It seems that two or three of the cases may well bear a close relationship to head injury, although not all of them do so. It is well recognized, in addition, that obsessive-compulsive disorders tend to arise in individuals who have compulsive personalities.

Predisposition

Individuals who have had psychological problems before head injury are more likely to show a variety of difficulties in adjustment subsequently. Nevertheless, the syndromes that have just been discussed are discrete and well identifiable and will ordinarily appear without having been present immediately before head injury. By contrast, there is an intriguing report by Malt et al.,[43b] who carefully studied accident victims with respect to their immediate premorbid state. They looked for psychiatric disorders on admission in terms of a DSM-III diagnosis, and these were confirmed by DSM-III and the ICD-9 evaluations. Of 112 patients, none had psychotic disorders, only 4 had depressive or dysthymic complaints, and 8 had anxiety conditions. Nineteen were substance abusers, and altogether only 42 patients (37%) had a prior psychiatric illness. Among those injured, no evidence was found for an accident-prone personality type. Thirty-one persons (28%) had a personality disorder according to DSM-III or ICD-9, of which antisocial personality disorder was the most common (12 patients). Two-thirds of the group with personality disorder overlapped with the individuals who had one of the other diagnoses, and approximately 9% did not. From this study, one might expect 46% of people involved in accidents to have had psychiatric problems before the accident, whereas one might only expect approximately one-sixth of individuals in the general population to have such problems as anxiety or depression. The implications of the frequency of personality disorder in this series compared with the general population are more difficult to estimate.

Outcome and Implications

Prognosis is assumed to be related to the extent of brain damage, but the contribution of the premorbid personality is obviously relevant. In all the psychiatric and neurological conditions discussed, treatment is in accordance with the usual lines of management for these different diagnoses, whether antidepressants or psychotherapy. Social rehabilitation is clearly of great importance, although it is not discussed here.

REFERENCES

1. Achte KA, Hillborn E, Aalberg V: Psychoses following war brain injuries. Acta Psychiatr Scand 45:1–18, 1979.
2. Allodi F: Assessment and treatment of torture victims: A critical review. J Nerv Ment Dis 179:4–11, 1991.
3. American Psychiatric Association: Diagnostic and Statistical Manual of Mental Disorders, 3rd ed (DSM-III). Washington, DC, American Psychiatric Association, 1980.
4. American Psychiatric Association: Diagnostic and Statistical Manual of Mental Disorders, 4th ed (DSM-IV). Washington, DC, American Psychiatric Association, 1994.
5. Askevold F: War sailor syndrome. Psychother Psychosom 27:133–138, 1976–1977.
6. Askevold F: The war sailor syndrome. Dan Med Bull 27:220–223, 1980.
7. Banks MH, Beresford SHZ, Morrell DC, et al: Factors influencing demand for primary medical care in women aged 20–40 years; a preliminary report. Int J Epidemiol 4:189–255, 1975.
8. Bonica JJ: The Management of Pain. Philadelphia, Lea & Febiger, 1953.
9. Buchsbaum M: The frontal lobes, basal ganglia and temporal lobes as sites for schizophrenia. Schizophren Bull 16:379–390, 1990.
10. Burstein A: Posttraumatic stress disorder in victims of motor vehicle accidents. Hosp Common Psychiatry 40: 295–297, 1989.
11. Cassidy JD, Carroll L, Coté P: Effect of eliminating compensation for pain and suffering on the outcome of insurance claims for whiplash injury. N Engl J Med 343: 1120, 2000.

12a. Cassidy JD, Carroll L, Coté P, Lemstra M, Berglund A, Nygren A: Effect of eliminating compensation for pain and suffering on the outcome of insurance claims for whiplash injury. N Engl J Med, 342:1179–1186, 2000.

12b. Clark AF, Davison K: Mania following head injury: A report of two cases and a review of the literature. Br J Psychiatry 150:841–844, 1987.

13. Cobb S, Lindemann E: Neuropsychiatric observations. Ann Surg 117:814–824, 1943.
14. Edwards JG: Psychiatric aspects of civilian disaster. BMJ 1:944–947, 1976.
15. Eitinger L: Concentration Camp Survivors in Norway and Israel. Oslo, Universitets Forlaget, 1964.
16. Eitinger L, Krell R, Rieck M: The Psychological and Medical Effects of Concentration Camps and Related Persecutions on Survivors of the Holocaust, a Research Bibliography. Vancouver, University of British Columbia Press, 1985.
17. Eitinger L, Strom A: Mortality and Morbidity After Excessive Stress; A Follow-up Investigation of Norwegian Concentration Camp Survivors. New York, Humanities Press, 1973.
18. Erichsen JE: On Railway and Other Injuries of the Nervous System. Philadelphia, Henry C Lea, 1867.
19. Erichsen JE: On Concussion of the Spine, Nervous Shock and Other Obscure Injuries to the Nervous System in Their Clinical and Medico-legal Aspects. A New and Revised Edition. New York, William Wood & Co, 1886.
20. Fahy TJ, Irving MH, Millac P: Severe head injuries: A six-year follow-up. Lancet 2:475–479, 1967.
21. Figley CR: Stress Disorders among Vietnam Veterans. Theory, Research and Treatment. New York, Brunner/Mazel, 1978.
22. Gould R, Miller BL, Goldberg MA, et al: The validity of hysterical signs and symptoms. J Nerv Ment Dis 174: 593–597, 1986.
23. Grant I, Alves W: Psychiatric and psychosocial disturbances in head injury. In: Levin HS, Grafman J, Eisenberg HM (eds): Neurobiological Recovery from Head Injury. Oxford, Oxford University Press, 1987, pp. 232–261.

24a. Graves R: Goodbye To All That. Harmondsworth, Penguin, 1960.

24b. Grimshaw C: Obsessional disorders and psychological illness. J Neurol Neurosurg Psychiatry 27:229–231, 1964.

25. Grinker RF, Spiegel JP. Men Under Stress. Philadelphia, McGraw-Hill, Blakiston, 1945.
26. Guttmann, E: Late effects of closed head injuries: Psychiatric observations. J Ment Sci 92:1–18, 1946.
27. Haas DC, Ross GS: Transient global amnesia triggered by mild head trauma. Brain 109:251–257, 1986.
28. Hésnard A: Les troubles nerveux et psychiques consecutifs aux catastrophes navales. Rev Psychiatrie 18: 139–151, 1914.
29. Hildingsson C, Wenngren BI, Bring G, et al: Oculomotor problems after cervical spine injury. Acta Orthop Scand 60:513–516, 1989.
30. Hodges RM: So-called concussion of the spinal cord. Boston Med Surg J 104:361, 1881.
31. International Classification of Diseases, 10th revision. Geneva, World Health Organization, 1992.
32. Jacome DE: Basilar artery migraine after uncomplicated whiplash injuries. Headache 26:515–516, 1986.
33. Khanna S, Srinath S: Symptomatic mania after minor head injury. Can J Psychiatry 30:236–237, 1985.
34. Khurana RK, Nirankari VS: Bilateral sympathetic dysfunction in post-traumatic headaches. Headache 26:183–188, 1986.
35. Kinston W, Rosser R: Disaster: Effects on mental and physical state. J Psychosom Res 18:437–456, 1974.
36. Kivol K: Re: Saskatchewan Government Insurance Study. Pain Res Manage 5:129–130, 2000.
37. Kuch K, Evans RJ, Watson CP et al: Accidents and chronic myofascial pain. Pain Clin 4:79–86, 1991.
38. Levav I, Abramson JH: Emotional distress among concentration camp survivors—a community study in Jerusalem. Psychol Med 14:215–218, 1984.

39a. Lishman WA: Brain damage in relation to psychiatric disability after head injury. Br J Psychiatry 114:373–410, 1968.
39b. Lishman WA: Organic Psychiatry: The Psychological Consequences of Cerebral Disorder, 2nd ed. Oxford, Blackwell, 1987.
40. Loftus EF: The reality of repressed memories. Am Psychol 48:518–537, 1993.
41. Magni G, Caldieron C, Rigatti-Luchini S, Merskey H: Chronic musculoskeletal pain and depressive symptoms in the general population. An analysis of the 1st national health and nutrition examination survey data. Pain 43:299–307, 1990.
42. Magni G, Moreschi C, Rigatti-Luchini S, Merskey H: Prospective study of the relationship between depressive symptoms and chronic musculoskeletal pain. Pain 56:289–297, 1994.
43a. Mairet A, Durante G: Du syndrome commotionnel. Presse Med 25:478–479, 1917.
43b. Malt U, Myhrer T, Bhikra G, et al: Psychopathololgy and accidental injuries. Acta Psychiatr Scand 76:261–271, 1987.
44a. Mayou R, Bryant B: Psychiatry of whiplash neck injury. Br J Psychiatry 180:441–448, 2002.
44b. McKeon J, McGuffin P, Robinson P: Obsessive-compulsive neurosis following head injury, a report of four cases. Br J Psychiatry 144:190–192, 1984.
45. McNally RJ, Bryant RA, Ehlers A: Does early psychological intervention promote recovery from post-traumatic stress? Psychol Sci Public Interest 4:45–79, 2003.
46. Mendelson G: Not "cured by a verdict." Effect of legal settlement of compensation claimants. Med J Aust 2: 219–230, 1982.
47. Merskey H: The importance of hysteria. Br J Psychiatry 149:23–28, 1986.
48. Merskey H: Regional pain is rarely hysterical. Arch Neurol 45:915–918, 1988.
49. Merskey H: Current perspectives—psychiatry and chronic pain. Can J Psychiatry 34:329–336, 1989.
50. Merskey H: Shell shock. In: Berrios GE, Freeman HL (eds): 150 Years of British Psychiatry. 1841–1991. London, Gaskell, 1991, pp 245–267.
51a. Merskey H: The Analysis of Hysteria: Understanding Conversion and Dissociation, 2nd ed. London, Gaskell, 1995.
51b. Merskey, H: Pain Disorder: Hysteria on somatization? Pain Res Manage 9:64–71, 2004.
52. Merskey H, Buhrich N: Hysteria and organic brain disease. Br J Med Psychol 48:359–366, 1975.
53. Merskey H, Teasell RW: The disparagement of pain: Social influences on medical thinking. Pain Res Manage 5(4)259–270, 2000.
54. Mott FW: The microscopic examination of the brains of two men dead of commotion cerebri (shell shock) without visible external injury. BMJ 2:612–615, 1917.
55. Myers JK, Weissman MM, Tischler GL, et al: Six-month prevalence of psychiatric disorders in three communities. Arch Gen Psychiatry 41:959–967, 1984.
56. Ofshe R, Watters E: Making Monsters: False Memories, Psychotherapy, and Sexual Hysteria. New York, Charles Scribner's Sons, 1994.
57. Oppenheim H: Die traumatischen neurosen. Berlin, Hirschwald, 1889.
58. Page HW: Injuries of the Spine and Spinal Cord without Apparent Mechanical Lesion and Nervous Shock in Their Surgical and Medico-Legal Aspects. London, J&A Churchill, 1883.
59. Pendergrast M. Victims of Memory. Incest Accusations and Shattered Lives. Hinesburg, VT: Upper Access Books, 1995.
60. Piper A, Merskey H: The persistence of folly: a critical examination of dissociative identity disorder. Part I: The excuses of an improbable concept. Part II: The defence and decline of multiple personality or dissociative identity disorder. Can J Psychiatry 49:592–600, 678–683, 2004.
61. Pond DA, Bidwell BH: A survey of epilepsy in 14 general practices. II. Social and psychological aspects. Epilepsia 1:285–299, 1959.
62. Putnam JJ: Recent investigations in the pathology of so-called concussion of the spine. Boston Med Surg J 109: 217–220, 1883.
63a. Rassmussen OV: Medical aspects of torture. Dan Med Bull 33(suppl 1):1–88, 1990.
63b. Riess H, Schwartz CE, Klerman GL: Manic syndrome following head injury: Another form of secondary mania. J Clin Psychiatry 48:30–31, 1987.
64. Romano JM, Turner JA: Chronic pain and depression: Does the evidence support a relationship? Psych Bull 97:18–34, 1985.
65. Sargant W, Shorvon HJ: Acute war neurosis. Arch Neurol Psychiatry 54:231–240, 1945.
66a. Shepherd JP, Qureshi R, Preston MS, et al: Psychological distress after assaults and accidents. BMJ 301:849–850, 1990.
66b. Shukla S, Cook BL, Mukherj S, et al: Mania following head trauma. Am J Psychiatry 144:93–96, 1987.
67. Sjaastad O: The war sailor syndrome: After-effects of extreme mental stress. An organic brain syndrome or pseudodementia? In: Rose FC (ed): Modern Approaches to the Dementias. Part II: Clinical Therapeutic Aspects. Basel, Karger, 1985, pp 94–114.
68. Slater E: Diagnosis of 'hysteria'. BMJ 1:1395–1399, 1965.
69. Southwick SM, Morgan PA III, Nicolaou AL, Charney TA: Consistency of memory for combat related traumatic events in veterans of Operation Desert Storm. Am J Psychiatry 154:173–177, 1997.
70. Starkstein SE, Pearlson GD, Boston J, et al: Mania after brain injury: A controlled study of causative factors. Arch Neurol 44:1065–1073, 1987.
71. Starkstein SE, Robinson RG, Price TR: Comparison of cortical and subcortical lesions in the production of poststroke mood disorders. Brain 110:1045, 1987.
72. Starkstein SE, Robinson RG, Price TR: Comparison of patients with and without poststroke major depression matched for size and location of lesion. Arch Gen Psychiatry 45:247, 1988.

73a. Unwin C, Blatchley N, Kokar W, et al: The health of United Kingdom servicemen who served in the Persian Gulf War. Lancet 353:169–178, 1999.
73b. von Economo C: Encephalitis Lethargica (Translated by Newman KO, 1930). London, Oxford University Press, 1929.
74. Walton GL: Possible cerebral origin of the symptoms usually classed under "railway spine." Boston Med Surg J 109:337–340, 1883.
75. Weisaeth L, Eitinger L: Research on PTSD and other post-traumatic reactions in European literature. PTSD Res Q 2:1–7, 1991.
76. Wessely S, Unwin C, Hotopf M, Hull L, Ismail K, Nicolaou AL, David A: Stability of recall of military hazards over time. Evidence from the Persian Gulf War of 1991. Br J Psychiatry 183:314–322, 2003.
77. Whitlock FA: Symptomatic Affective Disorders. A Study of Depression and Mania Associated with Physical Disease and Medication. Sydney, Academic Press, 1982.
78a. Wilson JP, Raphael B (eds): International Handbook of Traumatic Stress Syndromes. New York, Plenum, 1993.
78b. Yatham LN, Benbow AM, Jeffers AM: Mania following head injury. Acta Psychiatry Scand 77:359–360, 1988.
79. Young A: The Harmony of Illusions. Princeton, NJ, Princeton University Press, 1995.

Chapter 35

Posttraumatic Infections of the Central Nervous System

ALLAN R. TUNKEL
AND ALAN R. TURTZ

Infections that occur following trauma to the central nervous system (CNS) are associated with high morbidity and mortality if not recognized, diagnosed, and treated promptly. Even apparently minor trauma can lead to significant infection that may result in death. The aim of this chapter is to review the acute infectious complications following trauma to the CNS with emphasis on meningitis, brain abscess, and subdural empyema.

Meningitis

Epidemiology and Etiology

Bacterial meningitis may follow varying degrees of trauma, ranging from relatively minor injuries to penetrating injuries of the skull. The incidence of acute bacterial meningitis after head trauma ranges from 0.2% to 17.8%.[8,12,14,50,51,55,90] The presence of a leak of cerebrospinal fluid (CSF), manifested clinically as rhinorrhea or otorrhea, generally leads to an increase in the incidence of posttraumatic bacterial meningitis. Rhinorrhea and otorrhea most often occur after a basilar skull fracture and are definite signs of a dural and arachnoid tear.[57] In one study that examined the incidence of bacterial meningitis in 1587 head injury patients, the incidence was only 0.38%, but it increased to 18% and 9% when the head injury was complicated by otorrhea and rhinorrhea, respectively.[51] In another study at the Maryland Institute for Emergency Medical Service Systems, meningitis was found in 35 of 45 selected head trauma patients;[90] 26 of the patients had evidence of a CSF leak, and there was a 10-fold increased risk of meningitis if a CSF leak had occurred; rhinorrhea was more common than otorrhea and was associated with a higher risk of infection in this study. Another study showed that meningitis developed in 17% of 246 patients with rhinorrhea and 4% of 156 patients with otorrhea.[58] Others have also noted the development of bacterial meningitis after a CSF leak, with an incidence ranging from 3% to 50%[38,41,55,58,99] In addition, the longer the duration of the CSF leak, the greater the risk for the subsequent development of meningitis.[29,41] The types of head trauma that have been reported to lead to CSF leaks include accidental falls, motor vehicle accidents, blunt trauma, chopstick and arrow injuries, gunshot wounds, and military missile head wounds.[1,36,45,47,74]

The microorganisms responsible for posttraumatic bacterial meningitis depend upon the pathogenesis responsible for the initial trauma.[4,6,16,26,33,36,44,45,51,52,55,65,78,83,86] With basilar skull fracture and CSF rhinorrhea, *Streptococcus pneumoniae* is the microorganism usually isolated, although other pathogens (that are usually transient residents of the upper respiratory tract) may also be important etiological agents (e.g., *Haemophilus influenzae* and group A beta-hemolytic streptococci). Staphylococci and gram-negative bacilli are very rarely isolated after basilar skull fracture unless the patient has been hospitalized for a prolonged period or if the meningitis has occurred as a complication of penetrating trauma or open head wound. The best predictors of a nonpneumococcal etiology in patients with posttraumatic bacterial meningitis are the length of time between the injury and the onset of meningitis, the nature and extent of the cranial injury, and the severity of the accompanying injury.[45] If the meningitis occurs within 3 days in a patient after a closed head injury or nondepressed skull fracture, *S. pneumoniae* is almost always the causative pathogen. Meningitis caused by anaerobes[15] and *Candida*[13] has also been reported in patients following head injury.

Pathogenesis

There are several pathogenic mechanisms that may lead to the development of meningitis following head trauma. One mechanism is the development of a dural fistula that allows microorganisms to enter the subarachnoid space. The anterior cranial fossa is separated from the nasal cavity and paranasal sinuses chiefly by a thin layer of bone and loosely adherent dura. The adhesion between the bone and dura is most pronounced at the base of the skull.[29] The dura is most likely to rupture with a fracture of the cranial bone to which it adheres, leading to an avenue for CNS invasion by bacteria located in the auditory canal, nose, or oropharynx. The dural tear is likely to involve the delicate arachnoid and leads to a CSF fistula with resulting rhinorrhea and/or otorrhea. Pneumocephalus is a not uncommon finding in this circumstance. In addition, at the site of the fracture and the dural/arachnoid tear, the cerebral tissue, which is denuded of its dural covering, may form a hernia through the fracture line. This traumatic encephalocele may sustain or occlude the CSF fistula. It is the presence of the dural fistula, not the rhinorrhea or otorrhea, that increases the risk of bacterial meningitis.[54]

Meningitis can also occur by direct ingress of skin flora into the epidural space or subdural space if the dura is lacerated during trauma.[90] Fractures of the temporal region are less likely to produce suppuration of the dura and subsequent infection, although a fracture across a chronically infected mastoid bone with an inflamed dura may lead to the development of meningitis.[4]

Clinical Presentation

The clinical features of posttraumatic bacterial meningitis are similar to those seen in patients with acute bacterial meningitis from other causes. However, since the patient has suffered head trauma, which may lead to findings that are similar to those of meningitis, it is important to have a high index of suspicion in considering the diagnosis and performing appropriate diagnostic tests.[95] The only clinical finding that may signal the possibility of posttraumatic meningitis is a deterioration of the patient's level of consciousness. Other symptoms include headache, confusion, inappropriate behavior, fever, chills, myalgias, stiff neck, vomiting, seizures, and CSF leak. Signs may include alteration of consciousness in association with fever, nuchal rigidity, and findings related to the cranial injury. The inflammatory response associated with meningitis may also seal the CSF fistula, such that an occasional sign of meningitis may be the cessation of a CSF leak. In these patients, it is important to carefully monitor for CSF rhinorrhea or other evidence of a CSF leak.

Diagnosis

The diagnosis of meningitis rests on examination of CSF performed after lumbar puncture. However, it is important to note that lumbar CSF may not accurately reflect the presence of ventriculitis if the normal flow of CSF has been interrupted.[90] In patients with an abnormal neurological exam or suspected focal lesions, computed tomography (CT) scanning should be performed prior to lumbar puncture. If there is diffuse cerebral edema, a significant mass effect, or noncommunicating hydrocephalus, lumbar puncture may not be safe. In some cases, neurosurgical management requires the use of ventriculostomy, which makes CSF analysis straightforward. If no CSF specimen can be safely obtained, empiric antimicrobial therapy should be initiated based on the likely infecting pathogen (see below). Analysis of CSF in patients with bacterial meningitis usually reveals a neutrophilic pleocytosis (generally 1000–5000 cells/mm^3, although the range may be <100/mm^3 to greater than 10,000/mm^3), low glucose (CSF:serum ratio of ≤0.4), and elevated protein 100–500 mg/dl).[92,96] However, it is important to note that similar CSF alterations may be found following head trauma, subarachnoid hemorrhage, or surgery. If the CSF is hemorrhagic, the relative numbers of red blood cells (RBCs) and white blood cells (WBCs) should be determined using the following formula[92]:

$$\text{True WBC in CSF} = \text{Actual WBC in CSF} - \frac{\text{WBC in Blood} \times \text{RBC in CSF}}{\text{RBC in Blood}}$$

A Gram's stain should be performed on all CSF specimens, although the likelihood of visualizing the microorganism by Gram's stain depends upon the CSF concentration of microorganisms (97% positivity if ≥10^5 colony-forming units/ml are present) and the specific bacterial pathogen causing meningitis.[92] A *Limulus* lysate test, which detects small quantities of bacterial endotoxin, is positive in more than 90% of patients with meningitis caused by gram-negative bacteria, although a negative test is inconclusive and a positive test does not distinguish among specific gram-negative pathogens. Elevated CSF lactate concentrations may also be useful in differentiating bacterial from chemical meningitis.

Sinus radiographs or CT imaging studies in patients with posttraumatic bacterial meningitis may reveal air-fluid levels, and scinticisternography may help localize the region of the fistula even if the CSF leak is not active. A cisternogram combined with high-resolution CT may be useful to help localize a cranial base CSF leak.

Treatment

Empiric antimicrobial therapy for patients with posttraumatic bacterial meningitis depends upon the etiology of the head trauma and the likely microorganism colonizing the patient's nasopharynx.[95,96] Early posttraumatic meningitis from a basilar skull fracture with a CSF leak is almost always caused by *S. pneumoniae*, and empiric therapy with vancomycin plus a third-generation cephalosporin (either cefotaxime or ceftriaxone) should be initiated, based on the possibility that the pneumococcus may not be susceptible to penicillin G or the cephalosporins. This regimen will also treat the other likely infecting microorganisms that may be present in the nasopharynx (e.g., *H. influenzae* and group A beta-hemolytic streptococci) and may have subsequently invaded the subarachnoid space. Once a specific pathogen is isolated, antimicrobial therapy can be modified based on in vitro susceptibility testing.

Posttraumatic meningitis following penetrating trauma or in patients with prolonged hospitalization can also be caused by staphylococci and gram-negative bacilli (including *Pseudomonas aeruginosa*). Empiric antimicrobial therapy should include vancomycin (to treat the possibility of methicillin-resistant staphylococci) combined with either ceftazidime, cefepime, or meropenem.[92,96]

The presence of a CSF leak may also necessitate surgical intervention because persistent dural defects may lead to recurrent episodes of bacterial meningitis. In the vast majority of patients, posttraumatic CSF rhinorrhea ceases spontaneously, although 10% of leaks continue for longer than 1 month.[41] Several studies have shown that if the CSF leaks stops in less than 7 days, there is no difference in the incidence of meningitis if the dural defect is repaired or not, although the likelihood of developing bacterial meningitis is much greater in patients with persistent CSF leaks. One group found an incidence of meningitis of 5% if the leak was present for less than 7 days and 55% if it lasted for more than 7 days.[55] Another study found an incidence of meningitis of 11% and 88% in patients with CSF leaks less than or greater than 7 days, respectively.[70] In another study of patients with temporal bone fractures, patients with CSF fistulae persisting for more than 7 days had a significantly increased risk of developing meningitis (23%) compared with patients whose fistulae closed within 7 days (3%) (P = .001).[14] Therefore, surgical management of a CSF fistula is indicated if it persists for more than 7–10 days. Furthermore, in a review of the medical records of 51 patients with CSF leaks that persisted for 24 hours or longer after head trauma,[32] 28 patients (53%) had spontaneous resolution of the leakage at an average of 5 days and 23 patients (47%) required surgery;

3 of the 23 patients required additional surgery for continued leakage. These authors suggested that patients with CSF leaks that persist for more than 24 hours are at a risk for meningitis and that many will require surgery.

Prevention

The use of prophylactic antimicrobial therapy in patients with basilar skull fracture and CSF leak is controversial. The rationale for the use of prophylaxis is based on the premise that the wound is contaminated, leading to CSF exposure by potentially pathogenic microorganisms from the nasopharynx, nasal sinuses, or external auditory canal. One group recommended antimicrobial prophylaxis from the time of injury until 1 week after the CSF leak had ceased;[55] they found that meningitis developed in 22.2%(12 of 54) of patients who received no prophylaxis compared to 1% (1 of 95 patients) of those who received prophylaxis. Similarly, no cases of meningitis occurred in 300 patients with basilar skull fracture who received prophylactic antimicrobial therapy,[12] although no control group was included in this study. Furthermore, in another study of 51 patients with clinically evident CSF leakage,[32] the frequency of meningitis was 10% in patients who received antimicrobial prophylaxis compared to 21% in those who did not.

In contrast, other authors have not documented the benefits of prophylactic antimicrobial therapy. In one study in which a series of 61 patients and a literature review of 402 cases were analyzed,[58] there were no significant differences in the development of posttraumatic bacterial meningitis whether or not prophylactic antimicrobial therapy was administered. A similar lack of benefit for prophylactic antimicrobial therapy was found by others in the clinical setting.[40,42] Indeed, one study found a 37% incidence of posttraumatic bacterial meningitis in patients on prophylactic antimicrobial therapy,[70] and another study of 115 patients with CSF leakage also showed that use of prophylactic antimicrobial agents was associated with a greater incidence of meningitis ($P = .024$).[22]

Interpretation and comparison of the various studies examining this question are confounded by multiple variables including patient selection, choice of antimicrobial agents, and definition of infection. Although no prospective controlled trials have examined the efficacy of prophylactic antimicrobial agents in patients with basilar skull fracture, a published meta-analysis reviewed the available data.[97] In this meta-analysis, 1241 patients with basilar skull fracture were included; 719 received antimicrobial prophylaxis and 522 did not. Antimicrobial prophylaxis was found not to prevent meningitis in patients with basilar skull fracture, even in those with CSF leak.

In summary, the data are presently insufficient to make a recommendation regarding prophylactic antimicrobial therapy in all cases of basilar skull fracture with CSF leak. Antimicrobial use may not change the incidence of posttraumatic bacterial meningitis and may result in the selection and growth of resistant organisms. Once symptoms or signs of meningitis develop in patients with basilar skull fracture, an aggressive diagnostic and therapeutic approach should be initiated.

Brain Abscess

Epidemiology and Etiology

Brain abscess is a devastating infectious complication of traumatic head injury. The risk of brain abscess after traumatic brain injury is three times greater in patients with gunshot wounds or retained bone fragments, five times greater after multiple open brain injuries, and eight times more likely in patients with cranial wound complications (e.g., hematomas, fluid collections, wound infection, and CSF fistulas.[90] Wounds that involve the facial-orbital air sinuses are twice as likely to be complicated by brain abscess.

The incidence of brain abscess after penetrating head trauma has been studied in civilian and military populations. Reported series in civilians have noted an incidence of penetrating head trauma as a cause of brain abscess ranging from 2.5% to 10.9%. Predisposing conditions in this patient population include open depressed skull fractures,[44,80] dog bites,[2,49] rooster pecking,[7] tongue piercing,[62] arrow and spear wounds,[43] and injury from lawn darts, wooden sticks, bamboo fragments, and pencil tips (especially in children).[21,27,28,30,31,63,67,89,91] In military populations, various combat series have found an incidence of brain abscess after head trauma of 3% to 17%.[1,11,17,77,84,87]

The morbidity and mortality following posttraumatic brain abscess are high. A mortality rate of

54% was found in patients with brain abscess in a series on head trauma in soldiers in Vietnam[77] compared to a mortality rate of 5% in the non–brain abscess group; death was more likely if the abscess contained gram-negative bacilli. These data indicate the need for prompt medical and surgical therapy in patients with posttraumatic brain abscess (see below).[67,75]

The microorganisms isolated from patients with posttraumatic brain abscesses are variable. They include staphylococci (*Staphylococcus aureus* and coagulase-negative staphylococci), streptococci, gram-negative bacilli, and anaerobes.[69,79,93] The most frequently isolated microorganism is *S. aureus*.[77] However, the abscess is often polymicrobial, especially in patients with war injuries or after lawn dart injuries in children.[89,91] One case of a fatal brain abscess after rooster pecking yielded cultures positive for *Streptococcus bovis*, *Clostridium tertium*, and *Aspergillus niger*.[7] The contaminated microbial flora is important in regard to the microorganisms subsequently isolated from patients with posttraumatic brain abscess. In one study of craniocerebral missile wounds in Vietnam 2–4 hours after occurrence, 44 of 45 skin wounds were contaminated with mixed gram-positive cocci and gram-negative bacilli,[19] with staphylococci the primary microorganisms isolated. Only five brain wounds were contaminated in this report, indicating that many missile tracks are sterile, although bone chips were culture positive (all staphylococci) in 20% of cases. Therefore, while the initial trauma may result in a sterile wound, contaminated skin, clothes, and the local environment may then contaminate the brain tissue and lead to brain abscess formation.

Pathogenesis

The pathogenesis of brain abscess formation after head trauma is the result of direct implantation of infected material into the brain at the time of injury. Compound wounds of the head may lead to dural tears, providing a suitable background for brain abscess formation. Children are more likely than adults to develop brain abscess after injury with pencil tips or lawn darts because of the thinness of the incompletely ossified pediatric skull, such that even minor trauma can lead to serious injuries of the dura and brain;[28,89] the fragility of the orbital roof may permit intracranial penetration of objects with considerably less force than is needed elsewhere in the skull.

In persons who suffer missile wounds in the military, the initial insult may result in a wound that is sterile, presumably because the area is cauterized by the hot metallic fragment.[19] The entry site can then be contaminated by microorganisms from the skin, clothes, and environment. In addition, embedded bone and metallic fragments may serve as a nidus for infection, although this may be less likely to occur around a metallic than a bone fragment.[34,35]

Clinical Presentation

The symptoms and signs of a posttraumatic brain abscess may be insidious.[95] Because the abscess develops in a previously traumatized area of brain tissue, progressive neurological disease is rarely seen. Patients usually have fever, irritability, mental sluggishness, and/or headache of increased severity; seizure may be the presenting manifestation. Other symptoms relate to the specific brain abscess location. If the brain abscess ruptures into the ventricular system, devastating consequences may ensue. In one recent study of 33 consecutive patients with intraventricular rupture of brain abscess,[88] severe headaches and signs of meningeal irritation were prominent before rupture, with a rapidly deteriorating clinical condition developing within 10 days after the signs of meningeal irritation. This complication is often associated with a high mortality rate (up to 80% in some series).

Diagnosis

Computed tomography has revolutionized the diagnosis of brain abscess.[93] It characteristically reveals a hypodense center with a peripheral uniform ring enhancement following the intravenous injection of contrast material; this is surrounded by a variable hypodense area of brain edema. Magnetic resonance imaging (MRI) is now the diagnostic procedure of choice for patients with brain abscess, provided that there are no metal fragments in the brain or the eyes. Magnetic resonace imaging is more sensitive than CT and offers significant advantages in the early detection of cerebritis, cerebral edema with greater contrast between edema and adjacent brain, more conspicuous spread of inflammation into the ventricles and subarachnoid space, and earlier detection of satellite lesions. On T1-weighted MRI, the abscess capsule often appears as a discrete rim that is hypointense to isointense; contrast enhancement with the paramagnetic agent gadolinium diethylenetriaminepentaacetic acid provides the added advantage of clearly differentiating the central abscess, surrounding enhancing rim, and cerebral edema.

Treatment

Because of the likelihood of a polymicrobial brain abscess after head trauma of various causes (see above), antimicrobial therapy should be targeted against staphylococci, anaerobes, and gram-negative bacilli (including *P. aeruginosa*). Vancomycin, metronidazole, and either cefepime or ceftazidime should be used pending final culture results and in vitro susceptibility testing of isolated microorganisms.[93] Antimicrobial therapy is usually administered for 6–8 weeks in patients with bacterial brain abscess, often followed by oral antimicrobial therapy for 2–6 months if an appropriate agent or agents is available; however, the efficacy and necessity of this approach have not been firmly established.[64] Shorter courses (e.g., 3–4 weeks) may be adequate for patients who have undergone surgical excision of the abscess.

Most patients with bacterial brain abscess require surgical exploration for optimal therapy. The two procedures available are aspiration of the abscess after burr hole placement or complete excision after craniotomy; no prospective trial comparing the two procedures has ever been performed.[60,85] In one series, no abscess larger than 2.5 cm resolved without surgical therapy.[59] In the series from Vietnam,[77] once an abscess developed, excision in conjunction with further debridement and local antimicrobial irrigation were used. Others have used either excision or aspiration of posttraumatic brain abscess and have noted a favorable outcome with aggressive therapy.[60]

Prevention

Aggressive surgical therapy may be required at the time of initial head injury to decrease the likelihood of infectious complications.[90] In patients with open depressed skull fractures, elevation of the bone fragments and repair of the dura are generally performed. Bone fragments can be cleaned and replaced, except in the presence of preexisting infection. Replacement is possible even when the dura is torn and cannot be closed, as long as the contaminated wound bone fragments are adequately cleaned. Disposing of contaminated bone fragments and reconstructing the skull defect with metallic material, such as titanium mesh, has more recently been used in an attempt to reduce infection rates. Although surgery is usually performed soon after the trauma, acceptable results have been obtained even when definitive treatment was delayed beyond 48 hours.[44]

Some penetrating injuries (e.g., fractures involving the paranasal sinuses) require specific management to reduce the risk of brain infection. For example, a significant fracture involving the posterior wall of the frontal sinus may require surgery to cranialize the sinus, repair the dura, remove the mucosa to avoid mucocele formation, and obliterate the sinus opening to prevent a CSF leak.

In patients with a penetrating brain injury, debridement and removal of necrotic debris is important. The experience in World War II revealed that early exploration and debridement reduced the incidence of posttraumatic infection.[56] In patients with penetrating brain injury, careful removal of devitalized brain tissue with dural closure is indicated to prevent the development of intracranial infection.[37,84] Compared to thorough brain debridement and watertight dural closure, minimal debridements and nonwatertight dural closure give inferior results and can result in a vastly greater number of patients who require additional operations.[18]

Earlier studies suggested that in patients with penetrating brain injury, removal of all bone fragments was important to improve the outcome. In a review of 1221 cases of soldiers who sustained head injury in Vietnam, a 3% incidence of brain abscess was reported.[77] In this patient population, retained bone fragments were important precursors of brain abscess formation. In another study of soldiers who sustained a brain wound in Vietnam,[20] complete brain debridement with removal of all indriven bone and removal of accessible retained bone by reoperation was recommended; the authors noted that an individual indriven bone chip had a small likelihood of bacterial contamination if initial debridement was done early.

In contrast, more recent studies have recommended that in patients with penetrating brain injury, only accessible bone and/or metallic fragments should be removed during intracranial debridement.[3,37,84,98] In one series of 127 consecutive patients with missile brain wounds during the war in Croatia,[98] patients were never reoperated on because of a single retained bone fragment, although the authors did recommend reoperation in patients with a retained cluster of bone fragments. In a study of 160 war missile penetrating craniocerebral injuries in Croatia in which 21 skull base injuries were treated surgically,[84] the authors did not attempt to remove all retained metallic or bone fragments but only the accessible ones, and the presence of retained foreign bodies did not seem to increase the infection rate, except in cases with an indriven cluster of bone fragments or CSF leak; three cases of brain abscess were seen, for which repeat surgery was required. These findings were confirmed in another retrospective study from Croatia in 88 patients with missile brain wounds in which only accessible bone/metallic fragments were removed during intracranial debridement;[37] there were nine cases of brain abscess, and the presence of retained fragments was not responsible for an increased rate of infection. In a study of 60 missile injuries, retained bone fragments were found in 36.3% of cases on follow-up CT, but no patient developed a brain abscess.[82] In another series that examined CNS infections after missile wounds during the Iran-Iraq conflict, 137 of 587 patients with retained bone fragments were followed for a mean of 42 months, with no evidence of delayed infection.[1] Finally, in a study of 43 patients who survived low-velocity missile injuries of the brain during military conflicts with retained intracranial fragments,[9] suppurative sequelae were seen in 6 patients, with two of these progressing to brain abscess.

Despite these findings, there have been isolated case reports of patients who have developed brain abscesses many years after suffering traumatic brain injury with retained foreign bodies. One patient developed a *Pseudomonas* brain abscess after surviving a grenade explosion injury during the Korean War 47 years previously,[53] and another patient developed a brain abscess 52 years after sustaining a penetrating craniocerebral shrapnel injury.[61] Therefore, retained foreign material may rarely serve as a nidus for the later development of a brain abscess.

In soldiers in Vietnam, prophylactic antimicrobial agents were used routinely in patients with penetrating head injury,[77] which seemed to significantly reduce the frequency of infection in those with craniocerebral injuries. This approach has also been shown to be effective in more recent studies.[84] In one study, it was noted that the rate of cerebral abscesses following these injuries dropped significantly from 55% to 29% with the use of prophylactic antimicrobial agents.[11] With antimicrobial regimens and surgical techniques in the military experience, the post–gunshot wound infection rate is about 4% to 6% in most series.[11,87] One recent study of gunshot wounds in the civilian population identified an incidence of CNS infections of 8.5% in those who received antimicrobial therapy at the time of presentation,[25] although few of these patients received CNS-specific coverage or an extended duration of therapy.

Subdural Empyema

Epidemiology and Etiology

Subdural empyema is a collection of pus between the dura and arachnoid layers of the meninges.[81] Cases of subdural empyema can be seen after head trauma,[5,10,23,39,46,48,68,76,100] although this is an unusual complication. A variety of microorganisms have been reported in posttraumatic subdural empyema including staphylococci, streptococci, Enterobacteriaceae, and anaerobes. The pathogenesis is secondary to introduction of microorganisms directly into the subdural space; the infective process can spread widely beyond the subdural space, leading to meningitis, and can even extend into the brain itself, with subsequent intracerebral abscess formation. The overall mortality in patients with posttraumatic subdural empyema is unknown, although one report found no deaths in head trauma patients in whom the mortality from all causes was 17%.[68] However, since subdural empyema is a rare complication of head trauma, the actual mortality rate in this subset of patients is difficult to quantify.

Clinical Presentation

The symptoms and signs of subdural empyema relate to increased intracranial pressure, meningeal irritation, and focal neurological findings corresponding to the location of the infection.[23,24,46,73,81]

Seizures, and at times refractory status epilepticus, can also be associated with subdural empyema. The disease is usually severe and rapidly progressive when secondary to trauma, with the appearance of headache, vomiting, obtundation, fever, and signs of cerebral herniation; however, this fulminant presentation may not be seen in all patients with cranial subdural empyema following head trauma. In one review of 55 patients with traumatic cranial subdural empyema,[72] headache (84% of cases), fever (69% of cases), and neck stiffness (65% of cases) were the most common clinical features, with the mean time from initial trauma to presentation of 19 days (range, 4–60 days).

Diagnosis

Diagnostic procedures for cranial subdural empyema are either CT scan with contrast enhancement or MRI.[81,94] Neuroimaging by CT scan usually reveals a crescent or elliptically shaped area of hypodensity lying directly below the cranial vault or adjacent to the falx cerebri. After contrast administration, there is a fine, intense line of enhancement between the subdural collection and cerebral cortex. However, MRI provides greater clarity of morphological detail and may detect the presence of a subdural empyema not seen on CT; it is especially helpful in detecting subdural empyemas located at the base of the brain, along the falx cerebri, or in the posterior fossa. In addition, MRI can differentiate extra-axial empyemas from most sterile effusions and subdural empyemas, and is now considered to be the diagnostic procedure of choice for cranial subdural empyema.

Treatment

The optimal therapy of subdural empyema requires a combined medical and surgical approach. Surgical drainage is necessary to guide antimicrobial selection and to control increased intracranial pressure.[94] Empiric antimicrobial therapy with vancomycin, metronidazole, and either cefepime or ceftazidime is recommended pending culture results and in vitro susceptibility testing. Depending upon the patient's clinical response, parenteral antimicrobial therapy should be continued for 3–4 weeks after drainage, although there are no firm data to support a specific duration in patients with cranial subdural empyema.

The goals of surgical therapy are to achieve adequate decompression of the brain and to completely evacuate the empyema. The optimal surgical approach (i.e., craniotomy or burr hole drainage) is controversial. In one report, the efficacy of craniotomy versus CT-guided burr hole or craniectomy drainage was analyzed during the periods from 1983 to 1987 (189 patients) and from 1988 to 1997 (509 patients); craniotomy became the preferred method of drainage by these authors since 1988 because their experience suggested that at operation, the empyema collections were sometimes found to be more loculated, tenacious, and extensive than indicated by neuroimaging studies.[71] A significant improvement in outcome was demonstrated during the study period (71.4% had a good outcome from 1983 to 1987 compared to 86.1% from 1988 to 1997; $P = .001$). In the entire database, mortality rates were also lower in patients who underwent craniotomy (8.4%) compared to those who underwent drainage via burr holes (23.3%) or craniectomies (11.5%). The authors recommended limited drainage (via burr holes or craniectomy) only in patients with septic shock and in those with limited parafalcine collections. Regardless of the initial surgical approach, however, several studies have shown that a number of patients require reoperation; in one study, reoperation was required in one-half of the patients treated with burr hole drainage versus one-fifth of those treated with craniotomy.[66] Although the data were not specifically on patients with cranial subdural empyema following trauma, it is reasonable to follow this approach in patients who develop posttraumatic subdural empyema.

REFERENCES

1. Aarabi B, Taghipour M, Alibaii E, Kamgarpour A: Central nervous system infections after military missile head wounds. Neurosurgery 42:500–509, 1998.
2. Alpert G, Sutton LN: Brain abscess following cranial dog bite. Clin Pediatr 23:580, 1984.
3. Amirjamshidi A, Abbassioun K, Rahmat H: Minimal debridement or simple wound closure as the only surgical treatment in war victims with low-velocity penetrating head injuries. Indications and management protocol based upon more than 8 years follow-up of 99 cases from Iran-Iraq conflict. Surg Neurol 60:105–111, 2003.
4. Appelbaum E: Meningitis following trauma to the head and face. JAMA 173:1818–1822, 1960.
5. Bannister G, Williams B, Smith S: Treatment of subdural empyema. J Neurosurg 55:82–88, 1981.

6. Belardi FG, Pascoe JM, Beegle ED: *Pasteurella multocida* meningitis in an infant following occipital dog bite. J Fam Pract 14:778–782, 1982.
7. Berkowitz FE, Jacobs DWC: Fatal case of brain abscess caused by rooster pecking. Pediatr Infect Dis J 6:941–942, 1987.
8. Bernal-Sprekelsen M, Bleda-Vazquez C, Carrau RL: Ascending meningitis secondary to traumatic cerebrospinal fluid leaks. Am J Rhinol 14:257–259, 2000.
9. Bhatoe HS: Retained intracranial splinters: A follow-up study in survivors of low intensity military conflicts. Neurol India 49:29–32, 2001.
10. Borzone M, Capuzzo T, Rivano C, Tortoridonatei P: Subdural empyema: Fourteen cases surgically treated. Surg Neurol 13:449–452, 1980.
11. Brandvold B, Levi L, Feinsod M, George ED: Penetrating craniocerebral injuries in the Israeli involvement in the Lebanese conflict, 1982–1985. Analysis of a less aggressive surgical approach. J Neurosurg 72:15–21, 1990.
12. Brawley BW, Kelly WA: Treatment of basal skull fractures with and without cerebrospinal fluid fistulae. J Neurosurg 26:57–61, 1967.
13. Brenier-Pinchart MP, Leclercq P, Mallie M, Bettega G: *Candida* meningitis possibly resulting from a harpoon injury. Eur J Clin Microbiol Infect Dis 18:454–455, 1999.
14. Brodie HA, Thompson TC: Management of complications from 820 temporal bone fractures. Am J Otol 18: 188–197, 1997.
15. Brook I: *Prevotella intermedia* meningitis associated with cerebrospinal fluid leakage in an adolescent. Pediatr Infect Dis J 22:751–753, 2003.
16. Bryan CS, Jernigan FE: Posttraumatic meningitis due to ampicillin-resistant *Haemophilus influenzae*. J Neurosurg 51:240–241, 1979.
17. Cairns H, Calvert CA, Daniel P, Northcroft GB: Complications of head wounds with special reference to infection. Br J Surg Suppl 1:198–243, 1947.
18. Carey ME: The treatment of wartime brain wounds: Traditional versus minimal debridement. Surg Neurol 60: 112–119, 2003.
19. Carey ME, Young HF, Mathis JL, Forsythe J: A bacteriological study of craniocerebral missile wounds from Vietnam. J Neurosurg 34:145–154, 1971.
20. Carey ME, Young HF, Rish BL, Mathis JL: Follow-up study of 103 American soldiers who sustained a brain wound in Vietnam. J Neurosurg 41:542–549, 1974.
21. Chang CJ, Huang LT, Lui CC, Huang SC: Oral wooden stick injury complicated by meningitis and brain abscess. Chang Gung Med J 25:266–270, 2002.
22. Choi D, Spann R: Traumatic cerebrospinal fluid leakage: Risk factors and the use of prophylactic antibiotics. Br J Neurosurg 10:571–575, 1996.
23. Coonrad JD, Dans PE: Subdural empyema. Am J Med 53:85–91, 1972.
24. Dill SR, Cobbs CG, McDonald CK: Subdural empyema: Analysis of 32 cases and review. Clin Infect Dis 20:372–386, 1995.
25. Doherty PF, Rabinowitz RP: Gunshot wounds to the head: The role of antibiotics. Infect Med 21:297–300, 2004.
26. Downs NJ, Hodges GR, Taylor SA: Mixed bacterial meningitis. Rev Infect Dis 9:693–703, 1987.
27. Duffy GP, Bhandari YS: Intracranial complications following transorbital penetrating injuries. Br J Surg 56: 685–688, 1969.
28. Dujovny M, Osgood CP, Maroon JC, Jannetta PJ: Penetrating intracranial foreign bodies in children. J Trauma 15:981–986, 1975.
29. Einhorn A, Mizrahi EM: Basilar skull fractures in children: The incidence of CNS infection and the use of antibiotics. Am J Dis Child 132:1121–1124, 1978.
30. Fanning WL, Willett LR, Phillips CF, Wallman LJ: Puncture wound of the eyelid causing brain abscess. J Trauma 16:919–920, 1976.
31. Foy P, Scharr M: Cerebral abscesses in children after pencil-tip injuries. Lancet 2:662–663, 1980.
32. Friedman JA, Ebersold MJ, Quast LM: Post-traumatic cerebrospinal fluid leakage. World J Surg 25:1062–1066, 2001.
33. Gilbert VE, Beals JD, Natelson SE, Tyler WA: Treatment of cerebrospinal fluid leaks and gram-negative bacillary meningitis with large doses of intrathecal amikacin and systemic antibiotics. Neurosurgery 18:402–406, 1986.
34. Hagan RE: Early complications following penetrating wounds of the brain. J Neurosurg 34:132–141, 1971.
35. Hammon WM: Retained intracranial bone fragments: Analysis of 42 patients. J Neurosurg 34:142–144, 1971.
36. Hand WL, Sanford JP: Posttraumatic bacterial meningitis. Ann Intern Med 72:869–874, 1970.
37. Hecimovic I, Dmitrovic B, Kurbel S, et al: Intracranial infection after missile brain wound: 15 war cases. Zentralblatt Neurochir 61:95–102, 2000.
38. Henry RC, Taylor PH: Cerebrospinal fluid otorrhoea and otorhinorrhoea following closed head injury. J Laryngol Otol 92:743–756, 1978.
39. Hitchcock E, Andreadis A: Subdural empyema: A review of 29 cases. J Neurol Neurosurg Psychiatry 27:422–434, 1964.
40. Hoff JT, Brewin A, U HS: Antibiotics for basilar skull fracture. J Neurosurg 44:649, 1976.
41. Hyslop NE, Montgomery WW: Diagnosis and management of meningitis associated with cerebrospinal fluid leaks. In: Remington JS, Swartz MN (eds): Current Clinical Topics in Infectious Diseases, vol 3. New York, McGraw-Hill, 1982, pp 254–285.
42. Ignelzi RJ, VanderArk GD: Analysis of the treatment of basilar skull fractures with and without antibiotics. J Neurosurg 43:721–726, 1975.
43. Jacob OJ, Rosenfeld JV, Taylor RH, Watters DAK: Late complications of arrow and spear wounds to the head and neck. J Trauma 47:768–773, 1999.
44. Jennett B, Miller JD: Infection after depressed fracture of the skull: Implications for management of nonmissile injuries. J Neurosurg 36:333–339, 1972.
45. Jones SR, Luby JP, Sandford JP: Bacterial meningitis complicating cranial-spinal trauma. J Trauma 13:895–900, 1973.

46. Kaufman DM, Miller MH, Steigbigel NH: Subdural empyema: Analysis of 17 recent cases and review of the literature. Medicine (Balt) 54:485–498, 1975.
47. Kawamura S, Hadeishi H, Sasaguchi N, et al: Penetrating head injury caused by a chopstick—case report. Neurol Med Chir 37:332–335, 1997.
48. Khan M, Griebel R: Subdural empyema: A retrospective study of 15 patients. Can J Surg 27:283–288, 1984.
49. Klein DM, Cohen ME: *Pasteurella multocida* brain abscess following perforating cranial dog bite. J Pediatr 92:588–589, 1978.
50. Kral T, Zentner J, Vieweg U, et al: Diagnosis and treatment of basilar skull fractures. Neurosurg Rev 20:19–23, 1997.
51. Lau YL, Kenna AP: Post-traumatic meningitis in children. Injury 17:407–409, 1986.
52. Leblanc W, Heagarty MC: Posttraumatic meningitis due to *Haemophilus influenzae* type A. J Natl Med Assoc 75:995–1000, 1983.
53. Lee JH, Kim DG: Brain abscess related to metal fragments 47 years after head injury. Case report. J Neurosurg 93:477–479, 2000.
54. Leech PJ: Cerebrospinal fluid leakage, dural fistulae and meningitis after basal skull fractures. Injury 6:141–149, 1974.
55. Leech PJ, Paterson A: Conservative and operative management for cerebrospinal-fluid leakage after closed head injury. Lancet 1:1013–1016, 1973.
56. Lewin W: Gram negative meningitis following head wounds with a special reference to infection with coliform bacilli. Br J Surg 35:266–280, 1948.
57. MacGee EE: Cerebrospinal fluid fistula. In Vinken PJ, Bruyn GW (eds): Handbook of Clinical Neurology, vol 24: Injuries of the Brain and Skull, part II. Amsterdam, North-Holland, 1976, pp 183–199.
58. MacGee EE, Cauthen JC, Brackett CE: Meningitis following acute traumatic cerebrospinal fluid fistula. J Neurosurg 33:312–316, 1970.
59. Mamelak AN, Mampalam TJ, Obana WG, Rosenblum ML: Improved management of multiple brain abscesses: A combined surgical and medical approach. Neurosurgery 36:76–86, 1995.
60. Mampalam TJ, Rosenblum ML: Trends in the management of bacterial brain abscesses: A review of 102 cases over 17 years. Neurosurgery 23:451–458, 1988.
61. Marquardt G, Schick U, Moller-Hartmann W: Brain abscess decades after a penetrating shrapnel injury. Br J Neurosurg 14:246–248, 2000.
62. Martinello RA, Cooney EL: Cerebellar brain abscess associated with tongue piercing. Clin Infect Dis 36:e32–e34, 2003.
63. Maruya J, Yamamoto K, Wakai M, Kaneko U: Brain abscess following transorbital penetrating injury due to bamboo fragments—case report. Neurol Med Chir 42: 143–146, 2002.
64. Mathisen GE, Johnson JP: Brain abscess. Clin Infect Dis 25:763–781, 1997.
65. Matschke J, Tsokos M: Post-traumatic meningitis: Histomorphological findings, postmortem microbiology and forensic implications. Forens Sci Int 115:199–205, 2001.
66. Mauser HW, van Houwelingen HC, Tulleken CA: Factors affecting the outcome of subdural empyema. J Neurol Neurosurg Psychiatry 50:1136–1141, 1987.
67. Miller CF, Brodkey JS, Colonibi BJ: The danger of intracranial wood. Surg Neurol 7:95–103, 1977.
68. Miller ES, Dias PS, Uttley D: Management of subdural empyema: A series of 24 cases. J Neurol Neurosurg Psychiatry 50:1415–1418, 1987.
69. Miller JD: Infection after head injury. In: Vinken PJ, Bruyn GW (eds): Handbook of Clinical Neurology, vol 24: Injuries of the Brain and Skull, Part II. Amsterdam, North-Holland, 1976, pp 215–230.
70. Mincy JE: Posttraumatic cerebrospinal fluid fistula of the frontal fossa. J Trauma 6:618–622, 1966.
71. Nathoo N, Nadvi SS, Gouws E, van Dellen JR: Craniotomy improves outcomes for cranial subdural empyemas: Computed tomography-era experience with 699 patients. Neurosurgery 49:872–878, 2001.
72. Nathoo N, Nadvi SS, van Dellen JR: Traumatic cranial empyema: A review of 55 patients. Br J Neurosurg 14: 326–330, 2000.
73. Nathoo N, Nadvi SS, van Dellen JR, Gouws E: Intracranial subdural empyema in the era of computed tomography: A review of 699 cases. Neurosurgery 44: 529–535, 1999.
74. Neal G, Downing EF: Clostridial meningitis as a result of craniocerebral arrow injury. J Trauma 40:476–480, 1996.
75. Nielsen H, Gyldensted C, Harmsen A: Cerebral abscess. Aetiology and pathogenesis, symptoms, diagnosis and treatment—a review of 200 cases from 1935–1976. Acta Neurol Scand 65:609–622, 1982.
76. Renaudin JW, Frazee J: Subdural empyema—importance of early diagnosis. Neurosurgery 7:477–479, 1980.
77. Rish BL, Caveness WF, Dillon JD, Kistler JP, Mohr JP, Weiss GH: Analysis of brain abscess after penetrating craniocerebral injuries in Vietnam. Neurosurgery 9:535–541, 1981.
78. Roberts SR, Esther JW, Brewer JH: Posttraumatic *Pasteurella multocida* meningitis. South Med J 81:675–676, 1988.
79. Saez-Llorens XJ, Umana MA, Odio CM, McCracken GH Jr, Nelson JD: Brain abscess in infants and children. Pediatr Infect Dis J 8:449–458, 1989.
80. Sande GM, Galbraith SL, McLatchie G: Infections after depressed fracture in the west of Scotland. Scott Med J 25:227–229, 1980.
81. Silverberg AL, DiNubile MJ: Subdural empyema and cranial epidural abscess. Med Clin North Am 69:361–374, 1985.
82. Singh P: Missile injuries of the brain: Results of less aggressive surgery. Neurol India 51:215–219, 2003.
83. Spagnuolo PJ, Ellner JJ, Lerner PI, McHenry MC, Flatauer F, Rosenberg P, Rosenthal MS: *Haemophilus influenzae* meningitis: The spectrum of disease in adults. Medicine (Balt) 61:74–85, 1992.

84. Splavski B, Sisljagic V, Peric LJ, et al: Intracranial infection as a common complication following war missile skull base injury. Injury 31:233–237, 2000.
85. Stephanov S: Surgical treatment of brain abscess. Neurosurgery 22:724–730, 1988.
86. Swartz MN, Dodge PR: Bacterial meningitis—a review of selected aspects. N Engl J Med 272:725–731, 779–787, 842–848, 898–902, 1965.
87. Taha JM, Haddad PS, Brown JA: Intracranial infection after missile injuries to the brain: Report of 30 cases from the Lebanese conflict. Neurosurgery 29:864–868, 1991.
88. Takeshita M, Kawamata T, Izawa M, Hori T: Prodromal signs and clinical factors influencing outcome in patients with intraventricular rupture of purulent brain abscess. Neurosurgery 48:310–317, 2001.
89. Tay JS, Garland JS. Serious head injuries from lawn darts. Pediatrics 79:261–263, 1987.
90. Tenney JH: Bacterial infections of the central nervous system in neurosurgery. Neurol Clin 4:91–114, 1986.
91. Tiffany KK, Kline MW: Mixed flora brain abscess with *Pseudomonas paucimobilis* after a penetrating lawn dart injury. Pediatr Infect Dis J 7:667–669, 1988.
92. Tunkel AR: Bacterial Meningitis. Philadelphia: Lippincott Williams & Wilkins, 2001.
93. Tunkel AR: Brain abscess. In: Mandell GL, Bennett JE, Dolin R (eds): Principles and Practice of Infectious Diseases, 6th ed. Philadelphia, Elsevier Churchill Livingstone, 2005, pp 1150–1163.
94. Tunkel AR: Subdural empyema, epidural abscess, and suppurative intracranial thrombophlebitis. In Mandell GL, Bennett JE, Dolin R (eds): Principles and Practice of Infectious Diseases, 6th ed. Philadelphia: Elsevier Churchill Livingstone, 2005, pp 1164–1171.
95. Tunkel AR, Scheld WM: Acute infectious complications of head trauma. In: Braakman R (ed): Handbook of Clinical Neurology, vol 13: Head Injury. Amsterdam, Elsevier Science, 1990, pp 317–326.
96. Tunkel AR, Scheld WM: Acute meningitis. In: Mandell GL, Bennett JE, Dolin R (eds): Principles and Practice of Infectious Diseases, 6th ed. Philadelphia: Elsevier Churchill Livingstone, 2005, pp 1083–1126.
97. Villalobos T, Arango C, Kubilis P, Rathore M: Antibiotic prophylaxis after basilar skull fracture. Clin Infect Dis 27:364–369, 1998.
98. Vrankovic D, Splavski B, Hecimovic I, et al: Analysis of 127 war inflicted missile brain injuries sustained in northeastern Croatia. J Neurol Sci 40:107–114, 1996.
99. Wehrle PF, Mathies AW, Leedom JM: Management of bacterial meningitis. Clin Neurosurg 14:72–85, 1967.
100. Weinman D, Samarasinghe HHR: Subdural empyema. Aust NZ J Surg 41:324–330, 1972.

Chapter 36
Functional Symptoms and Signs in Neurology

JON STONE AND MICHAEL SHARPE

A 30-year-old woman presents to a clinical neurology service with a 3-month history of right leg weakness. Her problems began slowly after she tripped and hurt her ankle while running to the assistance of her daughter. The ankle pain resolved, but the weakness gradually got worse. She complains of a number of other recent symptoms including pain, fatigue, poor memory, and bowel disturbance. Her file is noticeably large, with previous medical contacts for hysterectomy, laparoscopy for abdominal pain, and rather brittle asthma. Now her husband has to help her dress and bathe, and she is receiving state disability benefits. She has seen an orthopedic specialist, who has confirmed that there is no evidence of bony or soft tissue injury. On examination she walks with her leg dragging behind her and her hip laterally rotated. There is marked inconsistency between power testing on the bed and ability when walking. She has a strongly positive Hoover's sign, and although only her arm and face are not symptomatic, she is surprised to find that on testing, temperature and vibration sense are altered on the right side of her body, with a midline split. Magnetic resonance imaging (MRI) of the brain and spine, lumbar puncture, neurophysiology, and other relevant tests are all normal. A diagnosis of functional paralysis is made.

Around one-third of all new patients presenting to neurologists in the United States, the United Kingdom, and Europe have symptoms that are not explained by neurological disease. These symptoms, such as dizziness, headache, weakness, blackouts, and numbness, appear to be genuinely experienced but have no apparent basis in disease.

In this chapter, we first summarize what is known (and not known) about the diagnosis and management of patients with these symptoms, paying particular attention to disabling symptoms such as functional paralysis and nonepileptic attacks. Secondly, we discuss the potential causes of functional symptoms, both general and specific, exploring particularly the relationship of these so-called functional symptoms to physical and emotional trauma.

Our perspective in writing this chapter is that of clinicians who work almost exclusively in National Health Service (NHS) clinical practice in the United Kingdom. Our approach therefore is a practical one, based on an assumption that the patient is truly experiencing the reported symptoms and is deserving of assessment. This practical and transparent approach, as we will explain, involves moving away from a purely psychogenic explanation toward a more complex model in which symptoms are seen as the result of reversible dysfunction of the nervous system—dysfunction that, in turn, may be brought about by psychological, biological and social factors.

Functional Somatic Symptoms—The Wider Picture

Symptoms and Disease

Around one-third to one-half of all new neurological outpatients have symptoms rated by the neurologist as largely or not at all explained by disease.[23,52,139,182] This is not a peculiarity of neurology. Similar proportions are found in a wide range of primary and secondary care settings.[139] Table 36.1 illustrates the many different functional somatic symptoms and syndromes found in different specialties, placing those found in neurology in context. Although persons with these symptoms and syndromes present to different specialties, there are striking similarities in their associated epidemiology and response to treatment.[224]

Patients present to doctors with symptoms, and doctors generally look for a disease to explain them. But disease is only one cause of symptoms (Fig. 36.1). Symptoms also arise from normal physiology (e.g., physiological tremor) and from psychological factors (e.g., paresthesia during a panic attack) and are shaped by cultural or other social factors (e.g., the existence of a welfare state, patient advocacy groups). This is also the case even when disease is the major determining cause of the symptoms.

Using this model, it becomes clearer that trying to decide in a dichotomous way whether symptoms are either due to disease or are psychogenic is probably the wrong way to look at the problem. Instead, we should be attempting to apportion the symptoms of each patient to a variety of causes. In some, disease will be an important factor; in others, it will be a minor factor or not present at all. A crucial consequence of this approach is that the patient does not have to have a genuine disease in order to have a genuine symptom. We discuss conscious simulation of symptoms and misdiagnosis later.

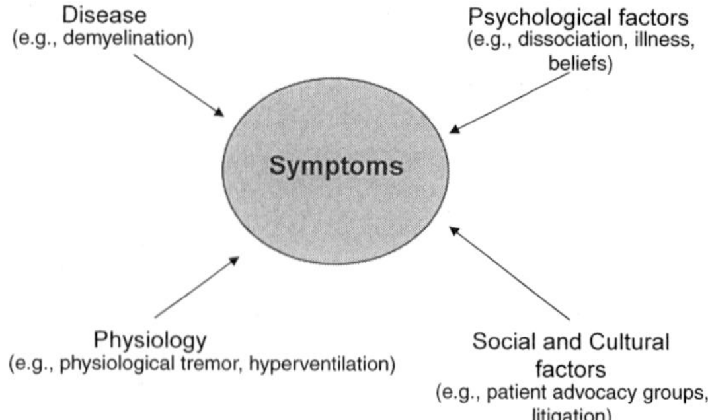

Figure 36.1. Disease is only one cause of symptoms.

Table 36.1. Examples of Functional Somatic Symptoms and Syndromes Found in Different Medical Specialties

Neurology	Functional weakness, nonepileptic attacks, hemisensory symptoms
Gastroenterology	Irritable bowel syndrome, nonulcer dyspepsia, chronic abdominal pain
Gynecology	Chronic pelvic pain, premenstrual syndrome
Otorhinolaryngology	Functional dysphonia, globus pharyngis
Cardiology	Atypical chest pain
Rheumatology	Fibromyalgia
Infectious diseases	(Postviral) chronic fatigue syndrome
Immunology	Multiple chemical sensitivity Syndrome

What Should We Call Them?

The many terms used to describe symptoms unexplained by disease is a reflection of the conceptual confusion in this area (Table 36.2). There are pure symptomatic labels (e.g., *chronic fatigue*), symptom syndromes (e.g., *chronic fatigue syndrome*), nondiagnoses that describe what the diagnosis isn't rather than what it is (e.g., *nonepileptic*

Table 36.2. Words Used to Describe Symptoms Unexplained or Largely Unexplained by Disease

Symptom descriptions	Low back pain, chronic fatigue
Symptom syndromes	Chronic fatigue syndrome, irritable bowel syndrome
Nondiagnoses	Nonepileptic attacks, nonorganic
Psychological etiology	Psychogenic, psychosomatic, all in your mind
	Conversion disorder, somatoform symptoms, somatization disorder
Physical etiology	Reflex sympathetic dystrophy, myalgic encephalomyelitis, chronic fatigue syndrome with immune dysfunction
Traumatic etiology	Chronic whiplash syndrome, shell shock, railway spine
Other	Hysteria, functional, fibromyalgia, dissociative symptoms

attacks, nonorganic, medically unexplained), diagnoses that imply a disease cause after all (e.g., *reflex sympathetic dystrophy*), and others that suggest a purely psychological cause (*psychogenic, psychosomatic, "all in your mind"*). There are some that don't fit into any of these categories: *hysteria* implies that the symptoms arise unconsciously; *functional* suggests that they relate to a problem in bodily function. Finally, there are diagnoses that are found in psychiatric glossaries but are rarely used by neurologists (e.g., *conversion disorder, dissociative disorder, somatization disorder*) and terms for situations in which the problem is thought to be consciously motivated (e.g., *factitious disorder, malingering*).

Getting the terminology right is important, as it reflects and influences how you think about the problem. It may also determine the way in which the patient reacts when you try to explain what is wrong.

There are a variety of official diagnostic disorders that have formed the basis for research in this area. In the DSM-IV, the American Psychiatric Association's diagnostic manual of psychiatric disorder,[4] a diagnosis of conversion disorder requires at least one motor or sensory neurological symptom other than pain and fatigue that causes distress, is not explained by disease, is not malingered, and is thought to relate to psychological factors. Somatization disorder is diagnosed when the neurological symptom is combined with four different pain symptoms, two gastrointestinal (GI) symptoms, and one sexual symptom occurring as a long-standing pattern of repeated medical presentation. In the World Health Organization's diagnostic manual, the International Classification of Disease-Revision 10 (ICD-10), there is a subtly different set of diagnoses including dissociative motor disorder (which includes paralysis and attacks that resemble epilepsy) and neurasthenia (pure fatigue state). Other terms to be aware of are *hypochondriasis*, which refers to a state of anxiety about personal health, *factitious disorder* (where symptoms are consciously simulated in order to gain medical care), and *malingering* (where the symptoms are simulated for clear financial or material gain).

As well as trying to decide which diagnostic label most accurately reflects the cause of the symptoms, there are also practical considerations. Many of the terms in Table 36.2 are known to be potentially offensive to patients. For example, over 40% of general outpatients equate the words *psychosomatic* and *hysterical* with "putting on" or "imagining" symptoms or "going mad"[191,198] (Fig. 36.2). We prefer to use the word *functional*, popular in the nineteenth and early twentieth centuries, to describe many of these symptoms because (1) it sidesteps

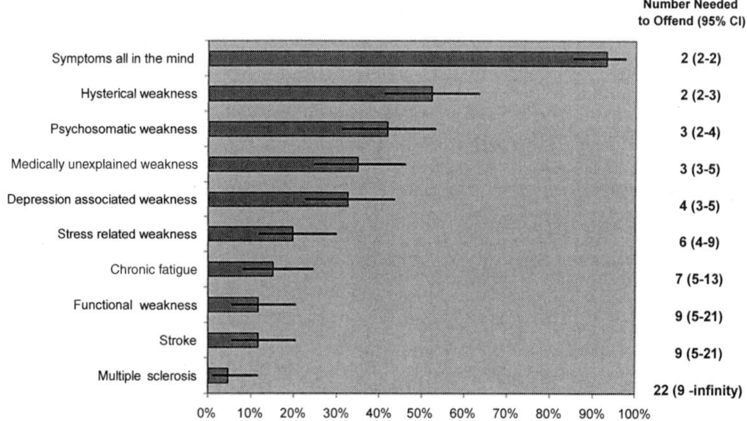

Figure 36.2. Many words we use to describe symptoms unexplained by disease are potentially offensive to patients. A study of 86 general neurology patients asked to imagine that they had a weak leg with normal tests and were being given a diagnosis. The figure illustrates the percentage who would equate the diagnosis with being mad, putting on symptoms, or imagining symptoms, along with the number needed to offend—the number of patients who have to be given the diagnosis before one is offended. (Reproduced with permission from the BMJ Publishing Group.[198])

unhelpful dualistic psychological/physical debates as well as unresolvable conscious/unconscious ones, (2) it leads to ways of thinking about treatment and restoring function that make sense to patients, and (3) it is not offensive. In the study mentioned above, it offended less than 10% of patients. This means that it can be used transparently—in the clinic letter copied for the patient, in leaflets, and in research articles. We recognize problems with it too; it is overly broad for some, it would probably acquire stigma if used widely again, and it introduces another dichotomy—that of function versus structure (although this seems to be a much more helpful one clinically).

How Common Are Functional Symptoms in Neurology?

Symptoms Unexplained by Disease in Neurological Practice

A number of studies have attempted to describe the proportion of patients attending neurological services who have symptoms unexplained by disease. Using case note criteria or doctor ratings, around one-third to one-half of all neurology patients fall into this category. This is a surprisingly robust finding that has been repeated in a number of studies in different countries.[23,52,139,182] These studies inevitably use a broader definition for the problem than that defined by conversion disorder and include patients with symptoms such as tension headache and dizziness.

Functional Motor and Sensory Symptoms

Population studies of functional symptoms such as paralysis, sensory disturbance, visual symptoms, and nonepileptic attacks (usually called *conversion disorder* or *hysteria*) are few, are often of poor quality, and vary considerably in the definitions they have used. Incidence rates of 5–10/100,000 are typical, with prevalence rates of 50–300/100,000.[1] To put this in perspective, these figures suggest that conversion disorder is at least as common as multiple sclerosis. The methodology used in most of these studies (looking for psychiatric diagnoses rather than just symptoms) probably means that most data are an underestimate of the clinical problem.

In neurological practice, estimates of the frequency of symptoms identified with conversion disorder are also few. One London neurologist diagnosed conversion hysteria in 4% of 7836 consecutive outpatients.[146] Many authors of similar studies do not mention functional symptoms at all, perhaps because they do not regard them as a neurological diagnosis.

The proportion of neurological inpatients reported to have conversion symptoms has varied from 1% to 18%.[48,123,131,172] One-third to one-half of patients with conversion disorder have paralysis as their main symptom.[199] A similar proportion have nonepileptic attacks, making these the two most common conversion symptoms.

More data exist about nonepileptic attacks, which characterize 10% to 20% of patients referred to a specialist epilepsy clinic with intractable seizures[181] and up to 50% of patients admitted to a hospital in apparent status.[80]

Functional movement disorders are increasingly recognized by movement disorders experts.[204] In the mid-twentieth century, dystonia was often misdiagnosed as psychogenic, and so this diagnosis has returned only cautiously. In recent series, however, patients with these symptoms comprise 6% of all new referrals to specialist movement disorder clinics.[204]

In conclusion, functional symptoms are probably the most common problem that any neurologist deals with. Even the more unusual functional neurological symptoms such as paralysis and nonepileptic attacks are relatively common in neurological practice.

Are Patients with Functional Symptoms Just the "Worried Well"?

Doctors tend to have a variety of reactions to the problem of symptoms unexplained by disease. Some believe that most of these patients are simply the worried well who are making a fuss about nothing. Some feel that many patients make up their symptoms to gain sympathy or financial benefit. Others view them all as psychiatrically unwell. Conversely, others believe that they all have a disease or a condition with a biological basis that has not been detected or described.

When patients with neurological symptoms unexplained by disease are compared to those whose symptoms are explained, they are found to have higher rates of distress and emotional disorder and just as much self-rated disability.[23] Their symptoms also tend to persist at follow-up, but these are rarely subsequently explained by a disease.[22,31,165] Studies like these raise the question "Are these patients *really* more disabled and distressed or is that just what they say?" This is a much harder question to answer. Disability and distress are by their very nature subjective. Ultimately, it is probably the patient's subjective view that matters most. Prognosis, misdiagnosis, and malingering are discussed in more detail later.

Taking a History from Someone with Functional Symptoms—A Practical Approach

If you suspect that a patient's presenting symptoms are functional, there are a number of ways in which history taking can be altered that are helpful not only in making the diagnosis, but also in making the consultation more efficient. These techniques are also likely to provide a platform for the explanation and management you provide. As we will explain later, for the patient with functional symptoms, a good assessment *is* actually the beginning of treatment. The following is a guide for taking the history of the patient with multiple and chronic functional symptoms. It can also be adapted for the patient with milder or less numerous symptoms.

"Drain the Symptoms Dry"

If you sense that your patient has many symptoms, the best way to start the consultation is often to ask the patient to help you make a complete list of them. Try to resist the urge to determine the features and onset of every symptom as you go. Instead, leave a few lines between each symptom on the list so that you can go back and discuss them later. The aim is to rapidly elicit the patient's current list of symptoms. This often has the effect of helping the patient unburden all the symptoms he or she has been concerned about. It also prevents new symptoms from cropping up later on in the consultation and gives you a much broader picture of the situation at the earliest stage. Fatigue, sleep disturbance, memory and concentration difficulties, and pain can be routinely inquired about at this stage without necessarily asking about mood, which we suggest should be left until later.

There is good evidence that the *more physical symptoms a patient presents with, the more likely it is that the primary presenting symptom will not be explained by disease*.[224] This means that a long list of symptoms should be a warning that the primary problem might be functional.

Asking about Disability

An easy way of assessing disability is to ask, "What's a typical day like for you?" Follow-up questions like "How much of the day do you spend in bed/asleep?" and "How often do you leave the house?" are sometimes more useful than the traditional disability questions about dressing and walking distance.

Finding Out More about Onset and Course

Although you often will want to take a more detailed history of certain symptoms, if a patient has had symptoms for many years it may be more helpful to get a general picture of the course of the illness by drawing a graph with time on the x-axis and severity on the y-axis (Fig. 36.3). For many patients. this is a useful and quick way of condensing, what may be a large amount of information into an understandable format—the line of the graph demonstrating how the illness has gradually worsened, cycled, or perhaps been static over the time period in question. Later on, other events can be added to the graph, such as an arrow indicating when the patient stopped working, other life events, or details of other medical interventions.

Asking about Dissociation

Dissociative symptoms such as depersonalization and derealization are not always familiar territory for neurologists. They are commonly experienced by healthy individuals, are induced deliberately by some people using psychoactive drugs, occur more commonly in patients with neurological disease such as epilepsy and migraine, and are particularly common in patients with functional symptoms, especially paralysis and nonepileptic attacks. The following statements give an indication of what sort of thing to look for: "I felt as if I was there, but not

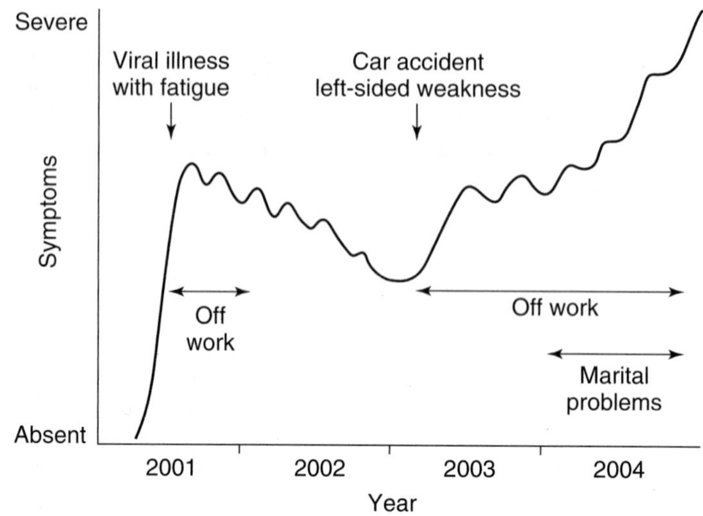

Figure 36.3. Using a graph to take a history from a patient with functional symptoms.

there, as if I was outside of myself"; "I was in a place all of my own"; "Things around me didn't feel real; it was like I was watching everything on television"; "My body didn't feel like my own"; "I couldn't see but I could hear everyone; I just couldn't reply."

Dissociative symptoms are useful to uncover for several reasons. Firstly, dissociation is sometimes the underlying explanation for the patient's complaints of dizziness. Secondly, dissociative symptoms are frightening to patients, who are often reluctant to describe them and relieved to discover that the symptom is common and does not indicate madness. Lastly, they can offer an extra way of explaining to patients the link between their experiences and the development of unusual symptoms such as a limb that no longer feels as if it is part of the body or the common reported sensation during a nonepileptic attack of being present but being unable to communicate with anyone.

Previous Medical and Other Interventions for These Symptoms/Illness

When given the opportunity, some patients will complain bitterly about a doctor who didn't listen to them or who told them that the condition was nothing serious. You don't need to agree with the patient's opinion of the previous doctor, but getting this information serves two useful purposes. Firstly, it can inform the way in which you deliver the diagnosis at the end of the consultation, and it orients you to which avenues of treatment (if any) are likely to be helpful. Secondly, by letting patients talk openly about previous disappointing medical encounters, you are implicitly showing them that you appreciate their experience of difficulty in having their symptoms taken seriously.

Asking about Illness Beliefs

It can be very helpful to ask patients for their own view of their symptoms. What do they think is causing them? What do they think should be done? Do they think the symptoms are irreversible or reversible? There is evidence from a number of studies that *patients with functional neurological symptoms are more likely to be convinced that their symptoms are caused by disease than are patients whose symptoms are due to disease.*[14,139] These questions are not particularly helpful diagnostically, but they help with rapport, prognostication, and orienting the explanation at the end. For example, if a patient goes to great lengths to explain to you that the problem is not psychological, this emphasizes the need for a careful approach in introducing psychological factors.

Past Medical History—Get the Notes

Apart from the overall number of symptoms, probably the only other general *diagnostic* red flag in the consultation is whether there is a previous history of functional symptoms. *The more functional symptoms the patient has had in the past, the more likely it is that the current symptom is also functional.*[224] There may be a history of one or more previous functional somatic symptoms (from Table 36.1) or of surgical operations related to them (hysterectomy at a young age, appendectomy, laparoscopy to investigate abdominal pain). Although it seems obvious, it can be vital to have access to accurate medical records in assessing someone with functional symptoms.

Stereotypical patients with functional symptoms may be highly forthcoming about their past medical history and bring with them a list of previous symptoms and investigations. In our experience, however, the majority of patients with a history of previous functional symptoms are much more reticent. This is sometimes because they have forgotten previous symptoms or normal investigations. More often, it is because they sense that the more they tell you about previous medical encounters that ended in no diagnosis, the more they worry (quite reasonably in many cases) that you will not take their current symptoms seriously. Asking specifically about time off work or school or asking the question "What would I find in your family doctor's notes?" can elicit extra information. Sometimes, things that patients tell you about their medical history (for example, that they were advised to have a hysterectomy or that the appendix was inflamed) may not be completely accurate, although the fault for this inaccuracy may not necessarily lie with the patient.[174a] Previous psychiatric diagnoses may be particularly likely to be unreported.

Comorbidity of Disease and Functional Symptoms

A large number of studies have suggested that functional neurological symptoms occur frequently in patients who also have established neurological disease. For example, in one study, 42% of patients with unexplained motor symptoms[31] had a comorbid neurological disease, half with a peripheral origin. In other studies of mixed functional symptoms, the range of disease comorbidity ranges from around 20% to 60%, although the method of case ascertainment has a large effect on these estimates.[9,43,57,88,97,108,110,115,123,129,130,151,166,226] The relationship between disease and coexisting functional symptoms is likely to be complex. Diseases of the nervous system can lead directly, via structural and functional changes in the brain, to emotional and personality changes that can leave some individuals susceptible to functional symptoms they otherwise would not have had. Having a disease of the nervous system is also a major life event, and it is also therefore not surprising if some patients react badly to it.

Asking about Emotional Symptoms and Stress

Having prioritized physical symptoms, disability, and the medical and social histories, now is a much better time to inquire about the patient's mood and other emotional symptoms. Rates of depression, anxiety, and panic are consistently higher in patients with functional symptoms than in those with disease. The patient may, however, be reluctant to talk about these symptoms. The key to successfully eliciting emotional symptoms is to frame the question in terms of the presenting symptom and avoid, at least initially, psychiatric words like *depression*, *anxiety*, and *panic*. For example:

Instead of asking "Have you been feeling depressed?", try "Do your symptoms ever make you feel down or frustrated? How much of the time?"

Instead of asking "Do you enjoy things any more?", try "How much of the time do your symptoms stop you from enjoying things? Is that most of the time? Do you still enjoy the things you can do?"

If you suspect that your patient has been having panic attacks or is agoraphobic, ask, "Do you ever have attacks where you have a lot of symptoms all at once? When do these happen? Is it when you're outside or in certain situations?"

Sometimes questions about stress need to be framed in a similar way. Rather than appearing to blame stress, ask, "Are there other things going on at home or at work that are making it even more difficult to cope with these symptoms?"

At first glance, this approach appears to involve pussyfooting around psychological issues. Why not just ask the patient directly about depression and anxiety? The stigma of psychiatric diagnoses is widespread in the general population, not just in patients with functional symptoms. For many normal people, anything psychological implies mental weakness or madness. Care in using terms initially avoids generating early hostility and means that important psychological aspects of the presentation can be questioned later when the patient is much more likely to accept it.

Modeling on Others

Although it is often suggested that patients copy or model the symptoms of friends and family,[106] there is little actual evidence for this in patients with functional neurological symptoms. Twenty-two percent of the patients in Crimlisk et al.'s study[31] had worked in medical or paramedical professions, which may have increased their scope for symptom modeling, but we do not know whether this rate exceeds the population norm. The specificity of this association has been examined only in one controlled study, which found that patients with functional visual loss were more frequently exposed to others with eye disease than were disease controls (67% vs. 28%).[90]

Psychiatric History

A full assessment of a patient with multiple functional symptoms requires a proper psychiatric history including questions about early life experiences and abuse. Unless you have a long time to spend with the patient, we suggest leaving these questions for subsequent consultations. The evidence from studies in primary care does not suggest that disclosure of important events such as abuse leads to an improved outcome.[173] The situation may be different in a psychotherapeutic environment, but in routine neurological practice, if blundered into too early, such disclosure might be detrimental to the therapeutic relationship.

Social History: Work, Money, the Law, and Marriage

An unpleasant job, being in a "benefit trap" (where money received as benefits is comparable to that earned at work), and involvement in a legal case (relevant to the symptom) are examples of powerful potential obstacles to recovery. While it is important to try not to leap to a judgment about the patient's motivation when these factors are present, they have important implications for treatment and prognosis. Similarly, an unhappy marital situation or loneliness may be relevant.

Examination

The diagnosis of functional neurological symptoms depends on demonstrating positive features in the examination, as well as on the absence of signs of organic disease. Fifty years ago, textbooks of nervous disease such as those of Purves-Stewart and Worster-Drought contained a large section on the positive physical manifestations of hysteria.[148] Although some can still be found, a lot of this information has been dropped from modern texts. Most of these signs relate to inconsistency, either internal (e.g., Hoover's sign reveals discrepancies in leg power) or external (e.g., tubular field defect is inconsistent with the laws of optics).

When considering any sign of functional weakness, it is important to remember the following caveats:

1. Functional signs usually depend on inconsistency, and as such do not distinguish hysterical from malingered problems.
2. The presence of a positive sign of functional symptoms does not exclude the possibility that the patient also has an organic disease.
3. All physical signs have limited sensitivity, specificity, and interrater reliability.

General Signs

La belle indifference

La belle indifference, or an apparent lack of concern about the nature or implications of disabling functional symptoms, is a clinical feature that continues to receive prominence in standard descriptions of conversion disorder. However, the evidence, such as it is, suggests that it is an unreliable clinical sign. The high rate of depression and anxiety found in studies of these patients is incompatible with a high proportion manifesting indifference. As Lewis and Berman observed,[115] "in marked contrast to their alleged indifference many hysterical patients manifest a deep interest . . . in describing their ailments."

Combining the results of studies published since 1966, most of which are of poor quality and uncontrolled, we have found that la belle indifference is reported in roughly the same proportion of patients with hysteria (around 20%)[9,24,43,87,115,151,175,219] as it is in patients with organic disease.[9,24,64,151,219] However, none of these studies have adequately operationalized the concept of la belle indifference. This is important because la belle indifference could be easily misdiagnosed in (1) patients who are making an effort to appear cheerful in a conscious attempt not be labeled as depressed; (2) patients with sensory signs they were unaware of (something Janet and Charcot emphasized, but that is not the same as indifference to disability); (3) patients who are concerned about a limb symptom when asked about it but appear absent-minded, apathetic, or distracted the rest of the time; and (4) patients whose symptoms are factitious (they may not be concerned since they know where the symptoms are arising from).[196]

The Laterality of the Symptoms

For many years, it has been accepted that functional motor and sensory symptoms are more common on the left side. Briquet himself had said so,[19] and a number of studies tailored to this question appeared to confirm it.[61,145,189] These data seemed to tie in nicely with a number of theories, including those suggesting a relationship with the *emotional right hemisphere*, a relationship to the *neglect* of right hemisphere lesions, or perhaps simply an asymmetry determined by the inconvenience of having a weak dominant hand.

We carried out a systematic review of the relevant literature published since 1965.[193] While studies that specifically set out to examine this issue (*headline studies*) often reported a positive answer, studies that reported laterality incidentally (*nonheadline studies*) did not find an asymmetry (Fig. 36.4).The net result from all studies combined suggested that while there may be a slight preponderance of left-sided symptoms over those on the right (about 55% for paralysis and 60% for sensory symptoms), a form of publication bias may account for most of this apparent asymmetry. The results of this study are backed up by a similar systematic analysis carried out in 1908 by Ernest Jones,[86] who found no lateralizing effect in 277 cases drawn from 164 articles. The diagnosis of functional weakness or sensory disturbance should therefore certainly not be made based on the side of the symptoms.

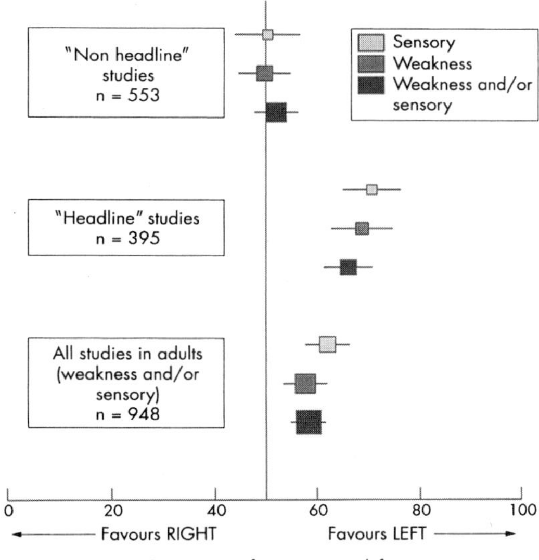

Figure 36.4. The laterality of functional weakness and sensory disturbance—a systematic review of all studies from 1965 to 2000 (*n* refers to number of subjects), demonstrating that studies in which laterality is specifically studied find a preponderance on the left, whereas those that report the data incidentally do not. (Reproduced with permission from the BMJ Publishing Group.[193])

Functional Weakness

Preliminary Observation

The assessment of the patient with functional weakness should begin as the patient gets up from the chair in the waiting room and not end until the patient leaves the consulting room (or the hospital). The primary objective is to look for evidence of *inconsistency*. It may be particularly helpful to watch the patient:

- Taking clothes off or putting them on.
- Removing something from and replacing it in a bag (e.g., a list of medications).
- Walking into the room, in comparison to walking out of the room or out of the building.
- Patients complaining of unilateral functional weakness in an arm often hold it conspicuously on their lap and use it less during the examination, like a patient with a stroke.

Hoover's Sign

Hoover's sign is probably the most useful test for functional weakness and the only one that has been subjected to scientific study with a neurological control group.[39,183,232] It is a simple, repeatable test, that does not require skilled surreptitious observation. The test relies on the principle that virtually all persons, whether they have a disease or not, extend their hip when flexing their contralateral hip against resistance. This finding is thought to be a result of the crossed extensor reflex, which enables normal walking and is present even in decorticate animals. The test, as described by Hoover in 1908,[77] can be performed in two ways:

1. Hip extension—In patients with functional weakness, a discrepancy can be observed between their voluntary hip extension (which is often weak) and their involuntary hip extension when the opposite hip is being flexed against resistance (which should be normal) (Fig. 36.5). When testing involuntary hip extension, it is important to ask the patient to concentrate hard on the good leg.
2. Hip flexion—The opposite test, in which hip flexion in the weak leg is tested while the examiner's hand is held under the good heel, is also described, although it has not been adequately evaluated. In this test, the absence of downward pressure in the good leg indicates a lack of effort transmitted to either leg.

Head described an additional variant in which the patient lies on the stomach and is asked to extend the good hip while hip flexion is tested in the weak leg.[72] Raimiste has described a similar phenomenon of simultaneous leg adduction and abduction,[150] which has been tested and elaborated by Sonoo[183] with promising results. Hip abduction, like hip extension and plantar flexion, appears to be a movement that is commonly weak in functional paralysis. Hoover also described a similar test in the arms in which elevation against resistance of an arm stretched out in front of the patient can produces downward pressure of the other arm. In practice, this test is much more difficult to use.[77]

False positives may occur due to (1) pain in the affected hip producing greater weakness on direct compared with indirect testing as a result of at-

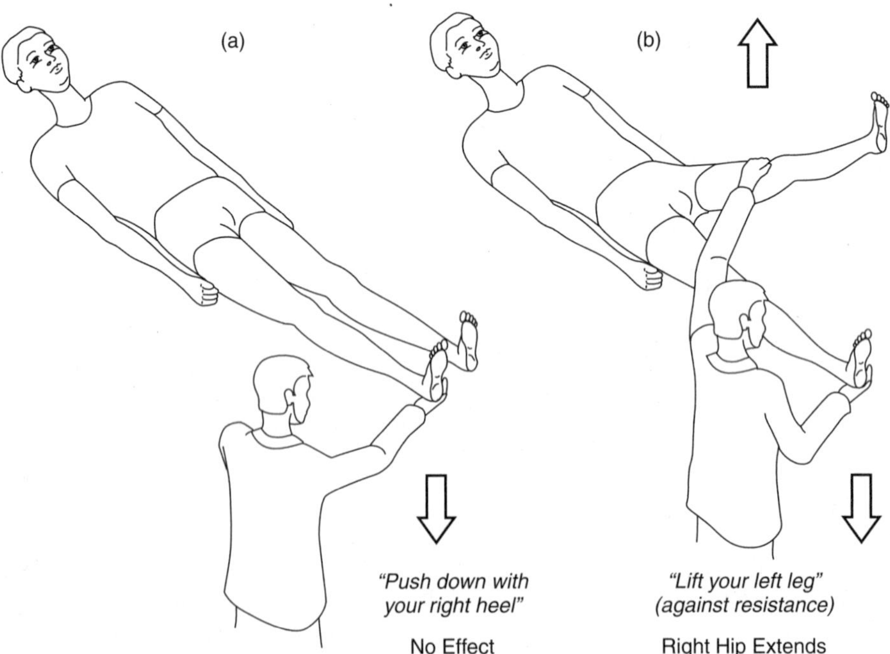

Figure 36.5. Hoover's sign. (a) Hip extension is weak when tested directly. (b) Hip extension is normal when the patient is asked to flex the opposite hip. (Reproduced with permission from the BMJ Publishing Group.[200])

tentional phenomena (related to pain rather than weakness); (2) neglect in the affected limb (so be more careful if the left side is weak); and (3) interpretation of mildly positive results related to the splinting effect of the test itself in normal people.

False negatives may occur if the patient does not concentrate sufficiently on flexing the good hip when you are testing involuntary extension of the weak hip. If so, ask the patient to look at the strong leg while testing it or ask why it has become weaker. Persistent failure to cooperate with a Hoover's test may be a marker of factitious disorder.

Hoover's test of hip extension has been evaluated in three small controlled studies[39,183,232] that suggest good sensitivity and specificity However, these numbers are still small, crucially none of the studies were blinded, and none mention the problem of neglect. They do, however, provide preliminary support for its use.

Collapsing Weakness

A common finding in functional weakness is *collapsing weakness*. This is the phenomenon in which a limb collapses from a normal position with a light touch (or, occasionally, even before your hand has touched the limb). Normal power can often be achieved transiently with encouragement. The instruction "At the count of three, stop me from pushing down" is often helpful in this respect. Another method for obtaining normal power is to gradually increase the force applied to the limb, starting extremely gently and building imperceptibly up to normal force. The intuitive explanation of collapsing weakness is that the patient simply isn't trying. While this is sometimes undoubtedly the case, in our experience the performance of most patients with functional weakness seems to worsen the more effort and attention they expend on the limb.

The problem with collapsing weakness is that, like Hoover's sign, it may also occur for reasons unrelated to the diagnosis. These include an inability to understand the instruction, pain in the relevant joint, being generally unwell, and a misguided eagerness of some patients to "help the doctor" or "convince the doctor" even though they actually have organic disease.

Collapsing or *give-way* weakness has been investigated neurophysiologically.[98,127,211] These studies have suggested the following abnormalities in patients with functional weakness: (1) the force generated by a limb at the point at which the examiner overcomes the muscle force can be unusually *high* when compared to the force generated by normal resistance;[211] (2) there may be significantly variable amounts of force in patients' limbs compared to those of controls;[98,127,211] and (3) they produce less force the slower the movement is.[98]

Collapsing weakness has been put to the test in one real life controlled clinical study and was found in 20% of patients with conversion disorder compared to 5% of patients with disease.[24] Gould et al.[64] found that of 30 patients with acute neurological pathology (mostly stroke), 10 had collapsing weakness, emphasizing the need for caution with this sign.

Functional Weakness of the Face, Pseudoptosis, and Wrong-Way Tongue Deviation

Pseudoptosis, or functional ptosis, is occasionally encountered, often in association with photophobia. Organic unilateral ptosis is usually associated with frontalis overactivity, whereas in pseudoptosis a *persistently* depressed eyebrow with a variable inability to elevate the frontalis and overactivity of the orbicularis is characteristic (Fig. 36.6). Given the rarity of pseudoptosis, it's always worth considering whether an underlying or coexistent problem such as blepharospasm or myasthenia gravis is present. Functional weakness of the lower half of the face is not described in recent literature, but we have seen striking cases.

In neurological hemiplegia the tongue may sometimes deviate toward the paretic side. Functional paralysis with tongue deviation toward the normal rather than the paretic side has been described,[93] again suggesting overactivity rather than underactivity of the affected side.

Other Signs of Functional Weakness

Cocontraction describes the contraction of an antagonist muscle (e.g., triceps) when the agonist muscle (biceps) is being tested. Knutsson and Martensson showed that in 12 patients with functional weakness, knee flexion was weaker than it would have been if they had just let the weight of the lower leg carry out the movement—indicating antagonist activation.[98]

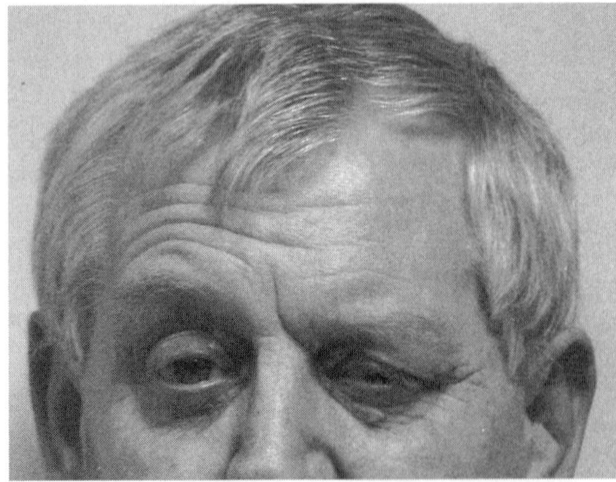

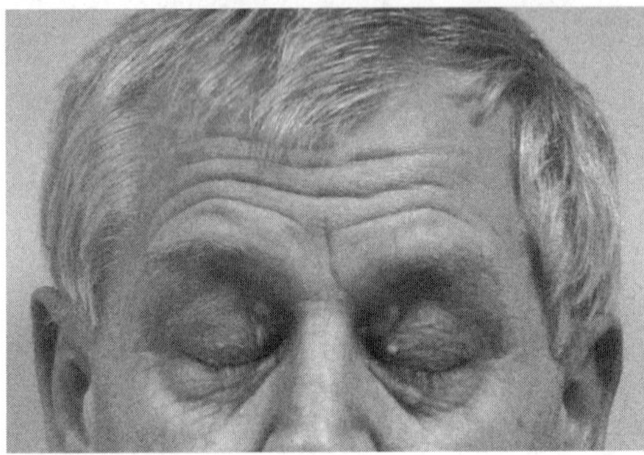

Figure 36.6. Pseudoptosis. This man presented with photophobia and difficulty elevating the right side of his forehead. The photograph shows his normal resting state (top) and normal movement of his forehead with his eyes shut (bottom). The problem was overactivity of his left orbicularis oculis with functional weakness of his left frontalis, which had been incorrectly interpreted as ptosis. It improved with gradual exposure to light. (Reproduced by permission from Blackwells Publishing.[190])

We do not advocate the use of the *arm drop*—dropping a supposedly paralyzed arm over the patient's face to see if he or she will protect themself from its fall (also described as a test on the unconscious patient). The arm must be so weak for this test to be interpretable that we suggest that it rarely adds information. A less aggressive variation is to look for an unusually slow, jerky descent of the arm from an outstretched position on to the lap. Occasionally, when this test is performed the arms remain inexplicably elevated, so called '*pseudo-waxy flexibility*, a phenomenon akin to that seen under hypnosis.

Finally, in patients with unilateral symptoms, it may also be worthwhile to pay particular attention to the *strength of the sternocleidomastod* (SCM). A recent study found that 80% of patients with functional hemiparesis had ipsilateral SCM weakness, whereas only 11% of vascular hemiparesis patients had weakness of the SCM (which is bilaterally innervated and so is rarely weak in upper motor neuron lesions).[41]

Using Sedation/Hypnosis

In the altered mental state induced by sedative drugs or hypnosis, patients with functional weakness may begin to move their limbs normally again. Using video to record this event can be a positive experience for a patient and a breakthrough in treatment in some cases. However, it may be dangerous to use sedation to obtain more history from your patient.

Important Absent Signs in Functional Weakness

We have emphasized the importance of looking for positive signs of functional weakness and sensory disturbance. The absence of certain specific signs is also important. Tone and reflexes should be normal, although pain may increase tone and there may be mild reflex asymmetry, particularly if there is attentional interference from the patient.[58,188] Clonus is not necessarily an organic sign. Pseudoclonus was well described in the late nineteenth and early twentieth centuries as a clonus with irregular and variable amplitude.[58,65] The plantar response may be mute on the affected side, particularly if there is marked sensory disturbance, but it should not be upgoing.

Functional Sensory Disturbance

The clinical detection and localization of sensory dysfunction in structural lesions is probably one of the least reliable areas of the neurological examination.[116] What evidence exists suggests that these signs are just as untrustworthy in the detection of functional symptoms.

Functional sensory disturbance may be noticed by the patient or, as is often the case, may be detected by the examiner and come as a surprise to the patient. It typically affects all sensory modalities, either in a hemisensory distribution ("I feel as if I'm cut in half") or affecting a whole limb. In the latter, sharply demarcated boundaries at the shoulder and at the groin are common.[59,82] If the trunk is involved, the front is more commonly involved than the back. Someone with functional weakness usually has functional sensory disturbance as well—perhaps suggesting a shared pathophysiology. While a number of functional sensory signs none appear to be specific and should not therefore be used to make a diagnosis.

Midline Splitting and the Hemisensory Syndrome

The hemisensory syndrome has been described for over a century and continues to be a well-known but rarely studied clinical problem in neurology (Fig. 36.7). The intensity of the sensory disturbance often varies, and while it may be complete, it is usually rather patchy, but with a distinct complaint from the patient that something is "not right" down one side.

Patients with hemisensory disturbance frequently complain of intermittent blurring of vision in the ipsilateral eye (asthenopia) and sometimes of ipsilateral hearing problems as well. Hemisensory symptoms are increasingly recognized in patients with chronic pain[120,164] and in patients diagnosed as having reflex sympathetic dystrophy.[214]

Recently, Toth has published a study of 34 outpatients with the hemisensory syndrome,[208] finding that the majority of patients improved at follow-up.

It has been commonly assumed that exact splitting of sensation in the midline cannot occur in organic disease. The reason usually given is that cutaneous branches of the intercostal nerves overlap from the contralateral side, so sensory loss should be paramedian—that is, 1 or 2 cm from the midline. But midline splitting can occur in thalamic stroke when a profound loss of several modalities in a manner similar to functional sensory loss can occur. Similar hemisensory disturbance can be provoked by hyperventilation[142] or hypnotic suggestion.[56] The finding of contralateral thalamic and basal ganglia hypoactivation in patients with this symptom using single photon emission computed

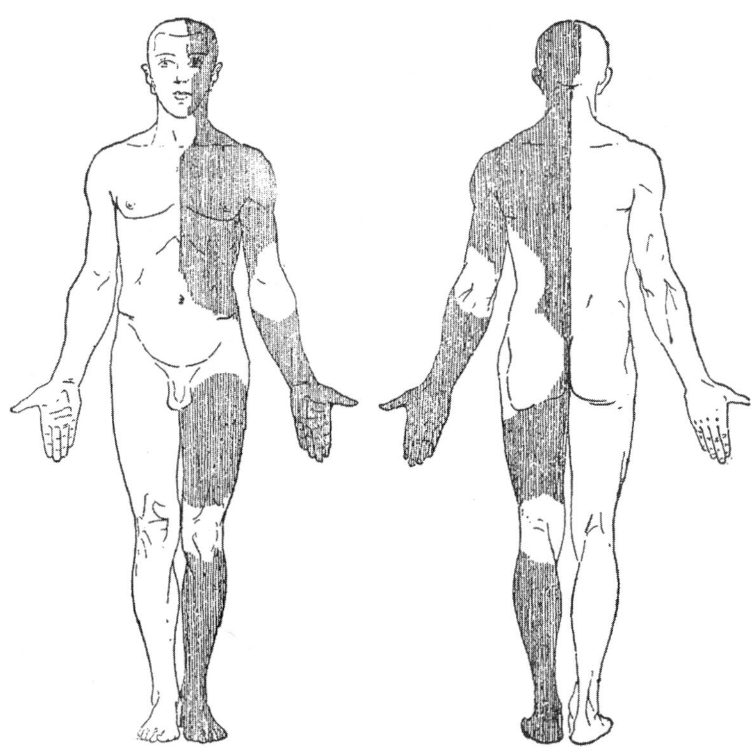

Figure 36.7. Hemisensory disturbance. (From Charcot JM: Clinical Lectures on Diseases of the Nervous System, vol 3. London, New Sydenham Society, 1889.)

tomography (SPECT) is also intriguing in this respect.[216] Chabrol et al. found midline splitting in 26% of 15 conversion disorder patients compared to 15% of 40 neurological controls, indicating its unreliablity.[24]

Splitting of Vibration Sense

There should be little difference in the sensation of a tuning fork placed over the left compared to the right side of the sternum or frontal bone, as the bone is a single unit and must vibrate as one. Toth found this sign in 68% of his sample.[208] However, other studies have found it frequently (70%,[64] 86%[163]) in patients with organic disease. The surprising conclusion at present must be that this test cannot be recommended.

Tests Involving Doctor Trickery

If you ask a patient to "Say 'yes' when you feel me touch you and 'no' when you don't" (originally described by Janet), the patient may indeed say "no" in the affected area. The problem is, firstly, that the patient may be using "no" to mean "not as much." Secondly, unless they a have learning disability, many patients will know (at least in hindsight) that they were being tricked. This makes this test unhelpful in situations where a therapeutic relationship is aimed for. Sensory examination of the hands while they are either crossed behind the back or interlocked and rotated on the chest (the Bowlus maneuver[35]) and forced choice procedures have been described in which testing is made sufficiently complicated that a systematic underperformance (performance worse than chance) can be detected.[133,202] These tests may have medicolegal uses but would also be positive in patients naively trying to convince the doctor that there is a problem.

Nonepileptic Attacks

There is considerably more evidence with which to approach the problem of the clinical diagnosis of nonepileptic attacks or pseudoseizures. As with functional weakness, the history may be suggestive, for example with a history of other functional symptoms[152,154] and contact with psychiatric services,[100] but will not be in itself diagnostic.

Semiology

Table 36.3 lists some of the signs that have been tested in studies of patients with both nonepileptic attacks and epilepsy. As the table demonstrates, there are no clinical signs of nonepileptic attacks that *never* occur in epilepsy, and apart from ictal electroencephalographic (EEG) abnormalities, there are no signs unique to epilepsy. For this reason, it is dangerous to use any of the signs listed in isolation to make a diagnosis. Despite considerable heterogeneity, attempts have been made to classify nonepileptic attacks into different types, for example attacks with excessive movement and attacks with atonia or swooning. Patients with more dramatic attacks may have a worse prognosis.[155] Further work using predictive models incorporating multiple signs are helping to make clinical diagnosis without videotelemetry more reliable.[66,100]

In this area, it is important to recognize that certain types of epilepsy, particularly frontal lobe seizures, can look bizarre. In addition, the term *nonepileptic attacks* may be confusing, as it is sometimes broadened to include any attacks, such as syncope and paroxysmal movement disorders, that are not epileptic.

Prolactin Measurement

Serum prolactin is often elevated 10–20 minutes after a generalized tonic clonic seizure and should be normal after a nonepileptic attack. However, a prolactin rise has also been demonstrated after syncope and may be normal after a partial seizure. The test can be useful, but in our experience it is often carried out badly in practice, with no baseline sample and a postictal specimen that is measured either too early or too late. For this reason, we do not advocate its use outside specialist units.

Electroencephalography and Videotelemetry

Electroencephalography with or without videotelemetry remains, the gold standard investigation for nonepileptic attacks. However, patients with partial epilepsy, particularly frontal lobe epilepsy, may not show any abnormalities on surface EEG recording when there is a deep ictal focus. In addition, some patients may not have attacks during monitoring.

Table 36.3. Attack Features That Can Help to Distinguish Nonepileptic Attacks from Epileptic Seizures

Observation	Nonepileptic Seizures	Epileptic Seizures
Situational onset	Occasional	Rare
Gradual onset	Common	Rare
Precipitated by stimuli (noise, light)	Occasional	Rare
Undulating motor activity	Common	Very rare
Asynchronous limb movements	Common	Rare
Purposeful movements	Occasional	Very rare
Rhythmic pelvic movements	Occasional	Rare
Opisthotonus, "arc de cercle"	Occasional	Very rare
Side-to-side head shaking	Common	Rare
Tongue biting (tip)	Occasional	Rare
Tongue biting (side)	Rare	Common
Prolonged ictal atonia	Occasional	Very rare
Ictal crying	Occasional	Very rare
Closed mouth in "tonic phase"	Occasional	Very rare
Vocalization during "tonic–clonic" phase	Occasional	Very rare
Closed eyelids	Very common	Rare
Convulsion >2 min	Common	Very rare
Resistance to eyelid opening	Common	Very rare
Pupillary light reflex	Usually retained	Commonly absent
Reactivity during "unconsciousness"	Occasional	Very rare
Lack of cyanosis	Common	Rare
Rapid postictal reorientation	Common	Rare

Source: Reprinted by permission from reference 152.

Using Placebo and Suggestion to Induce Attacks

Rather than waiting for an attack to occur during videotelemetry, various techniques have been described to induce attacks quickly, thus saving resources and allowing monitoring of the attack in highly controlled circumstances. One method, using a bolus of intravenous saline, given with the suggestion that it will bring on an attack, is controversial, as it can involve deception by the doctor (depending on how the procedure is explained to the patient). In these cases, the diagnosis may be made more quickly, which may be important in reducing the morbidity of a wrong diagnosis of epilepsy.[12] However, subsequent treatment may be more difficult, as the patient may, on reflection, realize that he or she was duped. Being honest and telling the patient that the injection is saline is an improvement, but an even better method is simply to use suggestion on its own, without props. McConigal et al.[128] have shown that a completely honest *suggestion protocol* can be effective in diagnosing nonepileptic attacks. In their randomized study, the diagnostic yield was doubled with this protocol, particularly for patients with a history of attacks in medical settings.

Functional or Psychogenic Movement Disorders

Making the diagnosis of a functional movement disorder can be one of the most difficult tasks in this area of neurology. Organic movement disorders are often bizarre, for example the *geste antagoniste* seen in dystonia and the intermittent nature of the paroxysmal movement disorders. Partly for this reason, movement disorders figure disproportionately in cases where structural disease has been misdiagnosed as functional. For this reason, a diagnosis of psychogenic movement disorder should only be made by a movement disorders specialist.

The following is a summary of some useful diagnostic features, but as with nonepileptic attacks, none of these features, perhaps with the exception of prolonged reversal after hypnosis/sedation, should be used in isolation to make a diagnosis. Further description of the features below can be found elsewhere,[204] and useful video material can be found accompanying a textbook on movement disorders.[171]

There are some general features common to all functional movement disorders. These include:

Rapid onset—Several series have remarked on the high frequency of history of sudden onset (70%–90% in three series), whereas this is more unusual in patients with organic movement disorder.

Variability—Variability in frequency, amplitude, or distribution may be obvious during an examination or during observation at other times. It must be remembered that all movement disorders vary to some degree and will get worse during times of stress or worry, so minor variability is not helpful.

Improvement with distraction—Distraction includes asking the patient to perform tests of mental concentration (e.g., serial subtraction) or physical tasks with the normal limbs (such as rapid alternating hand movements). The inverse, worsening with attention, may also occur. Again, organic movement disorders may be susceptible to these factors to a mild degree.

Laterality—In a systematic review of laterality, there was a preponderance of right-sided symptoms (68%).[193]

Tremor

Functional tremor normally affects the hand, but can be generalized or occur in unusual places such as the palate.[96,169] It is the most common form of functional movement disorder.

Entrainment

Distraction tasks are particularly useful in the diagnosis of functional or psychogenic tremor. In the specific distraction of *entrainment*, the patient is asked to make a rhythmic movement with the normal hand or foot. Either the normal limb entrains to the same rhythm as the abnormal side or, more commonly, the requested rhythmic movement is irregular or incomplete. There is reasonable evidence for the reliability of this test from several clinical and neurophysiological studies comparing patients with psychogenic tremor and organic tremor.[126,187,231] One study, measuring tremor using accelerometry, suggested that a requested tapping frequency of 3 Hz was more discriminant, and produced more variation, than a faster 5 Hz rate.[231]

Tremor Amplitude Change with Weights/Coactivation Sign

Although variability is not always abnormal in patients with psychogenic tremor, there is evidence that adding weights to the affected limb in patients can help to bring out variability. Patients with psychogenic tremor tend to have a greater tremor amplitude, whereas in those with organic tremor the tremor amplitude, tends to diminish.[37,231] Deuschl et al. have suggested that the reason for increased amplitude with weighting is coactivation of agonist and antagonist muscles, coining the term *coactivation sign*.[37]

Dystonia

Patients with hysterical contracture were extensively described (concurrently with descriptions of organic dystonia) in the literature from the late nineteenth and early twentieth centuries (Fig. 36.8). Later, many patients with organic dystonia were misdiagnosed as psychogenic,[45,112] particularly in the mid-twentieth century, when symbolic psychodynamic interpretations such as torticollis, representing a "turning away from responsibility," were prevalent. When this error was realized and the organic nature of dystonia was characterized, the diagnosis of psychogenic dystonia almost disappeared. Increasingly, the problem is once again being recognized.[50,174b,204] The diagnosis is difficult, but features to be aware of include an inverted foot or "clenched fist" onset in an adult,[179] a fixed posture that is apparently present during sleep, the presence of severe pain, and marked inconsistency. Inconsistency is a particularly difficult clinical judgment since so many of the dystonias can manifest in unusual and apparently selective and inconsistent ways, for example writer's cramp and the geste antagoniste.

The gold standard for the diagnosis is to demonstrate complete remission after administration of general anesthesia, suggestion, or placebo.[50] Such a procedure, if handled carefully, may also have a highly persuasive therapeutic effect. Even then, some types of organic dystonia may remit spontaneously so caution is warranted A high proportion of patients with psychogenic dystonia have had an injury to the affected limb.[11,104] We discuss the pos-

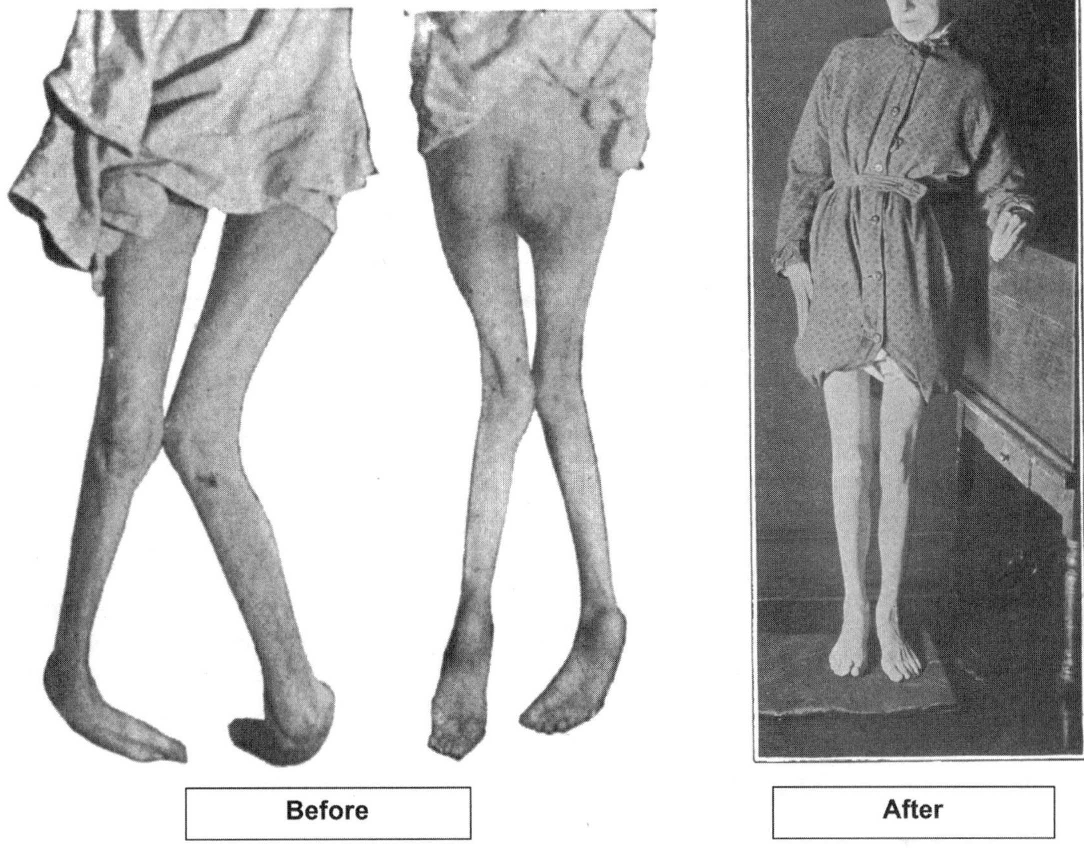

Figure 36.8. A patient with paraplegia and psychogenic/functional dystonia of 14 years' duration before and after treatment with psychotherapy (Reprinted from Purves-Stewart J, Worster-Drought C: The Psychoneuroses and Neuroses: Diagnosis of Nervous Diseases, 10th ed. Baltimore, Williams & Wilkins, 1952.)

sible reasons for this and the overlap with dystonia seen in complex regional pain syndrome later.

Other Movement Disorders

Psychogenic myoclonus is described as a myoclonus with variable amplitude and frequency.[138,205] It may be strikingly stimulus sensitive, for example to fluorescent lighting or with elicitation of deep tendon reflexes, in which case the latency between stimulus and jerk is often long and variable. Examination of the EEG for the premovement potential, or *Bereitschaftspotential*, may demonstrate the presence of this potential 1 second before the movement occurs. In myoclonus of organic origin there may be a cortical spike, but this typically occurs about 20 ms before the movement. This technique is laborious and requires numerous jerks to be successful.[20,203]

Psychogenic hemifacial spasm is described with clinical features similar to those of psychogenic dystonia.[201]

Rarely, *psychogenic parkinsonism* has been described.[105] Although stiffness may be present, this is usually not the same as rigidity. Other specific features include decreased stiffness with synkinetic movements, a hesitant gait pattern (described below), and dramatic responses during tests of postural instability, when inconsistency in limb movement may also be seen. Functional neuroimaging of the dopaminergic system is sometimes used in this scenario, although it is not known whether patients with psychogenic parkinsonism might also have abnormalities using this modality of imaging.

Psychogenic paroxysmal movement disorders that don't fit into any of the other categories, such as tongue protrusion, body stiffening, lurching, and running, are also reported.[204] These movements are sometimes similar to those seen during nonepileptic attacks but without altered awareness.

Functional Gait Disturbance

The functional hemiplegic gait has already been described. There have been several helpful case series describing other types of functional gait disturbance,[40,44,94,109] including one with video material.[71] General findings such as variability and improvement with distraction are important, but as with movement disorders, gait disturbances should be diagnosed with great caution, as they are also overrepresented in cases where structural disease has been misdiagnosed as functional.[197] As a very general rule, it is dangerous to leap to a diagnosis of a functional gait disorder simply because a particular gait looks bizarre or ridiculous. The main features have been described by Lempert et al.[109] and are summarized in the following subsections.

The Monoplegic/ Hemiplegic Gait

Unilateral functional weakness of a leg, if severe, tends to produce a characteristic gait in which the leg is dragged behind the body as a single unit, like a sack of potatoes (Fig. 36.9). The hip is either held in external or internal rotation so that the foot points inward or outward. This may be associated with a tendency to haul the leg onto an examination couch with both hands. This gait pattern was described as long ago as 1854 by Todd.[207]

Excessive Slowness

Patients with this gait have a dramatic delay in gait initiation without the subsequent improvement seen in parkinsonism. It is often associated with feet *sticking* to the ground.

Falling Toward or Away from the Doctor

Usually the pattern is a fall avoided by a clutching physician. Studies using sway magnetography in patients with functional dizziness have shown that they have greater amount of sway than patients with dizziness caused by disease.[55]

"Walking on Ice" Pattern

This is the gait pattern of a normal person walking on slippery ground, using cautious broad-based steps with decreased stride length and height, and stiff knees and ankles. The arms are sometimes abducted, as if the person is walking on a tightrope.

Uneconomic Postures with Waste of Muscle Energy

Patients use a gait with an eccentric displacement of the center of gravity, such as standing and walking with flexion of the hips and knees. This is often associated with fear of falling.

Sudden Knee Buckling

Patients usually prevent themselves from falling before they touch the ground. Knee buckling can occur in Huntington's chorea and cataplexy.

Pseudoataxia

This gait is characterized by crossed legs or by a general unsteadiness with sudden sidesteps.[40] A kinematic method of distinguishing this gait has been described.[122]

Other Symptoms

This brief summary of other symptoms (excluding cognition, pain, and fatigue) is given here to direct the interested reader to relevant literature.

Dizziness

A full discussion of how to determine whether dizziness is predominantly functional, and indeed whether such a distinction can be made, is outside the scope of this chapter but can be found elsewhere.[60] Making a diagnosis of functional dizziness requires expert knowledge of cardiovascular, vestibular, and central neurological disorders, including patterns of symptoms, such as momentary disequilibrium, which are not currently well characterized but are probably not functional in the sense of being driven by emotional or cognitive pro-

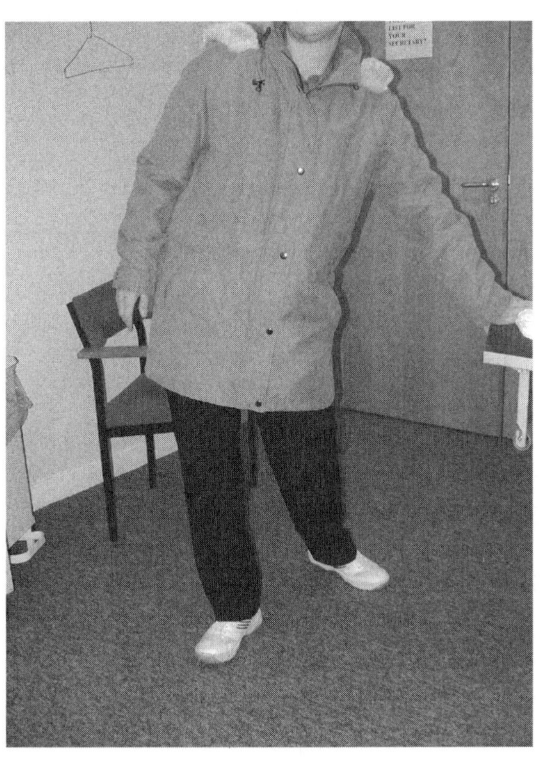

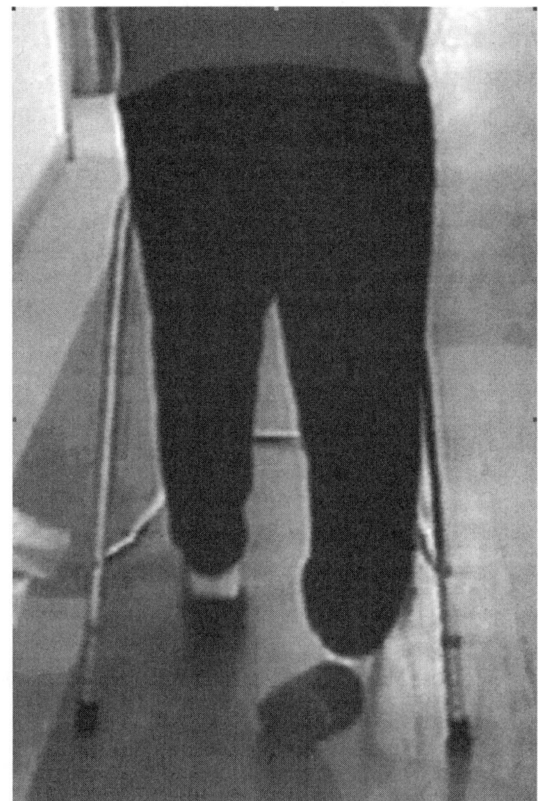

Figure 36.9. Functional monoplegic gait. In both cases the leg is dragged at the hip. External or internal rotation of the hip or ankle inversion/eversion is common. (Reproduced with permission from the BMJ Publishing Group.[200])

cesses. It is important to ask carefully for symptoms of depersonalization and derealization, which may be what the patient is referring to as giddiness. If this sensation exists all the time without other psychiatric or somatic problems, the patient may have depersonalization disorder.[7]

Anxiety and phobic avoidance of situations or head positions that bring on dizziness does not, by itself, indicate a psychogenic etiology. Dizziness is an anxiety-provoking symptom regardless of the cause, and avoidance of certain places may have different causes. For example, some people develop dizziness in the context of panic attacks primarily driven by a fear of embarrassment and being unable to escape from a place like a supermarket. In other people, the primary driver of dizziness is a physiological vestibular sensitivity to particular visual stimuli such as patterned lines or bright lights (sometimes called *visual vertigo*) that may be found in a supermarket. Rarely is the situation so black and white; most patients develop a complex interplay between their physical symptoms, emotions, and behavior. Disentangling it will often not be possible or even necessary. Asking the patient to hyperventilate to see if that reproduces the symptoms might appear a logical place to start, but this test has a high false positive rate (20% in one study[74]) in patients with known causes for dizziness and is probably unreliable.

A variety of terms have been used to describe the intersection of vestibular and psychogenic factors, including *phobic postural vertigo*, *excessive awareness of normal sensation*, and *space and motion discomfort*. With these patients, a full assessment of provoking stimuli and emotional symptoms can lead to useful tailored treatment in the form of vestibular rehabilitation and/or a cognitive behavioral approach without having to make an unhelpful distinction about whether the problem is in the mind or the brain.

Speech and Swallowing Symptoms

Dysarthria can sometimes accompany paralysis, and although very little has been written on this in recent times,[125] there are good descriptions in the older literature.[83a,148] Typically, the speech is slow and may resemble a stutter, or may be extremely slow, with long hesitations. Despite long gaps in the speech, it may be noticeable that these occur in the middle but not at the ends of sentences, and the patient will often still be difficult to interrupt. The emotional content of the speech may have a noticeable influence on its fluency, with anger often producing more fluency and discussion of the patient's emotional state leading to greater hesitation. Sometimes the speech will become telegrammatic, reduced to the main verbs and nouns in a sentence. In its extreme form, the patient may become mute. Just as the act of physical examination can make functional paralysis appear much worse, patients with functional dysarthria tend to be at their very worst when asked to repeat particular phrases.

Word-finding difficulty is a common symptom in anyone with significant fatigue or concentration problems and may compound a functional dysarthria. True dysphasia as a more severe functional symptom, however, is rare.

Dysphonia is a much more common functional speech complaint, and there is now quite a large literature outlining approaches to its diagnosis and management.[167] Often the clinical presentation is of whispering or hoarse speech that is initially thought to be laryngitis but that persists for months or years. The possibility of spasmodic adductor or abductor dysphonia must always be considered. A recent randomized trial of voice therapy suggests that this can be an effective treatment.[119]

Globus pharyngis or functional dysphagia also has a sizable literature. The patient normally complains of a sensation of a ball in the throat," and investigations do not reveal a cause. There remains controversy regarding how extensively patients with globus should be investigated before this diagnosis is made,[6,51] but there is no doubt that this most ancient of functional symptoms remains common.[34]

Visual Symptoms

Blurred vision, or asthenopia (meaning literally "tired eyes"), is commonly described by patients with functional weakness and sensory symptoms. Patients with this symptom usually describes intermittent blurring of vision that returns to normal if they screw up their eyes tight and then relax them again. Some of these patients have convergence or accommodative spasm, a tendency for the convergence reflex to be transiently overactive, either unilaterally or bilaterally.[168] In this situation, lateral gaze restriction can sometimes appear to be present, but the presence of miosis may help to confirm that the problem is convergence spasm.[210] Voluntary nystagmus is described and appears to be a "talent" possessed by about 10% of the population.[229]

The literature on functional visual acuity problems and the tests available to diagnose them are reviewed elsewhere.[10,18,92] Spiral or tubular fields are commonly seen clinically, are often asymptomatic, and can be elicited at the bedside. Keane has described functional hemianopia[91] as the *missing half defect*. Patients with functional hemianopia are typically found to have homonymous hemianopia with both eyes open and then, inconsistent with this, to have a monocular hemianopia in the affected eye with full fields in the normal eye—one of the clearest examples of *ideogenic* symptoms in this area of neurology.

Auditory Symptoms

The literature on functional deafness is smaller than that for visual symptoms. Basic tests for complete deafness relying on a startle response have been described, such as making a loud unexpected "clap" out of sight of the patient or seeing if the patient wakes to the sound of an alarm clock in the middle of the night.[220] In addition to audiometry, which relies on good cooperation from the patient, additional tests such as auditory brain stem evoked responses or evoked otoacoustic emissions may be necessary to fully investigate a patient with this symptom.[149]

Pseudocyesis

According to Evans, writing in 1984,[47] only 3 males and 100 females had been reported in the previous 45 years with the symptom of abdominal swelling imitating pregnancy. Pseudocyesis is the extreme end of what the French have labeled *couvade* ("to hatch"). Couvade simply refers to general symptoms of pregnancy such as nausea and weight gain. Estimates of its frequency vary widely. The psychotic delusion of pregnancy is also well reported in males and females. The mechanism of pseudocyesis must be something to do with exaggerated lordosis and persistent relaxation of abdominal muscles, but its well-studied presence in animals and its rarity in humans means that judgment must be reserved about its true nature.

Investigations

It should be remembered that positive evidence that symptoms are functional does not exclude the presence of coexisting disease. In many patients with disabling symptoms, a focused set of investigations may be unavoidable. Preferably these should be performed as quickly as possible, as protracted testing or minor abnormalities on these tests can maintain a focus on looking for disease rather than on rehabilitation. It may also be necessary to make two diagnoses—for example, one of an organic disease such as epilepsy and another of nonepileptic attacks.

Explaining the Diagnosis and Management

Explaining the Diagnosis

Most people who develop symptoms not unreasonably would like to know what is causing them. This may be a greater priority for patients than reassurance and treatment.[143] Explaining the diagnosis in a clear, logical, and nonoffensive way is a critical part of management and in many cases may be sufficient to allow resolution.

We have already outlined our own reasons, both pragmatic and scientific, for preferring to use the word *functional* in diagnoses such as *functional weakness* or *functional sensory disturbance*. At a first encounter, we explain the diagnosis to the patient using the following key points:

1. *Indicate that you believe the patient*: We pay particular attention to overcoming the patient's fear that the doctor doesn't believe them or thinks they are mad, imagining, or faking their symptoms. Sometimes simply saying, "I don't think you're mad, imagining, or putting on your symptoms" can be very effective.
2. *Explain what the patient doesn't have*: for example: "You do not have multiple sclerosis, epilepsy, etc."
3. *Explain what the patient does have*: for example, "You have 'functional weakness. This is a common problem. Your nervous system is not damaged, but it is not working properly. That is why you cannot move your arm."
4. *Emphasize that the condition is common*: for example, "I see a lot of patients with similar symptoms."
5. *Emphasize reversibility*: for example: "Because there is no damage, you have the potential to get better."
6. *Emphasize that self-help is a key part of getting better*: for example: "I know you didn't bring this on, but there are things you can do to help it get better."
7. *Metaphors and comparisons may be useful*: for example, "The hardware is alright, but there's a software problem"; "It's like a car/piano that's out of tune; all the parts are there, but they just aren't working right together"; "It's like a short circuit of the nervous system" [nonepileptic attacks];" It's like the opposite of phantom limb—they feel a limb that is not there; you cannot feel a limb that is."
8. *Show the patient his or her positive signs*: For example a patient (and the family) can be shown their own Hoover's sign or talked through a video of their nonepileptic attack. Explain how this confirms the diagnosis that the nervous system is working at some times but not at others.
9. *Introduce the role of depression/anxiety*: for example, "If you have been feeling low/worried, that will tend to make the symptoms even worse."
10. *Use written information*: Send the patient the clinic letter. Give the patient a leaflet.
11. *Talk to the family and friends*: Reinforce the diagnosis with family and friends.
12. *How to suggest using antidepressants*: for example, "We find that so-called antidepressants often help these symptoms even in patients who are not feeling depressed. They have wider actions than treating depression—for example, on energy, appetite, and sleep—and can reverse abnormalities in brain function. If you experience side effects, keep going for at least six weeks, as they may take time to wear off."
13. *How to make a psychiatric referral*: for example, "Dr X has a lot of experience and

interest in helping people like you to manage and overcome their symptoms. This referral does not mean I think that you are 'mad."

By medicalizing the diagnosis of functional symptoms, we run the risk of leaving patients with the impression that they have a neurological disorder over which they have no control. We acknowledge this risk, but our experience is that although these initial explanations are deliberately non-psychiatric, they allow the rapid development of a therapeutic relationship that permits the subsequent emergence and discussion of psychological factors that otherwise might never have taken place. When these factors do arise, we do not try to reattribute all the problems to a psychological cause, but we do emphasize that symptoms have multiple causes and that psychological factors may be making the symptoms worse. Making the referral to a psychiatrist is often much easier at the second appointment. Ideally, the psychiatrist will be someone experienced in managing patients who are focused on somatic symptoms, such as a specialist in psychosomatic medicine.

A detailed and systematic approach to explaining and managing functional symptoms in primary care that is based on these principles has been published.[53]

Further Management

In patients with mild symptoms, explanation and reassurance together with encouragement to resume normal activity may be sufficient to produce improvement. In those with more resistant symptoms, the following approaches may be helpful.

1. *Cognitive behavioral therapy (CBT)*—Evidence exists at systematic review level that CBT is moderately effective for a wide range of functional somatic symptoms.[101] An open trial of CBT for nonepileptic attacks[62] and a large, randomized trial involving patients with multiple severe functional somatic symptoms[17] have shown promising results, and a CBT approach to functional motor symptoms has been described.[25] In our own practice, we build on the implications of the *functional model* in longer-term treatment. This is in many ways simply a variant of the *rational persuasion* that Dubois and others used for such patients at the turn of the twentieth century.[42]
2. *Physical rehabilitation*—Patients with physical problems often need physical treatments to get better. Some of our best treatment successes have been accomplished by our experienced neurophysiotherapists, who combine hands-on physical treatments with suggestion and encouragement. Wade has reviewed the rehabilitation literature of functional paralysis and gait disorder.[217] Many studies report encouraging results, but none have been randomized and few have reported the long-term outcome.
3. *Antidepressants*—There is evidence from a systematic review that antidepressants are of moderate benefit in patients with functional symptoms, but there is no specific evidence for neurological symptoms.[140] The main problem in using them is one of implied psychiatric stigma and a perception that they are addictive or harmful, as discussed above.[192]
4. *Hypnosis and intravenous sedation*—Two small, randomized trials have examined the effect of hypnosis in patients with functional motor symptoms. For outpatients, 10 weeks of hypnosis produced a better outcome than that experienced by waiting list controls.[136] In the inpatient trial, both cases and controls improved equally with multidisciplinary input, and there was no extra effect from hypnosis.[135] Thus, it appears that hypnosis is better than doing nothing, but it is unclear whether it is superior to other interventions of similar intensity and duration. When expertise in hypnosis is not available, intravenous sedatives may be helpful in persuading some patients, with whom you already have a good relationship, that they can eventually make a recovery. We urge caution, however, in applying this potentially invasive procedure to all patients. The use of an interview after administration of intravenous sodium amytal was initially promoted as a method of uncovering the hidden psychic conflict causing the patient's symptom. More recently, *examination* under sedation, including the use of benzodiazepines,[46] has been used therapeutically to demonstrate to the neurologist, and by means of a video recording to the patient, that the apparently paralyzed limb can in fact move. White et al.[225] report positively on this technique in 11 patients with

functional locomotor disorders who had been disabled for several years. These methods merit more systematic study. Their potential for harm has not been evaluated.

5. *Other forms of psychotherapy*—For some patients, a more in-depth psychotherapy that addresses the antecedents of symptoms may be of value, but this has not been specifically evaluated in randomized trials.

Prognosis

Misdiagnosis

Doctors have always been concerned that their diagnosis of functional symptoms may be wrong and that the patient may eventually develop an organic disease that explains his sor her symptoms. Since the publication of an influential paper by Slater in 1965,[180] this has become part of conventional wisdom. Slater claimed that 61% of his cohort of patients with hysteria subsequently developed neurological disease. His analysis is flawed, however, and his conclusion that hysteria is a "delusion and a snare" is misleading.[165] Slater's views have now been refuted by several recent studies reporting rates of misdiagnosis of under 10% in patients assessed in regional and tertiary neurological centers.[165] We carried out a systematic review of the 26 studies relating to misdiagnosis of conversion symptoms/hysteria published since 1965.[197] We found a consistent misdiagnosis rate of around 4%–5% since 1970, before the advent of CT scanning (Fig. 36.10). Studies of varied functional symptoms in neurological outpatients have obtained similar results.[22,81] Any misdiagnosis of functional symptoms is unfortunate, but it must be seen in a wider perspective. Misdiagnosis is a fact of life in medicine, and a rate of 4% compares favorably with reported misdiagnosis rates for other neurological and psychiatric disorders. For example, reported rates of misdiagnosis in epilepsy vary from 26%[181] to 42%.[230] In a population-based study of 387 subjects diagnosed with multiple sclerosis, 17% subsequently turned out to be wrongly diagnosed, half because they had another neurological disorder and half because the symptoms were functional or psychological in origin.[70] Similar misdiagnosis rates have been reported in motor neuron disease (8%[33]) and schizophrenia (6%[84]).

This does not mean that the diagnosis of functional symptoms should be made complacently or never reviewed. We should remember that the reported studies were mostly of patients who had received extensive inpatient investigation in major neurological centers. However, it does suggest that misdiagnosis can no longer be used as a reason not to take functional symptoms seriously in their own right.

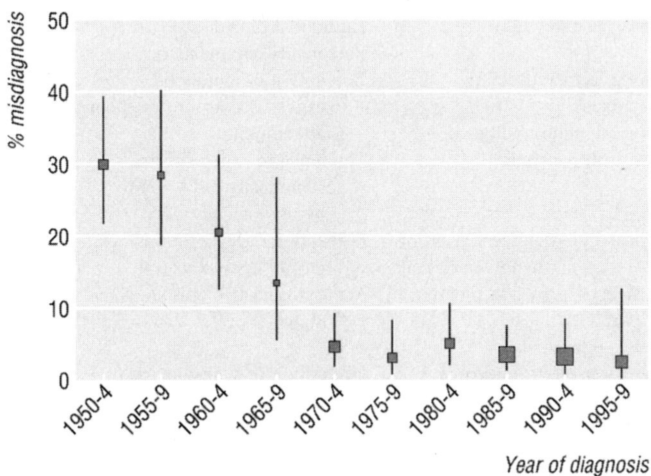

Figure 36.10. Systematic review of studies of the misdiagnosis of conversion symptoms (weakness, numbness, nonepileptic attacks, visual and auditory symptoms) (mean %, 95% exact binomial confidence intervals) published since 1965. Data points are plotted at the midpoint of 5-year intervals according to when the patients were diagnosed. The size of each point is proportional to the number of subjects at each time point (total n = 1466).[197]

Symptomatic Recovery and Other Measures of Outcome

Functional Symptoms in Neurology

While there are some data on individual symptoms, there are few data on the prognosis of functional symptoms as a whole in neurology. In an Edinburgh cohort study, over half of 66 patients with functional symptoms were unchanged or worse at 9-month follow-up.[22]

Functional Weakness and Sensory Symptoms

Around one-third to one-half of all patients with these symptoms remain symptomatic in the long term. Furthermore, long-term studies have also reported that many patients develop other symptoms suggestive of a diagnosis of somatization disorder[95,118,195] and have physical functioning similar to that of patients with multiple sclerosis. Sensory symptoms probably have a more benign prognosis than motor symptoms.[195,208] Long symptom duration and personality disorder are consistent predictors of poor recovery,[30,31] but there is also a subgroup of patients who appear to have a very good prognosis,. Interestingly, one study found that the presence of an Axis 1 psychiatric disorder (such as depression and anxiety) and a change in marital status (either a separation or a marriage) were positive prognostic factors.[31] Patients in that particular study were also found to frequently change their primary care physician and gain repeat referrals to neurology and other specialties even after a firm diagnosis had been made.[32]

Nonepileptic Attacks

In a review of 16 prognostic studies of patients with nonepileptic attacks, Reuber and Elger found that only around one-third were attack free at 3 years and one-third were still taking anticonvulsants.[152] Delay in diagnosis (indicating longer duration), personality disorder, and hypermotor attacks have been associated with a poorer outcome.

What Causes Functional Symptoms?

Table 36.4 summarizes a large, complex literature on the cause of functional symptoms. This is a problem that has been approached from many angles—biological, cognitive, psychoanalytic, psychological,

Table 36.4. A Scheme for Thinking About the Etiology of Functional Symptoms in Neurology with Examples

Factors	Biological	Psychological	Social
Acting throughout	Disease	Emotional disorder Personality/coping style	Life events and difficulties
Predisposing	Genetic factors affecting personality Biological vulnerabilities in nervous system?	Perception of childhood experience as adverse/poor attachment Tendency to express distress somatically rather than psychologically	Childhood neglect/abuse Poor family functioning
Precipitating	Abnormal physiological event or state (e.g., hyperventilation, sleep deprivation, sleep paralysis) Physical injury/pain	Perception of life event as negative, unexpected Acute dissociative episode/panic attack	Symptom modelling (via media or personal contact)
Perpetuating	Plasticity in central nervous system motor and sensory (including pain) pathways Deconditioning (e.g., lack of physical fitness in chronic fatigue, deconditioning of vestibular responsiveness in patients with dizziness who hold their heads still)	Perception of symptoms as being outside of personal control/due to disease Anxiety/catastrophization about cause of symptoms Not being believed Avoidance of symptom provocation (e.g., exercise in fatigue)	Fear of work/family responsibilities of being well The presence of a welfare system Social benefits of being ill Availability of legal compensation Stigma of mental illness

social, feminist, and historical—whereas a multifactorial approach seems to be the most appropriate one. In thinking about etiology, it is helpful to consider factors as predisposing, precipitating, and perpetuating. Many studies have examined the role of the factors shown in Table 36.1 and have found them to be more common in patients with functional neurological symptoms than in patients with similar symptoms caused by disease. However, most of these factors are common across all functional disorders, and we still do not know why some people develop unilateral paralysis, others have attacks that resemble epilepsy, and still others become profoundly tired.

Why and How Do Weakness, Numbness, or Nonepileptic Attacks Develop?

In this section we summarize the diverse, mostly speculative, literature that attempts to address this question and discuss the potential role of trauma and pain. In doing so, we must once again approach the problem from a number of different perspectives.

The Cognitive Perspective and the Importance of Panic, Dissociation, and Other Physiological Triggers

Ross Reynolds,[156] Charcot,[26] and others observed more than a century ago that ideas and suggestion could pay a central role in the formation of particular symptoms. Janet extended this notion further with the *idées fixes* and dissociation[82]. Here is a famous example:

> A man travelling by train had done an imprudent thing: while the train was running, he had got down on the step in order to pass from one door to the other, when he became aware that the train was about to enter a tunnel. It occurred to him that his left side, which projected, was going to be knocked slantwise and crushed against the arch of the tunnel. This thought caused him to swoon away but happily for him, he did not fall on the track, but was taken back inside the carriage, and his left side was not even grazed. In spite of this, he had a left hemiplegia. (Janet 1907[82])

Janet referred to the principal process in hysteria as a "retraction of the field of personal consciousness and a tendency to the dissociation and emancipation of the system of ideas and functions that constitute personality." In the example above, the idea of paralysis, brought on by terror of an imminent injury, has become dissociated from the patient's consciousness and is acting independently.

Dissociation and Panic

Dissociative symptoms are normal and common in the healthy population. They occur more frequently in patients with disease, particularly neurological and psychiatric conditions. For anyone who has not previously experienced them, or if they have only been experienced before in terrifying situations, they can be frightening.

In patients with nonepileptic attacks, the idea that dissociation occurs as a transient protective response during states of high arousal is an appealing one. It is also supported by our knowledge that animals can demonstrate freezing and cutting-off behavior in response to stress—the "rabbit in the headlights" effect.

There is some evidence that arousal before nonepileptic attacks has much in common with the arousal state seen in panic.[111,212] However, although some studies of patients with nonepileptic attacks have demonstrated higher rates of dissociation than in epilepsy, the differences are not dramatic[3,63] and other studies have failed to find any difference at all.[154] The questionnaires used in these studies, such as the Dissociative Experiences Scale, focus on cognitive symptoms (such as "absorption in a television program or movie") rather than somatic symptoms (such as "my body doesn't belong to me") and on persistent rather than episodic symptoms. This requires further investigation.

There has been even less systematic work examining dissociation in patients with functional paralysis, even though dissociation is a principal etiological factor in the ICD-10 classification. One study found a relationship between somatic and cognitive dissociative traits, hypnotizability, and child abuse in a cohort most of whom had functional motor symptoms.[158,159] Our experience is that during in-depth interviews, many patients report symptoms of panic just before the onset of functional paralysis. Specifically, they may report that they became "dizzy" (by which they often mean the dissociative symptoms of depersonalization or derealization) and have autonomic symptoms such as sweating, nausea, and breathing difficulties. Sometimes the patient either refuses to volunteer or genuinely didn't experience fear in association with other autonomic symptoms—so-called panic without fear.[102] This idea is not new. Savill comments on it in his 1909 book[170] extending the range of *attack types* at onset to include nonepileptic seizures, something we have also seen:

> If the patient is under careful observation at the time of onset, it will generally be found that cases of cerebral paresis, rigidity or tremor are actually initiated, about the time of onset, by a more or less transient hysterical cerebral attack. . . .
>
> Affirmative evidence on this point is not always forthcoming unless the patient was at the time under observation, or is himself an intelligent observer. I found affirmative evidence of this point in 47/50 cases of hysterical motor disorder which I investigated particularly. Sometimes there was only a 'swimming' in the head, or a slight syncopal or vertiginous attack, slight confusion of the mind, or transient loss of speech, but in quite a number there was generalised trepidation or convulsions. (Savill 1909[170])

Hyperventilation

Hyperventilation is another manifestation of arousal and may also occur at the onset of symptoms, either alone or in combination with panic and dissociation. The link between hyperventilation and unilateral sensory symptoms is well established both clinically[16,147] and experimentally,[56] but the mechanism for this remains unclear.[141]

More Studies of Attention and Arousal

Two older small studies found that patients with conversion symptoms had reduced habituation compared to 10 controls with anxiety, suggesting an impairment in attention.[78,103] Another study suggested that arousal was high even when la belle indifference was present.[157] The work of Roelofs et al. has suggested deficits in higher-level central initiation of movement with relative preservation of lower-level motor execution (as measured, for example, by reaction times) in patients with functional paralysis.[160,162] Detailed studies of attention in this patient group have been consistent with a high-level voluntary attentional deficit.[161] Spence has argued that functional paralysis is a disorder of action, drawing analogies with other disorders including depression and schizophrenia.[184]

The Development of Symptoms After Physiological Triggers

We tend to think of dissociation and paralysis, unlike abdominal bloating, as a symptom outside everyday experience and normal physiology. We have already discussed how common dissociative symptoms are in the healthy population (in fact, many people strive hard to develop dissociative symptoms using drugs or meditation). Paralysis too occurs in all of us during rapid eye movement (REM) sleep, when we are terrified (when it may occur with dissociation), when we are tired and our limbs feel like lead, or as a very transient protective response when we experience acute pain in a limb. We have seen patients who developed functional paralysis after surgery (who simultaneously experienced intense depersonalization as they came out of the anesthetic), a phenomenon also well described in nonepileptic attacks.[153] We have seen patients whose first experience of paralysis appeared to be an episode of undiagnosed sleep paralysis precipitated by depression and insomnia that later "snowballed" into more permanent non-sleep-related symptoms. Perhaps one of the most common routes to functional paralysis is that of a patient with mild chronic fatigue or pain who then becomes aware of an asymmetry of symptoms. For either biological or attentional reasons (but probably because of both), this asymmetry escalates over weeks and months until it appears more dramatically unilateral.

These are hypotheses regarding onset and they require testing, but it seems plausible that some of these more everyday causes of transient paralysis could be acting as triggers for more long-lasting symptoms in some patients.

The Social Perspective

As well as playing a role in attention, illness beliefs could influence symptom presentation through social means.[178] It has been suggested that patients respond to social pressures and expectations by choosing, either consciously or subconsciously, to present certain symptoms. The symptoms of paralysis or epileptiform attacks may be chosen because they are much more culturally acceptable presentations of ill health than depression and panic. A strong belief in or, less often, fear of a disease is a recurring theme in this patient group, a clinical impression confirmed by studies.[14] Conversely, the conviction that, whatever it is, it is not a psychological problem, is even more prevalent[194] and may reflect the socially determined stigma about psychological problems. The medical profession is also more interested in dramatic physical symptoms than emotional ones. The social dimension of functional symptoms in neurology is explored further in two recommended books.[177,221]

The Psychodynamic Perspective

In the twentieth century, psychodynamic theory was the dominant explanation for functional symptoms in neurology. This theory regards the symptoms as the result of mental conflict in a vulnerable individual, the mental conflict being resolved by the expression of physical symptoms—so-called primary gain. In addition to communicating distress that cannot be verbalized and escaping the conflict, the individual receives the status and advantage of being regarded as an invalid, so-called secondary gain. Some have regarded conversion hysteria purely as a form of communication. In this context, both paralysis and nonepileptic attacks can be seen as loss of function (one persistent, one intermittent) that communicates a conflict over action. The degree to which it is useful to interpret symptoms as symbolic (e.g., paralysis representing the helplessness experienced during abuse) is unclear.

While the hypothesis that conversion results from a transformation of distress into physical symptoms is clinically plausible for some patients, it is hard to test. The evidence shows that most patients have obvious *unconverted* emotional distress, as demonstrated by a number of studies that have found a greater prevalence of emotional disorder in patients with functional symptoms compared to controls with an equivalently disabling symptom caused by disease.[13] Further evidence against the conversion hypothesis is the poor sensitivity and specificity of la belle indifference as a clinical sign (see above). When emotional distress is apparently hidden, it is often the case that the patient is not *unaware* of his or her emotional symptoms; rather, the patient simply *does not want to tell a doctor* about them for fear of being labeled mentally ill. Wessely has made a plea for revision of DSM-IV criteria to a more practical and theoretical symptom-based classification,[223] which would entail removing the name *Conversion Disorder*. In our view, this would be a great step forward. At the same time, it would be foolish to abandon all of the things we have learned from psychoanalytic theory in doing so. Theories of development that integrate early life experiences with current behavior, such as attachment theory, may contribute to our understanding of functional symptoms.[27]

The Biological Perspective

Charcot believed that there must be a *dynamic* lesion in the brain to explain hysteria. Attempts to find neural correlates or biological ways of understanding these symptoms have appeared with increasing frequency, particular since the advent of functional neuroimaging, but we are still at an embryonic stage of understanding.

Transcranial Magnetic Stimulation and Evoked Responses

A number of studies have shown that transcranial magnetic stimulation (TMS) is normal in patients with functional weakness.[21] This suggests that TMS may be a useful adjunct in distinguishing organic from functional weakness.

An early study of functional hemianesthesia suggested that patients may have impaired standard evoked sensory responses in their affected limbs.[73] However, this was refuted by several even earlier[2] and later studies[67,79,89,113,114,137] including a recent study using magnetoencephalography.[76] Most recently, transiently absent scalp somatosensory evoked responses have been seen in two patients with conversion disorder who subsequently recovered.[227]

Of greater interest are the nature of P300 and other late components of the evoked response in patients with functional sensory loss. One study found that it was diminished in one patient with unilateral functional sensory loss but not in a subject feigning sensory loss,[117] and another found a reduction in P300 components in patients with hypnotically induced sensory loss.[186]

Functional Imaging

There is now a small body of work on the functional neuroimaging of functional motor and sensory symptoms complemented by work with hypnotic and feigning paradigms. These works are summarized in Table 36.5.

That the published data remain inconsistent is perhaps not surprising, as they were acquired from different experimental paradigms and in patients with varying symptom severity. Of note is the study by Vuilleimier et al.,[216] who performed SPECT scans on four patients with functional hemisensori-

Table 36.5. Studies of Functional Brain Imaging in Functional and Hypnotic Paralysis and Sensory Loss

First Author /Year		Subjects	Paradigm	Activations and Deactivations Seen
Conversion Disorder				
Tiihonen 1995[206]	1	Weak + Sensory (L)	SPECT before and after symptoms during electrical stimulation of left median nerve	Increased perfusion of right frontal lobe and hypoperfusion in right parietal lobe during symptomatic state compared to recovery.
Marshall 1997[124]	1	Paralysis (L)	PET. Attempted movement of leg against resistance	Activation of right anterior cingulate and orbitofrontal cortex.
Yazici 1998[228]	5	Gait (L+R)	SPECT	Predominantly left-sided temporal (4/5) and parietal (2/5) hypoactivation.
Spence 2000[185]	3	Paralysis (L+R)	PET. A hand joystick task of affected limb	Hysterical paralysis associated with deactivations in left dorsolateral prefrontal cortex during movements but not at rest. Feigners showed deactivation in right anterior frontal cortex regardless of laterality of weakness.
Vuilleimier 2001[216]	8	Weak+Sensory (L+R)	SPECT. Buzzers applied to all four limbs. Four patients had additional postrecovery	Reduced cerebral blood flow in the contralateral thalamus and basal ganglia. Less severe hypoactivation predicted recovery.
Mailis-Gagnon 2003[120]	4	Pain + Sensory (L+R)	fMRI scans, Sensory stimulation.	When stimulus not perceived—anterior cingulate activation. Deactivation in somatosensory, prefrontal, inferior frontal, and parietal cortex. Failure to activate thalamus and posterior cingulate.
Werring 2004[222]	5 7	Visual loss Controls	fMRI. 8 Hz visual stimulation	Reduced activation of visual cortices, with increased activation of left inferior frontal cortex, left insula-claustrum, bilateral striatum and thalami, left limbic structures, and left posterior cingulate cortex.
Hypnotically Induced (Hyp) and Feigned Paralysis				
Halligan 2000[68]	1	Hyp paralyzed (L)	PET. Attempted movement of paralyzed leg	Right anterior cingulate and right medial orbitofrontal cortex activation similar to that seen in the single patient described by Marshall et al.[124]
Ward 2003[218]	12 12	Hyp paralyzed (L) Feigned paralysis (L)	PET. Attempted movement of paralyzed leg	*Hypnotic Paralysis*: Activation of putamen bilaterally, left thalamus, right orbitofrontal cortex, left cerebellum, left supplementary motor area. *Feigned Paralysis*: Activation of right parietal operculum, left inferior frontal sulcus, right SMA, right ventral premotor cortex, bilateral cerebellum, left inferior parietal cortex.

PET, positron emission tomography; SMA, supplementary motor area; SPECT, single photon emission computed tomography.

motor symptoms during vibration of all four limbs. Scans taken while the symptom was present and after recovery demonstrated hypoactivation of the contralateral thalamus and basal ganglia during the symptomatic state (Fig. 36.11). Their within-subject design and the dose-response relationship between recovery and scan abnormality provide the most persuasive evidence in this area.

While activations on a scan do not tell us why the symptom is there (or even if it was fabricated or not), they do challenge conventional thinking about the problem.

Etiology—Conclusions

Recent studies based on cognitive neuroscience are leading the way to a more integrated cognitive neuropsychiatric approach to the problem of functional symptoms with a focus on mechanism rather than cause. But although they challenge conventional psychogenic models of causation, a purely biological interpretation of these data is just as unsatisfactory as a purely psychogenic theory of symptom formation. We suggest that the ideal is to maintain simultaneous multiple perspectives on the etiology of functional symptoms using a formulation individualized for each patient based on both the generic factors leading to vulnerability (Table 36.5) and the potential specific factors in symptom formation described above.

The Role of Trauma and Pain in Functional Symptoms in Neurology

The relevance of physical trauma, and its psychological correlates, in precipitating hysteria in vulnerable individuals was well understood by clinicians such as Charcot,[132] Page,[144] Oppenheim,[141] Fox,[58] and Janet[82] in the late nineteenth and early twentieth centuries. Lately, *trauma* and *shock* have acquired such a psychological flavor with respect to functional symptoms that the possibility that simple physical injury, even of a trivial nature, could be in itself a major factor in triggering hysterical symptoms has been lost.

In his book *Post-traumatic Neurosis: From Railway Spine to Whiplash,* Michael Trimble reminds us that the debate about whether trauma causes these symptoms via biological or psychological means has been going on for over 150 years.[209] In this section, we advance the argument, as others have done, that this is not an either/or question. We focus on our remit of examining functional symptoms, particularly weakness and movement disorder, but this discussion is relevant to all trauma-related symptoms and syndromes including chronic whiplash injury, low back pain–related leg symptoms, and complex regional pain.

The Frequency of Physical Trauma and Pain in Patients with Functional Motor Symptoms

Although little attention has been paid to it, the reported cases of functional weakness and movement disorder suggest that a surprising number were preceded by physical trauma. Several studies report series of patients with functional paraplegia *all of whom* developed their symptoms following injury.[8,38] Series of similar patients with functional motor symptoms can also be found from spinal units, where 80% have had a history of physical trauma.[5,75] Janssen found a 3% rate of functional paralysis following lumbar surgery,[83b] although the mechanism here could be related to the dissociative properties of a general anesthetic as much as pain. In patients with functional movement disorder, the presence of physical trauma is also consistently high, ranging from 20% to 60%.[37,49,96,99,104] The high frequency of sudden-onset symptoms in these series, ranging from 40% to 90%,[37,49,96,99] also suggests that some kind of ictus, painful, frightening, or dissociative, may be relevant to the symptom mechanism.

Rates of Functional Motor and Sensory Symptoms in Complex Regional Pain Syndrome

Looking at the problem from a different point of view, it is interesting to see how many patients with complex regional pain have symptoms of weakness or a movement disorder that might be said to be functional. Critics would point out that it is very hard to assess power in someone with a painful arm or leg, and there may be multiple reasons, already discussed, why a diagnosis of functional weakness could be incorrect. Motor symptoms, predominantly weakness, are, however, prominent in case series of reflex sympathetic dystrophy and complex regional pain. In Birklein et al.'s study, 79% of 145

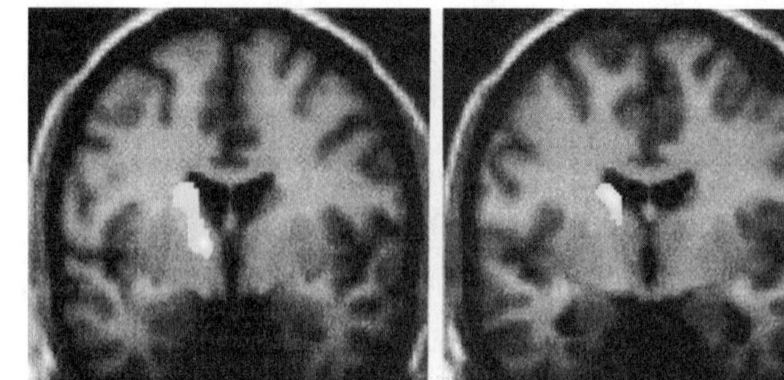
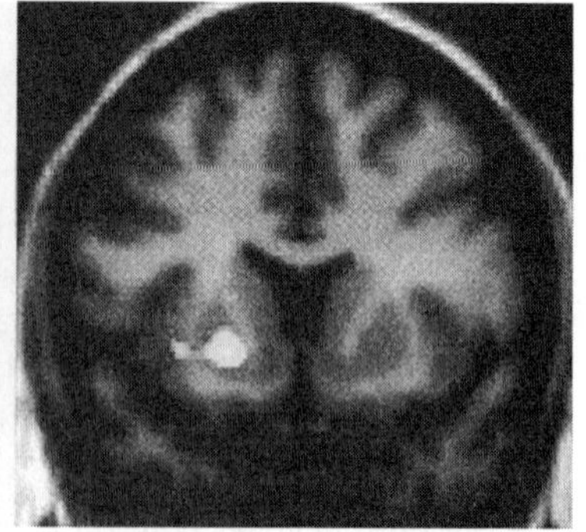

Figure 36.11. Hypoactivation of the contralateral thalamus, caudate, and putamen in four patients experiencing functional hemimotorsensory symptoms compared to recovery scans. (Reprinted by permission from Vuilliemier et al, Functional neuroanatomical correlates of hysterical sensorimotor loss. Brain 124:1077–1090, 2001.)

patients had weakness, mostly of the give-way variety, and 88% had sensory disturbance.[15] Veldman et al.[213] described over 829 patients with complex regional pain syndrome (CRPS) (type 1 with no nerve injury). Ninety-five percent had weakness, and 15% of these patients were so weak that they could not move the limb at all despite having a normal EMG. Movement disorders and sensory symptoms were also very common. When sensory signs and symptoms are actively sought in patients with other forms of chronic pain, they are remarkably common and often conform to a hemisensory or apparently nonanatomical distribution.[54,164]

There is evidence that much of the sensory disturbance and movement disorder seen in complex regional pain is similar to that seen in functional or psychogenic disorders.[36,214,215] In a study of 27 patients with CRPS type 1 and sensory symptoms, 50% of the patients had complete reversal of their hypoesthesia with placebo compared to none out of 13 patients with a nerve injury.[214] In another study, 15% of type 1 patients (n = 379) compared to 0% of type 2 patients—those with a nerve injury—(n = 307) had a movement disorder. The response to placebo was less dramatic, but nonetheless, three patients had their movement disorders abolished by placebo, and in another three patients all sensory, motor, and vasomotor phenomena typical of the condition were cured by cognitive psychotherapy.[215] Deuschl et al., studying the tremor associated with CRPS type 1, found that it had the neurophysiological qualities of an enhanced physiological tremor.[36]

Much of the debate about the physical signs in CRPS seems to arise, not from an impartial consideration of the symptoms, but from a desire to identify patients with CRPS as having something "genuine" compared to patients with functional weakness. If both conditions were considered equally genuine to begin with, this would go some way toward improving the quality of the debate.[36]

Potential Factors in the Relationship of Physical Trauma and Pain to Functional Symptoms

Just as a multifactorial model has to be used when thinking about the etiology of functional symptoms, the relationship between physical injury and presenting symptom is likely to be complex.

1. *Physical Injury and disease are potent causes of functional symptoms.* This is certainly true, as discussed on page 667 of this chapter.
2. *Immobility.* If pain leads to disuse of a limb, it stands to reason that there may be some local deconditioning of muscles and their nerve supply. Immobility is one factor that explains why the weakness seen in CRPS may become worse over time. Many authors believe that protection of a limb from pain, leading to a vicious circle of immobility and worsening symptoms, is one of the primary causes of CRPS.
3. *The shock of the injury.* There is a large literature on the relationship between physical injury, peri- and posttraumatic dissociation, and panic as they relate to PTSD but much less as they relate to physical symptom outcome and nothing at all as they might relate

to functional symptoms such as weakness. It seems reasonable to hypothesize, however, as has been done for over 100 years, that an actual or near-miss physical injury could lead to a fright or a nervous shock that in a vulnerable individual could be the trigger for a cascade of events leading to functional symptoms and disability. It also seems plausible, on the basis of the PTSD literature, to suggest that one of the reasons a physical injury, rather than just an emotional shock, could be powerful in a subgroup of these patients is that it is a reminder of past physical injuries sustained in neglectful or abusive circumstances. These ideas are not new in relation to functional somatic symptoms and were discussed widely from the nineteenth century on.

4. *Pain causes weakness and numbness.* Pain does not have to cause a shock to cause symptoms. It is well established that pain in itself causes a degree of weakness, which can be overcome only with effort.[107] There are plausible biological explanations for this phenomenon, which could act at many levels in the nervous system independently of emotional or conscious processing. Sensory information may be disrupted in a similar fashion but in the other direction.
5. *Attribution.* A patient who *already* has functional symptoms may experience a physical injury that provides a new reason for symptoms that were previously baffling and inexplicable to the sufferer. The injury may lead to distortion of memory about the nature of the symptoms before the accident.

Litigation

Another often quoted cause of the link between trauma and functional symptoms is the way that litigation can prolong the duration of the symptoms. There is no doubt that simulation in order to make money does occur, particularly in medicolegal scenarios (discussed in more detail below). Furthermore, very few of us would refuse the opportunity to make some money if it was suggested that we might be entitled to it. Leaving aside the financial motivation, compensation is a potent obstacle to recovery for several other reasons. Seeking compensation implicitly involves a commitment to (1) the idea that there is physical injury/damage; (2) the notion that someone else is to blame for the symptoms in the past and now; and (3) a desire on the patient's part to prove that he or she is actually unwell. Many patients with functional symptoms who are not seeking compensation share these feelings about their symptoms, often because they feel that no one believes them and that they are being accused of imagining their symptoms. It is hardly surprising that in the context of an injury, many would get involved with a legal process that is prepared to back them up and get them some money. These complex issues, and the negative role that lawyers and doctors can play, is discussed in detail by Andrew Malleson in his recent book *Whiplash and Other Useful Illnesses*.[121]

A Historical Perspective—Railway Spine, Shell Shock, and Whiplash

A historical viewpoint is essential to fully understand this area.[121,209] Railway spine in the nineteenth century, shell shock during the First World War, and whiplash in the second half of the twentieth century all started as organic disease concepts before debate about their nature ensued, in the first two cases ending in the conclusion that the problems were largely functional (with the third unresolved). Posttraumatic functional symptoms have been repeatedly rebranded with different labels, all of which implicitly blame the injury for the problem. The debates have focused on the same questions: Are these symptoms related to organic damage or not? If the trauma is relevant, is it the trigger in a vulnerable individual or could it happen to anyone? What is the role of simulation and compensation? These questions have tended to polarize opinion when a much more helpful approach would be to appreciate that there is such heterogeneity in the patients with these symptoms that no dogmatic standpoint is likely to be correct. We agree with Coombs-Knapp, writing about traumatic hysteria in 1895, who suggested that trauma should be considered just another etiological factor and that it was unhelpful to elevate it to a disease label.[29]

> Just as some men thought that, by proving there was no spinal concussion, they could disprove the existence of all these affections, so others, by showing that there was no 'traumatic neurosis', have slighted the real troubles. On the whole the introduction of the term has had a bad influence. . . . Hysteria,

neurasthenia . . . might all be classed as neuroses and they all may at times be of traumatic origin. (Coombs-Knapp 1895[29])

Malingering/Factitious Disorder in Relation to Paralysis and Sensory Loss

Although the diagnosis can be difficult, neurologists are generally good at telling whether symptoms are functional or associated with organic disease in that their diagnoses usually remain stable over time.[165,197] However, discriminating between consciously produced and unconsciously produced functional symptoms is far more difficult, if not impossible. The patient's awareness of control over symptoms is probably not an all-or-nothing phenomenon but rather lies on a continuum. It may also vary over time, so that a patient may begin an illness with little awareness about what is happening but gradually gain a degree of conscious control with time (or vice versa).

Doctors are almost certainly worse at detecting deception by a patient than we would like to think. A recent study where examiners were blind to whether subjects were feigning paralysis or genuinely experiencing it during a hypnotic state showed no better than chance performance.[218] Another study found that drama students simulating functional gait problems were more convincing than patients with genuine functional gait disturbance.[109] A search through the literature of the past 150 years does not help. Although there are some magnificent old books on malingering[28,85] and a couple of useful new ones,[69,121] none of them give any methods for detecting this reliably in patients with neurological symptoms. As Miller put it, the detection of malingering is "nothing more infallible than one man's assessment or what is probably going on in another man's mind."[134] Covert surveillance demonstrating a *major discrepancy* in function or a direct confession are probably the most reliable methods available in patients with neurological symptoms, but are rarely obtained other than as part of the lawyer's investigation in medicollegal disputes.[176]

Attempts have been made to detect a difference between malingered and hysterical neurological symptoms neurophysiologically—for example, Charcot's experiment showing that a volunteer was unable to simulate the same posturographic tracing as a patient with hysterical "catalepsy."[26] More recently, functional imaging of the brain has opened up new possibilities for detecting differences in intention and action that are not visible clinically. Two small studies do suggest that there may be differences, but they disagree on where in the brain these may reside.[185,218]

Among those patients who are consciously generating symptoms and signs, it is important to distinguish between those whose aim is to obtain medical care and those in pursuit of material gain. Behavior of the first kind is diagnosed as factitious disorder, a medical diagnosis analogous to that of deliberate self-harm, another conscious act. Those who simulate for financial or other material gain are malingerers and are not considered to have a medical condition.

After a bad experience of discovering that you have been deceived by a patient, it can be tempting to believe that a large proportion of patients with apparently functional symptoms are in fact factitious. The true proportion is unknown, but at times like this, it is useful to pose the following questions to yourself: Why do so many patients present such similar stories of bafflement and fear about their symptoms? Why do follow-up studies show persistence of symptoms in the majority over the long term? Why are patients with these symptoms so keen to have investigations to find an organic cause for their symptoms? If they were malingerers, they would know that this could weaken their case. When you see a patient clearly exaggerating a symptom or groaning heavily during an examination, is this exaggeration meant to deceive or to convince? Finally, it is useful to ask: Is it really a doctor's job to detect malingering anyway?

Conclusion

Functional symptoms, when grouped together, are one of the most common reasons for consulting a neurologist. It is no longer acceptable to view these symptoms as simply psychogenic. A much more complex model of causation and mechanism that takes into account biological, psychological, and social factors fits better with the available data. In making the diagnosis, which may not be easy, there are a number of positive signs that are as important as simply the absence of signs of disease. However, none should be used in isolation, and all must be interpreted in the overall context of the presentation. Always bear in mind the possibility that your patient may have both a functional *and* an organic disorder. If made by a neurologist, a diagnosis of functional symptoms is usually correct. Physical trauma has an important relationship with functional symptoms via several different mechanisms. The functional model allows a transparent explanation and interaction with the patient that can facilitate later physical and psychological treatments.

ACKNOWLEDGMENTS

We would like to thank our colleagues in Edinburgh, especially Dr. Adam Zeman, Dr. Alan Carson, and Professor Charles Warlow, for their valuable collaboration and support of this work.

REFERENCES

1. Akagi H, House A: The epidemiology of hysterical conversion. In: Halligan PW, Bass C, Marshall JC (eds): Contemporary Approaches to the Study of Hysteria: Clinical and Theoretical Perspectives. Oxford, Oxford University Press, 2001, pp 73–87.
2. Alajouanine T, Scherrer J, Barbizet J, Calvelt J, Verley R: Potentiels évoqués corticaux chez de sujets atteints de troubles somesthesiques. Rev Neurol 98:757, 1958.
3. Alper K, Devinsky O, Perrine K, Luciano D, Vazquez B, Pacia S, et al: Dissociation in epilepsy and conversion nonepileptic seizures. Epilepsia 38(9):991–997, 1997.
4. American Psychiatric Association: Diagnostic and Statistical Manual of Diseases, Text Revision, 4th ed. Washington, DC, American Psychiatric Association, 2000.
5. Apple DF Jr: Hysterical spinal paralysis. Paraplegia 27(6):428–431, 1989.
6. Back GW, Leong P, Kumar R, Corbridge R: Value of barium swallow in investigation of globus pharyngeus. J Laryngol Otol 114(12):951–954, 2000.
7. Baker D, Hunter E, Lawrence E, Medford N, Patel M, Senior C, et al: Depersonalisation disorder: Clinical features of 204 cases. Br J Psychiatry 182:428–433, 2003.
8. Baker JH, Silver JR: Hysterical paraplegia. J Neurol Neurosurg Psychiatry 50(4):375–382, 1987.
9. Barnert C: Conversion reactions and psychophysiologic disorders: A comparative study. Psychiatry Med 2(3): 205–220, 1971.
10. Beatty S. Non-organic visual loss. Postgrad Med J 75(882): 201–207, 1999.
11. Bhatia KP, Bhatt MH, Marsden CD: The causalgia-dystonia syndrome. Brain 116 (pt 4):843–851, 1993.
12. Bhatia M, Sinha PK, Jain S, Padma MV, Maheshwari MC: Usefulness of short-term video EEG recording with saline induction in pseudoseizures. Acta Neurol Scand 95(6):363–366, 1997.
13. Binzer M, Andersen PM, Kullgren G: Clinical characteristics of patients with motor disability due to conversion disorder: A prospective control group study. J Neurol Neurosurg Psychiatry 63(1):83–88, 1997.
14. Binzer M, Eisemann M, Kullgren G: Illness behavior in the acute phase of motor disability in neurological disease and in conversion disorder: A comparative study. J Psychosom Res 44(6):657–666, 1998.
15. Birklein F, Riedl B, Sieweke N, Weber M, Neundorfer B: Neurological findings in complex regional pain syndromes—analysis of 145 cases. Acta Neurol Scand 101(4): 262–269, 2000.
16. Blau JN, Wiles CM, Solomon FS: Unilateral somatic symptoms due to hyperventilation. BMJ 286(6371): 1108, 1983.
17. Bleichhardt G, Timmer B, Rief W: Cognitive-behavioural therapy for patients with multiple somatoform symptoms—a randomised controlled trial in tertiary care. J Psychosom Res 56(4):449–454, 2004.
18. Bose S, Kupersmith MJ: Neuro-ophthalmologic presentations of functional visual disorders. Neurol Clin 13(2):321–339, 1995.
19. Briquet P: Traité clinique et thérapeutique de l'Hysterie. Paris, JB Ballière, 1859.
20. Brown P, Thompson PD: Electrophysiological aids to the diagnosis of psychogenic jerks, spasms, and tremor. Mov Disord 16(4):595–599, 2001.
21. Cantello R, Boccagni C, Comi C, Civardi C, Monaco F: Diagnosis of psychogenic paralysis: The role of motor evoked potentials. J Neurol 248(10):889–897, 2001.
22. Carson AJ, Best S, Postma K, Stone J, Warlow C, Sharpe M: The outcome of neurology outpatients with medically unexplained symptoms: A prospective cohort study. J Neurol Neurosurg Psychiatry 74(7):897–900, 2003.
23. Carson AJ, Ringbauer B, Stone J, McKenzie L, Warlow C, Sharpe M: Do medically unexplained symptoms matter? A prospective cohort study of 300 new referrals to neurology outpatient clinics. J Neurol Neurosurg Psychiatry 68:207–210, 2000.
24. Chabrol H, Peresson G, Clanet M: Lack of specificity of the traditional criteria of conversion disorders. Eur Psychiatry 10:317–319, 1995.
25. Chalder T: Cognitive behavioural therapy as a treatment for conversion disorders. In: Halligan P, Bass C, Marshall JC (eds): Contemporary Approaches to the Study of Hysteria: Clinical and Theoretical Perspectives. Oxford, Oxford University Press, 2001, pp 298–311.
26. Charcot JM: Clinical Lectures on Diseases of the Nervous System. London, New Sydenham Society, 1889.
27. Ciechanowski PS, Walker EA, Katon WJ, Russo JE: Attachment theory: A model for health care utilization and somatization. Psychosom Med 64(4):660–667, 2002.

28. Collie J: Malingering. London, Arnold, 1913.
29. Coombs-Knapp P: General morbid states: Traumatic neuroses. In: Dercum FX (ed): Text-Book on Nervous Diseases by American Authors. Edinburgh and London: Young J Pentland, 1895, pp 169–170.
30. Couprie W, Wijdicks E-FM, Rooijmans H-GM, van Gijn J: Outcome in conversion disorder: A follow-up study. J Neurol Neurosurg Psychiatry 58:750–752, 1995.
31. Crimlisk HL, Bhatia K, Cope H, David A, Marsden CD, Ron MA: Slater revisited: 6 year follow-up study of patients with medically unexplained motor symptoms. BMJ 316(7131):582–586, 1998.
32. Crimlisk HL, Bhatia KP, Cope H, David AS, Marsden D, Ron MA: Patterns of referral in patients with medically unexplained motor symptoms. J Psychosom Res 49(3):217–219, 2000.
33. Davenport RJ, Swingler RJ, Chancellor AM, Warlow CP: Avoiding false positive diagnoses of motor neuron disease: Lessons from the Scottish Motor Neuron Disease Register. J Neurol Neurosurg Psychiatry 60(2): 147–151, 1996.
34. Deary IJ, Wilson JA, Kelly SW: Globus pharyngis, personality, and psychological distress in the general population. Psychosomatics 36(6):570–577, 1995.
35. DeJong R: Examination in Cases of Suspected Hysteria and Malingering: The Neurologic Examination. New York, Harper & Row, 1967, pp 989–1015.
36. Deuschl G, Blumberg H, Lucking CH: Tremor in reflex sympathetic dystrophy. Arch Neurol 48(12):1247–1252, 1991.
37. Deuschl G, Koster B, Lucking CH, Scheidt C: Diagnostic and pathophysiological aspects of psychogenic tremors. Mov Disord 13(2):294–302, 1998.
38. Dickson H, Cole A, Engel S, Jones RF: Conversion reaction presenting as acute spinal cord injury. Med J Aust 141(7):427–429, 1984.
39. Diukova GM, Liachovitskaia NI, Begliarova AM, Vein AM: Simple measurement of Hoover's test in patients with psychogenic and with organic pareses. Nevrolog Z 5(5):19–21, 2001.
40. Diukova GM, Stoliarova AV: [Psychogenic disorders of stance and gait as seen in videotaping]. Zh Nevrol Psikhiatr Im SS Korsakova 101(12):13–18, 2001.
41. Diukova GM, Stoliarova AV, Vein AM: Sternocleidomastoid (SCM) muscle test in patients with hysterical and organic paresis. J Neurol Sci 187(suppl 1):S108, 2001.
42. Dubois P: The Psychic Treatment of Nervous Disorders. New York, Funk & Wagnalls, 1909.
43. Ebel H, Lohmann T: Clinical criteria for diagnosing conversion disorders. Neurol Psychiatry Brain Res 3(4): 193–200, 1995.
44. Ehrbar R, Waespe W: Funktionelle Gangstörungen. Schweiz Med Wochenschr 122(22):833–841, 1992.
45. Eldridge R, Riklan M, Cooper IS: The limited role of psychotherapy in torsion dystonia. Experience with 44 cases. JAMA 210(4):705–708, 1969.
46. Ellis SJ: Diazepam as a truth drug. Lancet 336(8717):752–753, 1990.
47. Evans DL, Seely TJ: Pseudocyesis in the male. J Nerv Ment Dis 172(1):37–40, 1984.
48. Ewald H, Rogne T, Ewald K, Fink P: Somatization in patients newly admitted to a neurological department. Acta Psychiatr Scand 89(3):174–179, 1994.
49. Factor SA, Podskalny GD, Molho ES: Psychogenic movement disorders: Frequency, clinical profile, and characteristics. J Neurol Neurosurg Psychiatry 59(4):406–412, 1995.
50. Fahn S, Williams DT: Psychogenic dystonia. Adv Neurol 50:431–455, 1988.
51. Farkkila MA, Ertama L, Katila H, Kuusi K, Paavolainen M, Varis K: Globus pharyngis, commonly associated with esophageal motility disorders. Am J Gastroenterol 89(4):503–508, 1994.
52. Fink P, Hansen MS, Sondergaard L, Frydenberg M: Mental illness in new neurological patients. J Neurol Neurosurg Psychiatry 74(6):817–819, 2003.
53. Fink P, Rosendal M, Toft T: Assessment and treatment of functional disorders in general practice: The extended reattribution and management model—an advanced educational program for nonpsychiatric doctors. Psychosomatics 43(2):93–131, 2002.
54. Fishbain DA, Goldberg M, Rosomoff RS, Rosomoff H: Chronic pain patients and the nonorganic physical sign of nondermatomal sensory abnormalities (NDSA). Psychosomatics 32(3):294–303, 1991.
55. FitzGerald JE, Birchall JP, Murray A: Identification of non-organic instability by sway magnetometry. Br J Audiol 31(4):275–282, 1997.
56. Fleminger JJ, McClure GM, Dalton R: Lateral response to suggestion in relation to handedness and the side of psychogenic symptoms. Br J Psychiatry 136:562–566, 1980.
57. Folks DG, Ford CV, Regan WM: Conversion symptoms in a general hospital. Psychosomatics 25(4):285, 1984.
58. Fox CD: The Psychopathology of Hysteria. Boston: Richard G. Badger, Gorham Press, 1913.
59. Freud S: Quelques considerations pour une étude comparative des paralysies motrices organiques et hystériques. Arch Neurol 26:29–43, 1893.
60. Furman JM, Jacob RG: Psychiatric dizziness. Neurology 48(5):1161–1166, 1997.
61. Galin D, Diamond R, Braff D: Lateralization of conversion symptoms: More frequent on the left. Am J Psychiatry 134(5):578–580, 1977.
62. Goldstein LH, Deale AC, Mitchell-O'Malley SJ, Toone BK, Mellers JD: An evaluation of cognitive behavioral therapy as a treatment for dissociative seizures: A pilot study. Cogn Behav Neurol 17(1):41–49, 2004.
63. Goldstein LH, Drew C, Mellers J, Mitchell-O'Malley S, Oakley DA: Dissociation, hypnotizability, coping styles and health locus of control: Characteristics of pseudoseizure patients. Seizure 9(5):314–322, 2000.
64. Gould R, Miller BL, Goldberg MA, Benson DF: The validity of hysterical signs and symptoms. J Nerv Ment Dis 174(10):593–597, 1986.

65. Gowers WR: Hysteria. A Manual of Diseases of the Nervous System. London, Churchill, 1892, pp 903–960.
66. Groppel G, Kapitany T, Baumgartner C:. Cluster analysis of clinical seizure semiology of psychogenic nonepileptic seizures. Epilepsia 41(5):610–614, 2000.
67. Halliday AM: Computing techniques in neurological diagnosis. Br Med Bull 24(3):253–259, 1968.
68. Halligan PW, Athwal BS, Oakley DA, Frackowiak RS: Imaging hypnotic paralysis: Implications for conversion hysteria. Lancet 355(9208):986–987, 2000.
69. Halligan PW, Bass C, Oakley DA: Malingering and Illness Deception. Oxford, Oxford University Press, 2003.
70. Hankey GJ, Stewart-Wynne EG: Pseudo-multiple sclerosis: A clinico-epidemiological study. Clin Exp Neurol 24:11–19, 1987.
71. Hayes MW, Graham S, Heldorf P, de Moore G, Morris JG: A video review of the diagnosis of psychogenic gait: Appendix and commentary. Mov Disord 14(6): 914–921, 1999.
72. Head H: The diagnosis of hysteria. BMJ 1:827–829, 1922.
73. Hernández-Peón R, Chávez-Ibarra G, Aguilar E: Somatic evoked potentials in one case of hysterical anaesthesia. Electroencephalogr Clin Neurophysiol 15:889–892, 1963.
74. Herr RD, Zun L, Mathews JJ: A directed approach to the dizzy patient. Ann Emerg Med 18(6):664–672, 1989.
75. Heruti RJ, Reznik J, Adunski A, Levy A, Weingarden H, Ohry A: Conversion motor paralysis disorder: Analysis of 34 consecutive referrals. Spinal Cord 40(7):335–340, 2002.
76. Hoechstetter K, Meinck HM, Henningsen P, Scherg M, Rupp A: Psychogenic sensory loss: Magnetic source imaging reveals normal tactile evoked activity of the human primary and secondary somatosensory cortex. Neurosci Lett 323(2):137–140, 2002.
77. Hoover CF: A new sign for the detection of malingering and functional paresis of the lower extremities. JAMA 51(9):746–747, 1908.
78. Horvath T, Friedman J, Meares R: Attention in hysteria: A study of Janet's hypothesis by means of habituation and arousal measures. Am J Psychiatry 137(2): 217–220, 1980.
79. Howard JE, Dorfman LJ: Evoked potentials in hysteria and malingering. J Clin Neurophysiol 3(1):39–49, 1986.
80. Howell SJ, Owen L, Chadwick DW: Pseudostatus epilepticus. Q J Med 71(266):507–519, 1989.
81. Jacobs H, Russell WR: Functional disorders. A follow-up study. BMJ 2:346–349, 1961.
82. Janet P: The Major Symptoms of Hysteria. London, Macmillan, 1907.
83a. Janet P: The Troubles of Speech: The Major Symptoms of Hysteria. New York, Macmillan, 1907, pp 208–226.
83b. Janssen BA, Theiler R, Grob D, Dvorak J: The role of motor evolked potentials in psychogenic paralysis. Spine 20:608–611, 1995.
84. Johnstone EC, Macmillan JF, Crow TJ: The occurrence of organic disease of possible or probable aetiological significance in a population of 268 cases of first episode schizophrenia. Psychol Med 17(2):371–379, 1987.
85. Jones AB, Llewellyn LJ: Malingering or the Simulation of Disease. London, William Heinemann, 1917.
86. Jones E: Le côté affecté par l'hémiplégie hystérique. Rev Neurol 16:193–196, 1908.
87. Kapfhammer HP, Buchheim P, Bove D, Wagner A: Konverssionssymptome bei patienten im psychiatrischen konsiliardienst. Nervenarzt 63(9):527–538, 1992.
88. Kapfhammer HP, Dobmeier P, Mayer C, Rothenhausler HB: Konversionssyndrome in der Neurologie: Eine psyhopathologische und psychodynamische Differenzierung in Konversionsstörung, Somatisierungstörung und artifizielle Störung. Psychother Psychosom Med Psychol 48(12): 463–474, 1998.
89. Kaplan BJ, Friedman WA, Gravenstein D: Somatosensory evoked potentials in hysterical paraplegia. Surg Neurol 23(5):502–506, 1985.
90. Kathol RG, Cox TA, Corbett JJ, Thompson HS, Clancy J: Functional visual loss: II. Psychiatric aspects in 42 patients followed for 4 years. Psychol Med 13(2):315–324, 1983.
91. Keane JR: Hysterical hemianopia. The "missing half" field defect. Arch Ophthalmol 97(5):865–866. 1979.
92. Keane JR: Neuro-ophthalmic signs and symptoms of hysteria. Neurology 32(7):757–762, 1982.
93. Keane JR: Wrong-way deviation of the tongue with hysterical hemiparesis. Neurology 36(10):1406–1407, 1986.
94. Keane JR: Hysterical gait disorders: 60 cases. Neurology 39(4):586–589, 1989.
95. Kent DA, Tomasson K, Coryell W: Course and outcome of conversion and somatization disorders. A four-year follow-up. Psychosomatics 36(2):138–144, 1995.
96. Kim YJ, Pakiam AS, Lang AE: Historical and clinical features of psychogenic tremor: A review of 70 cases. Can J Neurol Sci 26(3):190–195, 1999.
97. Kligerman MJ, McKegney FP: Patterns of psychiatric consultation in two general hospitals. Psychiatry Med 2(2):126–132, 1971.
98. Knutsson E, Martensson A: Isokinetic measurements of muscle strength in hysterical paresis. Electroencephalogr Clin Neurophysiol 61(5):370–374, 1985.
99. Koller W, Lang A, Vetere-Overfield B, Findley L, Cleeves L, Factor S, et al: Psychogenic tremors. Neurology 39(8):1094–1099, 1989.
100. Kotsopoulos IA, de Krom MC, Kessels FG, Lodder J, Troost J, Twellaar M, et al: The diagnosis of epileptic and non-epileptic seizures. Epilepsy Res 57(1):59–67, 2003.
101. Kroenke K, Swindle R: Cognitive-behavioral therapy for somatization and symptom syndromes: A critical review of controlled clinical trials. Psychother Psychosom 69(4):205–215, 2000.
102. Kushner MG, Beitman BD: Panic attacks without fear: an overview. Behav Res Ther 28(6):469–479, 1990.
103. Lader M, Sartorius N: Anxiety in patients with hysterical

conversion symptoms. J Neurol Neurosurg Psychiatry 31(5):490–495, 1968.

104. Lang AE: Psychogenic dystonia: A review of 18 cases. Can J Neurol Sci 22(2):136–143, 1995.

105. Lang AE, Koller WC, Fahn S: Psychogenic parkinsonism. Arch Neurol 52(8):802–810, 1995.

106. Lazare A: Current concepts in psychiatry. Conversion symptoms. N Engl J Med 305(13):745–748, 1981.

107. Le Pera D, Graven-Nielsen T, Valeriani M, Oliviero A, Di Lazzaro V, Tonali PA, et al: Inhibition of motor system excitability at cortical and spinal level by tonic muscle pain. Clin Neurophysiol 112:1633–1641, 2001.

108. Lecompte D: Organic disease and associated psychopathology in a patient group with conversion symptoms. Acta Psychiatr Belg 87:662–669, 1987.

109. Lempert T, Brandt T, Dieterich M, Huppert D: How to identify psychogenic disorders of stance and gait. A video study in 37 patients. J Neurol 238(3):140–146, 1991.

110. Lempert T, Dieterich M, Huppert D, Brandt T: Psychogenic disorders in neurology: Frequency and clinical spectrum. Acta Neurol Scand 82(5):335–340, 1990.

111. Lempert T, Schmidt D: Natural history and outcome of psychogenic seizures: A clinical study in 50 patients. J Neurol 237(1):35–38, 1990.

112. Lesser RP, Fahn S: Dystonia: A disorder often misdiagnosed as a conversion reaction. Am J Psychiatry 135(3): 349–352, 1978.

113. Levy R, Behrman J: Cortical evoked responses in hysterical hemianaesthesia. Electroencephalogr Clin Neurophysiol 29(4):400–402, 1970.

114. Levy R, Mushin J: The somatosensory evoked response in patients with hysterical anaesthesia. J Psychosom Res 17(2):81–84, 1973.

115. Lewis WC, Berman M: Studies of conversion hysteria. Arch Gen Psychiatry 13:275–282, 1965.

116. Lindley RI, Warlow CP, Wardlaw JM, Dennis MS, Slattery J, Sandercock PA: Interobserver reliability of a clinical classification of acute cerebral infarction. Stroke 24(12):1801–1804, 1993.

117. Lorenz J, Kunze K, Bromm B: Differentiation of conversive sensory loss and malingering by P300 in a modified oddball task. NeuroReport 9(2):187–191, 1998.

118. Mace CJ, Trimble MR: Ten-year prognosis of conversion disorder. Br J Psychiatry 169(3):282–288, 1996.

119. MacKenzie K, Millar A, Wilson JA, Sellars C, Deary IJ: Is voice therapy an effective treatment for dysphonia? A randomised controlled trial. BMJ 323(7314):658–661, 2001.

120. Mailis-Gagnon A, Giannoylis I, Downar J, Kwan CL, Mikulis DJ, Crawley AP, et al: Altered central somatosensory processing in chronic pain patients with "hysterical" anesthesia. Neurology 60(9):1501–1507, 2003.

121. Malleson A: Whiplash and Other Useful Illnesses. Montreal, McGill-Queen's University Press, 2002.

122. Manto MU: Discrepancy between dysmetric centrifugal movements and normometric centripetal movements in psychogenic ataxia. Eur Neurol 45(4):261–265, 2001.

123. Marsden CD: Hysteria—a neurologist's view. Psychol Med 16(2):277–288, 1986.

124. Marshall JC, Halligan PW, Fink GR, Wade DT, Frackowiak RS: The functional anatomy of a hysterical paralysis. Cognition 64(1):B1–B8, 1997.

125. Matas M: Psychogenic voice disorders: Literature review and case report. Can J Psychiatry 36(5):363–365, 1991.

126. McAuley J, Rothwell J: Identification of psychogenic, dystonic, and other organic tremors by a coherence entrainment test. Mov Disord 19(3):253–267, 2004.

127. McComas AJ, Kereshi S, Quinlan J: A method for detecting functional weakness. J Neurol Neurosurg Psychiatry 46(3):280–282, 1983.

128. McGonigal A, Oto M, Russell AJ, Greene J, Duncan R: Outpatient video EEG recording in the diagnosis of non-epileptic seizures: A randomised controlled trial of simple suggestion techniques. J Neurol Neurosurg Psychiatry 72(4):549–551, 2002.

129. McKegney FP: The incidence and characteristics of patients with conversion reactions. I. A general hospital consultation service sample. Am J Psychiatry 124(4): 542–545, 1967.

130. Merskey H, Buhrich NA: Hysteria and organic brain disease. Br J Med Psychol 48(4):359–366, 1975.

131. Metcalfe R, Firth D, Pollock S, Creed F: Psychiatric morbidity and illness behaviour in female neurological in-patients. J Neurol Neurosurg Psychiatry 51(11):1387–1390, 1988.

132. Micale MS: Charcot and Les nevroses traumatiques: Scientific and historical reflections. J Hist Neurosci 4(2):101–119, 1995.

133. Miller E: Detecting hysterical sensory symptoms: An elaboration of the forced choice technique. Br J Clin Psychol 25(pt 3):231–232, 1986.

134. Miller H: Accident neurosis: Lecture 2. BMJ 1:992–998, 1964.

135. Moene FC, Spinhoven P, Hoogduin KA, Van Dyck R: A randomised controlled clinical trial on the additional effect of hypnosis in a comprehensive treatment programme for in-patients with conversion disorder of the motor type. Psychother Psychosom 71(2):66–76, 2002.

136. Moene FC, Spinhoven P, Hoogduin CA, Van Dyck R: A randomized controlled clinical trial of a hypnosis-based treatment for patients with conversion disorder, motor type. Int J Clin Exp Hypn 51:29–50, 2003.

137. Moldofsky H, England RS: Facilitation of somatosensory average-evoked potentials in hysterical anesthesia and pain. Arch Gen Psychiatry 32(2):193–197, 1975.

138. Monday K, Jankovic J: Psychogenic myoclonus. Neurology 43(2):349–352, 1993.

139. Nimnuan C, Hotopf M, Wessely S: Medically unexplained symptoms: An epidemiological study in seven specialities. J Psychosom Res 51(1):361–367, 2001.

140. O'Malley PG, Jackson JL, Santoro J, Tomkins G, Balden E, Kroenke K: Antidepressant therapy for unexplained symptoms and symptom syndromes. J Fam Pract 48(12):980–990, 1999.

141. Oppenheim H (Bruce A trans): Textbook of Nervous Diseases. Edinburgh, Schulze, 1911.
142. O'Sullivan G, Harvey I, Bass C, Sheehy M, Toone B, Turner S: Psychophysiological investigations of patients with unilateral symptoms in the hyperventilation syndrome. Br J Psychiatry 160:664–667, 1992.
143. Packard RC: What does the headache patient want? Headache 19(7):370–374, 1979.
144. Page HW: Injuries of the Spine and Spinal Cord without Apparent Mechanical Lesions. London, J.&A. Churchill, 1883.
145. Pascuzzi RM: Nonphysiological (functional) unilateral motor and sensory syndromes involve the left more often than the right body. J Nerv Ment Dis 182(2):118–120, 1994.
146. Perkin GD: An analysis of 7836 successive new outpatient referrals. J Neurol Neurosurg Psychiatry 52(4):447–448, 1989.
147. Perkin GD, Joseph R: Neurological manifestations of the hyperventilation syndrome. J R Soc Med 79(8):448–450, 1986.
148. Purves-Stewart J, Worster-Drought C: The Psychoneuroses and Psychoses: Diagnosis of Nervous Diseases, 10th ed. Baltimore, Williams & Wilkins, 1952, pp 661–758.
149. Qiu WW, Yin SS, Stucker FJ, Welsh LW: Current evaluation of pseudohypacusis: Strategies and classification. Ann Otol Rhinol Laryngol 107(8):638–647, 1998.
150. Raimiste J: Deux signes d'hèmiplegie organique du membre inférieur. Rev Neurol 17:125–129, 1912.
151. Raskin M, Talbott JA, Meyerson AT: Diagnosis of conversion reactions. Predictive value of psychiatric criteria. JAMA 197(7):530–534, 1966.
152. Reuber M, Elger CE: Psychogenic nonepileptic seizures: A review and update. Epilepsy Behaviour 4:205–216, 2003.
153. Reuber M, Enright SM, Goulding PJ: Postoperative pseudostatus: Not everything that shakes is epilepsy. Anaesthesia 55(1):74–78, 2000.
154. Reuber M, House AO, Pukrop R, Bauer J, Elger CE: Somatization, dissociation and general psychopathology in patients with psychogenic non-epileptic seizures. Epilepsy Res 57(2–3):159–167, 2003.
155. Reuber M, Pukrop R, Bauer J, Helmstaedter C, Tessendorf N, Elger CE: Outcome in psychogenic nonepileptic seizures: 1 to 10–year follow-up in 164 patients. Ann Neurol 53(3):305–311, 2003.
156. Reynolds JR: Paralysis and other disorders of motion and sensation dependent on idea. BMJ 1:483–485, 1869.
157. Rice DG, Greenfield NS: Psychophysiological correlates of la belle indifference. Arch Gen Psychiatry 20(2): 239–245, 1969.
158. Roelofs K, Hoogduin KA, Keijsers GP, Naring GW, Moene FC, Sandijck P: Hypnotic susceptibility in patients with conversion disorder. J Abnorm Psychol 111(2):390–395, 2002.
159. Roelofs K, Keijsers GP, Hoogduin KA, Naring GW, Moene FC: Childhood abuse in patients with conversion disorder. Am J Psychiatry 159(11):1908–1913, 2002.
160. Roelofs K, Naring GW, Keijsers GP, Hoogduin CA: Motor Imagery in conversion paralysis. Cognitive Neuropsychiatry 6(1):21–40, 2001.
161. Roelofs K, van Galen GP, Eling P, Keijsers GP, Hoogduin CA: Endogenous and exogenous attention in patients with conversion disorders. Cogn Neuropsychol 20(8):733–745, 2003.
162. Roelofs K, van Galen GP, Keijsers GP, Hoogduin CA: Motor initiation and execution in patients with conversion paralysis. Acta Psychol (Amst) 110(1):21–34, 2002.
163. Rolak LA: Psychogenic sensory loss. J Nerv Ment Dis 176(11):686–687, 1988.
164. Rommel O, Gehling M, Dertwinkel R, Witscher K, Zenz M, Malin JP, et al: Hemisensory impairment in patients with complex regional pain syndrome. Pain 80(1–2):95–101, 1999.
165. Ron M: The prognosis of hysteria/somatisation disorder. In: Halligan P, Bass C, Marshall JC (eds): Contemporary Approaches to the Study of Hysteria. Oxford, Oxford University Press, 2001, pp 271–281.
166. Roy A: Cerebral disease and hysteria. Compr Psychiatry 18(6):607–609, 1977.
167. Roy N: Functional dysphonia. Curr Opin Otolaryngol Head Neck Surg 11(3):144–148, 2003.
168. Rutstein RP, Daum KM, Amos JF: Accommodative spasm: A study of 17 cases. J Am Optom Assoc 59(7): 527–538, 1988.
169. Samuel M, Kleiner-Fisman G, Lang AE: Voluntary control and a wider clinical spectrum of essential palatal tremor. Mov Disord 19(6):717–719, 2004.
170. Savill TD: Lectures on Hysteria and Allied Vasomotor Conditions. London, Glaisher, 1909.
171. Sawle GV, Brown P: Movement Disorders in Clinical Practice. Oxford, Taylor and Francis, 1998.
172. Schiffer RB: Psychiatric aspects of clinical neurology. Am J Psychiatry 140(2):205–207, 1983.
173. Schilte AF, Portegijs PJ, Blankenstein AH, Der Horst HE, Latour MB, van Eijk JT, et al: Randomised controlled trial of disclosure of emotionally important events in somatisation in primary care. BMJ 323(7304):86, 2001.
174a. Schrag A, Brown RJ, Trimble MR: Reliability of self-reported diagnoses in patients with neurologically unexplained symptoms. J Neurol Neurosurg Psychiatry 75(4):608–611, 2004.
174b. Schrag A, Trimble M, Quinn N, Bhatta K: The syndrome of fixed dystonia: an evaluation of 103 patients. Brain 127(10): 2360–2372, 2004.
175. Sharma P, Chaturvedi SK: Conversion disorder revisited. Acta Psychiatr Scand 92(4):301–304, 1995.
176. Sharpe M: Malingering and psychiatric disorder. In: Halligan P, Bass C, Oakley DA (eds): Malingering. Oxford, Oxford University Press, 2002, pp 156–70.
177. Shorter E: From Paralysis to Fatiguie. New York, Free Press, 1992.
178. Showalter E: Hystories. London, Picador, 1997.

179. Simmons BP, Vasile RG: The clenched fist syndrome. J Hand Surg [Am] 5(5):420–427, 1980.
180. Slater ET: Diagnosis of 'hysteria'. BMJ 1:1395–1399, 1965.
181. Smith D, Defalla BA, Chadwick DW: The misdiagnosis of epilepsy and the management of refractory epilepsy in a specialist clinic. QJM 92(1):15–23, 1999.
182. Snijders TJ, de Leeuw FE, Klumpers UM, Kappelle LJ, van Gijn J: Prevalence and predictors of unexplained neurological symptoms in an academic neurology outpatient clinic—an observational study. J Neurol 251(1): 66–71, 2004.
183. Sonoo M: Abductor sign: A reliable new sign to detect unilateral non-organic paresis of the lower limb. J Neurol Neurosurg Psychiatry 73:121–125, 2004.
184. Spence SA: Hysterical paralyses as disorders of action. Cogn Neuropsychiatry 4(3):203–226, 1999.
185. Spence SA, Crimlisk HL, Cope H, Ron MA, Grasby PM: Discrete neurophysiological correlates in prefrontal cortex during hysterical and feigned disorder of movement. Lancet 355(9211):1243–1244, 2000.
186. Spiegel D, Chase RA: The treatment of contractures of the hand using self-hypnosis. J Hand Surg [Am] 5(5):428–432, 1980.
187. Spiegel J, Heiss C, Fruhauf E, Fogel W, Meinck HM: [Polygraphic validation of distraction tasks in clinical differential tremor diagnosis]. Nervenarzt 69(10):886–891, 1998.
188. Stam J, Speelman HD, van Crevel H: Tendon reflex asymmetry by voluntary mental effort in healthy subjects. Arch Neurol 46(1):70–73, 1989.
189. Stern DB: Handedness and the lateral distribution of conversion reactions. J Nerv Ment Dis 164(2):122–128, 1977.
190. Stone J: Pseudoptosis. Practical Neurol 2:364–365, 2002.
191. Stone J, Campbell K, Sharma N, Carson A, Warlow CP, Sharpe M: What should we call pseudoseizures? The patient's perspective. Seizure 12(8):568–572, 2003.
192. Stone J, Durrance D, Wojcik W, Carson A, Sharpe M: What do medical outpatients attending a neurology clinic think about antidepressants? J Psychosom Res 56(3):293–295, 2004.
193. Stone J, Sharpe M, Carson A, Lewis SC, Thomas B, Goldbeck R, et al: Are functional motor and sensory symptoms really more frequent on the left? A systematic review. J Neurol Neurosurg Psychiatry 73(5):578–581, 2002.
194. Stone J, Sharpe M, Deary I, Warlow C: Functional paresis: Paradoxes in illness beliefs and disability in 107 subjects (abstract). J Neurol Neurosurg Psychiatry 75: 518, 2003.
195. Stone J, Sharpe M, Rothwell PM, Warlow CP: The 12 year prognosis of unilateral functional weakness and sensory disturbance. J Neurol Neurosurg Psychiatry 74(5):591–596, 2003.
196. Stone J, Smyth R, Carson A, Warlow C, Sharpe M: *La belle indifference* in conversion symptoms/hysteria—a systematic review. Br J Psych (in press).
197. Stone J, Smyth R, Sharpe M, Carson A, Warlow C: The misdiagnosis of conversion symptoms (hysteria): A systematic review. BMJ 331(7523):989, 2005.
198. Stone J, Wojcik W, Durrance D, Carson A, Lewis S, MacKenzie L, et al: What should we say to patients with symptoms unexplained by disease? The "number needed to offend." BMJ 325(7378):1449–1450, 2002.
199. Stone J, Zeman A: Hysterical conversion—the view from clinical neurology. In: Halligan PW, Bass C, Marshall JC (ed): Contemporary Approaches to the Study of Hysteria. Oxford, Oxford University Press, 2001, pp 102–125.
200. Stone J, Zeman A, Sharpe M: Functional weakness and sensory disturbance. J Neurol Neurosurg Psychiatry 73(3):241–245, 2002.
201. Tan EK, Jankovic J: Psychogenic hemifacial spasm. J Neuropsychiatry Clin Neurosci 13(3):380–384, 2001.
202. Tegner R: A technique to detect psychogenic sensory loss. J Neurol Neurosurg Psychiatry 51(11):1455–1456, 1988.
203. Terada K, Ikeda A, Van Ness PC, Nagamine T, Kaji R, Kimura J, et al: Presence of *Bereitschaftspotential* preceding psychogenic myoclonus: Clinical application of jerk-locked back averaging. J Neurol Neurosurg Psychiatry 58(6):745–747, 1995.
204. Thomas M, Jankovic J: Psychogenic movement disorders: Diagnosis and management. CNS Drugs 18(7): 437–452, 2004.
205. Thompson PD, Colebatch JG, Brown P, Rothwell JC, Day BL, Obeso JA, et al: Voluntary stimulus-sensitive jerks and jumps mimicking myoclonus or pathological startle syndromes. Mov Disord 7(3):257–262, 1992.
206. Tiihonen J, Kuikka J, Viinamaki H, Lehtonen J, Partanen J: Altered cerebral blood flow during hysterical paresthesia. Biol Psychiatry 37(2):134–135, 1995.
207. Todd RB: Clinical Lectures on Paralyses: Diseases of the Brain, and Other Affections of the Nervous System. London, J Churchill, 1854.
208. Toth C: Hemisensory syndrome is associated with a low diagnostic yield and a nearly uniform benign prognosis. J Neurol Neurosurg Psychiatry 74(8):1113–1116, 2003.
209. Trimble MR: Post-traumatic Neurosis: From Railway Spine to Whiplash. Chichester, Wiley, 1981.
210. Troost BT, Troost EG: Functional paralysis of horizontal gaze. Neurology 29(1):82–85, 1979.
211. van der Ploeg RJ, Oosterhuis HJ: The "make/break test" as a diagnostic tool in functional weakness. J Neurol Neurosurg Psychiatry 54(3):248–251, 1991.
212. Vein AM, Djukova GM, Vorobieva OV: Is panic attack a mask of psychogenic seizures?—A comparative analysis of phenomenology of psychogenic seizures and panic attacks. Funct Neurol 9(3):153–159, 1994.
213. Veldman PH, Reynen HM, Arntz IE, Goris RJ: Signs and symptoms of reflex sympathetic dystrophy: Prospective study of 829 patients. Lancet 342(8878):1012–1016, 1993.
214. Verdugo RJ, Ochoa JL: Reversal of hypoaesthesia by

nerve block, or placebo: A psychologically mediated sign in chronic pseudoneuropathic pain patients. J Neurol Neurosurg Psychiatry 65(2):196–203, 1998.

215. Verdugo RJ, Ochoa JL: Abnormal movements in complex regional pain syndrome: Assessment of their nature. Muscle Nerve 23(2):198–205, 2000.
216. Vuilleumier P, Chicherio C, Assal F, Schwartz S, Skusman D, Landis T: Functional neuroanatomical correlates of hysterical sensorimotor loss. Brain 124:1077–1090, 2001.
217. Wade D: Rehabilitation for conversion symptoms. In: Halligan P, Bass C, Marshall JC (eds): Contemporary Approaches to the Study of Hysteria. Oxford, Oxford University Press, 2001, pp 330–346.
218. Ward NS, Oakley DA, Frackowiak RS, Halligan PW: Differential brain activations during intentionally simulated and subjectively experienced paralysis. Cogn Neuropsychiatry 8(4):295–312, 2003.
219. Weinstein EA, Lyerly OG: Conversion hysteria following brain injury. Arch Neurol 15(5):545–548, 1966.
220. Weintraub MI: Hysteria. A clinical guide to diagnosis. Clin Symp 29(6):1–31, 1977.
221. Wenegrat B: Theatre of Disorder: Patients, Doctors and the Construction of Illness. Oxford, Oxford University Press, 2001.
222. Werring DJ, Weston L, Bullmore ET, Plant GT, Ron MA: Functional magnetic resonance imaging of the cerebral response to visual stimulation in medically unexplained visual loss. Psychol Med 34(4):583–589, 2004.
223. Wessely S: Discrepancies between diagnostic criteria and clinical practice. In: Halligan P, Bass C, Marshall JC (eds): Contemporary Approaches to the Science of Hysteria. Oxford, Oxford University Press, 2001, pp 63–72.
224. Wessely S, Nimnuan C, Sharpe M: Functional somatic syndromes: One or many? Lancet 354(9182):936–939, 1999.
225. White A, Corbin DO, Coope B: The use of thiopentone in the treatment of non-organic locomotor disorders. J Psychosom Res 32(3):249–253, 1988.
226. Whitlock FA: The aetiology of hysteria. Acta Psychiatr Scand 43(2):144–162, 1967.
227. Yazici KM, Demirci M, Demir B, Ertugrul A: Abnormal somatosensory evoked potentials in two patients with conversion disorder. Psychiatry Clin Neurosci 58(2):222–225, 2004.
228. Yazici KM, Kostakoglu L: Cerebral blood flow changes in patients with conversion disorder. Psychiatry Res 83(3):163–168, 1998.
229. Zahn JR: Incidence and characteristics of voluntary nystagmus. J Neurol Neurosurg Psychiatry 41(7):617–623, 1978.
230. Zaidi A, Crampton S, Clough P, Fitzpatrick A, Scheepers B: Head-up tilting is a useful provocative test for psychogenic nonepileptic seizures. Seizure 8(6):353–355, 1999.
231. Zeuner KE, Shoge RO, Goldstein SR, Dambrosia JM, Hallett M: Accelerometry to distinguish psychogenic from essential or parkinsonian tremor. Neurology 61(4):548–550, 2003.
232. Ziv I, Djaldetti R, Zoldan Y, Avraham M, Melamed E: Diagnosis of "non-organic" limb paresis by a novel objective motor assessment: the quantitative Hoover's test. J Neurol 245(12):797–802, 1998.

Chapter 37

Physical Trauma, Psychological Stress, and Multiple Sclerosis

DOUGLAS S. GOODIN

It seems clear that physical trauma and/or psychological stress can either cause or exacerbate certain medical conditions. For example, trauma is known to precipitate seizures, headache, or focal neurological deficits in previously asymptomatic individuals. Similarly, psychological stress seems to be a factor in the development of some peptic ulcers, anxiety disorders, and other psychiatric states. In addition, trauma and/or stress have been suspected to have links to many other medical disorders. It is perhaps not surprising, therefore, that both physical trauma and psychological stress have been posited to be causal factors in either the onset or exacerbation of multiple sclerosis (MS). Indeed, this notion has been a conspicuous part of the lore of this illness dating back to its earliest clinical descriptions. For example, in 1879 Charcot suggested a relationship between MS and stress,[10] and in 1897 Mendel reported four cases of MS that followed severe skull or spinal injury.[49] Other early authors reached similar conclusions,[29,37] and in 1922 a commission of the Association of Nervous and Mental Diseases concluded that "in a small percentage of cases [multiple sclerosis] appears to be excited by trauma, but trauma cannot itself cause [it]."[15] Despite this conclusion, however, a lively debate about the relationship between MS and either trauma or stress has continued to the present.[1,22–24,32,43,44,60,61,75] There are several reasons for this continuing controversy. First is the reliance (by some) on the findings of small case series,[10,27,29,36,37,49,76] an experimental design, which is widely recognized as having a high likelihood of bias. Second, minor traumatic or stressful events are extremely common; thus, the co-occurrence of trauma or stress with various unrelated medical conditions is expected. For example, the annual incidence of injuries (of all types) in the United States has been estimated to be 33.2/100 persons/year,[73] a figure that almost certainly underestimates the incidence of truly minor traumatic injuries. Similarly, stress is a very common occurrence in the course of everyday living. Indeed, in three recent studies in MS,[2,3,9] the incidence of documented stressful life events exceeded four/person/year. Because of this high frequency of stress, any given MS attack will, on average, occur within 3–4 months of some traumatic or stressful life event; thus, even a well-designed retrospective case-control study may be contaminated by recall bias. As a result, prospectively acquired and controlled data are essential to the evaluation of any proposed relationship between these life events and MS.

It was not until the reports of McAlpine et al.[46–48] and Kurland and Westlund[41] in the 1940s and 1950s that the first controlled data became available.

However, despite a growing realization on the part of the medical community about the value of controlled data, case series suggesting a link between MS and trauma, often with a striking temporal relationship, continue to be reported.[34,50,66] Such case reports may be viewed by some as suggestive but most practitioners of *evidence-based medicine* would consider such reports by themselves highly unreliable. Nevertheless, if either traumatic injury or psychological stress could be linked to either MS onset or MS exacerbations, this would have important implications for practicing clinicians. Not only would this affect the recommendations made to patients (i.e., avoid, if possible, activities that risk physical injury or increase stress), but it would also substantially increase the value of this information as evidence in the resolution of medicolegal matters.[13,80] By contrast, if no such relationship exists, spurious lawsuits and unnecessarily conservative lifestyle recommendations could be avoided. The purpose of this chapter, therefore, is to review and to analyze the evidence linking MS to physical trauma and/or psychological stress.

Biological Plausibility of the Proposed Relationship

In medicine, the validity of any proposed causal relationship must be weighed, in large part, by the plausibility of the connection between the two events. For example, if, on the one hand, an MS episode occurred within days of a lunar eclipse, most physicians would not consider this observation as evidence of a causal connection between these two events. The reason, of course, is that there is no obviously plausible way to link these two events. If, on the other hand, a plausible theoretical basis for connecting the two events were developed, then the observation would carry considerably more weight. Therefore, the first question that requires consideration relates to the biological plausibility of the causal model. As in the example above, if there is no such biological plausibility, the epidemiological evidence of an association would need to be overwhelming in order for one to be convinced of a true association. In the case of MS, one possible connection that has been proposed is through the breakdown of the blood–brain barrier (BBB). This is an important early event in the development of an MS lesion[7,35,45,53,57,58] and is also a consequence of traumatic injury to the brain or spinal cord. Perhaps, as suggested by others,[57,58] the disrupted BBB exposes peripheral immune cells to normally sequestered central nervous system (CNS) antigens and thereby provokes an autoimmune response against certain myelin antigens such as myelin basic protein, proteolipid protein, myelin oligodendrocyte glycoprotein, or myelin-associated glycoprotein. Certainly, there is evidence that direct trauma can produce demyelination,[79] although whether this is immune-mediated is less clear.

Even if a causal relationship between trauma and MS onset is considered biologically plausible, however, there are certain observations suggesting that trauma is unlikely to account for a substantial percentage of MS cases. For example, although trauma can produce a shear injury to the CNS white matter, it generally also injures the cerebral cortex. In such a circumstance, the preferential (but not exclusive) involvement of the white matter would be difficult to rationalize. Similarly, because men (at all ages) are more likely to sustain traumatic injury than women,[73] the marked female preponderance of MS would be unanticipated.

Naturally, these considerations do not affect any potential relationship between trauma and MS exacerbation, although, even in this case, there are reasons to question the strength of any association. First, the biological plausibility outlined above seems to explain an abnormal initial response to sequestered antigens better than a subsequent response, especially in the circumstance where activated T lymphocytes can traffic easily through an intact BBB.[81] Second, in experimental allergic encephalomyelitis (EAE), the animal model of MS, the inflammatory lesions in heterotopic brain transplants have been demonstrated to occur selectively in the core of the transplant where the BBB is intact, rather than at the edges of the transplant where the BBB is disrupted.[38] Third, there is evidence that changes occur within the normal-appearing white matter that precede and predict the disruption of the BBB on magnetic resonance imaging (MRI).[18] This observation suggests that the breakdown of the BBB may not be the initial event in the development of an MS lesion. If this is so, the logical steps in biological plausibility outlined above would begin to unravel. Moreover, at least in EAE, there is evidence that the initial injury may be to the oligodendrocyte rather than to the myelin sheath directly.[67]

Consequently, in order to establish a causal connection between trauma or psychological stress and MS, there will need to be strong epidemiological evidence either from a prospective cohort study (comparing the incidence of MS onset or MS attacks in persons or patients with or without antecedent events) or from a well-designed retrospective case-control study (comparing prior histories of traumatic injury or stress in patients and matched controls). Each of these methods, however, has limitations,[28] and each raises other important questions. It is not clear, for example, how closely the onset of MS or the MS attack needs to follow the trauma or stress in order to link these two events but, clearly, some upper limit needs to be set. Most disruptions of the BBB peak early and fall off sharply with time. Thus, gadolinium enhancement on the MRI scan typically resolves within 3 months,[7,35,53] and this seems like a reasonable period in which to expect the effects of trauma to be manifested. Some authors, however, have considered either shorter or longer intervals, although most seem to agree that an interval beyond a year is not plausible.[6,27,29,34,36,37,45,46,49,50,61,71,72,76]

In addition, it is unclear which kinds of trauma or stress should be included in the analysis of these relationships. For example, although some authors have included minor traumatic events (e.g., dental procedures, minor abrasions, bruises) as examples of trauma in their studies,[46,47] the biological plausibility outlined earlier would not seem to be applicable to these circumstances. Consequently, in considering these issues, Poser reached the conclusion that "in order for trauma to be considered in aggravating or accelerating the course of the disease, there must be evidence of injury to the head, neck or back above the lumbo-sacral region."[57] Clearly, this is a sensible analytical approach. Moreover, because the biological plausibility is most convincing for the more serious traumatic injuries (in which the BBB is clearly disrupted), it also seems sensible to focus on the most severe events in assessing the relationship of trauma or stress to MS. To include potentially irrelevant minor injuries or minor stresses would likely dilute the power of the analysis. It also seems sensible to analyze different classes of traumatic injury or stress separately because different antecedent events will probably have different relationships with MS.

Because clinical studies often lack the statistical power to detect reliably a relationship between trauma or stress and MS, it is important to estimate from each study the confidence interval (CI) that provides a measure of the range of nonexcluded effect sizes. One approach, in a four-cell study design, is to calculate the odds ratio (OR), together with its 95% CI.[28] The OR provides both effect size and directional information. The effect size can also be expressed using the so-called **w**-statistic,[14] a statistic that can also be extended naturally to provide directional information for the two-cell goodness-of-fit case. In this circumstance, **w** ranges between –1.0 and +1.0, with **w** = 0.1 or **w** = –0.1 representing a small-sized effect; **w** = 0.3 or **w** = –0.3 representing a medium-sized effect; and **w** = 0.5 or **w** = –0.5 representing a large-sized effect.[14] From the critical value of the chi-square distribution (p =.05) above and below the experimental observation, a 95% CI around **w** can be constructed. Because many of the published clinical studies of trauma and MS have employed two-cell designs, this method has some advantages over the OR approach.

Physical Trauma and Multiple Sclerosis

McAlpine and coworkers reported the first controlled study of the effects of trauma on MS.[46–48] This retrospective case-control study involved interviewing 250 patients and 250 controls who were patients selected at random from admissions to the Middlesex Hospital. Controls were matched with patients with respect to sex and age at the time of the interview, although patients were interviewed about more remote events, which could well have introduced bias into this study. These authors reported a history of trauma within 3 months of MS onset in 36 patients (14.4%) compared to a similar history in only 13 controls (5.2%). Analyzed either as an OR or with the **w**-statistic, this difference is statistically significant; OR = 3.07 (CI = 1.58–5.94); **w** (two-cell) = 0.47 (CI = 0.22–0.71). By contrast, there was no apparent effect of trauma on MS exacerbations. There are, however, concerns about this study as reported, especially because peripheral trauma and dental procedures are included within the definition of trauma.[46–48] Moreover, the numbers of patients in these categories is not specified, so the impact of these presumably irrelevant types of trauma cannot be estimated. In consequence, this study provides only very weak evidence of any association between trauma and MS onset. It provides no evidence of a relationship between trauma and

MS exacerbation. Another early case-control study of 112 MS patients and 123 controls in Canada[41] reported no association between "head injuries causing unconsciousness" and the onset of MS (time frame not specified), although, again, this study provides only weak evidence against such an association between trauma and MS onset.

In 1968, a study of 36 MS patients and 72 matched controls reported that neither surgery (**w** = –0.03; CI = –0.26–0.20) nor moderately severe head trauma (**w** = 0.11; CI = –0.24–0.45) was significantly associated with MS onset.[4] In 1991, the final results of a prospective cohort study of 170 MS patients were reported.[6,71] Patients were followed monthly for an average of 5.2 years. The principal analysis considered those periods of time when the patients were at risk for an exacerbation because they had sustained a traumatic injury within the previous 3 months separately from those periods of time when they were not at risk because, during the previous 3 months, the patients had been free of trauma. The statistical analysis used a two-cell goodness-of-fit chi square test[14] that compared the observed exacerbations during the at-risk and not-at-risk periods to the expected number of such exacerbations based on the attack rate for both time periods combined. There was no significant difference between the actual and expected number of exacerbations, either for trauma as a whole or for any specific category of traumatic injury. The only exception was the possibility that electrical injury might aggravate MS, although even this observation is unreliable. Thus, this potential effect was only marginally significant ($p < .02$) and would not survive even the most modest adjustment for multiple comparisons. Moreover, it was based on a very small number of patients. The effect sizes and confidence intervals for different categories of trauma reported in this study were as follows: for trauma as a whole, **w** = 0.06 (CI = –0.07–0.19); for closed head injuries with and without loss of consciousness, **w** = 0.02 (CI = –0.20–0.24); and for major surgeries, **w** = –0.11 (CI = –0.34–0.12). As a result, this study effectively excludes anything more than a modest effect (**w** < 0.24) of trauma within the previous 3 months on MS exacerbations and, in fact, the actual findings are considerably more supportive of no association than they are of an association of this magnitude.

In 1993, the results of a population-based study were reported.[72] Both an incidence cohort of 225 new-onset MS cases occurring between 1905 and 1991 and a prevalence cohort of 164 MS patients as of December 1, 1991, were studied. These authors examined MS exacerbations occurring within a 1-year study period, divided into the 6-month period before (not-at-risk) and the 6-month period after (at-risk) traumatic injury. Their definition of trauma included both head trauma severe enough to produce skull fracture, loss of consciousness, focal neurological deficits, or posttraumatic amnesia and peripheral as well as spinal trauma severe enough to result in fractures. These authors also followed a cohort of 819 patients (aged 10–50 years) who had sustained head trauma (as defined above) to evaluate the probability of their developing MS within 10 years of their injury. They found only 39 patients with trauma in the prevalence cohort, and none of these patients had had an episode of head trauma during the average 19-year period during which they were followed. The authors also reported that in only 2 of the 819 patients who experienced head trauma (as defined above) did the trauma antedate the onset of MS, and in both instances the trauma was remote (3 and 21 years prior to MS onset).

For some analyses this study clearly lacks statistical power. For example, the incidence rate of MS in Olmsted County has been estimated to be 5.17 new cases/100,000 population/year.[75] If this is an accurate estimate, one would anticipate only 0.42 cases of MS developing in the 8190 person-years of follow-up represented by this study. Moreover, if only trauma within a year of MS onset is considered relevant, this study represents only 819 person-years of follow-up and only 0.042 new cases would be expected. Even if this estimated incidence is a substantial underestimate,[40] however, it is unlikely that the number of new cases of MS could ever be adequate to study the relationship between trauma and MS onset with such a small sample. Indeed, the necessity of extremely large sample sizes may preclude the use of a prospective study design to explore differences in MS incidence following some antecedent event.[28]

Nevertheless, certain results from this trial have important implications with regard to any possible relationship between serious head trauma and either MS onset or MS exacerbation. Thus, none of the 225 patients with new-onset MS in Olmsted County between 1905 and 1991 had serious head trauma in the year preceding the onset of their illness. This observation indicates that serious head trauma could be a factor related to MS onset in no more than 1.3% of cases (upper limit of the 95% CI, Poisson analysis). Consequently, at least 98.7% of cases must be caused by other factors. Similarly, none of the 164 patients in the prevalence cohort had even a single episode of head trauma within the 6-month period preceding an exacerbation during the average of 19 years in which these patients were followed. Even though the total number of exacerbations in this prevalence cohort is unknown, it seems almost certain that the actual number would be at least several hundred. Again, this observation indicates that the number of MS exacerbations that could conceivably be associated with antecedent head trauma is no more than a fraction of a percentage of the total number of exacerbations. As a consequence of these observations, this study effectively excludes anything even approaching the prevalence of either MS onset or MS exacerbation related to head trauma that is suggested by some of the uncontrolled case series reviewed earlier.

In a case-control study of 155 MS patients and matched controls, the occurrence of head trauma (severe enough to cause loss of consciousness) was analyzed in the two groups.[26] In this study, head trauma was not associated with a higher risk of MS (OR = 1.13; CI = 0.62–2.03). Considering only head trauma that occurred after age 15 and that, therefore, was the head trauma likely to have occurred within a year of MS onset, there was actually more head trauma in the controls than in the patients (OR = 0.59; CI = 0.22–1.58). This study, therefore, also provides reasonably good evidence against any association between moderately severe head trauma and MS onset.

There has also been interest, particularly from the medicolegal perspective, in the possible relationship between MS and trauma to the cervical spine of the type experienced by patients who sustain whiplash injuries. This notion was introduced originally by Brain and Wilkinson[8] in a case series of 16 MS patients who also had cervical spondylosis. Although the case histories of all 16 patients were reviewed, the pathological evidence in this paper is confined to the study of only 2 patients who came to autopsy. Nevertheless, these authors concluded from their study that the distribution of demyelinating lesions within the spinal cord "may have been a chance finding, but it is more likely that the site of demyelination was associated with the presence of the spondylotic bars. These bars may have caused interference with the blood supply of the cord or actual compression of the cord. It is quite likely that both these factors play a part."[8] To arrive at such a conclusion from this study, however, seems astonishing. First, the authors marshal no actual evidence from their study to support any of these statements. Nor do they provide any reasoned arguments to show how they reached these conclusions. Second, in both of the autopsied cases, the worst cord damage was removed from the actual level of maximum disk disease, so that the site of cervical pathology would seem to correlate rather poorly with the lesion location. Moreover, in a subsequent pathological study, Oppenheimer[55] examined the distribution of MS lesions within the cervical spinal cord in 18 MS patients who came to autopsy. Despite the fact that this paper is often cited in the debate regarding the role of whiplash injury in the exacerbation or onset of MS,[11,61] this case series was not a study of the relationship between MS lesions and either trauma or cervical spondylosis. In fact, only 3 of the 18 patients had severe degenerative changes in their cervical spine. More importantly, the actual findings in this study were thought to be at odds with the Brain and Wilkinson hypothesis.[8,55] Thus, Oppenheimer concluded that the Brain and Wilkinson hypothesis "loses its force" because the lesions of MS "do not appear to be related to points of compression by spondylotic bars."[55] Finally, in a recent paper by Chaudhuri and Behan,[12] the authors report on their experience about the relationship between minor whiplash injury (no patient had cervical vertebral fracture, dislocation, or spinal cord compression) and MS. However, not only does this study lack any control group for comparison, it also represents a series of highly selected patients who were specifically referred to Dr. Behan for the purpose of his medicolegal consultation regarding the possible relationship between their trauma and their MS. As a result, this group constitutes an extremely biased sample of the MS population. For this reason, the reported findings from this case series are unreliable There are other sources of potential bias as well. Thus, because the nature and severity of the injury were judged retrospectively over a period of 1 to 10 years, the study is also subject to substantial recall bias. As a result of these concerns, the strength of any scientific evidence provided by this study is quite low. Moreover, it is unclear how the authors concluded that certain symptoms, such as optic neuritis, osillopsia, and internuclear ophthalmoloplegia, could be precipitated by minor cervical trauma. These symptoms are generally thought to arise from CNS locations remote from the spinal cord and would be unexpected in a direct whiplash injury to the cord. Based on these considerations, therefore, none of these studies provide any evidence that minor cervical whiplash injury can either aggravate or cause MS.

In summary, therefore, on the basis of generally consistent and convincing evidence, it seems highly unlikely that trauma, especially head trauma or minor cervical whiplash injury, can precipitate either the onset or the exacerbation of MS. Moreover, even if such an association did exist in a few selected cases, the percentage of such cases must be extremely small and, because the frequency of minor traumatic injuries is so high in the general population,[73] it would never be possible to establish this relationship with any degree of medical probability in any individual case.

Psychological Stress and Multiple Sclerosis

The effect of psychological stress on either MS onset or MS exacerbation is more challenging to evaluate than the effect of physical trauma. In large part this is due to the lack of a clear biological plausibility for the proposed relationship, although, in the future, such a plausible model may well be developed. For example, there are known interactions between stress and the immune system that may well turn out to fit into such model. These potentially important interactions include the influence of the immune system on the distribution of T-cell subsets, the association of a disordered hypothalamic-pituitary-adrenal axis and MS, and/or the influence of stress-induced heat shock proteins on the disease pathogenesis.[17,19,20,64,65,74] However, several other factors, in addition to the lack of a plausible model, have also hampered research in this area.

First, there has been no consistent or agreed-upon measure of stress. This is not to suggest that some valid and reliable instruments do not exist. Rather, it is to suggest that authors in this field typically use different (i.e., individualized) instruments with different definitions of stress and different measures of severity. For example, in four of the more recent studies in this area,[2,3,9,51] multiple different instruments were used to assess stress, including self-report diaries, the life events and difficulties schedule (LEDS), a modified Holmes and Rahe social readjustment rating scale (SRRS), a hassles scale, and a profile of mood states. With such a diversity of analytic methods, cross-trial comparisons are often difficult, if not impossible.

Second, as discussed in connection with the possible relationship between MS and physical trauma, it seems likely that any relationship between psychological stress and MS will be different for different types and different degrees life stress, and this lack of uniformity complicates interpretation of the existing data. This is of particular concern in an area such as stress, where the possible variations are so numerous. For example, stress can be acute and self-limited, chronic and long-lasting, or somewhere in between. It can range in severity from a minor disruption of a person's life to a life-threatening or psychologically traumatic event.

Third, there is considerable variability in the actual impact that apparently similar life events (e.g., divorce, loss of employment, or the death of a loved one) have on different individuals. Fourth, there are concerns about the retrospective interview, a technique often used by studies in this area. These interviews, in which subjects are asked to remember and report on life events that preceded MS onset or an MS exacerbation, are prone to recall bias, even when the information is collected or completed close to, but not actually prior to, an event. As a consequence, there is a need to obtain truly prospective data in this area if an association between these life events and MS is to be confidently established.

Finally, there is a notion that there should be some evidence of a dose-response relationship between stress and MS (i.e., if a little stress is bad, then a lot of stress should be worse). This is certainly true in many, if not most, clinical conditions, where increasing the dose of exposure increases the likelihood of producing disease. For example, subdural hematomas are more likely to follow a head injury resulting in unconsciousness than a light tap on the head; high levels of ionizing radiation exposure are more likely to result in illness than a single dental X-ray; massive exposure to a pathogen is more likely to result in sickness than minimal exposure; and so forth. Although some authors have argued to the contrary,[51] this is a particularly important consideration in an area such as the relationship of stress to MS because the lack of a dose-response relationship (in the absence of a plausible model to explain such a finding) would seem to raise serious questions about the reliability of the study results. Certainly, if a dose-response relationship is absent (and there is no plausible model to explain its absence), the epidemiological evidence of an association would need to be both consistent and overwhelming.

Perhaps, as a consequence of difficulties such as these, the experience in the different controlled trials has been mixed. Thus, early controlled trials tended not to find a significant relationship between MS and stress,[5,62,63] whereas some of the more recent trials have reported positive associations.[2,3,9,21,25,52,77,78] Thus, for example, in 1982, Warren and colleagues[77] studied 100 MS patients and 100 matched controls. They interviewed both patients and controls about various life events that might or might not have occurred during the 2 years prior to disease onset. Using part of the Holmes and Rahe scale for stressful life events, these authors reported that 79% of the MS patients compared to only 54% of the controls had experienced "more unwanted stress than usual" in the 2-year study period ($p < .001$). They also found that patients had experienced three times as many stressful life events as controls[59] during the 2-year period.

In 1988, Franklin et al.[21] prospectively studied the relationship between exacerbations of MS and "stressful life events" (SREs) determined from the Psychiatric Epidemiology Research Interview. Fifty-five patients completed the study in which these interviews were administered at consecutive 4-month intervals until an exacerbation occurred. Twenty-five patients had exacerbations during an average of 20 months of follow-up. These 25 patients did not have significantly more SREs in the 6 months prior to an exacerbation (20.2 events) than the 30 control patients (17.2 events) during a comparable period of time. Exposure to "extreme events," by contrast, was marginally higher in the cases compared to the controls ($p < .05$). Thus, although this study provides only marginal evidence of an association between extreme stress and MS attacks, the findings suggest a possible dose-response relationship.

In 1989, Grant and coworkers[25] reported the results of a study of 39 MS patients and 40 matched controls. Both patients and controls were evaluated on the LEDS. The authors reported that in the 6 months prior to MS onset, 62% of the patients and only 15% of controls had experienced "severely threatening events" as defined by the LEDS ($p < .001$). This study may well suffer from recall bias but, again, it suggests a dose-response relationship.

In 1991, Warren and coworkers[78] interviewed 95 pairs of MS patients who were either in exacerbation or in remission using the General Health Questionnaire to measure emotional stress (a score of ≥5 on this scale defined emotional stress). These authors found that in the 3 months preceding an exacerbation, 56.8% of the patients had experienced intense, emotionally stressful events compared to only 28.4% of the patients who were in remission at the time of the interview ($p < .001$). This study is also prone to recall bias but suggests a dose-response relationship.

In 1993, Nisipeanu and Korczyn[54] reported on their experience during the 1991 Persian Gulf War, which was a period of extreme stress for the inhabitants of Israel. Among 32 MS patients (entered into a therapeutic trial), 3 experienced an exacerbation either in the 2 months of the war or in the 2 months thereafter. The calculated attack rate during this period was significantly lower ($p < .01$) than the prewar (also pretherapeutic trial) attack rate. However, the very brief time of observation, the small number of subjects studied, and, most importantly, the well-documented tendency for MS attack rates to drop spontaneously following entry into a therapeutic trial[62–64] raise important concerns about the validity of these findings. Nevertheless, the apparent absence of any dose-response relationship in this study is notable.

In 1997, Sibley[70] reported the final results of a prospective evaluation of life events preceding an exacerbation in 170 MS patients, determined as part of the previously described monthly questionnaire.[6,70,71] Analysis of the data indicated a marginally significant ($p < .02$) association between job and/or marital stress with the subsequent occurrence of MS exacerbation but no association with the death or serious illness of a close family member. Again, although this study provides some marginal evidence for an association between antecedent stress and MS exacerbations, the lack of a dose-response relationship is notable.

In 2000, Mohr and coworkers[51] published a prospective study of the relationship between psychological stress and new brain lesions found on MRI. These authors reported that following conflicts and disruption in routine (but not following major negative events, positive events, or daily hassles), there was an increase in the number of new MRI lesions after an 8-week lag ($p < .001$) but not after lags of 0, 4, or 12 weeks. Clearly, the use of MRI to identify disease activity in a prospective study represents an important advance in this area of inquiry. Nevertheless, there are concerns about this study, many of which relate to its preliminary nature. Thus, the period of 8 weeks was not an a priori prediction made by the authors based on theoretical considerations. Rather, this was an observation made after the fact. Also of note in this study are both the clear lack of a dose-response relationship, with major stressful events having no impact on MRI activity, and the lack of any clinical accompaniment to the reported MRI change. Importantly, however, these different observations (the 8-week lag and the lack of a dose-response relationship) will now become the a priori predictions in a new study that is currently underway; thus, each can be tested directly. Of course, these kinds of a priori predictions pose certain potential problems as well. For example, if the new study were to demonstrate an MRI effect at 4 or 12 weeks, or if there were an MRI effect from severely stressful events, the new evidence would have to be viewed as inconsistent with the old and, therefore, unconvincing.

In a 2003 study of the relationship between stress and MS, Buljevac et al.[9] identified 110 eligible patients, 37 of whom chose not to take part in the study because of the intense nature of the follow-up and another 13 of whom dropped out during the study. Thus, only 60 patients (55%) completed the trial. The authors collected weekly diaries on a variety of stressful events ranging from "stress related to a holiday" to "death of [a] close family member," excluding 48/505 (9.5%) of the events, which were thought to be "caused by multiple sclerosis itself." These authors reported that patients with stressful events in the preceding 4 weeks were more likely to experience a first or second exacerbation than patients without such events ($p = .01–.02$). No analysis of the relationship of stress severity to exacerbation is provided, although the authors note that there was no difference between the effect of a single event compared to multiple events in the prior 4 weeks. There are several sources of potential bias in these data. First, even though the patient diaries were filled out on Sunday each week, there is a substantial possibility of recall bias. For example, if an attack began prior to the Sunday assessment, it seems likely that patients, knowing the research hypothesis being tested, would report more stress in the previous week than if they had been symptom free during the prior week. In addition, the number of dropouts and excluded events might bias the findings. Most importantly, however, the 4-week (or shorter) lag between the stress and the clinical effect doesn't seem to mesh well with the study results of Mohr et al.,[51] which reported a 4- to 8-week lag between the stress and the measurable effect on gadolinium-enhanced MRI.

Also in 2003, Ackerman and colleagues[3] reported the results of a study of the relationship between stress and MS exacerbation in 50 patients (all women) followed for up to 1 year. Similar to the study of Buljevac et al.,[9] subjects completed a weekly questionnaire regarding life events, which may or may not have occurred in the previous week, and events were classified on a 4-point scale as either severe (levels 1 or 2) or nonsevere (levels 3 or 4). Again, events "potentially related to MS disease activity (e.g., losing a job following an MS attack) were excluded from analysis." The number of such excluded events is not clear from the publication but, in a preliminary analysis of the first 23 subjects from this trial,[2] 63% of severe events and 26% of total events were excluded.[23] These authors report that the risk of MS exacerbation in the 6 weeks following level 1 to 3 life events is greater compared to the risk with level 4 events ($p < .05$), but they found no difference in this association between severe and nonsevere events. Interestingly, no comparison seems to have been made between patients with and without any events. These authors also report that the density of life events (i.e., the number of events per week) was "positively correlated with the proportion of weeks ill with MS-exacerbations" ($p < .05$). Clearly, this trial has a substantial risk of bias arising from the possibility of recall bias, the exclusion of such a large proportion of life events, and the failure to compare the findings in patients with and without any life events in the preceding 6 weeks. More importantly, however, as discussed earlier, even the reported results from this trial do not seem to mesh well with those from earlier reports. Thus, the fact that both severe and nonsevere events are associated with MS exacerbations is at odds with the report of Mohr et al.,[51] and the finding that event density is associated with MS attacks is at odds with the findings of Buljevac et al.[9] Also, the 6-week (or shorter) lag between the life event and subsequent clinical event is probably inconsistent with the 4- to 8-week lag reported by Mohr et al.

In summary, although there is some evidence both for and against an association between antecedent stress and the onset or exacerbation of MS, the majority of the recent evidence tends to favor a relationship of stress and MS exacerbation rather than MS onset. However, even the recent data on the relationship between stress and MS exacerbation are inconclusive and apparently in conflict with respect to both the effect of the dose and the timing of the relationship. These apparent conflicts will need to be sorted out by future research, particularly in studies employing MRI as an objective measure of disease activity, before confidence can be placed in the relationship. Moreover, the strength of the favorable evidence (as it exists at present) must be tempered by the lack of a plausible biological model, by the lack of a uniform definition of stress or method of measurement, by the possibility of substantial recall bias from retrospectively acquired data, by the apparent inconsistency of the relationship among study findings, by the lack of any consistent dose-response relationship, and by the lack of conclusive prospective data. Thus, although a relationship between antecedent stress and MS is possible, there are insufficient data, at the present time, to establish such a relationship with any degree of reasonable medical probability.

REFERENCES

1. Ackerman KD: Relationship between multiple sclerosis exacerbations and stress. Psychosom Med 66:288–289, 2004.
2. Ackerman KD, Heyman R, Rabin BS, et al: Stressful life events precede exacerbations of multiple sclerosis. Psychosom Med 64:916–920, 2002.
3. Ackerman KD, Stover A, Heyman R, et al: Relationship of cardiovascular reactivity, stressful life events, and multiple sclerosis disease activity. Brain Behav Immun 17: 141–151, 2003.
4. Alter M, Speer J: Clinical evaluation of possible etiologic factors in multiple sclerosis. Neurology 18:109–115, 1968.
5. Antonovsky A, Leibowitz U, Medalie JM, et al: Reappraisal of possible etiologic factors in multiple sclerosis. Am J Public Health 58:836–848, 1968.
6. Bamford CR, Sibley WA, Thies C, Laguna JF, Smith MS, Clark K: Trauma as an aggravating factor in multiple sclerosis. Neurology 31:1229–1234, 1981.
7. Barnes D, Munro P, Youl B, et al: The longstanding MS lesion. Brain 114:1271–1280, 1990.
8. Brain R, Wilkinson M: The association of cervical spondylosis and disseminated sclerosis. Brain 80:456–478, 1957.
9. Buljevac D, Hop WCJ, Reedeker W, et al: Self reported stressful life events and exacerbations in multiple sclerosis: prospective study. Br Med J 327:646–651, 2003.
10. Charcot JM: Lectures on the Diseases of the Nervous System. London, New Sydenham Society. 1879, pp 157–222.
11. Chaudhuri MD, Behan PO: The relationship of multiple sclerosis to physical trauma and psychological stress: Report of the therapeutics and technology assessment subcommittee. Neurology 54:1393, 2000.
12. Chaudhuri MD, Behan PO: Acute cervical hyperextension-hyperflexion injury may precipitate and/or exacerbate symptomatic multiple sclerosis. Eur J Neurol 8:659–664, 2001.
13. Christie B: Multiple sclerosis linked with trauma in a court case. Br Med J 313:1228, 1996.
14. Cohen J: Statistical Power Analysis for the Behavioral Sciences, 2nd ed. Hillsdale, NJ, Erlbaum, 1988.
15. Dana CL: Multiple sclerosis and the methods of ecology. Res Pub Assoc Nerv Ment Dis 2:43–48, 1922.
16. Ebers GC: Multiple sclerosis: New insights from old tools. Mayo Clin Proc 68:711–712, 1993.
17. Fassbender K, Schmidt R, Mößner R, et al: Mood disorders and dysfunction of hypothalamic-pituitary-adrenal axis in multiple sclerosis: Association with cerebral inflammation. Arch Neurol 55:66–72, 1998.
18. Filippi M, Rocca MA, Martino G, Horsfield MA, Comi G: Magnetization transfer changes in the normal appearing white matter precede the appearance of enhancing lesions in patients with multiple sclerosis. Ann Neurol 43: 809–814, 1998.
19. Foley FW, Miller AH, Traugott U, et al: Psychoimmunological dysregulation in multiple sclerosis. Psychosomatics 29:398–403, 1988.
20. Foley FW, Traugott U, LaRocca NG, et al: A prospective study of depression and immune dysregulation in multiple sclerosis. Arch Neurol 49:238–244, 1992.
21. Franklin GM, Nelson LM, Heaton RK, et al: Stress and its relationship to acute exacerbations in multiple sclerosis J Neurol Rehabil 2:7–11, 1988.
22. Goodin DS: The relationship of multiple sclerosis to physical trauma and psychological stress: Report of the therapeutics and technology assessment subcommittee. Neurology 54:1394–1395, 2000.
23. Goodin DS: Relationship between multiple sclerosis exacerbations and stress. Psychosom Med 66:287–288, 2004.
24. Goodin DS, Ebers GC, Johnson KP, et al: The relationship of multiple sclerosis to physical trauma and psychological stress: Report of the therapeutics and technology assessment subcommittee. Neurology 52:1737–1745, 1999.

25. Grant I, Brown GW, Harris T, et al: Severely threatening events and marked life difficulties preceding onset or exacerbation of multiple sclerosis. J Neurol Neurosurg Psychiatry 52:8–13, 1989.
26. Gusev E, Boiko A, Lauer K, et al: Environmental risk factors in MS: A case-control study in Moscow. Acta Neurol Scand 94:386–394, 1996.
27. Harris W: The traumatic factor in organic nervous disease. BMJ 4:955–960, 1933.
28. Hibberd PL: Use and misuse of statistics for epidemiological studies of multiple sclerosis. Ann Neurol 36(S2): S218–S230, 1994.
29. Hoffmann J: Die multiple Sklerose des Centralnervensystems Deutsh Zts Nervenheilk 21:1–27, 1902.
30. IFNB MS Study Group: Interferon-beta-1b is effective in relapsing-remitting multiple sclerosis: Clinical results of a randomized double blind, placebo-controlled trial. Neurology 43:655–661, 1993.
31. Jacobs LD, Cookfair DL, Rudick RA, et al: Intramuscular interferon beta-1a for disease progression in relapsing multiple sclerosis. Ann Neurol 39:285–294, 1996.
32. Jellnick EH: Trauma and multiple sclerosis. Lancet 343: 1053–1054, 1994.
33. Johnson KP, Brooks BR, Cohen JA, et al: Copolymer I reduces relapse rate and improves disability in relapsing-remitting multiple sclerosis. Neurology 45:1268–1276, 1995.
34. Kelly R: Clinical aspects of multiple sclerosis. In: Vinken PJ, Bruyn GW, Koestier C (eds): Handbook of Clinical Neurology, vol 47. Amsterdam, Elsevier, 1985, pp 49–78.
35. Kermode AG, Thompson AJ, Tofts PS, et al: Onset and duration of the blood–brain barrier breakdown in multiple sclerosis. Neurology 40(suppl 1):377, 1990.
36. Keschner M: The effect of injuries and illness on the course of multiple sclerosis. Res Pub Assoc Nerv Ment Dis 28:533–547, 1950.
37. Klausner I: Ein Beitrag zur Aetiologie der multiplen Sklerose Arch Psychiatry Nervenk 34:841–868, 1901.
38. Knobler RL, Marini JC, Goldowitz D, Lublin FD: Distribution of the blood–brain barrier in heterotopic brain transplants and its relationship to the lesions of EAE. J Neuropathol Exp Neurol 51:36–39, 1992.
39. Kurland LT: Trauma and multiple sclerosis. Ann Neurol 36:S33–S37, 1994.
40. Kurland LT, Rodriguez M, O'Brien PC, Sibley WA: Physical trauma and multiple sclerosis. Neurology 44:1362–1364, 1994.
41. Kurland LT, Westlund KB: Epidemiologic factors in the etiology and prognosis of multiple sclerosis. Ann NY Acad Sci 58:682–701, 1954.
42. Lampert P, Carpenter S: Electron microscopic studies on the vascular permeability and the mechanism of demyelination in experimental allergic encephalomyelitis. J Neuropathol Exp Neurol 24:11–14, 1965.
43. Lauer K: Physical trauma and multiple sclerosis. Neurology 44:1360, 1994.
44. Lehrer GM: The relationship of multiple sclerosis to physical trauma and psychological stress: Report of the therapeutics and technology assessment subcommittee. Neurology 54:1393–1394, 2000.
45. Mathews W: Some aspects of the natural history. Pathophysiology. In: Mathews W (ed): McAlpine's Multiple Sclerosis, 2nd ed. Edinburgh, Churchill Livingstone, 1991.
46. McAlpine D: The problem of disseminated sclerosis. Brain 69:233–250, 1946.
47. McAlpine D, Compston, N: Some aspects of the natural history of disseminated sclerosis. Q J Med 21:135–167, 1952.
48. McAlpine D, Lumsden CE, Acheson ED: Multiple Sclerosis: A New Appraisal. Baltimore, Williams & Wilkins, 1965.
49. Mendel K: Tabes und multiple Sklerose in ihren Beziehungen zum Trauma Neurol Ctrbl 16:140–141, 1897.
50. Miller H: Trauma and multiple sclerosis. Lancet 1:848–850, 1964.
51. Mohr DC, Goodkin DE, Bacchetti P, et al: Psychological stress and the subsequent appearance of new brain lesions in MS. Neurology 55:55–61, 2000.
52. Mohr DC, Hart SL, Julian L, et al: Association between stressful life events and exacerbation in multiple sclerosis: A meta-analysis. Br Med J 328:731–735, 2004.
53. Nesbit GM, Forbes GS, Scheithauer BW, Okazzaki H, Rodriguez M: Multiple sclerosis: Histopathologic and MR and/or CT correlation in 37 cases at biopsy and three cases at autopsy. Neuroradiology 180:467–474, 1991.
54. Nisipeanu P, Korczyn AD: Psychological stress as a risk factor for exacerbation in multiple sclerosis. Neurology 43:1311–1312, 1993.
55. Oppenheimer DR: The cervical cord in multiple sclerosis. Neuropathol Appl Neurobiol 4:151–162, 1978.
56. Poser CM: A prospective study of physical trauma and multiple sclerosis. J Neurol Neurosurg Psychiatry 55:524, 1992.
57. Poser CM: The pathogenesis of multiple sclerosis: Additional considerations. J Neurol Sci 115(suppl):S3–S15, 1993.
58. Poser CM: The role of the blood–brain barrier in the pathogenesis of multiple sclerosis. In: Salvati S (ed): A Multidisciplinary Approach to Myelin Diseases II. New York, Plenum Press, 1994.
59. Poser CM: The role of trauma in the pathogenesis of multiple sclerosis: A review. Clin Neurol Neurosurg 96:103–110, 1994.
60. Poser CM: Physical trauma and multiple sclerosis. Neurology 44:1360–1362, 1994.
61. Poser CM: The relationship of multiple sclerosis to physical trauma and psychological stress: Report of the therapeutics and technology assessment subcommittee. Neurology 54:1393, 2000.
62. Pratt RTC: An investigation of the psychiatric aspects of disseminated sclerosis. J Neurol Neurosurg Psychiatry 14:326–336, 1951.
63. Rabins PV, Brooks BR, O'Donnell, et al: Structural brain correlates of emotional disorder in multiple sclerosis. Brain 109:585–597, 1986.
64. Raine CS, Wu E, Ivanyi J, et al: Multiple sclerosis: A

protective or a pathogenic role for heat shock protein 60 in the central nervous system. Lab Invest 75:109–123, 1996.

65. Reder AT, Lowy MT, Meltzer HY, Antel JP: Dexamethasone suppression test abnormalities in multiple sclerosis: Relation to ACTH therapy. Neurology 37:849–853, 1987.
66. Ridley A, Scharira K: Influence of surgical procedures on the course of multiple sclerosis. Neurology 11:81–82, 1961.
67. Rodriguez M, Scheithauer BW, Forbes G, Kelly PJ: Oligodendrocyte injury is an early event in lesions of multiple sclerosis. Mayo Clin Proc 68:627–636, 1993.
68. Sibley WA: Risk factors in multiple sclerosis—implications for pathogenesis. In: Crescenzi GS (ed): A Multidisciplinary Approach to Myelin Diseases, NATO Advanced Research Series. New York, Plenum Press, 1988, pp 227–232.
69. Sibley WA: A prospective study of physical trauma and multiple sclerosis: A reply. J Neurol Neurosurg Psychiatry 55:524, 1992.
70. Sibley WA: Risk factors in multiple sclerosis. In: Raine CS, McFarland HF, Tourtellotte WW (eds): Multiple Sclerosis: Clinical and Pathogenic Basis. London, Chapman and Hall, 1997, pp 141–148.
71. Sibley WA, Bamford CR, Clark K, Smith MS, Laguna JF: A prospective study of physical trauma and multiple sclerosis. J Neurol Neurosurg Psychiatry 54:584–589, 1991.
72. Siva A, Radhakrishnan K, Kurland LT, O'Brien PC, Swanson JW, Rodriguez M: Trauma and multiple sclerosis: A population-based cohort study from Olmsted County, Minnesota. Neurology 43:1878–1882, 1993.
73. U.S. Department of Human and Health Services: Types of Injuries and Impairments Due to Injuries. National Health Survey 1986. Series 10. Public Health Service (PHS) Washington, DC, 159 pp 8–26.
74. Van Nort JM: Multiple sclerosis: An altered immune response or an altered stress response. J Mol Med 74:285–296, 1996.
75. Visintainer PF: Physical trauma and multiple sclerosis. Neurology 44:1360, 1994.
76. Von Hoesslin R: Uber multiple Sklerose. Munich: JF Lehmans Verlag, 1934, pp 68–74.
77. Warren S, Greenhill S, Warren KG: Emotional stress and the development of multiple sclerosis: Case-control evidence of a relationship. J Chronic Dis 35:821–831, 1982.
78. Warren W, Warren, KG, Cockerill R: Emotional stress and coping in multiple sclerosis (MS) exacerbations. J Psychosom Res 35:37–47, 1991.
79. Waxman SG: Demyelination in spinal cord injury and multiple sclerosis: What can we do to enhance functional recovery? J Neurotrauma 9:S105–S117, 1992.
80. Weintraub MI: Trauma and multiple sclerosis: Medicolegal implications. Dev Med Child Neurol 30:407–408, 1988.
81. Wekerle SG: T-cell autoimmunity in the central nervous system. Intervirology 35:95–100, 1993.

Chapter 38
The Neurologist as Expert Witness

MICHAEL I. WEINTRAUB

Gentlemen of the jury, there are three kinds of liars: the common liar, the damned liar, and the scientific expert.

Judge William L. Foster

There is a witness everywhere.

Thomas Fuller (1654–1734)
Gnomoligia 1732, No. 4, 886

Thou shalt not bear false witness against thy neighbor.

Exodus 20:16

The American judicial system is sophisticated and complex. Thus, ideally, the courtroom is the arena to determine justice and provide compensation. It is essentially fault-based and adversarial. Injured claimants may bring a lawsuit in order to obtain financial compensation in state or federal courts. Both types of courts rely upon information and opinions provided by expert witness testimony to determine causality, permanence, disability, and so on. These opinions are offered on behalf of both plaintiffs and defendants, and the medical expert plays an indispensable role in determining the outcome of jury claims. Since medical expert testimony assumes such a central position, it is not surprising that testimonial abuse exists and that medical expertise is now a cottage industry. All medical societies have articulated positions and guidelines on the proper behavior and compensation of experts, and even the Supreme Court has attempted to address the issue of flawed and unreliable testimony in the *Daubert* decision.[13] Clarity and consistency are sought, and standards for credibility and reliability of testimony are being developed.[24] This chapter will explore the current status of expert witness testimony as well as the peer review process as it is evolving in this litigious society. The law is in flux and affects the neurologist.

Definition

The *Oxford English Dictionary* defines *expert* as "a person who has gained skill from experience" and "one whose special knowledge and skills causes him to be regarded as an authority." This definition is also incorporated in Federal Rule of Evidence (FRE) 702.[15] Although the FREs do not bind state courts, they have considerable influence and therefore the courts usually adopt similar rulings. Rule 702 specifically authorizes trial courts to admit relevant scientific testimony if it will assist judges or juries to "understand the evidence or to determine a fact in issue."

What Constitutes a Medical Expert?

In many states, any licenced physician can testify as an expert witness. Thus, a medical witness/expert may be a treating physician or a physician who has been retained solely for the purpose of providing expert testimony. In either scenario, the physician is obligated to make a truthful statement under oath and must be as impartial and objective as possible. The physician also needs to be familiar with all the issues in this specific matter. While the American Academy of Neurology (AAN)[3] suggests that a physician who is serving as an expert should have actual professional knowledge and experience in the practice or specialty in which the opinion is to be given, the reality is that the Illinois Appellate Court stated in a medical malpractice litigation: "Whether the expert is qualified to testify is not dependent on whether he is a member of the same specialty or subspecialty as the defendant, but rather, whether the allegations of negligence concern matters within his knowledge and observation."[7] Physicians must be licenced and familiar with the methods, procedures, and treatments in either the defendant physician's community or a similar community. A federal appeals court was even more specific. A medical expert need not be a specialist in the area concerned nor be practicing in the same field as the defendant.[34] The fact that the physician is not a specialist in the field for which he or she is giving an opinion is of no consequence, only the weight the jury may place on it. Numerous cross-examinations are considered the best safeguard for credibility, and ultimately the jury must resolve the issues.[38] Thus, nonneurologists can testify against neurological defendants in medical malpractice cases or, alternatively, neurologists can testify in nonneurological medical matters. The AAN has specific guidelines stating that experts must be in active practice and must not devote more than 20% of their time to testimony. They also must be knowledgeable about the topic and not accept contingency fees. Despite all of the above, states are tightening qualifications for expert witnesses. A handful of states, including Florida, Louisiana, and Nevada, approved bills in the past 2 years requiring a physician expert to generally have the same specialty as the doctor against whom he or she is testifying, according to the National Conference of State Legislatures.[5]

Legal Background

The courts have expressed concern regarding the standards for the admissibility of expert testimony. In 1923, the Frye test[19] held that expert testimony, based upon a scientific technique, is "inadmissable unless the technique is generally accepted in the scientific community." This standard was adopted in all federal courts and in most state courts. However, critics felt that genuine claimants were harshly and unfairly treated by this high standard. This led to passage of the Federal Rules of Evidence FRE in 1973 allowing for liberalization of admissibility. Specifically, FRE 702 allows admission of scientific testimony if it will assist judges or juries to understand complex issues. Rule 703 permits an expert to base an opinion on facts or data "perceived by or made known at or before the hearing." Rule 704 permits an expert to offer an opinion on the "ultimate" factual issue in a case, that is, causality. Rule 705 permits an expert to state an opinion without disclosing the data on which it is based. Thus, marginal testimony might be admitted and vigorous cross-examination will either discredit it. Rule 403 empowers the court to exclude testimony if its "probative value is substantially outweighed by the danger of unfair prejudice, confusion of the issues or misleading of the jury." After these FRE were adopted, some courts continued to rule based on Frye test admissibility of scientific evidence. The majority of state and federal courts, however, concluded that the Frye test was no longer applicable and that it relied on less rigorous standards. Obviously, this led to creative theories concerning causation, *junk science*, that did not reflect mainstream science, and, ultimately *junk justice*.[21,22] It also led to a burgeoning of lawsuits and the expert witness cottage industry.[41,45] Huge verdicts led to an insurance crisis.

In an effort to resolve the conflict among the lower federal courts as to the status of the Frye test, the U.S. Supreme Court agreed to hear an appeal from a federal circuit court decision in which the Frye test was applied to exclude expert testimony regarding the significance of epidemiological studies.[13] Specifically, in 1993 the Supreme Court in *Daubert v. Merrell Dow Pharmaceuticals, Inc.* compromised the Frye decision[19] and issued a new 4-point test for admissibility of scientific evidence to ensure that the testimony is "not only relevant but reliable." This constituted a new standard. Specifically, animal studies may not be relevant or reliable when applied to human conditions. In addition, (1) testimony and opinion have been tested using the scientific method; (2) information must be peer reviewed or published; (3) information must be evaluated for error; and (4) testimony must be directly relevant to the particular case. Specifically, the Supreme Court had the benefit of amicus briefs from 13 Nobel laureates, and from the American Academy of Science and many other scientific organizations. In a unanimous opinion, the Supreme Court rejected and reversed the decision that was based on alleged culture and animal studies and concluded that Bendectine was not responsible for birth defects. They rejected the expert's opinion of a reconfigured method of collecting epidemiological data. They stated that the Frye test had been superseded. They also suggested that FRE 702 should be based on the scientific method rather than on subjective beliefs or speculation. Reliability of data was the major concern, as well as the potential rate of error of the methodology. The Court provided careful judicial instructions indicating that judges need to serve as *gatekeepers* for scientific admissibility. If judges had problems, Rule 706 allowed them to appoint their own experts and Rule 403[16] empowered them to exclude biased, flawed, or misleading testimony. Two dissenting opinions stated the concern that judges would be encouraged to become "amateur scientists." On December 1, 2000, Rule 702 of FRE[15] was amended to indicate that (1) testimony is based on scientific facts or data, (2) the testimony is the product of reliable principles and methods, and (3) the witness has applied the principles and methods reliably to the facts of the case.[42]

Daubert in Practice

As noted, judges were given new responsibilities, but there has been criticism. For example, Gatowski and coworkers conducted a survey of 400 state court judges, seeking to assess their level of "scientific literacy" with respect to the *Daubert* criteria. They found that 5% demonstrated a clear understanding of falsify ability and 4% demonstrated a clear understanding of error rate. The overall majority of responding judges (96% of 251) indicated that they had not received instructions about general scientific methods and principles. Gatowski et al. concluded that many of the judges surveyed lacked the scientific literacy required by the *Daubert* decision and were unreliable gatekeepers when it came to the interpretation of scientific knowledge.[20] While Rule 706 exists, judges have rarely used it.

Another criticism of the *Daubert* decision has come from its uneven application and inconsistent results by judges, especially in state courts, where there is no obligation or requirement that *Daubert* be applied.[24] In fact, 19 states and the District of Columbia still adhere to the Frye general acceptance standard for the admission of novel scientific evidence. Three states have rejected both Frye and *Daubert* and favor their own admissibility guidelines. Thus, scientific admissibility is still "law in flux."[24,25,27,48]

False Testimony and the Expert Witness

Ideally, all physicians acting as expert witnesses under oath are expected to speak the truth and attempt to be impartial.[44,47,48] However, litigation is adversarial, and each side (plaintiff and defendant) retains those experts that agree with its opinion. Obviously, conflicting expert testimony occurs and the trial is often reduced to a "battle of the experts."[8,46–48] Flawed expert testimony (inaccurate or false representations) is often a charge heard after a decision is rendered. The Supreme Court has long recognized that the principal safeguard against errant expert testimony is the opportunity for opposing counsel to vigorously cross-examine the witness to demonstrate bias,[18] partisanship, or financial interest.[8,9,23,29]

Can Experts Who Testify Falsely Be Held in Contempt of Court?

There has been a call to punish "those who breach the standard of care in the practice of legal medicine."[10,11,17] The two legal maneuvers specifically designed to punish experts accused of testifying falsely are civil contempt and medical malpractice. In both scenarios, the courts have denied these motions, indicating that "flawed testimony" did not obstruct the court's orderly proceedings or ability to perform its duties. Courts have also held that testimony at trials is often conflicting and that expert witnesses often have opposite opinions. They believe that punitive action would violate the "concept of witness immunity."[23,31,36] This doctrine originated hundreds of years ago in English common law,[8,9] and immunity was important to ensure that witnesses would speak freely when giving testimony. Both the U.S. Supreme Court and numerous state courts have affirmed the concept of witness immunity for reasons of public policy. Lawsuits against experts for witness malpractice have generally led to rejection.[28,31] The courts have maintained their reluctance to take punitive action against an expert who has testified falsely.

Discipline by Professional Associations

In June 2001, the Seventh U.S. Circuit Court of Appeals held that a professional society, the American Academy of Neurological Surgery (AANS), could discipline a member for improper testimony.[6] Over the previous 15 years, the AANS has reviewed complaints against 50 members for potential misconduct in expert witness testimony and has suspended or expelled 10 members.[10] Only one brought a lawsuit against the association, and the district court, the appellate court and U.S. Court of Appeals all agreed that organizations have the right to review members behavior.[2] The AAN has specifically reviewed five potential cases from the years 2000 to 2003 with no disciplinary actions taken. The Expert Witness Program of the Florida Medical Association reviews expert testimony upon request by a member.[39b] There were 12 complaints regarding plaintiff testimony in 11 cases.[5] Organizations do not prohibit their members from acting as experts, but their opinions are considered the practice of medicine, and individuals can be held accountable by professional associations, states,[3] and licencing boards. The American Medical Association (AMA) has specifically passed Resolutions 121 and 216 stating[4,39] that physicians who provide statements on health-related issues, that is, malpractice or managed care, are to be considered as practicing medicine. The court system does not require physical presence as a prerequisite for a legal relationship. This opinion is also shared by the AMA and other specialty societies. The physician's opinion is tantamount to medical practice and is therefore under the purview of peer review.[30,32,40,45,46,48] This will ensure accountability. Various academies have specific guidelines for disciplining members. (AAN, Academy of Pediatrics, etc.).[3,12] Fear of lawsuits and their cost have led many organizations, such as the American Academy of American Association of Neuromuscular and Electrodiagnostic Medicine (AANEM) and the AAN, to be cautious. While the AMA is quite proactive and is willing to report individuals to state medical licensing boards, two states licensing boards (in North Carolina, District of Columbia) have succeeded in reprimanding or revoking a physician's medical license for giving false expert testimony.[10] Several others are contemplating similar actions. Only 7 of 36 specialty organizations that were reviewed by Milunsky[33] for their disciplinary policies spelled out the consequence of censure, suspension, and expulsion of members. Only four organizations indicated reporting procedures to the National Practitioner Data Bank (NPDB). Not all discipline by a specialty medical society must be reported to the NPDB. The American Society of Plastic Surgeons was among the first organizations to indemnify officers and committee members against any actions taken against them as a result of their having served in their various capacities. The AANS has expelled one of its members for giving false expert testimony,[1,6,11b] and the American College of Radiology as well as other specialty organizations possess the machinery to undertake similar action, but it is unclear if they will react due to fear of lawsuits and legal costs. In fact, trial lawyers argue that holding medical experts accountable is a form of witness intimidation and restraint of trade that is negatively affecting the legal system.[26] Recently, an ad hoc program created a new organization called the Coalition and Center for Ethical Medical Testimony (CCEMT), which collects expert testimony and shares the names of expert witnesses and examples of what they consider unethical testimony.

Use, Review Physicians, and Managed Care

In 1974, Congress passed the Employee Retirement Income and Security Act (ERISA),[14] which has essentially shielded managed care organizations from liability for negligent treatment for coverage decisions. States have been preempted from seeking damages due to the liberal interpretation taken by managed care organizations (MCOs). Courts have struggled with interpreting ERISA, and various decisions have been difficult to reconcile. Legislative resolution is necessary, and Congress has failed to act. The U.S. Supreme Court is currently considering whether ERISA can restrict state regulations of health maintenance organizations (HMOs) and managed care. This is of vital concern to physicians since an MCO decision to deny services to a patient, based on the decision of a house physician who has no direct patient contact and claims that the treatment and/or procedures are "not medically necessary," may expose the treating physician to liability and effectively shields the MCO from liability. The cases of *Pegram*[37] and *Moran*[35] demonstrated that ERISA is not a shield against liability for negligence.

Conclusion

Neither judges nor juries can truly or accurately assess the veracity of medical expert testimony.[41–43] Thus, misleading testimony must be examined by specialty societies. The inclination of the court system to discipline experts presenting false testimony does not extend to the AMA, specialty organizations, or state medical licencing boards. It is hoped that more proactive and aggressive surveillance programs will allow for accurate testimony and reduce testimonial abuse.

REFERENCES

1. Albert T: Ruling allows discipline over expert testimony. Am Med News 44(25):13, 2001.
2. Albert T: Neurosurgeon sues specialty society over suspension. Am Med News 44 (6):17, 2001.
3. American Academy of Neurology: Qualifications and guidelines for the physician expert witness. Neurology 39:9a, 1989.
4. American Medical Association Councils on Ethical and Judicial Affairs: §9,07, Medical Testimony In: Code of Medical Ethics. Chicago, American Medical Association, 2000, pp 210–212.
5. Andrews M: Making malpractice harder to prove. New York Times, December 21, 2003, p 8.
6. Austin V: *American Association of Neurological Surgeons*. 253.F.3d 967, Seventh Circuit 2001.
7. Barton V: *Chicago and North Western Transportation Co*. 757 NE 2d 533 (ILL App 2001).
8. Beresford HR: Containing partisan medical experts. J Child Neurol 10:170–173, 1995.
9. Beresford HR: Neurology and the Law: Private Litigation and Public Policy. Philadelphia, FA Davis, 1998.
10. Berlin L: Malpractice issues in radiology: Bearing false witness. Am J Radiol 180:1515–1521, 2003.
11a. Binder RL: Liability for the psychiatrist expert witness. Am J Psychiatry 159:1819–1825, 2002.
11b. Cohen, FL: The expert medical witness in legal perspective. J Legal Medicine 25:285–209, 2004.
12. Committee on Medical Liability, American Academy of Pediatrics: Guidelines for expert witness testimony in medical malpractice litigation. Pediatrics 109:974–979, 2002.
13. Daubert V. Merrell Dow Pharmaceuticals, 509 US 579 (1993).
14. Employee Retirement Income Security Act, US Code, Title 29, Section 1140 (ERISA).
15. Federal Rules of Evidence §§702-705, Pub Law #No. 93-595, 88 STAT 1926,1975.
16. Federal Rules of Evidence, Rule 403, 88 STAT 1926 (1975).
17. Flanagan D: U.S. Supreme Court decisions, expert testimony, and implant dentistry. J Oral Implantol 28:97–98, 2002.
18. Foster WL: Expert testimony—prevalent complaints and proposed remedies. Harvard Law Rev 11:169–186, 1898.
19. *Frye v. United States*, 293 F 1013 (DC Cir 1923).
20. Gatowski SI, Dobbin SA, Richardson JT, et al: Asking the gatekeepers: A national survey of judges on judging expert evidence in a post-Daubert world. Law Hum Behav 25:433–458, 2001.
21. Hagen MA: Whores of the Court: The Fraud of Psychiatric Testimony and the Rape of American Justice. New York, Regan Books, 1997.
22. Huber PW: Galileo's Revenge—Junk Science in the Courtroom. New York, Basic Books, 1991.
23. *Jones v. Lincoln Electric Company*. 188 F 3d 709 US App. Seventh Cir. 1999.
24. Kassirer JP, Cecil JS: Inconsistency in evidentiary standards for medical testimony. JAMA 288:1382–1387, 2002.
25. Kaufman HH: The expert witness: Neither Frye nor Daubert solved the problem: What can be done? Sci Justice 41:7–20, 2002.
26. Kleinman AY: When the medical expert is not an expert. Westchester Physician 15:1–10, 2003.

27. Kulich RJ, Driscoll J, Prescott JC, et al: The Daubert standard, a primer for pain specialists. Pain Med 4:75–80, 2003.
28. *LLMD of Michigan v. Jackson Cross Co.*, 740 A 2d 186 Pa 1999.
29. Matson JV: Effective Expert Witnessing: A Handbook for Technical Professionals. Chelsea, MI, Lewis, 1990.
30. McAbee GN: Peer review of medical expert witnesses. J Child Neurol 9:216–217, 1994.
31. McDowell CM: Authorizing the expert witness to assassinate character for profit: A re-examination of the testimonial immunity of the expert witness. Univ Memphis Law Rev 28:239–269, 1997.
32. McGraw WR, Taylor S: Judicial overview of expert testimony for independent medical examiners: A perspective from the bench. Disability Med 2:17–20, 2002.
33. Milunsky A: Lies, damned lies and medical experts: The abrogation of responsibility by specialty organizations and a call for action. J Child Neurol 18:413–419, 2003.
34. *Mitchell v. United States*, 141 F 3d 8 (US App. First Cir. 1980).
35. *Moran v. Rush Prudential HMO, Inc.* 230 F. 3d 959 (Seventh Cir. 2000), US 150 L.Ed. 2d, 749 (2001).
36. Norton ML: The physician expert witness and the U.S. Supreme Court—an epidemiologic approach. Med Law 21:435–449, 2002.
37. *Pegram v. Herdrich*, 530 U.S. 211 (2000).
38. *Preston v. Simmons*, 747 M.E. 2d, 1059 ILL App 2001.
39a. Report 18 of the Board of Trustees of the American Medical Association (1–98), Executive Summary: Expert Witness Testimony 7/5/02; 1–7.
39b. Sagsveen, M: American Academy of Neurology Policy on Expert Medical Testimony. Neurology 63:1555–1556, 2004.
40. Shields WD: Peer review of expert medical-legal testimony: A proposal for child neurology. J Child Neurol 7:237–239, 1992.
41. Weinstein JB: Improving expert testimony. Univer Richmond Law Rev 20:473–494, 1986.
42. Weinstein JB: The effect of Daubert on the work of federal trial judges. Shepard's Expert Sci Evidence 2:1–9, 1994.
43. Weinstein JB: Expert witness testimony: A trial judge's perspective. In: Weintraub MI (ed): Medical-legal issues facing neurologists. Neurol Clin North Am 17:355–362, 1997.
44. Weintraub MI: Expert witness testimony: A time for self-regulation. Neurology 45:855–858, 1995.
45. Weintraub MI: Physicians and managed care. N Engl J Med 332:1173–1174, 1995.
46. Weintraub MI: Expert witness under scrutiny. Lancet 349:1776, 1997.
47. Weintraub MI: Expert witness testimony: An update. Neurol Clin 17:363–369, 1999.
48. Weintraub MI: Standards for medical expert testimony. JAMA 88:2971–2972, 2002.

Part VIII

Iatrogenic Trauma

Chapter 39
Complications of Lumbar Puncture

RANDOLPH W. EVANS

Although neurologists often evaluate the surgical complications of other physicians, they are responsible for complications of the lumbar puncture, the quintessential neurological procedure. Headache is the most common complication, usually lasting for 1 week or less, occurring in up to 40% of patients after lumbar puncture. Other complications, including headaches lasting for 8 days to 1 year, cranial neuropathies, prolonged backache, nerve root injury, and meningitis, are rare, following perhaps 0.3% of lumbar punctures.[163] This chapter reviews historical aspects and the following complications of lumbar puncture: cerebral and spinal herniation, postdural puncture headache, cranial neuropathies, nerve root irritation, low back pain, stylet associated problems, infections, and bleeding complications (Table 39.1).

Table 39.1. Complications of Lumbar Puncture

Uncal or tonsillar herniation
Reversible tonsillar descent
Spinal coning in patients with rostral subarachnoid block
Postdural puncture headache
Cranial neuropathies
Nerve root irritation, herniation, and transection
Low back pain
Implantation of epidermal tumors
Infections
Bleeding complications
Intracranial bleeding
Traumatic lumbar puncture
Spinal hematomas
Other complications
Vasovagal syncope
Cardiac arrest
Seizures
Incorrect lab analysis of cerebrospinal fluid

Historical Aspects

Fluid or Ether?

Before the lumbar puncture procedure could be developed, an understanding of cerebrospinal fluid (CSF) circulation was necessary. The first written record of the CSF, in the Edwin Smith Surgical Papyrus, is in association with head injury from about seventeenth century B.C. Egypt. In the fifth century B.C., Hippocrates reported the presence of fluid around the brain that he believed was pathological. Galen (129–199 A.D.) described the cerebral ventricles, which he concluded were filled with *pneuma*, a gaseous substance. This misconception, which persisted until the early nineteenth century, arose because of the dissection technique in which decapitation resulted in draining out of CSF before the ventricular system was examined.[64]

A number of investigators were responsible for discovering the presence and circulation of the CSF. Valsalva was the first to describe fluid around the spinal cord in 1692.[126] The demonstration by Domeneco Cotugno (1735–1822) in 1764 of the CSF around the brain and spinal cord and in the ventricles received little attention (in the same publication, he described the anatomical basis of sciatica).[31] In 1783, Alexander Monro (1733–1817) rediscovered the open foramina between the lateral and third ventricles (previously described by Leonardo da Vinci in 1503) that are named after him.[64,101] Cotugno's findings were rediscovered in 1825 by François Magendie (1783–1855), who coined the term translated as CSF: *liquide céphalo-rachidien or cérébro-spinal*.[50] Magendie also described the outflow of fluid from the midline foramen of the fourth ventricle and, in 1865, Hubert von Luschka (1820–1875) wrote a detailed description of the fourth ventricle and the lateral foramina.[89] In 1872, Quincke injected red sulfide of mercury into various sites of the ventricles and subarachnoid spaces of living and dead animals, demonstrating the unidirectional flow from the ventricles and the connection between the cerebral and spinal subarachnoid spaces.[115]

The First Lumbar Puncture

In May 1891, Walter Essex Wynter (1860–1945), medical registrar at the Middlesex Hospital in London, reported the cases of four children: two in whom the skin and the theca were incised at L1 or L2 and two in whom the lamina was removed. A drainage tube was inserted in the subarachnoid space to remove CSF in the treatment of tubercular meningitis.[164] Wynter described the first procedure performed in February 1889: "No anaesthetic was needed; the child was supported in a sitting posture, a tiny incision was made in the skin beside the spine of the second lumbar vertebra, and a Southey's tube and trocar inserted till the point impinged against the lamina; the point was then directed slightly downwards and was pushed though the ligamentum subflavum and theca with an inclination towards the middle line. Clear fluid at once welled up into the tube on withdrawing the trocar, a fine indiarubber tube was arranged for continuous drainage, and the child put back to bed."

Heinrich Quincke (1842–1922), the chair of medicine at Kiel, performed the first percutaneous lumbar puncture in December 1890 on a 1¾-year-old boy (who was febrile and comatose, with a stiff neck and pneumonia), which he reported in April 1891 to the Tenth Congress of Internal Medicine at Wiesbaden: "Therefore I punctured the subarachnoidal sac in the lumbar area, passing a very fine cannula 2 cm deep between the third and fourth spinal arches, and drop by drop I drained a few cubic centimeters of watery-clear fluid . . . one could see clearly increases [in flow] with expiration and decreases with inspiration."[117] During a third lumbar puncture on the child, for the first time ever, he measured the opening pressure in a person: "The cannula was connected immediately to a narrow rectangular glass pipe with rubber tubing. With the patient in the horizontal partially prone position, the pressure at the opening was 13–15 cm water (equal to 10–11 mm mercury). With crying it was 20, decreased rapidly again to 15. . . ." He considered the opening pressure normal. The child subsequently recovered completely. On April 3, 1891, he performed the first percutaneous lumbar puncture on an adult: a 25-year-old man with a 17-month history of headaches and dizziness with findings of bilateral papilledema, bilateral eye muscle paresis, and ataxic gait. The opening pressure was 50 cm water.

Later, in September 1891, Quincke reported additional cases of five adults and five children and described his technique:

> The procedure is based on the anatomical and experimentally demonstrated facts that the cerebral and spinal subarachnoid spaces communicate with each other and with the cerebral ventricles. In adults the spinal cord extends only to the third lumbar vertebra, in children only to the second. The point of a puncture cannula introduced through the third or fourth lumbar intervertebral space therefore does not reach the spinal cord but ends up among the nerve roots of the cauda equina floating in the cerebrospinal fluid. I originally feared that the needle point might cause some injury to the cauda, but in this I was mistaken. . . . The appropriate diameter of the hollow needles varies from 0.6 to 1.2 mm. The wider needles were fitted with a stylet. . . . After removal of the stylet a conical adapter is fitted to the cannula and connected via a piece of rubber tubing to a glass tube that reads the pressure. The glass tube is then lowered, the required amount of fluid is collected, the cannula is removed and the site of the puncture covered with cotton and iodoform collodion. . . . The patient must rest in bed for 24 hours.[116]

This new procedure was quickly adopted. In an 1895 address before the New York Neurological Society, Jacoby stated: "When in 1891, . . . Quincke, . . . spoke of a method of withdrawing fluid . . . , it was little thought that within four years this procedure, which can not but be characterized as simple, would take its place among the recognized diagnostic methods in medicine, and possibly form the stepping-stone to local treatment of the brain and cord."[70]

Complications

With this widespread use of lumbar puncture, reports of complications appeared. In 1896, Fürbringer reported four deaths attributed to the procedure: one patient with a cerebellar abscess, one with a frontal tumor, and two with cerebellar tumors.[56] Also in 1896, Wentworth described headache caused by lumbar puncture in the presence of cerebral tumor,[161] and Jennings reported a needle breaking deep in the tissues of the back.[74]

The first description that I can find of postdural puncture headache is Bier's cases from 1898, reported in 1899.[12] With this article, August Bier (1861–1949), a colleague of Quincke at Kiel, was also the first to report the technique of spinal anesthesia. (Among other accomplishments, Bier devised the Bier regional block and invented the steel helmet for German troops during World War I.) He described the successful use of this spinal anesthesia with cocaine for one ischial and five lower extremity operations. Three of the six patients developed headache afterward. To investigate possible side effects of the procedure, Bier decided to have the procedure performed on himself by his assistant, Dr. Hildebrandt. After a successful lumbar puncture, the syringe did not fit the needle properly and the cocaine escaped. Immediately afterward Bier successfully performed spinal anesthesia on his assistant. Bier describes subsequent events:

> After these experiments on our own bodies we both went to dinner without any physical complaints. We drank wine and smoked several cigars. . . . [T]he next morning . . . I noticed a slight headache which increased during the course of the day. . . . Furthermore, I had the sensation of a very strong pressure in my head and felt slightly dizzy when I arose quickly from my chair. All these symptoms disappeared as soon as I lay down horizontally, but they returned when I arose. . . . I had to go to bed, and I stayed in bed for nine days, since all the described symptoms returned whenever I tried to arise. As soon as I lay down horizontally, however, I felt perfectly well.[48]

Hildebrandt also had postural headaches lasting for a few days. Bier explained the symptoms as follows: "I believe that the headaches and vomiting . . . must be viewed as the results of circulatory disturbances (hyperemia or anemia) in the central nervous system. Furthermore, the escape of a considerable amount of cerebrospinal fluid could bring about such effects." To prevent the headaches, Bier recommended strict bed rest.

In 1917, Dana reported that postdural puncture headaches were more common in young adults and women and that some patients did better if allowed to get up promptly after the procedure.[33] MacRobert, in 1918, argued that the headache results from the dural puncture, where "we have punctured a fibrous sac distended with fluid-made a hole in a stiff membrane that has no contractile tissue. . . . The spinal fluid is always under some pressure in its sac, so what is to prevent a continuous leakage into the epidural space in the spinal canal[?] . . . At the base of the brain this pad [of CSF] becomes a veritable cushion or water-bed. When the fluid leaks away through a hole in the lower end of this sac, the base of the brain loses its supporting fluid cushion."[93a] MacRobert also concluded that the headache resolves when the dural puncture hole heals, usually within a week.

Pappenheim, in 1925, described the dangers of lumbar puncture including the following: occasional cases of herniation in the presence of a brain tumor; nerve root irritation and low back pain; unilateral and bilateral abducens palsy, oculomotor palsy, and auditory disturbances; and headache.[110] Although he recommended bed rest for 24 hours afterward, he noted that some patients could get up immediately without developing a headache.

In 1926 Greene reported that a 22 G needle with a rounded, tapering, and sharp point caused less leakage than a standard 19 G needle with a cutting edge in an experiment with a dural sac from a cadaver.[59] He argued that the smaller blunt-tipped needle separated rather than cut the dural fibers, which are arranged in a longitudinal direction. He then performed a series of 215 consecutive lumbar punctures, nearly all in the office, using a 22 G blunt-tipped needle; only two patients developed headaches. Many of the patients went back to work without lying down. In 1930, Labat recommended that spinal anesthesia be performed with the bevel of the needle east or west of the middle line of the back, that is, parallel to the longitudinal dural fibers.[83]

Jacobaeus and Frumerie, in 1923, reported that intraspinal injection of 35 to 90 cc normal saline relieved postdural puncture headache.[69] In 1925, Alpers recommended treatment of less severe postdural puncture headaches with pituitary extract intramuscularly and intravenous saline for severe headaches.[4] Gormley, in 1960, invented the lumbar epidural blood patch and described relief of the postdural puncture headaches of seven patients (including himself when he developed a headache after a myelogram).[58] For an in-depth review of the history of post–lumbar puncture headaches and the epidural blood patch, see Harrington.[60]

Herniation Due to Lumbar Puncture

Brain Masses

Even in the presence of a brain neoplasm, abscess, or hematoma, uncal or tonsillar herniation leading to neurological deterioration or death is quite uncommon. When a complication occurs, it can be difficult to determine whether the lumbar puncture was responsible if deterioration is not immediate or if the procedure is performed on an obtunded or comatose patient who might have gotten worse or died in a short time anyway.[153]

Lubic and Marotta reported a total of 447 lumbar punctures performed on 401 patients with a variety of primary and metastatic neoplasms (including 14% in the temporal lobe and 18.5% in the posterior fossa).[88] Papilledema was present in 32% of the patients. A complication was observed in only one case where the patient became comatose 12 hours after the lumbar puncture.

Korein et al. reported lumbar punctures performed on 129 patients with papilledema or intracranial hypertension due to neoplasms, hematomas, encephalopathies, infection, and thrombosis with only one possible complication.[78] They combined the results of their study and six prior studies of lumbar puncture performed on 418 patients with papilledema including 83% with neoplasms and 17% with posterior fossa lesions. Possible complications occurred in only 1.2% of the patients.

Normal optic discs and a nonfocal examination do not, of course, ensure that a lumbar puncture can be performed without risk of herniation.[107,122] Even in cases of neoplasm and increased intracranial pressure, papilledema is present in only 48% of cases.[53] Fortunately, with the availability of computed tomography (CT) and magnetic imaging (MRI), the incidence of this complication has become even less.

Meningitis

Cerebral or cerebellar herniation can result from lumbar puncture performed on patients with meningitis. Rennick et al. reported a series of 445 children over 30 days old with a mean age of 2 years with bacterial meningitis.[121] Nineteen episodes of herniation occurred in the 17 children who had a lumbar puncture, with 12 of the episodes occurring within the first 12 hours after the procedure. Computed tomography scans performed at about the time of herniation were normal in 5 of the 14 episodes of herniation. The authors recommended that in a child with suspected meningitis and decerebrate or decorticate posturing, focal neurological signs, or no response to pain, antibiotics should be given but a lumbar puncture not performed even when a CT scan of the brain is normal.

Durando et al. reviewed 493 episodes of acute bacterial meningitis in 445 adults 16 years of age or older in whom lumbar puncture was performed in all cases.[43] In five, clinical signs of herniation developed within several minutes to several hours after lumbar puncture. They recommended obtaining a CT scan in patients with suspected meningitis and signs of increased intracranial pressure or focal findings on neurological examination before performing a lumbar puncture.

Hasblin et al. performed a prospective study of 301 adults with suspected meningitis, 78% of whom underwent CT before undergoing lumbar puncture.[63] Twenty-four percent had an abnormal CT scan and 5% had evidence of a mass lesion (two of the four patients with a mass lesion subsequently herniated). Clinical features at baseline associated with an abnormal finding on CT were an age of at least 60 years, immunocompromise, a history of central nervous system disease, and a history of seizure within 1 week before presentation, as well as the following neurological abnormalities: an abnormal level of consciousness, an inability to answer two consecutive questions correctly or to follow two consecutive commands, gaze palsy, abnormal visual fields, facial palsy, arm drift, leg drift, and abnormal language (e.g., aphasia). These criteria had a negative predictive value of 97%. Of the three patients who were misclassified with the use of these characteristics, only one had a mild mass effect, and all three patients underwent lumbar puncture without subsequent brain herniation. Hasblin et al. concluded that adults with none of these significant baseline characteristics are good candidates for immediate lumbar puncture since they have a low risk of brain herniation as a result of lumbar puncture. Patients who have any of the baseline clinical features should undergo CT after blood has been drawn for culture and empirical antibiotic therapy has been initiated. "Our findings should inspire confidence on the part of clinicians that the risk of lumbar puncture is negligible in such patients, even in those with a mild or moderate mass effect on CT of the head."

Subarachnoid Hemorrhage, Pseudotumor Cerebri, and "Acquired" Chiari I Malformation

When a CT scan is normal and subarachnoid hemorrhage is suspected, a lumbar puncture is the next appropriate procedure.[155] However, in cases of subarachnoid hemorrhage with hematoma and mass effect, lumbar puncture can be dangerous. Duffy described 55 patients who underwent lumbar puncture within 12 hours of the ictus of subarachnoid hemorrhage.[42] Seven patients had dramatic deterioration at the time of lumbar puncture with the needle still in place. Six of them were found to have clot with ventricular displacement on CT scan.

In patients with suspected pseudotumor cerebri with a normal MRI scan (preferably) or CT scan, lumbar puncture can be safely performed. There is, however, a case report of an obese 27-year-old woman with pseudotumor cerebri who underwent a lumbar puncture and had a respiratory arrest.[141] The MRI scan was normal except for low-lying cerebellar tonsils. Five years later, she developed headache and fever. She had two lumbar punctures within several hours. Within minutes of the second, she had a respiratory arrest and died a few days later without regaining consciousness. The presumption is that the respiratory arrest was due to the lumbar puncture performed in the presence of increased intracranial pressure and low-lying tonsils. There is a case report of another complication of lumbar puncture in a patient with a Chiari I malformation: the development after 2 weeks of oscillopsia and horizontal nystagmus with resolution of the eye signs following occipital craniectomy.[8]

There are two case reports of lumbar puncture resulting in reversible descent of the cerebellar tonsils below the foramen magnum.[100,128] In one case, a 27-year-old woman underwent two lumbar punctures within 1 month for evaluation of headache. The opening pressure was normal during the first lumbar puncture. An MRI scan after the second lumbar puncture was normal except for a small vascular formation in the posterior fossa. She then developed recurring postural headaches. Serial MRI scans showed descent of the tonsils to 9 mm, which on a follow-up scan 4 months later, as the headache improved, had ascended to 4 mm below the foramen magnum.[128] Reversible tonsillar descent has also been reported as a complication of overdraining CSF shunts[100,160] and spontaneous intracranial hypotension.[76,86,100]

Subarachnoid Block and Spinal Coning

Neurological deterioration may occur when lumbar puncture is performed below the level of a complete spinal subarachnoid block. Removing CSF below the level of the block may further decrease the differential below the low-pressure compartment below the block and the higher pressure above the block, resulting in spinal coning.[66] Epidural venous engorgement and reduction of spinal cord movement within the canal could also result in neurological impairment.[75] Hollis et al. reported a series of 50 patients who underwent a lumbar myelogram in the presence of a more rostral complete spinal subarachnoid block with most due to neoplasms.[66] Fourteen percent deteriorated: six patients showed significant neurological deterioration with increased paresis within 1 to 4 days after the procedure, and one deteriorated within 30 minutes. By contrast, in another 50 patients with similar lesions who underwent myelogram by C1-2 puncture, no deterioration was seen.

Postdural Puncture Headache

Characteristics

Post–lumbar puncture headache, which is more precisely termed *postdural puncture headache*

(PDPH), is the most common complication of lumbar puncture, occurring in up to 40% of patients after diagnostic lumbar puncture.[37] The headache begins within 48 hours in about 80% and within 72 hours in about 90% of patients.[82,91] The onset can be immediately after the lumbar puncture[97] or delayed for as long as 14 days.[148] The duration of the headache is less than 5 days in about 80%,[91] although it can persist for 12 months.[84]

The headache, which is always bilateral, may be a frontal, occipital, or generalized pressure or throbbing occuring in the upright position and decreasing or resolving when supine. The headache may also decrease when epigastric pressure is applied to compress the inferior vena cava while the patient is sitting.[123] (The physician pushes the right fist just beneath the right costal margin and places the left hand on the patient's back for 1 minute.) The headache worsens with head movement, coughing, straining, sneezing, and jugular venous compression.[86] The longer the patient is upright, the longer the time before the headache subsides when supine.[118,148] In the study of Lybecker et al., the headaches were reported as mild in 11%, moderate in 22%, and severe in 69%.[91] Additional symptoms were present in the following percentages: neck stiffness, 43%; nausea, 66%; vomiting, 27%; cochlear symptoms, 15%; and ocular symptoms, 12%. In another series, nausea was present in 22% and vomiting in 2%.[1]

Pathophysiology

The cause of PDPH is not entirely certain. The best explanation is low CSF pressure due to CSF leakage through a dural and arachnoid tear produced by the puncture that exceeds the rate of CSF production. Cerebrospinal fluid hypotension can produce headache and cranial nerve symptoms through downward descent of the brain and stretching of pain-sensitive structures including the dura, nerves (cranial nerves V, IX and X and the upper three cervical nerves), and bridging veins.[81,86] Secondarily, intracranial venous dilatation and increased brain volume occur as the veins passively dilate in response to decreased extravascular pressure.[37,81,118,152]

As a following section on risk factors demonstrates, even in the presence of low CSF pressure,[94] there is individual susceptibility or resistance to headache. This is the case in many other pain disorders (including raised intracranial pressure,[135] neural compression, etc.) where the presence of objective pathology unreliably correlates with pain complaints. There is a recent intriguing hypothesis that may explain some of the individual susceptibility to PDPH. Substance P levels in plasma (and presumably in CSF) increase after lumbar puncture.[137] Patients with low CSF substance P levels are three times more likely to develop PDPH than those with higher levels.[28] Thus, PDPH may be mediated by the release of substance P after lumbar puncture in those with low levels of substance P and receptor-mediated hypersensitivity.[28,137]

In rare cases, PDPH can be caused by pneumocephalus due to the lumbar puncture, which spontaneously resolves in a few days.[79]

Investigations

Investigations are uncommonly performed since PDPH can be easily diagnosed based upon the characteristic symptoms. A repeat lumbar puncture will usually demonstrate an opening pressure from 0 to 70 cm H_2O, although the pressure can be in the normal range, especially if the procedure is performed after a period of bed rest.[86] As in the case of other low-pressure headaches, the CSF analysis may be normal or can demonstrate a moderate, primarily lymphocytic pleocytosis, the presence of red blood cells, and elevated protein, which can even above 500 mg/dl.[100]

An MRI scan of the brain may reveal diffuse meningeal enhancement with gadolinium and also, in some cases, subdural fluid collections, which return to normal with resolution of the headache.[17,100,109] The diffuse meningeal enhancement on MRI may be explained by dural vasodilatation and a greater concentration of gadolinium in the dural microvasculature and in the interstitial fluid of the dura.[51] The pleocytosis and elevated protein in the CSF and the subdural fluid collections are probably due to decreased CSF volume and hydrostatic pressure changes resulting in meningeal vasodilation and vascular leak.[100] There are two case reports of abnormal dural venous sinus enhancement suggesting compensatory venous expansion.[7,132]

Lumbar MRI may also be abnormal following lumbar puncture.[6,68] In one study of 11 patients, all had evidence of CSF leakage ranging from 1 to 460 ml.[68]

Yousry et al. obtained cervical spine MRI studies on 11 patients with PDPH.[168] Findings were present in the following percentages: dilatation of the anterior internal vertebral venous plexus, 82%; spinal hygromas (probably subdural), 73%; and a retrospinal fluid collection at C1-C2, 36%. Similar findings were present in 20 patients with spontaneous intracranial hypotension headache.

Risk Factors for Postdural Puncture Headache

Patient Demographics (Table 39.2)

Postdural puncture headache occurs twice as often in women as in men.[41,82,118,148,149,156] The incidence is much less in children younger than 13 years[15,72] and adults older than 60[65,154] and has the highest incidence in the 18- to 30-year-old age group.[87] Possible explanations for the reduced incidence PDPH in children are the lower CSF pressure in children and the lower hydrostatic pressure when upright, allowing less CSF leakage.[72] The incidence is greater in patients with a smaller body mass index (wt/ht^2).[82] Younger female patients with a low body mass index may have the highest risk of developing PDPH.[82] Younger women may be at greater risk because of increased dural fiber elasticity, which could maintain a patent dural defect better than a less elastic dura.[87] Estrogens might also increase substance P receptor sensitivity.[137] Decreased dural fiber elasticity, a smaller epidural space, and decreased sensitivity of pain structures in the dura and blood vessels may explain the lower incidence in patients over age 60.[87] However, Vilming et al. found that in adults, age and body mass index did not influence the prevalence of PLPH.[156]

Table 39.2. Risk Factors for Developing Postdural Puncture Headache

Patient Demographics
Female gender
Age (greatest in the 18- to 30-year age range)
Smaller body mass index
Prior chronic or recurrent headaches
Prior postdural puncture headache
Lumbar Puncture Needle
Quincke needle
Larger-diameter needle
Perpendicular orientation of the bevel
Not reinserting the stylet

Patients with a headache before the lumbar puncture are at greater risk for PDPH[82,113] that is more severe and lasts longer than in those without preceding headache.[82] Clark et al. found that patients with chronic or recurrent headaches were three times as likely to develop PDPH as those without headaches.[28] Patients with a prior history of PDPH are also at increased risk.[92]

Diameter of the Quincke Needle

The incidence of PDPH decreases with a smaller diameter of the needle. This is consistent with the CSF leakage theory of PDPH: a smaller-diameter needle produces a smaller tear in the dura and less potential for leakage.[39] Using a standard or Quincke needle with a bevel tip, the incidence of PDPH decreases with higher-gauge needles as follows: 16–19 G, about 70%; 20–22 G, 20%–40%; and 24–27 G, 5%–12%.[37]

Orientation of the Bevel

Orientation of the bevel of the Quincke needle also influences the development of PDPH. The dural fibers run parallel to the long axis of the spine.[59] When the dura is punctured with the bevel perpendicular to the fibers, more fibers are severed than when the bevel is parallel to the fibers.[99] (However, Reina et al. found no significant difference in the size of the punctures in the parallel vs. perpendicular axes in a study using isolated dural sac from cadavers.[120] It is not certain whether traction on the dura or CSF pressure in vivo affects the size of the punctures.) Four studies of patients receiving spinal anesthesia have demonstrated a reduction in the incidence of PDPH by 50% or greater when the bevel is parallel rather than perpendicular.[92,99,105,143]

Thus, when using a Quincke needle, the bevel should be inserted parallel to the longitudinal dural fibers.[50] This description of the orientation of the bevel is confusing. Parallel insertion means that a plane passing through the flat part of the bevel, going through both edges of the bevel, is parallel to the long or vertical axis of the spine. If a lumbar puncture is performed with the patient in the lateral position, the face or flat portion of the bevel (on the same side of the needle as the notch in the hub for the stylet) should point up toward the physician. If the lumbar puncture is performed with the patient sitting, the bevel should be turned to the left or right. In any patient position, the face of the bevel and the notch in the hub should point in the direction of the patient's side, not toward the patient's head or feet.

Reinserting the Stylet Before Withdrawing the Needle

Strupp and Brandt valuated the effect on PDPH of reinserting or not reinserting the stylet before withdrawing the needle.[139] All the lumbar punctures were performed with a Sprotte 21 G needle. Postdural puncture headache developed in 16% of the 300 patients without reinsertion and in only 5% of the 300 patients with reinsertion. The authors hypothesize: "The reason for this difference may be that a strand of arachnoid enters the needle with the outflowing cerebrospinal fluid during diagnostic lumbar puncture; when the needle is removed, the strand may then be threaded back through the dural defect and produce prolonged cerebrospinal fluid leakage along the arachnoid."[139] Based upon the findings of this study, it seems reasonable to replace the stylet when using the Sprotte needle and the Quincke needle (although similar evidence for replacing the stylet is not available for the Quincke needle).

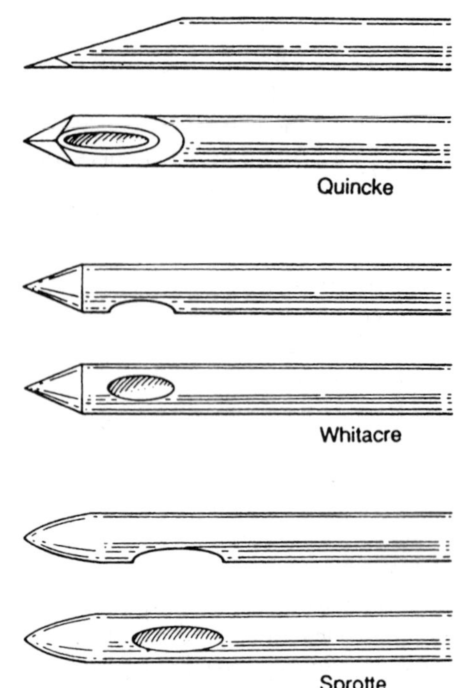

Figure 39.1. Three types of spinal needle tips: the Quincke, Whitacre, and Sprotte. (From Peterman SB: Postmyelography headache rates with Whitacre versus Quincke 22-guage spinal needles. Radiology 200:771–778, 1996, with permission.)

Atraumatic Needles

Pencil point or atraumatic needles such as the Whitacre[62] or Sprotte[138] (Fig. 39.1) may further reduce the incidence of PDPH as follows: 21 G Sprotte, 1.7%;[45] 22 G Sprotte, 2.6%;[45] and 22–24 G, atraumatic cone, about 2%.[37] The explanation is that the sharp-edged Quincke needle cuts dural fibers where the pencil point needle spreads the fibers.[112,140] In a study of 75 patients undergoing diagnostic lumbar puncture, the incidence of PDPH was 36% when the 22 G Quincke needle was used and 4% with the 22 G Sprotte needle.[18] In a study of 600 patients by Jager et al. who underwent diagnostic and/or therapeutic lumbar puncture with a Sprotte 21 G needle, only 3.6% reported PDPH.[71] In a study by Thomas et al. randomizing 101 patients using 20 G needles for diagnostic lumbar punctures, the incidence of moderate-severe headache was 25% when the Quincke needle was used and 16% when the Sprotte needle was used.[145] In a study by Strupp et al. of 230 patients using 22 G needles for diagnostic lumbar punctures, the incidence of PDPH was 24.4% with the Quincke needle and 12.2% with the Sprotte.[140] (The mean age of the cohort was about 40 years, about 64% of whom were females, which may have resulted in a higher rate of PLPH compared to other studies.)

When performing a diagnostic lumbar puncture, a flow rate of 2 ml/min is desirable unless only the opening pressure is going to be measured or if a small quantity of CSF is to be removed (or if you and your patient want to spend a lot of time together). Rapid pressure transduction to measure the opening pressure is also desirable. Carson and Serpell tested the characteristics of different brands and sizes of needles for rate of flow and time for CSF pressure transduction at CSF pressures of 12 and 24 cm.[26] Data on various needles are presented in Table 39.3. Needles with a diameter of less than 22 G may be satisfactory for spinal anesthesia[38] or myelography[113] but not for diagnostic lumbar puncture. Because there are variations in wall thickness and therefore in different internal diameters of the same gauge needles from different manufacturers, the flow rates and time for transduction of pressure were different with the same gauge needles from different manufacturers.[26]

Table 39.3. Mean Flow Rate in ml/hr and Seconds to Transduce 95.8% of Cerebrospinal Fluid (CSF) Pressure: Results for CSF Pressure of 12 cm CSF

Needle Brand and Gauge	ml/hr	Seconds to 95.8% of Pressure
Spinocan Quincke 20 G	133	43
Spinocan Quincke 22 G	30.4	225
Spinocan Quincke 25 G	10.5	336 to 83.3%
Becton Dickinson Quincke 22 G	40.6	168
Becton Dickinson Whitacre 22 G	47.6	121
Sprotte 24 G	17.9	269 to 83.3%
Sprotte 22 G	64.7	79
Sprotte 20 G	206	37

Source: Data from Carson D, Serpell M: Choosing the best needle for diagnostic lumbar puncture. Neurology 47:33–37, 1996.

The Sprotte 20 G is the best overall needle choice when both rapid pressure transduction and larger volumes of CSF are desired, with the Spinocan 20 G Quincke being second best.[26] The Sprotte 21 G needle also provides satisfactory pressure transduction and CSF flow. However, when considering CSF flow rate, pressure transduction time, and reduction of PLPH, the Sprotte 20 G, 21 G, and 22 G needles are all significantly advantageous compared to the standard Quincke 20 G needle.

A sharp, short introducer is provided with the Sprotte needle. The feel of the atraumatic needle during the procedure is different from the Quincke's sharp cutting edge, as it is necessary to push a little harder during insertion and the procedure is a little more difficult to perform than with the Quincke needle. Thomas et al. found that the failure rate in performing lumbar punctures with the Sprotte needle by house officers was 16% and was especially great in patients with high body mass indices.[145] When performing a lumbar puncture with a Sprotte needle, a Quincke needle should also be available in case of initial failure. The atraumatic needle is a little more expensive than the Quincke, but this difference is minor compared to the overall cost of the procedure, the cost of missed work with a PDPH, and the expense of an epidural blood patch, if needed.

Despite the evidence demonstrating the greatly reduced risk of PDPH with the Sprotte needle (especially in high-risk patients such as young adult females),[5,47] most U.S. neurologists are still performing diagnostic lumbar punctures with the Quincke needle. Most neurologists are either unfamiliar or only vaguely familiar with the atraumatic needles.[14]

Prevention of Postdural Puncture Headache Postprocedure

Contrary to the conventional wisdom still prevalent among many physicians and nurses, bed rest for up to 24 hours or various body positions, such as prone or head down, after the lumbar puncture do not reduce the incidence of PDPH compared to immediate ambulation.[23,30,35,37,127,158] In fact, prolonged recumbency following lumbar puncture may increase the risk of PDPH.[82,158] (In some cases, even after I explain the literature on this point to patients, if they develop a PDPH, a family friend who is a nurse or doctor asks them why they listened to the idiot neurologist: everyone knows bed rest is mandatory for at least X hours. Invariably, when I perform a lumbar puncture in the hospital, the nurse asks me how long bed rest will be required.) Intake of oral fluids following the lumbar puncture also does not prevent PDPH.[36] The report of the Therapeutics and Technology Assessment Subcommittee of the American Academy of Neurology concludes that "Class I and Class I data have not demonstrated that the duration of recumbency following a diagnostic LP influences the occurrence of PLPHA. There is no evidence that the use of increased fluids prevents PDPH."[47]

Treatment of Postdural Puncture Headache

For the many patients who do not relish the prospect of several days of bed rest, there are other effective treatments for PDPH (Table 39.4).

Oral and Intravenous Medications

The methylxanthines, caffeine and theophylline, may relieve PDPH. The mechanism may be blockade of cerebral adenosine receptors leading to intracerebral arterial constriction, resulting in decreased cerebral blood flow and intracranial pressure.[118] Oral caffeine, 300 mg every 4 to 6 hours (in tablet form or in beverages), is worth trying initially for PDPH,[87] although the relief may be transient. In a study of postpartum women with PDPH as a complication of epidural anesthetics, a single oral dose of 300 mg caffeine reduced headache intensity within 4 hours in 90% of patients,

Table 39.4. Treatments for Postdural Puncture Headaches

Initial or Mild Headache

Bed rest
Caffeine, 300 mg po every 6–8 hours or
Theophylline, 300 mg po every 8 hours

Moderate to Severe Headache Present for More Than 24 Hours

Bed rest
Caffeine sodium benzoate, 500 mg slow intravenous bolus
Epidural blood patch

with improvement persisting for 24 hours in 70%.[22] Intravenous caffeine sodium benzoate can substantially reduce PDPH. Sechzer and Abel reported that a slow intravenous bolus of 500 mg caffeine sodium benzoate may initially relieve headache in 75%.[131] However, permanent relief, including those who received a second bolus of caffeine after 2 hours, was reported in about 50%.[131] Although side effects from intravenous caffeine have not been described,[72,131] caution should be used in certain patients, such as those with coronary artery disease and seizure disorders.[27] In a pilot study, sustained release theophylline (281.7 mg) given orally three times per day also reduced the intensity of PDPH.[49]

There is one study reporting relief of PDPH in four out of six patients with a 6 mg subcutaneous injection of sumatriptan.[24] However, Connelly et al. found no benefit in a randomized study of 10 patients given the same subcutaneous drug compared to saline.[29]

Epidural Blood Patch

The epidural blood patch (EBP) is the most effective treatment for PDPH and is indicated for patients with moderate to severe headache present for more than 24 hours.[143] The success rate is about 85% after one injection and near 98% after a second.[1,125,143] The EBP is equally successful for treatment of PDPH in children and adolescents.[165,166] It is performed by slowly injecting 10 to 20 ml of the patient's blood into the lumbar epidural space either at the same interspace or at the interspace below the prior puncture.[25,106] Following the procedure, the patient should stay in the decubitus position for at least 1 hour and preferably for 2 hours to obtain maximum benefit.[95] Based upon a prospective study of 79 patients, Vilming et al. suggest that patients who have to lie in bed for more than half a day despite conservative treatment with analgesics and/or caffeine should be offered an EBP the next day.[157] Suffering and impairment are reduced when the decision is made at an early stage. However, prophylactic EBP at the time of the lumbar puncture does not appear to be effective.[10]

Based upon a serial MRI study, EBP has a mass effect that compresses the dural sac and displaces the conus medullaris and cauda equina.[9] The mass effect disappears after 7 hours. The main bulk of the clot occupied four or five vertebral levels with a thinner spread cephalad and caudad. The presumed mechanism of action is an immediate gelatinous tamponade of the dural hole.[106] Alternative hypotheses include a sudden increase in CSF pressure that antagonizes adenosine receptors and compression of the dural sac leading to activation of adrenergic, cholinergic, or peptidergic fibers.[118]

Side effects of EBP are usually mild and transient. In a retrospective study of 196 patients, the following percentages reported various side effects: 37%, pain at the site of injection; 12%, pain in the lower extremities; 10%, sensory disturbances in the lower extremities; 8%, walking disturbances; and 8%, weakness in the lower extremities.[143] The low back pain usually resolves within 1 to 3 days. Two cases of spinal subdural hematoma as a complication of immediate EBP have been reported.[144] Rare complications include bacterial meningitis, epidural abscess, arachnoiditis,[3] pneumocephalus,[80] and permanent paraparesis and cauda equina syndrome.[34]

Epidural injections with saline, dextran, fibrin glue, or opioids as alternative treatments to injections with blood are of unproven benefit.[151]

Cranial Neuropathies

Dysfunction of cranial nerves III, IV, V, VI, VII, and VIII has been reported after lumbar puncture.[55,104,146] The cranial neuropathies, which are usually transient, are presumably due to intracranial hypotension leading to traction on the nerves. In a large series of patients who had spinal anesthetics, .4% reported visual symptoms (including diplopia, blurred vision, spots before the eyes, photophobia, and scintillation) and .4% had auditory complaints (including dizziness, tinnitus, clogged-up and popping ears, and loss of hearing).[154] Both types of complaints were usually associated with typical postural headaches.

The most common cause of diplopia, abducens paresis, may follow as many as 1 in 400 lumbar punctures or spinal anesthesias and can be unilateral or bilateral.[104,146] The paresis usually occurs 4 to 14 days after the procedure and usually resolves over 4 to 6 weeks.[77,104] Fourth cranial nerve palsies, although rarely detected, may actually occur more frequently in association with sixth cranial nerve paresis.[77]

Reversible hearing loss, which can resolve within minutes following a lumbar EBP, may be symptomatic in up to 8% of patients.[20,90,98] Asymptomatic hearing loss is common after spinal anesthesia and occurs less often with a smaller-gauge needle.[52] Occasionally the hearing loss can be permanent.[98] The hearing loss is probably due to decreased CSF pressure that is transmitted by the cochlear aqueduct to the perilymph of the inner ear, causing a decrease in the perilymphatic pressure and endolymphatic hydrops.[90]

Nerve Root Irritation and Low Back Pain

During lumbar puncture, contact with the sensory roots causing transient electric shocks or dysesthesias is common, reported by 13% of patients in one series.[41] Permanent sensory and motor loss can rarely occur.[32] If the procedure is performed at the improper level, the spinal cord may be injured by the needle. Two cases of reflex sympathetic dystrophy following lumbar myelograms have been reported.[102]

Patients frequently complain of backache for several days after a lumbar puncture due to local trauma. In a study by Thomas et al., 61% of 97 patients reported low back pain 7 days after lumbar puncture with mild intensity in 37.1%, moderate intensity in 16.5%, and severe intensity in 7.2%.[145] The median duration of the pain was 72 hours. There was no difference in the occurrence of low back pain between the group who underwent lumbar puncture with the Quincke needle as compared with the Sprotte needle. Occasionally, the low back pain may persist for many months.

Atabaki et al. reported lumbar epidural CSF fluid collections revealed on MRI in three children with PDPH, low back pain, and lower extremity symptoms suggesting that the epidural collections can cause symptomatic root compression.[6] Rarely, if the needle is inserted beyond the subarachnoid space, the annulus fibrosis may be damaged and the intervertebral disc can herniate.[41] In addition, when the annulus fibrosis is punctured, there is also the possibility of introducing bacteria. Discitis and vertebral collapse may rarely ensue after a latency of 2 weeks to 3 months.[11]

Complications of Using or Not Using the Stylet

The stylet should always be used on insertion through the skin and the subcutaneous tissue. Rarely, a needle without a stylet may implant a plug of skin that can grow into an intraspinal epidermoid tumor.[96,120]

There are rare reports of nerve complications with both reinserting and not reinserting the stylet before removing the needle. Since a nerve root can rarely herniate through the dura due to aspiration by the needle during rapid withdrawal, the argument can be made that the stylet should be reinserted[134,150] or perhaps that the needle without the stylet should be slowly withdrawn. Conversely, there is a single case report of transection and withdrawal of a nerve filament due to replacement of the stylet (into a hollow needle with an end-hole-side-hole needle) following a lumbar myelogram.[167]

As described in the section on PDPH, replacing the stylet before withdrawing the needle significantly decreases the incidence of PDPH.

Infections

Lumbar puncture can cause infectious complications due to the following: a contaminated needle, such as contamination due to respiratory droplets; disseminating skin flora without adequate disinfection of the skin; performing a lumbar puncture when an infection is present in the area, such as cellulitis, furunculosis, or epidural abscess; and introducing blood in the subarachnoid space in the presence of bacteremia.[50,55] In patients with CSF leaks, lumbar puncture can reverse the flow gradient, produce retrograde spread of organisms from the nasopharynx through the dural leak, and result in meningitis.[85] In addition to bacterial meningitis, discitis (as described above),[11] lumbar epidural abscess, and spinal cord abscess rarely occur.[55]

Bacterial Meningitis

Bacterial meningitis is a rare complication of diagnostic lumbar puncture.[147] There are a number of reports of bacterial meningitis due to spread by droplets from the upper respiratory and oral flora to the needle and CSF during myelography. The responsible organisms include various *Streptococcus* species (*sanguis*, *viridans*, *salivarius*, *bovis*, Group G, and *pneumoniae*) and *Enterococcus fecalis*.[40,129] The Gram stain is often negative. In a retrospective study of neuroradiological procedures requiring lumbar puncture, the incidence of bacterial meningitis soon after a lumbar puncture was 0.2%.[40]

Bleeding Complications

A variety of bleeding complications may occur after lumbar puncture. Locations include intracranial and spinal subdural hematoma, intracranial and spinal subarachnoid hemorrhage, and spinal epidural hematoma.

Intracranial Bleeding

Intracranial subdural hematoma is a rare complication of lumbar puncture that can occur in healthy patients without bleeding disorders. A typical post–lumbar puncture headache is often but not always present initially.[159] The age of reported patients with subdural hematomas ranges from 22 to 79.[159] The subdural hematoma, which can be unilateral or bilateral, may be diagnosed after an interval ranging from 3 days to several months and can rarely be fatal.[57,61,103,159,162] The mechanism may be low CSF pressure resulting in traction on the meninges and tearing of dural vessels.[54,159] Similarly, traction on the basal blood vessels can rarely result in rupture of a saccular aneurysm and subarachnoid hemorrhage as a complication of lumbar puncture.[61] A subdural hematoma should be suspected when a persistent post–lumbar puncture headache lasts more than 1 week, when a headache recurs after initially resolving, if focal neurological symptoms or signs develop, or if the headache does not have the typical postural component.[159]

Traumatic Lumbar Puncture

A traumatic lumbar puncture, needle-induced blood in the CSF, occurs in 72% of diagnostic lumbar punctures, with the number of red blood cells (RBC)/mm^3 present in the following percentages of lumbar punctures: 1–5 RBC, 27%; 6–50 RBC, 21%; and >50 RBC, 24%.[19] The cause is usually puncture of the radicular vessels that accompany each nerve root along the length of its surface and only rarely from the epidural veins[19] (Fig. 39.2). Occasionally, the radiculomedullary artery of Adamkiewicz and the corresponding vein may be present in a lower than usual position and accompany the L3, L4, or L5 nerve roots where puncture could occur.[130]

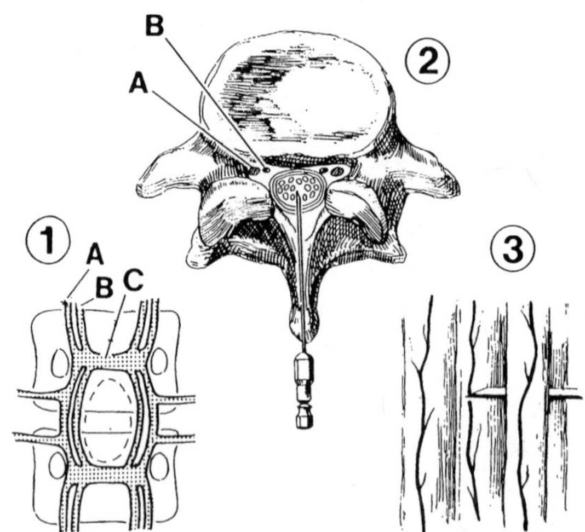

Figure 39.2. Sources of needle-induced blood in lumbar puncture. *1*, Anteroposterior view of lumbar venogram. (Adapted from Theron, J., and Moret J: Spinal Phlebography-Lumbar and Cervical Techniques. New York, Springer-Verlag, 1978, p. 27, with permission.) Lateral (*A*) and medial (*B*) longitudinal epidural veins, and (*C*) retrocorporeal anastomosis—the constant morphological patter and major components of the epidural venous system that lie anterior to the cord and away from the usual zone of entry of a lumbar puncture needle (dashed oval) into the vertebral canal. *2*, Path of a lumbar puncture needle into the crowded nerve roots of the cauda equina. *3*, Beveled edge of spinal needle, which may lacerate or impale radicular vessels that accompany each nerve root along the length of its surface. (From Breur AC, Tyler HR, Marzewski DJ, Rosenthal DS: Radicular vessels are the most probable source of needle-induced blood in lumbar puncture. Significance for the thrombocytopenic cancer patient. Cancer 49:2168–2172, 1982, with permission.)

Risk Factors for Spinal Hemorrhages

Thrombocytopenia, bleeding disorders, anticoagulation, and a difficult or bloody tap are all significant risk factors for spinal hemorrhages.[108] The standard recommendation is to perform a lumbar puncture, when the platelet count is not rapidly falling, only with a platelet count of 50,000 or greater,[50] although platelet counts of 20,000 or greater[19,44] and 100,000 or greater have also been recommended.[108] Most reports of spinal subarachnoid hematomas are in patients with platelet counts of less than 50,000,[108] although there is a report of a hematoma in a patient with relapsing lymphoblastic leukemia, a platelet count of 63,000, and normal prothrombin (PT) and partial thromboplastin times (PTT).[130]

In patients who are anticoagulated, adequate reversal (with protamine for those on heparin and vitamin K or fresh frozen plasma for those on warfarin) is mandatory before lumbar puncture. In patients with bleeding disorders, replacement therapy is indicated. For example, in one series, lumbar punctures were safely performed on 33 patients with hemophilia after pretreatment with clotting factor.[136] In questionable cases, a platelet count, international normalized ratio (INR), PT, PTT, and semplate bleeding time should be obtained before lumbar puncture. The international normalized ratio (INR), should be <1.5.

In one large study, preoperative antiplatelet therapy with aspirin or nonsteroidal anti-inflammatory medications and subcutaneous heparin on the operative day were not risk factors for spinal hematoma in patients undergoing spinal or epidural anesthesia.[67] However, anticoagulation with intravenous heparin following the lumbar puncture is a risk factor for spinal hemorrhage. Based upon a series of patients receiving heparin for cerebral ischemia after lumbar puncture, Ruff and Dougherty have recommended waiting at least 1 hour before anticoagulation.[124] However, there is one case report of a patient with cerebral ischemia who was placed on heparin 26 hours after a traumatic lumbar puncture and developed a spinal subarachnoid hematoma.[130]

Spinal Hematomas

Spinal subarachnoid hematoma, a rare complication of lumbar puncture, presents with severe low back and/or radicular pain followed within hours or days by progressive paraparesis, sensory loss, and sphincter disturbances.[130] Rarely, the spinal subarachnoid hematoma may rupture through the dura, resulting in a subdural collection as well.[13] The hematoma may be detected with myelography by cervical puncture followed by CT scan and MRI. Successful treatments include immediate decompressive laminectomy and hematoma evacuation as well as percutaneous hematoma aspiration.[130] Epidural hematomas[2,111,114] can also rarely occur after lumbar puncture with the same clinical presentation, risk factors, and treatment as spinal subarachnoid hematomas.[2,21,45]

Other Complications

A variety of other complications can occur.[55] Vasovagal syncope and cardiac arrest can result, as associated with any medical procedure. Hyperventilation during the procedure can result in multiple complaints including chest pain, dizziness, and paresthesias.[46a] Seizures have been reported in association with PDPH, although this may be due to concurrent caffeine administration.[16,133] Finally, results of the various types of CSF analysis from the laboratory can be incorrect and result in harm to the patient.[50]

Occasionally, family or friends who may be standing to observe the lumbar puncture may sustain injuries from vasovagal syncope.[46b] The injuries are usually but not always minor. Wide media coverage was given to a case in California where a man was allegedly asked to hold and steady his pregnant wife for an epidural anesthetic.[93b] Upon the sight of the needle, the man fainted and fell backwards striking his head on an aluminum cap molding at the base of the wall. He sustained a brain hemorrhage and died 2 days later. His wife sued the hospital and physician group for wrongful death. If a physician chooses to allow observers during a procedure, a warning might be issued about the possibility of vasovagal syncope and the observer(s) advised to remain seated during the procedure.

Summary

Before the first lumbar puncture, knowledge of the CSF pathways was essential. Galen's concept that pneuma, a gaseous substance, filled the ventricles was widely believed for 16 centuries until it was disproved by Cotugno in 1764 and Magendie in

1825. Wynter performed the first lumbar puncture via an incision of the skin and theca in February 1889. Quincke performed the first percutaneous lumbar puncture in December 1890. Death due to lumbar puncture performed on patients with cerebral neoplasms was first reported in 1896. In 1899, Bier reported the first cases of PDPH, including his own, as a complication of his new discovery, spinal anesthesia.

Multiple complications can occur after lumbar puncture including cerebral and spinal herniation, PDPH, cranial neuropathies, nerve root irritation, low back pain, stylet-associated problems, infections, and bleeding complications. Cerebral herniation in adults with lesions causing mass effect follows lumbar puncture in perhaps 1% of cases. Cerebral herniation is a significant risk of lumbar puncture in small children with suspected neurological symptoms who have focal neurological findings or are comatose. In a number of settings, lumbar puncture can result in reversible descent of the cerebellar tonsils. Spinal coning can occur in perhaps 14% of patients who undergo lumbar myelography in the presence of a more rostral subarachnoid block.

Postdural puncture headache occurs in up to 40% of patients. There are numerous demographic risk factors including female gender, the 18- to 30-year age range, small body mass index, and a history of prior headaches. The incidence of PDPH is greater the greater the diameter of the lumbar puncture needle. To reduce the incidence of PDPH, when using a Quincke needle, the flat portion or face of the bevel (on the same side of the needle as the notch in the hub for the stylet) should point in the direction of the patient's side, not toward the patient's head or feet. The Whitacre and Sprotte atraumatic needle can significantly reduce the incidence of PDPH. For diagnostic lumbar puncture, the Sprotte 20, 21, or 22 G needle may be preferred because of its excellent flow rate and rapid measurement of the opening pressure. When using a Quincke or atraumatic needle, the stylet should be replaced before removing the needle to decrease the incidence of PDPH. Bed rest for up to 24 hours, various body positions, and intake of oral fluids after the lumbar puncture do not reduce the incidence of PDPH. Depending upon its persistence and severity, PDPH can be treated with bed rest, oral caffeine and theophylline, intravenous caffeine, and a lumbar EBP.

Dysfunction of cranial nerves III, IV, V, VI, VII, and VIII has been reported after lumbar puncture. The most common cause of diplopia is abducens paresis, which follows 0.25% of the procedures. Dizziness and reversible hearing loss are fairly common.

During lumbar puncture, contact with the sensory roots causing transient electric shocks or dysesthesias occurs in about 13% of patients. Permanent motor and sensory loss can rarely occur. About 60% of patients complain of low back pain usually lasting for several days. Rarely, lumbar puncture can result in a herniated intervertebral disc.

A variety of infectious complications can occur including bacterial meningitis, discitis, lumbar epidural abscess, and spinal cord abscess. Bacterial meningitis is usually due to spread by droplets from the upper respiratory and oral flora to the needle and then to the CSF. The responsible organisms are usually of the streptoccal species.

Bleeding complications include intracranial and spinal subdural hematomas, intracranial and spinal subarachnoid hemorrhages, and spinal epidural hematoma. Traumatic lumbar puncture is usually due to puncture of the radicular vessels that accompany each nerve root along the length of its surface and only rarely from the epidural veins. Thrombocytopenia, bleeding disorders, and anticoagulation are risk factors for spinal hemorrhage.

REFERENCES

1. Abouleish E, de la Vega S, Blendinger I, Tio TO: Long-term follow-up of epidural blood patch. Anesth Analg 54:459–463, 1975.
2. Adler M, Comi AE. Walker AR: Acute hemorrhagic complication of diagnostic lumbar puncture. Pediatr Emerg Care 17:184–188, 2001.
3. Aldrete JA, Brown TL: Intrathecal hematoma and arachnoiditis after prophylactic blood patch through a catheter. Anesth Anal 84:233–234, 1997.
4. Alpers BJ: Lumbar puncture headache. Arch Neurol Psychiatry 14:806–812, 1925.
5. Armon C, Evans RW: Update: Assessment: Prevention of post-lumbar puncture headaches: report of the Therapeutics and Technology Assessment Subcommittee of the American Academy of Neurology. Neurology 65:510–512, 2005.
6. Atabaki S, Ochsenschlager D, Vezina G: Post-lumbar puncture headache and bachache in pediatrics: A case series and demonstration of magnetic resonance imag-

ing findings. Arch Pediatr Adolesc Med 153:770–773, 1999.

7. Bakshi R, Mechtler LL, Kamran S, et al: MRI findings in lumbar puncture headache syndrome: Abnormal dural-meningeal and dural venous sinus enhancement. Clin Imag 23:73–76, 1999.
8. Barton JJS, Sharpe JA: Oscillopsia and horizontal nystagmus with accelerating slow phases following lumbar puncture in the Arnold-Chiari malformation. Ann Neurol 33:418–421, 1993.
9. Beards SCD, Jackson A, Griffiths AG, Horsman EL: Magnetic resonance imaging of extradural blood patches: Appearances from 30 min to 18 h. Br J Anaesth 71:182–188, 1993.
10. Berrettini WH, Simmons-Alling S, Nurnberger JI Jr: Epidural blood patch does not prevent headache after lumbar puncture. Lancet 11:856–857, 1987.
11. Bhatoe HS, Gill HS, Kumar N, Biswas S: Post lumbar puncture discitis and vertebral collapse. Postgrad Med J 70:882–883, 1994.
12. Bier A: Versuche über Cocainisirung des Rückenmarkes. Deutsche Z Chir 51:361–369, 1899.
13. Bills DC, Blumbergs P, North JB: Iatrogenic spinal subdural haematoma. Aust NZ J Surg 61:703–706, 1991.
14. Birnbach DJ, Kuroda MM, Sternman D, Thys DM: Use of atraumatic spinal needles among neurologists in the United States. Headache 41:385–390, 2001.
15. Bolder PM. Post–lumbar puncture headache in pediatric oncology patients. Anesthesiology 65:696–698, 1986.
16. Bolton VE, Leicht CH, Scanlon TS: Postpartum seizure after epidural blood patch and intravenous caffeine sodium benzoate. Anesthesiology 70:146–149, 1989.
17. Bourekas EC, Jonathan SL, Lanzieri CF: Postcontrast meningeal MR enhancement secondary to intracranial hypotension caused by lumbar puncture. J Comput Assist Tomogr 19:299, 1995.
18. Braune H-J, Huffmann G: A prospective double-blind clinical trial, comparing the sharp Quincke needle (22G) with an "atraumatic" needle (22G) in the induction of post–lumbar puncture headache. Acta Neurol Scand 86:50–54, 1992.
19. Breuer AC, Tyler HR, Marzewski DJ, Rosenthal DS: Radicular vessels are the most probable source of needle-induced blood in lumbar puncture. Significance for the thrombocytopenic cancer patient. Cancer 49:2168–2172, 1982.
20. Broome IJ: Hearing loss and dural puncture. Lancet 341:667–668, 1993.
21. Bruyn GW: Epidural anaesthesia and haematoma. In: Frankel HL (ed): Handbook of Clinical Neurology, vol 17: Spinal Cord Trauma. Amsterdam, Elsevier, 1992, pp 137–145.
22. Camann WR, Murray RS, Mushlin PS, Lambert DH: Effects of oral caffeine on postdural puncture headache: A double-blind, placebo-controlled trial. Anesth Analg 70:181–184, 1990.
23. Carbaat PAT, van Crevel H: Lumbar puncture headache: Controlled study on the preventative effect of 24 hours bed rest. Lancet 2:1133–1135, 1981.
24. Carp H, Singh PJ, Vadhera R, Jayaram A: Effects of the serotonin-receptor agonist sumatriptan on postdural puncture headache: Report of six case. Anesth Analg 79:180–182, 1994.
25. Carrie LES: Postdural puncture headache and extradural blood patch (editorial). Br J Anaesth 71:179–180, 1993.
26. Carson D, Serpell M: Choosing the best needle for diagnostic lumbar puncture. Neurology 47:33–37, 1996.
27. Choi A, Laurito CE, Cunningham FE: Pharmacologic management of postdural puncture headache. Ann Pharmacother 30:831–839, 1996.
28. Clark JW, Solomon GD, deSenanayake P, Gallagher C: Substance P concentration and history of headache in relation to postlumbar puncture headache: Towards prevention. J Neurol Neurosurg Psychiatry 60:681–683, 1996.
29. Connelly NR, Parker RK, Rahimi A, Gibson CS: Sumatriptan in patients with postdural puncture headache. Headache 40:316–319, 2000.
30. Cook PT, Davies MJ, Beavis RE: Bes rest and postlumbar puncture headache. The effectiveness of 24 hours' recumbency in reducing the incidence of postlumbar puncture headache. Anaesthesia 445:389–391, 1989.
31. Cotugno D: De ischiade nervosa commentarius. Neapoli, Simonios, 1764.
32. Dahlgren N, Törnebrandt K: Neurological complications after anaęsthesia. A follow-up of 18,000 spinal and epidural anaesthetics performed over three years. Acta Ansesthesiol Scand 39:872–880, 1995.
33. Dana CL: Puncture headache. JAMA 68:1017, 1917.
34. Diaz JH: Permanent paraparesis and cauda equina syndrome after epidural blood patch for postdural puncture headache. Anesthesiology 96:1515–1517, 2002.
35. Dieterich M, Brandt T: Is obligatory bed rest after lumbar puncture obsolete? Eur Arch Psychiatry Neurol Sci 235:71–75, 1985.
36. Dieterich M, Brandt T: Incidence of post-lumbar puncture headache is independent of daily fluid intake. Eur Arch Psychiatry Neurol Sci 237:194–195, 1988.
37. Dieterich M, Perkin GD: Postlumbar puncture headache syndrome. In: Brandt T, Caplan LR, Dichland J, Diener HC, Kennard C (eds): Neurological Disorders: Course and Treatment. San Diego, CA, Academic Press, 1996, pp 59–63.
38. Dittmann M, Schäfer H-G, Renkl F, Greve I: Spinal anaesthesia with 29 gauge Quincke point needles and postdural puncture headache in 2,378 patients. Acta Anaesthesiol Scand 38:691–693, 1994.
39. Dittmann M, Schäfer H-G, Ulrich J, Bond-Taylor W: Anatomical re-evaluation of lumbar dura mater with regard to postspinal headache. Effect of dural puncture. Anaesthesia 43:635–637, 1988.
40. Domingo P, Mancebo J, Blanch L, Coll P, Martinez E: Iatrogenic streptococcal meningitis. CID 19:356–357, 1994.

41. Dripps RD, Vandam LD: Hazards of lumbar puncture. JAMA 147:1118–1121, 1951.
42. Duffy GP: Lumbar puncture in spontaneous subarachnoid haemorrhage. BMJ 285:1163–1164, 1982.
43. Durando ML, Calderwood SB, Weber DJ, et al: Acute bacterial meningitis. A review of 493 episodes. N Engl J Med 328:21–28, 1993.
44. Edelson RN, Chernik NL, Posner JB: Spinal subdural hematomas complicating lumbar puncture occurrence in thrombocytopenic patients. Arch Neurol 31:134–137, 1974.
45. Engelhardt A, Oheim S, Neundorfer B: Post–lumbar puncture headache: Experiences with Sprotte's atraumatic needle. Cephalagia 12:259, 1992.
46a. Evans RW: Neurologic aspects of hyperventilation syndrome. Semin Neurol 15(2):115–125, 1995.
46b. Evans RW: The risk of vasovagal syncope to family and friends observing a lumbar puncture. Headache, 2006, in press.
47. Evans RW, Armon C, Frohman EM, Goodin DS: Assessment: Prevention of post–lumbar puncture headaches: Report of the Therapeutics and Technology Assessment Subcommittee of the American Academy of Neurology. Neurology 55:909–914, 2000.
48. Faulconer A, Keys TE: August Karl Gustav Bier. In: Foundations of Anesthesiology, vol. II. Springfield, IL, Charles C. Thomas, 1965, pp 850–857 (translation from German)
49. Feuerstein TJ, Zeides A: Theophylline relieves headache following lumbar puncture: Placebo-controlled, double-blind pilot study. Klin Wochenschr 64:216–218, 1986.
50. Fishman RA: Cerebrospinal Fluid in Diseases of the Nervous System, 2nd ed. Philadelphia, WB Saunders, 1992.
51. Fishman RA, Dillon WP: Dural enhancement and cerebral displacement secondary to intracranial hypotension. Neurology 43:609–611, 1993.
52. Fog J, Wang LP, Sundberg A, Mucchiano C: Hearing loss after spinal anesthesia is related to needle size. Anesth Analg 70:517–522, 1990.
53. Forsyth PA, Posner JB: Headaches in patients with brain tumors: A study of 111 patients. Neurology 43:1678–1683, 1993.
54. Francia A, Parisi P, Vitale AM, Esposito V: Life-threatening intracranial hypotension after diagnostic lumbar puncture. Neurol Sci 22:385–389, 2001.
55. Frederiks JAM: Spinal puncture complications. In: Frankel HL (ed): Handbook of Clinical Neurology, vol 17: Spinal Cord Trauma, Amsterdam, Elsevier, 1992, pp 147–189.
56. Fürbringer P: Plötzliche Todesfalle nach Lumbalpunction. Centralblatt Innere Med 17:1–8, 1896.
57. Gaucher DJ, Perez JA: Subdural hematoma following lumbar puncture. Arch Intern Med 162:1904–1905, 2002.
58. Gormley JB: Treatment of postspinal headache. Anesthesiology 21:565–566, 1960.
59. Greene HM: Lumbar puncture and the prevention of postpuncture headache. JAMA 86:391–392, 1926.
60. Harrington BE: Postdural puncture headache and the development of the epidural blood patch. Anesth Pain Med 29:136–163, 2004.
61. Hart IK, Bone I, Hadley DM: Development of neurological problems after lumbar puncture. BMJ 296:51–52, 1988.
62. Hart JR, Whitacre RJ: Pencil-point needle in prevention of postspinal headache. JAMA 147:657–658, 1951.
63. Hasblin, R, Abrahams J, Jekel J, Quagliarello VJ: Computed tomography of the head before lumbar puncture in adults with suspected meningitis. N Engl J Med 345: 1727–1733, 2001.
64. Herndon RM: A brief history of the understanding of cerebrospinal fluid. In: Herndon RM, Brumback R (eds): The Cerebrospinal Fluid. Boston, Kluwer Academic, 1989, pp 1–13.
65. Hindley NJ, Jobst KA, King E, et al: High acceptability and low morbidity of diagnostic lumbar puncture in elderly subjects of mixed cognitive status. Acta Neurol Scand 91:405–411, 1995.
66. Hollis PH, Malis LI, Zappulla RA: Neurological deterioration after lumbar puncture below complete spinal subarachnoid block. J Neurosurg 64:253–256, 1986.
67. Horlocker TT, Wedel DJ, Schroeder DR, et al: Preoperative antiplatelet therapy does not increase the risk of spinal hematoma associated with regional anesthesia. Anesth Analg 80:303–309, 1995.
68. Iqbal J, Davis LE, Orrison WW: An MRI study of lumbar puncture headaches. Headache 35:420–422, 1995.
69. Jacobaeus H, Frumerie M: The leakage of spinal fluid after lumbar puncture and its treatment. Acta Med Scand 58:102, 1923.
70. Jacoby GW: Lumbar puncture and the subarachnoid spine. NY Med J 813–818, 1895.
71. Jager H, Krane M, Schimrigk K: Lumbar puncture—the post-puncture syndrome. Prevention with an "atraumatic" puncture needle, clinical observations. Schweiz Med Wochenschr 123:1985–1990, 1993.
72. Janssens E, Aerssens P, Alliet P, et al: Post-dural puncture headaches in children. A literature review. Eur J Pediatr 162:117–121, 2003.
73. Jarvis AP, Grenawalt JW, Fagraeus I: Intravenous caffeine for postdural puncture headache. Anesth Analg 65:313–321, 1986.
74. Jennings CG: A case of lumbar puncture of the subarachnoid space. Arch Pediatr 13:591–592, 1896.
75. Jooma R, Hayward RD: Upward spinal coning: Impaction of occult spinal tumours following relief of hydrocephalus. J Neurol Neurosurg Psychiatry 47:386–390, 1984.
76. Kasner SE, Rosenfeld J, Farber RE: Spontaneous intracranial hypotension: Headache with a reversible Arnold-Chiari malformation. Headache 35:557, 1995.
77. King RA, Calhoun JH: Fourth cranial nerve palsy following spinal anesthesia. J Clin Neuro-ophthalmol 7:20–22, 1987.
78. Korein J, Cravioto H, Leicach M: Reevaluation of lumbar puncture. A study of 129 patients with papilledema or intracranial hypertension. Neurology 9:290–297, 1959.

79. Kozikowski GP, Cohen SP: Lumbar puncture associated with pneumocephalus: Report of a case. Anesth Analg 98:524–526, 2004.
80. Krisanda TJ, Laucks SO: Pneumocephalus following an epidural blood patch procedure: An unusual cause of severe headache. Ann Emerg Med 23:129–131, 1994.
81. Kunkle EC, Ray BS, Wolff HG: Experimental studies on headache: Analysis of the headache associated with changes in intracranial pressure. Arch Neurol Psychiatry 49:323–358, 1943.
82. Kuntz KM, Kokmen E, Stevens JC, et al: Post–lumbar puncture headaches: Experience in 501 consecutive patients. Neurology 42:1884–1887, 1992.
83. Labat G: The trend of subarachnoid block. Surg Clin North Am 10:671–681, 1930.
84. Lance JW, Branch GB: Persistent headache after lumbar puncture. Lancet 343:414, 1994.
85. Lanska D, Lanska MJ, Selman WR: Meningitis following spinal puncture in a patient with a CSF leak. Neurology 39:306–307, 1989.
86. Lay CL, Campbell JK, Mokri B: Low cerebrospinal fluid pressure headache. In: Goadsby PJ, Silberstein SD (eds): Headache. Boston, Butterworth-Heinemann, 1997, pp 355–367.
87. Leibold RA, Yealy DM, Coppola M, Cantees KK: Post-dural-puncture headache: Characteristics, management, and prevention. Ann Emerg Med 22:1863–1870, 1993.
88. Lubic LG, Marotta JT: Brain tumor and lumbar puncture. Arch Neurol Psychiatry 72:568–572, 1954.
89. Luschka H: Die Adergeflechte der menschlichen Gehirnes. Berlin, G. Reimer, 1865.
90. Lybecker H, Andersen T: Repetitive hearing loss following dural puncture treated with autologous epidural blood patch. Acta Anaesthiol Scand 39:987–989, 1995.
91. Lybecker H, Djernes M, Schmidt JF: Postdural puncture headache (PDPH): Onset, duration, severity, and associated symptoms. Acta Anaesthesiol Scand 39:605–612, 1995.
92. Lybecker H, M<j>ller JT, May O, Nielsen HK: Incidence and prediction of postdural puncture headache. A prospective study of 1021 spinal anesthesias. Anesth Analg 70:389–394, 1990.
93a. MacRobert RG: The cause of lumbar puncture headache. JAMA 70:1350–1353, 1918.
93b. Man faints, dies after seeing epidural. Reuters July 7, 2005. Available at http://abcnews.go.com/Health/wireStory?id=918907.
94. Marshall J: Lumbar-puncture headache. J Neurol Neurosurg Psychiatry 13:71–74, 1950.
95. Martin R, Jourdain S, Clairoux M, Tétrault JP: Duration of decubitus position after epidural blood patch. Can J Anaesth 41:23–25, 1994.
96. McDonald JV, Klump TE: Intraspinal epidermoid tumors caused by lumbar puncture. Arch Neurol 43:936–939, 1986.
97. McSwiney M, Phillips J: Postdural puncture headache. Acta Anaesthesiol Scand 39:990–995, 1995.
98. Michel O, Brusis T: Hearing loss as a sequel of lumbar puncture. Ann Otol Rhinol Laryngol 101:390–394, 1992.
99. Mihic DN: Postspinal headache and relationship of needle bevel to longitudinal dural fibers. Regional Anesth 10:76–81, 1985.
100. Mokri B, Piepgras DG, Miller GM: Syndrome of orthostatic headaches and diffuse pachymeningeal gadolinium enhancement. Mayo Clin Proc 72:400–413, 1997.
101. Monro A: Observations on the Structure and Function of the Nervous System. Edinburgh, W Creech, 1783.
102. Morettin LB, Wilson M: Severe reflex algodystrophy (Sudeck's atrophy) as a complication of myelography: Report of two cases. AJR 110:156–158, 1970.
103. Newrick P, Read D: Subdural haematoma as a complication of spinal anaesthetic. Br. Med J 285:341–342, 1982.
104. Niedermuller U, Trinka E, Bauer G: Abducens palsy after lumbar puncture. Clin Neurol Neurosurg 104:61–63, 2002.
105. Norris MC, Leighton BL, DeSimone CA: Needle bevel direction and headache after inadvertent dural puncture. Anesthesiology 70:729–731, 1989.
106. Olsen KS: Epidural blood patch in the treatment of post-lumbar puncture headache. Pain 30:293–301, 1987.
107. Opeskin K, Anderson RM, Lee KA: Colloid cyst of the 3rd ventricle as cause of acute neurological deterioration and sudden death. J Paediatr Child Health 29:476–477, 1993.
108. Owens EL, Kasten GW, Hessel EA: Spinal subarachnoid hematoma after lumbar puncture and heparination: A case report, review of the literature, and discussion of anesthetic implications. Anesth Analg 65:1201–1207, 1986.
109. Pannullo S, Reich J, Posner J: Meningeal enhancement associated with low intracranial pressure. Neurology 42(suppl 3): 430, 1992.
110. Pappenheim M. The dangers of lumbar puncture. In: Pappenheim M (ed): Lumbar Puncture. New York, William Wood, 1925, pp 26–36.
111. Peltola J, Sumelahti ML, Kumpulainen T, et al: Spinal epidural haematoma complicating diagnostic lumbar puncture. Lancet 347:131, 1996.
112. Peterman SB: Postmyelography headache rates with Whitacre versus Quincke 22-gauge spinal needles. Radiology 200:765–770, 1996.
113. Peterman SB: Postmyelography headache: A review. Radiology 200:771–778, 1996.
114. Post MJD, Seminer DS, Quencer RM: CT diagnosis of spinal epidural hematoma. AJNR 3:190–192, 1982.
115. Quincke H. Zur physiologie der cerebrospinal Flüssigkeit. Arch Anat Physiol 153–177, 1872.
116. Quincke H: Die Lumbalpunction des Hydrocephalus. Berl Klin Wochenschr 28:929–933, 965–968, 1891. English translation from Toronto Hospital, Department of Anesthesia web site: http://auryn.ibme.utoronto.ca/casweb/s14d11.htm.
117. Quincke HI: Ueber hydrocephalus. Verhandlung des Congress Innere Medizin (X) 1891:321–339. English

translation from Wilkins RH: Neurosurgical Classics—XXXI. J Neurosurg 22:294–308, 1965.
118. Raskin NH: Lumbar puncture headache: A review. Headache 30:197–200, 1990.
119. Reina MA, Lopez A, Badorrey V, et al: Dura-arachnoid lesions produced by 22 gauge Quincke spinal needles during a lumbar puncture. J Neurol Neurosurg Psychiatry 75:893–897, 2004.
120. Reina MA, Lopez-Garcia A, Dittman M, de Andres JA, Blazquez MG: [Iatrogenic spinal epidermoid tumors. A late complication of spinal puncture.] Rev Esp Anestesiol Reanim 43:142–146, 1996.
121. Rennick G, Shann F, de Campo J: Cerebral herniation during bacterial meningitis in children. BMJ 306:953–955, 1993.
122. Richards PG, Towu-Aghantse E: Dangers of lumbar puncture. BMJ 292:605–606, 1986.
123. Roark GL, Abraham RA, Harris AP: SEPT sign: The use of the sitting epigastric pressure test for diagnosis of postdural puncture headaches. Anesthesiology 81(3A):A1016, 1994.
124. Ruff RL, Dougherty JH: Complications of lumbar puncture followed by anticoagulation. Stroke 12:879–881, 1981.
125. Safa-Tisseront V, Thormann F, Malassine P, et al: Effectiveness of epidural blood patch in the management of post-dural puncture headache. Anesthesiology 95: 334–339, 2001.
126. Sakula A: A hundred years of lumbar puncture: 1891–1991. J R Col Phys Lond 25:171–175, 1991.
127. Sand T, Myhr G, Stovner LJ, et al: Side effects after ambulatory lumbar iohexol myelography. Neuroradiology 31:49–54, 1989.
128. Sathi S, Stieg PE: "Acquired" Chiari I malformation after multiple lumbar punctures: Case report. Neurosurgery 32:306–309, 1993.
129. Schelkun SR, Wagner KF, Blanks JA, Reinert CM: Bacterial meningitis following pantopaque myelography. A case report and literature review. Orthopedics 8:73–76, 1985.
130. Scott EW, Cazenave CR, Virapongse C: Spinal subarachnoid hematoma complicating lumbar puncture: Diagnosis and management. Neurosurgery 25:287–293, 1989.
131. Sechzer PH, Abel L: Post-spinal anesthesia headache treated with caffeine. Evaluation with demand method. Part 1. Curr Ther Res 24:307–312, 1978.
132. Settipani N, Piccoli T, La Bella V, Piccoli F: Cerebral venous sinus expansion in post–lumbar puncture headache. Funct Neurol 19:51–52, 2004.
133. Shearer VE, Cunningham G, Wallace DH, Giesecke AH: Seizures following postdural puncture headache in postpartum women: A series with suggested etiology. Anesthesiology 75:A852, 1991.
134. Siddiqui TS, Buchheit WA: Herniated nerve root as a complication of spinal tap. J Neurosurg 56:565–566, 1982.
135. Silberstein SD, Marcelis J: Headache associated with changes in intracranial pressure. Headache 32:84–94, 1992.
136. Silverman R, Kwiatkowski T, Bernstein S, et al: Safety of lumbar puncture in patients with hemophilia. Ann Emerg Med 22:1739–1742, 1993.
137. Solomon GD, Clark JW, deSenanayake P, Kunkel RS: Hypersensitivity to substance P in the etiology of postlumbar puncture headache. Headache 35:25–28, 1995.
138. Sprotte G, Schedel R, Pajunk H, Pajunk H: Eine "atraumatische" Universalkanüle für einzeitige Regionalanaesthesien: Klinische Ergebnisse nach sechsjähriger Erprobung bei über 30,000 Regionalanaesthesien. Reg Anaesth 10:104–108, 1987.
139. Strupp M, Brandt T: Should one reinsert the stylet during lumbar puncture? N Engl J Med 336:1190, 1997.
140. Strupp M, Schueler O, Straube A, et al: "Atraumatic" Sprotte needle reduces the incidence of post–lumbar puncture headaches. Neurology 57:2310–2312, 2001.
141. Sullivan HC: Fatal tonsillar herniation in pseudotumor cerebri. Neurology 41:1142–1144, 1991.
142. Tarkkila PJ, Heine H, Tervo R-R: Comparison of Sprotte and Quincke needles with respect to postdural puncture headache and backkache. Reg Anesth 17:283–287, 1992.
143. Tarkkila PJ, Miralles JA, Palomaki EA: The subjective complications and efficiency of the epidural blood patch in the treatment of postdural puncture headache. Reg Anesth 14:247–250, 1989.
144. Tekkök IH, Carter DA, Brinker R: Spinal subdural haematoma as a complication of immediate epidural blood patch. Can J Anaesth 43:306–309, 1996.
145. Thomas SR, Jamieson DRS, Muir KW: Randomised controlled trial of atraumatic versus standard needles for diagnostic lumbar puncture. BMJ 321:986–990, 2000.
146. Thorsen G: Neurological complications after spinal anaesthesia. Acta Chir Scand 121(suppl):1–272, 1947.
147. Torres E, Alba D, Frank A, Diez-Tejedor E: Iatrogenic meningitis due to streptococcus salivarius following a spinal tap. CID 17:525–526, 1993.
148. Tourtellotte WW, Haerer AF, Heller GL, et al: Post–Lumbar Puncture Headaches. Springfield, IL, Charles C Thomas, 1964.
149. Tourtellotte WW, Henderson WG, Tucker RP, et al: A randomized, double-blind clinical trial comparing the 22 versus 26 gauge needle in the production of the post–lumbar puncture syndrome in normal individuals. Headache 12:73–78, 1972.
150. Trupp M: Stylet injury syndrome. JAMA 237:2524, 1977.
151. Turnbull DK, Shepherd DB: Post-dural puncture headache: Pathogenesis, prevention and treatment. Br J Anaesth 91(5):718–729, 2003.
152. Vadhera R, Suresh M, Gaynthri Y, et al: The relation of cerebral blood flow to postdural puncture headache. Anesthesiology 81(3A):A1168, 1994.
153. Van Crevel H, Hijdra A, deGans J: Lumbar puncture and the risk of herniation: When should we first perform CT? J Neurol 249:129–137, 2002.
154. Vandam LD, Dripps RD: Long-term follow-up of patients who received 10,098 spinal anestheticds. Syndrome of decreased intracranial pressure (headache and ocular and auditory difficulties). JAMA 161:586–591, 1956.

155. Vermeulen M, van Gijn J: The diagnosis of subarachnoid haemorrhage. J Neurol Neurosurg Psychiatry 53:365–372, 1990.
156. Vilming ST, Kloster R, Sandvik L: The importance of sex, age, needle size, height and body mass index in post-lumbar puncture headache. Cephalalgia 21:738–743, 2001.
157. Vilming ST, Kloster R, Sandvik L: When should an epidural blood patch be performed in post–lumbar puncture headache? A theoretical approach based on a cohort of 79 patients. Cephalalgia 25:523–527, 2005.
158. Vilming ST, Schrader H, Monstad I: Post-lumbar-puncture headache: The significance of body posture. A controlled study of 300 patients. Cephalalgia 8:75–78, 1988.
159. Vos PE, de Boer WA, Wurzer JAL, van Gijn J: Subdural hematoma after lumbar puncture: Two case reports and review of the literature. Clin Neurol Neurosurg 93: 127–132, 1991.
160. Welch K, Shillito J, Strand R, et al: Chiari I "malformation": An acquired disorder? J Neurosurg 55:604–609, 1982.
161. Wentworth AH: Discussion of lumbar puncture. Arch Pediatr 13:593, 1896.
162. Whiteley SM, Murphy PG, Kirollos RW, Swindells SR: Headache after dural puncture. BMJ 306:917–918, 1993.
163. Wiesel J, Rose DN, Silver AL, Sacks HS, Bernstein RH: Lumbar puncture in asymptomatic late syphilis. An analysis of the benefits and risks. Arch Intern Med 145:465–468, 1985.
164. Wynter WE: Four cases of tubercular meningitis in which paracentesis of the theca vertebralis was performed for the relief of fluid pressure. Lancet 1:981–982, 1891.
165. Ylonen P, Kokki H: Management of postdural puncture headache with epidural blood patch in children. Paediatr Anaesth 12:526–529, 2002.
166. Ylonen P, Kokki H: Management of postdural puncture headache with epidural blood patch in adolescents. Acta Anaesth Scand 46:794–798, 2002.
167. Young DA, Burney RE: Complication of myelography-transection and withdrawal of a nerve filament by the needle. N Engl J Med 285:156–157, 1971.
168. Yousry I, Forderreuther S, Moriggl B, et al: Cervical MR imaging in postural headache: MR signs and pathophysiological implications. Am J Neuroradiolol 22:1239–1250, 2001.

Chapter 40
Iatrogenic Nerve Injuries

ASA J. WILBOURN

The concept that healers could accidentally produce medical disorders in the course of diagnosing or treating their patients was recognized as early as 1700 B.C. Nonetheless, the term *iatrogenic* (from Greek: *iatros* = healer; *genic* = origin) was not used until the early twentieth century. By the 1970s, its meaning had been expanded considerably, so that it encompassed any type of adverse event experienced by any patient, caused by any health care provider, via either commission or omission.[39]

Iatrogenic peripheral nerve injuries are of two basic types: (1) those that affect the peripheral nervous system (PNS) in a generalized fashion, most often as a result of medications, and (2) those that affect it in a focal or regional manner, as a result of a multitude of devices, agents, and procedures. Only the latter type is discussed in this chapter; the former is reviewed extensively elsewhere.[31,53,55]

In regard to nongeneralized iatrogenic PNS disorders, little information is available concerning (1) their overall incidence among PNS lesions and (2) their relative incidence among the general category of iatrogenic disorders. Available data, however, suggest that they occur in rather significant numbers. Among "major peripheral nerve injuries" seen in 2000 patients at two hospitals in England over a 7-year period (1979–1986), nearly 200 (10%) were "the result of medical treatment."[6] In a more recent report from Germany, of 722 patients who underwent PNS surgery for various types of trauma, 126 (17%) had iatrogenic lesions.[83] In regard to brachial plexopathies, for which there are some comparative data, in two large series 7.4% and 9.5% were iatrogenic.[80,105]

An important point is that iatrogenic PNS injuries are not the province of any particular medical specialty. Although the majority occur perioperatively, and therefore are attributed to surgeons (especially orthopedists) and anesthesiologists, the members of almost every clinical specialty are at risk to some degree, because the etiologies are so diverse.[11,74] Many different PNS structures can be injured iatrogenically, at almost every point along their course and in a multitude of ways. Consequently, no attempt will be made in this chapter to discuss all of them. Instead, most of the more commonly encountered iatrogenic PNS lesions of this type, and their principal causes, will be reviewed.

Pathology/Pathophysiology

The large myelinated PNS axons—those that convey nerve impulses to the extrafusal muscle fibers for movement and to the spinal cord for appreciation of certain senses (vibration, position, light touch)—are quite limited in their ability, both pathologically and pathophysiologically, to respond to injury. Essentially, regardless of the type of insult (compression, traction, thermal, chemical, etc.), whenever the lesion is sufficiently severe it causes axon loss, and when it is less severe it produces focal demyelination. The small unmyelinated and lightly myelinated PNS fibers—those that conduct pain and temperature sensations to the spinal cord—have an even more limited repertoire of response to focal injury; they can either survive or undergo axon loss.[163]

Axon loss lesions affect the nerve fibers not only at the point of injury, but also along the entire segments distal to that site, due to the process of Wallerian degeneration. Initially after the focal injury, the degenerating distal segments can still conduct impulses, so there is a conduction block at the lesion site (labeled *axon discontinuity conduction block*). Within several days, however, degeneration is sufficiently advanced along the distal stumps that nerve impulses cannot traverse them, and the pathophysiological process characteristic of axon loss, that is, conduction failure, has supervened.[161]

Focal demyelinating lesions, in contrast to axon loss lesions, affect the nerve fibers solely at the injury site, without causing alterations along the distal segments. Focal demyelinating injuries often result in a disturbance of conduction, which is limited to the damaged segment of the axons and manifested as either conduction block or conduction slowing, depending upon the degree of myelin compromise (conduction block being a more severe process). With demyelinating conduction block, the nerve impulses cannot pass through the lesion site, so, from a functional point of view, the process is identical to conduction failure. Conversely, with conduction slowing, all the impulses ultimately reach their destinations, although, as they traverse the injured segment of nerve to do so, they are somewhat delayed.[161,163]

Of the three types of pathophysiology that occur with focal nerve lesions, only two of them, conduction failure and conduction block (due either to early denervation or, far more often, to focal demyelination), are significantly related to clinical symptoms: both can cause weakness, as well as impairment of certain sensory modalities (position, vibration, light touch), depending upon which type of nerve fibers, motor or sensory, is involved. Because conduction failure resulting from axon loss also affects unmyelinated axons, it produces deficits in pain and temperature sensation as well. In contrast to the substantial clinical changes described above, focal demyelinating slowing per se causes no clinical manifestations, motor or sensory, unless different degrees of slowing are present along different axons at the lesion site. In these instances, any functions that require action potentials to pass along the nerve fibers in synchronized volleys (e.g., vibration appreciation) may be compromised.[92,161,163]

Nearly all abrupt-onset focal nerve injuries and most gradual-onset ones cause either axon loss (with resulting conduction failure) or demyelinating conduction block. There are a few exceptions. Some subacute-onset ulnar neuropathies along the elbow segment (UN-ES) present with demyelinating focal slowing. The most conspicuous chronic focal nerve lesion that manifests demyelinating focal slowing, however, is median neuropathy distal to the wrist, or carpal tunnel syndrome (CTS).[33,161]

During the electrodiagnostic (EDX) examination, on nerve conduction studies (NCSs) both conduction block and conduction failure affect the amplitudes of the evoked responses, the former on stimulating proximal but not distal to the lesion, the latter on stimulating at any point along the nerve, either proximal to, at, or distal to the lesion. Conversely, demyelinating conduction slowing affects principally those components of the NCSs that measure the rate of impulse transmission, that is, the latencies and conduction velocities (CVs), and only when the involved nerve segment is between the stimulating and recording points. The latencies and CVs also can be affected to a modest degree by very severe lesions causing conduction block or conduction failure because of loss of conduction along the fastest-conducting fibers. However, the conduction slowing in these circumstances does not occur with sufficient consistency for diagnostic purposes. In many instances, more than 90% of the axons of a peripheral nerve may be either dead or have their conduction blocked, and yet the speed of conduction along the remaining fibers is still within the normal range.[161]

During the needle electrode examination (needle electromyography [EMG]) portion of the EDX assessment, both conduction block and conduction failure cause the voluntarily activated motor unit potentials (MUPs) to fire in reduced numbers on maximal patient effort, the degree of MUP dropout reflecting the severity of the lesion (i.e., the percentage of axons affected). In addition, fibrillation potentials are seen with axon loss injuries. (They often occur with predominantly demyelinating conduction block lesions as well due to coexisting axon loss involving a relatively small number of the fibers.) Moreover, with axon loss lesions of more than 5–6 months duration remodeling of the MUPs occurs, resulting in *chronic neurogenic MUP* changes. Focal demyelinating slowing, in contrast, has no effect on the needle EMG.[161,163]

Most iatrogenic peripheral nerve lesions are abrupt in onset. Moreover, they usually are severe enough that when they involve motor axons, clinical weakness is evident. Consequently, the pathology/pathophysiology underlying most of these injuries is axon loss/conduction failure or demyelination/conduction block. For practical purposes, therefore, excluding some perioperative UN-ES, demyelinating conduction slowing is not likely to be seen with any iatrogenic nerve lesion.[160]

Based on the above, it is obvious that on NCSs it is the amplitudes of the responses, and not their latencies or CVs, that are helpful in the diagnosis and localization of most iatrogenic nerve lesions.

Cranial Nerves

Although several cranial nerves, or their branches, can sustain iatrogenic injuries, only two of them do so with some frequency: the 7th, or facial, nerve (CN VII) and the 11th, or spinal accessory, nerve (CN XI). For this reason, only lesions of these two cranial nerves will be discussed in detail, although lesions of other nerves will be reviewed briefly.

Facial Nerve

The pathway that most of the facial nerve fibers traverse as they pass from the brain stem to the periphery can be divided into three segments: (1) intracranial, (2) infratemporal (i.e., within the temporal bone), and (3) extracranial. Iatrogenic facial nerve injuries can occur along any of these segments.[110]

Only a minority of iatrogenic lesions affecting this nerve occur intracranially. The most common cause for them is excision of acoustic neuromas. The principal site of iatrogenic facial neuropathies is infratemporal, and the most common cause is mastoidectomy. Often cholesteatomas are present, the result of chronic otitis media.[50,110] Other etiologies for infratemporal lesions include exostosis removal, tympanoplasty, stapes surgery, and removal of congenital deformities.[28,50] Many of these processes seriously distort the anatomy, thereby obscuring surgical landmarks; this situation is particularly likely to be encountered during revision surgery.[28,49,110,156] Extracranial facial nerve injuries result from a variety of causes, the most common surgical one being parotidectomy.[110] Branch lesions of the facial nerve characteristically occur with some extracranial injuries. The temporal branch may sustain damage during rhytidectomies.[86] The mandibular branch, specifically its marginal mandibular portion, can be injured during carotid endarterectomies and also by pressure exerted at the angle of the jaw by anesthesiologists during airway maintenance.[108]

Both immediate and delayed (up to 7 or more days after surgery) types of postoperative facial nerve involvement have been reported. However, as with almost all perioperative nerve injuries, the delay in these instances may refer to physician recognition of these complications, rather than to their actual onset.[41,49,50,156]

The principal clinical deficit seen with these injuries is paresis or paralysis of the facial muscles innervated by the damaged facial nerve fibers. These lesions may be partial or complete; the latter are of most concern, not only because the disfigurement and deficit are more severe, but also because recovery is less likely. Following chronic ear surgery, immediate facial weakness may represent the effects of the local anesthetic and resolve promptly.[58] However, weakness that persists for more than a day is caused by either demyelinating conduction block or axon loss, and many cases of the latter are due to nerve transection. Consequently, in marked contrast to idiopathic facial paralysis (Bell's palsy), in which the pathophysiology typically is conduction block (labeled *neurapraxia* clinically), with many of these lesions the pathophysiology is conduction failure, the result of fifth-degree neurotmesis axon loss lesions.[128,139,163] Consequently, reoperation and surgical repair of the facial nerve often is necessary. Under these circumstances, recovery frequently is incomplete and other *reanimation* surgical procedures are required.[49,58,110,156]

As with most PNS lesions, the EDX examination can be helpful in determining whether the pathology of the facial nerve injury is demyelination or axon loss and, if axon loss, its severity. The amplitudes of the facial motor NCS responses provide this information.[161] (In the otolaryngology literature, apparently because the authors were unaware of the voluminous material—including terminology—already available on the topic in the EMG literature, the standard facial motor NCS acquired a variety of names, including *electroneuronography* [ENoG], *neuromyography*, and *evoked electromyography*.)[41,131] Following presumably total axon loss lesions, needle EMG may reveal not only that some facial nerve fibers were spared, but also that reinnervation is occurring several weeks before it becomes clinically evident. It does the latter by demonstrating a few *reinnervational* MUPs in the paralyzed muscles.[33,163]

Vagus and Spinal Accessory Nerves

During the anterior cervical surgical approach to the cervical spine, popularized by Cloward, branches from the vagus cranial nerve (among others) can be damaged. The most common injury affects the recurrent laryngeal nerve, producing ipsilateral vocal fold paralysis, which manifests clinically as postsurgical dysphonia: hoarseness, cough, breathiness, and vocal fatigue. In most cases the right side is affected, the same side as the surgical approach. Although this approach is more popular than the left-sided one, the marked preponderance of right-sided involvement is attributed to the right recurrent laryngeal nerve, compared to the left, being shorter in overall length, having a shorter vertical rise, and traveling a more oblique course. The first two characteristics make it more susceptible to traction during the procedure, whereas the third one causes it to be more vulnerable to direct trauma. This postoperative deficit has been described as the single largest complication of anterior cervical spine surgery. It is a potent instigator of litigation. Because the pathology typically is axon loss, the symptoms are permanent in the majority of patients who experience them.[62,106,134,159]

Another complication of anterior cervical spine surgery caused by injury of cranial nerve fibers is postoperative dysphasia. This results from mechanical disruption of the fine nerve filaments passing to the pharyngeal constrictor muscles from the pharyngeal plexus (composed of branches from the glossopharyngeal, vagus, and spinal accessory cranial nerves). This complication also appears to be more prevalent with the right-sided approach.[15,134,160]

Spinal Accessory Nerve

After it becomes extracranial, the spinal portion of the spinal accessory nerve descends into the neck, in close proximity to the internal jugular vein. It passes deep to, and innervates, the sternocleidomastoid muscle and then surfaces on the posterior border of that muscle, at the junction of its upper and middle thirds. Next, the nerve passes obliquely posteroinferiorly in the posterior triangle of the neck, to reach the upper trapezius muscle, which it innervates. It then continues on an inferior course deep to that muscle. While traversing the posterior triangle of the neck, the spinal accessory nerve is quite vulnerable, being covered only by skin and fascia.[78,88,112,168]

Spinal accessory neuropathies are uncommon. Unfortunately, iatrogenic injury is the leading cause for them. In Kahn and Birch's series of 306 operated iatrogenic PNS lesions, accessory nerve injuries were the second most common: 53 (17%).[74] In one recently published surgical series by Kim and coworkers, dealing with 111 patients who had spinal accessory nerve lesions of all types, 103 of them (93%) had iatrogenic lesions.[77] The spinal accessory nerve can be irreparably damaged by radiation and by being resected during radial neck dissections. In both instances, these injuries are considered anticipated side effects rather than complications.[122,135] It can also be traumatized in the more superior neck, where it is near the sternocleidomastoid muscle, during several different procedures, most surgical, including carotid endarterectomies, cannulation of the internal jugular vein, removal of neck cysts, sternomastoid denervation to treat spasmodic torticollis, and placement of ventriculojugular shunts.[42,56,135] However, far more often, it is injured as it traverses the posterior triangle of the neck, typically during minor operations, such as biopsies or excisions of lymph nodes or other small masses (*lumpectomies*). In this neck region, the nerve is contiguous to a chain of lymph nodes and is quite near a branch of the transverse cervical artery. The exact cause of these lesions varies, but at least five mechanisms are possible: traction, transection, ligation (suturing), cauterization, and crushing (secondary to clamping).[116,168] The last three primarily occur because the nearby artery can be inadvertently punctured or transected during the procedure.

Denervation of the trapezius muscle causes drooping of the shoulder, weakness of shoulder elevation, and weakness of lateral elevation of the upper limb. Shoulder pain sometimes occurs; frequently it does not develop for several weeks.[79] One of the more impressive findings with these injuries, and the one that often first calls the attention of the patients to them, is the severe wasting of the upper trapezius muscle. This alters the contour of the neck and shoulder, particularly on the frontal view: the normal slope of the neck to the shoulder is lost, resulting in marked asymmetry.[78,88,168] The time interval between operation and the clinical recognition of these lesions varies greatly, from immediately to several months, depending mainly on whether pain is present and when it appears.

The pathology of these injuries almost invariably is axon loss, with resulting conduction failure. Only those lesions caused by two of the five possible etiologies—traction and crush—have any realistic possibility of resolving spontaneously. Certainly, transected or sutured nerves, and probably also those cauterized, are very unlikely to recover without surgical intervention.[160] Jensen and Rockwood pooled the data from a half dozen series and noted that only 7 of 62 patients (11%) recovered spontaneously and in only 2 of those (3% of the total) was the recovery complete.[64] These nerve lesions, similar to PNS lesions in general, should be operated on within the first 3 or, at most, 4 months after injury for optimal improvement to occur.[5,70,79,88,109,112,168] Among the large number of patients—111—recently reported by Kim and coworkers who underwent surgical repair of these lesions, more than three-fourths of them experienced favorable functional outcomes.[77]

The EDX examination readily demonstrates that these are axon loss injuries. Typically, the spinal accessory motor NCS response, recording from the upper trapezius muscle, is very low in amplitude or unelicitable on the involved side, while needle EMG of the affected trapezius muscle reveals fibrillation potentials and either absence or marked reduction in the number of MUPs that can be activated.

Roots

The roots, the very proximal portions of the PNS, may sustain iatrogenic injuries in a variety of ways. Relatively rare causes include direct trauma by needles inserted into the epidural or intraspinal canal regions for diagnostic or therapeutic purposes, chemicals injected for the same reasons, and radiation. The majority of iatrogenic radiculopathies, however, are related to various operative procedures performed on the spine and its contents. The root injury (or injuries) can occur preoperatively (because of delay in surgical decompression), intraoperatively, or postoperatively. Two generalizations are possible: (1) In most instances, the spinal cord is even more sensitive to the injurious agent than the roots, so often both PNS structures sustain damage together; nonetheless, at times, only the roots are affected. (2) Overall, the lumbosacral roots are affected more often than the cervical roots, and this increased incidence is independent of the fact that lumbar surgery is far more common than cervical surgery.[62,134]

Iatrogenic radiculopathies related to surgery may be direct or indirect. Direct causes include contusions, retraction (traction), lacerations, and electrocauterization. Direct injuries are more likely to occur during repeat operations, especially when extensive dissection of epidural scarring is required. Indirect causes, usually compressive, include postoperative hematomas; epidural abcesses; pseudomeningoceles due to dural tears; retained sponges; epidural scarring; impingement by hardware, particularly screws; and adhesive arachnoiditis. A few compressive causes essentially are unique to the specific surgical region, such as extrusion of bone grafts following cervical interbody fusions, and compression by autogenous fat graft replacements and failure to sufficiently relieve lumbar canal stenosis after lumbosacral procedures.[62,100,134]

Most of these radiculopathies are axon loss in type, and not all are amenable to surgical treatment, so prevention is stressed in the literature. A notable exception regarding underlying pathophysiology is the injury that results from pedicle screw malpositioning: it may be neurapractic in nature.[134]

One iatrogenic root lesion that merits special mention is the C5 radiculopathy that sometimes follows surgery for cervical compression myelopathy. Typically, the underlying problem is cervical spondylosis or ossification of the posterior longitudinal ligament. The surgical procedures performed include anterior interbody fusions (such as the Cloward procedure), subtotal corpectomies with bone grafts, multilevel cervical laminectomies, and cervical laminoplasties. Thus, both anterior and posterior approaches are responsible, particularly the latter. Following surgery, both radicular and spinal cord dysfunction can occur. Regarding the former, characteristically the C5 root is affected, with the motor component preferentially involved. Clinically, patients present with marked weakness of the deltoid and, more variably, the biceps muscles. The onset of weakness usually occurs after an initial phase of improvement, lasting several (4–6) hours to several (6–7) days. This delayed surgical complication is attributed to the malalignment of the spine related to graft complications, and especially to traction on the tethered extradural portion of the root caused by shifting (specifically posterior migration and expansion) of the spinal cord after decompression, combined with the relatively short length of the C5 root. The shoulder weakness caused by these lesions reportedly resolves, generally within 1 year of onset.[23,62,169]

The EDX examination of these root injuries characteristically reveals substantial axon loss (usually much more than is seen with the typical single compressive radiculopathy). This manifests, at least with recent-onset lesions, as abundant fibrillation potentials and prominent MUP dropout, along with low amplitude, or occasionally even absent, motor NCS responses when recording from muscles in the affected myotome. The sensory NCS responses in the involved dermatome, however, usually are normal—as they are with nearly all compressive radiculopathies—because the lesion is compromising the primary sensory root proximal to the dorsal root ganglia. An exception is the C5 root lesion that presents after surgery for cervical compression myelopathy; typically, it is due to extradural (i.e., postganglionic) injury of the root. Ironically, this cannot be demonstrated on sensory NCSs, because of the five roots composing the brachial plexus, no sensory NCS technique has been devised for assessing this root.[163]

Phrenic Nerve

Originating from the C3 through C5 spinal cord segments, the phrenic nerve is the most important derivative of the cervical plexus. It can sustain iatrogenic injury in the neck—for example, during internal jugular vein catheterization.[137] Far more often, however, it is damaged as it traverses the thorax to reach the diaphragm. Iatrogenic lesions, sometimes permanent, have occurred during a variety of intrathoracic operations performed on infants and young children, such as for repair of various congenital anomalies, especially around the esophagus.[93] Probably the single most common cause, however, is open heart surgery. While several etiological mechanisms have been proposed for these lesions, most authorities attribute them to hypothermic damage caused by the use of topical cold cardioplegia: iced saline slush placed into the pericardium to reduce myocardial oxygen consumption. Usually, the left phrenic nerve is affected. The symptoms range from none to relatively severe, the most common being lower lobe atelectasis and an elevated hemidiaphragm.[22,27,123,155,167]

In many patients, the lesions resolve within the first few months, consistent with demyelinating conduction block. However, in others they persist much longer, occasionally indefinitely, indicating that the underlying pathology is axon loss. These injuries have their greatest impact on patients with chronic obstructive pulmonary disease who undergo open heart surgery. Because their pulmonary reserve is already compromised, the addition of paralysis of a hemidiaphragm can have significant adverse clinical consequences.[18]

Phrenic nerve injury can be diagnosed by chest radiographs, diaphragmatic ultrasonography, phrenic NCSs, and diaphragmatic needle EMG.[27] Unfortunately, all of these techniques lack optimal sensitivity. The value of phrenic motor NCSs is substantially reduced for two reasons: (1) the responses consistently are quite small (usually less than 2 mV in amplitude) even in normal persons, because there is considerable distance between the recording electrodes and the diaphragm; (2) the side-to-side amplitudes obtained in normal persons show marked variations; as a result, the responses recorded from the uninvolved sides with possible unilateral partial phrenic nerve injuries cannot be used for comparison purposes.[140] Some investigators have attempted to use phrenic motor distal latencies for diagnosis.[27,123,167] However, the problem obviously is one of diaphragmatic weakness, and demyelinating conduction slowing does not cause weakness. Consequently, the prolonged phrenic distal latencies seen in these instances must be due to loss of impulse transmission along the fastest-conducting fibers, the result of either severe axon loss or demyelinating conduction block, rather than to demyelinating conduction slowing. For this reason, prolonged phrenic motor latencies are seen only with incomplete lesions and only then with some of the latter.[161,163]

Brachial Plexus

The brachial plexus is one of the largest, and certainly the most complex, of the PNS structures. It is also quite vulnerable to trauma. Most of the traumatic injuries it sustains, however, are not iatrogenic. Thus, among 100 consecutive lesions seen by Dubuisson and Kline, over a 3.5-year period, only 9 (9%) were iatrogenic.[32] Nonetheless, in one series concerned with perioperative nerve lesions, brachial plexopathies were the most common.[113]

The brachial plexus derives from the C5 through T1 roots and has the shape of a skewed triangle with its apex in the axilla. It has five components: five roots (C5-T1); three trunks (upper, middle, lower); six divisions (three anterior, three posterior); three cords (lateral, medial, posterior); and three to five terminal nerves (median, ulnar, radial, and sometimes musculocutaneous and axillary); the number varies with the reference source. Clinically, the brachial plexus is subdivided into two regions, supraclavicular and infraclavicular, based on the fact that when the upper extremity is at the side, the clavicle overlies its divisions. Thus, supraclavicular plexopathies involve the roots and trunks, whereas infraclavicular plexopathies affect the cords and terminal nerves.[162]

With one exception, the various iatrogenic brachial plexopathies are discussed in detail in Chapter 18, so the characteristics of each will not be reviewed here. Iatrogenic supraclavicular brachial plexopathies include obstetric paralysis, classic postoperative paralysis, post–median sternotomy lesions, and post–disputed thoracic outlet syndrome (TOS) surgery plexopathies;[14,20,44,45,59,61,99,103,105,113,117,126,129,144,145,157,162] they have also resulted from interscalene regional blocks, biopsies of masses at the base of the neck (often benign neoplasms of the upper trunk), cannulation of the internal jugular vein, and upper dorsal sympathectomies.[114,162] Noteworthy is that while only a few perioperative supraclavicular brachial plexopathies have occurred with sufficient frequency to merit a particular name (e.g., *post–median sternotomy lesions*), many more are encountered involving various portions of the roots and trunks. Iatrogenic infraclavicular brachial plexopathies include those occurring during shoulder arthroscopy and arthroplasty, glenohumeral reconstruction procedures, biopsies of axillary masses, transaxillary arterial bypass procedures, removal of infected axillary sweat glands, and following both axillary arteriograms and axillary regional blocks (the last two producing medial brachial compartment syndromes).[59,133,142,143,162] Infraclavicular lesions have also been caused by both surgical and nonsurgical compromise of the costoclavicular space. These include operations to correct Sprengel's deformity and to remove the midportion of the clavicle in adults. Probably the most common cause, however, has been nonsurgical: the ineffective treatment of midshaft clavicular fractures in adults using figure of eight bandages. This can result in displacement of fracture fragments and, later, in both nonunions and malunions (the latter often manifested as a hypertrophic callus at the fracture site (the *exuberant callus syndrome*).[52,71,96,162] (In Chapter 18, some of these are discussed under "Traumatic Thoracic Outlet Syndrome") Other nonsurgical causes for iatrogenic infraclavicular brachial plexopathies include crutch use and closed reductions of humeral head dislocations.[162] One iatrogenic brachial plexus lesion not discussed elsewhere is radiation-induced brachial plexopathy.

Radiation-Induced Brachial Plexopathy

These plexopathies typically are infraclavicular lesions, at least initially. Most of the patients are women who received radiation to lymph nodes in the axillary chain for breast cancer a few months to many years earlier. Recent reports indicate that patients who have received radiation are always at risk of developing this complication, regardless of the amount of time that has passed, such as 30 years.[66] One of the first symptoms is persistent paresthesias in the index or middle fingers. As time passes, the sensory disturbance spreads and weakness appears, the latter usually beginning most often in the pronator teres. Thus, both the early sensory and motor symptoms are in the distribution of the lateral cord or median terminal nerve. Once weakness appears, motor NCSs show prominent conduction blocks along the affected axons. Some patients, a distinct minority in our experience, experience severe pain as well. The disorder may plateau over varying periods but slow progression is the rule, usually leading ultimately to a useless arm, caused by marked sensory ataxia, and occasionally to a completely flail arm due to total denervation.[54,85,162]

There is no effective treatment for this type of brachial plexopathy, surgical or otherwise. This is particularly frustrating for two reasons: (1) until very late in their course, most of the deficits present are produced by a potentially reversible lesion, focal demyelination, and (2) these lesions are the by-product of earlier successful treatment of a potentially fatal disorder (i.e., carcinoma or lymphoma).[162]

Even in rather advanced cases, demyelinating conduction blocks usually are readily demonstrable on supraclavicular stimulation during motor NCSs while recording from median, musculocutaneous, ulnar, and radial nerve-innervated muscles. (It is pertinent to note that the demyelinating conduction blocks that occur with postradiation brachial plexopathies have a far different prognosis—that is, dismal—than those that follow acute injury; consequently, the clinical deficits they cause should not be referred to as *neurapraxia*.) Although the motor NCS responses often persist with advanced lesions, albeit low in amplitude, the sensory NCS responses eventually become unelicitable. Needle EMG shows fibrillation potentials, fasciculation potentials, and sometimes myokymic discharges, MUP loss, and, as time passes, progressively more prominent chronic neurogenic MUP changes.[166]

The neuroimaging study of choice is magnetic resonance imaging. Typically it reveals rather diffuse enhancement, unfortunately at times it cannot distinguish these changes from those caused by cancer.[160,162]

Lumbosacral Plexus

The lumbosacral plexus (or *pelvic plexus*) derives from the L1 through S4 roots. It supplies the hip girdle, lower limb, and pelvic floor. Traumatic injuries of the lumbosacral plexus of all types are quite uncommon compared to those of the brachial plexus. The principal iatrogenic lesions affecting this PNS plexus are maternal intrapartum lumbosacral plexopathy, injection injuries of various types, retroperitoneal hemorrhage in patients who are anticoagulated, and pelvic surgical procedures.[160] These are reviewed in Chapter 18. Radiation is another cause, however, not discussed elsewhere.

Radiation-Induced Lumbosacral Plexopathy

These lesions differ in many respects from their counterparts that affect the brachial plexus, beginning with the fact that the radiation usually was administered to treat pelvic neoplasms (e.g., lymphomas, genitourinary cancers) that relatively seldom invade the lumbosacral plexus directly (e.g., colorectal cancers). Also, these lesions frequently are bilateral, in part, because they are more likely to develop after intracavity irradiation (used to treat cervical and endometrial carcinomas) than external beam irradiation. Moreover, they often present with solely motor symptoms, specifically progressive limb weakness. Finally, the symptoms they cause may permanently stabilize at some point. In several other respects, however, their manifestations parallel those of radiation-induced brachial plexopathies. Thus, their incidence is related to the radiation dose; they may first become symptomatic years (more than three decades) after radiation therapy; paresthesias are a relatively common symptom; and while pain may occur at some time during their course in approximately half of the patients, usually it is not a prominent feature. Another similar feature is, regrettably, that there is no effective treatment. In regard to laboratory assessment, the EDX findings are identical to those seen with radiation-induced plexus lesions: (1) on NCSs, progressively lower amplitude motor and sensory responses; (2) on needle EMG, fibrillation potentials, fasciculation potentials, myokymic potentials, MUP loss, and progressively more prominent chronic neurogenic MUP changes, except that the changes frequently are bilateral. Neuroimaging studies (computed tomography, magnetic resonance imaging) apparently are much more effective in separating radiation damage from neoplasms than they are with brachial plexus lesions, presumably because often no abnormalities are noted in the lumbosacral plexus region when radiation is responsible.[30,124,154]

Mononeuropathies

Long Thoracic, Suprascapular, Axillary, and Musculocutaneous Nerves

The peripheral nerves that innervate the shoulder and upper arm regions sustain iatrogenic injuries less often than those that supply the forearm and hand, in relative as well as absolute terms. Thus, there are no instances of such lesions involving any of these nerves among the 126 iatrogenic cases in the surgical series reported by Kretschner and coworkers and only 11 instances (4%) (six musculocutaneous, five axillary) among the 306 iatrogenic neuropathies identified on 291 patients at operation by Khan and Birch.[74,83] However, 2 (4.3%) of the 46 pediatric upper extremity mononeuropathy cases seen by Jones were iatrogenic in nature.[67] Most of the lesions of this type occur during surgical procedures. The specific operations during which each of these nerves is most at risk are as follows: long thoracic nerve—first rib resections, scalenotomies, scalenectomies, thoracotomies, mastectomies, chest tube insertions, axillary node dissections, and transaxillary sympathectomies; suprascapular nerve—distal clavicular resections, rotator cuff tear repairs, radical neck dissections, and shoulder arthroscopies; axillary nerve—rotator cuff tear repairs, shoulder reconstruction procedures, shoulder arthroscopies, mastectomies, and other breast operations; musculocutaneous nerve—glenohumeral stabilization procedures, coracoid process transfer to treat clavicle instability, shoulder reconstruction procedures, and shoulder arthroscopies. (Of all these proximal nerves, the musculocutaneous is the one most frequently damaged during glenohumeral stabilization surgery performed to correct anterior shoulder dislocations.) Delayed injuries of these and other peripheral nerves have resulted from pseudoaneuryms forming when axillary arteries have been damaged by screws which came loose long after glenohumeral stabilization procedures.[17,24,40,48,81,83,89,120] Unrelated to a single surgical procedure, malpositioning on the operating table can produce both axillary and musculocutaneous neuropathies.[48,160,164] The claim that such malpositioning often causes long thoracic neuropathies[146] must be viewed with some caution, however, because this nerve is the one most frequently damaged by neuralgic amyotrophy, and few surgeons are aware that one of the major precipitating events for that disorder is an operative procedure of any type.

The lateral antebrachial cutaneous nerve, the sensory termination of the musculocutaneous nerve, can sustain iatrogenic injuries in isolation. (In fact, of all the nerves so far discussed, this is the only one in which the majority of focal lesions of it are iatrogenic.) Most of these occur near the elbow, and most are of the open type, even though some are not due strictly to operations per se. These include placement of arteriovenous shunts, insertion of the distal interlocking screw during humeral nailing, phlebotomies, and arterial catheterizations. The nerve lesions themselves most often occur during the procedures, but some are delayed in appearance when they are secondary to initial hematoma formation.[4,9,48,57,125,164]

The relatively rare nonoperative causes for iatrogenic injuries of these proximal peripheral nerves include chiropractic manipulation and use of a Milwaukee brace (long thoracic nerve), reduction of humeral head dislocations (axillary nerve), deep intramuscular injections into the posterior deltoid region (axillary nerve), use of tight figure of eight bandaging to treat clavicular fractures, as well as body casting (musculocutaneous nerve), and the medial brachial fascial compartment syndrome (axillary and especially musculocutaneous nerves)[48,67,142,143,164] (see below). The lateral antebrachial cutaneous nerve occasionally is injured by tourniquet paralysis. This occurs only in unusually severe cases and is always accompanied by simultaneous injuries to the radial, medial, and ulnar nerves.[158]

Radial Nerve

The radial nerve is a short nerve, extending only from the distal end of the axilla to the elbow before terminating as the posterior interosseous and superficial radial sensory nerves (PIN, SRSN). The preferential sites for iatrogenic injuries along the radial nerve and its terminal branches are as follows: radial nerve—at or near the spiral groove (RN-SG); posterior interosseous nerve—near the elbow; superficial radial nerve—near the wrist. In Khan and Birch's series of operated iatrogenic nerve lesions, injuries of the radial nerve and its two terminal branched were the most common, constituting 27% (55 of 206) of upper extremity and shoulder girdle lesions and 18% of all 306 lesions.[74]

Regarding lesions of the radial nerve proper, there are several iatrogenic causes. The nerve can be injured by various procedures used to treat fractures of the humerus. These include its being traumatized during placement of the distal locking screw during intramedullary nailing; entrapped at the fracture site following manipulation; crushed beneath the metal plate used to stabilize the fracture; and compressed by the callus that later forms at the site. In the last situation, the weakness that results is labeled *secondary paralysis* since it develops after, rather than at the time of, the fracture.[1,2,24,36,73,164] Improper positioning during surgical procedures, producing prolonged pressure on the nerve, is another cause. In two separate series, RN-SG was the third most common focal neuropathy seen in these situations.[29,113] Prolonged external compression also can be responsible for the development of these lesions in comatose patients; bilateral radial neuropathies, which are rarely encountered, have been observed under these circumstances.[101] With upper extremity tourniquet paralysis, there are two main presentations: radial nerve lesions alone and *tri-nerve paralysis*, with the radial, median, and ulnar nerves all injured at the tourniquet site at the midarm level.[84,158] Iatrogenic injuries of the RN-SG also result from misplaced intramuscular injections, specifically those intended for the deltoid muscle but given several inches farther distally along the limb, at the spiral groove.[137,158,164] These are relatively uncommon compared to sciatic nerve injection injuries. Nonetheless, 56 cases were reported in one published article,[43] and this etiology was responsible for 9% of the 81 upper arm radial neuropathies that required operation by Kline and Hudson.[79] (The mechanism of injury in these cases is similar to that responsible for sciatic injection injuries, and will be discussed below with that entity.) Causalgic pain, along with weakness and patchy sensory loss, is a near-constant symptom with injection injuries.[24]

The underlying pathology of iatrogenic RN-SG is variable and is determined by the etiology. Those pathologies associated with treatment of humeral fractures and with injections invariably are axon loss in type and often are very severe. While some of these, particularly among the fracture group, improve with conservative therapy, others often require surgical repair for optimal nerve regeneration. Conversely, those resulting from external compression, caused either by improper positioning during surgical procedures or by tourniquet use, characteristically consist of demyelinating conduction block. Consequently, recovery ultimately is complete with conservative treatment.[24,164] However, the RN-SG caused by tourniquet use, unlike that due to other types of compression, can persist for many months, occasionally nearly a year.[158] Regardless of their duration, surgery is not indicated for them unless substantial axon loss coexists (which is readily determined by the EDX examination); this rarely occurs.

If these lesions are extensive, the EDX examination can provide valuable information regarding their location, pathophysiology, and severity. Radial motor NCSs, recording extensor forearm, as well as radial sensory NCSs are necessary. Unlike many other main trunk peripheral nerve lesions, axon loss radial neuropathies can be localized quite satisfactorily by needle EMG because of the number of motor branches that arise from the nerve and their location. Nonetheless, needle EMG cannot establish the dominant type of pathophysiology present.[164]

Iatrogenic injuries of the PIN usually affect it near its origin, at the elbow region, and most are surgical. These include lipoma removals, resections of the humeral head, progressive scarring following humeral head resections, insertion or removal of metal plates for fracture treatment, and elbow arthroscopy. Historically (nearly 150 years ago), the first recorded nerve injection injuries affected this nerve, since the injection site was the extensor muscles of the proximal forearm. (The medication injected was ether.)[24,83,158,164] This nerve can also be damaged by casts.[83]

The SRSN sustains most of its traumatic injuries, including iatrogenic ones, distally near the wrist. The main iatrogenic causes are various operations, including K-wire placement, removal of ganglia and metal plates, and particularly tenosynovectomy to treat deQuervain's disease.[24,83,164] One nonsurgical cause produces a substantial number of serious injuries: venipuncture. Typically, this occurs at the lateral aspect of the distal wrist on attempts to cannulate the nearby vein. Based on their dissections of 33 cadaver forearms and wrists, Vialle and coworkers recently presented very compelling evidence that it is impossible to define a *safe zone* for venipuncture in this region because the crossing sites (one to three) of the SRSN over the cephalic vein tributaries are so variable.[147] In any case, these are a potent source of unremitting pain (and litigation).

The more distal fibers of both the PIN and the SRSN are injured with ischemic monomelic neuropathy.[160]

Median Nerve

Iatrogenic median nerve lesions occur principally at two locations: the elbow region and the wrist (i.e., at the carpal tunnel). Those at the elbow most often result from invasive diagnostic or therapeutic punctures in the antecubital fossa. These include venipunctures for blood drawing and infusions, as well as arterial punctures, both with needles and cannulas, for several functions, including intra-arterial blood gas measurements and cardiac catheterizations.[24,158,164] Two studies involving large populations of blood donors have indicated that serious neurological injuries (i.e., those that require physician consultation) have an incidence of approximately 1/20,000 to 1/26,700.[4,107] Various components of the median nerve can be injured during these procedures, either directly by the needle or indirectly due to formation of hematomas or pseudoaneurysms secondary to blood extravasation from the punctured blood vessel. Both the lateral and medial antebrachial cutaneous nerves are also at risk; they can be injured singly or in association with the median nerve during these procedures.[4,57] In our experience, with these procedures the main trunk of the median nerve, the motor branches supplying the pronator teres and flexor carpi radialis muscles, and the proximal anterior interosseous nerve can all be damaged, either singly or in various combinations. Almost invariably the underlying pathology is axon loss, at least when the symptoms are of more than a few days' duration. Typically, the main trunk lesions are incomplete; however, they frequently result in persistent causalgic pain in a median nerve sensory distribution in the hand.[79] Because the complaints are disproportionately severe compared to the clinical findings, patients may be labeled *symptom exaggerators* by physicians unfamiliar with this type of lesion. In this regard, Weir Mitchell observed almost 150 years ago that incomplete median nerve lesions at or proximal to the elbow are one of the two most common instigators of upper extremity causalgia, the other being incomplete brachial plexus lesions.[138]

Surgical exploration is indicated with many iatrogenic median neuropathies at the elbow. Even incomplete main trunk injuries may benefit from neurolysis for pain relief.[79]

The EDX examination can be quite helpful in determining the distribution and severity of axon loss present, particularly if median sensory NCS responses are recorded from the thumb, index finger, and middle finger, and if muscles innervated by both the main trunk and the anterior interosseous branch are assessed on needle EMG.

Iatrogenic median nerve injuries also can complicate the treatment of CTS. On occasion, during attempted injection of corticosteroid into the carpal tunnel, the medication is inadvertently injected into the median nerve itself.[91,141] The axon loss lesions produced are of variable severity, but at times they are very severe main trunk injuries. The majority of iatrogenic median nerve lesions at the wrist, however, are sustained during surgical release of the transverse carpal ligament. These have occurred with both open and endoscopic carpal tunnel release. Most of the open injuries are attributed to inappropriate incisions; small transverse incisions, at or near the distal wrist crease, appear to have an unusually high association with these complications.[19,72] Partial or complete severance of the following structures have occurred: (1) main trunk of median nerve, (2) palmar cutaneous branch, (3) recurrent motor branch, and (4) common and proper digital nerves.[8,72,79,90,102]

In addition to the above, the median nerve may be injured secondarily, in the postoperative period, following carpal tunnel release, by being anteriorly displaced during wrist flexion.[72] Another cause for these lesions at the wrist is removal of ganglia.[83]

Most iatrogenic median neuropathies at the wrist require reoperation, often with nerve repair, for optimal recovery.

Because these lesions cause axon loss, rather than the demyelinating focal slowing that typically is seen with CTS until late in its course, the EDX examination often can help determine both their location and their severity. (The major exceptions in this regard are the palmar cutaneous neuropathies, since that nerve is not assessed in most EMG laboratories.)

The median nerve can also be injured, along with the ulnar and radial nerves, with both tourniquet paralysis and ischemic monomelic neuropathy.[160]

Ulnar Nerve

Although iatrogenic lesions can occur along any portion of the ulnar nerve, for a variety of reasons most occur perioperatively and affect the elbow segment of the nerve (UN-ES). In two studies of perioperative nerve lesions in general, the ulnar nerve was the second and the fourth most involved nerve, respectively, after the brachial plexus in one series and the brachial plexus, radial nerve, and peroneal nerve in the other series.[29,113] Perioperative ulnar nerve lesions occur at an approximate rate of 1/2700 procedures performed under sedation or anesthesia (cardiac surgery excluded), and 9% are bilateral.[153] For many years, it has been assumed that these nerve injuries occur intraoperatively as the result of malpositioning of the patient on the operating table, inadequate padding of the elbow, or both.[13,25,113] Two precipitating causes have been mentioned with some frequency: first, having the forearm supinated during the procedure, either at the patient's side or abducted on an armboard; in these positions, the ulnar nerve is considered to be at increased risk due to direct pressure on it, either at the groove or over the cubital tunnel; second, having the elbow flexed to greater than 90°; this reportedly causes compression of the nerve within the cubital tunnel. In many instances, however, none of these predisposing factors is present during the surgical procedure and yet a perioperative UN-ES develops. Moreover, the duration of the surgery often has not been a major causative factor; many of these lesions have developed during relatively brief operations.[115,136,153] These facts, and other data that have surfaced over the past decade, have challenged the principal underlying concept regarding these lesions: that they occur during the surgical procedure. In particular, large retrospective studies revealed that the majority of patients who sustained perioperative UN-ES were men, who were either thin or obese rather than of normal body habitus, and who were hospitalized for more than 2 weeks. Moreover, patient positioning was not a factor, elbow protection was adequate, and often the patients did not develop their symptoms until some days (2–7) after their operations.[138,152,153] All of these points suggest that these lesions may actually develop in the early postoperative period, when these patients are under less scrutiny in regard to preventing excess pressure on their ulnar nerves at the elbow region.

The underlying nerve pathology/pathophysiology with this type of UN-ES is quite variable: demyelinating conduction slowing, demyelinating conduction block, and conduction failure due to axon loss have all been present, either alone or in various combinations.[163,164] This marked variability undoubtedly is responsible for the differences in prognosis reported with these lesions; while some investigators have noted no permanent residuals,[29,113] others have observed substantial long-term deficits, presumably due to severe axon loss.[37,97] In one large series, only 53% of patients were asymptomatic 1 year postoperatively.[153]

Because these iatrogenic lesions most often are presumed to have resulted from normal nerves being temporarily subjected to abnormal conditions, the role that surgery plays in their treatment is often questionable, particularly since they typically are nonprogressive.

A far less common cause for perioperative UN-ES is a nerve infarction developing during ulnar nerve transposition due to excess stripping away of the nutrient blood vessels. In this manner, often a lesion operated on for causing little more than intermittent paresthesias is converted to one producing marked, permanent sensory and motor deficits. Occasionally, the ulnar nerve sustains severe interoperative injury when a mass of unknown etiology is removed and proves to be a benign nerve tumor; this may occur at any point along the course of the nerve.[119,160]

Iatrogenic injuries of the ulnar nerve in the wrist and hand can result from the use of walkers and canes, as well as from treatments for CTS, such as endoscopic carpal tunnel release and corticosteroid injections.[137,160] They may also occur proximally (in the midarm) as a component of tourniquet paralysis and distally (mainly in the hand) as a component of ischemic monomelic neuropathy. With both of these lesions, however, almost invariably the median or radial nerves, or both, are also affected[160] (see below).

The EDX examination can detect all but the mildest UN-ESs, that is, those causing only intermittent paresthesias in a distal ulnar nerve distribution. It can, however, localize well only those in which at least some of the pathology is focal demyelination. Nonetheless, it can establish the severity of all UN-ESs, regardless of the underlying pathology. Ulnar nerve lesions in the hand usually are readily localized if the first dorsal interosseous, as well as the hypothenar muscles, is used as a recording site during ulnar motor NCSs.[33]

Ilioinguinal, Iliohypogastric, and Genitofemoral Nerves

All three of these nerves derive from the L1 root, with the ilioinguinal nerve sometimes receiving a contribution from the T12 root and the genitofemoral nerve constantly receiving a substantial contribution from the L2 root. These nerves are principally sensory in function, providing cutaneous sensation to the lower abdomen, inner thigh, and groin area (including some of the external genitalia). Most of the lesions involving them are iatrogenic, with traditional inguinal herniorrhaphies being the single most common cause. Other iatrogenic etiologies are lymph node dissections, appendectomies, orchiectomies, femoral artery punctures, scrotal herniorrhaphies, cesarean sections, and abdominoplasties.[69,83,104] Iliac bone harvesting for grafting purposes is another cause. Ironically, in most series, this is the single most common PNS complication associated with the anterior approach to cervical spine surgery.[134]

Diagnosing injuries of any type to these three nerves rests almost solely on the clinical history and examination because laboratory procedures, including the EDX examination, are essentially valueless.

Obturator Nerve

The obturator nerve derives from the L2-L4 roots via the lumbar plexus (anterior division). It passes through the obturator canal to reach the medial aspect of the thigh, where it innervates the thigh adductor muscles and provides cutaneous sensation to the proximal inner thigh. Iatrogenic injuries of this nerve are rare. No instances of obturator neuropathy occurred among the 126 iatrogenic PNS lesions reported by Kretschner et al., and only 2 of the 100 iatrogenic lower extremity nerve lesions operated on by Khan and Birch involved this nerve.[74,83] Nonetheless, it can be damaged during hip surgery, certain abdominal operations (e.g., oophorectomies, aortofemoral bypass) and various genitourinary procedures. Such nerve injuries have also been noted following vaginal deliveries (usually associated with forceps use).[69]

On EDX examination, obturator neuropathies present as denervation (i.e., fibrillation potentials, dropout of MUPs), seen on needle EMG, that is limited to the thigh adductor muscles.

Femoral Nerve

The femoral nerve derives from the L2-L4 roots via the lumbar plexus (posterior division). It enters the thigh by passing beneath the inguinal ligament and soon divides into a number of branches; its major motor contribution is to the quadriceps femoris muscle, while its major sensory component is the saphenous nerve.[137]

A disproportionate number of femoral nerve lesions are iatrogenic: 52 (42%) of 119 surgically treated cases in one series.[77] The mechanisms of injury are quite variable and include compression (particularly by retractors and hematomas), stretch, transection, ligation, and ischemia.[12,69,77,150] Both the intra- and extrapelvic portions of the femoral nerve may be affected. Probably the most common general cause of iatrogenic femoral nerve injuries is abdominal pelvic surgery, and the operation having the highest incidence of this complication is abdominal hysterectomy; this adverse outcome was first reported over a century ago.[150] Other such surgeries include abdominal colectomies, radical prostatectomies, and abdominal aorta repairs. The nerve can be stapled, sutured, or lacerated during these operations, but most of these intrapelvic injuries are attributed to the retractors used during the procedure, specifically, self-retaining retractors. The lateral blade of the retractor either exerts direct pressure on the nerve and psoas muscle or it compresses the nerve and muscle between it and the pelvic wall.[12,47,69] Contributory factors include (1) thin patients with poorly developed rectus abdominal muscles, (2) use of the Pfannenstiel incision, and (3) large retractor blades.[38,118] Perioperative femoral neuropathies also have occurred during renal transplantation. Various causes for these lesions have been proposed. Probably the most widely accepted is direct pressure on the nerves by retractor blades. Alternative theories have included nerve ischemia due to division of the iliolumbar artery and hematoma formation adjacent to the nerve.[65,94] A number of other operations, including laparoscopic procedures performed through the abdominal approach, have been complicated by femoral neuropathies, including rectal surgery (rectoplexy), appendectomies, ureterolithotomy, microsurgical tuboplasty, abdominal aneurysm repair, neoplasm removal, and lumbar sympathectomies.[63,69,150]

At or near the inguinal ligament, iatrogenic femoral nerve lesions have been sustained during both femoral and inguinal herniorrhaphies, particularly the latter, with the immediate causes being nerve transection, suture transfixation, and hematoma or pseudoaneurysm formation.[69,77] Hip arthroplastic procedures also can produce femoral nerve lesions at this level. The mechanisms of injury in these cases include damage from the methylmethacrylate bone cement (due to either direct thermal injury or encasement or compression of the nerve), cautery, hematoma formation, and especially retractor-caused compression injuries resulting from improper placement. Retractor injuries often occur during the lateral and anterolateral approaches to the hip joint and are particularly likely to be sustained during revision surgery. Other mechanisms include traction resulting from excessive leg lengthening and postoperative anterior dislocations.[60,69,132] Positioning is a another operative cause for femoral neuropathies occurring at this level. The femoral nerves and vessels are angulated sharply around the inguinal ligament whenever the lithotomy position is used. This can result in femoral nerve injuries, due either to compression of the nerve by the ligament, resulting from excess thigh flexion, or to traction on the nerve produced by excessive hip abduction and external rotation. These injuries occur during childbirth, vaginal hysterectomies, and prostatectomies. Both unilateral and bilateral lesions can occur under these circumstances.[51,69]

Diagnostic or therapeutic procedures performed on the nearby femoral artery, including aortofemoral bypass and femoral arterial puncture, also have produced femoral nerve injuries, either directly or indirectly, by causing hematomas or pseudoaneurysms.[136,151]

Patients receiving anticoagulant therapy can bleed into the substance of the psoas muscle, producing a lumbar plexopathy. They also can bleed within the iliacus muscle, and the hematoma that forms in the iliacus compartment, beneath the iliacus fascia, can compromise the femoral nerve alone. Of the three types of compartment syndrome that result from retroperitoneal bleeding and hematoma formation, the iliacus compartment syndrome is the most common.[69,137,170] The femoral nerve also can be injured by radiation directed to the inguinal region and by chemotherapy infused into the femoral artery, both to treat neoplasms.[69,137]

The clinical presentation of iatrogenic femoral neuropathies is quite variable, ranging from mild paresthesias to marked sensory and motor loss; moreover, either sensory or motor changes may appear in isolation. The most common motor symptom is buckling of the knee on attempted extension due to quadriceps muscle weakness; often this is initially noticed when the patient attempts to stand erect for the first time in the postoperative period. Pain is an inconstant symptom; however, it almost invariably occurs with compartment syndromes and typically is quite severe.[69]

Iliacus compartment hematomas can be diagnosed by computed tomography, ultrasound, and magnetic resonance imaging. Few of the other iatrogenic lesions that affect the femoral nerve can be detected with neuroimaging studies. The EDX examination generally is quite helpful in localizing these nerve lesions and, if they are axon loss in nature, in determining their severity. On femoral motor NCSs, the amplitudes of the responses obtained can be compared to those recorded from the contralateral normal side to determine the amount of axon loss that has occurred. On needle EMG, by demonstrating that abnormalities are strictly in a femoral nerve territory, the possibility that the symptoms are due to a lumbar plexopathy or L2-L4 radiculopathy is minimized. Where the EDX examination has the most difficulty is in establishing the type of pathophysiology present—focal demyelination versus axon loss/conduction failure—with lesions at the inguinal ligament; often it is difficult, on femoral motor NCSs, to determine whether the nerve is being stimulated distal to the lesion site, so whenever the NCS responses elicited are unelicitable or very low in amplitude, particularly within the first few weeks after onset, either process could be operative.[69]

Saphenous Nerve

This nerve derives from the femoral nerve. It is the largest sensory nerve in the body, supplying sensation to the medial aspect of the leg. The majority of injuries to it are iatrogenic. Most relate either to vein surgery—ligation, stripping, or harvesting (to be used as grafts during coronary artery bypass procedures)—or to operative knee procedures such as meniscectomies and arthroscopies. Other causes have been drain removals and excisions of exostoses.[69,83]

The diagnosis of these lesions characteristically rests solely on the history and clinical examination. The EDX examination generally is of no value because a reliable sensory NCS technique or assessing the saphenous nerve has not been devised.

Sciatic Nerve

The axons composing the sciatic nerve derive from the L4 through S2 roots. They traverse the sacral plexus, along with those axons that will form the inferior and superior gluteal nerves, the posterior femoral cutaneous nerve, and the pudendal nerve. The sciatic nerve leaves the pelvis through the greater sciatic foramen; it consists of two distinct nerve trunks: the lateral (or common peroneal) and the medial (or tibial). These are usually surrounded by a common sheath as they pass inferiorly in the thigh. Motor branches originate from them in the midthigh to supply the hamstrings muscles. The branch to the biceps femoris, short head (BF-SH), arises from the common peroneal portion, whereas the branches to the other three hamstrings muscles originate from the tibial portion of the nerve. Slightly proximal to the popliteal fossa, the two portions of the sciatic nerve generally grossly separate from each other; the common peroneal component passes anterolaterally, as well as inferiorly, to reach the fibular head, while the tibial component continues on a directly inferior course. The sciatic nerve innervates the hamstrings muscles and all the muscles in the lower extremity distal to the knee. It provides sensation to the entire lower extremity distal to the knee, except for a medial strip supplied by the saphenous nerve.[130,139]

Most iatrogenic sciatic neuropathies occur in the gluteal region and involve the proximal segment of the nerve. Two of the more common causes are total hip arthroplasty and misplaced intramuscular injections.[69]

Prospective studies have shown that the sciatic nerve is injured during total hip arthroplasty much more often than is clinically apparent.[69,130] A variety of mechanisms have been reported, including traction caused by intraoperative or postoperative hip dislocation, intraperative femoral shaft fracture, and intraoperative faulty limb positioning; compression due to trochanteric wiring or nerve sutures; thermal secondary to the methacrylate bone cement; and ischemia caused by gluteal compartment syndrome, the latter resulting from spontaneous bleeding in otherwise normal patients or in anticoagulated patients.[69,137] We also know of instances in which the nerve was ligated at the close of the operation. Overall, the majority of sciatic neuropathies associated with total hip arthroplasty are attributed to traction. Patients undergoing these surgical procedures for congenital hip dislocation and for revisions of prior total hip arthroplasties are considered to be at greater risk.[127,130,137] Nonetheless, in many instances, no specific etiology can be identified. Total hip arthroplasty also can result in the delayed (from 5 days to more than 5 years) appearance of iatrogenic sciatic neuropathies due to such factors as gluteal compartment syndromes developing, after the initiation of anticoagulation therapy, in the latter part of the first postoperative week; methylmethacrylate cement causing fibrosis around the nerve or forming a hard spur that penetrates the nerve; and breakage and subsequent migration of the trochanteric wire.[69,127,130,137]

Other causes for perioperative sciatic nerve lesions include pinning or nailing fractures of the neck of the femur, osteotomies, emaciated patients lying supine on operating tables, use of the lithotomy position for transvaginal surgery, and placing patients in sitting positions during neurosurgical procedures.[69,137]

Another major cause of iatrogenic sciatic neuropathies is misplaced gluteal muscle injections. The sciatic nerve is injured more often in this manner than any other PNS structure. Two recent series contained 131 and 370 lesions, respectively.[111,148] The principal sources for these injuries, as with all nerve injection injuries, are "carelessness combined with an appalling ignorance of elementary anatomy."[139] An important contributing cause with sciatic nerve lesions, at least in adults, is that the patients invariably are lean or frankly emaciated,[101] typically from inflammatory bowel disease or cancer. The incidence of these iatrogenic injuries is unknown and undoubtedly varies among countries and, at least in regard to North America, has varied considerably with time. Among Kline and Hudson's series of 54 operated patients with sciatic nerve injuries at the buttocks level, injection injury was responsible for 56% of them, the single largest category.[79] Nearly all of these lesions, at least in adults, result from the needle, which should have been inserted into the gluteal muscle mass in the superior lateral quadrant of the buttock, being inserted instead into the inferior medial area, where the sciatic nerve exits the pelvis. Although conceivably the nerve could be injured directly by the needle itself, due to penetration of its fascicles, in nearly all instances the damage results from the medication injected.[158] Most of these medications are composed of three elements: (1) a pharmacologically active compound, (2) a solvent, and (3) a buffering agent. Any one of these three components often has the potential to injure nerves.[16] The two most important factors in the occurrence and severity of any injection injury, including sciatic neuropathies, are the specific material injected and the precise location where it is placed; many medications damage the nerve only if they are deposited within the epineurium, whereas a few substances (such as paraldehyde) can cause injury just by being injected in the region of the nerve outside the epineurium.[158] Two different types of presentation have been reported in the literature: immediate and delayed. In the author's experience, the only delayed aspect of these injuries results from the failure of the medical personnel to recognize that they have occurred. Nonetheless, according to Kline and Hudson, in approximately 10% of patients, symptoms do not develop for several hours to even days after the injection; presumably, in these instances the medication was placed near, rather than within, the nerve or in a tissue plane from which it gravitated to invade the nerve.[79] Typically, the common peroneal component of the sciatic nerve is injured more severely than the tibial components. Although mild sciatic nerve injection injuries have been reported, in far too many instances the lesion is severe, and the symptomatology is dominated by the almost instantaneous onset—at least in awake, alert patients—of severe, burning pain in principally a superficial peroneal sensory nerve distribution, along with substantial weakness, the most prominent manifestation of which is footdrop.[69,158]

Proximal iatrogenic sciatic nerve lesions can also be due to hemorrhage into the gluteal space in anticoagulated patients, causing a gluteal compartment syndrome. With this disorder, increased intercompartmental pressure secondarily produces ischemic injury to the gluteal nerves within the compartment and compression injury of the sciatic nerve, which is outside the compartment but very near it. Typically, gluteal compartment syndromes present with the abrupt onset of rapidly progressive motor and sensory symptoms in gluteal and sciatic nerve distributions.[69,130,137] The diagnosis rests on the history, because both on clinical and EDX examinations, the abnormalities present often are indistinguishable from those of a very severe sacral plexopathy.

Sciatic nerve injuries have also resulted from closed reductions of hip dislocations. In the midthigh region, sciatic neuropathies can occur perioperatively as a manifestation of tourniquet paralysis.[158]

The pathophysiology with essentially all iatrogenic sciatic neuropathies, including those due to tourniquet paralysis, is axon loss. With most etiologies, the common peroneal component of the sciatic nerve tends to be more severely affected than the tibial component.[79,137] The location and severity of the lesion generally can be determined satisfactorily with EDX studies, particularly if the needle EMG is extensive and if certain additional NCSs are performed, such as peroneal motor, recording tibialis anterior, and superficial peroneal sensory studies.[69] Neuroimaging studies, such as, computed tomography or magnetic resonance imaging, can demonstrate a mass lesion if one is present—for example, with gluteal compartment syndrome (although the time expended obtaining such studies, when the lesions are developing, is far better spent in treating them on an emergency basis, thereby possibly preventing severe axon loss from occurring). However, neuroimaging studies generally have a relatively minor diagnostic role to play with iatrogenic sciatic neuropathies.[137]

Patients in whom the tibialis anterior muscle is totally denervated are very likely to have permanent impairment of foot dorsiflexion, since substantial proximodistal regeneration of the nerve from the lesion site rarely occurs because of the adverse time-distance factor. In contrast, the severe pain that typically accompanies these sciatic neuropathies (an exception being those caused by tourniquet paralysis, which are painless) often abates after about 8 months.

Common Peroneal Nerve

The sciatic nerve terminates by dividing, in the distal thigh, into the tibial and common peroneal nerves. The latter then passes to the fibular head, where it divides into deep and superficial branches.

Of all the lower extremity nerves, the common peroneal nerve, or its branches, has the highest frequency of iatrogenic injury. In Khan and Birch's series of 100 lower extremity iatrogenic nerve injuries, 36 involved this nerve.[74] Similarly, in Kretschner and coworkers' iatrogenic series, in which there were 67 lower extremity nerve lesions, 26 (39%) affected this nerve.[83] It also ranked second and fourth, respectively among all PNS structures most often injured perioperatively.[29,113]

The most common mechanism of injury is external compression. This occurs under a variety of circumstances. Perioperatively, these lesions are sustained when patients are positioned on their sides, or supine with supports beneath the knees. They also occur when patients are placed in the lithotomy position for childbirth or surgery, with their legs suspended by encircling straps at the knee level.[13,21,137] External compression injuries tend to equally affect both the deep and superficial components of the common peroneal nerve. The underlying pathophysiology may be demyelinating conduction block, axon loss/conduction failure, or a combination of the two; axon loss predominates, however. Thus, of 29 patients studied in the EDX laboratory with perioperative common peroneal neuropathies, axon loss was the dominant or sole process in more than 80%.[68]

Perioperative peroneal neuropathies also can occur during operations about the knee, such as total knee replacements, Baker cyst removal, proximal tibial osteotomies, vein stripping, gastrocnemius muscle release, and arthroscopic knee surgery (performed most often for meniscus repair or removal). With tibial osteotomies and arthroscopic knee surgery, frequently only the deep peroneal component of the common peroneal nerve is injured, and sometimes the motor innervation to the extensor hallucis muscle is selectively involved. These lesions are attributed to instrumentation injuries; typically at exploration, neuromas in continuity are found. In contrast, only tentative explanations have been proposed for the common peroneal nerve dysfunction that follows total knee arthroplasty. One of the more prevalent theories attributes these lesions to a combination of nerve traction caused by surgical correction of malalignment and nerve compression resulting from both soft tissue swelling and postoperative pressure dressings.[38,69,78a,82,121]

The majority of nonsurgical iatrogenic peroneal neuropathies occur in bedridden, emaciated patients. As with the majority of perioperative lesions, the cause is improper positioning, with undue pressure being placed on the common peroneal nerve at the fibular head. Less common nonoperative causes include leg braces, in which the upper edge of the brace is located just below the knee, tight bandages around the knee, and plaster casts; the last may be either below-knee or above-knee casts but, in either case, they compress the nerve at or near the fibular head.[137]

The most obvious symptom of both common and proximal deep peroneal neuropathies is footdrop, that is, weakness of foot dorsiflexion. With common peroneal neuropathies, in addition, weakness of foot eversion is also present, along with a sensory deficit over the anterolateral aspect of the leg and the dorsum of the foot. Paresthesias rarely occur, although an absence of normal sensation to touch is noted; in contrast to another iatrogenic PNS cause for footdrop, sciatic neuropathy, pain seldom is present.[68]

The EDX examination can readily demonstrate whether the lesion involves the common peroneal nerve or the proximal deep peroneal nerve. It also can disclose the type of pathophysiology present and the severity of the process. Optimal EDX studies require that additional NCSs be performed—peroneal motor, recording tibialis anterior muscle; superficial peroneal sensory—and that the needle EMG be rather extensive.[69]

While some of the common peroneal neuropathies caused by external compression are due to demyelinating conduction block that usually resolves promptly and should always be treated conservatively, others are due to axon loss. These also may recover spontaneously, but the time course is much slower. Typically, many months are required before foot dorsiflexion is restored. Moreover, occasionally spontaneous recovery does not occur, as with many of the peroneal nerve lesions that result from operations on the knee. Consequently, surgical exploration and nerve repair are indicated with many of these peroneal nerve lesions.[76,137]

Superficial Peroneal Nerve

This nerve arises at the fibular head when the common peroneal nerve terminates by forming it and the deep peroneal nerve. The superficial peroneal nerve has both substantial motor and sensory components. It innervates the peroneus longus and brevis in the lateral compartment of the leg and supplies sensation to most of the anterolateral aspect of the leg and dorsum of the foot. Motorwise, it is responsible for foot eversion. Causes of iatrogenic injuries of this nerve include osteotomies; removal of Baker cysts, plates, foreign bodies, and ganglia; and muscle excisions and ligament repairs.[83] Isolated axon loss lesions of this nerve, which nearly all iatrogenic injuries are, affect the amplitudes of the superficial peroneal sensory responses and, to some extent, the peroneal motor responses, recording tibialis anterior, on NCSs and produce signs of denervation in the peronei (longus and brevis) muscles on needle EMG.[33,163]

Tibial Nerve

This nerve originates in the distal thigh as one of the two terminal nerves of the sciatic nerve. It follows essentially a straight midline course distally in the leg, deep to the gastrocnemii, and terminates proximal to the medial ankle as the plantar and medial calcaneal nerves.[69,139] Tibial nerve injuries, including iatrogenic ones, are less common than peroneal nerve injuries, and approximately 25% of them occur proximal to the popliteal fossa, where the tibial nerve is nominally the medial component of the sciatic nerve.[69] In Kahn and Birch's series, which contained 100 lower extremity iatrogenic nerve lesions, the peroneal nerve was affected twice as often as the tibial: 36 times versus 17.[74]

Most iatrogenic lesions of the tibial nerve and its terminal branches are caused by orthopedic surgical procedures performed on or near the knee or ankle joints, such as arthroscopy and total knee replacements, and by vascular repairs. The nerve has been selectively infarcted during femoral arteriograms and has sustained severe damage when tendon strippers, seeking to obtain the tendons of plantaris muscles, have harvested long segments of it instead. On EDX examination, tibial nerve lesions, depending on their location, affect the following: (1) on NCSs, tibial motor responses and plantar responses; the sural NCS amplitude may be altered as well if the lesion is near the popliteal fossa; (2) on needle EMG, the gastrocnemii, flexor digitorum longus, tibialis posterior, and all intrinsic foot muscles except the exterior digitorum brevis.[69,160,163]

Similar to all other traumatic tibial neuropathies, particularly proximal ones, iatrogenic lesions often result in marked pain and hypersensitivity on the sole and heel of the foot, both following conservative treatment and after otherwise successful surgical repair.[69]

Sural Nerve

This cutaneous nerve forms in the distal posterior thigh; although the proximal common peroneal nerve contributes to it, the proximal tibial nerve is its major donor. It supplies cutaneous sensation to a narrow vertical strip on the posteromedial aspect of the leg, as well as the lateral aspect of the ankle and the lateral border of the sole. Although this nerve may be damaged at any point along its course, the most common site is distally, near the ankle. The most common iatrogenic cause by far is surgical biopsy done for diagnostic purposes. Another iatrogenic etiology in this region is ankle surgery (open or arthroscopic). Iatrogenic causes proximal to the ankle include knee arthroscopy, removal of Baker's cysts, vein surgery, hematoma evaluation, exostosis removal, and external compression such as from a cast.[69,83]

Almost all iatrogenic sural neuropathies manifest axon loss, so typically the sural NCS response with them is low in amplitude or unelicitable. However, this has no localizing value.

Multiple Mononeuropathies

Ischemic Monomelic Neuropathy

Multiple axon loss mononeuropathies can develop simultaneously in an extremity because of abrupt compromise of the arterial blood flow to that limb. This disorder, called *ischemic monomelic neuropathy* (IMN), characteristically results from proximal or midlimb occlusion of, or shunting of blood from, the major artery of the extremity.[165] Often IMN is iatrogenic. Nearly all reported cases of upper extremity IMN have occurred in diabetic patients with renal failure; the lesions have resulted from placement of arteriovenous shunts in their arms for dialysis purposes. Many instances of lower extremity IMN have developed after cannulation of the superficial femoral artery for cardiopulmonary bypass or intra-aortic balloon pump insertion. Also, lower extremity vascular procedures performed for advanced atherosclerotic disease occasionally have produced IMN.[87,165]

With IMN, the peripheral nerve fibers, both motor and sensory, in the more distal portion of the limb degenerate, progressively more severely distally. Typically, no abnormalities are found proximal to the elbow or knee. The most prominent symptom is severe, persistent burning pain in the hand or foot. Motor and sensory deficits are most severe in the most distal portion of the limb, regardless of peripheral nerve supply, and they shade proximally; weakness of the intrinsic muscles is much more obvious in the hand than in the foot.[87,92,165]

The striking distal-to-proximal gradient of axon loss and the uniform involvement at any given limb level, both characteristic features of IMN, appear obvious on an extensive EDX examination. The amplitudes of the responses are affected on motor and sensory NCSs, while fibrillation potentials and MUP loss are seen on needle EMG. The fact that multiple peripheral nerves are involved, and in a uniform manner at any given level, is much more apparent with upper extremity IMN, where abnormalities can be demonstrated in median, ulnar, and radial nerve distributions. With lower extremity IMN, in contrast, all the abnormalities are in a distal sciatic nerve distribution, except for sensory changes in a more distal saphenous nerve distribution; unfortunately, the latter nerve cannot be assessed reliably during the EDX examination.[165]

Even though IMN is due to distal nerve fiber infarction caused by limb ischemia, the arterial compromise typically already has been corrected by the time most patients are examined. An exception is the IMN that follows arteriovenous shunt placement. Even though it probably developed within a few hours after the shunt was created, often the shunts are removed to exclude the possibility of further nerve damage. The pain associated with IMN tends to persist for several months and then often resolves spontaneously. In the intervening period, it can usually be relieved by carbamazepine. A few patients have noted immediate relief of pain following sympathectomies.[165]

Tourniquet Paralysis

For more than a century, tourniquets have been used to produce a bloodless operative field during surgical procedures. There are two basic types of tourniquets: the inflatable, or pneumatic, type and the Esmarch band. These typically are placed about the arm, for hand and forearm surgery, and about the thigh, for foot and leg surgery. Occasionally, peripheral nerve injuries result from tourniquet use. These are referred to as *tourniquet paralysis* and have an estimated incidence of 1/8000 operations (1/5000 for the upper extremity and 1/13,000 for the lower extremity).[95] Although the cause of tourniquet paralysis continues to be debated—excess tourniquet pressure versus excess tourniquet time—much of the animal research data and nearly all the available patient data indicate that the peripheral nerve damage is due to excess pressure occurring beneath the tourniquet, causing shearing forces at the edges of the cuff.[46,158]

In 96% of patients with upper extremity tourniquet paralysis, one of three presentations is encountered: (1) simultaneous involvement of the radial, median, and ulnar nerves (seen in 60%); (2) involvement of the radial nerve alone (30%); or (3) simultaneous involvement of the radial, median, ulnar, and musculocutaneous nerves as well as the forearm cutaneous nerves (6%). Lower extremity tourniquet paralysis affects the sciatic nerve and occasionally the femoral nerve as well. Relatively subclinical involvement of the femoral nerve alone has been detected on perspective studies.[158] The characteristic underlying nerve pathophysiology with upper extremity tourniquet paralysis is demyelinating conduction block. Occasionally, however, axon loss supervenes. The focal demyelination that occurs with these lesions differs from that seen with most acute nerve injuries in that it can persist, unchanged, for many months.[158] For unclear reasons, lower extremity tourniquet paralysis typically presents solely with axon loss.

Clinically, tourniquet paralysis is predominantly a motor disorder. Typically, muscle paresis, if not complete paralysis, is found in the distribution of the affected nerve(s) distal to the tourniquet. In contrast, sensory abnormalities often are lacking. Moreover, when they are present, they characteristically are limited to large-fiber involvement, are restricted in their distribution (e.g., found only in the hand with upper extremity lesions), and resolve much sooner than do the motor abnormalities.[10,35,98]

The EDX examination is the only informative laboratory procedure with tourniquet paralysis. With upper extremity lesions it usually localizes the lesion precisely by demonstrating conduction blocks, on NCSs, with axilla and elbow stimulations of the affected nerves; with lower extremity lesions the localization is less precise (as is the etiology) because it only reveals axon loss along the distributions of the tibial and peroneal nerve fibers distal to the knee.[158]

Essentially all instances of upper extremity tourniquet paralysis are treated conservatively because almost all are due to focal demyelination, which will ultimately resolve completely. Most lower extremity ones are managed similarly because usually they are incomplete.

Medicolegal Aspects

All iatrogenic PNS injuries have medicolegal implications, to varying degrees, even though many of them are unavoidable and only a minority of them result from negligence. The principal problem often is not with the occurrence of the nerve damage itself but rather with the manner in which it is subsequently managed. Thus, the potential liability is not limited to those who allegedly are directly responsible for the injury, since it may also encompass medical personnel who interact with the patient only *after* the injury occurs. This most often pertains to severe axon loss lesions and specifically to the failure of medical personnel: (1) to promptly acknowledge that the injury happened and (2) to refer the patient to the appropriate surgeon, at the appropriate time, for evaluation and operative intervention if deemed necessary.[6,74,81] In this regard, almost invariably the central issue is unwarranted (and what proves to be highly inaccurate) optimism being expressed concerning the degree of spontaneous recovery that will be achieved and its time course. At least part of the overstated recovery potential of these lesions can be attributed to authoritative sources. Thus, the following sentence appeared in a textbook authored by an acknowledged expert in the field: "The most important aspect of these situations (i.e., iatrogenic nerve injuries) is that nearly always the damage can be rectified: the surgeon's knife, the tight plaster or errant needle almost never leads to nerve damage that cannot be substantially ameliorated"[2] Such comments, regrettably, are far more reassuring than they are accurate, because many of these lesions are marked by severe permanent symptoms, regardless of the therapy employed. Nonetheless, far too many physicians display this same unrealistic optimism after patients under their care sustain iatrogenic PNS lesions. Presumably, it is for this reason—their naive belief that the nerve injuries present will recover spontaneously and completely with the passing of time—that physicians much too often choose to merely observe these lesions for months, rather than to refer them to PNS surgeons during the time period (<6 months after injury) when operative repair could be most beneficial. In a 1991 article, Birch and coworkers noted that because of late referral, the diagnosis was delayed 6 months or more in nearly half of the iatrogenic PNS patients they saw.[6] The situation worsened over the next decade. In a 2001 article, Khan and Birch observed that delays in referral of patients with iatrogenic PNS lesions were now "the rule"and that the delay time had increased from 6 to 10 months.[74]

An appreciation of the type of nerve pathology present can prevent many of these injudicious predictions. Axon loss underlies most iatrogenic nerve lesions, particularly those that have persisted for more than 6–8 weeks (major exceptions: upper extremity tourniquet paralysis and radiation-induced brachial plexopathy).

Conversely, relatively few of them result from the type of short-lived demyelinating conduction block clinically labeled *neurapraxia*, which guarantees rapid, complete recovery. (Consequently, the use of that term is best avoided in these situations unless an EDX examination, performed 7 or more days after onset, has conclusively demonstrated that demyelination conduction blocks are responsible for the clinical deficits present.)

The amount of recovery achieved following iatrogenic axon loss lesions, with or without surgical intervention, often is uncertain. However, a few general statements can be made concerning this point. First, spontaneous recovery is more likely to occur with incomplete than with complete lesions. Moreover, it is a slow process (measured in months) and often is imperfect. Second, if operative intervention is required, it should be performed by a surgeon who specializes in PNS surgery, and it should be done within the first 3 or 4 months after injury if it is to yield optimal results; even with it, the ultimate recovery achieved almost invariably is imperfect.[7,59,79] An important point is that many iatrogenic PNS lesions need to be treated surgically, either to establish the diagnosis, to relieve pain, or to improve function. Thus, Kahn and Birch found that among 612 iatrogenic PNS lesions they examined over an 8-year period, 291 (48%) required operative exploration.[74]

Conclusions

Iatrogenic nerve lesions can complicate a large number of medical procedures. They can affect almost any portion of the PNS and can result from many different causes. Most often their underlying pathology is axon loss. For this reason, recovery with most of them typically is prolonged and suboptimal at times. In addition, in many instances there is no appreciable recovery without surgical intervention.

REFERENCES

1. Barton NJ: Radial nerve injuries. Hand 5:200–208, 1973.
2. Bateman JE: Trauma to Nerves in Limbs. Philadelphia, WB Saunders, 1962.
3. Bergqvist D: Peripheral nerve injuries associated with carotid endarterectomy. Semin Vasc Surg 4:47–53, 1991.
4. Berry PR, Wallis WE: Venepuncture nerve injuries. Lancet 1:1236–1238, 1977.
5. Bigliani LU, Perez-Sanz JR, Wolfe IN: Treatment of trapezius paralysis. J Bone Joint Surg 67A:871–877, 1985.
6. Birch R, Bonney G, Dowell J, Hollingdale J: Iatrogenic injuries of peripheral nerves. J Bone Jt Surg 73B:280–282, 1991.
7. Birch R, Bonney G, Wynn-Parry CB: Surgical Disorders of the Peripheral Nerves. London, Churchill-Livingstone, 1998.
8. Blair SJ: Avoiding complications for nerve compression syndromes. Orthop Clin North Am 19:125–130, 1988.
9. Blyth MJG, Macleod CMB, Asante OK, Kinninmouth AWG: Iatrogenic nerve injury with the Russell-Taylor humeral nail. Injury 34:227–228, 2003.
10. Bolton CF, McFarlane RM: Human pneumatic tourniquet paralysis. Neurology 28:787–793, 1978.
11. Bonney G: Iatrogenic injuries of nerves. J Bone Jt Surg 68B:9–13, 1986.
12. Brash RC, Bufo AJ, Kreienberg PF: Femoral neuropathy secondary to the use of a self-retaining retractor. Dis Colon Rectum 38:1115–1118, 1995.
13. Britt BA, Joy N, MacKay MB: Positioning trauma. In: Orkin FK, Cooperman LH (eds): Complications in Anesthesiology. Philadelphia, JB Lippincott, 1983, pp 646–670.
14. Brown KLB: Review of obstetrical palsies. Clin Plast Surg 11:181–187, 1984.
15. Buchholz DW: Dysphasia following anterior cervical spine surgery (editorial). Dysphasia 12:2–8, 1997.
16. Clark WK: Surgery for injection injuries of peripheral nerves. Surg Clin North Am 52:1325–1328, 1972.
17. Cofield RH: Total joint arthroplasty: The shoulder. Mayo Clin Proc 54:500–506, 1979.
18. Cohen AJ, Katz MG, Katz R, Mayerfeld D, Hauptman E, Schachner A: Phrenic nerve injury after coronary artery grafting: Is it always benign? Ann Thorac Surg 64:148–153, 1997.
19. Conolly WB: Pitfalls in carpal tunnel decompression. Aust NZ J Surg 48:421–425, 1978.
20. Cooper DE: Nerve injury associated with patient positioning in the operating room. In: Gelberman RH (ed): Operative Nerve Repair and Reconstruction, vol 2. Philadelphia, JB Lippincott, 1991, pp 1231–1242.
21. Cooper DE, Jenkins RS, Bready L, Rockwood CA: The prevention of injuries of the brachial plexus secondary to malposition of the patient during surgery. Clin Orthop 288:33–41, 1988.
22. Curtis JJ, Nawarawong W, Walls W, et al: Elevated hemidiaphragm after cardiac operations: Incidence, prognosis and relationship to the use of topical ice slush. Ann Thorac Surg 48:764–768, 1989.
23. Dai L, Ni B, Yuan W, Jia L: Radiculopathy in laminectomy for cervical compression myelopathy. J Bone Joint Surg 80B:846–849, 1998.
24. Dawson DM, Hallett M, Wilbourn AJ: Musculocutaneous axillary and suprascapular neuropathies; thoracic outlet syndromes; radial neuropathies. In: Dawson DM, Hallett M, Wilbourn AJ (eds): Entrapment Neuropathies, 3rd ed. Philadelphia, Lippincott-Raven, 1999, pp 335–368.
25. Dawson DM, Krarup C: Perioperative nerve lesions. Arch Neurol 46:1355–1360, 1989.
26. Della Santa D, Narakas A, Bonnard C: Late lesions of the brachial plexus after fracture of the clavicle. Ann Hand Surg 10:531–540, 1991.
27. DeVita MA, Robinson LR, Rehder J, Hattler B, Cohen C: Incidence and natural history of phrenic neuropathy occurring during open heart surgery. Chest 103:850–856, 1993.
28. Dew LA, Shelton C: Iatrogenic facial nerve injury: Prevalence and predisposing factors. Ear Nose Throat J 75: 724–729, 1996.
29. Dhuner K-G: Nerve injuries following operations: A survey of cases occurring during a six-year period. Anesthesiology 11:289–293, 1950.
30. Donaghy M: Lumbosacral plexus lesions. In: Dyck PJ, Thomas PK (eds): Peripheral Neuropathy, vol 2, 4th ed. Philadelphia, WB Saunders, 2005, pp 1375–1390.
31. Donofrio PD: Drug-related neuropathies. In: Brown WF, Bolton CF, Aminoff MJ (eds): Neuromuscular Function and Disease, vol 2. Philadelphia, WB Saunders, 2002, pp 1127–1141.
32. Dubuisson AS, Kline DG: Brachial plexus injury: A survey of 100 consecutive cases from a single service. Neurosurgery 51:673–683, 2002.
33. Dumitru D: Electrodiagnostic Medicine. Philadelphia, Hanley & Belfus, 1995.
34. Duncan MA, Lotze MT, Gerber LH, Rosenberg SA: Incidence, recovery and management of serratus anterior muscle palsy after axillary node dissection. Phys Ther 63:1243–1247, 1983.
35. Durkin MAP, Crabtree SD: Hazard of pneumatic tourniquet application. J R Soc Med 75:658–659, 1982.
36. Edwards P, Kurth L: Postoperative radial nerve paralysis caused by fracture callus. J Orthop Trauma 6:234–236, 1992.
37. Ekerot L: Postanesthetic ulnar neuropathy at the elbow. Scand J Plast Reconstr Surg 11:225–229, 1977.
38. Esselman PC, Tomski MA, Robinson LR, Zisfern J, Marks SJ: Selective deep peroneal nerve injury associated with arthroscopic knee surgery. Muscle Nerve 16: 1188–1192, 1993.

39. Faden, AJ: Iatrogenic neurological complications (editorial). Arch Neurol 51:1164–1165, 1994.
40. Fee HJ, McAvoy JM, Dainko EA: Pseudoaneurysm of the axillary artery following a modified Bristow operation: Report of a case and review. J Cardiovasc Surg 19:65–68, 1978.
41. Fisch U: Maximal nerve excitability testing vs. electroneuronography. Arch Otolaryngol 106:352–375, 1980.
42. Gatens PF, Mysiw WJ: Accessory nerve palsy—a hazard of ventriculojugular shunt surgery. Arch Phys Med Rehabil 64:484, 1983.
43. Gaur SC, Swarup A: Radial nerve injury caused by injections. J Hand Surg 21B:338–340, 1996.
44. Gilbert A, Tassin JL: Obstetrical palsy: A clinical, pathologic and surgical review. In: Terzis JK (ed): Microreconstruction of Nerve Injuries. Philadelphia, WB Saunders, 1987, pp 529–553.
45. Gilbert A, Whitaker I: Obstetrical brachial plexus lesions. J Hand Surg 16B:489–491, 1991.
46. Gilliatt RW: Physical injury to peripheral nerves. Mayo Clin Proc 56:361–370, 1981.
47. Goldman JA, Feldberg D, Dicker D, Samuel N, Dekel A: Femoral neuropathy subsequent to abdominal hysterectomy. A comparative study. Eur J Obstet Gynecol Reprod Biol 20:385–392, 1985.
48. Goslin KL, Krivickas LS: Proximal neuropathies of the upper extremity. Neurol Clin 17:525–548, 1999.
49. Graham MD: Prevention and management of iatrogenic facial palsy. Am J Otol 5:513, 1984.
50. Green JD, Shelton C, Brackmann DE: Iatrogenic facial nerve injury during otologic surgery. Laryngoscope 104: 922–926, 1994.
51. Hakim MA, Katirji MB: Femoral mononeuropathy induced by the lithotomy position: A report of 5 cases with review of the literature. Muscle Nerve 16:891–895, 1993.
52. Hansky B, Murray E, Minami K, Korfer R: Delayed brachial plexus paralysis due to subclavian pseudoaneurysm after clavicular fracture. Eur J Cardiothorac Surg 7:497–498, 1993.
53. Hargrave KR, Kothari MJ: Toxic neuropathies: Drugs. In: Katirji B, Kaminski HJ, Preston DC, Rulf RL, Shapiro BE (eds): Neuromuscular Disorders in Clinical Practice. Boston, Butterworth-Heinemann, 2002, pp 655–668.
54. Harper CM, Thomas JE, Casino TL, Litchy WJ: Distinction between neoplastic and radiation-induced brachial plexopathy with emphasis on the role of EMG. Neurology 39:502–506, 1989.
55. Herskowitz S, Sçhaumburg HH: Neuropathy caused by drugs: In: Dyck PJ, Thomas PK (eds): Peripheral Neuropathy, vol 2, 4th ed. Philadelphia, (Elsevier) WB Saunders, 2005, pp 2553–2558.
56. Hoffman JC: Permanent paralysis of the accessory nerve after cannulation of the internal jugular vein. Anesthesiology 58:583–584, 1983.
57. Horowitz SH: Peripheral nerve injury and causalgia secondary to routine venipuncture. Neurology 44:962–964, 1994.
58. House JW: Iatrogenic facial paralysis. Ear Nose Throat J 75:720–721, 1996.
59. Hudson AR, Tranmer B: Brachial plexus injuries. In: Wilkins RH, Rengachery SS (eds): Neurosurgery, vol 2. New York, McGraw-Hill, 1985, pp 1817–1832.
60. Hudson AR, Hunter GA, Waddell JP: Iatrogenic femoral nerve injuries. Can J Surg 22:62–66, 1979.
61. Hudson DA, Boone R, Sanpera I: Brachial plexus injury after median sternotomy. J Hand Surg 18A:282–284, 1993.
62. Huler KKH, Huler RJ: Neurologic complications of spinal surgery. In: Biller J (ed): Iatrogenic Neurology. Boston, Butterworth-Heineman, 1998, pp 105–174.
63. Infantino A, Fardin P, Pirone E, Masin A, Melega E, Cacciavillani M, Lise M: Femoral nerve damage after abdominal rectoplexy. Int J Colorectal Dis 9:32–34, 1994.
64. Jensen KL, Rockwood CA: Delayed primary repair of iatrogenic spinal accessory nerve injury. Clin Orthop Relat Res 336:116–121, 1997.
65. Jog MS, Turley JE, Berry H: Femoral neuropathy in renal transplantation. Can J Neurol Sci 21:38–42, 1994.
66. Johannsen S, Svensson H, Larson L-G, Denecamp J: Brachial plexopathy after postoperative radiotherapy of breast cancer patients. Acta Oncol 39:373–382, 2000.
67. Jones R: Pediatric neurology. In: Brown WF, Bolton CF (eds): Clinical Electromyography, 2nd ed. Boston, Butterworth-Heinemann, 1993, pp 695–758.
68. Katirji MB, Wilbourn AJ: Common peroneal mononeuropathy: A clinic and electrophysiologic study of 116 lesions. Neurology 38:1723–1728, 1988.
69. Katirji MB, Wilbourn AJ: Mononeuropathies of the lower limb. In: Dyck PJ, Thomas PK (eds): Peripheral Neuropathy, vol 2, 4th ed. Philadelphia, WB Saunders, 2005, pp 1487–1510.
70. Kauppila LA, Vastamaki M: Iatrogenic serratus anterior palsy; long-term outcome in 26 patients. Chest 109:31–34, 1996.
71. Kay SP, Eckardt JJ: Brachial plexus palsy secondary to clavicular non-union: Case report and literature review. Clin Orthop 206:219–222, 1986.
72. Kessler FB: Complications of the management of carpal tunnel syndrome. Hand Clin 2:401–406, 1986.
73. Kettelcamp DB, Alexander H: Clinical review of radial nerve injury. J Trauma 1967 7:424–432, 1967.
74. Khan R, Birch R: Iatrogenic injuries of peripheral nerves. J Bone Joint Surg 83B:1145–1148, 2001.
75. Kim DH, Cho Y-J, Trel RL, Kline DG: Surgical outcome of 111 spinal accessory nerve injuries. Neurosurgery 33:1106–1113, 2003.
76. Kim DH, Kline DG: Management and results of peroneal nerve lesions. Neurosurgery 39:312–320, 1996.
77. Kim DH, Morovic JA, Trel RL, Kline DG: Intrapelvic and thigh-level femoral nerve lesions: Management and outcomes in 119 surgically treated cases. J Neurosurg 100:189–996, 2004.
78. King RJ, Motta G: Iatrogenic spinal accessory nerve palsy. Ann R Coll Surg Eng 65:35–37, 1983.
78a. Kirgis A, Albrecht S: Palsy of the deep peroneal nerve after proximal tibial osteotomy. J Bone Jt Surg 72A:1180–1185, 1992.

79. Kline DG, Hudson AR: Nerve Injuries. Philadelphia, WB Saunders, 1995.
80. Kline DG, Judice DJ: Operative management of selected brachial plexus lesions. J Neurosurg 58:631–649, 1983.
81. Komurcii F, Zwolak P, Benditte-Klepetko H, Deutinger M: Management strategies for peripheral iatrogenic nerve lesions. Ann Plast Surg 54:135–139, 2005.
82. Krackow KA, Maar DC, Mont MA, Carroll C: Surgical decompression for peroneal nerve palsy after total knee arthroplasty. Clin Orthop 292:223–228, 1993.
83. Kretschner T, Antoniadis G, Braun V, Roth SA, Richter H-P: Evaluation of iatrogenic lesions in 722 surgically treated cases of peripheral nerve trauma. J Neurosurg 94:905–912, 2001.
84. Krivickas LS: Medial brachial fascial compartment syndrome versus tourniquet paralysis. In: Course E: Distinctive Regional Neuropathies [syllabus]. Rochester, MN, American Association of Electrodiagnostic Medicine, 2002, p 37.
85. Lederman RJ, Wilbourn AJ: Brachial plexopathy: Recurrent cancer or radiation? Neurology 34:1331–1335, 1984.
86. Leist FD, Masson JK, Erich JB: A review of 324 rhytidectomies, emphasizing complications and patient dissatisfaction. Plast Reconstruct Surg 59:525–529, 1977.
87. Levin KH: AAEE case report #19: Ischemic monomelic neuropathy. Muscle Nerve 12:791–795, 1989.
88. London J, London NJ, Kay SPJ: Iatrogenic accessory nerve injury. Ann R Coll Surg Eng 78:146–150, 1996.
89. Lynch NM, Cofield RH, Silbert PL, Hermann RC: Neurologic complications after total shoulder arthroplasty. J Shoulder Elbow Surg 5:53–61, 1996.
90. MacDonald RI, Lichtman DM, Hanlong JJ, Wilson JN: Complications of surgical release of carpal tunnel syndrome. J Hand Surg 3:70–76, 1978.
91. McConnell JR, Bush DC: Iatraneural steroid injection as a complication of carpal tunnel syndrome: A report of three cases. Clin Orthop 250:181–184, 1990.
92. McDonald WI: Physiological consequences of demyelination. In: Sumner A (ed): The Physiology of Peripheral Nerve Disease. Philadelphia, WB Saunders, 1980, pp 265–286.
93. Mearns AJ: Iatrogenic injury to the phrenic nerve in infants and young children. Br J Surg 64:558–560, 1977.
94. Meech PR: Femoral neuropathy following renal transplantation. Aust NZ J Surg 60:117–119, 1990.
95. Middleton RWS, Varian JP: Tourniquet paralysis. Aust NZ Surg 44:124–128, 1974.
96. Miller DS, Boswick JA: Lesions of the brachial plexus associated with fractures of the clavicle. Clin Orthop 64:144–149, 1964.
97. Miller RG, Camp PE: Postoperative ulnar neuropathy. JAMA 242:1636–1639, 1979.
98. Moldaver J: Tourniquet paralysis syndrome. Arch Surg 68:136–144, 1954.
99. Morin JE, Long R, Elleker MG, Eisen AA, Wynards E, Ralphs-Thibodean S: Upper extremity neuropathies following median sternotomy. Ann Thorac Surg 34:181–185, 1982.
100. Morris G: Adhesive arachnoiditis. In: Herkowitz HN, Garfin SR, Balderston RA, Eismont FJ, Bell GR, Wiesel SW (eds): The Spine, vol 2, 4th ed. Philadelphia, W.B. Saunders, 1999, pp 1705–1710.
101. Mumenthaler M, Schliack H: Peripheral Nerve Lesions. New York: Thieme Medical, 1991.
102. Murphey RX, Jennings JF, Wukich DK: Major neurovascular complications of endoscopic carpal tunnel release. J Hand Surg 19A:114–118, 1994.
103. Murray BE, Wilbourn AJ, Shields RW: The clinical and electrodiagnostic features of "classic" postoperative brachial plexopathy. Neurology 54(suppl 3):A48, 2000.
104. Nahabedian MY, Dellon AL: Outcome of the operative management of nerve injuries in the ilioinguinal region. J Am Coll Surg 184:265–268, 1997.
105. Narakas AO: The surgical treatment of traumatic brachial plexus lesions. Int Surg 6:521–527, 1980.
106. Netterville JL, Kowichak MJ, Courey MS, Winkle M, Assoff RH: Vocal fold paralysis following the anterior approach to the cervical spine. Ann Otol Rhinol Laryngol 105:85–91, 1996.
107. Newman BH, Waxman DA: Blood donation-related neurologic needle injury: evaluation of 2 years worth of data from a large blood center. Transfusion 36:213–215, 1996.
108. Nightingale PJ, Longreen A: Iatrogenic facial nerve paresis. Anesthesia 37:322–323, 1982.
109. Ogino T, Sugawara M, Minami A, Kato H, Ohnishi N: Accessory nerve injury: conservative or surgical treatment. J Hand Surg 16B:531–536, 1991.
110. Oliver P: Iatrogenic facial nerve paralysis. Surg Clin NA 60:629–635, 1980.
111. Orbach J, Aragones JH, Ruano D: The infrapiriformis syndrome resulting from intragluteal injection. J Neurol Sci 58:135–142, 1983.
112. Osgaard O, Eskesen V, Rosenorn J: Microsurgical repair of iatrogenic accessory nerve lesions in the posterior triangle of the neck. Acta Chir Scand 153:171–173, 1987.
113. Parks BJ: Postoperative peripheral neuropathies. Surgery 74:348–357, 1973.
114. Paschall RM, Mandel S: Brachial plexus injury from percutaneous cannulation of the internal jugular vein. Ann Emerg Med 12:112–114, 1982.
115. Perreault L, Drolet P, Farny J: Ulnar nerve palsy at the elbow after general anesthesia. Can J Anesth 39:499–503, 1992.
116. Petrera JE, Trojaborg W: Conduction studies along the accessory nerve and follow-up of patients with trapezius palsy. J Neurol Neurosurg Psychiatry 47:630–636, 1984.
117. Piatt JH: Neurosurgical management of birth injuries of the brachial plexus. Neurosurg Clin North Am 2:175–185, 1991.
118. Redfern AB, Zimmerman NB: Neurologic and ischemic complications of upper extremity vascular access for dialysis. J Hand Surg 20A:199–204, 1995.
119. Rengachery SS: Entrapment neuropathies. In: Wilkins RH, Rengachery SS (eds): Neurosurgery, vol 2, New York, McGraw-Hill, 1985, pp 1771–1795.
120. Richards RR, Hudson AR, Bertoia JT, Urbanik JR,

Waddell JP: Injury to the brachial plexus during Putti-Platt and Bristow procedures. Am J Sports Med 15:374–380, 1987.
121. Rodeo SA, Sobel M, Weiland AJ: Deep peroneal-nerve injury as a result of arthroscopic meniscectomy. J Bone Jt Surg 75A:1221–1224, 1993.
122. Roy PH, Beahrs OH: Spinal accessory nerve in radical neck dissections. Am J Surg 118:800–804, 1969.
123. Russell RI, Mulrey D, Laroche C, Shinebourne EA, Green M: Bedside assessment of phrenic nerve function in infants and children. J Thorac Cardiovasc Surg 101:143–147, 1991.
124. Rutcove SB, Sax TS: Lumbosacral plexopathies. In: Katirji B, Kaminski HJ, Preston DC, Rulf RL, Shapiro BE (eds): Neuromuscular Disorders in Clinical Practice. Boston, Butterworth-Heinemann, 2005, pp 907–915.
125. Sander HW, Conigliari M, Masdeu JC: Antecubital phlebotomy complicated by lateral antebrachial cutaneous neuropathy. N Engl J Med 339:2024, 1998.
126. Salvador JA: In discussion of: Morin JE, Long R, Elleker MG, et al: Upper extremity neuropathies following median sternotomy. Ann Thorac Surg 34:181–185, 1982.
127. Schmalzried TP, Amstutz HC, Dorey FJ: Nerve palsy associated with total hip replacement: Risk factors and prognosis. J Bone Jt Surg 73A:1074–1080, 1991.
128. Seddon H: Three types of nerve injury. Brain 66:236–288, 1943.
129. Seyfer AE, Grammer NY, Bogumill GP, Provost JM, Chandry U: Upper extremity neuropathies after cardiac surgery. J Hand Surg 10A:16–19, 1987.
130. Shields RW: Iatrogenic sciatic nerve injuries. In syllabus: 1990 AAEM Course D: Electrodiagnosis of Iatrogenic Neuropathies. Rochester MN, American Association of Electrodiag-nostic Medicine, 1990, pp 37–44.
131. Silverstein H, McDaniel AB, Hyman SM: Evoked serial electromyography in the evaluation of the paralyzed face. Am J Otology 6(suppl):80–87, 1985.
132. Simmons C, Izant TH, Rothman RH, Booth RE, Balderston RA: Femoral neuropathy following total hip arthroplasty. J Arthroplasty 6(suppl):559–566, 1991.
133. Smith DC, Mitchell DA, Peterson GW, Will AD, Mera SS, Smith LL: Medial brachial fascial compartment syndrome: Anatomical basis of neuropathy after transaxillary arteriography. Radiology 173:149–174, 1989.
134. Stambaugh JL, Simeone FA: Neurological complications in spine surgery. In: Herkowitz HN, Garfin SR, Balderston RA, Eismont FJ, Bell GR, Wiesel SW (eds): The Spine, vol 2, 4th ed. Philadelphia, W.B. Saunders, 1999, pp 1724–1732.
135. Starr DG, Cheng L, Loukota RA, Corrigan AM: Iatrogenic accessory nerve injury. Ann R Coll Surg Eng 78:399, 1996.
136. Steolting RK: Postoperative ulnar nerve paralysis: Is it a preventable complication? Anesth Analg 76:7–9, 1993.
137. Stewart JD: Focal Peripheral Neuropathies, 3rd ed. Philadelphia, Lippincott, Williams & Wilkins, 2000.
138. Stewart JD, Shantz SH: Perioperative ulnar neuropathies: A medical legal review. Can J Neurol Sci 30:15, 2003.
139. Sunderland S: Nerves and Nerve Injuries, 2nd ed. Edinburgh, Churchill-Livingstone, 1978.
140. Swenson MR, Rubenstein RS: Phrenic nerve conduction studies. Muscle Nerve 15:597–603, 1992.
141. Tavares SP, Giddens GEB: Nerve injury following steroid injection for carpal tunnel syndrome. J Hand Surg 21B:208–209, 1996.
142. Tsao B, Wilbourn A: The medial brachial fascial compartment syndrome following axillary arteriography. Neurology 61:1037–1041, 2003.
143. Tsao B, Wilbourn A: Infraclavicular brachial plexus injury following axillary regional block. Muscle Nerve 30: 44–48, 2004.
144. Vahl CF, Carl I, Muller-Vahl H, Struck E: Brachial plexus injury after cardiac surgery. J Thorac Cardiovasc Surg 102:724–729, 1991.
145. Vander Salm TV, Cereda J-M, Cutler BS: Brachial plexus injury following medial sterotomy. J Thorac Cardiovasc Surg 80:447–452, 1980.
146. Vastamaki M, Kauppila LI: Etiologic factors in isolated paralysis of the serratus anterior muscle: A report of 197 cases. J Shoulder Elbow Surg 2:240–245, 1993.
147. Vialle R, Pietin-Vialle C, Cronier P, Brillu C, Villapadierna F, Mercier P: Anatomic relationships between the cephalic vein and the sensory branches of the radial nerve: How can nerve lesions during vein puncture be prevented? Anesth Analg 93:1058–1061, 2001.
148. Villarejo FJ, Pascual AM: Injection injury of the sciatic nerve (370 cases). Childs Nerv Syst 9:229–232, 1993.
149. Wadsworth TG: The cubital tunnel and the external compression syndrome. Anesth Analg 53:303–308, 1974.
150. Walsh C, Walsh A: Postoperative femoral neuropathy. Surg Gyn Obstet 174:255–263, 1992.
151. Warfel BS, Marini SG, Lachmann EA, Nagler W: Delayed femoral nerve palsy following femoral vessel catheterization. Arch Phys Med Rehabil 74:1211–1215, 1993.
152. Warner MA, Warner DO, Matsumoto JY, et al: Ulnar neuropathy in surgical patients. Anesthesiology, 90:54–59, 1999.
153. Warner MA, Warner ME, Martin JT: Ulnar neuropathy: Incidence, outcome and risk factors in sedated or anesthetized patients. Anesthesiology 81:1332–1340, 1994.
154. Weber M: Lumbosacral plexopathies. In: Brown WF, Bolton CF, Aminoff MJ (eds): Neuromuscular Function and Disease, vol 1. Philadelphia, WB Saunders, 2002, pp 852–864.
155. Wheeler WE, Rubis LJ, Jones CW, Harrah JD: Etiology and prevention of topical cardiac hypothermia-induced phrenic nerve injury and left lower lobe atelectasis during cardiac surgery. Chest 88:680–683, 1985.
156. Wiet RJ: Iatrogenic facial paralysis. Otolarygnol Clin North Am 15:773–780, 1982.
157. Wilbourn AJ: Thoracic outlet syndrome surgery causing severe brachial plexopathy. Muscle Nerve 11:66–74, 1988.
158. Wilbourn AJ: Nerve injuries caused by injections and tourniquets. In syllabus: 1996 AAEM Plenary Session: Physical Trauma to Peripheral Nerves. Rochester, MN,

American Association of Electrodiagnostic Medicine, 1996, pp 15–33.
159. Wilbourn AJ: Peripheral nerve lesions complicating orthopedic procedures. Curr Opin Orthop 8:91–95, 1997.
160. Wilbourn AJ: Iatrogenic nerve lesions. Neurol Clin 16: 55–82, 1998.
161. Wilbourn AJ: Nerve conduction studies: Types, components, abnormalities, and value in localization. Neurol Clin 20:305–333, 2003.
162. Wilbourn AJ: Brachial plexus lesions. In: Dyck PJ, Thomas PK (eds): Peripheral Neuropathy, vol. 2, 4th ed. Philadelphia, WB Saunders, 2005, pp 1339–1373.
163. Wilbourn AJ, Ferrante MA: Clinical electromyography. In: Joynt RJ, Griggs RC (eds): Baker's Clinical Neurology on CD-ROM. Record 7692-8249. Philadelphia, Lippincott, Williams & Wilkins, 2000.
164. Wilbourn AJ, Ferrante MA: Upper limb neuropathies: Long thoracic (nerve to serratus anterior), suprascapular, axillary, musculocutaneous, radial, ulnar, and medial antebrachial cutaneous. In: Dyck PJ, Thomas PK (eds): Peripheral Neuropathy, vol. 2, 4th ed. Philadelphia, WB Saunders, 2005, pp 1463–1486.
165. Wilbourn AJ, Furlan A, Hulley W, Ruschhaupt W: Ischemic monomelic neuropathy. Neurology 33:447–451, 1983.
166. Wilbourn AJ, Levin KH, Lederman RJ: Radiation-induced brachial plexopathy: Electrodiagnostic changes over 13 years. Muscle Nerve 17:1108, 1994.
167. Wilcox PG, Pare PD, Pardy RL: Recovery after unilateral phrenic injury associated with coronary artery revascularization. Chest 98:661–666, 1990.
168. Wright TA: Accessory spinal nerve injury. Clin Orthop 108:15–18, 1975.
169. Yonenobu K, Hosono N, Iwasaki M, Asano M, Ono K: Neurologic complications of surgery for cervical compression myelopathy. Spine 16:1277–1282, 1991.
170. Young MR, Norris JW: Femoral neuropathy during anticoagulant therapy. Neurology 26:1173–1175, 1976.

Chapter 41

Complications of Stereotactic Brain Surgery

DOUGLAS KONDZIOLKA
AND L. DADE LUNSFORD

Stereotactic surgery refers to an image-guided neurosurgical procedure in which three-dimensional targeting is used to facilitate a diagnostic or therapeutic goal in the brain. A *surgical complication* is defined as an adverse event that occurs either during surgery or within a 30-day postoperative interval. Such a complication must arise as a direct consequence of the surgery or its associated administration of anesthesia or other medical care. Traditionally, stereotactic surgery uses a stereotactic head frame to register accurately high-resolution neurodiagnostic brain images for use in surgery. Most frame-based stereotactic procedures involve accessing brain targets using probes, electrodes, or catheters through small cranial openings. The use of closed-skull, single-treatment session irradiation to manage brain disease (stereotactic radiosurgery) is an important and increasingly used approach. Invisible radiation beams replace rigid surgical instruments. More recently, both frame-based and frameless stereotactic systems have proven helpful during conventional craniotomy procedures. These techniques use external cutaneous fiducial markers to correlate preoperative brain imaging with the surgical approach. Image-guided craniotomies are stereotactic procedures because of their use of a three-dimensional localizing system, but their postoperative complications are mainly those associated with the craniotomy itself rather than with the stereotactic technology. In this chapter, we discuss only those complications associated with stereotactic frame-based procedures that involve minimal or no opening of the cranial vault. These include diagnostic brain biopsy, cyst or abscess management, ablative movement disorder surgery, deep brain stimulation, and stereotactic radiosurgery.

Diagnostic Stereotactic Biopsy

Prior to 1980, stereotactic brain biopsy was usually performed using either freehand brain needle aspiration techniques or less sophisticated stereotactic devices. The target was localized by cerebral angiography, radioisotope scintigraphy, ventriculography, or early-generation computed tomography (CT), none of which provided high-resolution brain mapping. The field of stereotactic surgery was considered complex, risky, and "back room." Most patients who underwent these procedures were considered either too old or too medically ill to undergo the "preferred" craniotomy for resection of their brain lesion. A biopsy was frequently requested so that palliative chemotherapy or radiation therapy could be offered. Stereotactic technology did maintain a dominant role in functional neurosurgery with a history dating back to the 1940s.

With the advent of high-resolution CT and magnetic resonance imaging (MRI) over the past two decades, new stereotactic frame systems were introduced. The two most popular stereotactic devices in North America became the Leksell (Elekta Instruments, Atlanta, GA) and the Brown-Roberts-Wells (BRW) and later the Cosman-Roberts-Wells (CRW) (Radionics, Burlington, MA) systems. With the availability of spatially accurate brain parenchymal imaging (as CT quality improved), the role of stereotactic biopsy entered a renaissance. For the first time, brain lesions could be imaged and specific targets selected for sampling. The surgeon could choose a safe trajectory from the skull to the lesion that avoided critical brain regions, blood vessels, or the ventricular system. Most surgeons recognized that the bony opening needed to be only slightly larger than the diameter of the inserted probe. The opportunity to sample defined brain lesions through minute cranial openings with minimal brain exposure and confident instrument passage were the key elements to the reduction of complication rates for brain biopsy. The most significant complications of diagnostic stereotactic biopsy are hemorrhage and neurological deficits from injury to critical structures. Seizures and infection are rare.

Although the complication rate for stereotactic biopsy is low, varying from zero to 7%, a definite mortality rate exists for these procedures.[2,4,10,17,18,20] When complicated by a hemorrhage, insertion of the biopsy needle into critical areas of the brain can cause fatal injury. Seizures, although rare, can occur following a diagnostic biopsy. The direct relationship of the biopsy procedure itself to the onset of seizures, as well as the risk of development of chronic epilepsy, are not well understood. Infection is remarkably uncommon, and usually no hair is shaved. New or worsened neurological deficits secondary to tissue trauma or edema are also uncommon and are usually transient phenomena. Failure to obtain diagnostic tissue during biopsy varies among reported series, but in experienced centers nondiagnostic biopsy occurs in less than 10% of cases and can be related to the size and location of the lesion, the technique of surgery, and the nature of the lesion itself.

Successful stereotactic biopsy depends on appropriate patient selection, correct interpretation of imaging studies, proper selection of biopsy instruments and trajectory, judicious tissue sampling, and expert neuropathological evaluation. Complications are predictable when any of the aforementioned steps are not taken. These factors, addressed in order below, represent general principles for complication avoidance in all aspects of stereotactic brain surgery but are discussed within the context of diagnostic biopsy, the most common procedure (Fig. 41.1).

Selection of Patients for Brain Biopsy

Although lesions in nearly any brain location can be biopsied, the proper selection of appropriate patients for biopsy must be analyzed. Patients undergoing stereotactic biopsy should have lesions for which one or more plausible diagnoses are suspected but not confirmable by any other simpler means (e.g., an enhancing mass that could represent neoplasm, infarction, or infection). Furthermore, knowledge of the correct diagnosis should in some way alter the management of the patient, at the very least for appropriate counseling. Tumors, therefore, are among the most common lesions selected for stereotactic biopsy. Choices of surgical resection, radiation therapy, and chemotherapy will be influenced by the histological diagnosis of specific brain tumors. In contrast, for example, a patient with recently diagnosed metastatic bronchogenic adenocarcinoma who presents with multiple cerebral enhancing lesions (and no evidence of systemic infection) almost certainly has metastatic brain involvement of the underlying primary cancer. A stereotactic biopsy is not likely to alter the treatment plan. Some issues, however, are more controversial. Patients with rapidly progressive dementing or neurodegenerative illnesses, for example, sometimes present to neurosurgeons for brain biopsy, but only infrequently does obtaining brain tissue alter the management and prognosis of these patients. However, stereotactic biopsy remains important in the setting to rule out treatable disorders (e.g., vasculitis). Furthermore, if no discrete imaging abnormalities exist and a diagnosis might be achieved via meningeal or blood vessel biopsy, open brain sampling will be preferred over ster-

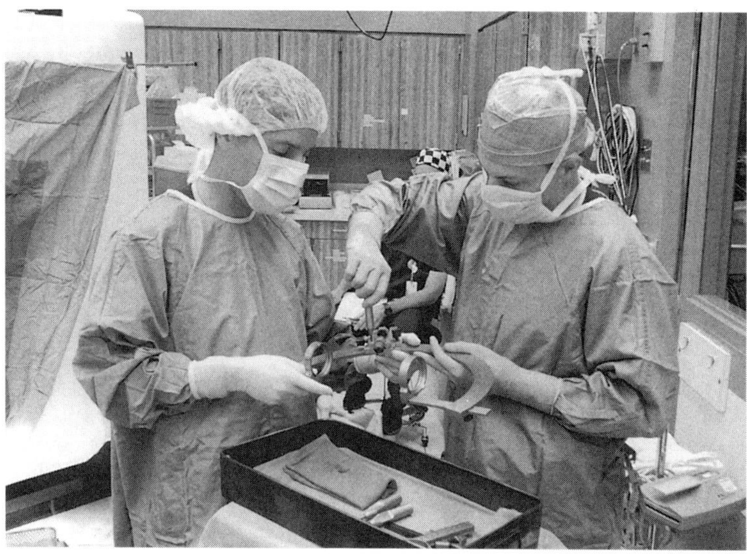

Figure 41.1. Preparation of the Leksell stereotactic frame during computed tomography stereotactic brain biopsy. All coordinates are checked three times prior to surgery.

eotactic brain biopsy. Patients with acquired immune deficiency syndrome (AIDS)–related brain lesions present similar challenges, since treatment of AIDS-related brain disease is not always possible or beneficial.

In addition to identifying patients who are likely to benefit from brain biopsy, an assessment of whether brain biopsy might be dangerous at the desired time of surgery should also be made. Patients with coagulopathies or thrombocytopenia must have these parameters corrected prior to the planning of a stereotactic brain biopsy. Patients with known liver disease are highly suspect. Normal coagulation function and a platelet count above 100,000/μl are desirable. Aspirin, warfarin, ticlodipine, and nonsteroidal anti-inflammatory drugs must be discontinued 5–7 days prior to stereotactic brain biopsy. Patients who require warfarin for cardiac valve prophylaxis may be converted to heparin-induced anticoagulation and the biopsy performed within a short 24-hour period of normalized coagulation function.

Patients whose lesions on CT or MRI appear to be highly vascular should be appropriately imaged to rule out the possibility that the lesion is a vascular malformation or aneurysm. A lesion that appears to be a small hemorrhagic tumor on a CT scan, for example, may have the characteristic appearance of a cavernous malformation on MRI. Diagnostic cerebral angiography may be necessary in rare cases to distinguish between a neoplasm and an arteriovenous malformation. It should be noted, however, that even tumors that have a propensity toward hemorrhage, such as glioblastoma multiforme or renal cell metastasis, can be safely biopsied with proper technique.

Lesions adjacent to vascular structures, such as pineal region tumors, can be biopsied with low surgical risk with proper attention to the regional anatomy. Lesions in the Sylvian fissure, posterior fossa, or third ventricular region may present a higher surgical risk from stereotactic biopsy. Such lesions are associated with a higher risk of hemorrhage because of their contiguity to pial or ependymal surfaces wherein lie important arterial or venous structures. Such cases often benefit from an experienced surgeon.[1,3,6,13,14] The type of imaging (CT versus MRI) should be chosen for clarity of lesion definition. Smaller slice thicknesses and intervals provide greater accuracy for target selection.

Judicious Brain Tissue Sampling

What portion of a brain lesion should be biopsied? Many brain lesions are inhomogeneous. Ring-enhancing lesions frequently require sampling of a portion of the enhancing rim to establish a diagnosis since the nonenhancing core may contain only necrotic debris with disrupted cytoarchitecture. Some cystic lesions, such as craniopharyngiomas, can be diagnosed simply by obtaining cyst fluid, but most often a sample of tissue from a solid portion of the lesion must be obtained. In order not to miss anaplastic regions of an otherwise benign tumor, Kelly has described taking a series of biopsies from one end of the tumor to the other.[10] While this has proved helpful in defining the nature of a general neoplasm, bleeding complications can be avoided by obtaining only as much tissue as necessary to make a diagnosis. As a general maxim, a negative biopsy is preferred to a negative outcome.

Depending on the lesion diameter, a single 8 to 10 mm long core biopsy specimen will contain both solid and necrotic tumor, useful in both diagnosis and grading of glial neoplasms. Cannulas that provide specimens 3–4 mm in length can be used in more critical brain locations if desired. If bleeding is encountered after a biopsy specimen is obtained, it is crucial to allow the blood to drain spontaneously out of the needle rather than to attempt to tamponade the bleeding in any way. This limits the volume of hematoma that otherwise would form in the brain. When this maneuver is used, hemorrhages are usually small and self-limited. Rarely, severe or persistent bleeding requires craniotomy to control. Chimowitz et al. reported that in three patients with intractable hemorrhage after stereotactic procedures, bleeding was controlled by instilling thrombin into the target site.[5] Injection of peroxide through the needle must be avoided since a catastrophic bubbling mass could result.

Hemorrhage during stereotactic surgery is easier to prevent than to treat. In addition to strategic planning to avoid major vessels, a normotensive (<150 systolic) blood pressure must be maintained throughout surgery. A frequent cause of intraoperative episodic hypertension is bladder distention often brought about by the contrast-enhanced scan. Sedation should be provided to patients who are anxious or restless. Children under 13 years of age often have surgery under general anesthesia.

Selection of Biopsy Instrumentation and Trajectory

For virtually all stereotactic approaches we use twist-drill craniostomy for cerebral access. We puncture the dura with a blunt-tip 1.9 mm diameter probe; some coagulate the dura with monopolar cautery touched to the probe. The side-cutting aspiration needle is preferred for biopsy. Other options include biopsy cup forceps (bronchoscopy type) and spiral needle devices. We prefer the Sedan-type aspiration cannulas of 2.1–2.5 mm outer diameter that safely provide adequate brain samples for histological analysis. Disposable biopsy cannulas are now available with a 2.1 mm outer diameter and an 8 mm side-coring opening. Although Apuzzo et al. preferred the cup forceps biopsy technique, we are hesitant to use it because of poor tactile feedback between tissue and blood vessels.[2] Selection of the type of biopsy instrument is less important than its proper use.

The biopsy trajectory is chosen such that important gyri, white matter tracts, and blood vessels are avoided whenever possible. A general principle in choosing a safe trajectory is to traverse as few pial and ependymal surfaces as possible en route to the target. Pial and ependymal surfaces harbor the blood vessels that lead to intraoperative hemorrhages. It is surprising that for the most part the blood vessels within a tumor are unusual sources of hemorrhage. The biopsy needle should enter the brain via a gyrus rather than a sulcus. This is easy to plan using current imaging techniques. Passage of the needle into a gyrus to obtain a specimen from an underlying white matter abnormality requires traversing only a single pial surface, whereas a pathway through a sulcus may enter and exit the pia several times where two pial surfaces are closely apposed.

Advances in planning stereotactic biopsy trajectories include sophisticated software packages. Surgiplan (Elekta Instruments, Atlanta, GA) is a computer program that enables the surgeon to view coronal, sagittal, and *probe-view* image reconstructions that show the exact location of the biopsy device at each level through the brain. This program allows the surgeon to refine trajectory planning such that important structures can be avoided. Careful attention to imaging information all the way from the skull to the target is important in reducing the risks of stereotactic biopsy. Using the techniques described above, the authors reported an evaluation of 500 patients who underwent a stereotactic biopsy. Forty patients (8%) had some hemorrhage on immediate postbiopsy imaging, and neurological deficits developed in six (1.2%). One patient died. The risk of hemorrhage correlated with the degree to which the platelet count was lower than 150,000/mm.[37]

Proper Neuropathological Evaluation

Expert neuropathological evaluation begins with careful handling and preparation of tissue in the operating room. Because of the necessarily small tissue volumes obtained at stereotactic biopsy, each piece is important. Samples should not be wiped off the biopsy instrument by hand with a cloth or gauze, since this traumatizes and disrupts the tissue. Small volumes of tissue deposited into large volumes of saline for transportation may also damage the cytoarchitecture of the tissue or make it difficult to retrieve. The preferred technique for biopsy specimen handling is to remove the tissue from the biopsy instrument with a 22-gauge needle and place in an empty petri dish. Here the specimen can be clearly seen and separated from any associated blood clot. The neurosurgeon should take an active role in presenting the tissues to the neuropathologist (who should come to the operating room). At that time, the clinical question is reviewed as well as the patient's history and imaging findings. We demonstrate on the scans the exact location from which each specimen was obtained. The neuropathologist provides input as to whether samples should be sent for culture, placed in formalin prior to paraffin embedding, or placed in glutaraldehyde for electron microscopic analysis. At times, all of these tests may be important to yield the final diagnosis. On average, two or three specimens are obtained. At our center, which contains a dedicated intraoperative CT scanner, a postoperative CT scan confirms the diagnostic site and absence of bleeding after biopsy.

Our ability to reach a diagnosis from small samples is related to the skills of a neuropathologist who is familiar with evaluating and interpreting small biopsy specimens. The main goal of the intraoperative neuropathology consultation is to determine whether or not potentially diagnostic tissue is present. The final diagnosis is frequently suggested during this initial phase of tissue evaluation, but it is reserved for the permanent sections. Making use of a *touch* preparation allows the neuropathologist to determine whether abnormal or diagnostic tissue is present intraoperatively and also conserves the tissue for permanent sections. Pollack et al. have refined the technique of diagnosis from touch preparations and in many cases prefer them to frozen sections, which are more time- and tissue-consuming.[19] Smear preparations of limited size are also popular to minimize tissue use.

Fluid Cavity Aspiration

Neurosurgeons occasionally are requested to drain cystic lesions within the brain. Cerebral abscesses and tumors or developmental cysts may be drained for either diagnostic or therapeutic purposes. Like diagnostic stereotactic biopsy, these procedures are rarely associated with the risk of hemorrhage, neurological deficit, seizures, or diagnostic failure. The principles of patient selection, target selection, and complication avoidance are the same as those for diagnostic stereotactic biopsy with some specific considerations.

Brain abscesses (>3 cm in average diameter), in addition to being aspirated, should be drained. In most instances, about one-half to two-thirds of the calculated volume of purulent material should be allowed to drain spontaneously from the abscess. Gentle aspiration may be required if the fluid is tenacious. Overzealous aspiration of pus can lead to hemorrhage from a friable and vascular abscess cavity wall. The remainder of the pus should be allowed to drain through a closed-system external catheter that will drain the abscess cavity over the next 1 to 3 postoperative days. This may prevent reaccumulation of pus and abscess recurrence. The catheter should be placed so that the drainage bag will remain in a dependent portion. The catheter length should be chosen so that it will not extend into a critical location when the abscess volume has diminished. Great care should be taken not to allow an abscess cavity to communicate with the ventricular system; this should be carefully thought out in the trajectory planning stage of the operation.

Nonpurulent cystic fluid collections in the brain may be drained to make a diagnosis or relieve mass effect. Craniopharyngioma cysts can be diagnosed and often definitively treated in one setting by sampling the fluid (to identify cholesterol crystals) and instilling a radioactive isotope (P32) to destroy the epithelial lining. The soft tissue penetrance of the isotope is limited and is associated with minimal morbidity even when the injection dose is 200 to 250 Gy. Glial tumor cysts are sometimes treated by aspiration, but they frequently require repeated aspirations or placement of an indwelling catheter for periodic drainage. Stereotactic intracavitary radiation may also be of benefit. Colloid cysts of the third ventricle, when filled with a low-density, low-viscosity fluid, can often be definitively treated by a single aspiration.[12] The complications of cyst aspiration and drainage are similar to those of diagnostic stereotactic biopsy.

Movement Disorder Surgery

In the 1990s, a resurgence in thalamotomy and pallidotomy occurred to treat patients with movement disorders. Recently, deep brain stimulation (DBS) of the thalamus, subthalamus, or globus pallidus has been used widely for Parkinson's disease, essential tremor, and dystonia. While thalamotomy was selected to affect primarily the tremor component of Parkinson's disease, pallidotomy emerged as a procedure that addressed not only tremor, but also rigidity, bradykinesia, and dopamine-induced dyskinesias. Leksell first evaluated stereotactic lesions in the pallidum in the late 1950s. After the introduction of levodopa in the late 1960s, progress with his concepts largely subsided until the early 1990s. Laitinen reevaluated pallidotomy in a modern series of patients.[16] He emphasized the ability of pallidotomy to complement levodopa therapy by ameliorating the drug-induced movements (dyskinesia).

Complications of pallidotomy and thalamotomy can occur in several ways.[9,11,16] Both procedures are designed to create defined lesions in deeply seated and critically located brain nuclei. Hemorrhage is the primary concern in both procedures. Fortunately, because the electrode is small and no tissue is removed during such procedures, the hemorrhage rate is low. Neurological deficits may be produced by the lesion itself. The most common neurological deficits following pallidotomy include visual field deficit, hemiparesis, and dysarthria. Such symptoms are usually temporary. The close approximation of the globus pallidus interna to the internal capsule and optic tract is the basis for these deficits. Radiofrequency lesion generation causes focal tissue necrosis surrounded by a zone of edema. This peripheral edema may cause transient deficits. Whenever a probe is inserted into the brain, abscess formation is possible; this was reported in a single patient in Iacono et al.'s series.[9] Seizures resulting from pallidotomy have yet to be reported. The most common side effects after thalamotomy include limb or facial numbness or weakness.

The mainstays of complication avoidance for thalamotomy and pallidotomy surgery are appropriate patient selection and target planning, the use of test lesions and visual evoked potential monitoring (pallidotomy), physiological evaluation, careful intraoperative neurological examinations, and judicious lesion generation.

Selection of Parkinson's Disease Patients for Surgery

The appropriate candidate for surgery is a patient with Parkinson's disease who has exhausted maximal medical therapy but nevertheless remains symptomatic with tremor, rigidity, bradykinesias, and dopamine-induced dyskinesias. Patients with tremor only may be best treated by thalamic surgery. Patients with parkinsonism secondary to other *Parkinson's plus* syndromes, because of the underlying differences in pathophysiology, are not thought to be appropriate candidates. Signs of autonomic, cerebellar, and extraocular movement dysfunction may signal that potential patients have some other disease process such as Shy-Drager syndrome, olivopontocerebellar atrophy, or progressive supranuclear palsy, each of which would make the patient less likely to respond to surgery.

Ideally, patients undergoing surgery should have the capacity for rehabilitation, either in a formal program or at home, as this affords them the best opportunity to benefit from their procedure. Patients who will necessarily return to a sedentary environment after surgery may have symptomatic improvement but may not make functional gains following surgery. Severe dementia is a contraindication for surgery.

Patients with bleeding diatheses, major intercurrent medical problems, and severe structural brain abnormalities (with distorted anatomy) are not acceptable candidates for surgery unless their medical condition is optimized. Radiosurgery may be appropriate for such patients. Poorly controlled hypertension is thought to increase the risk of hemorrhage during open surgery. Patients with preexisting ipsilateral hemianopsia have a relative contraindication to pallidotomy since the complication of contralateral hemianopsia would be unacceptable to them.

Physiological Testing

Some surgeons use microelectrode recording to identify pallidal, thalamic, or subthalamic neurons, borders, and regional structures. Others use macroelectrode-based stimulation. With stimulation, parameters include a 90–150 microsecond pulse wave, 50–100 Hz, and use of 0–3 V. If stimulation causes a capsular response with markedly increased tone and dysarthria at less than 1.5 V, most surgeons move the electrode farther away from the internal capsule (either lateral or more anterior). If a capsular response is achieved at or above 2 V, then this threshold usually is safe for lesioning. Identification of visual phosphenes during stimulation is an indication that the electrode should be moved away from the optic tract.

Lesioning During Pallidotomy

Prior to formal pallidotomy, we create a test lesion using a 1 × 3 mm electrode (45°C is delivered for 30 seconds). This lesion usually is temporary and reversible. If no deficits are identified on clinical examination and with (VEP), then a permanent lesion is created at 70°–80°C for 60 seconds, usually at two or three locations in the globus pallidus interna. Each lesion created by the 3 mm electrode is spaced at 2 mm increments in the superior-inferior axis. The patient is monitored clinically during each lesioning for strength, speech, and the appropriate clinical response off medications. If any adverse reaction is identified, lesion generation is stopped. If the patient's level of consciousness changes, then an immediate CT scan is performed. Five percent of patients have had transient dysarthria lasting for 1–3 weeks. This may be related to perilesional edema in the early period after surgery. We have had one patient who developed a hemorrhage close to the pallidotomy site (requiring surgical evacuation) and other who developed a superficial hemorrhage under twist drill exposure.

Deep Brain Stimulation

Deep brain stimulating (DBS) electrode systems have been used for the management of intractable tremor and other movement disorders. In the United States, general approval first was granted by the Food and Drug Administration for use in the thalamus. Deep brain stimulation systems could be used for patients with Parkinson's disease–related tremor and for essential tremor. Recently, approval was granted for placement of the system into the subthalamic nucleus or globus pallidus for the treatment of Parkinson's disease. Other patients have received DBS systems for the management of tremor related to multiple sclerosis, dystonia, and selected neuropsychiatric disorders. In past years, DBS was used for the management of intractable pain.

Placement of a DBS system requires precise stereotactic guidance, intraoperative physiological testing (for adult patients), attachment of the electrode lead to the burr hole, connection of the electrode lead to a cable, and tunneling of the cable into the upper chest region where a pulse generator is placed into a subcutaneous pocket (Fig. 41.2). Thus, insertion of the hardware is an extensive procedure and involves placement, connection, and fixation of numerous components. Each of these components is at risk for breakage, malfunction, infection, migration, erosion, or other problems. We reviewed data from consecutive thalamic DBS procedures performed over the initial 2-year period at two institutions and studied factors contributing to hardware-related complications. The average length of surgery was 4.1 hours, and patients had an average follow-up of 29 months. Stimulation proved effective for all patients who had placement of a thalamic stimulator. A total of 23 hardware problems were noted (34% of procedures in 27% of patients). The most common problem was breakage of the electrode lead in its extracranial location (n = 10). Immediate symptoms included loss of tremor control and paresthesias. All of these breakages were proximal to the connector and were most commonly found in the cervical area (8 of 10). System infection (n = 7) was diagnosed by clinical symptoms of fever and signs of erythema and purulent exudate. The subcutaneous pocket in the upper chest was believed to be the initial site of infection in four of these patients, one patient had obvious purulence from the cranial incision, and two patients had infection believed to be from erosion of the connector. Bacterial cultures usually yielded skin flora. Management of infections involved removal of the entire system, except when the infection involved only the pulse generator. There was one patient with migration of the cranial lead (the lead had pulled out), one patient with development of a chronic

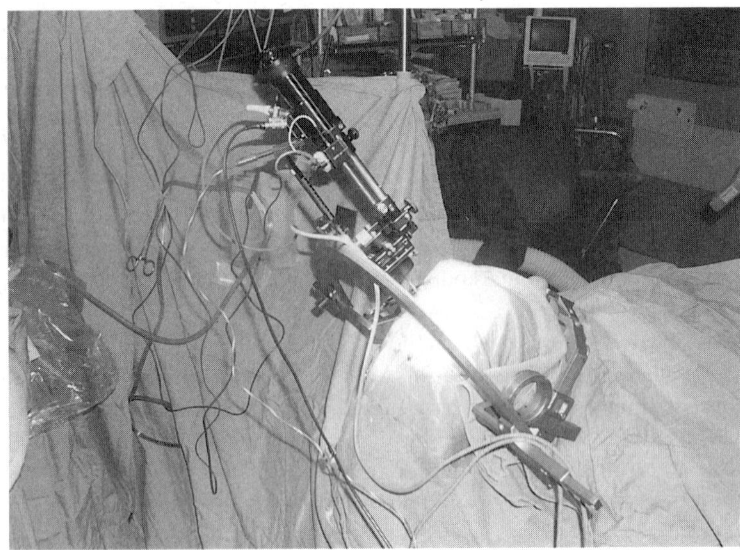

Figure 41.2. Operative setup during deep brain stimulation of the subthalamus in a patient with Parkinson's disease. The microelectrode array is attached to the arc of the stereotactic frame.

subdural hematoma below the burr hole site, one patient with a defective battery system (early battery depletion in less than 1 year), and one patient with a defective connector.[15] As experience increased, the frequency of complications decreased.

Stereotactic Radiosurgery

Radiosurgery is an increasingly used technique for the management of selected patients with vascular malformations, brain tumors, and functional disorders. Single-session radiation delivery with stereotactic guidance provides precise irradiation of a defined intracranial target. Stereotactic radiosurgery is performed with the model C or 4C Leksell Gamma Knife (Elekta Instruments) at the University of Pittsburgh (Figs. 41.3 and 41.4). The desired antitumor biological effects are cessation of tumor cell division and delayed blood vessel occlusion. Radiosurgery has been evaluated extensively in terms of clinical results, complications, and cost effectiveness.

The complications of stereotactic radiosurgery are based on the radiation dose delivered, the brain region targeted, and prior patient history (such as receipt of prior radiation therapy). Radiation-related complications can be either early or delayed. The early complications of radiosurgery are rare and consist only of mild headache or occasional nausea lasting for several hours after the procedure. Delayed complications occur 3 months to 3 years following radiosurgery and include both cranial nerve deficits and deficits associated with brain injury. In the radiosurgery of acoustic neuromas, currently we have seen a 1%–3% chance of delayed facial or trigeminal neuropathy (usually mild) that occurred a mean 6–9 months following radiosurgery. The dose tolerance of the optic nerve and chiasm has been investigated and is considered by many to be a conservative 8–9 Gy. Thus, for tumors of the parasellar region, we limit the dose received by the chiasm. Using this approach, we have not detected visual complications in any patient treated during the past 7 years. Special techniques of beam blocking or beam shaping are effective in reducing the dose received by normal structures surrounding the brain target.

Delayed vascular effects can include thrombosis and ischemia. These are most prominent in the management of patients with vascular malformations of the brain where regional brain edema can occur prior to vascular malformation obliteration. It is not known whether obliteration of the malformation itself causes this response or if it is a direct response of radiation. Up to 3% of the patients in our series of vascular malformations developed permanent morbidity after radiosurgery. The oc-

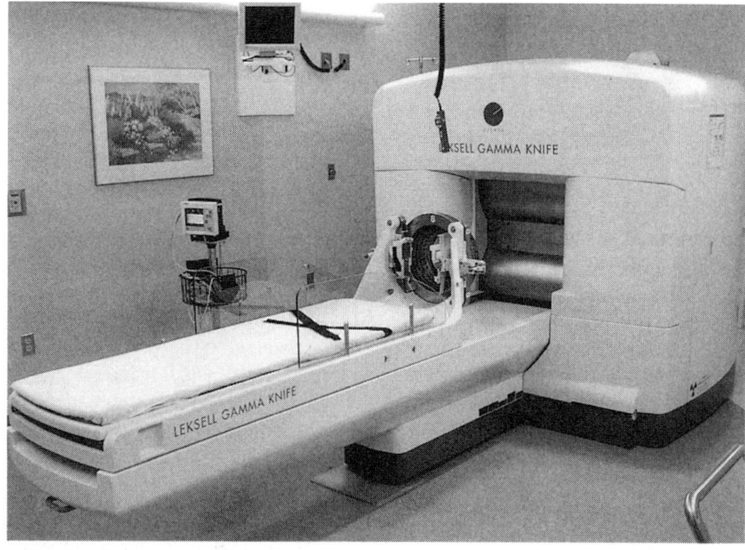

Figure 41.3. Leksell Model C Gamma Knife® at the University of Pittsburgh.

currence of radiation necrosis is rare. We usually select a radiation dose associated with less than a 3% chance of permanent necrosis based on lesion volume.[8]

Radiation-associated malignancy after radiosurgery is rare. We have not seen such a patient in our experience with 7400 procedures. We believe that the chance for malignant transformation 5 to 30 years later is less than 1:1000. This reduced risk of delayed oncogenesis may be one advantage of stereotactic radiosurgery as an alternative to conventional fractionated radiation therapy.

Complication avoidance in radiosurgery is dependent upon proper patient selection, the use of high-resolution neuroimaging for dose planning, the creation of a conformal dose plan that fits the lesion margin precisely, the selection of a safe yet effective radiation dose, and proper education of

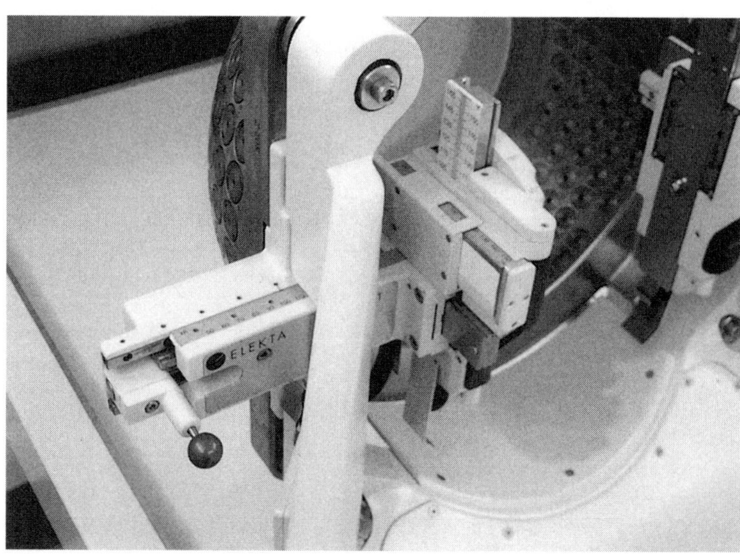

Figure 41.4. The automatic positioning system (APS) of the Leksell Gamma Knife allows robotic movement to the different radiation isocenters.

the patient and family as to the realistic expectations of radiosurgery.

Summary

Stereotactic neurosurgery is a minimally invasive management strategy for patients with brain tumors, vascular malformations, and functional disorders. With proper attention to the guidance provided by high-resolution neuroimaging, the use of advanced computer workstations, and proper use of surgical tools, surgical morbidity should be low. Patients and referring physicians must be informed about the results and expectations of stereotactic surgery. As these techniques become more and more common in the neurosurgical armamentarium, proper attention to the details of these approaches must be maintained.

REFERENCES

1. Abernathy CD, Camacho A, Kelly PJ: Stereotaxic suboccipital transcerebellar biopsy of pontine mass lesions. J Neurosurg 70:195–200, 1989.
2. Apuzzo MLJ, Chandrasoma PT, Cohen D, Zee CS, Zelman V: Computed imaging stereotaxy: Experience and perspective related to 500 procedures applied to brain masses. Neurosurgery 20:930–937, 1987.
3. Apuzzo MLJ, Chandrasoma PT, Zelman V, Gianotta SL, Weiss MH: Computed tomographic guidance stereotaxis in the management of lesions of the third ventricular region. Neurosurgery 15:502–508, 1984.
4. Bernstein M, Parrent AG: Complications of CT-guided stereotactic biopsy of intra-axial brain lesions. J Neurosurg 81:165–168, 1994.
5. Chimowitz MI, Barnett GH, Palmer J: Treatment of intractable arterial hemorrhage during stereotactic brain biopsy with thrombin. J Neurosurg 74:301–303, 1991.
6. Coffey RJ, Lunsford LD: Stereotactic surgery for mass lesions of the midbrain and pons. Neurosurgery 17:12–18, 1985.
7. Field M, Witham T, Flickinger J, Kondziolka D, Lunsford LD: Comprehensive assessment of hemorrhage risks and outcomes after stereotactic brain biopsy. J Neurosurg 94:545–551, 2001.
8. Flickinger JC: An integrated logistic formula for predictions of complications after radiosurgery. Int J Radiat Oncol Biol Phys 17:879–885, 1989.
9. Iacono RP, Shima F, Lonser RR, Kuniyoshi S, Maeda G, Yamada S: The results, indications, and physiology of posteroventral pallidotomy for patients with Parkinson's disease. Neurosurgery 36:1118–1127, 1995.
10. Kelly PJ: Tumor Stereotaxis. Philadelphia, WB Saunders, 1991.
11. Kondziolka D, Bonaroti EA, Lunsford LD: Pallidotomy for Parkinson's disease. Contemp Neurosurg 18:1–7, 1996.
12. Kondziolka D, Lunsford LD: Stereotactic management of colloid cysts: Factors predicting success. J Neurosurg 75:45–51, 1991.
13. Kondziolka D, Lunsford LD: Stereotactic biopsy for intrinsic lesions of the medulla through the long axis of the brainstem: Technical considerations. Acta Neurochir 128: 89–91, 1994.
14. Kondziolka D, Lunsford LD: Results and expectations of image-guided brainstem biopsy. Surg Neurol 43:558–562, 1995.
15. Kondziolka D, Whiting D, Germanwala A, Oh M: Hardware-related complications after placement of thalamic deep brain stimulator systems. Stereotact Funct Neurosurg 79:228–233, 2002.
16. Laitinen LV, Bergenheim AT, Hariz MI: Leksell's posteroventral pallidotomy in the treatment of Parkinson's disease. J Neurosurg 76:53–61, 1992.
17. Lunsford LD, Martinez AJ: Stereotactic exploration of the brain in the era of computed tomography. Surg Neurol 22:222–230, 1984.
18. Ostertag CB, Mennel HD, Kiessling M: Stereotactic biopsy of brain tumors. Surg Neurol 14:275–283, 1980.
19. Pollack IF, Martinez A, Hall W, Lunsford LD. Touch preparations in the rapid intraoperative analysis of central nervous system lesions: A comparison with frozen sections and paraffin embedded sections. Mod Pathol 1:378–384, 1988.
20. Voges J, Schroder R, Treuer H, Pastyr O, Schlegel W, Lorenz WJ, Sturm V: CT-guided and computer assisted stereotactic biopsy: Technique, results, indications. Acta Neurochir 125:142–149, 1993.

Chapter 42

Iatrogenic Complications of Spine Surgery

ANIL NANDA, SATISH RUDRAPPA, AND PRASAD VANNEMREDDY

Spine surgery is changing with introduction of newer imaging techniques, diagnostic protocols, and treatment methods including biocompatible implants. With refined diagnostic methods and surgical techniques, the spine surgeon is now faced with a rapidly changing educational substrate. In the United States alone, 400,000 lumbar surgeries are performed annually and an estimated $3 billion was spent on spine fusion procedures in 2003. From time to time, different series are published describing complications following spinal surgery in varied contexts. Spine surgeons need constant updates on the topic of complications encountered with newer and evolving techniques. In this chapter, we will discuss iatrogenic complications related to all spine surgeries. The complications common to all levels of the spine are presented first, followed by some problems specific to different spinal segments (Table 42.1). The secondary iatrogenic complications of spine surgeries such as deep vein thrombosis, thromboembolism, pneumonia, and so on are not included in this chapter.

Table 42.1. Common Complications of Spine Surgery

Dural laceration, cerebrospinal fluid leaks, and pseudomeningocele
Worsening of neurological deficits
Hematoma formation
Graft displacement and hardware-related problems
Vascular injuries
Postoperative discitis

Common Complications of Spine Surgery

Dural Laceration, Cerebrospinal Fluid Leaks, and Pseudomeningoceles

Dural tears and cerebrospinal fluid (CSF) leaks are the most common complications of spine surgeries. If unnoticed or treated in a timely fashion, this can lead to infection, pseudoarthrosis and nerve irritation.

Unlike lumbar disc surgery,[106] cervical disc surgery is more direct, with no distraction of the root or thecal sac during the procedure. For this reason, CSF leak is a rare phenomenon in cervical disc surgery. It is commonly seen in removal of ossification of the posterior longitudinal ligament (OPLL) by the anterior approach when the ossified portion involves part of the dura. Other procedures in which this problem is noted include (1) making a burr hole in the suboccipital region or (2) passing a wire through the foramen magnum region in occipitocervical fusions and, (3) in inexperienced hands, during muscle separation from the lamina, especially in cases of subluxation or dislocations.

Dural tear can be encountered in lumbar surgeries (1) during excision of the ligamentum flavum with a Kerrison punch; (2) during nerve root retraction, especially with large central disc herniation or a calcified disc; and (3) during insertion of bone grafts/cages with posterior lumbar interbody fusion (PLIF).[52]

Postsurgical pseudomeningocele (PSPM) forms when CSF extravasates through a dura-arachnoid tear, becoming encysted within the wound. Its incidence is less than 0.1% with intervertebral disc surgery.[94]

The patient's complaints closely resemble those of an intervertebral disc prolapse with symptoms of low back pain or occasional radicular symptoms, or they can present with wound swelling associated with low-pressure headache. This diagnosis is usually reached 2–3 years postsurgery. Magnetic resonance imaging (MRI) confirms the diagnosis.

Treatment

Intraoperative detection of the CSF leak is important. A mere dural tear may not have a CSF leak as long as the arachnoid is intact. A small, rugged tear at the shoulder of the root or close to the root canal can be controlled using a small, fat plug and Gelfoam. This rarely requires any suturing. A thorough watertight closure is mandatory, and the patient may be kept prophylactically in the prone position with empirical coverage by acetazolamide or furosemide for a week or more, depending upon the response.

A midline or paramedian tear of the dura and arachnoid necessitates placement of a couple of regular dural sutures using dural substitute or primary dura. No harm is done if the tear has to be widened for better closure of the dura. In principle, the torn arachnoid membrane has to be placed back inside the dura. Postoperative management may be similar to that of other intradural surgeries in these cases.

The risk of CSF leak increases in patients who have repeated surgery when there is a dural tear. These patients need to be monitored carefully for wound inspection and systemic manifestation of infection. The scar tissue in these patients delays normal healing, and a neglected CSF leak could result in pseudomeningocele.

An occasional patient requires surgical repair of pseudomeningocele with dural substitutes.[46] The double breasting technique while suturing the wound reduces the dead space and recollection.

Worsening of Neurological Deficits

Recent operative techniques using magnification and improved illumination have contributed to a reduction in operative morbidity and mortality. Better understanding of position-related spinal dynamics and refined anesthetic methods has also reduced the incidence of neurological deterioration. Routine intraoperative electrophysiological monitoring helps to prevent or identify neurological deterioration during operative procedures. However, both radicular and cord injuries occur at different rates. Flynn reported a 1.3% rate of radicular dysfunction and a 3.3% rate of worsening myelopathy.[23,110]

Radicular injuries are more common than cord injuries. For unknown reasons, the C5 root is very sensitive to minor trauma during surgery. This is noted even in patients with simple decompressive laminectomy and laminoplasty.[78,81] Paralysis of the deltoid and biceps brachii muscles is an exclusive feature of deterioration in the nerve root group. Causes of this paralysis include misalignment of the spine related to graft complications and a tethering effect on the nerve root following major shifting of the spinal cord after decompression. This complication may be avoided by performing selective foraminotomy in addition to posterior central canal decompression. Preexisting subclinical C5 root compression is a cause of C5 palsy after posterior cervical decompression for myelopathy.[80]

The causes of deterioration of cord function include direct spinal cord injury during surgery, misalignment of the spine associated with graft placement, extrusion, implant failure, and epidural hematoma. However, cord injury can also occur when the patient has severe canal stenosis, during drilling of the adherent portion of the OPLL over the dura (producing heat and vibration), and sublaminar wire insertion.

Precautionary measures such as intubation while the patient is awake, proper positioning of the patient, intraoperative monitoring with an image intensifier before induction and during spinal fusion, and/or fixation help to prevent most complications.[76]

Table 42.2 focuses on common causes of neurological worsening, and we suggest a few points regarding prevention.

In the *lumbar region*, the spinal cord usually ends at the lower part of the body of L1 or the upper part of the body of L2. Fortunately, most elective surgeries done in the lumbar region are below this level. A familiar neurological problem encountered with lumbar surgery is radiculopathy, which usually occurs at the level of L4-5. Thus, many patients present with footdrop. This is observed with simple microdiscectomy or, more commonly, with injury secondary to a fractured medial wall of the pedicle by screws.[108] With extension of the pedicle screw to the thoracolumbar region, the chances of injury to the conus or cauda equina increase.[47,58] These patients usually present with bilateral lower limb weakness, with involvement of both proximal and distal muscle groups (in varying proportions), sensory loss below L1, and bowel and bladder involvement with sluggish deep tendon reflexes in the lower limbs.

The prognosis following spinal surgery, irrespective of the level of the spine, varies with the persistence of the impinging elements (e.g., screw, bony fragments), age of the patient, comorbid factors, nature of employment, and postoperative rehabilitation.[60] However, strict adherence to anatomical landmarks while inserting the screws, use of magnification, and good illumination with either a loop or a microscope will significantly reduce these complications.

Other causes of neurological deficits in the lumbar region include slipping of the drill over the root or rootlet injuries associated with dural tear, blind insertion of the Kerrison punch, rongeurs in and around the roots, excessive coagulation of epidural vessels around the nerve roots, and root injury during insertion of a bone graft or cage.

Hematoma Formation

The anterior approach to the cervical spine is usually done through the well-defined avascular plane between the carotid sheath/sternomastoid laterally and the trachea/esophagus medially. Two arteries (superior and inferior thyroid arteries) that connect the carotid sheath with the midline structures are at risk when excessive lateral retraction is applied or during dissection with electrocautery. If there

Table 42.2. Common Causes of Neurological Worsening in Cervical Surgery

Cause	Prevention
Excessive neck manipulation during anesthetic induction	Preoperative assessment of active flexion and extension of the neck
Brachial plexus stretching during positioning	Keep the shoulder lax during taping
Excessive use of monopolar cautery during longus coli dissection	Have orientation of root exit zone and minimize the use of monopolar cautery
Poor illumination and magnification during osteophyte/ subposterior longitudinal ligament removal	Appropriate knowledge about the use of microscope
Excessive use of bipolar coagulation near the root sleeve during discectomy	Control epidural bleeding by packing with Surgicel
Blind insertion of curette to remove the osteophyte	Use high-speed drill with diamond bits of appropriate size irrigation. Use a *pencil grip* on the drill
Overdistraction and rapid distraction of the vertebral spreaders in the presence of multilevel osteophytes	Slow, progressive spreading
Improper placement of grafts	Place the graft under appropriate distraction and use locking plates
Improper placement of pilot holes for screws	Use image intensifier and rescue screws if abnormal position of the screws is noticed
Epidural or subcutaneous plane hematoma formation	Meticulous hemostasis and suction drain use

is any injury to these vessels, it is usually noticed intraoperatively and coagulated. It can sometimes present postoperatively as anterior neck swelling secondary to hematoma or increased sanguinous output from inserted drains.

An acute collection can compromise the airway, necessitating emergency removal of clots. Hematoma formation may be seen with multilevel corpectomies, in patients who had epidural venous bleeding during corpectomy (which usually opens up during distraction before graft placement), excision of diseased bone (e.g., primary or secondary bone tumor), and in patients with reoperation. It is safer to keep a suction drain in the cavity in such cases prior to closure. There are anecdotal reports of pseudoaneurysm formation in the inferior thyroid arteries secondary to thermal/mechanical injury.[22]

Hematoma collection in *lumbar surgery* is proportional to the type of surgery done. In the case of a simple microdiscectomy, there may be no collection at all, whereas with long-segment spinal stabilization, PLIF, and surgery for bone tumors or vascular malformations, the collection can be quite significant. Hematoma collection can be significantly reduced by decreasing levels of exposure, strict subperiosteal dissection of the muscle, waxing of the laminectomy sites, coagulation or compression of the epidural vessels, and meticulous closure of the muscle layers. Perioperative use of cell savers is useful in the above instances. Meticulous hemostasis significantly reduces the chances of epidural fibrosis and further complications. Use of postoperative suction drains decreases such collections, indirectly facilitating wound healing and thereby reducing the chances of wound infection.

Graft Displacement and Hardware-Related Problems

Graft migration rates proportionately increase with levels of fusion. Cervical corpectomies involving a fusion ending at the C7 vertebral body are associated with a higher rate of graft migration. Long-segment anterior cervical plates have been used to reduce the incidence of graft displacement and migration but have been shown to increase the risk of early failure because of screw dislodgment.

Vertebral fracture and graft extrusion requiring revision developed in 14% of 22 patients of Epstein[19] without plates within 24 hours of surgery, whereas neither of these problems occurred in the other 22 patients with plates. Similarly, Wang et al.[107] studied 249 consecutive patients who underwent one- to five-level anterior cervical corpectomies with strut grafting using autogenous bone grafts (iliac crest or fibula). Sixteen patients experienced graft migration during the postoperative period, and 14 had procedures involving a corpectomy of C6 with a fusion extending inferiorly to the C7 vertebral body. The authors demonstrated that a greater number of vertebral bodies removed and a longer graft increased the frequency of graft displacement. Corpectomies involving a fusion at the C7 vertebral body were associated with a higher rate of graft migration. Sasso et al.[83] reiterated that the failure rate could be as high as 71% after three-level fixed-plated anterior cervical corpectomy and fusion (ACF) reconstruction compared to a 6% failure rate with a two-level ACF.[40]

An early failure rate is higher with screws that are incorrectly locked to the plate and with the use of a peg-in-hole-type bone grafting technique. Anterior cervical plating and bone grafting alone after a three-level cervical corpectomy for various spinal disorders appear to afford inadequate stability in the early postoperative period, regardless of the immobilization method.[102] The use of a junctional plate anteriorly, along with posterior segmental fixation and fusion, may prevent or decrease the incidence of graft dislodgment after a long-segment cervical reconstruction procedure.[105] The use of additional screws to the graft weakens the graft. Recent literature suggests single-stage 360 degree fusion[83,102] for patients undergoing three or more levels of corpectomy, when there is significant osteoporosis or weak bone with malignancy or infection, and with active smoking.

Since 10% of the graft settles by 6 weeks, graft placement intraoperatively under cervical traction reduces the chances of loosening and displacement. Experience with artificial disc placement is ongoing. Clinical trials using the charite III prosthesis are ongoing.[38]

Some case illustrations follow.

Case 1: A 34-year-old male was admitted with a history of neck pain radiating to both upper extremities. Upon investigation, he was found to have a herniated disc at C3 and C4. An anterior cervical discectomy with bone graft placement was performed. The patient, however, returned after 6 weeks with recurrence of symptoms. Radiological evaluation revealed a broken and displaced bone graft (Fig. 42.1*A*). A second procedure with reinforcement with a screw plate construct restored the graft position and spine curvature (Fig. 42.1*B*). This case illustrates the indications for spine fixation after discectomy in some instances where the removal of posterior osteophytes and a posterior longitudinal ligament might induce instability when the load on the spine motion segment exceeds the limits of bone graft resilience.

Case 2: A 53-year-old female patient underwent anterior cervical discectomy with fusion and fixation for spondylitic radiculopathy. She returned to the clinic after 4 weeks with complaints of dysphagia and sensory radiculopathy. Cervical spine X-rays revealed dislodged screws and an unstable construct at C5 and C6 (Fig. 42.2*A*). She underwent implant extrication but with injury to the trachea and esophagus that required repair in the otolaryngology unit. The recovery was uneventful, and cervical spine X-rays revealed no instability on follow-up (Fig. 42.2*B*). Implant failures, as this case illustrates, relate to the metal as well as the bone. In postmenopausal women especially, bone strength is questionable and screws may not lodge securely.

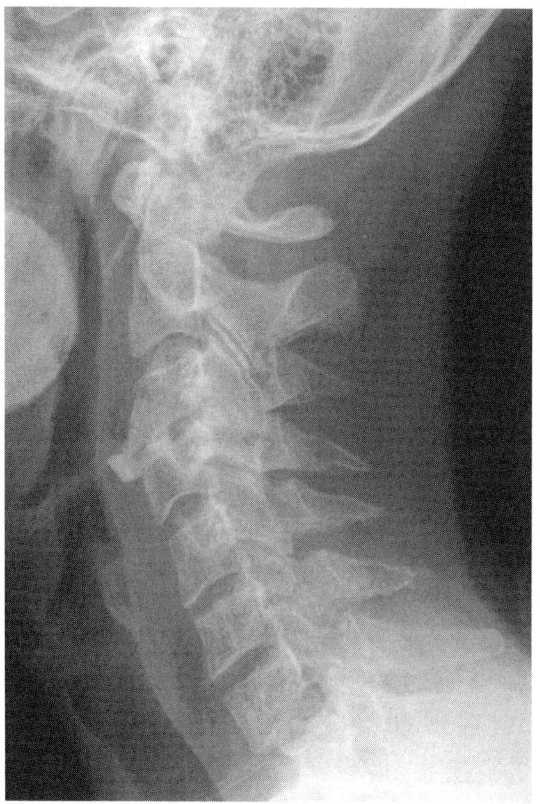

Figure 42.1A. An anterior cervical discectomy with bone graft placement was performed. The patient returned after 6 weeks with recurrence of symptoms. Radiological evaluation revealed the broken and displaced bone graft.

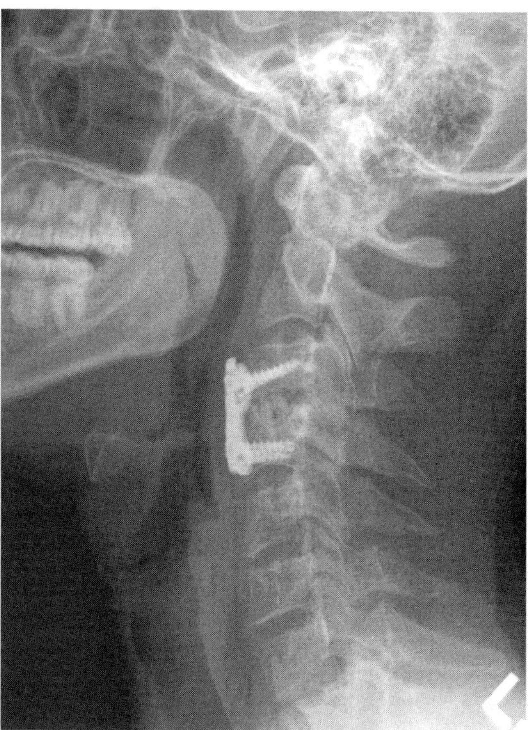

Figure 42.1*B*. A second procedure with reinforcement with a screw plate construct restored the graft position and spine curvature.

Malpositioning of the Plate and Screws

The exact incidence of malpositioning of the plate or screws in cervical surgeries is not clearly documented in the literature. Such malpositioning can lead to graft failure, displacement and migration, and injury of adjacent structures (especially the esophagus).[30] This condition is often noted in patients with long-segment anterior cervical fusion and/or fixation without posterior instrumentation, noncorrection of preexisting kyphosis, smokers, osteoporotic/diseased bone, and noncompliant orthotic usage.

Use of properly sized plates and correct positioning of the screws usually prevents such complications. During the procedure, the removal of any malpositioned screws should be followed by drilling

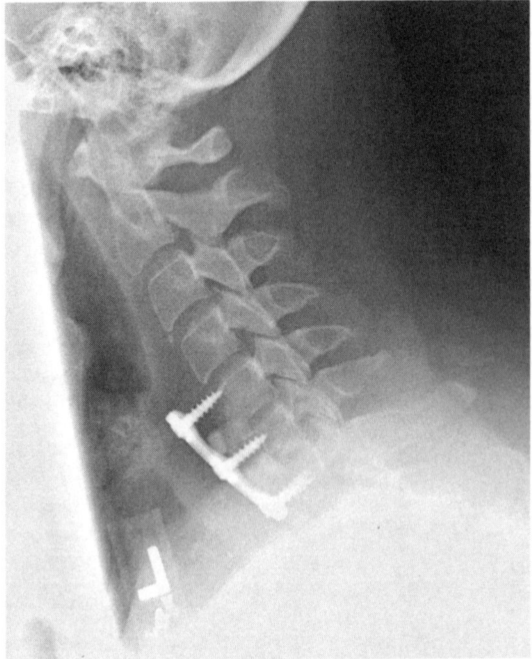

Figure 42.2A. A 53-year-old female patient underwent anterior cervical discectomy with fusion and fixation for spondylitic radiculopathy. She returned to the clinic after 4 weeks with complaints of dysphagia and sensory radiculopathy. Cervical spine X-rays revealed dislodged screws and an unstable construct at C5 and C6.

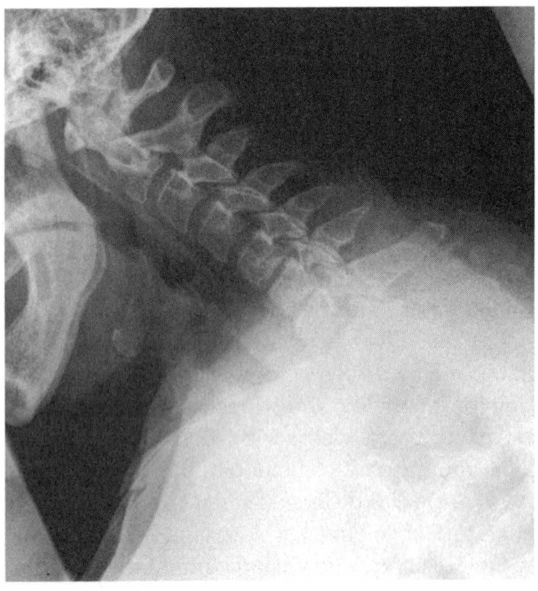

Figure 42.2*B*. The patient underwent implant extrication but with injury to the trachea and esophagus that required repair in the otolaryngology unit. The recovery was uneventful, and cervical spine X-rays revealed no instability on follow-up.

of new pilot holes and placement of rescue screws. Plugging the previously drilled hole with bone chips will help to hold reinserted screws more securely. Essential factors in the success of this surgery include proper selection of the patient, surgical procedure counseling, and postoperative use of orthotics.

Pedicle Screw–Related Complications

The use of pedicle screw fixation for various disorders of thoracic and lumbar spine with instability has progressively increased since King used the first transfacet screw in 1944. Watkins was credited with developing the posterolateral fusion technique in 1953. Modifications of this technique are used today. Biomechanical studies have suggested that pedicle screws are superior to other posterior fixation techniques, providing increased rigidity and construct stiffness.[3] This increased rigidity allows for shorter construct lengths and a shorter duration of external immobilization. Often screw placement becomes difficult with altered spine curvatures following trauma, disease, or scarring around the root canal. However, pedicle screw fixation has an acceptable complication rate and is a safe, reliable technique in experienced hands.[20,21]

Various factors contribute to complications with pedicle screw insertion. Some of the factors reported are (1) the site of fusion, (2) the number of levels included, (3) association with kyphoscoliosis, (4) age of the patient, (5) osteoporosis, (6) implant features, and (7) experience of the spinal surgeon[50,79] (Table 42.3).

Screws that are malpositioned medially or inferiorly place the nerve root at risk as they course around the pedicle. Most perioperative difficulties can be mitigated by thorough preoperative evalua-

Table 42.3. Methods to Prevent Graft Migration in Cervical Surgery

Proper selection of patients
Appropriate shaping of graft to fit into the corpectomy site
Placement of graft in accordance with the normal lordotic curve of the cervical spine
Placement of graft after adequate distraction of adjacent vertebral bodies

Table 42.4. Pedicle Screw–Related Complications

Perioperative complications—screw misplacement, nerve root impingement, cerebrospinal fluid leak, pedicle fracture, blood loss, neurological complications
Postoperative complications—deep wound infection, screw loosening, rod-screw disconnection
Hardware failures
Junctional problems

tion, adequate exposure, and attention to anatomical landmarks during screw insertion and fixation of the implant. Tactile feedback while making the pilot hole and inserting screws is essential to avoid complications. Percutaneous insertion of pedicle screws in the lumbar spine is a safe and reliable technique but is technically demanding. Screw placement in the thoracic spine can be extremely challenging due to the smaller size and more complex three-dimensional morphology of the thoracic pedicle.[97] At the thoracic level, pedicular size is widely variable, ranging from the smallest mean transverse diameter of 4.5 mm at T4 to the largest mean transverse diameter of 7.8 mm at T12. The other reason that thoracic pedicle screw insertion is complicated is its proximity to the thoracic pleura, nerve roots, and the spinal cord itself. In several published series,[62] cortical violations have been reported in up to 15%–50% of screws placed with standard fluoroscopic techniques, with a significantly higher rate of cortical perforation in the midthoracic spine. Medial errors are less forgiving in the thoracic spine because there is less mobility of the spinal cord than that of the nerve roots in the cauda equina. Lateral perforations of the pedicular cortex are potential threats to the pleural cavity and great vessels. There is segmental variability from left to right. Though pedicle screw insertion in the thoracolumbar spine with the use of lateral plain radiography alone is safe and effective, different authors have used stereotactic image guidance with varied success. Cases of reducible spondylolisthesis at L5–S1 without anterior support were found to be especially prone to screw breakage. To avoid screw breakage and subsequent loss of correction, anterior fusion through either posterior or anterior lumbar interbody fusion (PLIF or ALIF) techniques is advocated.[45]

Perioperative use of electrophysiological monitoring techniques such as somatosensory evoked potentials or electroneurography and nerve conduction velocity studies are reliable and useful diagnostic methods that provide intraoperative information about the functional integrity of neural structures. Persisting root irritation or neurological deficit demand implant revision/removal.

Vascular Injuries in Spine Surgery

Vertebral Artery Injury

Vertebral Artery Injury During Anterior Cervical Procedures

Vertebral artery injury during anterior cervical procedures is rare,[15,16,63] occurring in 0.3% of cases. The true incidence remains unknown and underreported.[44] Injury to the artery during cervical discectomy was first reported in 1973, and Smith et al.[95] reported a series of 10 cases among 1195 cases of anterior cervical surgery. Most cases of vertebral artery injury were treated with hemostatic packing. Occlusion of a single vertebral artery is well tolerated but, unlike patients having aneurysm surgery, those undergoing anterior cervical surgery will not have preoperative angiography to determine the dominant artery, subjecting them to irreversible ischemic damage. Accurate preoperative evaluation of the cervical MRI scan is necessary[18] to identify tortuosity and atherosclerotic change of the vertebral artery, to maintain a strict midline plane, and to minimize lateral dissection below the longus colli muscle. This will prevent inadvertent injury of the vertebral arteries.

If treated only with packing, vertebral artery injury can lead to fistula formation, as well as hemorrhagic and embolic complications. Golfinos et al.[31] have advocated reconstruction of the artery by exposing the artery proximal and distal to the injury site.

Vertebral Artery Injury in Posterior Cervical Surgery

Vertebral artery injury in posterior cervical surgery can occur with transarticular screw insertion and during lateral mass plating, as well as during exposure over the superior part of the posterior ring of atlas.[68]

When patients require transarticular screw fixation, it is important for them to undergo preoperative thin-slice (2 mm) computed tomography (CT) scanning through C1-2 with sagittal and coronal reconstruction to determine the course of the vertebral artery and its relation to the bone anatomy of the pars interarticularis of C-2.[1] During surgery, it is better to expose the C2 pars along with the C1-2 joint so that the exact path of the screw is visualized (along with the use of fluoroscopy). If brisk bleeding occurs during the procedure, it indicates vertebral artery bleeding. Placement of the screw usually stops such bleeding, but no attempt should be made to place the contralateral screw.

Different trajectories used by Magerl, Anderson, and An screws pose varying threats to the nerve roots. Xu et al.[109] found that the overall percentage of nerve violation was significantly higher with the Magerl and Anderson techniques than with the An technique. The screw trajectory should be directed toward the wider, thicker upper lateral part of the lateral mass rather than the waist (middle thinner part). Graham et al.[33] reported a 1.8% per screw risk of radiculopathy following a 6.1% rate (10 out of 164 lateral mass screws) of screw malposition. They found no vertebral artery or spinal cord injury. There are no reports in the literature on whether to abandon the procedure on the opposite side if there is brisk bleeding on the side of the procedure in case of lateral mass plating.

In both of the above cases, if bleeding is controlled with the screws, there is always a chance of arteriovenous fistula formation, which should be investigated during follow-up.

Vascular Injury Complicating Lumbar Spine Surgery

Several thousand procedures on prolapsed lumbar discs are performed each year. Injury to the abdominal vasculature during these procedures is uncommon. Fewer than 100 cases have been reported so far.[6,25,32,73]

The exact incidence is difficult to calculate, although Harbison[39] reported on accumulated data from different surgeons. Gurdjian et al.[36] reported 2 deaths in 1176 cases of lumbar disc surgery; one of them was due to laceration of the inferior vena cava. Papadoulas et al.[64] proposed an incidence of 1–5 in 10,000 disc operations

The anatomical basis for this injury was described in 1945 by Linton and White,[53] who described the danger of removing the ruptured intervertebral disc material due to the close anatomical proximity of aortic and iliac vessel injuries to the anterior longitudinal ligament opposite the L4/5 disc space. The aortic bifurcation and common iliac vessels lie just anterior to this disc space. Injury to either of the iliac arteries or the veins can result in breach of the intervening anterior longitudinal ligament that might be weak, perforated, or degenerated. The abdominal aorta and inferior vena cava are at risk at the L3/4 disc space, and an aortocaval fistula might result. Since the L4-5 level is the one most commonly explored, the highest number of injuries are described with surgery at this level.[73] Most often, the common iliac artery or vein is injured, depending upon the variable anatomical relationship with the spinal column.

Most vascular injuries are reported to occur within a few centimeters of the aortic bifurcation, although injuries to internal and external iliac arteries are also reported.[39] The most common mode of injury involves the use of the pituitary rongeur. Predisposing factors like degenerative changes, rents in the anterior longitudinal ligament, vascular anomaly, previous surgery, and scar formation with or without previous surgery, along with incorrect positioning of the patient, are described as contributory conditions.[7,25]

Severe retroperitoneal hemorrhage was reported to occur in 24 cases following lumbar disc surgery.[73] Arterial injury was recorded in 19 of them, and 3 had inferior vena cava injury. The most common vessel involved was the left common iliac artery. All cases were diagnosed intraoperatively or in the immediate postoperative period. In spite of the urgent laparotomy and corrective procedures, 7 of 24 patients died; only in 14 patients could repair be performed. Raptis et al.[73] collected 46 cases by 1994; the most common level was L4-5 again, and the vessels involved most often were the right common iliac artery and vein. Fourteen of these cases were diagnosed at admission, and others presented as much as 8 years later. Not all cases present with significant bleeding with shock, as noted by Jarstfer and Rich[43] in 71% of cases there was no significant bleeding in their review, although 22% had hypotension. Intraoperatively, our experience has been similar in present cases. The most common procedure was fistula repair with or without sympathectomy.[89] In eight cases, four-vessel ligation with sympathectomy was performed. There is no case in which a nonsurgical procedure was advocated for correction of the lesion. To our knowledge, there are very few instances in the literature where an endovascular procedure has been employed for successful treatment of iatrogenic injury to the abdominal vessels in cases of lumbar disc disease.[51]

The overall mortality in the 70 cases reviewed by Raptis et al.[73] was 14%; it was higher with hemorrhagic complications (7/24) compared to fistula formation (3/46). Harbison[39] reported a rate as high as 61%. Delay in diagnosis and treatment accounted for the reported high mortality. Prompt diagnosis and intervention are suggested by many authors to reduce the mortality to 24%.[93] In many cases, bleeding from the operative site is not profuse and can easily be stopped,[25] sometimes delaying the appropriate investigation in the postoperative period. Pelvic vein thrombosis in some of these cases might well be due to direct injury to the iliac veins, and only a detailed investigation in suspected cases will reveal the exact incidence of vascular trauma in lumbar disc surgery.[72] Limited excision of herniated nucleus pulposus remains a safe and successful procedure.

Vascular Injury Secondary to the Anterior Lumbar Approach

Vascular injury is commonly seen in anterior lumbar interbody fusion surgery involving either the hypogastric-midline-transperitoneal approach or the minimally invasive muscle-sparing retroperitoneal approach.[48] Frequently, the left iliac or common femoral arteries are involved, especially at the L4-5 level. Common Iliac veins are also more prone to injury when placing the cages or during the application of cage insertion devices. Veins have thin walls, and bleeding from them is harder to control than arterial injury.

In addition, ALIF surgery might become complicated due to thromboembolism and vasospasm.[49] Intraoperative monitoring of lower limb blood flow by measuring toe oxygen saturation with a pulse oximeter can be helpful in making an early diagnosis.

Postoperative Discitis

Disc space infection or discitis, an infection of the intervertebral disc with contiguous subchondral vertebral osteomyelitis, most frequently follows previous intervertebral disc surgery or arises by hematogenous dissemination.[17,70] Direct contamination during surgery is far more frequent than hematogenous contamination. Apart from bacterial factors, immunological mechanisms are implicated. The majority of such cases are located in the lumbosacral spine and rarely in the cervical spine. The most common organism isolated is *Staphylococcus aureus*. Two major types of postoperative discitis have been described: *septic* discitis and *avascular* or *chemical* discitis. This complication may occur with superficial or deep wound infection.

Clinical findings include localized back pain and fever. Most patients mention that their previous radicular pain is significantly diminished; however, they complain of new, severe low back pain in the lumbar spine that is worsened by movement and vibration. In addition, they may complain of muscle cramps in the legs. Straight-leg raising becomes much more limited than before surgery.

Blood tests show a sharp rise in the leukocyte count and the erythrocyte sedimentation rate. Confirmation is obtained by blood culture or culture of material obtained from the involved disc space. Percutaneous discal biopsy is an important way of distinguishing septic from chemical discitis. Commonly, as previously mentioned, *Staphylococcus* is the causative agent; others are *Streptococcus*, *Candida*, and *Mycobacterium*. Microbiological analysis of the CT-guided percutaneous aspiration specimens was positive in 39 of 43 patients proven to have active infections, with four false-negative and no false-positive cases (sensitivity, 91%; specificity, 100%) in a recent report.[13]

Typical plain radiographic findings are narrowing of the affected disc space and end plate resorption, which usually appear 3–4 weeks after the initial symptoms. Various isotope studies using technetium-99 with leukocytes and monoclonal antibodies, as well as ciprofloxacin, have been employed to identify skeletal infection at different stages.[29,86] Single photon emission computed tomography (SPECT) and positron emission tomography (PET) also have been useful in the diagnostic workup.[12,98] In the early phase, CT may show hypodense disc material in the affected disc space, which may be the first radiological sign of discitis. The CT scan will also show anterior paravertebral soft tissue swelling with obliteration of paravertebral fat planes, fragmentation or erosion of vertebral end plates, and a paravertebral fluid collection (abscess).

An MRI scan will substantiate the CT findings. However, an MRI scan alone is insufficient for the diagnosis of early discitis and is unreliable as the sole method for distinguishing septic from aseptic discitis in the early postoperative stage.[24] Nevertheless, it is helpful in differentiating discitis from recurrent disc herniation, which clinically mimics it. Nerve root displacement and nerve root enhancement caused by recurrent disc herniation may strengthen the indication for repeat discectomy. Contrast enhancement and signal changes in the intervertebral disc or the vertebral end plates are not specific for spondylodiscitis, since these are also seen in asymptomatic patients. However, absence of Modic type 1 changes, of contrast enhancement of the disc, or of enhancing paravertebral soft tissues suggests that the patient does not have spondylodiscitis. Magnetic resonance imaging appears to be more useful for exclusion than for confirmation of postoperative spondylodiscitis.[104]

Due to the negative findings of neuroradiological studies in the acute stage, recognition of the typical syndrome is very important for diagnosis. Treatment consists of antimicrobial therapy (broad spectrum with antistaphylococcal therapy), spinal immobilization, and surgical intervention in selected circumstances. Przybylski and Sharan[69] concluded that single-stage debridement, arthrodesis, and internal fixation can be effective in the treatment of postoperative discitis and vertebral osteomyelitis. A 6-week course of postoperative intravenous antibiotics may be sufficient in patients with few risk factors. The harvesting of iliac autograft through the same operative exposure may not increase the risk of secondary infection. The exact duration of antibiotic therapy is debatable, but an average of 12 weeks with additional antibiotic therapy for 2 weeks after normalization of the erythrocyte sedimentation rate is recommended in high-risk patients. Patients with discitis have a good prognosis, but residual back pain, limited spinal mobility, and neurological deficits may persist. Identification of *Mycobacterium* or a fungus on cultures would indicate initiation of appropriate medical treatment.

Complications Specific to Cervical Spine Surgeries

Cervical spine surgery became the most common spine surgery after its initial introduction by Cloward in 1958. It comprises about 10% to 15% of the total number of surgeries in any neurosurgical practice. Proper understanding of the anatomy and technicalities of such surgery greatly reduces the complication rates.

Cervical spine surgery complications can be divided into (1) those occurring with anterior spine surgery (Table 42.5), (2) those related to posterior spine surgery, and (3) those secondary to instrumentation.

Incidence of Complications of Cervical Spine Surgery

The incidence of various complications related to cervical surgery varies in the literature. Some complications are well reported, while others are underreported (Table 42.6).

Dysphagia

The incidence of dysphagia was higher in patient-reported series than in surgeon-reported series, suggesting that postoperative dysphagia is more common than was previously thought. The reported incidence ranges from 1.7% to 60%.[10,103]

Dysphagia in patients undergoing anterior cervical surgery can be classified as (1) transient, (2) delayed, or (3) structurally induced.

Transient dysphagia usually occurs within 48 hours of surgery, and most patients undergoing anterior cervical surgery complain of this problem. It is usually related to postoperative edema of the pharyngeal structures secondary to long periods of retraction, trauma during intubation, and so on. It usually subsides without any sequelae.

Delayed dysphagia (nonstructural) usually appears after 48 hours and can sometimes be severe and chronic. It is postulated to be secondary to damage of the nerve supplying the pharyngeal muscles. It is commonly attributed to forceful

Table 42.5. Complications of Anterior Cervical Surgery

Common Complications	Less Frequent Complications
Dysphagia	Hypoglossal nerve injury
Recurrent laryngeal nerve palsy	Phrenic nerve injury
Vertebral artery injury	Sympathetic chain injury
Esophageal injury	Stroke

Table 42.6. Major Complications of Cervical Spine Surgery

Complication	Average Incidence
Anterior bone graft failure	2.10%
Posterior bone graft failure	0.30%
Cerebrospinal fluid leak	0.40%
Recurrent laryngeal nerve injury	0.20%
Cervical nerve root injury	0.60%
Quadriplegia	0.40%
Infection	0.50%

Source: Data from Zeidmaan et al: Trends and complications in cervical spine surgery: 1989–1993. J Spinal Disord 10(6):523–526, 1997.

retraction, surgical manipulation, and aggressive use of monopolar diathermy. No single nerve is indicated but one important nerve often cited as a possible cause is the vagus nerve, which supplies all the pharyngeal muscles except the stylopharyngeous.[92] Whether mechanical retraction disrupts the neural supply of the esophagus or induces a state of dysmotility is unknown.

Structurally induced dysphagia is usually related to hematoma, esophageal perforations, scarring, and protrusion of the graft/implant.[66,90,91] Most of these patients commonly complain of difficulty in swallowing solids. Treating the appropriate cause will relieve the dysphagia.

The pattern of dysfunction in swallowing can be recognized by thorough clinical assessment and radiological investigation. Predominant impairment of a specific stage of swallowing may suggest a particular etiology.[26] Impaired pharyngeal swallowing suggests disruption of the connections between the pharyngeal plexus and the pharyngeal muscles during retraction. On the other hand, difficulty in the oral stage of swallowing points to the possibility of damage to the hypoglossal nerve.

Evaluation of Patients with Dysphagia

The complication of severe dysphagia following anterior cervical fusion necessitates the prompt exclusion of potentially reversible surgical complications. Early recognition of severe swallowing deficits requires particular attention to the nutritional state of the patient. A multidisciplinary approach involving speech pathology and otolaryngology evaluation is helpful.

Patients should be initially evaluated with a plain radiograph to rule out structurally induced dysphagia.[96] If delayed dysphagia is suspected, a barium swallow study is initially conducted. If necessary, manometry and esophagoduodenoscopy can be used.

Treatment

Treatment options in cases of chronic dysphagia (nonstructural) include consultation with a speech pathologist to develop specific swallowing maneuvers and cricopharyngeal myotomy in severe, protracted dysphagia. Occasionally, dilatation of the esophagus can also be used to reduce the severity of symptoms. In some instances, open repair is helpful.[74]

Recurrent Laryngeal Nerve Injury

The incidence of recurrent laryngeal nerve injury is less than 1%. The incidence also varies with the type of procedure. The incidence of recurrent laryngeal nerve (RLN) symptoms was 2.1% with anterior cervical discectomy, 3.5% with corpectomy, 3% with instrumentation, and 9.5% with reoperative anterior surgery. There was a significant increase in the rate of injury with reoperative anterior fusion. There was no association between the side of the approach and the incidence of RLN symptoms.[5]

Most reports mention that RLN injury commonly occurs while operating from the right side rather than the left side because of typical anatomical variation between the two sides. On the right side, the RLN leaves the main trunk of the vagus nerve and passes anterior to and under the subclavian artery. It then ascends in the tracheoesophageal groove. It frequently bifurcates before entering the larynx. On the left side, the RLN again descends parallel to the carotid but then passes under and posterior to the aorta at the ligamentum arteriosum. It ascends up into the neck in the tracheoesophageal groove before its division. Injury of the RLN is commonly noted in surgery below the C6 level.

The commonly implicated causes of RLN injury are direct surgical trauma, nerve division, ligature or pressure, stretch-induced neuropraxia, and postoperative edema. Direct trauma to the nerve during the anterior cervical approach is unlikely if properly performed, as the dissection occurs in the fascial plane medial to the sternocleidomastoid muscle and carotid sheath structures. This keeps the approach lateral to the trachea, the esophagus, and the RLN. The more common cause noticed is injury caused by the endotracheal tube (ET), which in some series was reported to be as high as 7.5%. The ET exerts pressure against the RLN as it enters the larynx. The compression usually happens between the thyroid lamina and the ET.[14] Prolonged pressure by the ET decreases mucosal and neuronal capillary blood flow, thus increasing the risk of nerve injury.[41] Deflating the cuff immediately after placing the retractor prevents this problem. According to a report by Apfelbaum et al.,[2] the most common cause of vocal cord paralysis after anterior cervical spine surgery is compression of the RLN within the endolarynx.[57] Monitoring of ET cuff pressure and release after retractor placement may prevent injury to the RLN during anterior cervical spine surgery.

Stretch neuropraxia is commonly seen with surgery around the lower levels of the cervical spine. It is found that whenever the retractors are opened more than 30 mm or more during surgery, the chances of RLN injury are highest. However, in routine anterior cervical operative settings, retractor opening is no more than 25 mm. The width of the opening is limited by the placement of the retractor blades under the longus coli muscles. During surgery in the lower cervical and upper thoracic spine (substernal or transsternal), identifying the nerve in the lower part of the neck during dissection, freeing it from adjacent structures, and visualizing it while applying the retractors will minimize further injury.

Minimal use of monopolar cautery and relaxation of the retractors during prolonged surgery prevent the occurrence of these injuries. Unilateral injury is often temporary and takes several months to improve. If there is no recovery, unilateral injuries are usually well compensated. There are anecdotal reports of devastating bilateral injuries. It is always advisable to note vocal cord movement preoperatively in every patient undergoing resurgery. If there is any injury to the vocal cord during previous surgery, it is better to go through the same incision rather than the opposite side (Table 42.7).

Table 42.7. Methods to Prevent Vocal Cord Paralysis

Careful dissection and surgical technique
Proper retractor placement beneath the bodies of the longus coli muscles away from the tracheoesophageal groove
Intermittent release of retraction of the retractors
Deflation of the endotracheal cuff after retractor placement
Minimal use of monopolar cautery around the nerve

Esophageal Injury

Esophageal perforation following anterior cervical spine surgery is an uncommon but potentially devastating complication. Esophageal injury may occur either as a result of sharp dissection (especially in the upper cervical region, where the hypopharynx is thinner) or from laceration by the sharp teeth of the self-retaining retractors. Use of a drill in corpectomy without creation of the initial gutter in the vertebral bodies sometimes leads to entanglement of the soft tissues in the drill bit, pulling this toward the esophagus and eventually leading to esophageal injury. During the postoperative period, esophageal injury is related to graft/implant-related complications (Table 42.8). Thus, complications may occur during surgery, early in the postoperative period or several months later.[37]

The most frequent clinical symptoms with esophageal injury are neck and throat pain, odynophagia, dysphagia, hoarseness, and aspiration. The most common clinical findings are elevated temperature, localized induration and neck tenderness, crepitus or subcutaneous air in the neck and anterior chest wall, unexplained tachycardia, and blood in the nasogastric tube if the patient has progressed to the stage of mediastinitis (Table 42.9).

Persistent dysphagia, especially associated with odynophagia following anterior cervical spine surgery, should be evaluated for graft/implant-related complications.[54] The presence of air in the fascial planes of the neck and increasing soft tissue swelling on the postoperative X-ray suggest esophageal

Table 42.8. Causes of Esophageal Injury

Sharp dissection near the hypopharynx
Sharp tooth of the retractors
Inappropriate use of drill during corpectomy
Graft/implant impingement on the esophagus

Source: Glaudinez et al: Esophageal perforations after anterior cervical surgery. J Spinal Disord 13(1): 77–84, 2000.

Table 42.9. Clinical Features of Esophageal Injury

Neck or throat pain
Odynophagia
Dysphagia
Hoarseness
Aspiration pneumonia
Mediastinitis

perforation. This diagnosis can be confirmed by contrast esophagography with a high accuracy rate.[61]

The treatment of esophageal perforation depends upon the severity of the problem, the patient's general condition, and the presence of any complications. If this complication occurs preoperatively, it should be corrected in the same setting before tissue edema develops. Asymptomatic extrusion of the graft compressing the esophagus should be reexplored.

Patients presenting with external fistula and abscess formation require wound debridement and removal of the graft and implant. Patients with a large esophageal defect require reinforcement using the sternocleidomastoid muscle flap.[26] It is better to delay oral feeding for at least 4–6 weeks after healing is demonstrated radiologically.[42] Early recognition and proper management of postoperative esophageal fistulas prevent further major complications.

Hypoglassal Nerve Injury

Hypoglassal nerve injury is occasionally noticed with surgery of the upper cervical spine. This usually occurs when there is an oblique incision along the chin to expose the C1-3 area. So far, only two cases have been reported.[88] In both, the patients presented in the immediate postoperative period with dysphagia and dysphonia, and in both, hypoglossal injury persisted as permanent palsy. The authors advise careful identification and protection of the nerve during dissection as an important factor in preventing these injuries.

The other cause of hypoglossal injury is a long transarticular screw projecting beyond the anterior cortex of the lateral mass of C1 and impinging on the hypoglossal nerve in the anterior neck. Proper use of fluoroscopy and avoiding drilling beyond the upper border of the C1 anterior arch with lateral fluoroscopy (to select the appropriate length for the transarticular screw) can prevent this complication.

Phrenic Nerve Injury

Phrenic nerve injury is very seldom encountered. It can be caused by stretch injury of the C4 nerve root, and sometimes this stretch can involve the anterior horn cells at the same level.[27] Occasionally there may be bilateral injury leading to long-term ventilator support. Phrenic nerve injuries are noticed mainly on postoperative chest X-rays that show the lax dome of the diaphragm and on fluoroscopy that shows decreased diaphragm movement.

Stroke

Most symptomatic cervical spondylotic patients requiring discectomy or vertebrectomy present in their 40s–60s or later. There is a significant association between this age range and progressive atherosclerotic disease of the vessels of the neck.[64] Occasionally there is a chance of embolic displacement of atherosclerotic plaque during preoperative preparation of the neck or overretraction during surgery. There are case reports in which patients developed significant stroke secondary to this complication.

Injury to the Cervical Sympathetic Chain

This is a rare entity and results in Horner's syndrome. It is usually secondary to transection of the sympathetic chain or to stretching lateral to the longus colli muscles.[99]

For completion of cervical spine surgery complications, Table 42.10 details common complications following C1–C2 fixation.

Complications Specific to Lumbar Spine Surgeries

Lumbar discectomy is a common surgical procedure to relieve preoperative sciatic pain with a physician-reported good outcome of 85% to 95%. However, postoperatively, up to 40% of patients have persistent limitations in activity. Some reports

Table 42.10. Complications Related to Posterior Surgery of the Cervical Spine.

Complications	Occipital-Cervical Fusion	Atlantoaxial Cable Fixation	C1-2 Transarticular Fixation	Lateral Mass Fixation	Prevention
Cerebrospinal fluid leak	+++	+	+	+	Proper burr holeplacement, meticulous use of monopolar cautery
Venous hemorrhage	++	++	+++	+	Proper coagulation and pressure compression
Vertebral artery injury	+	+	++++	+++	Preoperative computed tomography scan, good trajectory of pilot hole
Worsening of neurological deficits	++++	++	++		Proper dissection technique
Malpositioning of rod/screw/plate	++		++	++++	Use image intensifier for pilot hole
Nerve root injury	++		+++	++++	Use image intensifier for pilot hole, C2 proper dissection, less use of monopolar cautery
Wound infection/ dehiscence	+++	+	+	+	Meticulous closure technique
Hematoma formation	+	+	+	+	Proper hemostasis
Hypoglossal injury			++		Use screw of appropriate length
Graft displacement	+++	++			Proper fixation of graft with wires

cite complication rates as high as 15% to 30%.[11,56] The main causes of failed back syndrome are recurrent disk herniation, postsurgical granulation tissue/epidural fibrosis, central or lateral bony spinal stenosis, and/or accelerated degeneration of the treated motion segment with or without instability following discectomy. Spondylodiscitis, arachnoiditis, and pseudomeningocele are other less frequent etiologies.[84,100] Another important complication associated with ALIF apart from vascular injury is retrograde ejaculation.[77]

The recent additions of minimally invasive surgery including lumbar disc removal with endoscopy, percutaneous lumbar disc decompression using laser (PLDD),[59] percutaneous interbody fixations, and fusion;[55] minimally invasive transforaminal lumbar interbody fusion;[85] and various prosthetic materials for disc replacement[8,37,101] have all added new dimensions to the hitherto more commonly encountered failed back surgery syndrome. Series with large populations are yet to be published on these techniques for evaluation of the risk-benefit ratio. However, according to the recent literature, minimally invasive nucleotomy currently is the state-of-the-art treatment for symptomatic disc prolapses.[71]

Epidural fibrosis

Discectomy after laminectomy is always known to produce some fibrosis, but few patients develop clinical symptoms. Epidural fibrosis (EF) is a natural consequence of normal postoperative healing that can cause symptoms by tethering the nerve roots. Identification of fibrosis as the cause of recurring lumbar or sciatic pain requires a good clinical history and selective physical examination. Patients with extensive epidural scarring have been shown to be 3.2 times more likely to experience recurrent radicular pain than those with less extensive epidural scarring.[4] The association between epidural scar and activity-related pain was analyzed by BenDebba et al.[4] at 6-month follow-up, when successful surgical excision of protruding disc material should have eliminated chronic pain. Logistic regression analysis demonstrated a significant association (p = .02, odds ratio = 0.7) whereby the odds of extensive scar decreased by 30% for every 31% decrease in activity-related pain score. In addition, those patients receiving Adhesion Control in a Barrier Gel (ADCON-L; Gliatech, Cleveland, OH) at surgery developed significantly less scar in the months following operation ($p = .01$ 6 and 12 months postoperatively). Magnetic resonance imaging is the imaging technique of choice.[34,35] In patients operated on for unilateral single-level lumbar disc hernias, implantation of closed-suction drainage into the operation site results in less formation of EF radiologically and yields a better clinical outcome.[87] Various other methods have been tried to prevent its occurrence, including the use of fat grafts. Recently, ADCON-L has been used in clinical settings to inhibit EF. Cell culture analysis demonstrated that ADCON-L blocked the ingrowth of fibroblasts and thus minimized the formation of peridural fibrotic scar, improving the postoperative outcome.[67] If reoperation is necessary due to residual disc or lateral stenosis, the absence of EF will facilitate surgery.[9] Barriers composed of carboxymethylcellulose (CMC) and polyethylene oxide (PEO) (Oxiplex; FzioMed, Inc., San Luis Obispo, CA) are being studied for their ability to reduce epidural adhesion formation in rabbit laminotomy and laminectomy models.[74]

Retrograde Ejaculation

The incidence of retrograde ejaculation in men after anterior lumbosacral spinal surgery is reported to range from 0.42% to 5.9%. A transperitoneal approach to the lumbar spine at L4-L5 and L5-S1 has a 10 times greater likelihood of causing retrograde ejaculation in men than a retroperitoneal approach.[82]

Direct access to the L5-S1 disc through the middle of the plexus puts the elements of the superior hypoglossal plexus at higher risk than if they are gently retracted to the right side. The hypogastric plexus typically courses over the left iliac vessel and the surface of the sacral promontory to reach the anterior surface of the sacrum. To expose the intervertebral disc without damaging the plexus, the posterior peritoneum should be opened carefully on the right or left side of the bifurcation, elevating the presacral tissue from the periosteum and sweeping it from the front of the sacrum as a block. Precautionary measures include avoiding dissecting through the plexus, cutting transversely across, or using cautery during dissection.

Patients should be informed of the risk of retrograde ejaculation preoperatively. Many surgeons do not recommend the transabdominal approach in male patients because of this risk. One-fourth of such retrograde ejaculation resolves. Some patients even experience impotence, which is nonorganic in nature.

REFERENCES

1. Apfelbaum RI: Screw fixation of the upper cervical spine: Indications and techniques. Contemp Neurosurg 16(7): 1–8, 1994.
2. Apfelbaum RI, Kriskovich MD, Haller JR: On the incidence, cause, and prevention of recurrent laryngeal nerve palsies during anterior cervical spine surgery. Spine 25(22): 2906–2912, 2000.
3. Belmont PJ Jr, Klemme WR, Dhawan A, Polly DW Jr: In vivo accuracy of thoracic pedicle screws. Spine 26(21): 2340–2346, 2001.
4. BenDebba M, Augustus van Alphen H, Long DM: Association between peridural scar and activity-related pain after lumbar discectomy. Neurol Res 21(suppl 1):S37–S42, 1999.
5. Beutler WJ, Sweeney CA, Connolly PJ: Recurrent laryngeal nerve injury with anterior cervical spine surgery risk with laterality of surgical approach. Spine 26(12):1337–1342, 2001.
6. Bingol H, Cingoz F, Yilmaz AT, Yasar M, Tatar H: Vascular complications related to lumbar disc surgery. J Neurosurg 100(3 Suppl):249–253, 2004.
7. Bolesta MJ: Vascular injury during lumbar diskectomy associated with peridiskal fibrosis: Case report and literature review. J Spinal Disord 8(3):224–227, 1995.
8. Brantigan JW, Neidre A, Toohey JS: The Lumbar I/F Cage for posterior lumbar interbody fusion with the variable screw placement system: 10-year results of a Food and Drug Administration clinical trial. Spine J 4(6):681–688, 2004.
9. Brotchi J, Pirotte B, De Witte O, Levivier M: Prevention of epidural fibrosis in a prospective series of 100 primary lumbo-sacral discectomy patients: Follow-up and assessment at re-operation. Neurol Res 21(suppl 1):S47–S50, 1999.
10. Buchholz DW: Editorial: dysphagia following anterior cervical spine surgery. Dysphagia 12:10, 1997.
11. Caspar W, Campbell B, Barbier DD, Kretschmmer R, Gotfried Y: The Caspar microsurgical discectomy and comparison with a conventional standard lumbar disc procedure. Neurosurgery 28(1):78–86; discussion 86–87, 1991.
12. Chacko TK, Zhuang H, Nakhoda KZ, Moussavian B, Alavi A: Applications of fluorodeoxyglucose positron emission tomography in the diagnosis of infection. Nucl Med Commun 24(6):615–624, 2003.
13. Chew FS, Kline MJ: Diagnostic yield of CT-guided percutaneous aspiration procedures in suspected spontaneous infectious diskitis. Radiology 218(1):211–214, 2001.
14. Clvo JW: True vocal cord paralysis following intubation. Laryngoscope 95:1352–1358, 1985.
15. Coric D, Branch CL Jr, Wilson JA, Robinson JC: Verte-

bral artery injury in the posterior cervical surgeries. J Neurosurg 85(2):340–343, 1996.
16. Daentzer D, Deinsberger W, Boker DK: Vertebral artery complications in anterior approaches to the cervical spine: Report of two cases and review of literature. Surg Neurol 59(4):300–309, 2003.
17. Ebeling U, Reichenberg W, Reulen HJ: Results of microsurgical lumbar discectomy: Review on 485 patients. Acta Neurochir (Wien) 81(1–2):45–52, 1986.
18. Ebraheim NA, Lu J, Hamna SP, Yeasting RA: Anatomic basis of the anterior surgery on the cervical spine: Relationships between uncus-artery-root complex and vertebral artery injury. Surg Radiol Anat 20(9)389–392, 1998.
19. Epstein NE: The value of anterior cervical plating in preventing vertebral fracture and graft extrusion after multilevel anterior cervical corpectomy with posterior wiring and fusion: Indications, results, and complications. J Spinal Disord 13(1):9–15, 2000.
20. Esses SI, Sachs BL, Dreyzin V: Complications associated with the technique of pedicle screw fixation: A selected survey of ABS members. Spine 18(15):2231–2238, 1993.
21. Faraj AA, Webb JK: Early complications of spinal pedicle screw. Eur Spine J 6(5):324–326, 1997.
22. Fielding J: Complications of anterior cervical disk removal. Clin Orthop 284:10–13, 1992.
23. Flynn TB: Neurologic complications of anterior cervical interbody fusion. Spine 7:536–539, 1982.
24. Fouquet B, Goupille P, Jattiot F, Cotty P, Lapierre F, Valat JP, Amouroux J, Benatre A: Discitis after lumbar disc surgery. Features of "aseptic" and "septic" forms. Spine 17(3):356–358, 1992.
25. Fruhwirth J, Koch G, Amann W, Hauser H, Flaschka G: Vascular complications of lumbar disc surgery. Acta Neurochir (Wien) 138(8):912–916, 1996.
26. Fuji T, Kuratsu S, Shirasaki N, Harada T, Tatsumi Y, Satani M, et al: Oesophagocutaneous fistula after anterior cervical spine surgery and successful treatment using a sternocleidomastoid muscle flap. A case report. Clin Orthop 267:8–13, 1991.
27. Fujibayashi S, Shikata J, Yoshitomi H, Tanaka C, Nakamura K, Nakamura T: Bilateral phrenic nerve palsy as a complication of anterior decompression and fusion for cervical ossification of the posterior longitudinal ligament. Spine 26(12):E281–E286, 2001.
28. Gaudinez RF, English GM, Gebhard JS, Brugman JL, Donaldson DH, Brown CW: Esophageal perforations after anterior cervical surgery. J Spinal Disord 13(1):77–84, 2000.
29. Gemmel F, De Winter F, Van Laere K, Vogelaers D, Uyttendaele D, Dierckx RA: 99mTc ciprofloxacin imaging for the diagnosis of infection in the postoperative spine. Nucl Med Commun 25(3):277–283, 2004.
30. Geyer TE, Foy MA: Oral extrusion of a screw after anterior cervical spine plating. Spine 26:1814–1816, 2001.
31. Golfinos JG, Dickman CA, Zabramski JM, Sonntag VK, Spetzler RF: Repair of vertebral artery injury during anterior cervical decompression. Spine 19(22):2552–2556, 1994.
32. Goodkin R, Laska LL: Vascular and visceral injuries associated with lumbar disc surgery: Medicolegal implications. Surg Neurol 49(4):358–370; discussion 370–372, 1998.
33. Graham AW, Swank ML, Kinard RE, Lowery GL, Dials BE: Posterior cervical arthrodesis and stabilization with a lateral mass plate: Clinical and computed tomographic evaluation of lateral mass screw placement and associated complications. Spine 21(3):323–328; discussion 329, 1996.
34. Grane P: The postoperative lumbar spine: A radiological investigation of the lumbar spine after discectomy using MR. Acta Radiol Suppl 414:1–23, 1998.
35. Grane P, Josephsson A, Seferlis A, Tullberg T: Septic and aseptic post-operative discitis in the lumbar spine—evaluation by MR imaging. Acta Radiol 39(2):108–115, 1998.
36. Gurdjian ES, Ostrowski AZ, Hardy WG, Lindner DW, Thomas LM: Results of operative treatment of protruded and ruptured lumbar discs based on 1176 operative cases with 82 per cent follow-up of 3 to 13 years. J Neurosurg 18:783–791, 1961.
37. Guyer RD, Delamarter RB, Fulp T, Small SD: Complication of cervical spine injury In: Rothman - Simeone (eds): The Spine, 4th ed. Philadelphia, WB Saunders, 1999, pp 540–552.
38. Guyer RD, McAfee PC, Hochschuler SH, Blumenthal SL, Fedder IL, Ohnmeiss DD, Cunningham BW: Prospective randomized study of the Charite artificial disc: Data from two investigational centers. Spine J 4(6 suppl): 252S–259S, 2004.
39. Harbison SP: Major vascular complications of intervertebral disc surgery. Ann Surg 140(3):342–348, 1954.
40. Hee HT, Majd ME, Holt RT, Whitecloud TS 3rd, Pienkowski D: Complications of multilevel cervical corpectomies and reconstruction with titanium cages and anterior plating. J Spinal Disord Tech 16(1):1–8, 2003.
41. Heeneman H: Vocal cord paralysis following approaches to the anterior cervical spine. Laryngoscope 83:17–21, 1973.
42. Jamjoom ZA: Pharyngo-cutaneous fistula following anterior cervical fusion. Br J Neurosurg 11:69–74, 1997.
43. Jarstfer BS, Rich NM: The challenge of arteriovenous fistula formation following disk surgery: A collective review. J Trauma 16(9):726–733, 1976.
44. Jenis LG, Leclair WJ: Late vascular complication with anterior cervical discectomy and fusion. Spine 19(11): 1291–1293, 1994.
45. Jutte PC, Castelein RM: Complications of pedicle screws in lumbar and lumbosacral fusions in 105 consecutive primary operations. Eur Spine J 11(6):594–598, 2002.
46. Kaar GF, Briggs M, Bashir SH: Thecal repair in postsurgical pseudomeningocoele. Br J Neurosurg 8(6):703–707, 1994.
47. Katonis P, Christoforakis J, Kontakis G, Aligizakis AC,

Papadopoulos C, Sapkas G, Hadjipavlou A, Katonis G: Complications and problems related to pedicle screw fixation of the spine. Clin Orthop (411):86–94, 2003.

48. Kotilainen E, Alanen A, Erkintalo M, Valtonen S, Kormano M: Association between decreased disc signal intensity in preoperative T2-weighted MRI and a 5-year outcome after lumbar minimally invasive discectomy. Minim Invasive Neurosurg 44(1):31–36, 2001.
49. Kulkarni SS, Lowery GL, Ross RE, Ravi Sankar K, Lykomitros V: Arterial complications following anterior lumbar interbody fusion: Report of eight cases. Eur Spine J 12(1):48–54, 2003.
50. Kumano K, Hirabayashi S, Ogawa Y, Aota Y: Pedicle screws and bone mineral density. Spine 19(10):1157–1161, 1994.
51. Lee KH, Park JH, Chung JW, Han JK, Shin SJ, Kang HS: Vascular complications in lumbar spinal surgery: Percutaneous endovascular treatment. Cardiovasc Intervent Radiol 23(1):65–69, 2000.
52. Lin PM: Posterior lumbar interbody fusion technique: Complications and pitfalls. Clin Orthop Relat.Res. (193): 90–102, 1985.
53. Linton RR, White PD: Arteriovenous fistula between the right common iliac artery and the inferior vena cava: Report of a case of its occurrence following an operation for ruptured intervertebral disc with cure by operation. Arch Surg 50:6–13, 1945.
54. Loop FD, Groves LK: Collective review, esophageal perforations. Ann Thorac Surg 10:571–587, 1970.
55. MacMillan M: Computer-guided percutaneous interbody fixation and fusion of the L5–S1 disc: A 2-year prospective study. J Spinal Disord Tech 18(suppl):S90–S95, 2005.
56. Maroon JC, Onik G, Vidovich DV: Percutaneous discectomy for lumbar disc herniation. Neurosurg Clin North Am 4(1):125–134, 1993.
57. Mazumdar DP, Deopujari CE, Bhojraj SY: Bilateral vocal cord paralysis after anterior cervical discoidectomy and fusion in a case of whiplash cervical spine injury: a case report. Surg Neurol 53(6):586–588, 2000.
58. McLain RF: Surgical approach to lumbar spine. In: Fryameyer JW (ed): The Adult Spine: Principles and Practices. Philadelphia, Lippincot-Raven, 1997, pp 1736–1737.
59. McMillan MR, Patterson PA, Parker V: Percutaneous laser disc decompression for the treatment of discogenic lumbar pain and sciatica: A preliminary report with 3-month follow-up in a general pain clinic population. Photomed Laser Surg 22(5):434–438, 2004.
60. Moreland DB, Asch HL, Clabeaux DE, Castiglia GJ, Czajka GA, Lewis PJ, Egnatchik JG, Cappuccino A, Huynh L: Anterior cervical discectomy and fusion with implantable titanium cage: Initial impressions, patient outcomes and comparison to fusion with allograft. Spine J 4:184–191, 2004.
61. Newhouse KE, Lindsey RW, Clark CR, Lieponis J, Murphy J: Esophageal perforation following anterior cervical spine injury. Spine 14:1051, 1989.
62. Odgers CJ 4th, Vaccaro AR, Pollack ME, Cotler JM: Accuracy of pedicle screw placement with the assistance of lateral plain radiography. J Spinal Disord 9(4):334–338, 1996.
63. Oga M, Yuge I, Terada K, Shimizu A, Sugioka Y: Tortuosity of the vertebral artery in patients with cervical spondylotic myelopathy: Risk factor for the vertebral artery injury during anterior cervical decompression. Spine 21(9):1085–1089, 1996.
64. Papadoulas S, Konstantinou D, Kourea HP, Kritikos N, Haftouras N, Tsolakis JA: Vascular injury complicating lumbar disc surgery: A systematic review. Eur J Vasc Endovasc Surg 24(3):189–195, 2002.
65. Pollard ME, Little PW: Changes in carotid artery blood flow during anterior cervical spine surgery. Spine 27(2): 152–155, 2002.
66. Pompili A, Canitano S, Caroli F, Caterino M, Crecco M, Raus L, et al: Asymptomatic esophageal perforation caused by late screw migration after anterior cervical plating: Report of a case and review of relevant literature. Spine 27:E499–E502, 2002.
67. Porchet F, Lombardi D, de Preux J, Pople IK: Inhibition of epidural fibrosis with ADCON-L: Effect on clinical outcome one year following re-operation for recurrent lumbar radiculopathy. Neurol Res 21(suppl 1):S51–S60, 1999.
68. Prabhu VC, France JC, Voelker JL, Zoarski GH: Vertebral artery pseudoaneurysm complicating posterior C1-2 transarticular screw fixation: Case report. Surg Neurol 55(1):29–33, 2001.
69. Przybylski GJ, Sharan AD: Single-stage autogenous bone grafting and internal fixation in the surgical management of pyogenic discitis and vertebral osteomyelitis. J Neurosurg Spine 94(1):1–7, 2001.
70. Puranen J, Makela J, Lahde S: Postoperative intervertebral discitis Acta Orthop Scand 55(4):461–465, 1984.
71. Putzier M, Schneider SV, Funk JF, Tohtz SW, Perka C: The surgical treatment of the lumbar disc prolapse: Nucleotomy with additional transpedicular dynamic stabilization versus nucleotomy alone. Spine 30(5):E109–E114, 2005.
72. Quigley TM, Stoney RJ: Arteriovenous fistulas following lumbar laminectomy: The anatomy defined. J Vasc Surg 2(6):828–833, 1985.
73. Raptis S, Quigley F, Barker S: Vascular complications of elective lower lumbar disc surgery. Aust NZ J Surg 64(3):216–219, 1994.
74. Reid RR, Dutra J, Conley DB, Ondra SL, Dumanian GA: Improved repair of cervical esophageal fistula complicating anterior spinal fusion: Free omental flap compared with pectoralis major flap. Report of four cases. J Neurosurg 100(1 suppl):66–70, 2004.
75. Rodgers KE, Robertson JT, Espinoza T, Oppelt W, Cortese S, diZerega GS, Berg RA: Reduction of epidural fibrosis in lumbar surgery with Oxiplex adhesion barriers of carboxymethylcellulose and polyethylene oxide. Spine J 3(4):277–283; discussion 284, 2003.

76. Rundshagen I, Schroder T, Prichep LS, John ER, Kox WJ: Changes in cortical electrical activity during induction of anaesthesia with thiopental/fentanyl and tracheal intubation: A quantitative electroencephalographic analysis. Br J Anaesth 92(1):33–38, 2004.
77. Sagdic K, Ozer ZG, Senkaya I, Ture M: Vascular injury during lumbar disc surgery: Report of two cases; a review of the literature. Vasa 25(4):378–381, 1996.
78. Sakaura H, Hosono N, Mukai Y, Ishii T, Yoshikawa H: C5 palsy after decompression surgery for cervical myelopathy: Review of the literature. Spine. 28(21):2447–2451, 2003.
79. Sanden B, Olerud C, Petren-Mallmin M, Johansson C, Larsson S: The significance of radiolucent zones surrounding pedicle screws: Definition of screw loosening in spinal instrumentation. J Bone Joint Surg Br 86(3): 457–461, 2004.
80. Sasai K, Saito T, Akagi S, Kato I, Ohnari H, Iida H: Preventing C5 palsy after laminoplasty. Spine 28(17):1972–1977, 2003.
81. Sasao L, Saito T, Akagi S, Kato I, Ohnari H, Iida H: Preventing C5 palsy after laminoplasty. Spine 28:1972–1977, 2003.
82. Sasso RC, Kenneth Burkus J, LeHuec JC: Retrograde ejaculation after anterior lumbar interbody fusion: Transperitoneal versus retroperitoneal exposure. Spine 29(1): 106–107, 2004.
83. Sasso RC, Ruggiero RA Jr, Reilly TM, Hall PV: Early reconstruction failures after multilevel cervical corpectomy. Spine 15:140–142, 2003.
84. Schumacher HW, Wassmann H, Podlinski C: Pseudomeningocele of the lumbar spine. Surg Neurol 29(1):77–78, 1988.
85. Schwender JD, Holly LT, Rouben DP, Foley KT: Minimally invasive transforaminal lumbar interbody fusion (TLIF): Technical feasibility and initial results. J Spinal Disord Tech 18(suppl):S1–S6, 2005.
86. Sciuk J, Brandau W, Vollet B, Stucker R, Erlemann R, Bartenstein P, Peters PE, Schober O: Comparison of technetium 99m polyclonal human immunoglobulin and technetium 99m monoclonal antibodies for imaging chronic osteomyelitis. First clinical results. Eur J Nucl Med. 18(6):401–407, 1991.
87. Sen O, Kizilkilic O, Aydin MV, Yalcin O, Erdogan B, Cekinmez M, Caner H, Altinors N: The role of closed-suction drainage in preventing epidural fibrosis and its correlation with a new grading system of epidural fibrosis on the basis of MRI. Eur Spine J 2005 May; 14(4): 409–414 Epub 2004 Nov 4.
88. Sengupta DK, Grevitt MP, Mehdian SM: Hypoglossal nerve injury as a complication of anterior surgery to the upper cervical spine. Eur Spine J 8:78–80, 1999.
89. Serrano Hernando FJ, Paredero VM, Solis JV, Del Rio A, Lopez Parra JJ, Orgaz A, Aroca M, Tovar A, Paredero del Bosque V: Iliac arteriovenous fistula as a complication of lumbar disc surgery: Report of two cases and review of literature. J Cardiovasc Surg (Torino) 27(2):180–184, 1986.
90. Sharma RR, Sethu AU, Lad SD, Turel KE, Pawar SJ: Pharyngeal perforation and spontaneous extrusion of the cervical graft with its fixation device: A late complication of C2-C3 fusion via anterior approach. J Clin Neurosci 8:464–468, 2001.
91. Shenoy SN, Raja A: Delayed pharyngo-esophageal perforation: Rare complication of anterior cervical spine surgery. Neurol India 51(4):534–536, 2003.
92. Shun Lee SK, Lee GYF, Wong GTH: Prolonged and severe dysphagia following anterior cervical surgery J Clin Neurosci 11(4):424–427, 2004.
93. Smith DW, Lawrence BD: Vascular complications of lumbar decompression laminectomy and foraminotomy: A unique case and review of the literature. Spine 16(3): 387–390, 1991.
94. Smith MD, Bolesta MJ, Leventhal M, Bohlman HH: Postoperative CSF fistula associated with erosion of the dura: Finding after anterior resection of the OPLL. J Bone Joint Surg Am 74(2):270–277, 1992.
95. Smith MD, Emery SE, et al: Vertebral artery injury during anterior decompression of the cervical spine. J Bone Joint Surg 79:161–173, 1993.
96. Stewart M, Johnston RA, Stewart I, Wilson JA: Swallowing performance following anterior cervical spine surgery. Br J Neurosurg 9(5):605–609, 1995.
97. Suk SI, Kim WJ, Lee SM, Kim JH, Chung ER: Thoracic pedicle screw fixation in spinal deformities: Are they really safe? Spine 26(18):2049–2057, 2001.
98. Swanson D, Blecker I, Gahbauer H, Caride VJ: Diagnosis of discitis by SPECT technetium-99m MDP scintigram. A case report. Clin Nucl Med 12(3):210–211, 1987.
99. Tew JM, Mayfield FH: Complications of surgery of the anterior cervical spine. Clin Neurosurg 23:424–434, 1976.
100. Tronnier V, Schneider R, Kunz U, Albert F, Oldenko P: Postoperative spondylodiscitis: Results of a prospective study about the etiology of spondylodiscitis after operation for lumbar disc herniation. Acta Neurochir (Wien) 117(3–4):149–152, 1992.
101. Tropiano P, Huang RC, Girardi FP, Cammisa FP Jr, Marnay T: Lumbar total disc replacement: Seven to eleven-year follow-up. J Bone Joint Surg Am 87-A(3):490–496, 2005.
102. Vaccaro AR, Falatyn SP, Scuderi GJ, Eismont FJ, McGuire RA, Singh K, Garfin SR: Early failure of long segment anterior cervical plate fixation. J Spinal Disord 11(5): 410–415, 1998.
103. Vanderveldt HS, Young MF: The evaluation of dysphagia after anterior cervical spine surgery: a case report. Dysphagia 18(4):301–304, 2003.
104. Van Goethem JW, Parizel PM, van den Hauwe L, Van de Kelft E, Verlooy J, De Schepper AM: The value of MRI in the diagnosis of postoperative spondylodiscitis. Neuroradiology 42(8):580–585, 2000.
105. Vanichkachorn JS, Vaccaro AR, Silveri CP, Albert TJ: Anterior junctional plate in the cervical spine. Spine 23(22):2462–2467, 1998.
106. Vogelsang H, Stolke D: Pseudomeningoceles—a rare

complication following lumbar intervertebral disk operation. Neurochirurgia (Stuttg) 27(3):73–77, 1984.

107. Wang JC, Hart RA, Emery SE, Bohlman HH: Graft migration or displacement after multilevel cervical corpectomy and strut grafting. Spine 28(10):1016–1021; discussion 1021–1022, 2003.

108. Wiesner L, Kothe R, Schulitz KP, Ruther W: Clinical evaluation and computed tomography scan analysis of screw tracts after percutaneous insertion of pedicle screws in the lumbar spine. Spine 25(5):615–621, 2000.

109. Xu R, Haman SP, Ebraheim NA, Yeasting RA: The anatomic relation of lateral mass screws to the spinal nerves: A comparison of the Magerl, Anderson, and An techniques. Spine 24(19):2057–2061, 1999.

110. Yonenobu K, Hosono N, Iwasaki M, Asano M, Ono K: Neurologic complications of surgery for cervical compression myelopathy. Spine 16(11):1277–1282, 1991.

111. Zeidman SM, Ducker TB, Raycroft J: Trends and complications in cervical spine surgery: 1989–1993. J Spinal Disord 10(6):523–526,1997.

complication following lumbar intervertebral disk operation. Neurochirurgia (Stuttg) 27(3):73–77, 1984.
107. Wang JC, Hart RA, Emery SE, Bohlman HH: Graft migration or displacement after multilevel cervical corpectomy and strut grafting. Spine 28(10):1016–1021; discussion 1021–1022, 2003.
108. Wiesner L, Kothe R, Schulitz KP, Ruther W: Clinical evaluation and computed tomography scan analysis of screw tracts after percutaneous insertion of pedicle screws in the lumbar spine. Spine 25(5):615–621, 2000.
109. Xu R, Haman SP, Ebraheim NA, Yeasting RA: The anatomic relation of lateral mass screws to the spinal nerves: A comparison of the Magerl, Anderson, and An techniques. Spine 24(19):2057–2061, 1999.
110. Yonenobu K, Hosono N, Iwasaki M, Asano M, Ono K: Neurologic complications of surgery for cervical compression myelopathy. Spine 16(11):1277–1282, 1991.
111. Zeidman SM, Ducker TB, Raycroft J: Trends and complications in cervical spine surgery: 1989–1993. J Spinal Disord 10(6):523–526,1997.

Index

Note: Page numbers followed by f and t refer to figures and tables, respectively.